Primer on KIDNEY DISEASES

5th Edition

Editor

Arthur Greenberg, MD
Division of Nephrology
Department of Medicine
Duke University Medical Center
Durham, North Carolina

Associate Editors

Alfred K. Cheung, MD
Professor of Medicine, University of Utah and
Veterans Affairs, Salt Lake City Healthcare System

Thomas M. Coffman, MD
James R. Clapp Professor of Medicine
Chief, Division of Nephrology
Duke University Medical Center
Durham, North Carolina

Ronald J. Falk, MD
DJ Thurston Professor of Medicine
Director, UNC Kidney Center
Chief, Division of Nephrology and Hypertension
University of North Carolina
Chapel Hill, North Carolina

J. Charles Jennette, MD
Department of Pathology and Laboratory Medicine
University of North Carolina
Chapel Hill, North Carolina

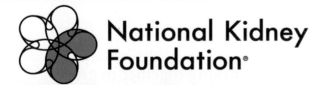

National Kidney Foundation®

SAUNDERS

ELSEVIER

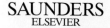

1600 John F. Kennedy Blvd.
Ste 1800
Philadelphia, PA 19103-2899

PRIMER ON KIDNEY DISEASES   ISBN: 978-1-4160-5185-5

Copyright © 2009, 2005, 2001, 1998, 1994 by National Kidney Foundation.

Notice

Knowledge and best practice in this field are constantly changing. As new research and experience broaden
our knowledge, changes in practice, treatment and drug therapy may become necessary or appropriate.
Readers are advised to check the most current information provided (i) on procedures featured or (ii) by the
manufacturer of each product to be administered, to verify the recommended dose or formula, the method
and duration of administration, and contraindications. It is the responsibility his or her relying on his or her
own experience and knowledge of the patient, to make diagnoses, to determine dosages and the best
treatment for each individual patient, and to take all appropriate safety precautions. To the fullest extent of
the law, neither the Publisher nor the Authors assumes any liability for any injury and/or damage to persons
or property arising out of or related to any use of the material contained in this book.

The Publisher

Library of Congress Cataloging-in-Publication Data
Primer on kidney diseases / editor, Arthur Greenberg; associate editors, Alfred K. Cheung... [et al.]. — 5th ed.
  p. ; cm.
Includes bibliographical references and index.
ISBN 978-1-4160-5185-5
1. Kidneys—Diseases. 2. Nephrology. I. Greenberg, Arthur, 1950– II. Cheung, Alfred K.
  [DNLM: 1. Kidney Diseases. 2. Kidney—pathology. WJ 300 P953 2009]

RC902. P75 2009
612.6'1–dc22   2008022961

Acquisitions Editor: Adrianne Brigido
Developmental Editor: Angela Norton
Publishing Services Manager: Frank Polizzano
Senior Project Manager: Peter Faber
Design Direction: Steven Stave
Cover Designer: Lou Forgione

Printed in China

Last digit is the print number: 9   8   7   6   5   4   3   2

Primer on Kidney Diseases

Contributors

Sharon Adler, MD
Professor of Medicine,
David Geffen School of Medicine at UCLA,
Los Angeles, California;
Chief, Division of Nephrology and Hypertension,
Harbor-UCLA Medical Center,
Torrance, California

Horacio J. Adrogué, MD
Professor of Medicine,
Baylor College of Medicine;
Chief of Nephrology and Hypertension,
The Methodist Hospital,
Houston, Texas

Nidhi Aggarwal, MD
Post-Doctoral Clinical Fellow
Columbia University
New York Presbyterian Hospital
New York, New York

Michael Allon, MD
Professor of Medicine,
Division of Nephrology,
University of Alabama at Birmingham,
Birmingham, Alabama

Sharon Anderson, MD
Professor of Medicine,
Division of Nephrology and Hypertension,
Oregon Health and Science University,
Chief, Medical Service,
Portland VA Medical Center,
Portland, Oregon

Sharon Phillips Andreoli, MD
Byron P. and Frances D. Hollet Professor of Pediatrics,
Indiana University Medical Center,
James Whitcomb Riley Hospital for Children,
Indianapolis,
Indiana

Gerald B. Appel, MD
Professor of Clinical Medicine,
Columbia University College of Physicians
and Surgeons;
Director of Clinical Nephrology,
Columbia University Medical Center of the NY-
Presbyterian Hospital,
New York, New York

Vicente Arroyo, MD
Professor of Medicine,
University of Barcelona;
Director, Institute of Digestive and Metabolic Diseases,
Hospital Clinic,
Barcelona, Spain

Phyllis August, MD, MPH
Ralph A. Baer
Professor of Research in Medicine,
Weill Medical College of Cornell,
Attending Physician,
New York Presbyterian Hospital,
New York, New York

George L. Bakris, MD
Professor of Medicine,
University of Chicago, Pritzker School of Medicine,
Director, Hypertentive Diseases Unit,
Univeristy of Chicago Hospitals,
Chicago, Illinois

James E. Balow, MD
Professor of Medicine,
Uniformed Services University of the Health Sciences,
Chief, Kidney Disease Section and Clinical Director,
National Institute of Diabetes and Digestive
and Kidney Diseases,
National Institutes of Health,
Bethesda, Maryland

Srinivasan Beddhu, MBBS
Associate Professor of Medicine,
University of Utah School of Medicine,
Staff Physician,
VA Healthcare System,
Salt Lake City, Utah

Jeffrey S. Berns, MD
Professor of Medicine and Pediatrics,
University of Pennsylvania School of Medicine,
Hospital of the University of Pennsylvania,
Philadelphia, Pennsylvania

Joseph V. Bonventre, MD, PhD
Director, Renal Division,
Brigham and Women's Hospital;
Robert H. Ebert Professor of Medicine
and Health Sciences and Technology,
Harvard Medical School;
Director, Division of Helath Sciences,
Harvard Medical School-MIT;
Brigham and Women's Hospital,
Harvard Institutes of Medicine,
Boston, Massachusetts

Larissa Braga, MD, MPH
Assistant Professor,
Department of Radiology-University of Nebraska
Medical Center,
Omaha, Nebraska

Josephine P. Briggs, MD
Director, National Center for Complementary
and Alternative Medicine,
National Institute of Health,
Bethesda, Maryland

Maria Luiza Caramori, MD, MS, PhD
Assistant Professor,
Division of Endocrinology and Diabetes,
Department of Medicine,
University of Minnesota,
Minneapolis, Minnesota

Daniel C. Cattran, MD, FRCP(C)
Professor of Medicine
University of Toronto;
Senior Research Scientist,
Toronto General Hospital Research Institute,
Toronto, Ontario, Canada

Arlene B. Chapman, MD
Professor of Medicine,
Department of Medicine,
Renal Division,
Emory University School of Medicine,
Atlanta, Georgia

Glenn M. Chertow, MD, MPH
Chief, Division of Nephrology,
Department of Medicine,
Stanford University School of Medicine,
Palo Alto, California

Alfred K. Cheung, MD
Professor of Medicine,
Division of Nephrology and Hypertension,
University of Utah;
Staff Physician,
Veterans Affairs Salt Lake City Healthcare System,
Salt Lake City, Utah

Kerry C. Cho, MD
Fellowship Program Director,
Assistant Clinical Professor,
Division of Nephrology,
Department of Medicine,
University of California,
San Francisco, California

Thomas M. Coffman, MD
James R. Clapp Professor of Medicine,
Chief, Division of Nephrology,
Duke University Medical Center,
VA Medical Center,
Durham, North Carolina

Peter J. Conlon, MD, FRCPi
Professor Nephrology,
Royal College of Surgeons of Ireland,
Beaumont Hospital, Dublin, Ireland

Jeffrey J. Connaire, MD
Assistant Professor of Medicine,
University of Minnesota Medical School,
Hennepin County Medical Center,
Minneapolis, Minnesota

Gary Curhan, MD, ScD
Associate Professor of Medicine,
Harvard Medical School;
Associate Professor of Epidemiology,
Harvard School of Public Health;
Assistant Physician,
Renal Unit and General Medicine Unit,
Massachusetts General Hospital,
Boston, Massachusetts

Paula Dennen, MD
Assistant Professor of Medicine,
Department of Medicine,
Nephrology and Critical Care Medicine,
Denver Health,
Denver, Colorado

Thomas D. DuBose, Jr., MD, MACP
Tinsley R. Harrison Professor
and Chair of Internal Medicine,
Professor of Physiology and Pharmacology,
Wake Forest University School of Medicine;
Chief of Internal Medicine Service,
North Carolina Baptist Hospital,
Winston-Salem, North Carolina

David H. Ellison, MD
Head, Division of Nephrology and Hypertension,
Professor of Medicine, Physiology, and Pharmacology,
Oregon Health and Science University,
Portland, Oregon

Michael Emmett, MD
Chairman,
Department of Internal Medicine,
Baylor University Medical Center,
Dallas, Texas

Ronald J. Falk, MD
Doc J. Thurston Professor of Medicine,
University of North Carolina School of Medicine;
Director, UNC Kidney Center,
Chief, Division of Nephrology and Hypertension,
University of North Carolina,
Chapel Hill, North Carolina

Javier Fernández, MD
Barcelona Medical School,
Liver Unit Hospital Clinic,
Barcelona, Spain

Catherine M. Goeddeke-Merickel, MS, RD, LD
Nutrition and Kidney Disease,
Clinical Consultant and Advanced Practice Dietitian,
Private Practice,
Maple Grove, Minnesota

D. Jordi Goldstein-Fuchs, DSc, RD, RN
Kidney Nutrition Specialist,
Sparks and Fallon Dialysis,
Reno, Nevada

Arthur Greenberg, MD
Division of Nephrology,
Department of Medicine,
Duke University Medical Center,
Durham, North Carolina

Martin C. Gregory, BM, BCh, PhD
Professor of Medicine,
University of Utah Health Sciences Center,
Salt Lake City, Utah

Antonio Guasch, MD
Associate Professor of Medicine, Renal Division,
Emory University, Atlanta, Georgia

Lakshman Gunaratnam, MD, MSc
Instructor in Medicine,
Harvard Medical School;
Fellow, Renal Division,
Brigham and Women's Hospital,
Boston, Massachusetts

William L. Henrich, MD, MACP
Dean of the School of Medicine,
Vice President for Medical Affairs,
University of Texas Health Science Center, San Antonio,
San Antonio, Texas

Friedhelm Hildebrandt, MD
Professor of Pediatrics and Human Genetics,
Doris Duke Distinguished Clinical Scientist;
Frederick G.L. Huetwell Professor for the Cure
and Prevention of Birth Defects,
University of Michigan,
Ann Arbor, Michigan

Ronald J. Hogg, MB, ChB, DCH
Professor of Pediatrics,
Texas A&M University,
College Station, Texas;
Chief, Pediatric Nephrology,
Scott and White Hospital,
Temple, Texas

Jean L. Holley, MD
Clinical Professor of Medicine,
University of Illinois, Urbana-Champaign;
Nephrologist, Carle Clinic,
Carle Clinic and Carle Foundation Hospital,
Urbana, Illinois

Chi-yuan Hsu, MD, MSc
Associate Professor, Division of Nephrology,
University of California-San Francisco,
San Francisco, CA

Alastair J. Hutchison, MD, FRCP
Clinical Director of Renal Medicine, Manchester,
Institute of Nephrology and Transplantation, The Royal,
Infirmary, Manchester, United Kingdom

A. David Jayne, MD, FRCP
Department of Medicine,
University of Cambridge,
Renal Unit,
Addenbrooke's Hospital,
Cambridge, United Kingdom

J. Charles Jennette, MD
Brinkhous Distinguished Professor
and Chair, Department of Pathology
and Laboratory Medicine,
School of Medicine,
University of North Carolina;
Chief of Pathology and Laboratory Medicine Services,
University of North Carolina Hospitals,
Chapel Hill, North Carolina

Wladimiro Jiménez, PhD
Associate Professor of Medicine,
University of Barcnelona,
Head of Service of Biochemistry
and Molecular Genetics,
Hospital Clinic, Barcelona, Spain

Bertram L. Kasiske, MD,
Director of Nephrology, Hennepin County
Medical Center; Professor of Medicine,
University of Minnesota College of Medicine,
Minneapolis, Minnesota

Nitin Khosla, MD
University of California at San Diego
San Diego, California

Paul E. Klotman, MD
Professor and Chair, Samuel Bronfman
Department of Medicine,
Mount Sinai School of Medicine,
New York, New York

Eugene C. Kovalik, MD, CM, FRCP(C), FACP
Associate Professor of Medicine,
Department of Medicine,
Duke University Medical Center,
Durham, North Carolina

Jean-Paul Kovalik, MD, PhD
Division of Endocrinology,
Metabolism and Nutrition,
Department of Medicine,
Duke University School of Medicine,
Durham, North Carolina

Michelle Whittier Krause, MD, MPH
Associate Professor of Medicine,
University of Arkansas for Medical Sciences;
Staff Physician,
Central Arkansas Veteran's Healthcare System,
Little Rock, Arkansas

Wilhelm Kriz, MD
Professor of Anatomy and Developmental Biology,
University of Heidelberg,
Medical Faculty Mannheim,
Mannheim, Germany

Andrew S. Levey, MD
Dr. Gerald J. and Dorothy R. Friedman,
Professor of Medicine,
Tufts University School of Medicine;
Chief, William B. Schwartz Division of Nephrology,
Tufts Medical Center,
Boston, Massachusetts

Fang-Ying Lin, MD
Assistant Professor of Medicine,
Division of Nephrology,
University of Texas Health Science Center
at San Antonio
San Antonio, Texas

Stuart Linas, MD
Professor of Medicine,
Department of Renal Disease and Hypertension,
University of Colorado Health Science Center;
Chief of Nephrology,
Denver Health,
Denver, Colorado

Nicolaos E. Madias, MD
Maurice S. Segal, MD Professor of Medicine,
Tufts University School of Medicine,
Chairman, Department of Medicine,
Caritas St. Elizabeth's Medical Center,
Boston, Massachusetts

Roslyn B. Mannon, MD
Professor of Medicine and Surgery,
University of Alabama at Birmingham,
Director of Research,
Alabama Transplant Center,
Birmingham, Alabama

Diego R. Martin, MD, PhD
Professor and Director of MRI,
Department of Radiology,
Emory University School of Medicine,
Atlanta, Georgia

Gary R. Matzke, PharmD, FCP, FCCP
Associate Dean for Clinical Research and Public Policy,
Professor of Pharmacy and Medicine,
School of Pharmacy,
Virginia Commonwealth University,
Richmond, Virginia

Michael Maver, MD
Professor and Co-Director,
Pediatric Neprology,
Department of Pediatrics,
University of Minnesota,
Minneapolis, Minnesota

Rory McQuillan, MB, BCH BAO, MRCPi
Beaumont Hospital,
Beaumont, Dublin, Ireland

Ankit N. Mehta, MD
Department of Internal Medicine,
Baylor University Medical Center,
Dallas, Texas

Catherine M. Meyers, MD
Director, Inflammatory Renal Disease Program,
Kidney, Urologic, and Hematologic Diseases Division,
National Institute of Diabetes, Digestive,
and Kidney Diseases,
National Institute of Healthl; Medical Staff
Nephrologist, NIDDK/Warren G. Magnuson
Clinical Center,
Bethesda, Maryland

Alain Meyrier, MD
Professor of Medicine (Emeritus),
University René Descartes Medical School,
Consultant Nephrologist,
Hôpital Broussais-Georges Pompidou,
Paris, France

Sharon M. Moe, MD
Professor of Medicine,
Vice-Chair for Research,
Department of Medicine,
Indiana University,
Indianapolis, Maryland

Marianne Monahan, MD
Division of Infectious Diseases,
Department of Medicine,
Mount Sinai School of Medicine,
New York, New York

Narayana S. Murali, MD
Instructor in Medicine,
Mayo Clinic College of Medicine,
Rochester, Minnesota

Cynthia C. Nast, MD
Professor of Pathology,
David Geffen School of Medicine at UCLA,
Professor of Pathology,
Cedars-Sinai Biomedical Science Program,
Los Angeles, California

Karl A. Nath, MD
Professor of Medicine,
Department of Internal Medicine,
Mayo Clinic College of Medicine,
Rochester, Minnesota

Lindsay E. Nicolle, MD, FRCPC
Professor, Department of Internal Medicine,
Medical Microbiology,
University of Manitoba,
Winnipeg, Manitoba,
Canada

John F. O'Toole, MD
Assistant Professor,
Case Western Reserve University School of Medicine,
Metro Health Medical Center,
Cleveland, Ohio

Biff F. Palmer, MD
Professor of Internal Medicine,
Director, Renal Fellowship Training Program,
University of Texas Southwestern Medical Center,
Dallas, Texas

Roberto Pisoni, MD
Division of Nephrology and Dialysis,
Azienda Ospedaliera Ospedali Riuniti di Bergamo;
Research Coordinator,
'Mario Negri' Institute of Pharmacological Research,
Bergamo, Italy

Tiina Podymow, MD
Division of Nephrology,
McGill University Health Center,
Royal Victoria Hospital,
Montreal, Quebec, Canada

Charles D. Pusey, DSc, FRCP
Professor of Medicine,
Imperial College of Medicine,
Honorary Consultant Physician,
Hammersmith Hospital,
London, United Kingdom

L. Darryl Quarles, MD
Summerfield Endowed Professor of Nephrology,
University of Kansas Medical Center,
Kansas City, Kansas

Maya K. Rao, MD
Division of Nephrology and Hypertension,
Oregon Health & Science University,
Portland, Oregon

Giuseppe Remuzzi, MD, FRCP
Director, Division of Nephrology and Dialysis,
Azienda Ospedaliera Ospedali Riuniti di Bergamo,
Research Coordinator,
'Mario Negri' Institute for Pharmacological Research,
Bergamo, Italy

Eberhard Ritz, MD
Department of Internal Medicine, Nierenzentrum
Ruperto-Carola-University Heidelberg, Heidelberg,
Germany

Akber Saifullah, MD
Research Fellow,
Indiana University School of Medicine,
Indianapolis, Maryland

Alan D. Salama, MBBS, PhD, FRCP
Senior Lecturer, Imperial College London;
Consultant Nephrologist,
Hammersmith Hospital,
London, United Kingdom

Paul W. Sanders, MD
Professor of Medicine, Departments of Medicine and
Physiology and Biophysics, Division of Nephrology,
University of Alabama-Birmingham,
Chief, Renal Section,
Department of Veterans Affairs Medical Center,
Veterans Affairs Medical Center
Birmingham, Alabama

Mark J. Sarnak, MD, MS
Associate Professor of Medicine,
Department of Medicine,
Tufts University School of Medicine,
Associate Director Research Training Program,
Division of Nephrology,
Tufts Medical Center,
Boston, Massachusetts

Steven J. Scheinman, MD
Senior Vice President,
Dean, College of Medicine,
Professor of Medicine and Pharmacology,
SUNY Upstate Medical University,
Syracuse, New York

Arrigo Schieppati, MD
Division of Nephrology and Dialysis,
Azienda Ospedaliera Ospedali Riuniti di Bergamo;
Research Coordinator,
'Mario Negri' Institute for Pharmacological Research,
Bergamo, Italy

Jürgen B. Schnermann, MD
Chief, Kidney Disease Section
National Institute of Diabetes, and Digestive
and Kidney Diseases,
National Institutes of Health,
Bethesda, Maryland

Richard C. Semelka, MD
Professor of Radiology,
Director of MR service,
Vice-Chair of Clinical Research,
Department of Radiology,
University of North Carolina at Chapel Hill,
Chapel Hill, North Carolina

Lesley A. Stevens, MD, MS
Assistant Professor of Medicine,
Tufts University School of Medicine,
Attending Nephrologist,
Tufts Medical Center, Boston, Massachusetts

Nicholas Stoycheff, MD
William B Schwartz Division of Nephrology,
Tufts-New England Medical Center,
Boston, Massachusetts

Harold M. Szerlip, MD
Professor and Vice Chair, Department of Medicine,
Medical College of Georgia, Augusta, Georgia

Nadine D. Tanenbaum, MD
Assistant Professor Division of Nephrology,
Washington University of St. Louis School of Medicine,
St. Louis, Missouri

Howard Trachtman, MD
Professor of Pediatrics,
Albert Einstein College of Medicine, Bronx, New York,
Chief, Division of Nephrology,
Schneider Children's Hospital of North Shore-LIJ
Health System,
New Hyde Park, New York

Joseph G. Verbalis, MD
Professor of Medicine,
Program Director, General Clinical
Research Center, Georgetown
University Medical School,
Chief, Division of Endoerinology and
Metabolism, Georgetown University Hospital,
Washington, DC

Anand Vardhan, MD
Consultant Nephrologist,
The Royal Infirmary,
Manchester, United Kingdom

Daniel E. Weiner, MD, MS
Assistant Professor of Medicine,
Tufts University School of Medicine,
Boston, Massachusetts

Christopher S. Wilcox, MD, PhD
George E. Schreiner Professor of
Nephrology and Director,
Georgetown University Center for
Hypertension, Kidney and Vascular Disorders,
Department of Medicine
Georgetown University,
Chief of Division of Nephrology and Hypertension,
Department of Medicine,
Georgetown University Medical Center,
Washington, DC

Jay B. Wish, MD
Professor of Medicine,
Case Western Reserve University,
Medical Director, Hemodialysis Services,
University Hospitals Case Medical Center,
Cleveland, Ohio

Christina M. Wyatt, MD
Assistant Professor,
Division of Nephrology,
Department of Medicine,
Mount Sinai School of Medicine,
New York, New York

Fuad N. Ziyadeh, MD
Professor of Medicine and Biochemistry,
Chairman, Department of Internal Medicine,
Associate Dean for Academic
Affairs/Faculty of Medicine,
American University of Beirut,
Beirut, Lebanon

Christopher S. Wilcox, MD, PhD
George E. Schreiner Professor of
Nephrology, and Director,
Georgetown University Center for
Hypertension, Kidney, and Vascular Disorders,
Department of Medicine,
Georgetown University,
Chief, Division of Nephrology and Hypertension,
Department of Medicine,
Georgetown University Medical Center,
Washington, DC

Jay B. Wish, MD
Professor of Medicine,
Case Western Reserve University,
Medical Director, Hemodialysis Service/Acute,

Christina M. Wyatt, MD
Assistant Professor,
Division of Nephrology,
Department of Medicine,
Mount Sinai School of Medicine,
New York, New York

Fuad N. Ziyadeh, MD
Professor of Medicine and Biochemistry,
Chairman, Department of Internal Medicine,
Associate Dean for Academic,
Affairs, Faculty of Medicine,
American University of Beirut,
Beirut, Lebanon

Preface

The goal of this fifth edition of the *Primer* is the same as that of the first: to provide a comprehensive but accessible summary of kidney and electrolyte disorders suitable for students, residents, fellows, and practitioners. Again, authors were asked to provide a consensus view of the topic, and the chapters were each read by at least two editors to assure balance and uniformity of coverage. An updated list of key references rather than detailed citations follows the text of each chapter.

While the depth of coverage and intended readership of the book have not changed, Nephrology surely has. A comparison of this edition of the *Primer* with the first, published in 1993, gives us a snapshot of how the substance of Nephrology and even its lexicon have changed in the last fifteen years. In the first two editions, the chapter on progression of chronic kidney disease (*chronic renal failure* then) included a figure illustrating several phases of declining function linked to a curve showing the hyperbolic relationship between serum creatinine and GFR. Terms like chronic renal insufficiency and renal failure were widely used, with meaning and import that varied with the chapter and context. Not until the fourth edition in 2005 was Chronic Kidney Disease (CKD) staging introduced. Much copy editing was required during the preparation of that edition to bring the *Primer* into compliance with the new and more precise terminology for reduced kidney function and CKD that is now widely accepted. Stratification and stage specific management have become routine features of the care of patients with progressive kidney damage. In this edition, the Risk-Injury-Failure-Loss-Endstage (RIFLE) classification of Acute Kidney Injury (AKI) and Outcome makes its debut even as we struggle with what to do with terms like Acute Renal Failure (ARF). Perhaps by the time of the next edition, we will learn how this standardized approach to severity of injury, hopefully combined with the use of new biomarkers of early injury, change the approach to detection, prevention, and treatment of AKI.

Understanding of the genetic and molecular basis of structural kidney disease has expanded remarkably. The first edition did not discuss causes of hereditary focal segmental glomerulosclerosis (FSGS). In the fourth edition, a new chapter summarizing in one place the emerging knowledge of the genetic basis of structural kidney disease appeared. When selecting what to include in the current edition, we omitted that superb chapter because the field had already outgrown it. Instead, the now well-established gene defects are included in the chapters on individual disorders. This decision recognizes that the genetic defects have become essential to an understanding of the pathophysiology of FSGS like many other structural disorders. The chapter on polycystic kidney disease (PKD) in the first edition was largely descriptive, although mention was made of the recently discovered PKD gene. This edition discusses the gene products of the two PKD genes in detail and explains how their absence contributes to cyst formation. The chapter describes the potentially useful interventions being tested or soon to be tested in clinical trials.

What else have we learned since the *Primer* first appeared? This edition introduces readers to the specific vasopressin receptor antagonists, the first truly new treatment of hyponatremia in a generation, although we don't know yet how best to employ these aquaretic agents. The role of renin-angiotensin-aldosterone system inhibition in limiting progression of CKD has been proven. CKD and albuminuria are now known to be prominent and independent risk factors for cardiovascular disease, but we still need to learn how best to intervene. One could go on and on. Of course, the book is not a history. Most readers will use it as an updated reference on pathophysiology and for help with clinical problems. The essence of a primer is brevity. The editors and authors have kept these goals in mind throughout the preparation of the *Primer*. We sincerely hope readers will agree.

Finally, a few words of acknowledgment. The authors sent us expertly written summaries of their topic and responded graciously to any requests for revision. Associate Editors Alfred Cheung, Tom Coffman, Ron Falk, and Charles Jennette gave generously of their time to assure that the chapters would be accurate and on message. I am most grateful for all of these contributions and especially for the hard work behind them.

Arthur Greenberg, MD
Durham, NC

Contents

Structure and Function of the Kidneys and Their Clinical Assessment

CHAPTER 1

Overview of Kidney Function and Structure

Josephine P. Briggs, Wilhelm Kriz, and Jurgen B. Schnermann

BASIC CONCEPTS

Functions of the Kidney

The main functions of the kidneys can be categorized as follows:

1. *Maintenance of body composition:* The kidney regulates the volume of fluid in the body; its osmolarity, electrolyte content, and concentration; and its acidity. It achieves this regulation by varying the amounts of water and ions excreted in the urine. Electrolytes regulated by changes in urinary excretion include sodium, potassium, chloride, calcium, magnesium, and phosphate.

2. *Excretion of metabolic end products and foreign substances:* The kidney excretes a number of products of metabolism, most notably urea, and a number of toxins and drugs.

3. *Production and secretion of enzymes and hormones:*
   a. Renin is an enzyme produced by the granular cells of the juxtaglomerular apparatus that catalyzes the formation of angiotensin from a plasma globulin, angiotensinogen. Angiotensin is a potent vasoconstrictor peptide and contributes importantly to salt balance and blood pressure regulation.
   b. Erythropoietin, a glycosylated protein comprising 165 amino acids that is produced by renal cortical interstitial cells, stimulates the maturation of erythrocytes in the bone marrow.
   c. 1,25-Dihydroxyvitamin D_3, the most active form of vitamin D_3, is formed by proximal tubule cells. This steroid hormone plays an important role in the regulation of body calcium and phosphate balance.

In later chapters of this *Primer*, the pathophysiologic mechanisms and consequences of derangements in kidney function are discussed in detail. This chapter reviews the basic anatomy of the kidney, the normal mechanisms for urine formation, and the physiology of sodium, potassium, water, and acid-base balance.

The Kidney and Homeostasis

Numerous functions of the body proceed optimally only when body fluid composition and volume are maintained within an appropriate range. For example,

- Cardiac output and blood pressure are dependent on optimal plasma volume.

- Most enzymes function best over rather narrow ranges of pH and ionic concentrations.
- Cell membrane potential depends on the potassium ion (K^+) concentration.
- Membrane excitability depends on the calcium ion (Ca^{2+}) concentration.

The principal job of the kidneys is the correction of perturbations in the composition and volume of body fluids that occur as a consequence of food intake, metabolism, environmental factors, and exercise. In healthy people, such perturbations are typically corrected within a matter of hours so that, in the long term, body fluid volume and the concentrations of most ions do not deviate much from normal set points. In many disease states, however, these regulatory processes are disturbed, resulting in persistent deviations in body fluid volume or ionic concentrations. Understanding these disorders requires an understanding of the normal regulatory processes.

The Balance Concept

A central theme of physiology of the kidneys is understanding the mechanisms by which urine composition is altered to maintain the body in balance. The maintenance of stable body fluid composition requires that appearance and disappearance rates of any substance in the body balance each other. Balance is achieved when

Ingested amount + Produced amount =
Excreted amount + Consumed amount

For a large number of organic compounds, balance is the result of metabolic production and consumption. However, electrolytes are not produced or consumed by the body, so balance can only be achieved by adjusting excretion to match intake. Hence, when a person is in balance for sodium, potassium, and other ions, the amount excreted must equal the amount ingested. Because the kidneys are the principal organs where regulated excretion takes place, urinary excretion of such solutes closely follows the dietary intake.

Body Fluid Composition

To a large extent, humans are composed of water. Adipose tissue is low in water content; therefore, in obese people, the fraction of body weight that is water is lower than in lean individuals. As a consequence of their slightly greater fat

TABLE 1-1 Bedside Estimates of Body Fluid Compartment Volumes

REMEMBER	EXAMPLE FOR 60-Kg PATIENT
TBW = 60% × Body weight	60% × 60 kg = 36 L
Intracellular water = 2/3 of TBW	⅔ × 36 L = 24 L
Extracellular water = 1/3 of TBW	⅓ × 36 L = 12 L
Plasma water = 1/4 of Extracellular water	¼ × 12 L = 3 L
Blood volume = Plasma water ÷ (1 – Hct)	3 L ÷ (1 − 0.40) = 5 L

Hct, hematocrit; TBW, total body water.

TABLE 1-2 Typical Ionic Composition of Plasma and Intracellular Fluid

CONSTITUENT	PLASMA (mEq/L)	INTRACELLULAR FLUID (mEq/L)
Cations		
K^+	4	150
Na^+	143	12
Ca^{2+} (ionized)	2	0.001
Mg^{2+}	1	28
Total cations	150 mEq/L	190 mEq/L
Anions		
Cl^-	104	4
HCO_3^-	24	10
Phosphates	2	40
Protein	14	50
Other	6	86
Total anions	150 mEq/L	190 mEq/L

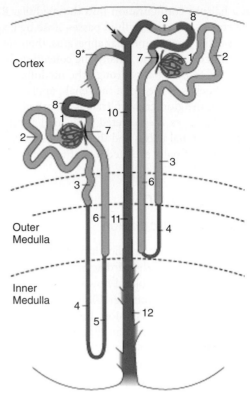

FIGURE 1-1 Organization of the nephron. The human kidney is made up of approximately 1 million nephrons, two of which are shown schematically here. Each nephron consists of the following parts: glomerulus (1), proximal convoluted tubule (2), proximal straight tubule (3), thin descending limb of the loop of Henle (4), thin ascending limb (5), thick ascending limb (6), macula densa (7), distal convoluted tubule (8), and connecting tubule (9). Several nephrons coalesce to empty into a collecting duct, which has three distinct regions: the cortical collecting duct (10), the outer medullary collecting duct (11), and the inner medullary collecting duct (12). As shown, the deeper glomeruli give rise to nephrons with loops of Henle that descend all the way to the papillary tips, whereas the more superficial glomeruli have loops of Henle that bend at the junction between the inner and outer medulla.

content, women contain a lower percentage of water on average than men—about 55% instead of 60%. Useful round numbers to remember for bedside estimates of body fluid volumes are given in **Table 1-1**. Typical values for the ionic composition of the intracellular and extracellular fluid compartments are given in **Table 1-2**.

KIDNEY STRUCTURE

The kidneys are two bean-shaped organs that lie in the retroperitoneal space, each weighing about 150 g. The kidney is an anatomically complex organ consisting of many different types of highly specialized cells, which are arranged in a highly organized, three-dimensional pattern. The functional unit of the kidney is the *nephron;* each nephron consists of a glomerulus and a long tubule, which is composed of a single layer of epithelial cells. There are approximately 1 million nephrons in one human kidney (**Fig. 1-1**). The nephron is segmented into distinct parts—proximal tubule, loop of Henle, distal tubule, and collecting duct—each with a typical cellular appearance and special functional characteristics.

The nephrons are packed together tightly to make up the kidney parenchyma, which can be divided into regions. The outer layer of the kidney is called the *cortex;* it comprises all of the glomeruli, much of the proximal tubules, and some of

the more distal portions as well. The inner section, called the *medulla,* consists largely of the parallel arrays of the loops of Henle and the collecting ducts. The medulla is formed into seven to nine cone-shaped regions, called *pyramids,* which extend into the renal pelvis. The tips of the medullary pyramids are called *papillae.* The medulla is important for concentration of the urine; the extracellular fluid in this region of the kidney has a much higher concentration of solutes than the plasma does, as much as four times higher, with the highest solute concentrations at the papillary tips.

The process of urine formation begins in the glomerular capillary tuft, where an ultrafiltrate of plasma is formed. The filtered fluid is collected in Bowman's capsule and enters the renal tubule to be carried over a circuitous course, successively modified by exposure to the sequence of specialized tubular epithelial segments with different transport functions. The proximal convoluted tubule, which is located entirely in the renal cortex, absorbs approximately two thirds of the glomerular filtrate. Fluid remaining at the end of the proximal convoluted tubule enters the loop of Henle, which dips down in a hairpin configuration into the medulla. Returning to the cortex, the tubular fluid passes close by its parent glomerulus at the juxtaglomerular apparatus, then enters the distal convoluted tubule and, finally, the collecting duct. The collecting duct courses back through the medulla, to empty into the renal pelvis at the tip of the renal papilla. Along the tubule, most of the glomerular filtrate is absorbed, but some additional substances are secreted. The final product, the *urine,* enters the renal pelvis and then the ureter, collects in the bladder, and is finally excreted from the body.

RENAL CIRCULATION

Anatomy of the Circulation

The renal artery, which enters the kidney at the renal hilum, carries about one fifth of the cardiac output; this represents the highest tissue-specific blood flow of all larger organs in the body (about 350 mL/min per 100 g tissue). As a consequence of this generous perfusion, the renal arteriovenous O_2 difference is much lower than that of most other tissues (and blood in the renal vein is noticeably redder in color than that in other veins). The renal artery bifurcates several times after it enters the kidney and then breaks into the arcuate arteries, which run, in an archlike fashion, along the border between the cortex and the outer medulla. As shown in **Figure 1-2**, the arcuate vessels give rise, typically at right angles, to interlobular arteries, which run to the surface of the kidney. The afferent arterioles supplying the glomeruli come off the interlobular vessels.

Two Capillary Beds in Series

The renal circulation is unusual in that it breaks into two separate capillary beds: the glomerular bed and the peritubular capillary bed. These two capillary networks are arranged in series, so that all of the renal blood flow passes through both. As blood leaves the glomerulus, the capillaries coalesce into the efferent arteriole, but almost immediately the vessels bifurcate again to form the peritubular capillary network. This second network of capillaries is the site where the fluid reabsorbed by the tubules is returned to the circulation. Pressure in the first capillary bed, that of the glomerulus, is rather high (40 to 50 mm Hg), whereas pressure in the peritubular capillaries is similar to that in capillary beds elsewhere in the body (5 to 10 mm Hg).

About one fourth of the plasma that enters the glomerulus passes through the filtration barrier to become the glomerular filtrate. Blood cells, most of the proteins, and about 75% of the fluid and small solutes stay in the capillary and leave the glomerulus via the efferent arteriole. This postglomerular blood, which has a relatively high concentration of protein and red cells, enters the peritubular capillaries, where the high osmotic pressure resulting from the high protein concentration facilitates the reabsorption of fluid. The peritubular capillaries coalesce to form venules and, eventually, the renal vein.

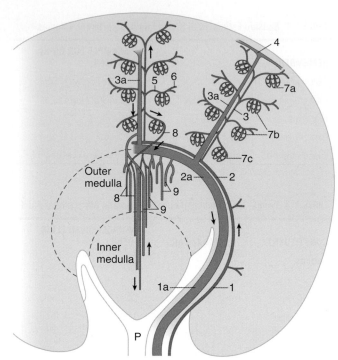

FIGURE 1-2 Organization of the renal vascular system. The renal artery bifurcates soon after entering the kidney parenchyma and gives rise to a system of arching vessels that run along the border between the cortex and the medulla. In this diagram, the vascular elements surrounding a single renal pyramid are shown. The human kidney typically has seven to nine renal pyramids. Here the arterial supply and glomeruli are shown in red, and the venous system is shown in blue. The peritubular capillary network that arises from the efferent arterioles is omitted for the sake of simplicity. The vascular elements are named as follows: interlobar artery and vein (1 and 1a); arcuate artery and vein (2 and 2a); interlobular artery and vein (3 and 3a); stellate vein (4); afferent arteriole (5); efferent arteriole (6); glomerular capillaries from superficial (7a) midcortex (7b), and juxtamedullary (7c) regions; and juxtamedullary efferent arterioles supplying descending vasa recta (8) and ascending vasa recta (9).

Medullary Blood Supply

The blood supplying the medulla is also postglomerular. Specialized peritubular vessels, called vasa recta, arise from the efferent arterioles of the glomeruli nearest the medulla (the juxtamedullary glomeruli). Like medullary renal tubules, these vasa recta form hairpin loops that dip into the medulla.

GLOMERULUS

Structure

The structure of the glomerulus is shown schematically in **Figure 1-3** and in a photomicrograph in **Figure 1-4**. The glomerulus is a ball consisting of capillaries, which are lined by endothelial cells. The capillaries are held together by a stalk of cells called the *mesangium,* and the outer surface of the capillaries is covered with specialized epithelial cells called *podocytes.* Podocytes are large, highly differentiated cells that form an array of lacelike foot processes over the outer layer of the glomerular capillaries. The foot processes of adjacent podocytes interdigitate, and a thin, membranous

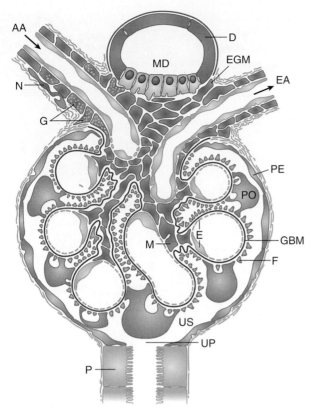

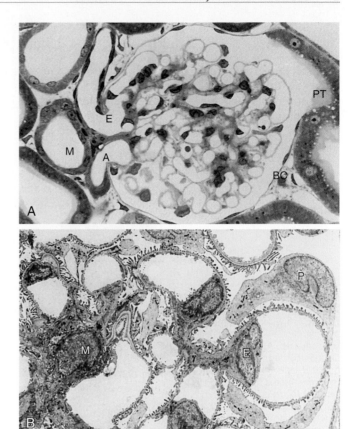

FIGURE 1-3 Schematic diagram of a section of a glomerulus and its juxtaglomerular apparatus. AA, afferent arteriole; D, distal tubule; E, endothelial cell; EA, efferent arteriole; EGM, extraglomerular mesangial cell; F, podocyte foot process; G, juxtaglomerular granular cell; GBM, glomerular basement membrane; M, mesangial cell; MD, macula densa; N, sympathetic nerve endings; P, proximal tubule; PE, parietal epithelial cell; PO, epithelial podocyte; UP, urinary pole; US, urinary space.

FIGURE 1-4 Structure of the glomerulus. **A,** Light micrograph of a glomerulus, showing the afferent arteriole (A), efferent arteriole (E), macula densa (M), Bowman's capsule (BC), and beginning of the proximal tubule (PT). The typical diameter of a glomerulus is about 100 to 150 μm, which is just visible to the naked eye (400X). **B,** Higher-power view of glomerular capillary loops, showing the epithelial podocyte (P), endothelial cells (E), and mesangial cells (M) (4,000X).

structure called the *slit diaphragm* connects adjacent podocyte foot processes. A structure called *Bowman's capsule* acts as a pouch to capture the filtrate and direct it into the beginning of the proximal tubule.

Glomerular Filtration Barrier

Urine formation begins at the glomerular filtration barrier. The glomerular filter through which the ultrafiltrate has to pass consists of three layers: the fenestrated endothelium, the intervening glomerular basement membrane, and the podocyte slit diaphragm (**Fig. 1-5**). This complex "membrane" is freely permeable to water and small dissolved solutes, but retains most of the proteins and other larger molecules, as well as all blood particles. The main determinant of passage through the glomerular filter is molecular size. A molecule such as inulin (5 kDa) passes freely through the filter, and even a small protein such as myoglobin (16.9 kDa) filters through to a large extent. Substances of increasing size are retained with increasing efficiency until, at a size about 60 to 70 kDa, the amount passing through the filter becomes very small. Some albumin escapes through the glomerular filtration barrier, but it is normally reabsorbed in the proximal tubule.

Function of the podocyte is critical for maintaining the integrity and selectivity of the glomerular filtration barrier.

Podocyte dysfunction causes increased protein excretion in the urine and a condition called *nephrotic syndrome,* which is discussed in detail in later chapters. Genetic studies, primarily in children with congenital proteinuric states, have established the identity of a number of the proteins critical for normal function of the podocyte. The podocyte is a terminally differentiated cell, with little capacity for division or cell repair. Injury to the podocyte is increasingly recognized as a key mechanism in many chronic kidney diseases.

Filtration by the Glomerulus

Filtrate formation in the glomerulus is governed by Starling forces, the same forces that determine fluid transport across other blood capillaries. The glomerular filtration rate (GFR) is equal to the product of the net ultrafiltration pressure (P_{net}), the hydraulic permeability (L_p), and the filtration area:

$$GFR = L_p \times Area \times P_{net}$$

The effective filtration pressure (P_{net}) is the difference between the hydrostatic pressure difference and the osmotic pressure difference across the capillary loop:

$$P_{net} = \Delta P - \Delta \Pi = (P_{GC} - P_B) - (\Pi_{GC} - \Pi_B)$$

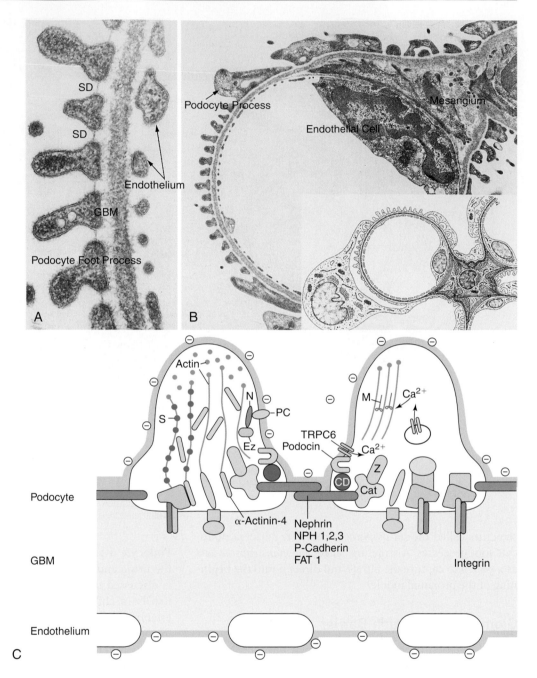

FIGURE 1-5 Structure of the glomerular capillary loop and the filtration barrier. **A,** The glomerular filtration barrier consisting of endothelial cells, glomerular basement membrane (GBM), and the slit diaphragms (SD) between podocyte foot processes (34,000X). **B,** A single capillary loop showing the endothelial and foot process layers and the attachments of the basement membrane to the mesangium. Pressure in the glomerular capillary bed is substantially higher than in other capillaries. As shown in the diagrammatic insert, the mesangium provides the structural supports that permit the cells to withstand these high pressures (13,000X). **C,** Schematic diagram of the filtration barrier and two podocyte foot process. GBM, glomerular basement membrane. Ez, ezrin; FAT1, FAT tumor suppressor homolog 1; M, myosin; N, NERF2; NPH, nephrin; PC, podocalyxin; S, synaptopodin; TRPC6, transient receptor potential- channel 6.

where P is hydrostatic pressure, Π is osmotic pressure, and the subscripts GC and B refer to the glomerular capillaries and Bowman's space, respectively. Changes in GFR can result from changes in the permeability/surface area product ($L_p \times$ Area) or from changes in P_{net}. One factor influencing P_{net} is the resistance in the afferent and efferent arterioles. An increase in resistance in the afferent arteriole (before blood gets to the glomerulus) decreases P_{GC} and GFR, whereas an increase in resistance as blood exits through the efferent arteriole tends to increase P_{GC} and GFR. Changes in P_{net} can also occur as a result of an increase in renal arterial pressure, which tend to increase P_{GC} and GFR. Obstruction of the tubule increases P_B and decreases GFR, and a decrease in plasma protein concentration tends to increase GFR.

Determination of the Glomerular Filtration Rate

GFR is measured by determining the plasma concentration and excretion of a marker substance that meets the following requirements:

1. The substance must be neither absorbed nor secreted by the renal tubules.
2. The substance should be freely filterable across the glomerular membranes.
3. The substance is not metabolized or produced by the kidneys.

Inulin, a large sugar molecule with a molecular weight of about 5000 Da, meets these requirements and is the classic marker substance infused to measure GFR. It follows from the requirements listed that, if P_{in} is the plasma concentration of inulin, U_{in} is the urinary concentration of inulin, and V is the urine flow rate,

$$\text{Filtered amount of inulin} = GFR \times P_{in}$$
$$\text{Excreted amount of inulin} = U_{in} \times V$$

Because the filtered amount of inulin is equal to the excreted amount of inulin,

$$GFR \times P_{in} = U_{in} \times V$$

Therefore,

$$GFR = \frac{U_{in} \times V}{P_{in}}$$

Other molecules with similar properties have been developed, including iothalamate and iohexol, and these compounds can be administered to patients to measure GFR. Creatinine is an endogenous substance that, although not a perfect GFR marker, is handled by the kidney in a similar way, so that its plasma concentration can be used to estimate GFR. The clearance of creatinine is slightly greater than GFR (15% to 20%) because some creatinine is secreted; therefore, the excreted amount exceeds the amount filtered. Cystatin is another endogenous substance that is cleared by the kidney in rough proportion to the level of GFR; plasma levels of cystatin have also been used to estimate GFR. The estimation of GFR is discussed in more detail in Chapter 2.

GFR is dependent on body size, age, and physiologic state. Typical normal values for GFR in adults are 100 mL/min for women and 120 mL/min for men. Values in children increase with growth and depend on age. A high-protein diet and high salt intake increase GFR, and GFR increases markedly with pregnancy (see Chapter 50). GFR decreases with a low-protein diet and declines steadily with age (see Chapter 51).

Juxtaglomerular Apparatus

Tightly adherent to every glomerulus, in between the entry and the exit of the arterioles, is a plaque of distal tubular cells called the *macula densa,* which is part of the juxtaglomerular apparatus. This cell plaque is in the distal tubule, at the very terminal end of the thick ascending limb of the loop of Henle, just before its transition to the distal convoluted tubule. This is a special position along the nephron, because at this site the salt concentration is quite variable. Low rates of flow result in a very low concentration of NaCl at this site, 15 mEq/L or less, whereas at higher flow rates the salt concentration increases to 40 to 60 mEq/L. The NaCl concentration at this site regulates glomerular blood flow through a mechanism called *tubuloglomerular feedback:* An increase in salt concentration causes a decrease in glomerular blood flow.

The other unique cells that make up the juxtaglomerular apparatus are the renin-containing juxtaglomerular granular cells. Renin secretion is also regulated locally by salt concentration in the tubule at the macula densa. In addition, the granular cells have extensive sympathetic innervation, and renin secretion is controlled by the sympathetic nervous system.

TUBULAR FUNCTION: BASIC PRINCIPLES
Epithelial Transport along the Renal Tubule

The glomerular filtrate undergoes a series of modifications before becoming the final urine. These changes consist of removal (absorption) and addition (secretion) of solutes and fluid (**Fig. 1-6**).

1. *Absorption,* the movement of solute or water from tubular lumen to blood, is the predominant process in the renal handling of Na^+, Cl^-, H_2O, bicarbonate (HCO_3^-), glucose, amino acids, protein, phosphates, Ca^{2+}, Mg^{2+}, urea, uric acid, and other molecules.
2. *Secretion,* the movement of solute from blood or cell interior to tubular lumen, is important in the renal handling of H^+, K^+, ammonium ion (NH_4^+), and a number of organic acids and bases.

Many specialized membrane proteins participate in the movement of substances across cell membranes along the renal tubule. Some of the important membrane transport mechanisms, together with examples of substances that use these mechanisms and proteins that are important for these processes, are listed in **Table 1-3**. A variety of mechanisms exist to regulate the activity of membrane proteins.

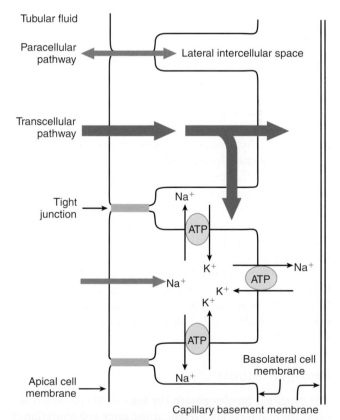

FIGURE 1-6 General scheme for epithelial transport. The driving force for solute movement is primarily generated by the action of sodium-potassium adenosine triphosphatase (Na^+,K^+-ATPase) in the basolateral membrane. Solutes and water can move either through a paracellular pathway between cells *(red arrows)* or through a transcellular transport pathway *(blue arrows),* which requires movement across both luminal and basolateral membranes. ATP, adenosine triphosphate. (From Koeppen BM, Stanton BA: Renal Physiology. St. Louis, CV Mosby, 1992.)

TABLE 1-3 Types of Membrane Transport Mechanisms Used in the Kidney

MECHANISM	EXAMPLES OF SUBSTANCES	EXAMPLES OF TRANSPORT PROTEIN
Facilitated or carrier-mediated	Glucose, urea	GLUT1 carrier, urea carrier
Active transport (pumps)	Na^+, K^+, H^+, Ca^{2+}	Na^+ K^+-ATPase, H^+-ATPase, Ca^{2+}-ATPase
Coupled transport Cotransport	Cl^-, glucose, amino acids, formate, phosphates	NKCC2
Countertransport	Bicarbonate, H^+	Cl^-/HCO_3^- exchanger (AE1), Na^+/H^+ antiporter (NHE3)
Osmosis	H_2O	Water channels (aquaporins)

ATPase, adenosine triphosphatase; GLUT1, glucose transporter 1; NKCC2, Na^+-K^+-$2Cl^-$ cotransporter.

Sometimes activity is altered by insertion or removal of the transport protein from the membrane, processes known, respectively, as endocytosis and exocytosis. Other proteins may undergo alterations in physical confirmation, triggered for example by phosphorylation or dephosphorylation, that result in changed channel activity or transport affinities.

As shown in **Figures 1-7** through **1-10,** one of the more striking characteristics of the renal tubule is its dramatic cellular heterogeneity. Early renal anatomists recognized that there are marked differences in the appearance of the cells of the proximal tubule, loop of Henle, and distal tubule. We now know that these nephron segments also differ markedly in function, distribution of important transport proteins, and responsiveness to drugs such as diuretics.

Most epithelial cells in the kidney and in other organs possess a single primary cilium. New attention has focused on the importance of cilia because of the discovery that genetic defects in cilial proteins are associated with the development of renal cysts. There is growing evidence that cilia play a role in determining epithelial shape and in the regulation of intracellular cell calcium by shear stress. Cilia may also participate in the regulation of tubular function by flow rate. The role of the cilium in cystic diseases of the kidney is discussed in more detail in Chapters 42 and 43.

Proximal Tubule

The proximal tubules absorb the bulk of filtered small solutes. These solutes are present at the same concentration in proximal tubular fluid as in plasma. Approximately 60% of the filtered Na^+, Cl^-, K^+, Ca^{2+}, and H_2O and more than 90% of the filtered HCO_3^- are absorbed along the proximal tubule. This is also the segment that normally reabsorbs virtually all the filtered glucose and amino acids, via Na^+-dependent cotransport. An additional function of the proximal tubule is

phosphate transport, which is regulated by parathyroid hormone. In addition to these reabsorption functions, secretion of solutes also occurs along the proximal tubule. The terminal portion of the proximal tubule, the S3 segment or pars recta, is the site of secretion of numerous organic anions and cations, a mechanism used by the body for elimination of a number of drugs and toxins. The proximal tubule (**Fig. 1-7**) has a prominent brush border, extensive interdigitated basolateral infoldings, and large prominent mitochondria, which supply the energy for sodium-potassium adenosine triphosphatase (Na^+,K^+-ATPase).

Loop of Henle

The loop of Henle consists of the terminal or straight portion of the proximal tubule, thin descending and ascending limbs, and a thick ascending limb and is important for generation of a concentrated medulla and for dilution of the urine. The thick ascending limb is often called the diluting segment, because transport along this water-impermeable segment results in development of a dilute tubular fluid. The thick ascending limb is also a major site of Mg^{2+} reabsorption along the nephron. The principal luminal transporter expressed in this segment is the Na^+-K^+-$2Cl^-$ cotransporter (NKCC2), which is the target of diuretics such as furosemide. The morphology of the loop of Henle epithelia is illustrated in **Figure 1-8**.

Distal Nephron

The distal nephron, which includes the distal convoluted tubule, the connecting tubule, and the cortical and medullary collecting duct, is the portion of the nephron where final adjustments in urine composition, tonicity, and volume are made. Distal segments are the sites where critical regulatory hormones such as aldosterone and vasopressin regulate acid and potassium excretion and determine final urinary concentrations of K^+, Na^+, and Cl^-. Both the distal convoluted tubule and the connecting tubule have well-developed basolateral infoldings with abundant mitochondria, like the proximal tubule; they are easily distinguished from the latter by the lack of brush border (**Fig. 1-9**). The distal convoluted tubule is the principal site of action of thiazide diuretics.

The collecting duct cells are cuboidal, and their basolateral folds do not interdigitate extensively. When there is a sizable osmotic gradient and water moves across this epithelium, the spaces between cells become wide. The collecting duct changes in its appearance as it travels from the cortex to the papillary tip (**Fig. 1-10**). In the cortex, there are two different cell types in the collecting duct: principal cells and intercalated cells. Principal cells are the main site of salt and water transport, and intercalated cells are the key site for acid-base regulation. The medullary collecting duct in its most terminal portions comes increasingly to resemble the tall cells typical of transitional epithelium that lines the bladder.

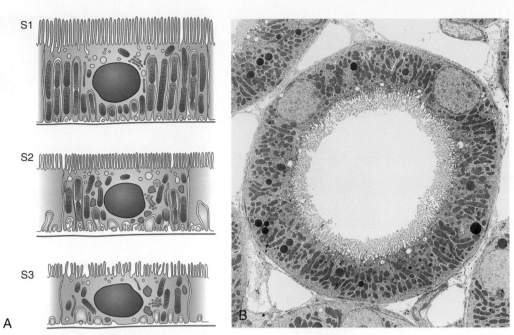

FIGURE 1-7 Proximal tubule. The proximal tubule consists of three segments: S1, S2, and S3. **A,** Schematic diagrams of the typical cells from these three segments. **B,** A cross-section of the S1 segment. The S1 begins at the glomerulus and extends for several millimeters before the transition to the S2 segment. The S3 segment, which is also called the proximal straight tubule, descends into the inner medulla. The proximal tubule is characterized by a prominent brush border, which increases the membrane surface area about 40-fold. The basolateral infoldings, which are lined with mitochondria, are interdigitated with the basolateral infoldings of adjacent cells (in the diagrams, processes that come from adjacent cells are shaded). These adaptations are most prominent in the first parts of the proximal tubule and are less well developed later along the proximal tubule (2,300 X).

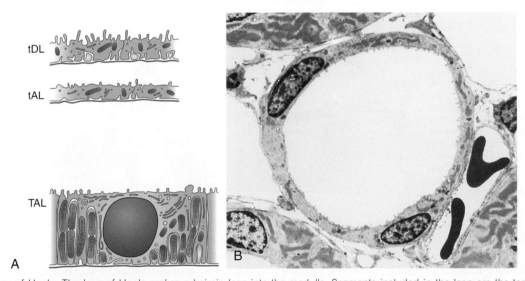

FIGURE 1-8 Loop of Henle. The loop of Henle makes a hairpin loop into the medulla. Segments included in the loop are the terminal portion of the proximal tubule, the thin descending (tDL) and thin ascending (tAL) limbs, and the thick ascending limb (TAL). **A,** Schematic drawings of cell morphology. **B,** A cross-section through the tDL in the outer medulla. The thin limbs, as their names suggest, are shallow epithelia without the prominent mitochondria of more proximal segments. The thick limb, in contrast, is a taller epithelium with basolateral infoldings and well-developed mitochondria. This segment is water impermeable; transport along this segment is important for generation of interstitial solute gradients and a low salt concentration and to dilute fluid in the tubular lumen (3,000 X).

SALT AND VOLUME REGULATION

Absorption of Sodium

Because of its high extracellular concentration, large amounts of Na^+ and its accompanying anions are present in the glomerular filtrate, and the absorption of this filtered Na^+ is, in a quantitative sense, the dominant work performed by the renal tubules. The amount of Na^+ absorbed by the tubules is the difference between the amount of Na^+ filtered and the amount excreted:

$$Na^+ \text{ absorption} = \text{Filtered } Na^+ - \text{Excreted } Na^+$$

or

$$Na^+ \text{ absorption} = (GFR \times P_{Na}) - (V \times U_{Na})$$

FIGURE 1-9 Distal convoluted tubule. The distal convoluted tubule is customarily divided into two parts: the true distal convoluted tubule (DCT) and the connecting tubule (CT), where cell morphology is somewhat more similar to that of the collecting duct. **A,** Schematic diagrams of cell morphology. **B,** Cross-section of DCT (3,000 X).

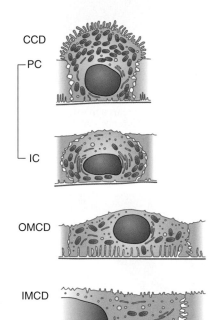

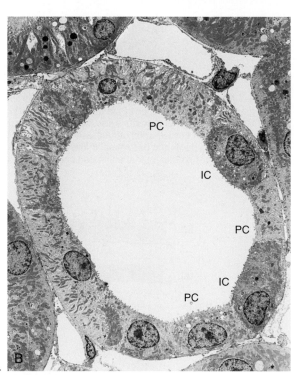

FIGURE 1-10 Collecting duct. **A,** Schematic appearance. **B,** Cross-section. The collecting duct changes its morphology as it travels from cortex to the medulla. In the cortex there are two cell types: principal cells (PC) and intercalated cells (IC). CCD, cortical collecting duct; IMCD, inner medullary collecting duct; OMCD, outer medullary collecting duct (3,000 X).

where U_{Na} is the urinary Na^+ concentration and P_{Na} is the plasma Na^+ concentration. With a GFR of 120 mL/min and a plasma Na^+ concentration of 145 mEq/L, 17.4 mEq of Na^+ is filtered every minute, or about 25,000 mEq (575 g) of Na^+ per day. Because only about 100 to 250 mEq of Na^+ is excreted per day (this reflects the average intake provided by a typical Western diet), one can estimate that the tubule reabsorbs somewhat more than 99% of the filtered Na^+. The fractional excretion of Na^+ (FE_{Na}) is defined as the fraction of filtered Na^+ excreted in the urine. Using creatinine as a GFR estimate, FE_{Na} is calculated as follows:

$$FE_{Na} = \frac{\text{Excreted } Na^+}{\text{Filtered } Na^+} = \frac{U_{Na} \times V}{P_{Na} \times GFR}$$

$$= \frac{U_{Na} \times V}{P_{Na} \times (U_{Cr}/P_{Cr} \times V)} = \frac{U_{Na}/P_{Na}}{U_{Cr}/P_{Cr}}$$

where UCr and PCr are the urinary and plasma concentrations of creatinine, respectively.

FE_{Na} is usually less than 1%. However, this value depends on Na^+ intake and can vary physiologically from almost 0% at extremely low intakes to about 2% at extremely high intakes. FE_{Na} can also exceed 1% in disease states in which the tubular transport of Na^+ is impaired (e.g., in most cases of acute renal failure).

Mechanisms of Sodium Ion Absorption

Tubular Na^+ absorption is a primary active transport process driven by the enzyme Na^+,K^+-ATPase. In renal epithelial cells, as in most cells of the body, this pump translocates Na^+ out of cells (and K^+ into cells) and thereby lowers the intracellular Na^+ concentration (and elevates intracellular K^+ concentration). A key for the generation of net Na^+ movement from tubular lumen to blood is the asymmetrical distribution of this enzyme; it is present exclusively in the basolateral membrane (the blood side) of all nephron segments, but not in the luminal membrane. Delivery of Na^+ to the pump sites is maintained by Na^+ entry into the luminal side of the cells along a favorable electrochemical gradient. Because Na^+ permeability of the luminal membrane is much higher than that of the basolateral membrane, Na^+ entry is fed from the luminal Na^+ pool. The asymmetrical permeability results from the presence of a variety of transport proteins or channels located exclusively in the luminal membrane.

A number of these luminal transporters are the target molecules for diuretic action. Principal entry mechanisms for Na^+ and Cl^- in the various nephron segments are as follows:

1. *Early proximal tubule:* Na^+-dependent cotransporter, Na^+/H^+ exchanger (NHE3)
2. *Late proximal tubule:* Na^+/H^+ exchanger, Cl^--anion exchanger
3. *Thick ascending limb:* NKCC2 cotransporter (furosemide-sensitive carrier)
4. *Distal convoluted tubule:* Na^+/Cl^- cotransporter (NCCT) (thiazide-sensitive carrier)
5. *Collecting duct:* epithelial Na^+ channel (ENaC) (amiloride-sensitive channel)

Regulation of Salt Excretion

Because Na^+ salts are the most abundant extracellular solutes, the amount of sodium in the body (the total body sodium) determines the extracellular fluid volume. Therefore, excretion or retention of Na^+ salts by the kidneys is critical for the regulation of extracellular fluid volume. Disturbance in volume regulation, particularly enhanced salt retention, is common in disease states. The sympathetic nervous system, the renin-angiotensin-aldosterone system, atrial natriuretic peptide, and vasopressin represent the four main regulatory systems that change their activity in response to changes in body fluid volume. These changes in activity mediate the effects of body fluid volume on urinary Na^+ excretion.

Sympathetic Nervous System

A change in extracellular fluid volume is sensed by stretch receptors on blood vessels, principally those located on the low-pressure side of the circulation in the thorax (e.g., vena cava, cardiac atria, pulmonary vessels). A decreased firing rate in the afferent nerves from these volume receptors enhances sympathetic outflow from cardiovascular medullary centers. Increased renal sympathetic tone enhances renal salt reabsorption and can decrease renal blood flow at higher frequencies. In addition to its direct effects on kidney function, increased sympathetic outflow promotes the activation of another salt-retaining system, the renin-angiotensin system.

Renin-Angiotensin System

Renin is an enzyme that is formed by and released from granular cells in the wall of renal afferent arterioles near the entrance to the glomerulus. These granular cells are part of the juxtaglomerular apparatus (see **Fig. 1-3**). Renin is an enzyme that cleaves angiotensin I from angiotensinogen, a large circulating protein made principally in the liver. Angiotensin I, a decapeptide, is converted by angiotensin-converting enzyme to the biologically active angiotensin II. Renin catalyzes the rate-limiting step in the production of angiotensin II, and therefore it is the plasma level of renin that determines the concentration of angiotensin II in plasma. There are three principal mechanisms that control renin release:

1. *Macula densa mechanism:* The term "macula densa" refers to a group of distinct epithelial cells located in the wall of the thick ascending limb of the loop of Henle, where it makes contact with its own glomerulus. At this location, the NaCl concentration is between 30 and 40 mEq/L and varies as a direct function of tubular fluid flow rate (i.e., it increases when the flow rate is high and decreases when it is low). A decrease in NaCl concentration at the macula densa strongly stimulates renin secretion, and an increase inhibits it. The connection to the regulation of body fluid volume results from the dependence of the flow rate past the macula densa cells on the body sodium content. The flow rate is high in states of sodium excess and low in sodium depletion.
2. *Baroreceptor mechanism:* Renin secretion is stimulated by a decrease in arterial pressure, an effect believed to be mediated by a "baroreceptor" in the wall of the afferent arteriole that responds to pressure, stretch, or shear stress.
3. *β-Adrenergic stimulation:* An increase in renal sympathetic activity or in circulating catecholamines stimulates renin release through β-adrenergic receptors on the juxtaglomerular granular cells.

Angiotensin II has direct and indirect effects that promote salt retention. It enhances Na^+ reabsorption in the proximal tubule (through stimulation of Na^+/H^+ exchange), and, because it is a potent renal vasoconstrictor, it may reduce GFR by reducing glomerular capillary pressure or plasma flow. Angiotensin II affects salt balance indirectly by stimulating the production and release of the steroid hormone aldosterone from the zona glomerulosa of the adrenal gland.

Aldosterone

Aldosterone acts on the collecting duct to augment salt reabsorption, largely by increasing the activity of the sodium channel, ENaC, and thereby increasing salt absorption. A second important action of aldosterone in the kidney is the stimulation of K^+ secretion. This effect is not dependent on angiotensin; rather, high K^+ stimulates the secretion of aldosterone directly. In the distal nephron, these two effects of aldosterone are not always coupled, and recent evidence suggests that a family of kinases, called WNK kinases, may participate in switching the distal nephron response to allow either maximal NaCl reabsorption (in hypovolemia) or maximal K^+ secretion (in hyperkalemia). The first evidence that these kinases are important functional molecular switches came from genetic studies in patients with a Mendelian form of hypertension accompanied by hyperkalemia called pseudohypoaldosteronism type II.

Atrial Natriuretic Factor

Atrial natriuretic factor (ANF) is a peptide hormone that is synthesized by atrial myocytes and released in response to increased atrial distention. As a result, ANF secretion is increased in volume expansion and inhibited in volume depletion. The main cause of the ANF-induced natriuresis is an inhibition of Na^+ reabsorption along the collecting duct, but an increase in GFR may sometimes play a contributory role.

Vasopressin or Antidiuretic Hormone

Vasopressin or antidiuretic hormone (ADH) is regulated primarily by body fluid osmolarity. However, in states in which intravascular volume is depleted, the set point for vasopressin release is shifted, so that, for any given plasma osmolarity, vasopressin levels are higher than they would be normally. This shift promotes water retention to aid in restoration of body fluid volumes.

WATER AND OSMOREGULATION

Regulation of Body Fluid Osmolarity

When water intake is low or water is lost from the body (e.g., in hypotonic fluids such as sweat), the kidneys conserve water by producing a small volume of concentrated urine. In dehydration, urine production is less than 1 L/day (<0.5 mL/min), and the osmotic concentration of the urine (U_{osm}) may reach 1200 mOsm/kg H_2O. When water intake is high, urine flow may increase to as much as 14 L/day (10 mL/min), with an osmolality substantially lower than that of plasma (75 to 100 mOsm/kg). These wide variations in urine volume and osmotic concentration do not obligatorily affect the excretion of the daily solute load. For example, the daily solute excess of about 1200 mOsm may be excreted in 12 L of urine (U_{osm} = 100 mOsm/L) or in 1 L (U_{osm} = 1200 mOsm/L). The hormone responsible for the regulatory changes in urine volume and tonicity is ADH (vasopressin).

Role of Antidiuretic Hormone in Osmolarity Regulation

ADH is a nonapeptide produced by neurons located in the supraoptic and paraventricular nuclei of the hypothalamus. It is stored in and released from granules in nerve terminals that are located in the posterior pituitary (neurohypophysis). The release of ADH is exquisitely sensitive to changes in plasma osmolality (P_{osm}), with increases in P_{osm} above a threshold of about 285 mOsm/kg leading to increases in ADH secretion and plasma ADH concentration. As has been pointed out, the actual set point for release depends on body fluid volume as well.

The most important function of ADH is the regulation of water permeability of the distal portions of the nephron, particularly the collecting duct. As shown schematically in **Figure 1-11**, ADH binds to receptors in the basolateral membrane of collecting duct cells. This activates adenylate cyclase to form cyclic adenosine monophosphate (cAMP). The latter molecule activates a protein kinase, which leads to the phosphorylation of undefined proteins. Phosphorylation causes membrane fusion of vesicles that contain preformed water channels. The result is an increase in water permeability of the apical (luminal) membrane of collecting duct cells. On removal of ADH, water channels are rapidly removed from the apical membrane by endocytosis.

Tubular Water Absorption

At each point along the nephron, the osmotic pressure of the tubular fluid is lower than that in the interstitial space. This transtubular osmotic pressure difference provides the driving force for tubular water reabsorption. The rate of fluid absorption in a given nephron segment is determined by the magnitude of this gradient and the osmotic water permeability of the segment. Even though the osmotic pressure difference across the proximal tubule epithelium is small (3 to 4 mOsm/L), the rate of fluid absorption is high, because this segment has a very high water permeability. In contrast, osmotic gradients across the thick ascending limb may be as high as 250 mOsm/L, and yet virtually no water flows across this segment because it is highly water impermeable. This segment dilutes the urine, because it absorbs Na^+ and Cl^- without water.

In contrast to the constancy of water conductivity in the proximal tubule and the thick ascending limb, water permeability in the collecting duct is highly variable and is controlled by the influence of ADH. When ADH is absent, water permeability and water absorption are low, and the hypotonicity generated in the thick ascending limb persists along the collecting duct. As a consequence, a dilute urine

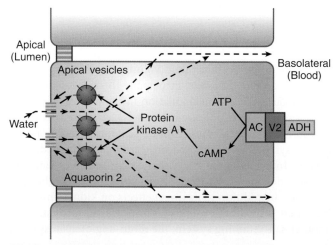

FIGURE 1-11 Mechanism of action of antidiuretic hormone (ADH) on the collecting duct. ADH combines with a basolateral receptor (V2), which is coupled with adenylate cyclase (AC). Generation of cyclic adenosine monophosphate (cAMP) leads to activation of protein kinase A, which in turn phosphorylates the water channel, aquaporin 2. The vesicles containing aquaporin are then inserted into the luminal membrane, increasing water permeability ATP, adenosine triphosphate.

is excreted. When ADH is present, the collecting duct becomes quite water permeable, and water is reabsorbed until the tubular fluid in the collecting duct equilibrates with the hypertonic interstitium. In this situation, the final urine is osmotically concentrated and has a low volume.

Medullary Hypertonicity

To allow osmotically driven water absorption, the osmotic concentration in the medullary interstitium must be slightly higher than that in the collecting duct lumen. For example, when a final urine with an osmolality of 1200 mOsm/kg is excreted, the medullary interstitium at the tips of the papillae must be a little higher than 1200 mOsm/kg. The generation of such a unique extracellular environment is achieved by the countercurrent multiplication system of the renal medulla, which consists of the countercurrent arrangement of descending and ascending limbs of the loops of Henle.

Countercurrent Multiplication

By passing through two adjacent tubes with flow in opposite directions, the tubular fluid can attain an osmotic concentration difference in the longitudinal axis of the system that by far exceeds that seen at each level along it. This principle of countercurrent multiplication requires energy expenditure and the presence of unique differences in membrane characteristics between the two limbs of the system.

The countercurrent multiplier represented by the loops of Henle is believed to generate an osmotic gradient for the following reasons:

1. Active NaCl transport across the ascending limb (the so-called single effect of the countercurrent system) generates an osmotic difference between the tubular fluid and the surrounding local interstitium.
2. Low water permeability in the ascending limb prevents dissipation of this gradient.
3. High water permeability in the descending limb permits equilibration of descending limb contents with the surrounding local interstitium.

The mechanism by which such a system can result in progressive increases in osmotic concentration along the corticopapillary axis is shown in **Figure 1-12**. In step 1 (time zero), the fluid in the descending and ascending limbs and in the interstitium is iso-osmotic to plasma. In step 2, NaCl is absorbed from the ascending limb into the interstitium until a gradient of 200 mOsm/kg is reached. In step 3, the fluid in the descending limb equilibrates osmotically with the interstitium by water movement out of the tubule. In step 4, the hypertonic fluid is presented to the thick ascending limb with an increased solute concentration in the region near the tip of the system. Active NaCl transport along the ascending limb again establishes a 200 mOsm/kg gradient (step 5), thereby increasing the interstitial concentration and (by water abstraction) the descending limb concentration (step 6). Note that concentrations near the tip are now higher than those near the base. Continued operation of such a mechanism gradually results in the generation of a gradient of hypertonicity, with the highest osmolarities at the papillary tip (step 7). The tubular fluid leaving the ascending limb of the loop of Henle countercurrent multiplier is hypotonic, but the medullary interstitium has been osmotically "charged."

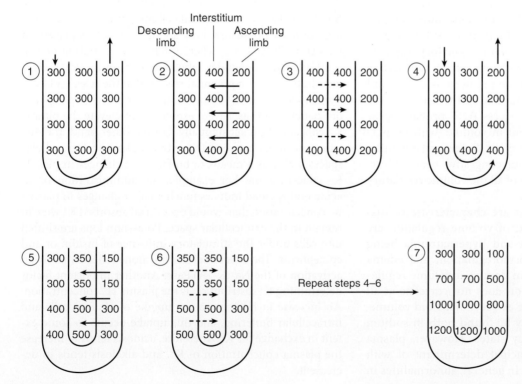

FIGURE 1-12 The process of countercurrent multiplication. See text for description. (From Koeppen BM, Stanton BA: Renal Physiology. St. Louis, CV Mosby, 1992.)

Because the collecting ducts on their way to the papillary tip return to the hypertonic medullary environment, their content can be concentrated by water flow along an osmotic gradient.

Role of Urea in the Countercurrent Mechanism

In addition to Na^+ and Cl^-, urea is the other major solute concentrated in the renal medulla. Urea enters the medulla by reabsorption across the collecting duct. Marked differences in permeability to urea allow reabsorption to proceed only across the terminal portions of the medullary collecting duct. In the early portions of the collecting duct, urea permeability is low, and reabsorption of urea cannot occur. Because water leaves the tubule under the influence of ADH, the urea staying behind is progressively concentrated. As a consequence, a substantial urea gradient develops, providing the driving force for urea reabsorption when the permeability to urea permits it. The contribution of urea accumulation to osmotic water absorption along the inner medullary collecting duct must be sizable, because urea accounts for about half of inner medullary tonicity. Therefore, a reduction in urea synthesis due to reduced protein intake markedly impairs the concentrating ability of the kidneys.

Comparison Between Volume Regulation and Osmoregulation

Osmoregulation is under the control of a single hormonal system, ADH, whereas volume regulation is under the control of a set of redundant and overlapping control mechanisms. Lack or excess of ADH results in defined and rather dramatic clinical syndromes of excess water loss or water retention. In contrast, a defect in a single volume regulatory mechanism generally results in more subtle abnormalities, because of the redundant regulatory capacity from the other mechanisms. Therefore, excess aldosterone results in a mild volume retention followed by escape and return to normal Na^+ excretion, due to the action of the other mechanisms. Similarly, excess ANF probably produces only a modest decrement in volume, with no persistent abnormality in Na^+ excretion. Severe salt-retaining states, such as liver cirrhosis or congestive heart failure, are characterized by activation of all the volume regulatory mechanisms.

Finally, the symptoms that are characteristic of disorders of osmoregulation and of volume regulation are different, with hyponatremia and hypernatremia being the hallmarks of deranged osmoregulation, and edema or hypovolemia resulting from deranged volume regulation. Plasma Na^+ concentration does not correlate at all with total body sodium or the extracellular fluid volume. In fact, a low serum Na^+ may be found both in sodium excess and sodium deficiency states. However, plasma Na concentration is the principal determinant of with extracellular fluid osmolarity. In general, abnormalities in Na^+ concentration arise from defects in osmoregulation, not volume regulation.

REGULATION OF BODY FLUID POTASSIUM AND ACIDITY

Both potassium and hydrogen ions are present in body fluids at low concentrations, about 4 to 4.5 mEq/L for K^+ and about 40 mEq/L for H^+. Both ions show a number of features:

1. Relatively small deviations in either the K^+ or the H^+ concentration can be life-threatening, and therefore the regulation of K^+ and H^+ requires control systems with high sensitivity and precision.
2. Constancy of both the K^+ and the H^+ concentration over the long term is achieved by regulated excretion of these ions in the urine. However, in both cases, other mechanisms exist that provide immediate protection against excessive deviations of plasma concentrations from normal.
3. Regulation in the renal excretion of both K^+ and H^+ is caused to a large extent by variation in the secretion of these ions by collecting ducts. The principal cell of the collecting duct is the cell type responsible for regulated K^+ secretion; the intercalated cell is the cell type responsible for H^+ secretion (see **Fig. 1-10**).
4. The rate of both K^+ secretion and H^+ secretion is increased by aldosterone.
5. A primary derangement of K^+ balance can cause an acidity disturbance, and a primary acidity disturbance can derange K^+ homeostasis.

Regulation of Body Fluid Potassium

Distribution of Potassium Ion in the Body

K^+ is mostly an intracellular ion, owing to the presence of Na^+,K^+-ATPase in virtually all cell membranes. Of the 3500 mEq of body potassium, only about 1% to 2% is present in the extracellular space, where it has a concentration of 4 to 5 mEq/L. The remainder (about 98%) is intracellular. This distribution poses a potential risk, in that the release of even a small amount of K^+ from intracellular stores (e.g., insulin deficiency, cell lysis, severe exercise) can elevate the plasma K^+ concentration substantially. On the other hand, the distribution of K^+ between the extracellular and intracellular spaces serves as a means to buffer acute changes in plasma K^+ concentration. For example, the administration of an acute oral K^+ load induces much smaller changes in plasma K^+ concentration than would occur if all absorbed K^+ were to remain in the extracellular space. Potassium ions are shifted into cells under the stimulatory influence of insulin or and epinephrine. The effect of either hormone reflects mainly an activation of the Na^+,K^+-ATPase. Another important factor determining K^+ distribution is the plasma H^+ concentration. An increase in H^+ ions causes uptake of H^+ into cells and intracellular buffering, and this uptake occurs to some extent in exchange for K^+. Therefore, acidosis tends to increase the plasma concentration of K^+, and alkalosis tends to decrease it.

Renal Handling of Potassium

Potassium ion homeostasis requires the excretion of an amount equivalent to the daily K^+ intake (50 to 150 mEq). This represents a fractional K^+ excretion (FE_K) of about 10%, much higher than the FE_{Na}. About 60% to 70% of filtered K^+ is absorbed along the proximal tubule, and further reabsorption of K^+ takes place in the thick ascending limb of the loop of Henle; only about 10% of filtered K^+ enters the distal tubule. Along the collecting duct, K^+ is both secreted and absorbed. Collecting duct K^+ secretion increases when dietary K^+ intake is elevated. When dietary intake is low, collecting duct K^+ secretion virtually ceases, and absorption is dominant. Therefore, although K^+ absorption along the proximal tubule and the loop of Henle does not change very much depending on intake, collecting duct K^+ secretion is variable, and this variability accounts almost completely for the variation in urinary K^+ excretion.

Mechanisms of Potassium Ion Secretion

K^+ secretion across the collecting duct epithelium utilizes the transcellular route. K^+ uptake across the basolateral membrane is driven by Na^+,K^+-ATPase, which elevates the intracellular K^+ concentration to a level above electrochemical equilibrium. K^+ can then move along a favorable gradient from cell interior to tubule lumen, utilizing potassium channels in the luminal membrane.

Three major variables determine the rate at which K^+ is secreted by collecting duct cells:

1. Changes in the activity of Na^+,K^+-ATPase affect uptake and thereby change the intracellular K^+ concentration. An increase in pump activity increases intracellular K^+ levels and tends to stimulate K^+ secretion.
2. Changes in the electrochemical gradient affect the driving force for K^+ movement across the luminal membrane. Either an increase in intracellular K^+ concentration or in the transepithelial potential difference (lumen-negative) will increase the driving force and will tend to increase K^+ secretion.
3. Changes in the permeability of the luminal membrane determine the amount of K^+ that can be secreted for a given driving force. An increase in luminal K^+ conductance increases K^+ secretion.

Regulation of Potassium Ion Excretion

Plasma K^+ Concentration

One important determinant of K^+ excretion is the plasma K^+ concentration. For example, the change in K^+ excretion that occurs after an increase in dietary K^+ intake is mediated by an increase in plasma K^+. The effect of plasma K^+ on secretion is induced partly by a direct effect on the intracellular K^+ concentration.

Aldosterone

At any level of plasma K^+, the secretion of K^+ also depends on the plasma aldosterone level. Aldosterone enhances K^+ secretion by activation of Na^+,K^+-ATPase and by an increase in permeability of the luminal membrane to K^+. Aldosterone is partly responsible for the diet-induced increase in K^+ excretion, because its production and secretion are directly stimulated by the plasma K^+ concentration. This effect is independent of angiotensin.

Tubular Flow Rate

An increase in tubular flow rate past the K^+-secreting cells stimulates K^+ secretion, and a decrease reduces K^+ secretion. The K^+ concentration gradient across the apical membrane increases when delivery of fluid increases. In addition, increased flow has been found to increase K^+ permeability, perhaps mediated by changes in the deflection of the cilia on tubular cells.

Distal Sodium Delivery

When more Na^+ is delivered to the distal nephron, if reabsorption increases, the net electrical charge in the lumen becomes more negative. This favorable electrochemical gradient tends to increase urinary K^+ secretion.

Hydrogen Ions

A decrease in H^+ concentration in alkalotic states causes a stimulation of K^+ secretion. This effect is mediated by the increase in intracellular K^+ concentration that occurs in alkalosis.

Diuretics and Potassium Ion Excretion

Diuretics increase the tubular flow rate. Agents, such as loop diuretics and thiazides, that inhibit absorption of NaCl and water in segments that precede the collecting duct (NaCl in the loop of Henle and water in the distal tubule) increase the flow of fluid past the collecting duct cells, which causes increased K^+ secretion. In addition, diuretics cause volume depletion, which stimulates aldosterone secretion.

Regulation of Body Fluid Acidity

Basic Considerations

Maintenance of the extracellular pH at approximately 7.4 depends on the operation of buffer systems that accept protons (H^+) when they are produced and liberate protons when they are consumed. The state of the demand on total body buffering can be determined by assessing the behavior of the HCO_3^-/CO_2 system, which is the major extracellular buffer. The law of mass action for this buffer system states the following:

$$pH = 6.1 + \log \frac{\left[HCO_3^-\right]}{\left[CO_2\right]}$$

where brackets indicate the concentration of a substance. Because the $[CO_2]$ equals the solubility coefficient multiplied by the partial pressure of carbon dioxide (P_{CO_2}), the equation can be rewritten as

$$pH = 6.1 + \log \frac{\left[HCO_3^-\right]}{0.03 \times P_{CO_2}}$$

This, the familiar Henderson-Hasselbach equation, tells us that pH constancy depends on a constant ratio between the concentrations of the two buffer components. If this ratio increases, because either HCO_3^- increases or CO_2 decreases, the pH will increase (alkalosis). If the ratio decreases, because either HCO_3^- decreases or CO_2 increases, the pH will decrease (acidosis). Regulation of HCO_3^- is mainly a function of the kidneys, and regulation of CO_2 is a respiratory function.

The regulation of HCO_3^- concentration by the kidneys consists of two main components:

1. *Absorption of HCO_3^-:* Because of the high GFR and because plasma HCO_3^- concentrations are also relatively high (24 mEq/L), large amounts of HCO_3^- are filtered. Retrieval of this filtered HCO_3^- is essential for acid-base balance. This process of renal HCO_3^- absorption does not add new HCO_3^- to the blood but merely prevents a loss of filtered HCO_3^- into the urine. Therefore, renal HCO_3^- absorption cannot correct an existing metabolic acidosis.

2. *Excretion of H^+:* Under normal dietary conditions, approximately 40 to 80 mmol of H^+ is generated daily (mostly sulfuric acid from the metabolism of sulfur-containing amino acids). This H^+ is buffered and therefore consumes HCO_3^-. The kidneys must excrete this H^+ to regenerate the HCO_3^- pool; this second task can therefore be viewed as generation of "new" HCO_3^-.

Mechanisms of Bicarbonate Absorption

Filtered HCO_3^- (about 4300 mEq/day) is efficiently absorbed by the renal tubules, predominantly the proximal tubules, and under normal acid-base conditions very little HCO_3^- is found in the urine. As a rule, all tubular HCO_3^- absorption is the consequence of H^+ secretion, and not of direct absorption of HCO_3^- ions. H^+ is continuously generated inside the cells from the dissociation of H_2O (or from the reaction of CO_2 with H_2O) and transported into the lumen. In the lumen, secreted H^+ combines with filtered HCO_3^- to form carbonic acid, which is broken down to CO_2 and H_2O in a reaction that is catalyzed by a carbonic anhydrase located in the apical brush border membrane. CO_2 and H_2O are then absorbed passively. The OH^- generated in the cell during this process combines with CO_2 to form HCO_3^-, a reaction catalyzed by a cytosolic carbonic anhydrase. HCO_3^- exits across the basolateral side of the cell and returns to the blood in association with Na^+. The net balance of this process can be expressed as follows:

2. The second mechanism is a primary active transport of H^+. An H^+-ATPase has been found in the luminal membrane of one class of intercalated collecting duct cells. There is also some evidence for the presence of an H^+, K^+-ATPase similar to that found in parietal cells of the gastric mucosa. Active H^+ transport is responsible for the secretion of smaller amounts of H^+ than Na^+/H^+ exchange, but it can proceed against a steeper gradient.

There are also at least two mechanisms for the transport of HCO_3^- across the basolateral membrane. The movement of HCO_3^- can be coupled to the movement of Na^+, and this is the major exit mechanism in the proximal tubule. In the collecting duct, HCO_3^- exit occurs predominantly through a basolateral Cl^-/HCO_3^- exchanger (equivalent to the band 3 protein of red cells, AE1).

Bicarbonate Secretion

Although net HCO_3^- transport for the whole kidney is always in the reabsorptive direction, certain intercalated cells in the cortical portion of the collecting duct can actually secrete HCO_3^-. These bicarbonate-secreting cells have a polarity that is the reverse of the proton-secreting cells; that is, they possess a basolateral H^+-ATPase and probably a luminal Cl^-/HCO_3^- exchanger. HCO_3^- secretion may be important during consumption of a diet providing base equivalents and for the correction of metabolic alkalosis.

Excretion of Protons (Formation of New Bicarbonate Ions)

Urinary acid excretion cannot, to any significant extent, occur as free H^+. The minimum urinary pH in humans is about 4.5, corresponding to an H^+ concentration of only 0.03 mEq/L. Because some 40 to 80 mEq of H^+ must be excreted each day, it is clear that most H^+ ions must be excreted in a bound or buffered form. Excretion of bound H^+ is achieved in two ways: by the titration of luminal nonbicarbonate buffers and by the renal synthesis and excretion of ammonium ions.

Titratable Acidity

Binding of secreted H^+ to filtered nonbicarbonate buffer anions leads to the formation and excretion of urinary titratable

$$H_2O + CO_2 \leftarrow H_2CO_3 \leftarrow HCO_3^- + H^+ \leftarrow H_2O \rightarrow OH^- + CO_2 \rightarrow HCO_3^- + Na^+$$

| tubular lumen | cell interior | blood |

Specific transport proteins in renal epithelial cells cause the H^+ and HCO_3^- to move in the right directions. Two different mechanisms, both located in the apical membrane, are responsible for the movement of protons into the tubular fluid.

1. The first mechanism is an Na^+/H^+ exchanger (NHE3) that is driven by the Na^+ gradient and is found in the proximal tubule. In terms of milliequivalents transported, it contributes most to HCO_3^- absorption.

acidity. (Titratable acidity is defined as the number of moles of NaOH that must be added to bring the urine back to pH 7.4.) The ability to buffer H^+ depends on its dissociation constant (pK) and the quantity of buffer. Under normal conditions, only the $HPO_4^{2-}/H_2PO_4^-$ buffer is present in amounts sufficient to act as an intratubular H^+ acceptor. This buffer pair has a pH of 6.8 and is excreted at a daily rate of about 50 mmol. Applying the Henderson-Hasselbalch equation for the phosphate buffer (pH = 6.8 + log $[HPO_4^{2-}]/[H_2PO_4^-]$),

TABLE 1-4 Effect of Tubular Acidification on Buffering Capacity*

LOCATION	pH	HPO_4^{2-} (mmol/day)	$H_2PO_4^-$ (mmol/day)	H^+ BUFFERED (mmol/day)
Filtrate	7.4	40	10	0
End of proximal tubule	6.8	25	25	15
Urine	4.8	0.5	49.5	39.5

and considering only that fraction of total phosphate that is actually excreted (about 25% to 30% of the filtered phosphate load), the relationships shown in **Table 1-4** can be calculated.

This tabulation shows that the buffer capacity of HPO_4^{2-} can be fully utilized if the intratubular pH is lowered sufficiently. In some situations, other urinary buffers become important. In diabetic ketoacidosis, large amounts of β-hydroxybutyrate are excreted (e.g., 300 mmol/L). Even though this buffer component has a pK of 4.8, it carries up to 150 mmol H^+ per liter.

Ammonium Excretion

The second form of bound H^+ in the urine is ammonium. The excretion of NH_4^+ is equivalent to generation of HCO_3^- or excretion of H^+. The major source of urinary ammonium is glutamine, which is formed in the liver from glutamate and extracted from the blood by uptake mechanisms in the luminal and basolateral membranes of renal proximal tubule cells. Ammonium is generated in the proximal tubule by a metabolic pathway that degrades glutamine to glutamate and further to α-ketoglutarate; this yields $2NH_4^+$ and $2HCO_3^-$ (rather than NH_3, CO_2, and H_2O). Whereas the NH_4^+ ions are secreted through distinct transport pathways into the lumen of the proximal tubule, the new HCO_3^- ions are added to the blood HCO_3^- pool.

It is essential for the NH_4^+ that is formed by renal proximal tubules to be preferentially secreted into the tubular lumen and then excreted in the urine. If the generated NH_4^+ were to be absorbed by the renal tubular epithelium (or secreted preferentially into the blood), it would be used to form urea (H_2NCONH_2). Ureagenesis forms protons that would consume the produced bicarbonate and thereby negate the net base production. This is shown in the following reactions:

$$2NH_4^+ + CO_2 \rightarrow urea + H_2O + 2H^+$$

or

$$2NH_4^+ + 2HCO_3^- \rightarrow urea + CO_2 + 3H_2O$$

Urinary H^+ excretion in the form of NH_4^+ is on the order of 40 to 50 mmol/day. Renal NH_4^+ formation and excretion are greatly enhanced in metabolic acidosis. Failure of the proximal tubules to generate NH_4^+ is the main reason that metabolic acidosis occurs in chronic kidney disease.

Regulation of Proton Secretion
Intracellular pH

Systemic pH changes, whether caused by changes in plasma HCO_3^- (metabolic) or by changes in Pco_2 (respiratory), alter H^+ secretion (and therefore HCO_3^- absorption). Intracellular

acidification (e.g., in acidosis) stimulates H^+ secretion, and intracellular alkalinization (alkalosis) inhibits it.

Aldosterone

In addition to affecting Na^+ absorption and K^+ secretion, aldosterone stimulates H^+ secretion by the collecting ducts.

Potassium

Changes in plasma K^+ concentration can affect H^+ secretion, in part by changing the intracellular pH. For example, hypokalemia increases intracellular acidity and stimulates H^+ ion secretion. Although the effect of hypokalemia alone is relatively small, a marked stimulation of H^+ secretion results when hypokalemia occurs with high plasma aldosterone levels. In this situation, which can happen in primary hyperaldosteronism or with the administration of diuretics, metabolic alkalosis may be generated by the kidneys.

RENAL HANDLING OF GLUCOSE AND AMINO ACIDS

An important function of the renal tubule is retrieval of the glucose and amino acids that are present in glomerular filtrate and would be lost to the body if they were not reabsorbed. To a large extent, this is a function of the proximal tubule, and disordered glucose and amino acid transport is characteristic of diseases that disturb proximal tubular function.

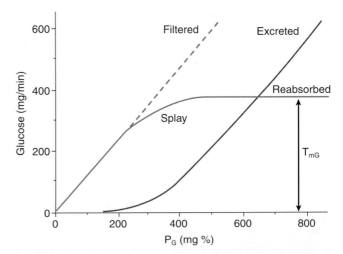

FIGURE 1-13 A typical filtration curve for renal glucose reabsorption. At plasma glucose concentrations less than approximately 200 mg/dL, the filtered glucose is completely reabsorbed, and no glucose is excreted in the urine. When the plasma glucose concentration exceeds this level, the filtered load of glucose exceeds the transport capacity of the tubule, and glucose appears in the urine. P_G, plasma glucose; T_{mG}, tubular transport maximum for glucose.

Glucose transport by the proximal tubule occurs via a transport protein present in the luminal membrane that carries a glucose molecule together with a sodium ion, the glucose-sodium cotransporter. This transporter uses the sodium concentration gradient (the concentration of Na^+ is higher outside the cell) to drive the movement of glucose into the cell. Glucose then diffuses out of the cell across the basolateral membrane, a process facilitated by a second carrier protein. The resulting reabsorption process is highly efficient. In normal circumstances, almost all of the filtered glucose is removed from the proximal tubule fluid, and, as a result, glucose is virtually absent from urine.

When the plasma glucose concentration rises, increasing amounts of glucose are filtered, and at a certain point the filtered load of glucose exceeds the capacity of the proximal transport mechanisms. This maximum reabsorption rate is called the *tubular transport maximum for glucose* (T_{mG}).

When glucose delivery exceeds the T_{mG}, the excess glucose is excreted in the urine (**Fig. 1-13**).

Many of the same principles apply to the reabsorption of amino acids, another function of the proximal tubule. Amino acid absorption is also highly effective: For most amino acids, less than 1% of the amount filtered escapes into the urine. A number of different luminal and basolateral transport proteins are needed to remove the amino acids from the glomerular filtrate. A specific transporter carries the dibasic amino acids, L-arginine and L-lysine, and another carrier is responsible for removal of the acidic amino acids from the tubular fluid. There also are luminal transporters that, like the sodium-glucose cotransporter, exploit the sodium concentration gradient for cotransport of certain amino acids together with sodium. Other carrier molecules in the basement membrane facilitate the exit of amino acids from the cell.

BIBLIOGRAPHY

Brater DC: Diuretic therapy. N Engl J Med 339:387-395, 1998.

Durvasula RV, Shankland SJ: Podocyte injury and targeting therapy: An update. Curr Opin Nephrol Hypertens 15:1-7, 2006.

Giebisch GH: A trail of research on potassium. Kidney Int 62: 1498-1512, 2002.

Giebisch G, Windhager E: The urinary system. In Boron WF, Emile L, Boulpaep EL (eds): Medical Physiology: A Cellular and Molecular Approach. Section VI. Philadelphia, WB Saunders, 2003, pp 735-875.

Guyton AC, Hall JE: Unit V: The body fluids and kidney. In Guyton AC, Hall JE: Textbook of Medical Physiology, 11th ed. Philadelphia, Elsevier, 2006.

Jefferson JA, Shankland SJ: The molecular mechanisms of proteinuria. In Mount DB, Pollak MR (eds): Molecular and Genetic Basis of Renal Disease. Philadelphia, Saunders Elsevier, 2007.

Kahle KT, Ring AM, Lifton RP: Molecular physiology of the WNK kinases. Annu Rev Physiol 70:329-355, 2008.

Lifton RP: Genetic dissection of human blood pressure variation: Common pathways from rare phenotypes. Harvey Lect 100: 71-101, 2004.

Meyer TW, Hostetter TH: Uremia. N Engl J Med 357:1316-1325, 2007.

Pavenstadt H, Kriz W, Kretzler M: Cell biology of the glomerular podocyte. Physiol Rev 83:253-307, 2003.

Rose BD, Post T, Rose B: Clinical Physiology of Acid-Base and Electrolyte Disorders, 5th ed. New York, McGraw-Hill, 2001.

Schrier RW: The sea within us: Disorders of body water homeostasis. Curr Opin Investig Drugs 8:304-311, 2007.

Shayman JA: Renal Physiology. Philadelphia, JB Lippincott, 1995.

Singla V, Reiter JF: The primary cilium as the cell's antenna: Signaling at a sensory organelle. Science (New York) 313:629-633, 2006.

Stanton BA, Koeppen BM: The kidney. In Berne RM, Levy MN, Koeppen BM, Stanton BA (eds): Physiology, 5th ed. Section VII. St. Louis, CV Mosby, 2004, pp 621-716.

Stevens LA, Coresh J, Greene T, Levey AS: Assessing kidney function: Measured and estimated glomerular filtration rate. N Engl J Med 354:2473-2483, 2006.

CHAPTER 2

Clinical Evaluation of Kidney Function

Chi-yuan Hsu

DEFINITION OF CHRONIC KIDNEY DISEASE

This chapter discusses the evaluation of kidney function in clinical practice. The approach taken is largely influenced by the National Kidney Foundation Kidney Disease Outcomes Quality Initiative (K/DOQI) Clinical Practice Guidelines for Chronic Kidney Disease (CKD).

The National Kidney Foundation criteria for diagnosis of CKD are as follows:

1. Kidney damage for 3 months or longer, as defined by structural or functional abnormalities of the kidney, with or without decreased glomerular filtration rate (GFR), manifested by either pathologic abnormalities or markers of kidney damage (including abnormalities in composition of the blood or urine or in imaging tests), *or*
2. Glomerular filtration rate less than 60 mL/min/1.73 m² for 3 months or longer, with or without kidney damage.

CKD is further divided into stages 1 to 5, as shown in **Table 2-1**. For further details regarding the rationale behind the definition and staging of CKD, see Chapter 53.

GLOMERULAR FILTRATION RATE: THE KEY PARAMETER

GFR is generally accepted as the best overall index of kidney function and is the most important parameter to determine in the clinical evaluation of kidney function. The level of GFR correlates well, albeit not perfectly, with the likelihood of developing complications of kidney disease, such as cardiovascular disease, anemia, hyperphosphatemia, and uremic symptoms.

A chronically low GFR (<60 mL/min/1.73 m²) is by itself sufficient to make the diagnosis of CKD, regardless of the presence or absence of other markers of kidney damage.

GFR is the rate at which fluid is filtered across the glomerular basement membrane into the renal tubules. Measured GFR is the sum of all the single-nephron GFRs in both kidneys. It is possible for a disease to reduce the number of nephrons but for GFR to be relatively preserved because of a compensatory increase in single-nephron GFR. However, it is not feasible to measure nephron number or single-nephron GFR in humans, so overall GFR remains the cornerstone of the clinical evaluation of kidney function.

Historically, the gold standard for measurement of GFR has been clearance of the small molecule, inulin. Inulin has been considered an ideal filtration marker because it is freely filtered in the glomerulus and neither reabsorbed nor secreted by the tubule. Because of this, and because *clearance* is defined as the volume of plasma cleared entirely of a substance in a unit of time, the clearance rate of inulin equals the GFR. Direct measurement of GFR using inulin clearance is cumbersome, because it requires intravenous infusion and timed urine collection. In research studies, GFR has been measured by clearance of iothalamate, another small molecule that can be radiolabeled. Although simpler than inulin clearances, iothalamate clearance measurements are also impractical for routine clinical use.

WHY NOT USE SERUM CREATININE ALONE TO EVALUATE KIDNEY FUNCTION?

In routine clinical practice, the serum creatinine concentration (SCr) has been the most commonly used parameter to evaluate kidney function. The small molecule creatinine (molecular weight, 113 Da) is endogenously produced by muscles and excreted by the kidneys. Therefore, a reduction in GFR leads to an increase in SCr. The measurement of SCr is easy and cheap, and no urine collection is needed. Nonetheless, the National Kidney Foundation CKD Guidelines explicitly recommend that clinicians "should not use SCr as the sole means to assess the level of kidney function." The reasons for this recommendation are several.

One problem is that creatinine clearance rate (CrCl) is not identical to GFR, because creatinine is not only filtered in the glomeruli but, in contrast to inulin, also actively secreted by renal tubules. As a result, CrCl tends to overestimate GFR, especially when the GFR is low. More importantly, SCr often

TABLE 2-1	The Five Stages of Chronic Kidney Disease as Defined by the National Kidney Foundation	
STAGE	**DESCRIPTION**	**GFR (mL/min/1.73 m²)**
1	Kidney damage with normal or ↑ GFR	≥90
2	Kidney damage with mild ↓ GFR	60-89
3	Moderate ↓ GFR	30-59
4	Severe ↓ GFR	15-29
5	Kidney failure	<15 or dialysis

GFR, glomerular filtration rate.
From National Kidney Foundation K/DOQI Clinical Practice Guidelines for Chronic Kidney Disease: Evaluation, classification, and stratification. Am J Kidney Dis 39(Suppl 1):S1-S266, 2002.

does not reflect underlying GFR, because SCr is a function not only of CrCl (which reflects kidney function) but also creatinine production (which largely reflects muscle mass and, to a lesser extent, dietary meat intake). Therefore, the same SCr can represent very different underlying GFRs in individuals because of differences in muscle mass.

A clinically practical solution to this problem is to use the SCr to estimate kidney function via equations that include parameters that correlate with muscle mass, such as age, sex, race, and body size. Numerous such equations have been proposed, but the two endorsed by the National Kidney Foundation as being most valid are the Cockcroft-Gault equation and the Modification of Diet in Renal Disease study (MDRD) equation.

The Cockcroft-Gault equation estimates CrCl (in milliliters per minute) for a male patient from the age (in years), weight (in kilograms), and SCr (in milligrams per deciliter):

The Cockcroft-Gault equation estimates creatinine clearance (mL/min):

$$= [(140 - \text{age in yrs}) \times \text{weight (in kg)} (\times 0.85 \text{ if female}) / 72] / \text{SCr (in mg/dL)}$$

The abbreviated version of the MDRD equation estimates GFR (mL/min/1.73m²):

$$= 186 \times [\text{SCr (in mg/dL)}]^{-1.154} \times [\text{age (in yrs)}]^{-0.203} \times [0.742 \text{ if female}] \times [1.212 \text{ if black}]$$

If the patient is female, the value is multiplied by 0.742; if he or she is black, it is multiplied by 1.212.

An example is illustrative. A 20-year-old black man with proteinuria, hematuria, and an SCr of 1.8 mg/dL for 3 or more months is estimated to have a GFR of 62 mL/min/1.73 m² using the MDRD equation. However, by the same equation, the same stable SCr of 1.8 mg/dL in an 80-year-old white woman with proteinuria and hematuria corresponds to an underlying GFR of only 29 mL/min/1.73 m². The former patient would be classified as having stage 2 CKD and the latter as having stage 4 CKD. In other words, SCr alone does not adequately assess GFR.

Particularly among elderly patients, who are at higher risk for kidney disease, the absolute SCr can be misleadingly low despite substantial reductions in GFR, due to decreased muscle mass and consequent decreased creatinine production. In such patients, the SCr may rise, for example, from 0.5 to 1.0 mg/dL over 5 years because of kidney disease, but this rise may be missed by clinicians because the SCr remains in the "normal reference range." In actuality, this doubling of SCr signifies the approximate halving of GFR.

Other clinical scenarios in which changes in SCr within the "normal reference range" may represent major disease events include young women with progression of lupus nephritis and wasted cancer patients receiving nephrotoxic medications. It is clear from this discussion that, for SCr, the laboratory normal reference range has the potential to be misleading.

THE ROLE OF 24-HOUR URINE COLLECTIONS

Timed (24-hour) urine collections have long been used clinically to measure CrCl and, hence, GFR. However, the National Kidney Foundation CKD Guidelines also recommend against this common practice, because studies have shown that a single 24-hour urine collection often does not provide a better estimate of GFR then the estimation equations do.

Figure 2-1 shows the results of one such study. In this pilot investigation for the African American Study of Kidney Disease and Hypertension (AASK), SCr, 24-hour urine CrCl, and iodine 125–labeled iothalamate clearance were measured in 118 men and women. Compared with ¹²⁵I-iothalmate clearance as the gold standard, the GFR estimated from the 24-hour urine CrCl was less precise than that estimated from the Cockcroft-Gault equation.

The notorious difficulties in obtaining reliable 24-hour urine specimens most likely account for the imprecision of this test. In other words, errors resulting from undercollection or overcollection of urine introduce significant mistakes in the calculated CrCl. It is difficult even in the research setting to obtain reliable 24-hour urine collections, and in clinical practice this is even less likely.

FIGURE 2-1 A single 24-hour urine collection is less precise than equations in estimating the glomerular filtration rate. There is less variability in the scatter plot of creatinine clearance estimated using the Cockcroft-Gault equation vs. the gold standard of ¹²⁵I-iothalmate clearance (left panel) compared with the scatter plot of 24-hour urinary creatinine clearance vs. ¹²⁵I-iothalmate clearance (right panel). (From Coresh J, Toto RD, Kirk KA, et al: Creatinine clearance as a measure of GFR in screens for the African-American Study of Kidney Disease and Hypertension pilot study. Am J Kidney Dis 32:32-42, 1998.)

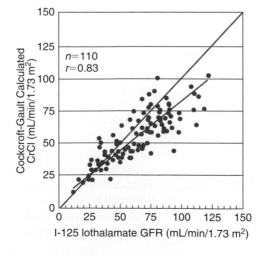

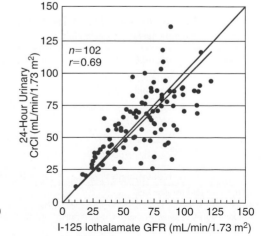

CAVEATS IN THE ESTIMATION OF GLOMERULAR FILTRATION RATE

Several caveats must be kept in mind when applying SCr-based equations to the estimation of GFR in clinical practice. First, the patient's SCr must be in a steady state. When the level of SCr is changing, such as during acute kidney injury (AKI), the GFR values obtained using the Cockcroft-Gault or the MDRD equation are grossly inaccurate. It may be possible under those circumstances to model the GFR from the rate and pattern of change in SCr, using complex mathematical models that are beyond the scope of usual clinical practice. An extreme case illustration is the patient who has just undergone bilateral nephrectomy. The SCr may be 1.5 mg/dL immediately after the operation, but the GFR is zero.

Second, a variety of conditions have been known to artifactually increase or decrease SCr without affecting GFR. Some substances (e.g., certain cephalosporins) interfere with the measurement of SCr. Others reduce renal tubular creatinine secretion and, hence, CrCl without affecting GFR. Two well-known substances that inhibit the tubular secretion of creatinine are cimetidine and trimethoprim. Of course, these considerations are relevant not only for GFR estimation equations but also when SCr alone is used to assess kidney function.

Finally, for patients with unusual body compositions or extremes of body size, SCr-based equations are likely to give invalid estimates of GFR because of alterations in the usual relationship between muscle mass and parameters such as age, sex, and weight. Examples include patients with hepatic cirrhosis, limb amputation, spinal cord injury, or morbid obesity, as well as athletes such as weight lifters who have an increased muscle mass. For such patients, multiple 24-hour urine collections (to reduce inaccuracies in collection) may be the best practical way to evaluate GFR. Ancillary markers of kidney function, such as blood urea nitrogen (BUN), may also provide clinically useful hints regarding the degree of kidney function impairment.

RECENT DEVELOPMENTS

Since the fourth edition of this *Primer*, there has been a flurry of research activity regarding the estimation of GFR. A consensus has emerged that the MDRD equation underestimates GFR in patients with normal underlying GFR. One reason is that the MDRD equation was derived and validated in a population of individuals with known parenchymal kidney disease and diminished GFR. Many laboratories now automatically compute estimated GFR using the MDRD equation with each SCr measurement. A recommended strategy to avoid the underestimation of GFR in those patients with actually normal GFR is to report numeric estimated GFR values only if the estimates are less than 60 mL/min/1.73 m² and to report all others as "greater than 60 mL/min/1.73 m²." Even with this precaution, there will still be individuals whose true GFR is greater than 60 ml/min/1.73 m² who

are misclassified as having CKD because their estimated GFR is less than 60 mL/min/1.73 m². The likelihood of this false-positive result depends on the person being tested and the pretest probability that the person indeed has CKD as judged by other clinical indicators. From a clinical and public health perspective, missing cases of CKD due to the poor sensitivity of SCr is arguably a worse problem than overdiagnosing CKD among healthy individuals using estimating equations.

Another important development has been the general acceptance that calibration of SCr measurements is critically important for accurate GFR estimation. Any fixed differences in SCr measurement between laboratories (e.g., 0.3 mg/dL) would have a disproportionately large impact among patients without significant SCr elevation, compared to those with substantially elevated SCr. This is another factor contributing to the greater inaccuracy of the MDRD equation, especially among subjects with low or normal SCr values. It should be noted that this same systematic error exists when timed urine collections are used to evaluate kidney function. The National Kidney Disease Education Program has launched the Creatinine Standardization Program to address interlaboratory variation in creatinine assay calibration, in order to provide more accurate estimates of GFR. The plan is for clinical laboratories to establish and maintain SCr assays that are calibrated against isotope dilution mass spectrometry (IDMS). These standardized SCr values could then be used with the re-expressed MDRD equation to eliminate calibration bias—for example:

$$\text{Estimated GFR (mL/min/1.73m}^2)$$
$$= 175 \times [\text{standardized SCr}]^{-1.154} \times (\text{age})^{-0.203}$$
$$\times [0.742 \text{ if female}] \times [1.212 \text{ if black}].$$

A third development worth noting is that there has been considerable interest in using cystatin C as an alternative or complementary marker to creatinine for the estimation of GFR. Many studies have now shown that serum cystatin C levels correlate better than SCr with direct measures of GFR such as iothalamate clearance. Interest in cystatin C was greatly stimulated by studies showing that it is a stronger predictor of risk of death and cardiovascular events than is SCr. There remains controversy about whether this improved predictive value occurs because the cystatin C level is a better measure of kidney function or because it correlates with some other disease processes. Nonetheless, there is general agreement that the association between serum cystatin C level and GFR is much less influenced by age, gender, and variations in body composition than SCr, because its production is not as affected by these parameters. Use of serum cystatin C may be particularly advantageous in patients with higher GFR levels. Several equations have been proposed to estimate GFR from the cystatin C concentration or from the combination of cystatin C and SCr, in addition to other variables. This is an active area of research that will undoubtedly refine the ability to evaluate GFR in the future.

EVALUATION OF PROTEINURIA

Proteinuria is the second most important parameter in the clinical evaluation of kidney function for several reasons. First, for many patients with early kidney disease, the GFR is normal and there is no upward trend in SCr. In these subjects, proteinuria may be the only sign of kidney damage. The best-known example is classic diabetic nephropathy, in which the development of albuminuria precedes reduction in GFR. Persistent proteinuria is diagnostic of CKD regardless of GFR level. Epidemiologic studies estimate that more than 10 million adults in the United States have an estimated GFR greater than 60 mL/min/1.73 m² but persistent albuminuria as evidenced by abnormally high urine albumin-to-creatinine ratios (stages 1 and 2 CKD). This is a larger number than those with GFR less than 60 mL/min/1.73 m² (stages 3 to 5 CKD).

Second, proteinuria is the single most important risk factor for future loss of kidney function. Numerous studies have shown that patients with increased proteinuria are at the highest risk for further loss of GFR. The reason, according to one popular hypothesis, is that proteinuria in and of itself causes kidney damage. Another view holds that proteinuria is mostly a marker for severity of underlying kidney disease and glomerular hyperfiltration (see Chapter 52 for the pathophysiology and consequences of hyperfiltration). Importantly, interventions that reduce proteinuria, such as blood pressure control, also retard the progression of kidney disease. Therefore, it is important to be able to easily and accurately quantify proteinuria over time in patients under treatment.

Third, among patients with CKD, proteinuria is an important and independent risk factor for cardiovascular disease and mortality. It may be that leakage of protein into the urine reflects generalized endothelial damage and capillary injury (see Chapter 59).

RANDOM URINE SAMPLES VERSUS 24-HOUR URINE COLLECTIONS TO QUANTIFY PROTEINURIA

Many clinicians are familiar with dipstick urinalysis and 24-hour urine collection assessments of proteinuria. The former, however, provides only a relatively crude quantification, and, because it measures protein concentration, it is affected by the overall state of urine concentration or dilution. The latter assessment is susceptible to the same overcollection and undercollection errors that plague 24-hour urine quantification of CrCl (see earlier discussion). The hassle and inconvenience to patients of collecting 24-hour urine specimens, especially with instructions to store the collection in a home refrigerator, are also disadvantages.

The National Kidney Foundation CKD Guidelines recommend that, under most circumstances, random ("spot") untimed urine samples should be used to detect and monitor proteinuria. The Guideline authors concluded from their review of the literature that it is usually not necessary to obtain a timed urine collection. This recommendation is supported by data such as that shown in **Figure 2-2** from a study of

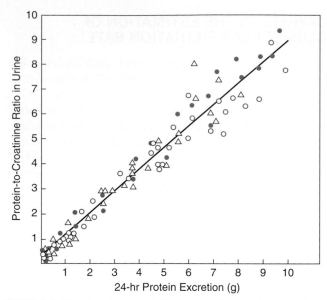

FIGURE 2-2 There is a close correlation between the protein-to-creatinine ratio in a random urine sample and the 24-hour urinary protein excretion. The linear regression parameters are $y = 0.87x + 0.33$; $r = .96$; $n = 101$. Solid circles represent ambulatory outpatients, open circles represent ambulatory inpatients, and open triangles represent bed-bound inpatients. (From Schwab SJ, Christensen RL, Dougherty K, Klahr S: Quantitation of proteinuria by the use of protein-to-creatinine ratios in single urine samples. Arch Intern Med 147:943-944,1987.)

101 ambulatory, hospitalized, and bed-bound patients encompassing a wide range of age, SCr, amount of proteinuria, and underlying cause of kidney disease. A random urine specimen and a 24-hour urine collection were obtained on the same day for each patient. A strong correlation was found between the unitless urine protein-to-creatinine ratio and the 24-hour urine protein concentration measured in grams. In this study, all patients who excreted more than 3.0 g of protein in 24 hours had a protein-to-creatinine ratio that exceeded 3.0; and, all patients who excreted less than 0.2 g of protein had a protein-to-creatinine ratio less than 0.2.

The underlying physiologic and mathematical reason that the unitless urine protein-to-creatinine ratio is numerically very similar to the 24-hour proteinuria measured in grams is that most people produce and excrete approximately 1 g of creatinine every day. Therefore, when both urine protein and urine creatinine are reported in identical units (e.g., mg/dL), the urine protein-to-creatinine ratio can be considered as the excretion rate of urinary protein in grams relative to the excretion of 1 g of creatinine.

CAVEATS IN THE ESTIMATION OF PROTEINURIA

Several caveats must be kept in mind when applying the spot urine protein-to-creatinine ratio to evaluate proteinuria in clinical practice. Again, the kidney function must be in a steady state, and the patient must not have progressing AKI. For patients who generate much less than 1 g of creatinine a day (e.g., a severely malnourished elderly patient), the urine protein-to-creatinine ratio would imply that daily protein excretion is greater than it is. Conversely, for individuals who generate much more than 1 g of creatinine a day (e.g., a young male body builder), the urine protein-to-creatinine ratio would imply that daily protein excretion is less than what a complete 24-hour urine collection would reveal.

A further caveat in the interpretation of proteinuria as a marker of parenchymal kidney disease is that there are numerous causes of transient proteinuria, including vigorous exercise, fever, and poor glycemic control among diabetic patients. If possible, proteinuria should be measured in the absence of such conditions. Persistence of proteinuria over several measurements is a more robust indicator of CKD than a single determination, and a 3-month period for assessment is recommended by the National Kidney Foundation CKD Guidelines.

OTHER SIGNS OF CHRONIC KIDNEY DISEASE

In addition to chronically reduced GFR and persistent proteinuria, other diagnostic criteria for CKD include hematuria or pyuria originating in the kidney parenchyma, glycosuria in the absence of hyperglycemia, and other kidney abnormalities defined by radiologic or pathologic studies.

EVALUATING KIDNEY FUNCTION IN ACUTE KIDNEY INJURY

As alluded to previously, SCr-based equations cannot be used to estimate GFR in AKI. Historically, AKI has been defined as an acute rise in SCr. Some patients also show other signs of kidney dysfunction, such as low urine output, hyperkalemia, or metabolic acidosis. There has been no universal agreement on the rate of decline in GFR that constitutes AKI.

Several attempts have been made recently to standardize the definition of AKI. In 2004, the Acute Dialysis Quality Initiative (ADQI) proposed the "RIFLE" criteria, which take into account both acute changes in SCr and urine output.

The acronym RIFLE stands for *R*isk of renal dysfunction, *I*njury to the kidney, *F*ailure of kidney function, *L*oss of kidney function, and *E*nd-stage kidney disease.

More recently, the Acute Kidney Injury Network (AKIN) proposed the following diagnostic criteria for AKI: an abrupt (within 48 hours), absolute increase in SCr of at least 0.3 mg/dL or an increase of at least 50% above baseline or documented urine output of less than 0.5 mL/kg/hr for at least 6 hours.

Many of the limitations of using SCr alone to evaluate kidney function in CKD also apply in AKI. For example, for any acute GFR decrement, those individuals who have greater muscle mass and generate more creatinine are more likely to show a greater increase in SCr than those who generate less creatinine. This may be one reason for some reports of a higher incidence of AKI in hospitalized men than in women. Similarly, an increase in SCr of 0.5 mg/dL from 1.0 to 1.5 mg/dL reflects a greater absolute GFR reduction than does a similar increase in SCr from 4.0 to 4.5 mg/dl.

In AKI, the BUN level is sometimes useful diagnostically. The K/DOQI CKD Guidelines, as well as the ADQI and AKIN definitions, place relatively little emphasis on BUN level as an index of kidney function, because the BUN, even more than the SCr, is influenced by numerous non–kidney-related factors. For example, independent of GFR, lower protein intake will lower urea generation and BUN. Likewise, increased catabolism (e.g., sepsis, use of corticosteroids) will elevate BUN. In AKI, the ratio of BUN to SCr has been used as a guide for differentiating the potential etiologies. A BUN/SCr ratio of more than 20:1 (when both are expressed in milligrams per deciliter) suggests reduced kidney perfusion as the cause of acute renal failure. This is because urea (molecular weight, 60 Da) is not only filtered in the glomerulus but also reabsorbed in the renal tubules, and this reabsorption increases with reduced renal perfusion and low urine flow rate, even without a change in GFR.

There is great interest in the development of novel biomarkers for AKI, but none has yet been introduced into clinical practice.

BIBLIOGRAPHY

Bellomo R, Ronco C, Kellum JA, et al: Acute renal failure—Definition, outcome measures, animal models, fluid therapy and information technology needs: The Second International Consensus Conference of the Acute Dialysis Quality Initiative (ADQI) Group. Critical Care 8:R204-R212, 2004.

Coresh J, Toto RD, Kirk KA, et al: Creatinine clearance as a measure of GFR in screens for the African-American Study of Kidney Disease and Hypertension pilot study. Am J Kidney Dis 32:32-42, 1998.

Hsu CY, Chertow GM, Curhan GC: Methodological issues in studying the epidemiology of mild to moderate chronic renal insufficiency. Kidney Int 61:1567-1576, 2002.

Levey AS, Coresh J, Greene T, et al: Expressing the Modification of Diet in Renal Disease Study equation for estimating glomerular filtration rate with standardized serum creatinine values. Clin Chem 53:766-772, 2007.

Molitoris BA, Levin A, Warnock DG, et al; on behalf of the Acute Kidney Injury Network: Improving outcomes from acute kidney injury. J Am Soc Nephrol 18:1992-1994, 2007.

Moran SM, Myers BD: Course of acute renal failure studied by a model of creatinine kinetics. Kidney Int 27:928-937, 1985.

National Kidney Foundation K/DOQI Clinical Practice Guidelines for Chronic Kidney Disease: Evaluation, classification, and stratification. Am J Kidney Dis 39(Suppl 1):S1-S266, 2002.

Schwab SJ, Christensen RL, Dougherty K, Klahr S: Quantitation of proteinuria by the use of protein-to-creatinine ratios in single urine samples. Arch Intern Med 147:943-944, 1987.

Shlipak MG, Sarnak MJ, Katz R et al: Cystatin C and the risk of death and cardiovascular events among elderly persons. N Engl J Med 352:2049-2060, 2005.

Stevens LA, Coresh J, Greene T, Levey AS. Assessing kidney function—measured and estimated glomerular filtration rate. N Engl J Med 354:2473-2483, 2006.

CHAPTER 3

Urinalysis

Arthur Greenberg

The microscopic examination of the urine sediment is an indispensable part of the evaluation of patients with impaired kidney function, proteinuria, hematuria, urinary tract infection, or nephrolithiasis. The relatively simple chemical tests performed in the routine urinalysis rapidly provide important information about a number of primary kidney and systemic disorders. Examination of the urine sediment provides valuable clues about the renal parenchyma. The dipstick tests can be automated, and flow cytometry can be used to identify some cells in the urine. However, mechanized tests cannot detect unusual cells or distinguish among casts. There is no substitute for careful examination of the urine under the microscope. This task must not be delegated; it should be performed personally. Experience in examining the urine is valuable; studies show both that a urinalysis performed by a nephrologist is more likely to aid in reaching a correct diagnosis than a urinalysis reported by a clinical chemistry laboratory and that urinalysis performed by physicians without special training is inaccurate. The features of a complete urinalysis are listed in **Table 3-1**.

TABLE 3-1 Routine Urinalysis
APPEARANCE
Specific Gravity
Chemical Tests (Dipstick)
pH
Protein
Glucose
Ketones
Blood
Urobilinogen
Bilirubin
Nitrites
Leukocyte esterase
Microscopic examination (formed elements)
Crystals: urate; calcium phosphate, oxalate, or carbonate; triple phosphate; cystine; drugs
Cells: leukocytes, erythrocytes, renal tubular cells, oval fat bodies, transitional epithelium, squamous cells
Casts: hyaline, granular, red blood cell, white blood cell, tubular cell, degenerating cellular, broad, waxy, lipid-laden
Infecting organisms: bacteria, yeast, *Trichomonas*, nematodes
Miscellaneous: spermatozoa, mucous threads, fibers, starch, hair, and other contaminants

SPECIMEN COLLECTION AND HANDLING

Urine should be collected with a minimum of contamination. A clean-catch midstream collection is preferred. If this is not feasible, bladder catheterization is appropriate in adults; the risk of contracting a urinary tract infection after a single catheterization is negligible. Suprapubic aspiration is used in infants. In the uncooperative male patient, a clean, freshly applied condom catheter and urinary collection bag may be used. Urine in the collection bag of a patient with an indwelling bladder catheter is subject to stasis, but a sample suitable for examination may be collected by withdrawing urine from above a clamp placed on the drainage tube.

The chemical composition of the urine changes with standing, and the formed elements degenerate over time. The urine is best examined when fresh, but a brief period of refrigeration is acceptable. Because bacteria multiply at room temperature, bacterial counts from unrefrigerated urine are unreliable. High urine osmolality and low pH favor cellular preservation. These two characteristics of the first voided morning urine give it particular value in cases of suspected glomerulonephritis.

PHYSICAL AND CHEMICAL PROPERTIES OF THE URINE

Appearance

Normal urine is clear, with a faint yellow tinge due to the presence of urochromes. As the urine becomes more concentrated, its color deepens. Bilirubin, other pathologic metabolites, and a variety of drugs may discolor the urine or change its smell. Suspended erythrocytes, leukocytes, or crystals may render the urine turbid. Conditions associated with a change in the appearance of the urine are listed in **Table 3-2**.

Specific Gravity

The specific gravity of a fluid is the ratio of its weight to the weight of an equal volume of distilled water. The urine specific gravity is a conveniently determined but inaccurate surrogate for osmolality. Specific gravities of 1.001 to 1.035 correspond to an osmolality range of 50 to 1000 mOsm/kg. A specific gravity near 1.010 connotes isosthenuria, with a urine osmolality matching that of plasma. Relative to osmolality, the specific gravity is elevated when dense solutes

TABLE 3-2 Selected Substances That May Alter the Physical Appearance or Odor of the Urine

COLOR CHANGE	SUBSTANCES
White	Chyle, pus, phosphate crystals
Pink/red/brown	Erythrocytes, hemoglobin, myoglobin, porphyrins, beets, senna, cascara, levodopa, methyldopa, deferoxamine, phenolphthalein and congeners, food colorings, metronidazole, phenacetin, anthraquinones, doxorubicin, phenothiazines
Yellow/orange/brown	Bilirubin, urobilin, phenazopyridine urinary analgesics, senna, cascara, mepacrine, iron compounds, nitrofurantoin, riboflavin, rhubarb, sulfasalazine, rifampin, fluorescein, phenytoin, metronidazole
Brown/black	Methemoglobin, homogentisic acid (alcaptonuria), melanin (melanoma), levodopa, methyldopa
Blue or green, green/brown	Biliverdin, *Pseudomonas* infection, dyes (methylene blue and indigo carmine), triamterene, vitamin B complex, methocarbamol, indican, phenol, chlorophyll, propofol, amitriptyline, triamterene
Purple	Infection with *Escherichia coli, Pseudomonas, Enterococcus,* others
ODOR	**SUBSTANCE OR CONDITION**
Sweet or fruity	Ketones
Ammoniac	Urea-splitting bacterial infection
Maple syrup	Maple syrup urine disease
Musty or mousy	Phenylketonuria
"Sweaty feet"	Isovaleric or glutaric acidemia or excess butyric or hexanoic acid
Rancid	Hypermethioninemia, tyrosinemia

such as protein, glucose, or radiographic contrast agents are present.

Three methods are available for specific gravity measurement. The hydrometer is the reference standard, but it requires a sufficient volume of urine to float the hydrometer as well as equilibration of the specimen to the hydrometer calibration temperature. The second method is based on the well-characterized relationship between urine specific gravity and refractive index. Refractometers calibrated in specific gravity units are commercially available and require only a drop of urine. Finally, the specific gravity may also be estimated by dipstick.

The specific gravity is used to determine whether the urine is or may be concentrated. During a solute diuresis accompanying hyperglycemia, diuretic therapy, or relief of obstruction, the urine is isosthenuric. In contrast, with a water diuresis caused by overhydration or diabetes insipidus, the specific gravity is typically 1.004 or lower. In the absence of proteinuria, glycosuria, or iodinated contrast administration, a specific gravity of more than 1.018 implies preserved concentrating ability. Measurement of specific gravity is useful in differentiating between prerenal azotemia and acute tubular necrosis (ATN) and in assessing the import of proteinuria observed in a random voided urine sample. Because the protein indicator strip responds to concentration of protein, the significance of a borderline reading depends on the overall urine concentration.

Chemical Composition of the Urine

Routine Dipstick Methodology

The urine dipstick is a plastic strip to which paper tabs impregnated with chemical reagents have been affixed. The reagents in each tab are chromogenic. After timed development, the color on the paper segment is compared with a chart. Some reactions are highly specific. Others are sensitive to the presence of interfering substances or extremes of pH. Discoloration of the urine with bilirubin or blood may obscure the color changes.

pH

The pH test pads use indicator dyes that change color with pH. The physiologic urine pH ranges from 4.5 to 8. The determination is most accurate if done promptly, because growth of urea-splitting bacteria and loss of carbon dioxide raise the pH. In addition, bacterial metabolism of glucose may produce organic acids and lower pH. These strips are not sufficiently accurate to be used for the diagnosis of renal tubular acidosis.

Protein

Protein measurement uses the protein-error-of-indicators principle. The pH at which some indicators change color varies with the protein concentration of the bathing solution. Protein indicator strips are buffered at an acid pH near their color change point. Wetting them with a protein-containing specimen induces a color change. The protein reaction may be scored from trace to 4+ or by concentration. Their equivalence is as follows: trace, 5 to 20 mg/dL; 1+, 30 mg/dL; 2+, 100 mg/dL; 3+, 300 mg/dL; 4+, greater than 2000 mg/dL. Highly alkaline urine, especially after contamination with quaternary ammonium skin cleansers, may produce false-positive reactions.

Protein strips are highly sensitive to albumin but less so to globulins, hemoglobin, or light chains. If light-chain proteinuria is suspected, more sensitive assays should be used. With acid precipitation tests, an acid that denatures protein is added to the urine specimen, and the density of the precipitate is

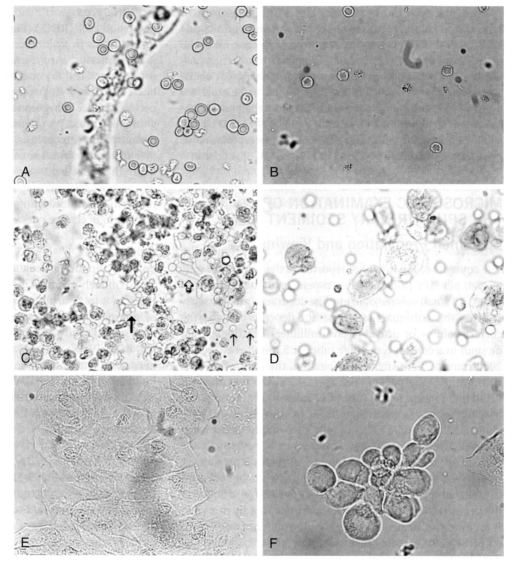

FIGURE 3-1 Cellular elements in the urine. In this and subsequent figures, all photographs were made from unstained sediments and, except as specified, photographed at ×400 original magnification. **A,** Nondysmorphic red blood cells. They appear as uniform, biconcave disks. **B,** Dysmorphic red blood cells from a patient with immunoglobulin A nephropathy. Their shape is irregular, with membrane blebs and spicules. **C,** Urine obtained from a patient with an indwelling bladder catheter. Innumerable white blood cells as well as individual *(small arrows)*, budding *(single thick arrow)*, and hyphal *(open arrow)* forms are present. **D,** Renal tubular epithelial cells. Note the variability of shape. The erythrocytes in the background are much smaller. **E,** Squamous epithelial cells. **F,** Transitional epithelial cells in a characteristic clump.

Hyaline Casts

Hyaline casts (**Fig. 3-2A**) consist of the protein alone. Because their refractive index is close to that of urine, they may be difficult to see, requiring subdued light and careful manipulation of the iris diaphragm. Hyaline casts are nonspecific. They occur in concentrated normal urine as well as in numerous pathologic conditions.

Granular Casts

Granular casts (see **Fig. 3-2B**) consist of finely or coarsely granular material. Immunofluorescence studies show that fine granules derive from altered serum proteins. Coarse granules may result from degeneration of embedded cells. Granular casts are nonspecific but are usually pathologic. They may be seen after exercise or with simple volume depletion and as a finding in ATN, glomerulonephritis, or tubulointerstitial disease.

Waxy Casts

Waxy casts or broad casts (see **Fig. 3-2C**) are made of hyaline material with a much greater refractive index than hyaline casts—hence, their waxy appearance. They behave as if they

were more brittle than hyaline casts and frequently have fissures along their edge. Broad casts form in tubules that have become dilated and atrophic due to chronic parenchymal disease.

Red Blood Cell Casts

RBC casts indicate intraparenchymal bleeding. The hallmark of glomerulonephritis, they are seen less frequently with tubulointerstitial disease. RBC casts have been described along with hematuria in normal individuals after exercise. Fresh RBC casts (see **Fig. 3-2D**) retain their brown pigment and consist of readily discernible erythrocytes in a tubular cast matrix. Over time, the heme color is lost, along with the distinct cellular outline. With further degeneration, RBC casts are hard to distinguish from coarsely granular casts. RBC casts may be diagnosed by the company they keep: They appear in a background of hematuria with dysmorphic red cells, granular casts, and proteinuria. Occasionally, the evidence for intraparenchymal bleeding is a hyaline cast with embedded red cells. These have the same pathophysiologic implication as RBC casts.

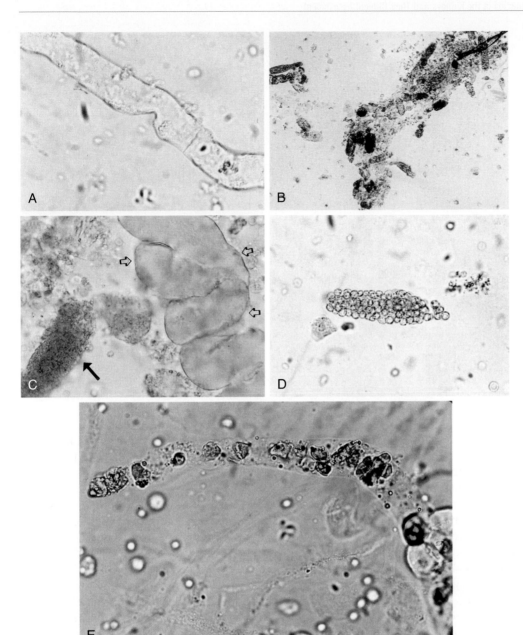

FIGURE 3-2 Casts. **A,** Hyaline cast. **B,** Muddy brown granular casts and amorphous debris from a patient with acute tubular necrosis (original magnification ×100). **C,** Waxy cast *(open arrows)* and granular cast *(solid arrow)* from a patient with lupus nephritis and a telescoped sediment. Note background hematuria. **D,** Red blood cell cast. Background hematuria is also present. **E,** Tubular cell cast. Note the hyaline cast matrix.

White Blood Cell Casts

WBC casts consist of WBCs in a protein matrix. They are characteristic of pyelonephritis and are useful in distinguishing that disorder from lower urinary tract infection. They may also be seen with interstitial nephritis and other tubulointerstitial disorders.

Tubular Cell Casts

Tubular cell casts (see **Fig. 3-2E**) consist of a dense agglomeration of sloughed tubular cells or just a few tubular cells in a hyaline matrix. They occur in concentrated urine but are more characteristically seen with the sloughing of tubular cells that occurs with ATN.

Bacteria, Yeast, and Other Infectious Agents

Bacillary or coccal forms of bacteria may be discerned even on an unstained urine sample. Examination of a Gram stain preparation of unspun urine allows estimation of the bacterial count. One organism per HPF of unspun urine corresponds to 20,000 organisms per cubic millimeter. Individual and budding yeasts and hyphal forms occur with *Candida* infection or colonization. *Candida* organisms are similar in size to erythrocytes, but they are greenish spheres, not biconcave disks. When budding forms or hyphae are present, yeast cells are obvious (see **Fig. 3-1C**). *Trichomonas* organisms are identified by their teardrop shape and motile flagellum.

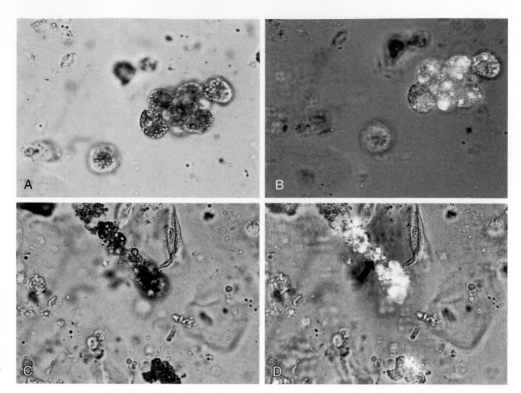

FIGURE 3-3 Lipid. **A,** Oval fat bodies, as seen by bright-field illumination. **B,** Same field as in **A,** viewed under polarized light. **C,** Lipid-laden cast, bright-field illumination. **D,** Same field as in **C,** viewed under polarized light. Arrow points to characteristic Maltese cross.

Lipiduria

In the nephrotic syndrome with lipiduria, tubular cells reabsorb luminal fat. Sloughed tubular cells containing fat droplets are called oval fat bodies. Fatty casts contain lipid-laden tubular cells or free lipid droplets. By light microscopy, lipid droplets appear round and clear with a green tinge. Cholesterol esters are anisotropic; cholesterol-containing droplets rotate polarized light, producing a "Maltese cross" appearance under polarized light. Triglycerides appear similar by light microscopy, but they are isotropic. Crystals, starch granules, mineral oil, and other urinary contaminants are also anisotropic. Before concluding that anisotropic structures are lipid, the observer must compare polarized and bright-field views of the same object (**Fig. 3-3**).

Crystals

Crystals may be present spontaneously, or they may precipitate with refrigeration of a specimen. They can be difficult to identify because they have similar shapes; the common urinary crystals are described in **Table 3-3**. The pH is an important clue to identity, because solubility of a number of urinary constituents is pH dependent. The three most distinctive crystal forms are cystine, calcium oxalate, and magnesium ammonium (triple) phosphate. Cystine crystals are hexagonal plates that resemble benzene rings. Calcium oxalate crystals (**Fig. 3-4A**) are classically described as "envelope shaped," but, when viewed as they rotate in the urine under the microscope, they appear bipyramidal. Coffin lid–shaped triple phosphates (see **Fig. 3-4B**) are rectangular with beveled ends. Oxalate (see **Fig. 3-4C**) may also occur in

dumbbell-shaped crystals. Urate may have several forms, including rhomboids (see **Fig. 3-4D**) or needles (see **Fig. 3-4E**).

Characteristic Urine Sediments

The urine sediment is a rich source of diagnostic information. Occasionally, a single finding (e.g., cystine crystals) is pathognomonic. More often, the sediment must be considered as a whole and interpreted in conjunction with clinical and other laboratory findings. Several patterns bear emphasis.

In the acute nephritic syndrome, the urine may be pink or pale brown and turbid. Blood and moderate proteinuria are detected by dipstick analysis. The microscopic examination shows RBCs and RBC casts as well as granular and hyaline casts; WBC casts are rare. In the nephrotic syndrome, the urine is clear or yellow. Increased foaming may be noted because of the elevated protein content. In comparison with the sediment of nephritic patients, the nephrotic sediment is bland. Hyaline casts and lipiduria with oval fat bodies or lipid-laden casts predominate. Granular casts and a few tubular cells may also be present, along with a few RBCs. With some forms of chronic glomerulonephritis, a "telescoped" sediment is observed (see **Fig. 3-2C**). This term refers to the presence of the elements of a nephritic sediment together with broad or waxy casts, indicative of tubular atrophy and dipstick findings of heavy proteinuria. In pyelonephritis, WBC casts and innumerable WBCs are present, along with bacteria. In lower tract infections, WBC casts are absent. The sediment in ATN (see **Fig. 3-2B**) shows tubular cells, tubular cell casts, and muddy brown granular casts. The typical urinary findings in individual kidney disorders are discussed in their respective chapters.

TABLE 3-3 Common Urinary Crystals

DESCRIPTION	COMPOSITION	COMMENT
Crystals Found in Acid Urine		
Amorphous	Uric acid Sodium urate	Cannot be distinguished from amorphous phosphates except by urine pH; may be orange tinted by urochromes.
Rhomboid prisms	Uric acid	
Rosettes	Uric acid	
Bipyramidal	Calcium oxalate	Also termed "envelope-shaped."
Dumbbell-shaped	Calcium oxalate	
Needles	Uric acid Sulfa drugs Radiographic contrast material	Clinical history provides useful confirmation Sulfa may resemble sheaves of wheat; urate and contrast crystals are thicker.
Hexagonal plates	Cystine	Presence may be confirmed with nitroprusside test.
Crystals Found in Alkaline Urine		
Amorphous	Phosphates	Indistinguishable from urates except by pH.
"Coffin lid" (beveled rectangular prisms)	Triple (magnesium ammonium) phosphate	Seen with urea-splitting infection and bacteriuria.
Granular masses or dumbbells	Calcium carbonate	Larger than amorphous phosphates.
Yellow-brown masses with or without spicules	Ammonium biurate	—
Platelike rectangles, fan-shaped, starburst	Indinavir	Causes nephrolithiasis or renal colic. In vitro solubility increased at very low pH. The lowest urine pH achievable in vivo may not actually be acid enough to lessen crystalluria.

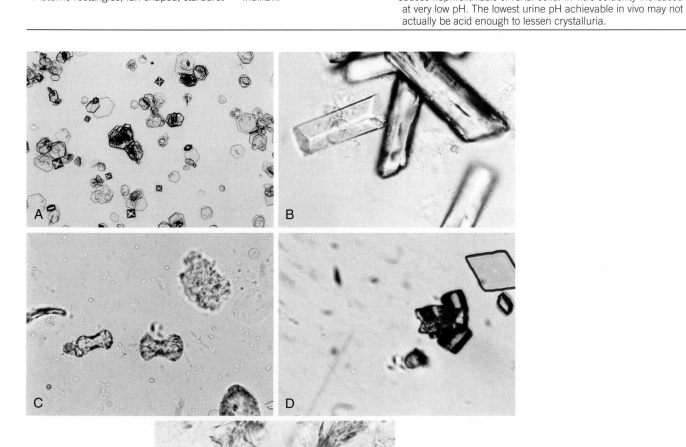

FIGURE 3-4 Crystals. **A,** Hexagonal cystine and bipyramidal or envelope-shaped oxalate. **B,** Coffin lid–shaped triple phosphate. **C,** Dumbbell-shaped oxalate. **D,** Rhomboid urate. **E,** Needle-shaped urate. (**A,** Courtesy of Dr. Thomas O. Pitts.)

BIBLIOGRAPHY

Birch DF, Fairley KF, Becker GJ, Kincaid-Smith P: A Color Atlas of Urine Microscopy. New York, Chapman & Hall, 1994.

Braden GL, Sanchez PG, Fitzgibbons JP, et al: Urinary doubly refractile lipid bodies in nonglomerular renal disease. Am J Kidney Dis 16:332-337, 1988.

Canaris CJ, Flach SD, Tape TG, et al: Can internal medicine residents master microscopic urinalysis? Results of an evaluation and teaching intervention. Acad Med 78:525-529, 2003.

Fairley KF, Birch DF: Hematuria: A simple method for identifying glomerular bleeding. Kidney Int 21:105-108, 1982.

Fassett RG, Owen JE, Fairley J, et al: Urinary red-cell morphology during exercise. Br Med J 285:1455-1457, 1982.

Fogazzi GB, Cameron JS: Urinary microscopy from the seventeenth century to the present day. Kidney Int 50:1058-1068, 1996.

Fogazzi GB, Ponticelli C, Ritz E: The Urinary Sediment: An Integrated View, 2nd ed. Oxford, Oxford University Press, 1999.

Fogazzi GB, Verdesca S, Carigali G: Urinalysis: Core curriculum 2008. Am J Kidney Dis 51: 1052-1067, 2008.

Foot CL, Fraser JF: Uroscopic rainbow: Modern matula medicine. Postgrad Med 82:126-129, 2006.

Graff L: A Handbook of Routine Urinalysis. Philadelphia, JB Lippincott, 1983.

Henry JB, Fuller CE, Threatte GA: Basic examination of the urine. In Henry JB (ed): Clinical Diagnosis and Management by Laboratory Methods, 20th ed. Philadelphia, WB Saunders, 2001, pp 367-402.

Kincaid-Smith P: Haematuria and exercise-related haematuria. Br Med J 285:1595-1597, 1982.

Kopp JB, Miller KD, Mican JM, et al: Crystalluria and urinary tract abnormalities associated with indinavir. Ann Intern Med 127:119-125, 1997.

Raymond JR, Yarger WE: Abnormal urine color: Differential diagnosis. South Med J 81:837-841, 1988.

Rutecki GJ, Goldsmith C, Schreiner GE: Characterization of proteins in urinary casts: Fluorescent-antibody identification of Tamm-Horsfall mucoprotein in matrix and serum proteins in granules. N Engl J Med 284:1049-1052, 1971.

Schumann GB, Harris S, Henry JB: An improved technic for examining urinary casts and a review of their significance. Am J Clin Pathol 69:18-23, 1978.

Stamey TA, Kindrachuk RW: Urinary Sediment and Urinalysis. A Practical Guide for the Health Professional. Philadelphia, WB Saunders, 1985.

Tsai JJ, Yeun JY, Kumar VA, Don BR: Comparison and interpretation of urinalysis performed by a nephrologist versus a hospital-based clinical laboratory. Am J Kidney Dis 46:820-829, 2005.

Voswinckel P: A marvel of colors and ingredients: The story of urine test strips. Kidney Int 46(Suppl):3-7, 1994.

CHAPTER 4

Hematuria and Proteinuria

David Jayne

Hematuria and proteinuria are signs of disease of the kidney or urinary tract. The accessibility of urine testing and the insidious nature of many kidney diseases that develop without overt symptoms emphasize the clinical importance of urinalysis, both in screening and in monitoring of kidney pathology. Early detection of kidney disease plays a key role in preventing its progression to end-stage renal disease. Regular urine testing is undertaken during pregnancy, for insurance medical evaluations, and in individuals who are at high risk for renal disease, such as patients with diabetes mellitus; the utility of routine urine testing for healthy children or adults has not been determined. Similarly, the reliability of urine testing for the detection of renal and urinary tract disease has not been robustly addressed.

A pragmatic approach to the evaluation of hematuria and proteinuria will alert the clinician to the need for further investigation and referral. For the nephrologist managing kidney disease, the detection of abnormal levels of hematuria and proteinuria should trigger a systematic approach aimed at achieving a definitive diagnosis. This process requires understanding of the techniques of urine testing, the significance and deficiencies of urinary abnormalities, and the pathophysiology of hematuria and proteinuria.

HEMATURIA

Definition

Hematuria means the abnormal presence of erythrocytes in urine. The erythrocytes may be of normal morphology or damaged; they may originate from any site in the urinary tract, from the glomerular basement membrane (GBM) to the distal urethra. Hematuria at low levels that does not change the appearance of urine and is detected only by microscopy or dipstick analysis is termed *microscopic hematuria*. Higher levels of hematuria may stain the urine red or give it a smoky-brown appearance, that of *macroscopic hematuria*. True hematuria must be distinguished from urine discolored by other pigments—either proteinaceous material, such as hemoglobin or myoglobin, or other substances, including food dyes and drugs such as rifampicin. Proteinaceous pigment appears in the urine if it is filtered from the circulation by the glomerulus and will also be detected in the urine as proteinuria.

Erythrocytes appear in the urine at very low levels in healthy individuals but may increase after vigorous physical activity, so-called joggers' nephritis. Normal levels are less than 13,000/mL of uncentrifuged urine. After resuspension of centrifuged, freshly voided urine, two or fewer erythrocytes per high-powered field (HPF) are seen by light microscopy (×400). Urethral or bladder trauma due to catheterization or urethral contamination from menstruation increases the number or erythrocytes in the urine and makes it impossible to determine whether pathologic levels of hematuria are present.

Erythrocyturia is quantified crudely by urine dipsticks, or more accurately by counting the number of erythrocytes per HPF of centrifuged urine by light microscopy. In addition to the descriptions of microscopic (i.e., covert) and macroscopic hematuria, it is important to note whether hematuria is transient, intermittent, or persistent; is associated with other symptoms such as dysuria; is "symptomatic" versus "asymptomatic", or is associated with proteinuria (**Table 4-1**). If hematuria is the only urinary abnormality. it is termed *isolated* hematuria. Such associations reflect the underlying cause and contribute to the eventual diagnosis.

Detection and Assessment

Hematuria is detected either by microscopy or by urine dipstick. Direct microscopy is preferable, because it is less prone to error and permits ready quantitation and because it allows confirmation of erythrocyturia, assessment of red blood cell (RBC) morphology, and detection of RBC casts. Furthermore, microscopy may detect other abnormalities, including leukocyturia and microorganisms. RBC morphology is of

TABLE 4-1 Initial Approach to Hematuria

Genuine erythrocyturia (i.e., not hemoglobinuria/ myoglobinuria)?	Presence of erythrocytes confirmed by microscopy
Microscopic or macroscopic?	Visible change in color of urine
Intermittent or sustained?	—
Accompanied by proteinuria?	Proteinuria >1000 mg/24 hr
Associated with menstruation or catheterization?	—
Associated with infection?	Pyuria or nitrites, or positive urine microscopy or culture for microorganisms

deduced from urine examination (see **Table 4-2**), with the major division being between glomerular and nonglomerular hematuria.

Investigation of Glomerular Hematuria

The causes of glomerular hematuria can be viewed in three categories (see **Table 4-3**). History and examination should provide evidence to support multisystem and "other" causes and may identify underlying causes for secondary glomerulonephritis, such as malignancy or chronic infection. Investigations should be directed to defining the severity of the renal disease, exploring the immunopathogenesis of immune-mediated renal disease, detecting extrarenal features of inflammatory disease, and diagnosing other causes of glomerular hematuria (**Table 4-4**). Proteinuria should be quantified and assessed for light chains and glomerular filtration rate, either estimated from serum creatinine or directly measured. Renal imaging, typically by ultrasound, defines the renal anatomy, identifies evidence of chronic renal disease, and helps exclude causes of nonglomerular hematuria. It is also an essential prerequisite for renal biopsy. Renal ultrasound Doppler examination of the renal artery and vein detects renal vein thrombosis, a cause of nonglomerular hematuria.

Immunologic investigations aim to identify serologic abnormalities associated with an underlying diagnosis of glomerulonephritis. Patients with glomerular hematuria of unknown cause require antinuclear antibodies (ANA), anti–neutrophil cytoplasmic antibodies (ANCA), complement levels, and protein electrophoresis. Anti-GBM antibodies should be requested if RBC casts, deteriorating renal function, or lung hemorrhage is present. A positive ANA result should be followed by a search for related autoantibodies, such as anti–double-stranded DNA, which has greater specificity for lupus nephritis; anti-Ro (SSA) and anti-La (SSB) in Sjögren's syndrome; and anti-SCL70 or anti-RNA polymerase III in scleroderma. ANCA positivity requires confirmation by detection of autoantibodies to proteinase 3 (PR3-ANCA) or myeloperoxidase (MPO-ANCA), which are closely associated with pauci-immune, necrotizing glomerulonephritis found in the context of a primary systemic vasculitis or as an isolated entity (termed renal-limited vasculitis) (see Chapter 23).

Reduced complement levels indicate an immune complex pathogenesis, such as occurs in systemic lupus erythematosus (SLE), but, if ANA is negative, other causes should be sought. In cryoglobulinemia, rheumatoid factor is elevated, cryoglobulins are measured by the cryocrit, and a monoclonal gammopathy may be present. Unexplained hypocomplementemia requires further investigation for C3 nephritic factor and defects of factor H. Rheumatoid factor is also elevated in some cases of infection-associated glomerulonephritis, as well as in rheumatoid arthritis (see Chapter 22). Serum immunoglobulin estimation and electrophoresis can detect monoclonal gammopathies associated with multiple myeloma and cryoglobulinemia (see Chapter 27). Total IgG is usually elevated in SLE and in Sjögren's syndrome but may be depressed due to renal excretion in the nephrotic syndrome. IgA levels may be elevated in IgA nephropathy or in Henoch-Schönlein purpura. The antiphospholipid syndrome can cause a thrombotic microangiopathy, and the presence of a lupus anticoagulant is suggested by a prolonged activated partial thromboplastin time or the presence of anticardiolipin antibodies.

The hematuria of crescentic glomerulonephritis is accompanied by proteinuria typically greater than 100 mg/dL (2+), and the presence of RBC casts with a rising serum creatinine indicates that the syndrome of rapidly progressive glomerulonephritis is present (see Chapter 16). Serologic analysis for ANCA, anti-GBM antibodies, or ANA is often positive, reflecting the more common causes of this presentation. Renal ultrasonography shows normal-sized kidneys which may display exaggerated corticomedullary differentiation, reflecting the intensity of the inflammation. IgA nephropathy, minimal change disease, and focal segmental glomerulosclerosis are not usually associated with serologic abnormalities. Low complement and C3 nephritic factor may be found in membranoproliferative glomerulonephritis (MPGN) type I, and low complement levels and defects in factor H may be present in MPGN type II and dense deposit disease. This histologic pattern is also found in

TABLE 4-4 Laboratory Investigation of Glomerular Hematuria

DIAGNOSIS	RELEVANT ABNORMAL INVESTIGATIONS
Membranoproliferative glomerulonephritis (MPGN)	C3/C4, C3 nephritic factor, cryoglobulins, hepatitis B/C
Anti–GBM disease	Anti-GBM antibodies, chest radiograph
Fibrillary and immunotactoid glomerulopathy	Electrophoresis, C3/C4, calcium, bone marrow, skeletal survey
Systemic lupus erythematosus	ANA, anti-dsDNA, ENAs, C3/C4, anti-cardiolipin
Vasculitis (Wegener's granulomatosis, microscopic polyangiitis, Churg-Strauss angiitis)	ANCA (C-ANCA/PR3-ANCA or P-ANCA/MPO-ANCA)
Thrombotic microangiopathy	Anti-cardiolipin, lupus anticoagulant
Hereditary	
Alport's disease	Audiometry
Fabry's disease	Plasma alpha-galactosidase A activity
Infection-associated glomerulonephritis	
HIV nephropathy	HIV
Poststreptococcal glomerulonephritis	ASO, anti-DNAase, C3/C4, rheumatoid factor
Infective endocarditis	Echocardiography, C3/C4, rheumatoid factor

ANA, antinuclear antibodies; ANCA, antineutrophil cytoplasmic antibody; ASO, antistreptolysin O; C3/C4, third and fourth components of complement; c-ANCA, cytoplasmic ANCA; anti-DNAase, anti–deoxyribonuclease; anti-dsDNA, anti–double-stranded (native) DNA; ENAs, extractable nuclear antigens; anti-GBM, anti–glomerular basement membrane; HIV, human immunodeficiency virus; MPO-ANCA, autoantibodies to myeloperoxidase; P-ANCA, perinuclear ANCA; PR3-ANCA, autoantibodies to protease 3.

cryoglobulinemia. Fibrillary glomerulonephritis is associated with amyloidosis, monoclonal gammopathies, and other causes.

An elevated C-reactive protein is consistent with acute inflammation in glomerulonephritis but may also be caused by infection, and microbiologic studies should include urine and blood cultures. Chronic viral infection due to hepatitis B or hepatitis C should be excluded, and human immunodeficiency virus (HIV) should be considered if risk factors are present. The erythrocyte sedimentation rate is of less value, because it is influenced by anemia, hypoproteinemia, and biochemical abnormalities that are frequently present in glomerular disease. Poststreptococcal nephritis, more common in children, is associated with a raised antistreptolysin O titer (ASO) and elevated anti-DNAase antibodies. If an infection-associated glomerulonephritis is suspected, echocardiography is essential to exclude endocarditis, and thoracoabdominal computed tomographic (CT) scanning should be considered to detect occult abscesses. Infectious causes of glomerulonephritis vary among geographical areas and ethnic communities; tuberculosis, malaria, hantavirus, arboviruses, and other infections may also need to be considered.

The association of glomerular hematuria with hearing loss should raise suspicion of Alport's syndrome, especially if there is a family history of renal disease. The presence of angiokeratomas is diagnostic for Fabry's disease, the presence of which can be confirmed by measurement of plasma α-galactosidase A activity.

The investigation of glomerular hematuria typically leads to consideration of renal biopsy. This offers a high chance of a histologic description of the glomerular pathology by light microscopy, immunofluorescence, and electron microscopy, which, in combination with evidence from the history, examination, and serological testing, permits a formal diagnosis. Indications for renal biopsy vary among centers, and the potential risks of this procedure need to be balanced against the advantages of obtaining a histologic description. For glomerular hematuria with only low levels of proteinuria, the most likely histologic diagnoses are thin basement membrane disease and IgA nephropathy. Because these conditions either have no specific therapy or the role of specific therapy is controversial, the decision whether to proceed to renal biopsy will be influenced by the value attached to knowledge of the result.

Indeterminate hematuria, in which features of both glomerular and nonglomerular hematuria are present, requires both the investigation of glomerular hematuria, as described here, and investigation of the lower urinary tract.

Investigation of Nonglomerular Hematuria

In nonglomerular hematuria (**Table 4-5**), the history and physical examination should focus on symptoms and signs of urinary tract disease, including constitutional disturbances, abdominal or flank pain, lower abdominal pain, dysuria, urinary frequency, and incontinence. A family history may

TABLE 4-5 Investigation of Nonglomerular Hematuria

DIAGNOSIS	RELEVANT ABNORMAL INVESTIGATIONS
Renal Causes	
Tubulointerstitial disorders	Renal biopsy
Hypersensitivity tubulointerstitial nephritis	Eosinophils in urine (Hansel's stain)
Sjögren's syndrome	ANA, Anti-Ro (SSA), Anti-La (SSB)
Vascular disorders	
Scleroderma renal crisis	RNA polymerase III, SCL-70 (anti-topoisomerase)
Polyarteritis nodosa	Mesenteric or renal angiography
Renal embolism or arterial or venous thrombosis	Doppler ultrasound, angiography
Arteriovenous malformation	Angiography
Neoplasias (e.g., renal cell carcinoma, Wilms' tumor, leukemia, lymphoma, metastatic disease)	Ultrasound, CT, MR, biopsy, urine cytology
Papillary necrosis (causes include diabetes mellitus, sickle cell anemia, analgesic abuse, and obstructive uropathy)	CT, MR
Infections (e.g., pyelonephritis, tuberculosis, hantavirus, BK virus in transplants)	Microbiology, urine cytology, renal biopsy
Hereditary (e.g., polycystic kidney disease, medullary sponge kidney)	Genetic evaluation, urine calcium
Trauma	CT, MR
Urinary tract causes	
Neoplasias (e.g., transitional cell carcinoma; carcinoma of bladder, prostate, or urethra)	CT, MR, cytology, cystoscopy, ureteroscopy, PSA
Calculi	Ultrasound, CT, stone evaluation (including urine calcium, phosphate, oxalate, uric acid, cysteine, parathyroid hormone)
Infections—bacterial, fungal or parasitic (e.g., *Schistosoma hematobium*)	Microscopy and culture; ova and parasites
Vascular Malformations	Cystoscopy, ureteroscopy
Extra–urinary tract inflammation	CT
Hypersensitivity cystitis or urethritis	Cystoscopy, ureteroscopy
Urinary obstruction	Ultrasound

ANA, antinuclear antigen; CT, computed tomography; MRI, magnetic resonance imaging; PSA, prostate-specific antigen.

suggest renal stone disease. Abdominal or flank masses may be palpable in polycystic kidney disease or renal tumors. A hemorrhagic diathesis will be apparent from a history of anticoagulant use or from detection of thrombocytopenia or deranged clotting. Sickle cell anemia causes papillary necrosis and hematuria which is typically painless (see Chapter 41).

Urine microscopy and culture reveals most urinary bacterial infections. Infection with *Mycobacterium tuberculosis* in the urinary tract can be difficult to isolate despite culture of multiple early morning urine specimens. Further investigations are needed, including tuberculin skin testing and thoracoabdominal CT scanning. Parasitic infection with *Schistosoma hematobium* is restricted to those who have traveled to or lived in endemic areas; it is diagnosed by detection of ova and parasites in the urine.

If renal stone disease is suspected, a renal metabolic screen is performed with biochemical analysis of timed urine collections to identify hypercalciuria, hyperuricosuria, or hyperoxaluria (see Chapter 47). Urine microscopy can identify renal crystals, which are seen, for example, with urate stones. Renal stones may coexist with urinary tract infection. Renal or urinary tract malignancy is more likely in smokers, in those with a history of constitutional disturbance and weight loss, and in those with exposure to certain drugs and toxins, such as analgesics, cyclophosphamide, and aniline dyes. Urine cytology and prostate-specific antigen tests in older men should be requested. Cystoscopy is indicated, even if cytology results are negative, for unexplained nonglomerular hematuria. The indications for cystoscopy are more restricted in children, because lower urinary tract tumor as a cause of unexplained hematuria is rare, and investigation should focus on structural renal and ureteric abnormalities detected by ultrasound, metabolic abnormalities including hypercalciuria and hyperuricosuria, and thin membrane glomerulopathy.

Imaging investigations aim to localize the site of bleeding through systematic investigation of the whole length of the urinary tract. Ultrasonography, followed by contrast-enhanced CT scanning or magnetic resonance imaging (MRI), is most widely used to identify pathology and has largely replaced intravenous pyelography. Noncontrast CT is the preferred approach for detection of stones in the kidneys or ureters. If cystoscopy and imaging fail to reveal a cause for nonglomerular hematuria, there should be consideration of intrarenal tumors and arteriovenous malformations, which may be detected by conventional angiography or magnetic resonance angiography with gadolinium enhancement.

Gross hematuria with red-stained urine with or without blood clots requires urgent investigation. Causes such as trauma or renal biopsy may be obvious, but in their absence, imaging followed by cystoscopy is necessary. Bleeding from the urethra or prostate is more likely to be confined to the first 10 to 50 mL of the voided specimen, whereas bleeding from the urinary bladder or higher will be equally present throughout urination. Blood is irritating to the urinary bladder and urethra and can cause pain, dysuria, and frequency.

Blood clots in the ureter may cause colic, and, like clots in the bladder, may lead to urinary obstruction.

The majority of pathologies resulting in nonglomerular hematuria will be identified by these studies. If no cause is recognized and the hematuria persists, a repeated cycle of investigation should be considered, along with rarer causes of hematuria such as factitious hematuria and loin-pain hematuria syndrome. Those with ongoing unexplained hematuria should continue under follow-up in case serious underlying pathology emerges.

PROTEINURIA

Because proteinuria is a marker of both active renal inflammation and renal injury, it has important roles in the detection, diagnosis, and monitoring of renal disease. If proteinuria is heavy, the urine may appear frothy, and symptoms of the nephrotic syndrome, such as ankle edema, may be present.

Normal and Abnormal Values for Proteinuria

In health, small amounts of protein of glomerular and tubular origin are excreted, averaging 80 mg/24 hr (**Table 4-6**). Proteinuria greater than 200 mg/24 hr is regarded as abnormal. Protein excretion rates increase on standing, are higher in children and adolescents, and increase with exercise and fever. The majority of protein excretion occurs while the person is ambulant. Pressor agents, such as angiotensin and norepinephrine, increase proteinuria. If proteinuria is sufficiently high to cause hypoalbuminemia—the nephrotic syndrome—it is referred to as *nephrotic range* proteinuria and is typically higher than 3000 mg/24 hr. Proteinuria in the range between 200 and 3000 mg/24 hr is readily detected by urine dipstick and is termed *overt* or *subnephrotic range* proteinuria.

Composition of Urine Proteins

Urinary protein includes protein filtered by the glomerulus that is not reabsorbed in the tubules, protein secreted by the renal tubules (including Tamm-Horsfall protein), and protein secreted into the urine by the lower urinary tract, for example in association with injury or inflammation (including secreted IgA). Incomplete glomerular protein, partially degraded in the renal tubules, may also appear in the urine and may not be detected by assays for complete protein such as the immunoreactive tests for albumin. Approximately 50% of urine protein is from the glomerulus; the composition of urine protein is described in **Table 4-6**.

Albumin is the predominant protein filtered by the glomerulus and therefore is the most consistent marker of glomerular pathology. However, in health, albumin comprises only a minority of urinary proteinuria. Proteins crossing the GBM are largely reabsorbed and degraded by the renal tubules through endocytosis. This process has a preference for cationic proteins and only limited capacity for albumin; therefore, minor glomerular abnormalities result

TABLE 4-6 **Protein Composition of Normal Urine**

PLASMA PROTEINS	EXCRETION (mg/day)
Plasma Proteins	
Albumin	12
Immunoglobulin G	3
Immunoglobulin A	1
Immunoglobulin M	0.3
Light chains	
κ	2.3
λ	1.4
β-Microglobulins	0.12
Other plasma proteins	20
All plasma proteins	*40*
Nonplasma Proteins	
Tamm-Horsfall protein	40
Other non–renal-derived proteins	<1
All nonplasma proteins	*40*
Total Proteins	80 ± 24 (SD)

From Glassock R: Proteinuria. In Massry SG, Glassock RJ (eds): Textbook of Nephrology, 3rd ed. Baltimore, Williams & Williams, 1995.

in an increase in albuminuria. Physiologic albumin excretion is 4 to 15 μg/min or 6 to 20 mg/day, and values greater than 30 mg/day are abnormal. Microalbuminuria refers to albumin excretion in the range of 20 to 200 μg/min, or 30 to 300 mg/24 hr, a range that for total protein would be regarded as normal or minimal. This equates to a urinary albumin-to-creatinine ratio of 17 to 250 mg/g for men and 25 to 355 mg/g for women.

Detection and Quantification

Urine testing by reagent strip is the most widely used technique for detection of abnormal levels of proteinuria. Paper strips impregnated with an indicator dye, such as tetra-bromophenol blue or bromocresol green, undergo a color change with albumin in the concentration range of 20 to 300 mg/dL. They give a semiquantitative read-out but primarily detect albumin and are insensitive to other urinary proteins, such as globulins (e.g., Bence Jones protein) and underestimate urine protein levels when nonalbumin proteins are present. Quantification is influenced by urine concentration, with dilute urine giving falsely low results. False-positive results can occur with strongly alkaline urine, which overwhelms the buffer on the strip, and in the presence of certain drugs (tolbutamide, cephalosporins, and radiocontrast agents). These dipsticks are insufficiently sensitive to detect microalbuminuria. Test strips specifically designed to detect microalbuminuria are available for that purpose and should be used for screening diabetic patients. Screening for proteinuria with regular dipsticks is advised in hypertension, in established diseases such as SLE when nephritis may occur, and, perhaps most importantly, in the evaluation of any

patient with unexplained symptoms or signs of disease. The presence of proteinuria is an independent risk factor for the development of end-stage renal disease in those who are at risk for cardiovascular disease and in those with a reduced glomerular filtration rate. Although routine population screening of urine is performed in some countries, it is not supported by scientific studies.

Laboratory-based techniques, including the biuret reaction and turbidimetry utilizing acetic acid or sulfosalicylic acid, detect lower levels of proteinuria, down to 5 mg/dL, and react equally to albumin and globulins. Therefore, a borderline or negative result by dipstick testing and a positive result by turbidimetry or other laboratory technique indicate the presence of globulins, such as light chains. They may also be influenced by drugs, including nonsteroidal anti-inflammatory drugs and cephalosporins, and radiocontrast agents.

The measurement of protein content in a timed urine collection has been the standard method for quantification of proteinuria. The inaccuracies in urine collection, especially when performed at a patient's home, and the inconvenience of transporting large volumes of urine have made the estimation of the protein content in a smaller urine sample more attractive. An adjustment for urinary concentration is made by relating the urine protein concentration (mg/dL) to the urine creatinine concentration (mg/dL) in the protein-to-creatinine ratio, measured as mg/mg or g/g. An abnormal protein-to-creatinine ratio is one that is greater than 0.2 mg/dL (protein) per 1.0 mg/dL creatinine, or 0.2 mg/mg or g/g. The albumin-to-creatinine ratio is measured in a similar fashion. The most consistent results are obtained from the first voided urine in the morning, but the test can be applied to a random sample obtained in the clinic.

The physiologic excretion of protein by the kidneys increases with upright posture, known as *orthostatic proteinuria*. Therefore, ambulant samples carry the possibility of detecting orthostatic proteinuria, and high results require confirmation by comparison with recumbent samples or a timed 24 hour collection. Variable creatinine excretion between women and men and among ethnic groups needs to be considered in the establishment of normal ranges. The clinical utility and accuracy of the protein-to-creatinine ratio has been validated in several clinical settings, including screening for diabetic nephropathy and for proteinuria in pregnant women and in children. The correlation of the protein-to-creatinine ratio with measured collections is less exact in nephrotic range proteinuria, but precise quantification in this setting is less important. It is important to distinguish between the protein-to-creatinine ratio and the albumin-to-creatinine ratio, because the latter will not detect nonalbumin proteinuria.

Further laboratory examination, such as immunoelectrophoresis of urine or nephelometry using specific antibodies, may be used to determine the chemical nature of excreted proteins. Comparison of the albumin concentration to that of other urinary proteins will reflect the selectivity of glomerular proteinuria, which is influenced by the underlying glomerular pathology. *Selective* proteinuria refers to glomerular proteinuria that is predominantly albumin; in contrast, *nonselective* proteinuria implies the presence in appreciable concentration of other plasma proteins, especially immunoglobulins.

Causes of Abnormal Proteinuria

Abnormal proteinuria can originate from (1) glomerular pathology, (2) tubular pathology, (3) overflow of an abnormal plasma protein, or (4) pathologic protein secretion from the urinary tract. Identification of the source of proteinuria has direct diagnostic significance and determines the approach to evaluation. The many causes of proteinuria are listed under these four categories in **Table 4-7**. Certain diseases can causes proteinuria in more than one category, and the diagnostic evaluation builds on this initial classification.

Glomerular proteinuria arises when excess protein crosses the GBM and overwhelms the capacity for tubular reabsorption. The GBM is a high-capacity ultrafiltration membrane, and proteins can pass across by convection or by diffusion down a concentration gradient. Mutations of podocyte cell surface proteins, such as nephrin and podocin, or of podocyte intracellular proteins that contribute to the integrity of the membrane, result in proteinuria. The membrane is negatively charged due to heparin sulfate in the glomerular endothelial wall, and this prevents similarly charged proteins, such as albumin, from passing across. Therefore, glomerular pathology that impairs the ability of the GBM to maintain its charge results in proteinuria. When overt glomerular injury is absent, as in minimal change nephropathy, proteinuria is largely comprised of albumin (selective proteinuria). As more damage to the GBM occurs, such as in proliferative glomerulonephritis or focal glomerulosclerosis, larger proteins, including immunoglobulins (nonselective proteinuria) make a greater contribution to the proteinuria. In addition to quantification of proteinuria, evaluation of the proportions of albumin and immunoglobulins in the urine is of diagnostic significance; it also influences the prognosis and permits monitoring of therapy, as has been demonstrated in membranous glomerulonephritis.

Nephrotic range proteinuria implies proteinuria of glomerular origin of sufficient severity to cause the clinical nephrotic syndrome, with hypoalbuminemia, hypercholesterolemia, and fluid retention. Individuals vary in the severity of proteinuria necessary to induce the nephrotic syndrome, reflecting factors such as hepatic albumin synthesis rate and dietary status. This occurs with proteinuria greater than 3000 mg/24 hr (nephrotic range proteinuria), but proteinuria may exceed 20,000 mg/24 hr.

Detection of albuminuria between 30 and 300 mg/24 hr (microalbuminuria) is a very useful and predictive screening test for diabetic nephropathy, reflecting early glomerular injury by diabetes mellitus (see Chapter 25). Microalbuminuria is also of prognostic value for renal and patient survival in chronic kidney disease and in cardiovascular disease.

TABLE 4-7 Causes of Proteinuria according to Pathophysiology

Glomerular Proteinuria

Primary glomerular disease
   Minimal change glomerulopathy
   Immunoglobulin A nephropathy
   Focal and segmental glomerulosclerosis
   Membranous glomerulonephritis
   Membranoproliferative glomerulonephritis
   Fibrillary and immunotactoid glomerulopathy
   Crescentic glomerulonephritis

Secondary glomerular disease
   Multisystem disease: SLE, vasculitis, amyloid, scleroderma
   Metabolic disease: diabetes mellitus, Fabry's disease
   Neoplasia: myeloma, leukemia, solid tumors
   Infections: bacterial, fungal, viral, parasitic
   Drugs, toxins and allergens: gold, penicillamine, lithium, NSAID, penicillin
   Familial: congenital nephrotic syndrome, Alport's syndrome, nephronophthisis
   Other: toxemia of pregnancy, transplant nephropathy, reflux nephropathy

Glomerular proteinuria without renal disease: exercise-induced, orthostatic, febrile proteinuria

Tubular Proteinuria

Drugs and toxins
   Luminal injury: light chain nephropathy, lysozyme (myelogenous leukemia)
   Exogenous: heavy metals (lead, mercury, cadmium), tetracycline
   Aristolochic acid (Balkan nephropathy)

Tubulointerstitial nephritis
   Hypersensitivity (drug, toxin)
   Multisystem: SLE, Sjögren's syndrome, tubulointerstitial nephritis with uveitis

Other: Fanconi's syndrome

Overflow Proteinuria

Myeloma, light chain disease, amyloidosis, hemoglobinuria, myoglobinuria

Tissue Proteinuria

Acute inflammation of urinary tract

Uroepithelial tumors

NSAID, nonsteroidal anti-inflammatory drug; SLE, systemic lupus erythematosus.

Tubular proteinuria results from a failure to absorb proteins normally filtered or secreted by the renal tubules due to tubular pathology such as Dent's disease, Lowe's syndrome, hereditary nephritis, tubulointerstitial nephritis, or heavy metal poisoning. It comprises alpha and beta globins, including α-microglobulin and β_2-microglobulin detectable either by specific immunoassay or by urine protein electrophoresis, appearing in the alpha and beta fractions. Albumin is usually present in addition, and proteinuria in the range of 200 to 2000 mg/24 hr is seen. Glomerular and tubular proteinuria may coexist as glomerular pathologies and often progress to cause tubular injury, in which case albumin contributes a greater proportion to the proteinuria.

Overflow proteinuria occurs when the filtered load of a plasma protein present at pathologic concentrations exceeds the reabsorptive capacity of the renal tubules. In hemolytic anemia, free hemoglobin not bound to haptoglobin appears in the urine, and in rhabdomyolysis, greatly increased plasma levels of myoglobin result in myoglobinuria. These proteins discolor the urine and are detected by specific reagents. Monoclonal gammopathies can result in monoclonal light chains or immunoglobulins in the urine. Their identity is confirmed by a monoclonal band on urine immunoelectrophoresis. Quantities of excreted protein in overflow proteinuria reflect the severity of the underlying pathology; they may be minor, or they may reach nephrotic range proteinuria.

Proteinuria occurring secondary to disease of the urinary tract is of relatively low concentration, up to 0.5 g/g (500 mg/24 hr), and may contain secreted IgA in inflammatory conditions. It is likely to be accompanied by nonglomerular hematuria and is best detected by urine electrophoresis.

Evaluation of Proteinuria

First, the presence of proteinuria on a screening test, such as a urine testing strip, requires confirmation by laboratory measurement in a controlled urine sample, either a protein-to-creatinine ratio from an early morning urine specimen or a 24-hour collection. Next, the proteinuria is quantified and classified into one of the four categories presented earlier. Finally, other investigations contribute to a definitive diagnosis (**Table 4-8**).

Initial Confirmation

Possible causes of false-positive results of testing strips should be considered, along with the clinical status of the patient when the sample was obtained. Vigorous exercise, fever, or the use of pressor agents increases proteinuria. Repeated positivity on dipstick testing requires confirmation and quantification in the laboratory by measurement of the protein-to-creatinine ratio or of proteinuria in a timed urine collection. A normal albumin excretion rate does not exclude tubular or overflow causes with nonalbumin proteins. Similarly, a discrepancy with a borderline or low-positive dipstick test and clearly abnormal measured protein excretion suggests nonalbumin proteinuria that is not detected well by the dipstick. If the protein excretion exceeds 200 mg/24 hr,

then evaluation should consider the identification of the cause. The initial step is urine microscopy on a freshly voided sample to assess erythrocytes and leucocytes and erythrocyte casts. Glomerular hematuria with proteinuria points to an underlying glomerular or tubular pathology. In these circumstances, sequential quantification of proteinuria plays a role in the monitoring of the disorder.

Preliminary Investigation

A thorough history should identify exposure to toxic agents or drugs, family history of renal disease, symptoms of renal disease, or symptoms of extrarenal disease in multisystem autoimmunity. Examination should evaluate the blood pressure, fluid balance, and cardiac status and look for signs associated with renal disease. After quantification of the proteinuria with classification into nephrotic or non-nephrotic range and assessment as to the likely origin, glomerular or nonglomerular, the kidney function (glomerular filtration rate) should be estimated from the serum creatinine. A complete blood count with white cell differential and biochemical studies including serum albumin, globulins, cholesterol, calcium, phosphate, uric acid, and liver function tests should be obtained. If the patient is at risk, serologic testing for hepatitis B, hepatitis C, HIV, or syphilis is necessary. A urinary tract ultrasound study defines the renal size and identifies structural abnormalities in the kidney or urinary tract. Immunologic studies including ANA, ANCA, complement levels, rheumatoid factor, cryoglobulins, and serum protein electrophoresis should be requested as appropriate.

Definitive Evaluation

If the proteinuria is less than 2000 mg/24 hr and is not accompanied by hematuria or other symptoms or signs, the kidneys are symmetrical and of normal size, and immunologic studies are normal, the patient may be observed for several months before further investigation is planned. Orthostatic proteinuria without other features of disease should be reassessed at infrequent intervals but does not require further investigation. The presence of this benign entity can be confirmed by comparing the protein content of a split 24-hour urine collection, with urine produced during the day (while ambulatory) and the urine produced at night (while recumbent) collected in separate containers. If there is further evidence of disease or if proteinuria persists, then renal biopsy should be considered if the proteinuria is of glomerular or tubular origin and its cause is not evident. Indications for renal biopsy vary and are not robustly evidence based. In adults, nephrotic range proteinuria in the absence of systemic disease (idiopathic nephrotic syndrome) is an indication for biopsy. Proteinuria greater than 1000 mg/24 hr that is accompanied by other features of disease or that is persistent after several months of observation typically requires a renal biopsy. Proteinuria in the range of 200 to 1000 mg/24 hr usually indicates a need for repeated observation. In patients with SLE, histologic class correlates poorly with urinary abnormalities, and a renal biopsy proteinuria threshold of 500 mg/24 hr has been advocated (see Chapter 24).

TABLE 4-8 Evaluation of Proteinuria Based on Type

ORIGIN OF PROTEINURIA	INVESTIGATIONS
Glomerular	Quantify by protein-to-creatinine ratio or 24-hr protein excretion Measure serum albumin and cholesterol Serology workup as in Table 4-3 Plasma and urine protein electrophoresis
Tubular	Alpha microglobulin, retinol-binding protein β_2-Microglobulin-to-albumin ratio Heavy metal screen Plasma and urine electrophoresis
Abnormal plasma proteins	Serum protein electrophoresis Urine protein electrophoresis and Bence Jones protein Erythrocyte hemolysis Reticulocyte count, blood film Lactate dehydrogenase Haptoglobins

In hypertensive nephropathy, renal size is usually reduced and low-level proteinuria is common. Nephrotic range proteinuria occurs rarely and is difficult to distinguish from other causes of the nephrotic syndrome without a biopsy. Similarly, diabetic nephropathy causes variable levels of proteinuria. In the patient with long-standing diabetes and a history of progressive microalbuminuria, renal biopsy is not justified; evaluation of the acute development of nephrotic syndrome in a diabetic is more complex. Most of these patients are found to have diabetic nephropathy on biopsy, but a minority have nondiabetic glomerular disease. The diabetic with no history of proteinuria who presents with proteinuria in the range of 0.5 to 3.0 g/g (500 to 3000 mg/24 hr) should be investigated for glomerular hematuria, impaired renal function, and circulating immunologic abnormalities (ANA, complement levels, and protein electrophoresis). If any of these additional factors are present, renal biopsy should be considered.

Immunologic studies identify circulating autoantibodies, abnormal complement levels, and pathologic immunoglobulins or immune complexes. The specificity of ANAs for SLE is increased by the presence of anti–double-stranded DNA antibodies or antibodies to extractable nuclear antigens, especially Ro, Sm, or RNP. Isolated proteinuria is not a sign of active vasculitis, but proteinuria accompanied by hematuria with a positive ANCA, confirmed by a positive PR3-ANCA or MPO-ANCA, is strongly suggestive of microscopic polyangiitis or Wegener's granulomatosis. Low complement levels imply complement consumption by immune complexes and, in the context of proteinuria, suggest an immune complex glomerulonephritis, either as a primary process or in the setting of a systemic disease (see **Table 4-7**). Although rheumatoid factor has a low specificity for renal disease, its presence in the evaluation of proteinuria is associated with cryoglobulinemia and infection-associated glomerulonephritis.

Glomerular disease can be associated with malignancy, especially in older patients. If malignancy is detected at the time of the initial presentation with proteinuria, renal biopsy is not justified; however, in older patients, occult malignancy may become apparent after more detailed investigation or during follow-up. Bone marrow examination and skeletal survey should be considered in overflow proteinuria due to abnormal light chains or if there is other evidence of myeloma. Fibrillary glomerulopathy is associated with amyloidosis, connective tissue disease, and monoclonal gammopathies and may cause the nephrotic syndrome. Carcinoma (e.g., of the colon, stomach, lung, breast) is associated with membranous and membranoproliferative glomerulonephritis. Hodgkin's disease and non-Hodgkin's lymphoma are associated with minimal change nephropathy. Appropriate screening or diagnostic studies, such as detection of occult gastrointestinal bleeding, CT scanning of the chest, mammography, and prostate examination, are indicated if a renal biopsy discloses one of these forms of glomerulonephritis.

Myoglobinuria in the absence of evidence of muscle injury requires evaluation for drug toxicity or inherited muscle enzyme deficiency. Hemoglobinuria can be caused by intravascular hemolysis, such as occurs in the erythrocyte membrane abnormality of paroxysmal nocturnal hemoglobinuria. Proteinuria may also be the presenting feature of inherited renal disease, such as Fabry's disease.

Patients with tubular proteinuria require a careful search for heavy metal intoxication (cadmium, lead, antimony) and for systemic disease, including Sjögren's syndrome and malignancy. Tubular proteinuria can be quantified and monitored by assessment of the ratio of the excretion rate of β_2-microglobulin to that of albumin. Rarely, egg albumin or other protein is added to the patient's urine (factitious proteinuria) and is readily detected by urine electrophoresis.

BIBLIOGRAPHY

Cohen RA, Brown RS: Microscopic hematuria. N Engl J Med 348:2330-2338, 2003.

Fairley K, Birch DF: A simple method for identifying glomerular bleeding. Kidney Int 21:105-108, 1982.

Fogazi GB, Ponticelli C, Ritz E: The Urinary Sediment: An Integrated View, 2nd ed. Oxford, Oxford University Press, 1999.

Gaspari F, Perico N, Remuzzi G: Timed urine collections are not needed to measure urine protein excretion in clinical practice. Am J Kidney Dis 47:8-14, 2006.

Grossfeld GD, Litwin MS, Wolf JS, et al: Evaluation of asymptomatic microscopic haematuria in adults: The American Urological Association best practice policy. Part 1: Definition, detection, prevalence and etiology. Urology 57:599-603, 2001.

Grossfeld GD, Litwin MS, Wolf JS, et al: Evaluation of asymptomatic microscopic haematuria in adults: The American Urological Association best practice policy. Part 2: Patient evaluation, cytology, voided markers, imaging, cystoscopy, nephrology evaluation and follow-up. Urology 57:604-610, 2001.

Hogg RJ, Furth S, Lemley KV: National Kidney Foundation's Kidney Disease Outcomes Quality Initiative Clinical Practice Guidelines for Chronic Kidney Disease in children and adolescents: Evaluation, classification and stratification. Pediatrics 111:1416-1421, 2003.

National Kidney Foundation: Clinical Practice Guidelines for Chronic Kidney Disease: Evaluation Classification and Stratification. Part 4: Definition and classification of stages of chronic kidney disease. Am J Kidney Dis 39(Suppl 1):46-75, 2002.

CHAPTER 5

Imaging the Kidneys

Larissa Braga, Diego R. Martin, and Richard C. Semelka

KIDNEY IMAGING TECHNIQUES

The spectrum of kidney abnormalities is very broad. Therefore, this chapter highlights only the most important disorders and recent critical topics related to imaging methods. Technological advances have resulted in less invasive imaging methods. With the growing range of imaging methods available, the selection of the optimal method to provide the most accurate diagnosis in a particular case is not always obvious. Not every imaging modality is available at every health care facility. Therefore, interaction among clinicians and radiologists at the level of selection of studies is often essential.

Abdominal Radiography and Intravenous Urography

Plain radiographs of the abdomen previously were the mainstay of the evaluation of kidney stones. In recent years, they have been superseded by non–contrast-enhanced computed tomography (CT). Nonetheless, plain radiographs are sometimes still valuable to evaluate kidney size and morphology, and especially to follow stones that are known to be present. The advantage of the use of plain films in this setting is the considerably lower radiation dose (0.01 versus 5 mSv), compared with a CT study. Difficulty distinguishing kidney stones from other radiopacities in the abdomen is, however, commonly encountered with plain radiographs.

Intravenous urography was formerly the primary imaging modality used to evaluate kidney stones and hydronephrosis. Like CT, this method uses iodinated contrast and carries the risk of ionizing radiation exposure. This technique has been largely replaced by ultrasonography (US), multiphase CT studies, and new methodologies such as magnetic resonance urography (MRU).

Ultrasonography

Gray-scale US has been the preferred method for screening of kidney abnormalities. It is inexpensive, can be performed at the bedside, does not emit radiation, and is performed without intravenous contrast. In addition, it provides an excellent guide for biopsies, because it is easily manipulated and is able to provide multiplanar images.

Gray-scale US provides accurate measurement of overall kidney size, evaluates parenchymal thickness, identifies hydronephrosis, and is able to differentiate solid from simple cystic lesions. Differentiation between solid and complex cystic lesions can be challenging by US, and often further studies, such as CT or magnetic resonance imaging (MRI), are performed to achieve the final diagnosis. Sensitivity for visualization of a renal calculus depends on the size of the calculus. The reflection of the ultrasound wave causes posterior acoustic shadowing, which indicates the presence of the calculus. The ureter is not well visualized by US, unless it is dilated. The urinary bladder wall and the bladder contents, as well as bilateral urine jets, are often well demonstrated. Patients with long-term prostatic enlargement may have a bladder with trabeculated walls and increased postvoid residual volume (normal, ≤50 mL); these features are well demonstrated by US. As a drawback, however, US is operator dependent and is adversely affected by large body habitus and overlying bowel gas.

Doppler US is often performed as part of a gray-scale examination to evaluate the blood flow in the kidney vessels. Resistive index is a parameter used to evaluate vascular compliance and resistance. In adult patients, a value greater than 0.70 is considered abnormal; however, elderly patients may have an elevated resistance index without clinical findings, most likely due to small vessel disease. The morphology of Doppler waveforms can be indicative of renal artery stenosis. Loss of the early systolic peak of the waveforms is suggestive of up to 60% luminal stenosis of the main renal artery. As a downside, Doppler US is hampered by respiratory movements in addition to large body habitus and overlying bowel gas.

Computed Tomography

Spiral CT, using either single-detector or multidetector CT, has been widely used to assess the urinary tract. Multidetector computed tomography (MDCT) obtains multiple slices in a single rotation. The advantages of MDCT over single-detector CT are thinner slices that allow for three-dimensional reconstructions, fewer artifacts, and shorter scan times. The major drawback of MDCT is the potentially higher radiation dose, compared with single-slice CT, if very thin sections are acquired.

CT without contrast has become the study of choice to detect renal calculi. In addition, CT is unmatched in its ability to detect calcified nonobstructing kidney stones as small as 2 mm that lie along the course of the ureters.

A good delineation of the renal vasculature and iliac vessels, a crucial step in the planning process for kidney transplantation in both donors and recipients, can be achieved by CT angiography (CTA). CTA images are obtained with MDCT, which is able to acquire thinner slices with faster scanning, and CTA is considered slightly superior to magnetic resonance angiography (MRA) for evaluation of the renal vasculature. Conventional angiography, which often requires the injection of the contrast directly into the artery or vein of interest and is therefore much more invasive, has been gradually supplanted by CTA and MRA.

Magnetic Resonance Studies

MRI is advantageous over either CT or US, because it provides a superior definition of internal structure and better characterization of lesions, through the acquisition of multiple sequences, in various planes (transverse, sagittal, and coronal), and the use of intravenous gadolinium-containing contrast. Solid structures (i.e., liver, spleen, pancreas, kidneys, adrenal glands, uterus, ovaries, and prostate) enhance to a greater extent on postcontrast images with MRI compared to CT. Enhancement features are distinctive for each organ and are influenced by the length of time between contrast injection and image acquisition.

Protocols for imaging the kidneys with MRI vary somewhat among institutions. In general, kidneys are imaged using T2-weighted and T1-weighted images before contrast administration, followed by dynamic postcontrast T1-weighted images. Fluids appear hyperintense on T2-weighted images; therefore, coronal T2-weighted images provide good visualization of the ureters throughout their course and of the urinary bladder. T1-weighted precontrast and postcontrast sequences are valuable to depict and characterize kidney abnormalities, including malignancies and complex cysts.

The lack of radiation emission with MRI is an important advantage over CT. Women during pregnancy may particularly benefit from MRI rather than CT, especially if repeated examinations are necessary, such as for follow-up of suspicious malignant disease.

MRA is a study dedicated to evaluating the caliber and anatomy of the vessels; it is especially useful when there is suspicion of renal artery stenosis. Functional MRU is a new modality that is able to provide physiologic information apart from anatomy, including renal blood flow and glomerular filtration rate (GFR) (**Fig. 5-1**). It has the advantage over CT and nuclear renal scintigraphy of not utilizing radiation.

Radionuclide Studies

Nuclear scintigraphy evaluates renal perfusion and anatomy and quantifies kidney function. Agents with different mechanisms of action are available to image the kidneys. They are selected based on the clinical setting and the diagnostic. The most frequently used agents are technetium 99mL–Labeled pentetate (^{99m}Tc-DTPA), succimer (^{99m}Tc-DMSA), and mertiatide (^{99m}Tc-MAG3). Obstructive uropathy, hypertension, and evaluation of differential function between the two kidneys are some of the clinical indications for which

nuclear scintigraphy is most valuable. However, radiation is a concern in nuclear scintigraphy, especially in monitoring the applications for which follow-up studies are needed.

KIDNEY ABNORMALITIES
Renal Cysts

Renal cysts are often found incidentally during an imaging investigation. They can be structurally divided into simple (**Fig. 5-2**) and complex forms. The Bosniak classification system has been widely used to categorize cystic lesions based on the likelihood of malignancy. Although this system is tailored to CT, studies have shown that it can be extrapolated to MRI.

US is the preferred method to differentiate cystic from solid lesions because of its ease of performance and lower costs. However, MRI is superior in characterizing a lesion as cystic or solid, information that can be especially useful for evaluation of complex cystic lesions that have been classified as indeterminate by US. Because of its higher costs, MRI should be reserved for specific clinical settings, such as further evaluation of complex cysts or ruling out an additional or contralateral kidney malignancy in a patient with a report of an indeterminate lesion on US.

Autosomal Dominant Polycystic Kidney Disease

Imaging features of autosomal dominant polycystic kidney disease (ADPKD) may differ according to the severity of the disease (**Fig. 5-3**). Imaging methods may be applied to assess disease progression, with visualization of kidney enlargement due to cyst development or increased cyst size. Severe cases of ADPKD show massively enlarged kidneys with distorted architecture and multiple cysts of various sizes. Recent studies have demonstrated an inverse linear correlation between kidney volume and GFR. For patients with ADPKD, CT and MRI are the preferred methods to calculate kidney volume, an assessment that is not feasible with US, especially in the presence of massively enlarged kidneys. The depiction of early malignancy in the setting of moderate or severe ADPKD is challenging by any imaging method because of the presence of multiple cysts and distorted kidney architecture.

Kidney Infection and Abscess

Most patients with a clinical diagnosis of pyelonephritis have normal imaging studies. Severe cases may demonstrate enlarged kidneys due to interstitial infiltration and edema, heterogeneous contrast enhancement due to edema and vasospasm, and thickening of the perinephric fascia and septa in the perinephric space (also called fat stranding) due to inflammatory reaction. These findings are best appreciated by CT and MRI.

The diagnosis of renal abscess by US or CT without contrast is challenging, because abscesses may mimic complex

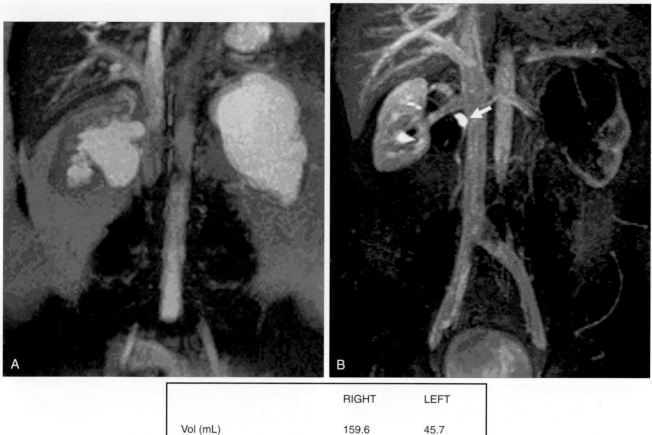

	RIGHT	LEFT
Vol (mL)	159.6	45.7
RBF (mL/sec)	6.3	1.0
RBF (mL/min)	379.5	62.2
RBF/Vol (min^{-1})	2.38	1.36
GFR/Vol (min^{-1})	0.37	0.13
Fitration Fraction	0.16	0.1
GFR (mL/min)	59 (91%)	6 (9%)
Total GFR = 65 mL/min		

C

FIGURE 5-1 Magnetic resonance studies of a patient with unexplained bilateral hydronephrosis. **A,** Coronal T2-weighted image shows bilateral hydronephrosis, moderate on the right and severe on the left side. **B,** Coronal post-gadolinium contrast-enhanced three-dimensional gradient echo maximum intensity projection taken 10 minutes after contrast administration shows excretion only from the right kidney. Note that the proximal ureter *(arrow)* is positioned anterior to the medial border of the fluid-filled structure that is well shown on **A. C,** The summary of quantitative information derived from the gadolinium-enhanced magnetic resonance urography demonstrates that the function of the right kidney is within normal limits, whereas the left kidney is markedly impaired. GFR, glomerular filtration rate; RBF, renal blood flow.

cysts. The hallmark of an abscess is the presence, around a cystic lesion, of a thick wall that enhances after administration of contrast material and can be readily detected on postcontrast CT or MRI. Necrotic kidney cancer may appear similar to an abscess, including the enhancement with contrast, but the presence of prominent perinephric stranding favors a diagnosis of abscess. The clinical history is also important to establish the nature of the lesion.

Nephrolithiasis

Noncontrast CT is now the gold-standard diagnostic test for nephrolithiasis. The use of contrast is undesirable in this disorder, because both contrast materials and kidney stones appear hyperdense on CT images (**Fig. 5-4**). On gray-scale US, a calculus may appear as a hyperechoic structure and, based on the size of the concretion, may

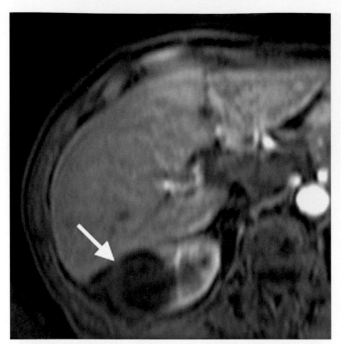

FIGURE 5-2 T1-weighted early phase magnetic resonance image shows a simple cyst *(arrow)* in the mid-pole of the right kidney.

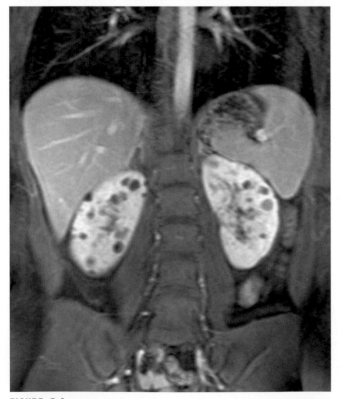

FIGURE 5-3 Coronal T1-weighted magnetic resonance image in a patient with early-stage autosomal dominant polycystic kidney disease (ADPKD) shows multiple cysts.

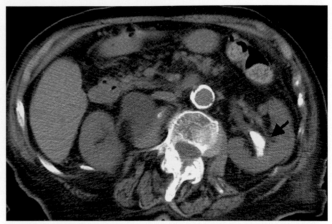

FIGURE 5-4 Computed tomography without contrast demonstrates a hyperdense calculus *(black arrow)* in the left kidney.

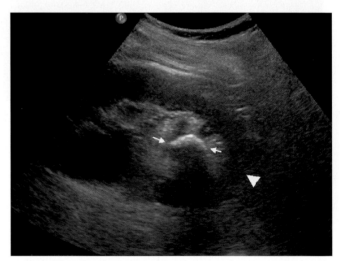

FIGURE 5-5 Gray-scale ultrasonography shows a hyperechoic area *(arrows)* with shadowing located in the inferior pole of the left kidney *(arrowhead)*, compatible with calculus.

Collecting System Dilatation or Obstruction

Evaluation of the dilated collecting system is a common clinical scenario. US has been employed as a morphologic tool, whereas CT, MRI, and scintigraphy studies all provide dynamic information after the administration of an intravenous agent. Radionuclide scanning before and after administration of a diuretic (*furosemide renogram*) can help distinguish between a collecting system that is dilated due to obstruction and a collecting system that is patulous but unobstructed. In the former case, excretion of scintigraphic contrast material after administration of the diuretic is delayed. In the latter, excretion of "cold" urine in response to the diuretic rapidly clears the collecting system of contrast material. Evaluation by a retrograde approach is commonly employed in pediatric patients. Fluoroscopic voiding cystography with iodinated contrast and scintigraphic voiding cystography are two common techniques.

demonstrate shadowing (**Fig. 5-5**). Not uncommonly, calcified vessels and small stones have a similar appearance on US. MRI is not an ideal method for evaluation of nephrolithiasis, because calcification is not well depicted by this method.

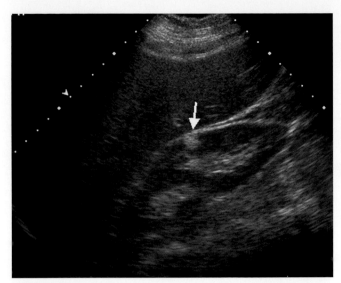

FIGURE 5-6 Gray-scale ultrasonography exhibits a small hyperechoic area *(arrow)* in the anterior aspect mid-pole of the kidney, consistent with angiomyolipoma.

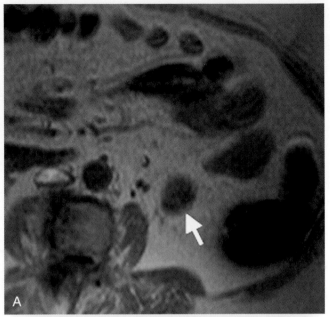

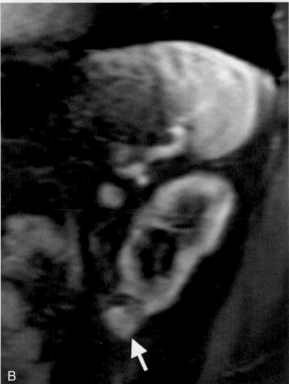

FIGURE 5-7 Transverse T1-weighted precontrast (**A**) and sagittal T1-weighted late-phase fat-suppressed postcontrast (**B**) magnetic resonance images demonstrate a renal cell carcinoma in the inferior pole of the left kidney *(arrow)*.

Kidney Trauma and Infarct

CT is the imaging method of choice in the setting of kidney trauma. Intravenous contrast must be administered, in the absence of any contraindication, to achieve superior delineation of structures. The presence and extension of subcapsular and perirenal hematomas, as well as parenchymal lacerations, are well depicted by CT. Infarct often occurs during kidney trauma because of thrombosis, and CTA is a reliable method to assess artery patency. MRI is superior to CT to follow up kidney trauma in patients who are not acutely ill, because it provides a multiplanar view of the affected area and vessels without exposing the patient to radiation. Limited US can be useful to follow up resolution of perinephric fluid collections. CTA and MRA are preferred over Doppler US to evaluate vessel stenosis.

Kidney Neoplasms

The increasing number of imaging examinations is leading to a higher detection of incidental kidney tumors. In a significant number of cases, the distinction between benign and malignant lesions can be made based on imaging characteristics. Angiomyolipomas with predominantly fat tissue have negative Hounsfield numbers on CT, appearing hypodense, whereas on US, they appear hyperechoic (**Fig. 5-6**). MRI using out-of-phase or fat-suppressed techniques is very effective at demonstrating fat in Angiomyolipomas. Oncocytomas may exhibit a central scar ("spoke wheel"), a highly suggestive sign that can be demonstrated by any imaging method. The degree of tumor enhancement by iodinated contrast on CT or by gadolinium on MRI is a valuable finding suggestive of malignancy, as in the case of renal cell carcinomas, which are hypervascular tumors (**Fig. 5-7**; see **Fig. 5-6**). However, small renal cell carcinomas can be missed on CT images, depending on the timing of the contrast administration. Regarding tumor staging, especially in late stages of disease, MRI is superior to CT or US. MRI scans in the sagittal and coronal planes are both superb for demonstrating the extension of the tumor into the renal vein and inferior vena cava (**Fig. 5-8**; see **Fig. 5-7**). Small (<5 mm) lung metastases are better shown on CT than on MRI. Bone metastases are generally better shown on MRI than on CT. Positron emission tomography (PET) using fluorine 18–labeled fluorodeoxyglucose

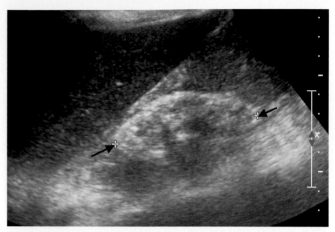

FIGURE 5-9 Gray-scale ultrasonography demonstrates a kidney *(black arrows)* decreased in size, measuring approximately 6 cm in length (normal, about 10 cm) and with loss of corticomedullary differentiation, consistent with chronic kidney disease.

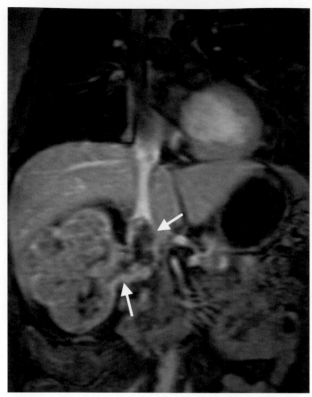

FIGURE 5-8 Coronal T2-weighted magnetic resonance image exhibits tumor invasion into the right renal vein and inferior vena cava *(arrows)*.

(FDG), called FDG PET, blends the information obtained by CT and radionuclide scanning; however, the role of FDG PET in the urinary tract has not been established.

Radiofrequency ablation and cryoablation have been employed as alternative (minimally invasive) therapeutic choices for small kidney tumors when a surgical approach is contraindicated. Either MRI or CT is an effective imaging method to evaluate the success of the procedure, because residual or recurrent tumors show enhancement after contrast administration within a hypointense (MRI) or hypodense (CT) ablated cavity.

Kidneys of Patients with End-Stage Renal Disease

Patients undergoing long-term dialysis may develop multiple small, simple cysts, predominantly in the renal cortex. Cysts are often well depicted by US, but solid lesions must be evaluated carefully, because dialysis patients are prone to develop malignancies in the kidneys. Imaging in ESRD for detection of malignancy, particularly by US, is limited because of the reduction in kidney size and poor differentiation between the cortex and the medulla (**Fig. 5-9**). In these cases, MRI is considered the method of choice; the enhancement after contrast administration is a crucial feature for detection and characterization of malignancies. In chronically failed kidneys, MRI shows better enhancement of parenchyma and kidney masses than does CT. However, gadolinium contrast

must be used with caution in patients with GFR less than 30 mL/min, because of the risk of nephrogenic systemic fibrosis (see later discussion).

Kidney Transplantation

CTA is an effective, noninvasive method to evaluate renal vessels from donors and recipients before transplantation. CTA can depict vascular disorders such as aneurysms, stenosis, thrombosis, and arteriovenous fistulas. MDCT provides greater information than single-detector CT, such as better delineation of vessels and three-dimensional images. Currently, because the slice thickness is smaller with CT compared to MRI, small intrarenal branches may be better shown with CT. Mural calcification may be more problematic on CT than on MRI scans, because the brightness of calcium may obstruct visualization of the vessel lumen on CT, whereas the darkness of calcium on MRI does not interfere with visualization (**Fig. 5-10**).

US plays an important role in the follow-up of patients after kidney transplantation. Size and characteristics (simple or complex) of perinephric fluid collections such as hematomas, urinomas, and lymphoceles are well demonstrated on US. In addition, Doppler US is able to evaluate the resistance index in the main and small branches of renal arteries (**Fig. 5-11**). An elevated resistance index (>0.80) has been considered a predictive factor for transplant failure.

Gadolinium and Nephrogenic Systemic Fibrosis

Gadolinium, a paramagnetic contrast medium, has been widely utilized in MRI studies for almost two decades. Nephrogenic systemic fibrosis (NSF) is characterized by progressive skin fibrosis, particularly of the distal extremities. The association between the use of gadolinium with the development of NSF 1 to 3 months later, which has been reported in

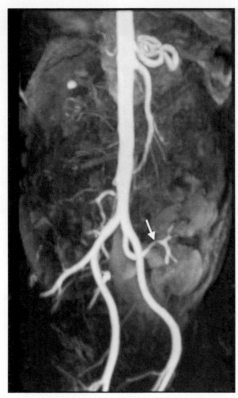

FIGURE 5-10 Magnetic resonance angiography after kidney transplantation demonstrates renal artery stenosis *(arrow).* Note typical allograft location in the pelvis, with artery anastomosed to the internal iliac artery.

recent studies, is a critical topic for radiologists and nephrologists. We recommend careful use of gadolinium in patients with GFR lower than 30 mL/min, and only if the information to be gained is essential. Informed consent, use of a minimum dose of gadolinium, avoidance of multiple dosing of gadolinium, and selection of agents less commonly associated with NSF are recommended. Hemodialysis promptly removes gadolinium from the circulation, but it is not currently recommended for patients not already on dialysis. No study has examined whether prompt dialysis obviates the development of NSF, although early dialysis may be prudent. Our experience suggests that early dialysis may lessen the severity of NSF.

It is important to emphasize that the interests of the patient should come first when choosing the appropriate imaging method. MRI is still considered the imaging method of choice in many circumstances to evaluate kidney functional impairment. Contrast-induced nephropathy secondary to iodinated contrast agents used in CT may in fact be as serious a condition as NSF. Its risk is highest in patients with impaired kidney function, but it can occur with any level of kidney function, including normal function. Nephrotoxicity from CT contrast and its prevention in patients at increased risk are discussed in Chapter 34.

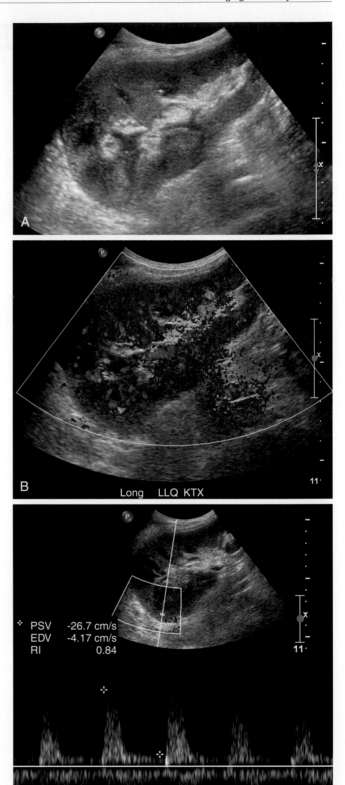

FIGURE 5-11 A, Gray-scale ultrasonography after kidney transplantation demonstrates a normal-appearing allograft. **B,** There is good perfusion by Doppler ultrasonography (red indicates arterial flow and blue venous flow). **C,** However, the resistance index (RI = 0.84) in the arcuate artery is mildly elevated (arterial pulse waveforms are shown at the bottom of the figure).

BIBLIOGRAPHY

Bosniak MA: The current radiological approach to renal cysts. Radiology 158:1-10, 1986.

Grantham JJ, Chapman AB, Torres VE: Volume progression in autosomal dominant polycystic kidney disease: The major factor determining clinical outcomes. Clin J Am Soc Nephrol 1: 148-157, 2006.

Israel GM, Hindman N, Bosniak MA: Evaluation of cystic renal masses: Comparison of CT and MR imaging by using the Bosniak classification system. Radiology 231:365-371, 2004.

Kanal E, Barkovich AJ, Bell C, et al: ACR guidance document for safe MR practices. AJR Am J Roentgenol 188:1-27, 2007.

Radermacher J, Mengel M, Ellis S, et al: The renal arterial resistance index and renal allograft survival. N Engl J Med 349: 115-124, 2003.

Rule AD, Torres VE, Chapman AB, et al: Comparison of methods for determining renal function decline in early autosomal dominant polycystic kidney disease: The Consortium of Radiologic Imaging Studies of Polycystic Kidney Disease cohort. J Am Soc Nephrol 17:854-862, 2006.

Semelka RC, Shoenut JP, Magro CM, et al: Renal cancer staging: Comparison of contrast-enhanced CT and gadolinium-enhanced fat-suppressed spin-echo and gradient-echo MR imaging. J Magn Reson Imaging 3:597-602, 1993.

Stavros AT, Parker SH, Yakes WF, et al: Segmental stenosis of the renal artery: Pattern recognition of tardus and parvus abnormalities with duplex sonography. Radiology 184:487-492, 1992.

Tublin ME, Bude RO, Platt JF: The resistive index in renal Doppler sonography: Where do we stand? [Review]. AJR Am J Roentgenol 180:885-892, 2003.

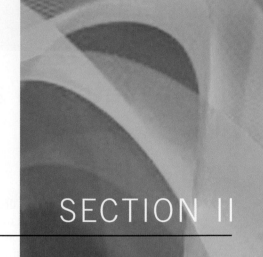

Acid-Base, Fluid, and Electrolyte Disorders

CHAPTER 6

Hyponatremia and Hypo-osmolar Disorders

Joseph G. Verbalis

The incidence of hyponatremia depends on the patient population and the criteria used to define hyponatremia. Hospital incidences of 15% to 22% are common if hyponatremia is defined as any serum sodium concentration ($[Na^+]$) of less than 135 mEq/L, but in most studies only 1% to 4% of patients have a serum $[Na^+]$ lower than 130 mEq/L, and fewer than 1% have a value lower than 120 mEq/L. Recent studies have confirmed prevalences from 7% in ambulatory populations to 28% in acutely hospitalized patients. The elderly are particularly susceptible to hyponatremia, with reported incidences as high as 53% among institutionalized geriatric patients. Although most cases are mild, hyponatremia is important clinically because (1) acute severe hyponatremia can cause substantial morbidity and mortality; (2) mild hyponatremia can progress to more dangerous levels during management of other disorders; (3) general mortality is higher in hyponatremic patients with a wide range of underlying diseases; and (4) overly rapid correction of chronic hyponatremia can produce severe neurologic deficits and death.

DEFINITIONS

Hyponatremia is of clinical significance only when it reflects corresponding hypo-osmolality of the plasma. Plasma osmolality (P_{osm}) can be measured directly by osmometry and is expressed as milliosmoles per kilogram of water (mOsm/kg H_2O). P_{osm} also can be calculated from the serum $[Na^+]$, measured in milliequivalents per liter (mEq/L), and the glucose and blood urea nitrogen (BUN) levels, both expressed as milligrams per deciliter (mg/dL):

$$P_{osm} = \left(2 \times Serum\left[Na^+\right]\right) + Glucose/18 + BUN/2.8$$

Both methods produce comparable results under most conditions, as does simply doubling the serum $[Na^+]$. However, total osmolality is not always equivalent to *effective osmolality*, which is sometimes referred to as the *tonicity* of the plasma. Solutes that are predominantly compartmentalized to the extracellular fluid (ECF) are effective solutes, because they create osmotic gradients across cell membranes, leading to osmotic movement of water from the intracellular fluid (ICF) to ECF compartments. In contrast, solutes that freely permeate cell membranes (urea, ethanol, methanol) are not effective solutes, because they do not create osmotic gradients across cell membranes and therefore are not associated with secondary water shifts. Only the concentration of effective solutes in plasma should be used to determine whether clinically significant hypo-osmolality is present. In most cases, these effective solutes include sodium and its associated anions and glucose (but only in the presence of insulin deficiency, which allows the development of an ECF/ICF glucose gradient); they do not include urea nitrogen, a solute that freely penetrates cells.

Hyponatremia and hypo-osmolality are usually synonymous, but with two important exceptions. First, *pseudohyponatremia* can be produced by marked elevation of serum lipids or proteins. In such cases, the concentration of Na^+ per liter of serum water is unchanged, but the concentration of Na^+ per liter of serum is artifactually decreased because of the increased relative proportion occupied by lipid or protein. Although measurement of serum or plasma $[Na^+]$ by ion-specific electrodes currently used by most clinical laboratories is less influenced by high concentrations of lipids or proteins than is measurement of serum $[Na^+]$ by flame photometry, such errors nonetheless still occur. However, because direct measurement of P_{osm} is based on the colligative properties of only the solute particles in solution, the measured P_{osm} will not be affected by increased lipids or proteins.

Second, high concentrations of effective solutes other than Na^+ can cause relative decreases in serum $[Na^+]$ despite an unchanged P_{osm}; this commonly occurs with hyperglycemia. Misdiagnosis can be avoided again by direct measurement of P_{osm} or by correcting the serum $[Na^+]$ by 1.6 mEq/L for each 100 mg/dL increase in blood glucose concentration above 100 mg/dL (although recent studies have suggested that 2.4 mEq/L may be a more accurate correction factor).

PATHOGENESIS

The presence of significant hypo-osmolality indicates excess water relative to solute in the ECF. Because water moves freely between the ICF and ECF, this also indicates an excess of total body water relative to total body solute. Imbalances between water and solute can be generated initially either by *depletion* of body solute more than body water or by *dilution* of body solute due to increases in body water more than body solute (**Table 6-1**). However, this distinction represents an oversimplification, because most hypo-osmolar states include variable components of both solute depletion and water retention. For example, isotonic solute losses occurring during an acute hemorrhage do not produce hypo-osmolality until the subsequent retention of

TABLE 6-1 Pathogenesis of Hypo-osmolar Disorders

Depletion (Primary Decreases in Total Body Solute + Secondary Water Retention)*

Renal Solute Loss
Diuretic use
Solute diuresis (glucose, mannitol)
Salt-wasting nephropathy
Mineralocorticoid deficiency

Nonrenal Solute Loss
Gastrointestinal (diarrhea, vomiting, pancreatitis, bowel obstruction)
Cutaneous (sweating, burns)
Blood loss

Dilution (Primary Increases in Total Body Water ± Secondary Solute Depletion)†

Impaired Renal Free Water Excretion

Increased Proximal Reabsorption
Hypothyroidism

Impaired Distal Dilution
Syndrome of inappropriate antidiuretic hormone secretion (SIADH)
Glucocorticoid deficiency

Combined Increased Proximal Reabsorption and Impaired Distal Dilution
Congestive heart failure
Cirrhosis
Nephrotic syndrome

Decreased Urinary Solute Excretion
Beer potomania

Excess Water Intake
Primary polydipsia
Dilute infant formula

*Virtually all disorders of solute depletion are accompanied by some degree of secondary retention of water by the kidneys in response to the resulting intravascular hypovolemia; this mechanism can lead to hypo-osmolality even when the solute depletion occurs via hypotonic or isotonic body fluid losses.
†Disorders of water retention primarily cause hypo-osmolality in the absence of any solute losses, but in some cases of SIADH, secondary solute losses occur in response to the resulting intravascular hypervolemia and can further aggravate the hypo-osmolality. (However, this pathophysiology probably does not contribute to the hyponatremia of edema-forming states such as congestive heart failure and cirrhosis, because in these cases, multiple factors favoring sodium retention result in an increased total body sodium load.)
Modified from Verbalis JG: The syndrome of inappropriate antidiuretic hormone secretion and other hypoosmolar disorders. In Schrier RW (ed): Diseases of the Kidney. Philadelphia, Lippincott Williams & Wilkins, 2007, pp 2214-2248.

water from ingested or infused hypotonic fluids causes a secondary dilution of the remaining ECF solute. Nonetheless, this concept has proved useful because it provides a framework for understanding the diagnosis and treatment of hypo-osmolar disorders.

DIFFERENTIAL DIAGNOSIS

The diagnostic approach to hypo-osmolar disorders should include a careful history (especially concerning medications); physical examination with emphasis on clinical assessment of the ECF volume status and a thorough neurologic evaluation; measurement of serum or plasma electrolytes, glucose, BUN, creatinine, and uric acid; calculated and/or directly measured P_{osm}; and determination of simultaneous urine sodium and osmolality. Although prevalences vary according to the population being studied, a sequential analysis of hyponatremic patients admitted to a large university teaching hospital revealed that approximately 20% were hypovolemic, 20% had edema-forming states, 33% were euvolemic, 15% had hyperglycemia-induced hyponatremia, and 10% had renal failure. Consequently, euvolemic hyponatremia generally constitutes the largest single group of hyponatremic patients found in this setting. A definitive diagnosis is not always possible at the time of presentation, but an initial categorization based on the patient's clinical ECF volume status allows a determination of the appropriate initial therapy in most cases (**Fig. 6-1**).

Decreased Extracellular Fluid Volume (Hypovolemia)

Clinically detectable hypovolemia, determined most sensitively by careful measurement of orthostatic changes in blood pressure and pulse rate, usually indicates some degree of solute depletion. Elevation of the BUN and uric acid concentration are useful laboratory correlates of decreased ECF volume. Even isotonic or hypotonic volume losses can lead to hypo-osmolality if water or hypotonic fluids are ingested or infused as replacement. A low urine sodium concentration (U_{Na}) in such cases suggests a nonrenal cause of the solute depletion, whereas a high U_{Na} suggests renal causes of solute depletion (see **Table 6-1**). Diuretic use is the most common cause of hypovolemic hypo-osmolality, and thiazides are more commonly associated with severe hyponatremia than are loop diuretics such as furosemide.

Although diuretics represent a prime example of solute depletion, the pathophysiologic mechanisms underlying the hypo-osmolality are complex and have multiple components, including free water retention. Many patients do not manifest clinical evidence of marked hypovolemia, in part because ingested water has been retained in response to non-osmotically stimulated secretion of arginine vasopressin (AVP), as is generally true for all disorders of solute depletion. To further complicate diagnosis, the U_{Na} may be high or low depending on when the last diuretic dose was taken. Consequently, any suspicion of diuretic use mandates careful consideration of this diagnosis. A low serum $[K^+]$ is an important clue to diuretic use, because few other disorders that cause hyponatremia and hypo-osmolality also produce appreciable hypokalemia. Whenever the possibility of diuretic use is suspected in the absence of a positive history, a urine screen for diuretics should be done.

Most other causes of renal or nonrenal solute losses resulting in hypovolemic hypo-osmolality will be clinically apparent, although some cases of salt-wasting nephropathies (e.g., chronic interstitial nephropathy, polycystic kidney disease, obstructive uropathy, Bartter's syndrome) or mineralocorticoid deficiency (e.g., Addison's disease) can be challenging to diagnose during the early phases.

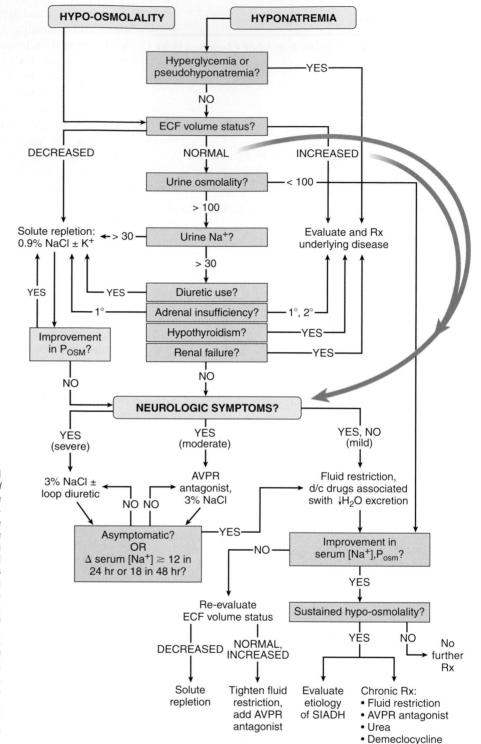

FIGURE 6-1 Algorithm for evaluation and therapy of hypo-osmolar patients. The *gold arrow* in the center emphasizes that the presence of central nervous system dysfunction due to hyponatremia should always be assessed immediately, so that appropriate therapy can be started as soon as possible in symptomatic patients even while the outlined diagnostic evaluation is proceeding. Values for osmolality are in mOsm/kg H_2O, and those referring to serum Na^+ concentration are in mEq/L. Δ, change (in concentration); 1°, primary; 2°, secondary; AVPR, arginine vasopressin receptor; d/c, discontinue; ECF, extracellular fluid volume; P_{osm}, plasma osmolality; Rx, treatment; SIADH, syndrome of inappropriate antidiuretic hormone secretion. (Modified from Verbalis JG: The syndrome of inappropriate antidiuretic hormone secretion and other hypoosmolar disorders. In Schrier RW (ed): Diseases of the Kidney. Philadelphia, Lippincott Williams & Wilkins, 2007, pp 2214-2248.)

Normal Extracellular Fluid Volume (Euvolemia)

Virtually any disorder associated with hypo-osmolality can manifest with a hydration status that appears normal by standard methods of clinical evaluation. Because clinical assessment of ECF volume status is not very sensitive, normal or low levels of serum BUN and uric acid are helpful laboratory correlates of relatively normal ECF volume.

Conversely, a low U_{Na} suggests a depletional hypo-osmolality secondary to ECF losses with subsequent volume replacement by water or other hypotonic fluids; as discussed earlier, such patients may appear euvolemic by all the usual clinical parameters used to assess hydration status. Primary dilutional disorders are less likely in the presence of a low U_{Na} (<30 mEq/L), although this pattern can occur in hypothyroidism.

A high U_{Na} ($\geq$30 mEq/L) generally indicates a dilutional hypo-osmolality such as the *syndrome of inappropriate antidiuretic hormone secretion (SIADH)* (see **Table 6-1**). SIADH is the most common cause of euvolemic hypo-osmolality in clinical medicine. The criteria necessary for a diagnosis of SIADH remain essentially as defined by Bartter and Schwartz in 1967 (**Table 6-2**), but several points deserve emphasis.

First, true ECF hypo-osmolality must be present, and hyponatremia secondary to pseudohyponatremia or hyperglycemia must be excluded. Second, the urinary osmolality (U_{osm}) must be inappropriate for the low P_{osm}. This does not require that U_{osm} must be greater than P_{osm}, but merely that the urine must not be maximally dilute (i.e., U_{osm} must be >100 mOsm/kg H_2O in adults).

Second, U_{osm} need not be inappropriately elevated at all levels of P_{osm} but simply at some level of P_{osm} less than 275 mOsm/kg H_2O, because, in patients with a *reset osmostat*, AVP secretion can be suppressed at some level of P_{osm}, resulting in maximal urinary dilution and free water excretion at plasma osmolalities below this level. Although some consider a reset osmostat to be a separate disorder rather than a variant of SIADH, such cases nonetheless illustrate that some hypo-osmolar patients can exhibit an appropriately dilute urine at some, although not all, plasma osmolalities.

Third, clinical euvolemia must be present to diagnose SIADH, and this diagnosis cannot be made in a hypovolemic or edematous patient. Importantly, this does not mean that patients with SIADH cannot become hypovolemic for other reasons, but in such cases it is impossible to diagnose the underlying SIADH until the patient is rendered euvolemic.

TABLE 6-2 Criteria for the Diagnosis of Syndrome of Inappropriate Antidiuretic Hormone Secretion (SIADH)

Essential Criteria

1. Decreased effective osmolality of the extracellular fluid (P_{osm} <275 mOsm/kg H_2O)

2. Inappropriate urinary concentration (U_{osm} >100 mOsm/kg H_2O with normal renal function) at some level of plasma hypo-osmolality

3. Clinical euvolemia, as defined by the absence of signs of hypovolemia (orthostasis, tachycardia, decreased skin turgor, dry mucous membranes) or hypervolemia (subcutaneous edema, ascites)

4. Elevated urinary sodium excretion despite a normal salt and water intake

5. Normal thyroid, adrenal, and renal function

Supplemental Criteria

6. Abnormal water load test (inability to excrete at least 80% of a 20 mL/kg water load in 4 hr and/or failure to dilute U_{osm} to <100 mOsm/kg H_2O)

7. Plasma vasopressin (AVP) level inappropriately elevated relative to plasma osmolality

8. No significant correction of serum sodium concentration ([Na^+]) with volume expansion but improvement after fluid restriction

Modified from Verbalis JG: The syndrome of inappropriate antiduretic hormone secretion and other hypoosmolar disorders. In Schrier RW (ed): Diseases of the Kidney. Philadelphia, Lippincott Williams & Wilkins, 2007, pp 2214-2248.

The fourth criterion, renal salt wasting, has probably caused the most confusion regarding SIADH. The importance of this criterion lies in its usefulness in differentiating hypo-osmolality caused by a decreased effective intravascular volume (in which case renal Na^+ conservation occurs) from dilutional disorders in which urinary Na^+ excretion is normal or increased due to ECF volume expansion. However, U_{Na} can also be high in renal causes of solute depletion, such as diuretic use or Addison's disease, and, conversely, patients with SIADH can have a low urinary Na^+ excretion if they subsequently become hypovolemic or solute depleted—conditions sometimes produced by imposed salt and water restriction. Consequently, although high urinary Na^+ excretion is generally the rule in patients with SIADH, its presence does not necessarily confirm this diagnosis, nor does its absence rule out the diagnosis.

The final criterion emphasizes that SIADH remains a diagnosis of exclusion, and the absence of other potential causes of hypo-osmolality must always be verified.

Glucocorticoid deficiency and SIADH can be especially difficult to distinguish, because either primary or secondary hypocortisolism can cause elevated plasma AVP levels and, in addition, has direct renal effects to prevent maximal urinary dilution. Therefore, no patient with chronic hyponatremia should be diagnosed as having SIADH without a thorough evaluation of adrenal function, preferably via a rapid adrenocorticotropin (ACTH) stimulation test. (Acute hyponatremia of obvious origin, such as postoperatively or in association with pneumonitis, may be treated without adrenal testing as long as there are no other clinical signs or symptoms suggestive of adrenal dysfunction.) Many different disorders have been associated with SIADH, and these can be divided into several major etiologic groups (**Table 6-3**).

Some cases of euvolemic hyponatremia do not fit particularly well into either a dilutional or a depletional category. Chief among these is the hyponatremia that sometimes occurs in patients who ingest large volumes of beer with little food intake for prolonged periods, called *beer potomania*. Even though the volume of fluid ingested may not seem sufficiently excessive to overwhelm renal diluting mechanisms, in these cases free water excretion is limited by very low urinary solute excretion, resulting in water retention and dilutional hyponatremia. However, because such patients have very low sodium intakes as well, it is likely that relative depletion of body Na^+ stores also is a contributory factor to the hypo-osmolality in some cases.

Increased Extracellular Fluid Volume (Hypervolemia)

The presence of hypervolemia, as detected clinically by the presence of edema or ascites or both, indicates whole body sodium excess, and hypo-osmolality in these patients suggests a relatively decreased effective intravascular volume or pressure leading to water retention as a result of both elevated plasma AVP levels and decreased distal delivery of glomerular filtrate. Such patients usually have a low U_{Na} because of secondary hyperaldosteronism, but under certain conditions the U_{Na} may be elevated (e.g., glucosuria in diabetics, diuretic therapy). Hyponatremia generally does not occur until fairly advanced stages of diseases such as congestive heart failure, cirrhosis, and nephrotic syndrome, so the diagnosis is usually not difficult. Renal failure can also cause retention of both sodium and water, but in that case, the factor limiting excretion of excess body fluid is not decreased effective circulating volume but rather decreased glomerular filtration.

It should be remembered that, even though many edema-forming states have *secondary* increases in plasma AVP levels as a result of decreased effective arterial blood volume, nonetheless they are not classified as SIADH, because they fail to meet the criterion of clinical euvolemia (see **Table 6-2**).

TABLE 6-3 Common Causes of the Syndrome of Inappropriate Antidiuretic Hormone Secretion (SIADH)

Tumors

Pulmonary/mediastinal (bronchogenic carcinoma, mesothelioma, thymoma)

Non-chest (duodenal carcinoma, pancreatic carcinoma, ureteral/prostate carcinoma, uterine carcinoma, nasopharyngeal carcinoma, leukemia)

Central Nervous System Disorders

Mass lesions (tumors, brain abscesses, subdural hematoma)

Inflammatory diseases (encephalitis, meningitis, systemic lupus, acute intermittent porphyria, multiple sclerosis)

Degenerative/demyelinative diseases (Guillain-Barré, spinal cord lesions)

Miscellaneous (subarachnoid hemorrhage, head trauma, acute psychosis, delirium tremens, pituitary stalk section, transphenoidal adenomectomy, hydrocephalus)

Drugs

Stimulated AVP release (nicotine, phenothiazines, tricyclic antidepressants)

Direct renal effects and/or potentiation of AVP antidiuretic effects (desmopressin, oxytocin, prostaglandin synthesis inhibitors)

Mixed or uncertain actions (ACE inhibitors, carbamazepine and oxcarbazepine, chlorpropamide, clofibrate, clozapine, cyclophosphamide, 3,4- methylenedioxymethamphetamine ["Ecstasy"], omeprazole, serotonin reuptake inhibitors, vincristine)

Pulmonary Diseases

Infections (tuberculosis, acute bacterial or viral pneumonia, aspergillosis, empyema)

Mechanical/ventilatory (acute respiratory failure, COPD, positive-pressure ventilation)

Other

AIDS and AIDS-related complex

Prolonged strenuous exercise (marathon, triathalon, ultramarathon, hot-weather hiking)

Postoperative state

Senile atrophy

Idiopathic

ACE, angiotensin-converting enzyme; AIDS, acquired immunodeficiency syndrome; AVP, vasopressin; COPD, chronic obstructive pulmonary disease. Modified from Verbalis JG: The syndrome of inappropriate antidiuretic hormone secretion and other hypoosmolar disorders. In Schrier RW (ed): Diseases of the Kidney. Philadelphia, Lippincott Williams & Wilkins, 2007, pp 2214-2248.

Although it can be argued that this represents a semantic distinction, nonetheless it is important because it allows segregation of identifiable etiologies of hyponatremia that are associated with different methods of evaluation and therapy.

Several situations can cause hyponatremia because of acute water loading in excess of renal excretory capacity. Primary polydipsia can cause hypo-osmolality in a small subset of patients with some degree of underlying SIADH, particularly psychiatric patients with long-standing schizophrenia who are taking neuroleptic drugs or, even more rarely, patients with normal kidney function in whom the volumes ingested exceed the maximum renal free water excretory rate of approximately 500 to 1000 mL/hr.

Endurance exercising, such as marathon or ultramarathon racing, has been associated with sometimes fatal hyponatremia, primarily as a result of ingestion of excessive amounts of hypotonic fluids during the exercise, exceeding the water excretory capacity of the kidney. This has been called *exercise-associated hyponatremia* (EAH). Many athletes with EAH have been shown to meet diagnostic criteria for SIADH, which serves to further decrease their free water excretory capacity during exercise. Although the stimuli to AVP secretion during endurance excise have not been fully elucidated, potential candidates include baroreceptor activation, nausea, cytokine release from muscle rhabdomyolysis, and exercise itself. Most cases of EAH are associated with weight gain reflecting the excess water retention, but patients are usually classified as clinically euvolemic, because water retention alone without sodium excess, as observed in these patients, does not generally produce clinical manifestations of hypervolemia such as edema or ascites.

CLINICAL MANIFESTATIONS OF HYPONATREMIA

Hypo-osmolality is associated with a broad spectrum of neurologic manifestations, ranging from mild, nonspecific symptoms (e.g., headache, nausea) to more significant deficits (e.g., disorientation, confusion, obtundation, focal neurologic deficits, seizures). In the most severe cases, death can result from respiratory arrest after tentorial herniation with subsequent brainstem compression. This neurologic symptom complex, termed *hyponatremic encephalopathy,* primarily reflects brain edema resulting from osmotic water shifts into the brain due to the decreased effective P_{osm}. Significant symptoms generally do not occur until the serum $[Na^+]$ falls to less than 125 mEq/L, and the severity of symptoms can be roughly correlated with the degree of hypo-osmolality. However, individual variability is marked, and the level of serum $[Na^+]$ at which symptoms will appear cannot be accurately predicted for any individual patient.

Furthermore, several factors other than the severity of the hypo-osmolality also affect the degree of neurologic dysfunction. Most important is the period over which hypo-osmolality develops. Rapid development of severe hypo-osmolality is frequently associated with marked neurologic symptoms, whereas gradual development over several days or weeks is often associated with relatively mild symptomatology despite achievement of an equivalent degree of hypo-osmolality. This occurs because the brain can counteract osmotic swelling by secreting intracellular solutes, both electrolytes and organic osmolytes, via a process called *volume regulation*. Because this is a time-dependent process, rapid development of hypo-osmolality can result in brain edema before adaptation can occur; with slower development of hypo-osmolality, brain cells can lose solute sufficiently rapidly to prevent the development of brain edema and subsequent neurologic dysfunction.

Underlying neurologic disease also can significantly affect the level of hypo-osmolality at which central nervous system symptoms appear. For example, moderate hypo-osmolality is usually not of major concern in an otherwise healthy patient, but it can precipitate seizure activity in a patient with underlying epilepsy. Non-neurologic metabolic disorders (e.g., hypoxia, hypercapnia, acidosis, hypercalcemia) similarly can affect the level of P_{osm} at which central nervous system symptoms occur. Recent studies have suggested that some patients may be susceptible to a vicious cycle in which hypo-osmolality-induced brain edema causes noncardiogenic pulmonary edema, and the resulting hypoxia and hypercapnia then further impair the ability of the brain to volume-regulate, leading to more brain edema with neurologic deterioration and death in some cases. Other clinical studies have suggested that menstruating women and young children may be particularly susceptible to the development of neurologic morbidity and mortality during hyponatremia, especially in the acute postoperative setting. The true clinical incidence and underlying pathophysiologic mechanisms responsible for these sometimes catastrophic cases remains to be determined.

Finally, the issue of whether mild to moderate hyponatremia is truly "asymptomatic" has been challenged by preliminary studies showing subtle defects in cognition and gait stability in hyponatremic patients that appear to be reversed by correction of the hyponatremia. Confirmation of these findings in larger numbers of subjects would have significant import for the treatment of chronic hyponatremia.

TREATMENT

Despite some continuing controversy about the optimal speed of correction of osmolality in hyponatremic patients, there is now a relatively uniform consensus about appropriate therapy in most cases (see **Fig. 6-1**). If any degree of clinical hypovolemia is present, the patient should be considered to have a solute depletion–induced hypo-osmolality, which should be treated with isotonic (0.9%) NaCl at a rate appropriate for the estimated volume depletion. If diuretic use is known or suspected, this therapy should be supplemented with potassium (30 to 40 mEq/L) even if the serum $[K^+]$ is not low, because of the propensity of such patients to have total body potassium depletion.

Most often, the hypo-osmolar patient is clinically euvolemic, but several situations dictate a reconsideration of potential solute depletion even in the patient without clinically apparent hypovolemia. These situations include a decreased U_{Na} (<30 mEq/L), any history of recent diuretic use, and any suggestion of primary adrenal insufficiency. Whenever a reasonable likelihood of depletion, rather than dilution, hypo-osmolality exists, it is appropriate to treat initially with a trial of isotonic NaCl. If the patient has SIADH, no harm will have been done with a limited (1 to 2 L) saline infusion, because such patients will excrete excess NaCl without significantly changing their P_{osm}. However, this therapy should be abandoned if the serum $[Na^+]$ does not improve, because longer periods of continued isotonic NaCl infusion can worsen the hyponatremia by virtue of cumulative water retention.

Treatment of euvolemic hypo-osmolality varies depending on the presentation. If all criteria for SIADH are met except that the U_{osm} is low, the patient should simply be observed, because this presentation may represent spontaneous reversal of a transient form of SIADH. If there is any suspicion of either primary or secondary adrenal insufficiency, glucocorticoid replacement should be started immediately after completion of a rapid ACTH stimulation test. Prompt water diuresis after initiation of glucocorticoid treatment strongly supports glucocorticoid deficiency, but the absence of a quick response does not negate this diagnosis, because several days of glucocorticoid therapy is sometimes required for normalization of P_{osm}.

Hypervolemic hypo-osmolality is usually treated initially by diuresis and other measures directed at the underlying disorder. Such patients rarely require any therapy to increase P_{osm} acutely but often benefit from varying degrees of sodium and water restriction to reduce body fluid retention.

In any case of significant hyponatremia, one is faced with the question of how quickly the P_{osm} should be corrected. Although hyponatremia is associated with a broad spectrum of neurologic symptoms, sometimes leading to death in severe cases, too rapid correction of severe hyponatremia can produce *pontine and extrapontine myelinolysis*, a brain demyelinating disease that also can cause substantial neurologic morbidity and mortality. Clinical and experimental results suggest that optimal treatment of hyponatremia must entail balancing the risks of hyponatremia against the risks of correction for each patient. Several factors should be considered: the severity of the hyponatremia, the duration of the hyponatremia, and the patient's symptomatology. Neither sequelae from hyponatremia itself nor myelinolysis after therapy is very likely in a patient whose serum $[Na^+]$ is 120 mEq/L or greater, although significant symptoms can develop even at higher serum $[Na^+]$ levels if the rate of fall of P_{osm} has been very rapid. The importance of duration and symptomatology relate to how well the brain has volume-regulated in response to the hyponatremia, and, consequently, the degree of risk for demyelination with rapid correction. Cases of acute hyponatremia (arbitrarily defined as hyponatremia of 48 hours' duration or less) are usually symptomatic if the hyponatremia is severe (i.e., ≤125 mEq/L). These patients are at greatest risk from neurologic complications due to the hyponatremia itself and the serum [Na⁺] should be corrected to higher levels promptly. Conversely, patients with more chronic hyponatremia (>48 hours in duration) who have minimal neurologic symptoms are at little risk from complications of hyponatremia itself but can develop demyelination after rapid correction. There is no indication to correct the serum [Na⁺] in these patients rapidly, and slower-acting therapies, such as fluid restriction, should be used.

Although these extreme situations have clear treatment indications, most patients have hyponatremia of indeterminate duration and varying degrees of milder neurologic impairment. This group presents the most challenging treatment decision, because the hyponatremia has been present sufficiently long to allow some degree of brain volume regulation but not enough to prevent some brain edema and neurologic symptomatology. Most authors recommend prompt treatment for such patients because of their symptoms, but with methods that allow a *controlled and limited correction* of their hyponatremia. Reasonable correction parameters consist of a rate of correction of serum [Na⁺] in the range of 0.5 to 2 mEq/L/hr, as long as the total magnitude of correction does not exceed 12 mEq/L over the first 24 hours and 18 mEq/L over the first 48 hours of correction. Treatments for individual patients should be chosen within these limits, depending on their symptomatology. For patients who are only moderately symptomatic, one should proceed at the lower recommended limit of 0.5 mEq/L/hr; in those who manifest more severe neurologic symptoms, initial correction at a rate of 1 to 2 mEq/L/hr would be more appropriate.

Controlled corrections of hyponatremia can be accomplished with hypertonic (3%) NaCl solution given via continuous infusion, because patients with euvolemic hypoosmolality (e.g., SIADH) usually will not respond to isotonic NaCl. An initial infusion rate can be estimated by multiplying the patient's body weight, in kilograms, by the desired rate of increase in serum [Na⁺] in milliequivalents per liter per hour. For example, in a 70-kg patient, an infusion of 3% NaCl at 70 mL/hr will increase serum [Na⁺] by approximately 1 mEq/L/hr, whereas infusing 35 mL/hr will increase serum [Na⁺] by approximately 0.5 mEq/L/hr.

Furosemide (20 to 40 mg IV) should be used to treat volume overload, in some cases anticipatorily in patients with known cardiovascular disease. Alternatively, AVP receptor antagonists (often referred to as "vaptans") can be used to increase the serum [Na⁺] by stimulating renal free water excretion, or *aquaresis*, thereby leading to increased serum [Na⁺] in the majority of patients with hyponatremia due to SIADH, congestive heart failure, or cirrhosis. Although the optimal use of AVP receptor antagonists in any setting has not yet been fully determined, the agent conivaptan has been approved by the U.S. Food and Drug Administration (FDA) and has been shown to reliably raise serum [Na⁺] beginning as early as 1 to 2 hours after administration; conivaptan permits normalization of serum [Na⁺] in most hyponatremic patients over a 2- to 4-day course of treatment. Despite the attractiveness of using an aquaretic agent to correct hyponatremia, insufficient data are available from clinical trials to know whether equivalently rapid correction can be achieved in patients with acute, severe hyponatremia with aquaretics compared with hypertonic saline; consequently, such patients should initially be corrected with infusion of 3% NaCl, as described earlier. (Theoretically, both treatments could be used initially; the hypertonic saline could then be stopped after the serum [Na⁺] has been increased by a few millimoles per liter, with the remainder of the first-day correction being accomplished by the AVP receptor antagonist–induced aquaresis.) However, until this or other approaches have been shown to be effective, monotherapy with AVP receptor antagonists should be limited to symptomatic hyponatremic patients in whom the neurologic symptoms are not deemed to be of life-threatening severity.

Patients with diuretic-induced hyponatremia usually respond well to isotonic NaCl and do not require 3% NaCl. However, such patients frequently have an electrolyte-free water diuresis once their ECF volume deficit has been corrected, because correction removes the hypovolemic stimulus to AVP secretion, resulting in a more rapid correction of the serum [Na⁺] than that predicted from the rate of saline infusion. Regardless of the initial rate of correction chosen, acute treatment should be interrupted once any of three end points is reached: (1) the patient's symptoms are abolished, (2) a safe serum [Na⁺] (typically, 120 mEq/L) has been achieved, or (3) a total magnitude of correction of 18 mEq/L has been achieved. It follows from these recommendations that serum [Na⁺] levels must be carefully monitored at frequent intervals (at least every 4 hours) during the active phases of treatment, in order to adjust therapy so that the correction stays within these guidelines. Regardless of the therapy or rate initially chosen, it cannot be emphasized too strongly that it is necessary to correct the P_{osm} acutely only to a safe range, rather than completely to normal levels. In some situations, patients may spontaneously correct their hyponatremia via a water diuresis. If the hyponatremia is acute (e.g., psychogenic polydipsia with water intoxication), such patients do not appear to be at risk for subsequent demyelination; however, if the hyponatremia has been chronic (e.g., hypocortisolism, diuretic therapy), intervention should be considered to limit the rate and magnitude of correction of serum [Na⁺], such as administration of desmopressin 1 to 2 μg IV or infusion of hypotonic fluids to match urine output, using the same end points as for active corrections.

Treatment of chronic hyponatremia entails choosing among several suboptimal therapies. One important exception is those patients with the reset osmostat syndrome; because the hyponatremia of such patients is not progressive but rather fluctuates around their reset level of serum [Na⁺], no therapy is generally required. For most other cases of mild to moderate SIADH, fluid restriction represents the least toxic therapy and is the treatment of choice. It should always be tried as the initial therapy, with pharmacologic intervention reserved for refractory cases in which the degree of fluid restriction required to avoid hypo-osmolality is so severe that the patient is unable, or unwilling, to maintain it. In general, the higher the U_{osm}, indicating higher plasma AVP levels, the less likely it is that fluid restriction will be successful. If pharmacologic treatment is necessary, the preferred drug at present is the tetracycline derivative demeclocycline, which causes nephrogenic diabetes insipidus, thereby decreasing the urine concentration. The effective dose of demeclocycline ranges from 600 to 1200 mg/day; several days of therapy are necessary to achieve maximum effects, so one should wait 3 to 4 days before increasing the dose. Demeclocycline can cause reversible nephrotoxicity, especially in patients with cirrhosis; renal function should be monitored, and the medication should be stopped if increasing azotemia occurs. Several other drugs can decrease AVP hypersecretion in selected cases, including diphenylhydantoin, opiates, and ethanol, but responses are unpredictable.

There is currently no ideal therapeutic agent for chronic dilutional hyponatremias, but this situation is likely to change in the near future, with the development of oral AVP receptor antagonists for chronic outpatient use. Several nonpeptide molecules that selectively antagonize the AVP V_2 receptor are currently in late stages of clinical trials and have proved to be effective at correcting hyponatremia by maintaining increased free water excretion in patients with SIADH, congestive heart failure, or cirrhosis over prolonged periods (30 days). Once approved by the FDA for clinical use, such drugs will probably become the treatment of choice for chronic dilutional hyponatremia, although their efficacy in some cases may be limited by associated increases in AVP concentration and the increased thirst that counteract the induced free water diuresis in cases of a reset osmostat. Despite many unanswered questions about their optimal use, the new class of aquaretic AVP receptor antagonists promise to initiate a new era in the treatment of hyponatremia.

BIBLIOGRAPHY

Anderson RJ, Chung H-M, Kluge R, et al: Hyponatremia: A prospective analysis of its epidemiology and the pathogenetic role of vasopressin. Ann Intern Med 102:164-168, 1985.

Ayus JC, Arieff AI: Pulmonary complications of hyponatremic encephalopathy: Noncardiogenic pulmonary edema and hypercapnic respiratory failure. Chest 107:517-521, 1995.

Ayus JC, Arieff AI: Chronic hyponatremic encephalopathy in postmenopausal women: Association of therapies with morbidity and mortality. J Am Med Assoc 281:2299-2304, 1999.

Bartter FC, Schwartz WB: The syndrome of inappropriate secretion of antidiuretic hormone. Am J Med 42:790-806, 1967.

Greenberg A, Verbalis JG: Vasopressin receptor antagonists. Kidney Int 69:2124-2130, 2006.

Hawkins RC: Age and gender as risk factors for hyponatremia and hypernatremia. Clin Chim Acta 337:169-172, 2003.

Renneboog B, Musch W, Vandemergel X, et al: Mild chronic hyponatremia is associated with falls, unsteadiness, and attention deficits. Am J Med 119:71-78, 2006.

Rosner MH, Kirven J: Exercise-associated hyponatremia. Clin J Am Soc Nephrol 2:151-161, 2007.

Schrier RW: Pathogenesis of sodium and water retention in high-output and low-output cardiac failure, nephrotic syndrome, cirrhosis and pregnancy. N Engl J Med 319:1065-1072. 1127–1134, 1988.

Sterns RH: Severe symptomatic hyponatremia: Treatment and outcome. A study of 64 cases. Ann Intern Med 107:656-664, 1987.

Sterns RH, Cappuccio JD, Silver SM, Cohen EP: Neurologic sequelae after treatment of severe hyponatremia: A multicenter perspective. J Am Soc Nephrol 4:1522-1530, 1994.

Verbalis JG: Vasopressin V2 receptor antagonists. J Mol Endocrinol 29:1-9, 2002.

Verbalis JG: How does the brain sense osmolality? J Am Soc Nephrol 18:3056-3059, 2007.

Verbalis JG: The syndrome of inappropriate antidiuretic hormone secretion and other hypoosmolar disorders. In Schrier RW (ed): Diseases of the Kidney. Philadelphia, Lippincott Williams & Wilkins, 2007, pp 2214-2248.

Verbalis JG, Goldsmith SR, Greenberg A, et al: Hyponatremia treatment guidelines 2007: Expert panel recommendations. Am J Med 120:S1-S21, 2007.

Zerbe R, Stropes L, Robertson G: Vasopressin function in the syndrome of inappropriate antidiuresis. Annu Rev Med 31:315-327, 1980.

CHAPTER 7

Hypernatremia

Paula Dennen and Stuart Linas

Dysnatremias, or abnormalities of serum sodium concentration, include both hyponatremia and hypernatremia. These electrolyte abnormalities occur in a wide spectrum of patient populations, ranging from infants to the elderly and from outpatients to the critically ill. Their occurrence is common, and diagnosis and appropriate management of these disorders can decrease the associated morbidity and mortality. This chapter focuses on hypernatremia.

It is important to recognize that a patient's fluid and electrolyte balance is dynamic, and therefore management must include frequent assessment of the individual's response to therapy. Close monitoring can facilitate early recognition of unanticipated clinical changes and avoid potential complications of treatment.

DEFINITIONS

Normal serum sodium concentration ($[Na^+]$) is 135 to 145 mEq/L. This range is generally maintained despite large individual variations in salt and water intake. Hypernatremia is defined as a $[Na^+]$ greater than 145 mEq/L and reflects cellular dehydration. It is *always* a water problem and *sometimes* a salt problem as well. There is no predictable relationship between serum $[Na^+]$ (a measure of osmolality and tonicity) and total body salt or volume status. To be more specific, whereas hypernatremia confirms the presence of a relative water deficit, the isolated laboratory finding of a serum $[Na^+]$ greater than 145 mEq/L does not reveal anything about a person's volume status. Hypernatremia can occur in the context of hypovolemia, euvolemia, or hypervolemia.

Dehydration and Volume Depletion

Although the term "dehydration" is commonly used to describe a person's volume status, this use is incorrect. Dehydration does not equal volume depletion. In fact, *dehydration* is a description of water balance, whereas *volume depletion* refers to a person's sodium balance. These two clinical scenarios may coexist but should not be confused and, importantly, the two terms should not be used interchangeably. In hypernatremia, cells become dehydrated and shrink because of water movement from the intracellular to the extracellular space.

Hyperosmolality and Hypertonicity

Hypernatremia always reflects a hyperosmolar state, whereas the reverse is not always true. For example, hyperosmolality may also be a consequence of severe hyperglycemia or elevated blood urea nitrogen (BUN), as is seen in acute or chronic kidney failure. Furthermore, hyperosmolality does not necessarily mean hypertonicity. For example, uremia is a hyperosmolar but not a hypertonic state. Urea can freely cross cell membranes, unlike sodium, and therefore contributes to osmolality but not tonicity. In contrast to urea, sodium, which is unable to freely cross cell membranes, is an effective osmole and is the primary electrolyte that affects plasma osmolality. In hypernatremia, a hypertonic state, sodium is an effective osmole causing water to flow from the intracellular to the extracellular space.

BACKGROUND

It's all about water. A more accurate term for hypernatremia might be "hypoaquaremia," because it quite literally means a state in which there is too little water in the intravascular space and, as a consequence, in the intracellular space. To begin any discussion of hypernatremia (or hyponatremia), it is important to understand that dysnatremias are actually disorders of water homeostasis.

Water distributes throughout all body compartments, two thirds in the intracellular and one third in the extracellular compartment. Three quarters of the water in the extracellular compartment is located in the interstitial space, and one quarter is in the intravascular space. Water is lost (or gained) in the same proportions as it is distributed throughout all body compartments. Pure water loss does not affect plasma volume status or hemodynamics significantly until very late, because of the normal distribution of water throughout all body compartments. For example, for every 1 L of water deficit, only approximately 80 mL is lost from the intravascular (plasma) compartment.

EPIDEMIOLOGY

The incidence of hypernatremia ranges from less than 1% to more than 3% of all hospitalized patients. Hypernatremia among nonhospitalized adults is primarily a disease of the

60

elderly and of those with mental illness or impaired sensorium. Most patients with hypernatremia on admission to the hospital have concomitant infections. Hypernatremia that is present on hospital admission is treated earlier than hypernatremia that develops during the hospital course, most likely because of increased attention paid to volume status on hospital admission.

So-called hospital-acquired hypernatremia is seen in patients who are, on average, younger than those with hypernatremia on admission and have an age distribution similar to that of the general hospitalized population. Hospital-acquired hypernatremia is largely iatrogenic, resulting from inadequate and/or inappropriate fluid prescription. It results from a combination of decreased access to water and disease processes that may increase insensible losses or interfere with the thirst mechanism. About half of patients with hospital-acquired hypernatremia are intubated and therefore have no free access to water. Of the remaining 50%, most have altered mental status.

Patients at highest risk for hospital-acquired hypernatremia are those at the extremes of age (infants and the elderly), those with altered mental status, and those without access to water (i.e., intubated or debilitated patients). Furthermore, in addition to the impaired thirst and decreased urinary concentrating ability that accompany advanced age, elderly patients have a lower baseline total body water content, making smaller changes more clinically relevant. Hypernatremia in nursing home residents has been identified as a marker of poor care.

CLINICAL MANIFESTATIONS

Signs

Signs of hypernatremia depend, in part, on the cause and severity of the hypernatremia. Abnormal subclavicular and forearm skin turgor and altered sensorium are commonly found in patients with hypovolemic or euvolemic hypernatremia, whereas patients with hypervolemic hypernatremia typically have classic signs of volume overload, such as elevated neck veins and edema.

Symptoms

Clinical symptoms related to hypernatremia can be attributed to cellular dehydration (cell shrinkage) due to the loss of intracellular water. Loss of intracellular water occurs throughout the body, but the primary symptoms are neurologic. The severity of neurologic symptoms is more dependent on the rate of rise in serum $[Na^+]$ than on the absolute value. Polyuria and polydipsia are frequently the presenting symptoms of diabetes insipidus (DI) with or without the presence of hypernatremia.

Neurologic symptoms comprise a continuum that begins with fatigue, lethargy, irritability, and confusion and progresses to seizures and coma. Additional symptoms of hypernatremia include anorexia, nausea, vomiting, and generalized muscle weakness. Altered mental status can be both a cause and an effect of hypernatremia and consequently can be difficult to distinguish clinically. Additionally, cellular dehydration (cell shrinkage) can lead to rupture of cerebral veins due to traction, which results in focal intracerebral and subarachnoid hemorrhages; this occurs more often in infants than in adults.

PATHOPHYSIOLOGY

A sound understanding of the normal physiology of salt and water balance is integral to the understanding and management of dysnatremias. The intracellular and extracellular body compartments exist in osmotic equilibrium. The development of hypernatremia is most commonly the result of increased water losses in the setting of inadequate intake, but it may also occur as a consequence of excessive sodium intake.

Regulation of plasma $[Na^+]$ is dependent on changes in water balance. Sodium is the primary determinant of plasma osmolality. Normal plasma osmolality (P_{osm}) is between 280 and 285 mOsm/kg. If the P_{osm} varies by 1% to 2% in either direction, normal physiologic mechanisms are in place to return the P_{osm} to normal. In the case of hypernatremia or hyperosmolality, receptor cells in the hypothalamus detect increases in P_{osm}; in response, they stimulate thirst, to increase water intake, and simultaneously stimulate the release of antidiuretic hormone (ADH), to limit renal water losses (by increasing water reabsorption in the collecting duct). Under normal conditions, the body is able to maintain the serum osmolality under tight control. The goal of "normonatremia" is to avoid changes in cellular volume and thereby prevent potential disruptions in cellular structure and function. The body's normal physiologic defense against hypernatremia is twofold: renal conservation of water and an endogenous thirst stimulus.

As with other electrolyte disturbances, the pathophysiology of hypernatremia can be easily categorized into two phases, an initiation phase and a maintenance phase. Simply stated, the initiation or generation phase must be caused by a net water loss or, less commonly, a net sodium gain. For hypernatremia to exist as anything more than a transient state, there must be a maintenance phase, defined necessarily by inadequate water intake.

Water metabolism is controlled primarily by arginine vasopressin (AVP) or ADH, as it is commonly termed. ADH is produced in the hypothalamus (supraoptic and paraventricular nuclei) and is stored in and secreted by the posterior pituitary. ADH release can be stimulated by either increases in plasma osmolality or decreases in mean arterial pressure or blood volume. In the setting of hypernatremia, the primary stimulus for the release of ADH comes from osmoreceptors located in the hypothalamus. ADH acts on the vasopressin (V_2) receptors in the collecting duct to cause increased water reabsorption from the tubular lumen via insertion of aquaporin 2 channels.

The kidney's primary role in hypernatremia is to maximally concentrate the urine, to prevent further loss of electrolyte-free fluid. For the kidney to do so, the following must occur: (1) development of a concentrated medullary interstitium, (2) presence of ADH to stimulate insertion of aquaporin 2 channels into the apical membranes of the collecting duct, and (3) ability of the collecting duct cells to respond to ADH.

In a steady state, water intake must equal water output. Obligatory renal water loss is directly dependent on solute excretion and urinary concentrating ability. If a person has to excrete, for example, 700 mOsm of solute per day (primarily Na^+, K^+, and urea) and the maximum urinary osmolality (U_{osm}) is 100 mOsm/kg, then the minimum urine output requirement will be 7 L. However, if the kidney is able to concentrate the urine to a U_{osm} of 700 mOsm/kg, urine output would need to be only 1 L.

Thirst, on the other hand, is an ADH-independent mechanism of defense against hypertonicity. Like ADH release, thirst is stimulated by osmoreceptors located in the hypothalamus. The intense thirst stimulated by hypernatremia may be impaired or absent in patients with altered mental status or hypothalamic lesions and in the elderly. It is important to note that patients with moderate to severe increase in electrolyte-free water losses may maintain eunatremia due to the powerful thirst mechanism. For example, a patient with partial nephrogenic DI due to a history of lithium use may have a normal serum $[Na^+]$ if given free access to water but may become quite symptomatic (with marked hypernatremia) if circumstances prevent this free access (e.g., acute hospitalization for altered mental status).

Although ADH activity is a pivotal physiologic defense against hyperosmolality, only an increase in water intake can replace a water deficit. An increase in ADH activity in collecting tubules can only help to prevent or decrease ongoing water losses. Therefore, it is the combination of both ADH-dependent and ADH-independent mechanisms that is integral to the body's efforts to protect against hypernatremia or hyperosmolality.

The brain has multiple defense mechanisms designed to protect it from the adverse effects of cellular dehydration. As the serum $[Na^+]$ rises, water moves from the intracellular to the extracellular space in order to return the serum osmolality to the normal range. Almost immediately, there is an increase in the net leak of serum electrolytes (primarily Na^+ and K^+) into the intracellular space, which increases intracellular osmolality. Additionally, there is an increased production of cerebrospinal fluid, with movement into the interstitial areas of the brain. Within the subsequent approximately 24 hours, the brain cells produce organic solutes (e.g., amino acids, trimethylamines, myoinositol), referred to as *osmolytes* or *idiogenic osmoles,* in an effort to draw water back into the cells. The increase in intracellular osmolality restores intracellular volume, thereby decreasing the adverse clinical impact of hypernatremia (i.e., cellular dehydration). The increase in transcellular transport of electrolytes is somewhat transient, because, over time, it interferes with normal cellular function. Cellular adaptation by the production of idiogenic osmoles requires days to reach full effect. Idiogenic

osmoles clearly serve a protective role, but removal of them is also slow (days) when isotonicity has been re-established. The clinical implication of the slow removal of these idiogenic osmoles is that correction of hypernatremia (hypertonicity) must be slow, to avoid cellular swelling or cerebral edema.

DIAGNOSTIC APPROACH AND PATHOGENESIS

Hypernatremia most commonly results from the combination of increased water loss and decreased water intake. However, it may also be a consequence of an increased sodium load. Any clinical condition associated with increased water loss or decreased water intake predisposes to hypernatremia. Generally speaking, for hypernatremia to occur, the rate of water excretion must exceed that of water intake. An exception to this basic principle, occurring less commonly, is hypernatremia secondary to sodium loading. Insensible losses include any water loss from the skin or respiratory tract. Examples of conditions that lead to increases in insensible losses include fever, burns, open wounds, and hyperventilation.

Hypernatremia is due to an imbalance of water homeostasis. Despite the fact that hypernatremia *always* represents inadequate total body water, there may also be a concomitant salt disturbance. After taking a thorough clinical history and doing a complete physical examination, the first decision point in the evaluation of any patient with hypernatremia is to determine the patient's volume status (**Fig. 7-1**). Hypernatremia can be seen in patients who are hypovolemic, euvolemic, or hypervolemic.

Hypovolemic Hypernatremia

Hypovolemic hypernatremia describes the individual who is both salt and water depleted because of the loss of hypotonic fluids (**Table 7-1**). These individuals have sustained losses of both sodium and water but with a relatively greater loss of water. They usually manifest typical signs of volume depletion, such as tachycardia and orthostatic hypotension. The most common example of hypovolemic hypernatremia in hospitalized patients is hyperglycemia with an osmotic diuresis. Determination of the urine sodium concentration (U_{Na}) can help distinguish between renal losses, such as from diuretics or osmotic diuresis (U_{Na} >20 mEq/dL), and extrarenal losses, such as from diarrhea or vomiting (U_{Na} <20 mEq/dL).

Euvolemic Hypernatremia

Euvolemic hypernatremia refers to those conditions associated with a loss of electrolyte-free fluid, or pure water loss (see **Table 7-1**). These patients have a normal total body sodium (and are therefore euvolemic), but they are depleted in total body water. As in the evaluation of hypovolemic hypernatremia, euvolemic hypernatremia can be further categorized into renal and extrarenal causes. In this case, urine osmolality (U_{osm}) is often more helpful than U_{Na}. U_{osm} is a measure

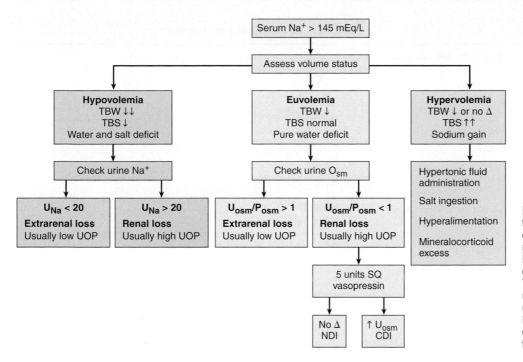

FIGURE 7-1 Diagnostic approach to hypernatremia. Δ, change; CDI, central diabetes insipidus; NDI, nephrogenic diabetes insipidus; P_{osm}, plasma osmolality; SQ, subcutaneous; TBS, total body salt; TBW, total body water; U_{Na}, random urine sodium concentration; UOP, urine output; U_{osm}, urine osmolality. Refer to Table 7-1 for further details on the specific causes of hypernatremia in each category.

of ADH levels and function. A low U_{osm} is consistent with renal losses and therefore with low ADH levels or function (DI), whereas a high U_{osm} suggests extrarenal losses of free water and intact secretion of and response to ADH.

Etiologies of DI may be central (**Table 7-2**), nephrogenic, or gestational. The key diagnostic step in determining a central versus a nephrogenic cause is based on the response to exogenous hormone replacement (i.e., vasopressin). A finding of no change in U_{osm} after administration of exogenous vasopressin is diagnostic of nephrogenic DI. However, it is important to remember that central or nephrogenic DI may be partial: either ADH is present but in insufficient quantity (partial central DI) or there is an incomplete response to ADH in the collecting duct (partial nephrogenic DI).

Gestational or pregnancy-related DI should be evident from the clinical history, but the manifestations are similar to those of nephrogenic DI, in that there is no change in U_{osm} with exogenous vasopressin, due to the presence of placental vasopressinase. However gestational DI responds to desmopressin acetate (dDAVP), a synthetic analogue of ADH, because dDAVP is unaffected by vasopressinase.

Nephrogenic DI can be either hereditary (genetic defect of the V_2 receptor gene or aquaporin water channel) or acquired. Acquired nephrogenic DI may be reversible and includes any clinical condition in which the kidney is unable to maximally concentrate the urine. The most common cause of acquired nephrogenic DI is chronic lithium use. The mechanism of lithium-induced nephrogenic DI includes both a decrease in density of V_2 receptors and decreased expression of aquaporin 2 channels. Hypercalcemia, hypokalemia, and severe malnutrition are other common examples of reversible nephrogenic DI. Hypercalcemia can induce a reversible nephrogenic DI through inhibition of the reabsorption of sodium in the loop of Henle, which impairs the generation of an adequate gradient and reduces concentrating ability.

Additionally, dysregulation of the aquaporin 2 channel can be seen with hypercalcemia. Hypokalemia causes nephrogenic DI by decreasing collecting tubule responsiveness to ADH. Decreased protein intake leads to decreased urea production and, therefore, a decreased medullary gradient with inability to maximally concentrate the urine.

A high U_{osm} suggests extrarenal losses as the cause of euvolemic hypernatremia. In order to generate a high U_{osm}, the kidney must be able to concentrate the urine, an ability that requires intact ADH-dependent mechanisms. Insensible losses are the primary source of electrolyte-free water loss in this subgroup of patients. Increased insensible losses occur via the skin (burns, sweat) or respiratory tract (tachypnea) or both.

Finally, patients with hypodipsia or adipsia may develop euvolemic hyponatremia. Most often, they have normally functioning kidneys but lack adequate water intake. These patients typically have a high U_{osm} and low urine output. Idiopathic hypodipsia occurs, but identification of an impaired thirst mechanism as the primary disorder causing hypernatremia should lead to a more thorough neurologic investigation to rule out the presence of hypothalamic tumors or disorders. An impaired thirst mechanism or limited access to water in the setting of DI can result in severe hypernatremia and can be life-threatening.

Hypervolemic Hypernatremia

Hypervolemic hypernatremia is caused by sodium gain and is the least common type of hypernatremia (see **Table 7-1**). Total body sodium is uniformly increased, but total body water may be increased or unchanged, depending on the cause. An increase in extracellular volume should be readily identifiable on clinical examination. This clinical presentation is usually iatrogenic, resulting from hypertonic fluid

TABLE 7-1 Causes of Hypernatremia

Hypovolemic Hypernatremia (TBW ⇊, TBS ↓, water and salt deficit)

Renal Loss (urine [Na+] >20 mEq/dL)

Loop diuretics
Post-AKI diuresis
Post-obstructive diuresis
Osmotic diuresis (hyperglycemia, mannitol, urea)

Extrarenal Loss (urine [Na+] <20 mEq/dL)

Gastrointestinal (vomiting, diarrhea, nasogastric suctioning,
    enterocutaneous fistula)
Skin (sweating, burns)

Euvolemic Hypernatremia (TBW ↓, TBS normal, pure water deficit)

Renal Loss (Uosm/Posm <1)

Diabetes Insipidus (ADH-dependent mechanism)
    Central diabetes insipidus
        Lack of ADH release, complete or partial (see Table 7-2 for
        causes)
    Nephrogenic diabetes insipidus (hereditary)
        X-linked recessive (defect in vasopressin V_2 receptor or
        aquaporin channel)
        Unresponsive to ADH, complete or partial
    Gestational diabetes insipidus
        Peripheral degradation of ADH
        Vasopressinase-mediated
Acquired Nephrogenic Diabetes Insipidus (urinary concentrating
defect, ADH-independent)
    Electrolyte disturbances (hypercalcemia, hypokalemia)
    Drug-induced (lithium, demeclocycline, amphotericin B, foscarnet,
    methoxyflurane, V_2 receptor antagonists)
    Chronic kidney disease (e.g., medullary cystic disease, sickle cell
    disease, amyloidosis, Sjögren's syndrome)
    Malnutrition (decreased medullary gradient)

Extrarenal Loss (U_{osm}/P_{osm} >1)

Increased Insensible Loss
    Cutaneous (fever, sweating, increased ambient temperature,
    burns)
    Respiratory (tachypnea)
Decreased Intake
    Primary hypodipsia (hypothalamic or osmoreceptor dysfunction,
    advanced age)
    Reset osmostat
    Decreased access to water (altered mental status, iatrogenic)
Shift
    Water Loss into Cells (seizures, severe exercise)

Hypervolemic Hypernatremia TBW ↓ or no △, TBS ↑↑

Increased Sodium Intake

Excessive Na+ administration (saline or bicarbonate)
Hyperalimentation (total parenteral nutrition)
Salt ingestion
Inadvertent substitution of salt for sugar in infant formula
Mineralocorticoid excess
Hypertonic dialysis

ADH, antidiuretic hormone; AKI, acute kidney injury; P_{osm}, plasma osmolality;
TBS, total body sodium; TBW, total body water; U_{osm}, urine osmolality.

TABLE 7-2 Central Diabetes Insipidus

Congenital (autosomal dominant or recessive)
Trauma
Neurosurgery
Primary or secondary CNS tumors
Infiltrative disorders (e.g., sarcoidosis, tuberculosis)
Hypoxic encephalopathy (post–cardiac arrest, Sheehan's syndrome)
Bleeding
Infection (meningitis, encephalitis)
Aneurysm
Idiopathic

CNS, central nervous system.

An example of *relative* hypervolemic hypernatremia is the hemodynamically stable hypernatremic patient with acute respiratory distress syndrome (ARDS) and an elevated central venous pressure (greater than a target of <4 mm Hg). This *relative* hypervolemic hypernatremic state is both a water and a salt problem. Commonly, the physician might be concerned that administration of the free water necessary to correct the serum [Na+] (e.g., 3 L) would cause the patient to become fluid overloaded. This would be in direct contrast to the goal of a net negative fluid balance for optimal management of ARDS. However, because of the normal distribution of water, less than 10% of the amount given as 5% dextrose in water (D5W) or through a feeding tube (i.e., <300 mL for administration of 3 L) would remain in the vascular space; therefore, the fluid administration would not materially affect the patient's volume status. Additionally, it is imperative to understand that further diuresis to obtain a net negative sodium balance will exacerbate the hypernatremia, increasing free water urinary losses, and therefore must be considered in calculating the free water deficit.

TREATMENT

Treatment goals of hypernatremia include both replacement of the free water deficit and prevention or reduction of ongoing water loss. The amount, route, and rate of replacement depend on the severity of symptoms, rate of onset, concurrent clinical conditions, and volume status. Volume resuscitation is always a priority, no matter how severe the hypernatremia. Depletion of extracellular fluid in the setting of hemodynamic instability should always be corrected with normal saline before the water deficit is addressed. It is important to focus on the treatment of hypernatremia, because frequently the complications of hypernatremia result not from the electrolyte disturbance itself but from inappropriate correction or treatment. Management of hypernatremia should include identification of the underlying cause in addition to correction of the hypertonic state. Treatment of hypernatremia can, most often, be broken down into the following seven steps (**Table 7-3**).

administration (saline or bicarbonate), and reflects a gain of sodium without an appropriate gain of water. Excess mineralocorticoid activity can also cause hypervolemic hypernatremia and, in the absence of typical iatrogenic risk factors, should alert the clinician to evaluate for potential causes of mineralocorticoid excess.

TABLE 7-3 Approach to the Treatment of Hypernatremia

Step 1. Determine volume status.

Step 2. Calculate free water deficit.

Step 3. Choose a replacement fluid.

Step 4. Determine rate of repletion.

Step 5. Estimate ongoing "sensible" losses.

Step 6. Estimate ongoing "insensible" losses.

Step 7. Determine underlying cause, if possible.

Step 1. Determine volume status. Evaluation of the patient's volume status is a critical first step for both appropriate diagnosis and treatment of hypernatremia. This information should be obtained through a thorough history and physical examination.

Step 2. Calculate free water deficit. Before initiating therapy, it is both prudent and appropriate to quantify the deficit and develop a treatment plan for the individual patient. Calculation of the water deficit represents only a snapshot in time. If it were possible to prevent any further water losses, insensible or otherwise, the calculated water deficit would be the amount that must be administered to normalize the serum [Na$^+$], as shown in *Formula 1:*

$$\text{Water deficit} = \text{TBW} \times \left(\text{Plasma}\left[\text{Na}^+\right]/140 - 1\right)$$

$$= \left(0.5 \text{ or } 0.4\right) \times \text{lean body weight} \times \left(\text{Plasma}\left[\text{Na}^+\right]/140 - 1\right)$$

where the lean body weight is expressed in kilograms. Note that, although TBW is normally considered to be 60% of lean body weight in men or 50% in women, in the setting of hypernatremia, a water-depleted state, it is reasonable to use 50% and 40%, respectively (because the TBW is estimated to be decreased by approximately 10%). The final term in the equation, (Plasma [Na$^+$]/140 − 1), may be replaced by the target serum [Na$^+$]. For example, if the current [Na+] is 160 mEq/L and the goal is to reduce this concentration by 10 mEq/L in 24 hours, then 150 mEq/L may be substituted. This method may be used to calculate the water deficit for any target serum [Na$^+$].

Step 3. Choose a replacement fluid. The choice of fluid for repletion of a free water deficit depends on the clinical assessment of volume status. Specifically, a key decision is whether the deficit is the result of a pure water loss, requiring only water repletion, or a hypotonic fluid loss, which requires both water and salt repletion. Generally, patients with a pure water loss should be repleted with the use of enteral free water (oral or nasogastric tube) or by intravenous administration of D5W. Hypovolemic hypernatremic patients should be repleted with a combination of salt and water. This correction may be accomplished by the administration of 0.2% or 0.45% saline or with the use of separate intravenous solutions, one for water repletion and one for repletion of the salt deficit. The potential advantage of using two separate infusions is the avoidance of continued salt repletion after the volume deficit has been corrected. One important caveat in the selection of an appropriate solution is the priority of

volume repletion in hemodynamic instability when isotonic saline is the most appropriate choice.

The *route of repletion* must also be determined. As with nutritional repletion, the enteral route for repletion of free water is preferable; however, it is not always an option, because patients commonly have altered mental status. Water can be repleted through a nasogastric tube if gut function is not compromised. One reason that the enteral route is preferable for repletion of free water is to avoid administration of the dextrose that is required to provide water through the intravenous route. Dextrose has the potential to increase serum osmolality via hyperglycemia, and this can contribute to additional renal clearance of electrolyte-free water due to an osmotic diuresis. Most commonly, correction of the free water deficit will be done, at least initially, via the intravenous route.

Step 4. Determine rate of repletion. The rate of correction of serum [Na$^+$] is recommended to be approximately 0.5 mEq/L/hr, or a decrease of 10 to 12 mEq/L in a 24-hour period. There have not been any human studies performed to substantiate the appropriateness of this rate. However, based on animal studies, this reflects the observed rate of cerebral de-adaptation, or the rate at which the brain is able to shed electrolytes and idiogenic osmoles acquired in the adaptive response to cellular dehydration. An important exception to this recommended rate of correction occurs in acutely symptomatic

patients who have seizures or acute obtundation potentially requiring intubation for airway protection. In these circumstances, the rate of correction can be 1 to 2 mEq/L/hr initially, with the overall rate still not to exceed the recommended 10 to 12 mEq/L in 24 hours. Furthermore, acute symptoms suggest that the hypernatremia developed rapidly and, consequently, the brain has not had time to adapt. If adaption to hypernatremia has not yet occurred, the risk that cerebral edema will complicate rapid correction is minimal. If the duration of hypernatremia is unknown, the clinician should err on the side of caution and avoid rapid correction. However, if the onset is known to be acute (i.e., developing within the last 12 hours), the serum [Na$^+$] can be corrected more quickly, because brain adaptation does not occur this rapidly.

The calculation of water deficit shown in step 2 (*Formula 1*) is particularly useful for hypernatremia caused by pure water losses. However, practically speaking, and in multiple observational studies, hypovolemia is present in more than 50% of cases of hyponatremia. For this reason, it is frequently necessary to replace both water and sodium deficits, and the use of 0.2% or 0.45% saline may be appropriate. (**Table 7-4** lists the sodium concentrations of commonly used intravenous fluids.) *Formula 2* can be clinically useful for *predicting the change in serum [Na$^+$]* that will occur with infusion of a particular fluid, and, accordingly, choosing an appropriate rate of infusion.

$$\Delta\left[\text{Na}^+\right]_s = \frac{\left[\text{Na}^+\right]_{inf} - \left[\text{Na}^+\right]_s}{\text{TBW} + 1}$$

Palevsky PM: Hypernatremia. Semin Nephrol 18:20, 1998.

Rose BD, Post TW: Clinical Physiology of Acid-Base and Electrolyte Disorders, 5th ed. New York, McGraw-Hill, 2001, pp 775-784.

Shoker AS: Application of the clearance concept to hyponatremic and hypernatremic disorders: A phenomenological analysis. Clin Chem 40:1220, 1994.

CHAPTER 8

Metabolic Acidosis

Harold M. Szerlip

Metabolic acidosis describes a process in which nonvolatile acids accumulate in the body. For practical purposes, this can result from either the addition of protons or the loss of base. The consequence of this process is a decline in the major extracellular buffer, bicarbonate, and, if unopposed, a decrease in extracellular pH. Depending on the existence and the magnitude of other acid-base disturbances, however, the extracellular pH may be low, normal, or even high. Normal blood pH is between 7.38 and 7.42, corresponding to a hydrogen ion concentration of 42 to 38 nmol/L.

Metabolic acidosis results in a compensatory increase in minute ventilation; respiratory compensation begins promptly. A decrease in pH sensitizes the peripheral chemoreceptors, triggering an increase in minute ventilation. Because increased ventilation is a compensatory mechanism stimulated by the acidemia, it never returns the pH to normal. The expected partial pressure of carbon dioxide (P_{CO_2}) for any given degree of metabolic acidosis can be predicted from the bicarbonate ion concentration using Winters' formula:

$$P_{CO_2} = \left(1.5 \times \left[HCO_3^-\right]\right) + 8 \pm 2.$$

OVERVIEW OF ACID-BASE BALANCE

In order to maintain extracellular pH within the normal range, the daily production of acid must be excreted from the body (**Fig. 8-1**). Most of this acid production results from the metabolism of dietary carbohydrates and fats. Complete oxidation of these metabolic substrates produces carbon dioxide and water. The 15,000 mmol of CO_2 produced daily are efficiently exhaled by the lungs and are therefore known as *volatile acid*. As long as ventilatory function remains normal, this volatile acid does not contribute to changes in acid-base balance. *Nonvolatile* or *fixed acids* are produced by the metabolism of sulfate- and phosphate-containing amino acids. In addition, incomplete oxidation of fats and carbohydrates results in the production of small quantities of lactate and other organic anions, which, when excreted in the urine, represent loss of base. Individuals consuming a typical meat-based diet produce approximately 1 mmol/kg/day of hydrogen ions. Fecal excretion of a small amount of base also contributes to total daily acid production.

The kidney is responsible not only for excretion of the daily production of fixed acid but also for reclamation of the filtered bicarbonate. Bicarbonate reclamation occurs

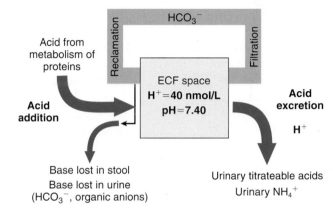

FIGURE 8-1 Maintenance of acid-base homeostasis requires that the addition of acid to the body be balanced by excretion of acid. Production of fixed nonvolatile acid occurs mainly through the metabolism of proteins. A small quantity of base also is lost in the stool and urine. Acid excretion occurs in the kidney through the secretion of H+ buffered by titratable acids and NH_3. Bicarbonate filtration and reclamation by the kidney is normally a neutral process. ECF, extracellular fluid.

predominantly in the proximal tubule, mainly through the Na^+/H^+ exchanger. Active transporters in the distal tubule secrete hydrogen ion against a concentration gradient. Although urinary pH can fall to as low as 4.5, this, by itself, would account for little acid excretion. For instance, to excrete 100 mmol of H^+ into unbuffered urine at a minimum urine pH of 4.5 would require a daily urine volume of 5000 L. Fortunately, urinary phosphate and creatinine help buffer these protons, allowing the kidney to excrete approximately 40% of the daily fixed acid load as titratable acids, so called because they are quantitated by titrating the urine pH back to that of plasma, 7.4. In addition, renal excretion of acid is supported by ammoniagenesis. NH_3 is generated in the proximal tubule by the deamidation of glutamine to glutamate, which is subsequently deaminated to yield NH_3 and α-ketoglutarate. The enzymes responsible for these reactions are up-regulated by acidosis and hypokalemia. Hyperkalemia reduces ammoniagenesis; NH_3 builds up in the renal interstitium and passively diffuses into the tubule lumen along the length of the collecting duct, where it is trapped by H^+.

Under conditions of increased acid production, the normal kidney can increase acid excretion, primarily by augmenting NH_3 production. Renal acid excretion varies directly with the rate of acid production. Net renal acid excretion is equal

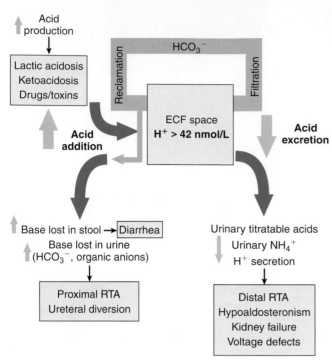

FIGURE 8-2 Metabolic acidosis can result from increased acid production, increased loss of base in stool or urine, or decreased H⁺ secretion in the distal tubule. The causes of these processes are shown. ECF, extracellular fluid; RTA, renal tubular acidosis.

TABLE 8-1 Tests of Renal Acid Excretion
Urine pH (enhanced by furosemide)
NH₄⁺ excretion
Urine NH₄⁺
Urine anion gap
Urine osmole gap
Urine Pco₂ with Bicarbonate Loading
Fractional excretion of HCO₃⁻

to the sum of titratable acids and ammonium ion excreted, minus any secreted bicarbonate ion:

$$\text{Net renal acid excretion} = \left(TA + NH_4^+\right) - HCO_3^-$$

Therefore, the causes of metabolic acidosis can be divided into four broad categories: (1) overproduction of fixed acids, (2) increased extrarenal loss of base, (3) decrease in the kidney's ability to secrete hydrogen ions, and (4) inability of the kidney to reclaim the filtered bicarbonate (**Fig. 8-2**).

EVALUATION OF URINARY ACIDIFICATION

The cause of metabolic acidosis often is evident from the clinical situation. However, because the kidney is responsible for reclamation of filtered HCO_3^- and excretion of the daily production of fixed acid, to evaluate a metabolic acidosis it may be necessary to assess whether the kidney is appropriately able to reabsorb HCO_3^-, secrete H⁺ against a gradient, and excrete NH_4^+ (**Table 8-1**). The simplest test is to measure urine pH. Although urine pH can be measured with the use of a dipstick, the lack of precision of this technique prevents its use to make clinical decisions. Ideally, the urine should be collected under oil and the pH measured using a pH electrode. Under conditions of acid loading, urine pH should be less than 5.5. A pH higher than 5.5 usually reflects impaired distal hydrogen ion secretion. Measuring the pH after a challenge with the loop diuretic

furosemide increases the sensitivity of this test by providing Na⁺ to the distal tubule for reabsorption. The reabsorption of Na⁺ creates a negative electrical potential in the lumen and enhances H⁺ secretion. It is important, however, to rule out urinary infections with urea-splitting organisms, which increase pH. An elevated urine pH may also be misleading in conditions associated with volume depletion and hypokalemia, as can occur in diarrhea. In contradistinction to furosemide, volume depletion with decreased sodium delivery to the distal tubule impairs distal H⁺ secretion. Furthermore, hypokalemia, by enhancing ammoniagenesis, raises the urine pH.

Because renal excretion of NH_4^+ accounts for the majority of acid excretion, measurement of urine NH_4^+ provides important information. Urinary NH_4^+ excretion can be decreased by a variety of mechanisms, including a primary decrease in ammoniagenesis by the proximal tubule, as seen in chronic kidney disease (CKD), and decreased trapping in the distal tubule, secondary to either decreased H⁺ secretion or increased delivery of HCO_3^- (which preferentially buffers H⁺, making it unavailable to form NH_4^+). Direct measurement of NH_4^+ is not usually readily available in clinical laboratories, but an estimate of NH_4^+ excretion is easily obtained by calculating the urine anion gap (UAG) or the urine osmole gap (**Fig. 8-3**). If, as is usually the case, the anion balancing the charge of the NH_4^+ is chloride (Cl^-), the UAG should be negative, because the Cl^- is greater than the sum of Na⁺ and K⁺:

$$UAG = \left(Na^+ + K^+\right) - Cl^-$$

Although measurement of the UAG in conditions of acid loading is often reflective of NH_4^+ excretion, the presence of anions other than Cl^- such as keto anions or hippurate (see **Fig. 8-3**), makes it a less reliable assessment of NH_4^+ than the urine osmole gap, which is calculated from the measured urine osmolality (U_{osm}) as follows:

$$\text{Urine osmole gap} = U_{osm} - \left[2\left(Na^+ + K^+\right) + \text{Urea nitrogen}/2.8 + \text{Glucose}/18\right]$$

The osmole gap is made up primarily of NH_4 salts, and half of the gap represents NH_4^+. An osmole gap greater than 100 mmol/L signifies normal NH_4^+ excretion.

Another test of distal H⁺ ion secretory ability is measurement of urine Pco₂ during bicarbonate loading. Distal delivery of HCO_3^- in the presence of a normal H⁺ secretory

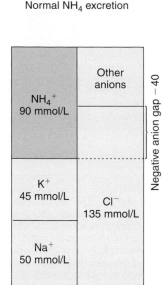

Normal NH$_4$ excretion

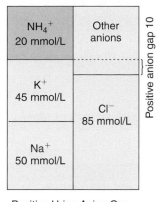

Decreased NH$_4$ excretion

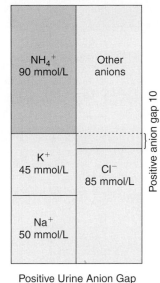

Normal NH$_4$ excretion
Increased organic anions

A — Negative Urine Anion Gap

B — Positive Urine Anion Gap

C — Positive Urine Anion Gap

FIGURE 8-3 In the presence of acidemia, the kidney increases NH$_4^+$ excretion. The urine anion gap (UAG) is an indirect method for estimating urine NH$_4^+$. If the accompanying anion is chloride (**A**), the UAG will be negative, reflecting the large quantity of NH$_4^+$ in the urine: UAG = (Na$^+$ + K$^+$) − Cl$^-$. A decrease in NH$_4^+$ secretion occurs when ammoniagenesis is diminished, H$^+$ secretion is impaired, or there is delivery of HCO$_3^-$ to the distal tubule. In these cases, the UAG will be inappropriately positive (**B**). If anions other than Cl$^-$ are excreted (e.g., ketones, hippurate), the UAG will be positive despite increased NH$_4^+$ excretion (**C**), because these anions are not used in calculation of the gap.

capacity results in elevated Pco$_2$ in the urine; if there is a secretory defect, urine Pco$_2$ does not increase. Accurate measurement of urine Pco$_2$ requires that the urine be collected under oil to prevent the loss of CO$_2$ into the air.

COMPLICATIONS OF ACIDOSIS

Although it has been accepted that a decrease in extracellular pH has detrimental effects on numerous physiologic parameters and should be aggressively treated, this dogma has been challenged. The proponents of treatment argue that acidemia depresses cardiac contractility, blocks activation of adrenergic receptors, and inhibits the action of key enzymes. Uncontrolled clinical studies are not easy to interpret because of the difficulties in separating the effects of the acidosis from the effects of the underlying illness. Most controlled studies investigating the role of acidosis on cellular processes have been done in isolated cells or organs; therefore, the effects of acidemia on whole-body physiology and their applicability to humans are unclear.

The effect of pH on cardiac function has been strongly debated. Cardiac output is determined by multiple components, and it is the sum of the effects on these individual components that determines the net effect of acidemia on cardiac function. Myocardial contractile strength and changes in vascular tone determine cardiovascular performance, and the relative contributions of each in the context of acidemia remain to be clarified. Because of differing effects of acidemia on contractile force, vascular tone, and sympathetic discharge, it is difficult to predict what will happen to cardiac output from studies using isolated myocytes or perfused hearts.

It has been shown that cardiac output and the rate of development of left ventricular force increase during continuous infusion of lactic acid. In addition, fractional shortening of the left ventricle, as assessed by transthoracic echocardiography, appears to be normal even in cases of severe acidemia. The pH at which cardiac output and blood pressure fall remains unclear.

APPROACH TO ACID-BASE DISORDERS

Complete evaluation of acid-base status requires a routine electrolyte panel, measurement of serum albumin, and arterial blood gas analysis. The traditional approach to the diagnosis of metabolic acidosis relies on calculation of the anion gap (AG) in plasma, with metabolic acidoses accompanied by an elevated AG being viewed separately from those in which the AG is normal—so-called hyperchloremic metabolic acidosis (**Fig. 8-4**). The AG is defined as the difference between the concentration of the major cation, sodium, and the sum of the concentrations of the major anions, chloride and bicarbonate:

$$AG = \left[Na^+\right] - \left(\left[Cl^-\right] + \left[HCO_3^-\right]\right)$$

Because the concentration of potassium changes minimally, its contribution is ignored for convenience. Obviously, electrical neutrality must exist, and the sum of the anions must equal the sum of the cations. The gap results because anions such as sulfate, phosphate, organic anions, and especially the weak acid proteins are present but are not measured on the routine chemistry panel. Because there are fewer unmeasured cations, it seems on examination of a chemistry panel that cations exceed anions, creating an AG. The normal AG is 8 ± 4 mEq/L. Any increase in the AG, even in the face of a normal or frankly alkalemic pH, represents accumulation of acids and the presence of an acidosis. In many cases, the anions that make up the gap are not easily identifiable.

The one caveat in using the AG is to recognize that the normal gap is predominantly composed of the negative charge on albumin. If hypoalbuminemia is present, the AG must be corrected for the serum albumin concentration. For

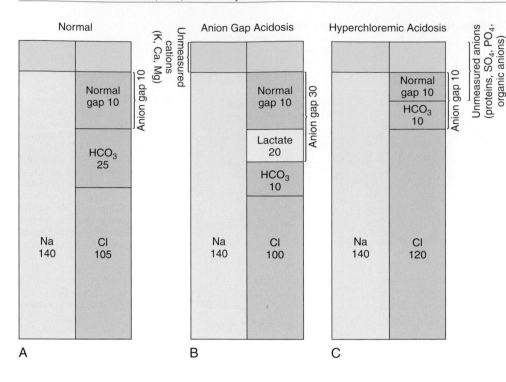

FIGURE 8-4 A, The anion gap (AG) is equal to $[Na^+] - ([Cl^-] + [HCO_3^-])$, which is equal to the unmeasured anions minus the unmeasured cations. **B,** In an AG acidosis, there is a decrease in $[HCO_3^-]$ and an increase in organic anions (e.g., lactate), which results in an elevated AG. **C,** In a hyperchloremic acidosis, there is a decrease in $[HCO_3^-]$ and an increase in $[Cl^-]$, with no change in the AG.

each 1 g/dL decrease in serum albumin, the calculated AG should be increased by 2.5 mEq/L. Therefore, the formula for the corrected AG (AG_c) is

$$AG_c = AG + 2.5(4 - Serum\ albumin)$$

If the AG is not corrected, the presence of a metabolic acidosis may be masked. This is especially true in critically ill patients, who typically have decreased serum albumin levels.

ANION GAP ACIDOSIS

As previously described, an increased AG represents the accumulation of nonchloride acids. AG acidosis can be divided into four major categories (**Table 8-2**): (1) lactic acidosis, (2) ketoacidosis, (3) toxins/drugs, and (4) severe kidney failure. In all but the last group, the accumulation of acids is caused by their overproduction. These acids dissociate into protons, which are quickly buffered by HCO_3^- and their respective conjugate bases, the unmeasured anions. As long as these anions are retained in the body and not excreted, they contribute to the elevation in the AG.

Lactic Acidosis

Lactic acidosis is a common AG acidosis, and it is by far the most serious of all AG acidoses. Anaerobic metabolism of glucose (glycolysis) occurs in the extramitochondrial cytoplasm and produces pyruvate as an intermediary. If this were the end of the glycolytic process, there would be a net production of two protons and a metabolically unsatisfactory reduction of nicotinamide adenine dinucleotide (NAD) to NADH. However, pyruvate rapidly undergoes one of two metabolic fates: (1) under anaerobic conditions, because of

the high NADH/NAD ratio, pyruvate is quickly reduced by lactate dehydrogenase to lactate—releasing energy, consuming a proton, and decreasing the NADH/NAD ratio, thereby allowing for continued glycolysis; or(2) in the presence of oxygen, pyruvate diffuses into the mitochondria and, after oxidation by the pyruvate dehydrogenase (PDH) complex, enters the tricarboxylic acid cycle, where it is completely oxidized to carbon dioxide and water. Neither of these pathways results in the production of H^+. However, during glycolysis, glucose metabolism produces two molecules of lactate and two molecules of adenosine triphosphate (ATP). It is the hydrolysis of ATP ($ATP \rightarrow ADP + H^+ + P_i$) that releases protons. Therefore, acidosis does not occur because of the production of lactate but because, under hypoxic conditions, the hydrolysis of ATP is greater than ATP production. Therefore, the buildup of lactate is a surrogate marker for ATP consumption during hypoxic states.

Although lactate production averages about 1300 mmol/day, serum lactate levels are normally less than 1 mmol/L, because lactate is either reoxidized to pyruvate and enters the tricarboxylic acid cycle or is utilized by the liver and kidney via the Cori cycle for gluconeogenesis. Increased concentration of lactate can therefore result from decreased oxidative phosphorylation, increased glycolysis, or decreased gluconeogenesis. Lactate levels between 2 and 3 mmol/L are frequently found in hospitalized patients. Some of these patients will go on to develop frank acidosis, but others will have no adverse events. *Lactic acidosis is defined as the presence of a lactate level of greater than 5 mmol/L.*

There is a poor correlation among arterial pH, calculated AG, and serum lactate levels, even in those patients with a serum lactic acid concentration greater than 5 mmol/L.

TABLE 8-2 Causes of Anion Gap Acidosis
Lactic acidosis
Type A
Type B
D-Lactic acidosis
Ketoacidosis
Diabetic ketoacidosis
Alcoholic ketoacidosis
Starvation ketosis
Toxins/Drugs
Methanol
Ethylene glycol
Salicylate
Kidney failure (with severe reduction in the glomerular filtration rate)

TABLE 8-3 Causes of Lactic Acidosis
Type A
Generalized seizure
Extreme exercise
Shock
Cardiac arrest
Low cardiac output
Severe anemia
Severe hypoxemia
Carbon monoxide poisoning
Type B
Sepsis
Thiamine deficiency
Uncontrolled diabetes mellitus
Malignancy
Hypoglycemia

Drugs/toxins
  Ethanol
  Metformin
  Zidovudine
  Didanosine
  Stavudine
  Lamivudine
  Zalcitabine
  Salicylate
  Propofol
  Niacin
  Isoniazid
  Nitroprusside
  Cyanide
  Catecholamines
  Cocaine
  Acetaminophen
  Streptozotocin
  Pheochromocytoma
  Sorbitol/fructose
  Malaria

Inborn errors of metabolism
Other
Hepatic failure
Respiratory or metabolic alkalosis
Propylene glycol
D-Lactic acidosis

Approximately 25% of patients with serum lactate levels between 5 and 9.9 mmol/L have a pH greater than 7.35, and as many as half have an AG of less than 12.

Lactic acidosis has been traditionally divided into types A and B (**Table 8-3**). Type A, or hypoxic lactic acidosis, results from an imbalance between oxygen supply and oxygen demand. In type B lactic acidosis, oxygen delivery is normal, but oxidative phosphorylation is impaired. Type B is seen in patients who have inborn errors of metabolism or who have ingested drugs or toxins. It has become increasingly clear, however, that lactic acidosis is often caused by the simultaneous existence of both hypoxic and nonhypoxic factors, and in many cases it is difficult to separate one from the other. For example, hereditary partial defects in mitochondrial metabolism or age-related declines in cytochrome IV complex activity may result in lactic acidosis with a lesser degree of hypoxia than in patients without such defects. Even in cases of shock in which tissue oxygen delivery is obviously inadequate, decreased portal blood flow and reduced hepatic clearance of lactate contribute to the acidosis. Similarly, in sepsis there is a decrease in both tissue perfusion and the ability to utilize oxygen. Therefore, this division based solely on cause is largely of historical and conceptual interest.

The presence of lactate acidosis is considered a poor prognostic sign. Studies have found that the probability of survival decreases precipitously as lactate levels increase above 2.0 to 2.5 mmol/L. It remains unclear, however, whether the blood lactate level is an independent contributor to mortality or whether it represents an epiphenomenon confounded by the severity of the patient's illness. Just as important to prognosis is the body's ability to metabolize lactate after restoration of tissue perfusion. Patients who are able to reduce their lactate by half within 18 hours of resuscitation have a significantly greater chance of survival. In all likelihood, the inability to metabolize lactate is a surrogate marker for organ dysfunction.

Type A Lactic Acidosis

Lactic acidosis is commonly observed in conditions in which oxygen delivery is inadequate, such as low cardiac output, hypotension, severe anemia, and carbon monoxide poisoning. States of hypoperfusion are more prone to the accumulation of lactate than hypoxemic states. In the latter situation, tissue oxygenation is often preserved by compensatory mechanisms such as increased cardiac output, augmented red blood cell production, and a reduced affinity of hemoglobin for oxygen. In all cases of type A lactic acidosis, oxygen is unavailable to the mitochondria, and pyruvate, unable to enter the tricarboxylic acid cycle, is reduced to lactate.

Type B Lactic Acidosis
Sepsis
Although sepsis is frequently associated with hypotension and a related type A lactic acidosis, lactic acidosis also may develop during sepsis even if oxygen delivery and tissue perfusion appear to be unimpeded. It has been postulated that, in sepsis, there is both an overproduction of pyruvate and an inhibition of PDH activity (the rate-limiting factor in oxidative phosphorylation). Because of the increased NADH/NAD ratio, pyruvate is rapidly reduced to lactate. Dichloroacetate, an activator of the PDH complex, lowers lactate levels significantly, suggesting that tissue oxygenation is adequate to support oxidative phosphorylation.

Drugs
Numerous drugs and toxins can cause lactic acidosis. The biguanide derivatives phenformin and metformin are recognized causes of lactic acidosis. Phenformin was withdrawn from the United States market in 1976 because of the high frequency of occurrence of lactic acidosis in association with its use. Both of these agents bind to complex 1 of the mitochondrial respiratory chain, inhibiting its activity. Metformin, a newer biguanide, has a markedly lower incidence of lactic acidosis than phenformin, possibly because it is less lipid soluble and therefore has limited ability to cross the mitochondrial membrane and bind to the mitochondrial complex. Almost all reported cases of metformin-associated lactic acidosis have occurred in patients with underlying CKD. It has been suggested that the present incidence of lactic acidosis in diabetics is no greater than the incidence of lactic acidosis before the introduction of metformin, so that the association of metformin with lactic acidosis is mere "guilt by association." However, a causative role is suggested by the observations that metformin inhibits the respiratory chain in isolated metochondria and that the incidence of lactic acidosis approaches zero when the drug is prescribed according to recommendations.

Lactic acidosis is being increasingly recognized in patients with human immunodeficiency virus (HIV) infection who are taking nucleoside reverse-transcriptase inhibitors. These agents, particularly stavudine, but also zidovudine, didanosine, and lamivudine, have been associated with severe lactic acidosis, often with concomitant hepatic steatosis. Nucleoside analogues inhibit mitochondrial DNA polymerase-γ. This causes mitochondrial toxicity and a decrease in oxidative phosphorylation, resulting in both lipid accumulation within the liver and decreased oxidation of pyruvate. Of note, hyperlactatemia without frank lactic acidosis is often present in patients taking these medications. What converts these mild elevations in lactate levels into frank lactic acidosis is not known.

Salicylate intoxication often produces lactic acidosis. This occurs both because the salicylate-induced respiratory alkalosis stimulates lactate production and because of the inhibitory effects of salicylates on oxidative metabolism. Ethanol ingestion may cause mild elevations in lactate levels secondary to impaired hepatic conversion of lactate to glucose. In addition, the metabolism of ethanol increases the NADH/NAD ratio, favoring the conversion of pyruvate to lactate. Concomitant thiamine deficiency, as is often seen in alcohol abusers, may exacerbate the acidosis.

Vitamin Deficiency
Deficiency of thiamine, a cofactor for PDH, also can result in lactic acidosis. Patients requiring total parental nutrition may develop thiamine deficiency if not supplemented with this vitamin. During a national shortage of parenteral vitamin preparations, numerous cases of lactic acidosis occurred due to inadequate thiamine supplementation.

Systemic Disease
Diabetes is often associated with lactic acidosis. Even under basal conditions, patients with diabetes have mildly elevated lactate levels. This is thought to be secondary to decreased PDH activity caused by free fatty acid oxidation by liver and muscle. Lactate increases even more during diabetic ketoacidosis (DKA), possibly secondary to decreased hepatic clearance. This accumulation of lactate contributes to the elevated AG present in ketoacidosis.

Malignancy
Lactic acidosis has been detected in patients with acute, rapidly progressive hematologic malignancies such as leukemia or lymphoma. Lactate levels usually parallel disease activity. The increased blood viscosity and microvascular aggregates that are frequently found in acute leukemia cause regional hypoperfusion. Overproduction of lactate may also result from a large tumor burden and rapid cell lysis.

Alternate Sugars
The use of sorbitol or fructose intravenously, as irrigants during prostate surgery, or in tube feedings, can cause lactic acidosis. The metabolism of these sugars consumes ATP, inhibiting gluconeogenesis and stimulating glycolysis, leading to the accumulation of excess lactate.

Propylene Glycol
Propylene glycol is a common vehicle for many drugs, including topical silver sulfadiazine and intravenous preparations of nitroglycerin, diazepam, lorazepam, phenytoin, etomidate, and trimethoprim-sulfamethoxazole, among others. Although it is considered relatively safe, many case reports have appeared demonstrating toxicity. Approximately 40% to 50% of administered propylene glycol is oxidized by alcohol dehydrogenase to lactic acid. Toxic patients commonly develop an unexplained AG acidosis with increased serum osmolality. Considering that patients receiving many of the medications solubilized with propylene glycol frequently have other possible causes for their acidosis, it is important to be aware of this iatrogenic cause for the acidosis. Correction of the metabolic abnormalities quickly follows discontinuation of the medication.

D-*Lactic Acidosis*
An unusual form of AG acidosis results from accumulation of the D-isomer of lactate. Unlike the lactate produced by glycolysis in animals, which is the L-isomer, colonic bacteria

produce the D-isomer. Overproduction of D-lactate occurs in patients with short-bowel syndrome and is usually precipitated by a high carbohydrate intake. Increased delivery of carbohydrates by the to the shortened bowel and an overgrowth of bacteria are responsible for this overproduction. Because D-lactate is not detected on the routine assay, which measures only L-lactate, diagnosis requires a high clinical suspicion. Patients typically present with mental status changes, ataxia, and nystagmus. Treatment consists of an oral fast with intravenous nutrition and restoration of gut flora to normal through the administration of oral antibiotics. In severe cases, hemodialysis can decrease the concentration of D-lactate.

Treatment of Lactic Acidosis

The treatment of lactic acidosis is fraught with controversy. The most important step is treatment of the underlying cause. In cases of sepsis, restoring oxygenation via mechanical ventilation and restoring perfusion via pressors or inotropes are of paramount importance, although these interventions do not always improve the lactic acidosis. In some patients with medication-induced lactic acidosis, withdrawal of the offending agent may be sufficient. There are anecdotal case reports of successful use of riboflavin or L-carnitine to treat lactic acidosis associated with nucleoside analogues in patients with acquired immunodeficiency syndrome.

Often these measures fail, and the clinician is faced with the decision of whether to give sodium bicarbonate in an effort to increase serum pH. There are several potential problems with this approach. First, as previously discussed, it is not clear to what extent acidosis is deleterious and therefore whether normalization of the pH is of any benefit. Also, increasing the pH may actually increase lactic acid production. Sodium bicarbonate is often given as a hypertonic solution, which can lead to hypernatremia and cellular dehydration. Perhaps most important is the possibility that the administration of HCO_3^- can cause a paradoxic decrease in intracellular pH despite an increase in extracellular pH. Bicarbonate combines with hydrogen, forming carbonic acid, which is then converted to CO_2 and water. Therefore, the P_{CO_2} increases with titration of acid by bicarbonate and rapidly diffuses into cells, causing acidification, while the bicarbonate remains extracellular. For these reasons, it is difficult to recommend the use of bicarbonate for the treatment of a low serum pH alone. If the serum pH is less than 7.1, however, many clinicians opt for treatment, despite the lack of supporting data, because a further small decline in serum bicarbonate can have a profound effect on serum pH.

Other buffers may be better tolerated insofar as they buffer hydrogen ions without increasing CO_2. One such buffer is tris-hydroxymethyl aminomethane (THAM), a biologically inert amino acid that can buffer both CO_2 and protons. It does not lead to production of CO_2 and therefore works well in a closed system. The protonated molecule is excreted by the kidney and should be used cautiously in patients with kidney failure. Potential side effects include hyperkalemia, hypoglycemia, ventilatory depression, and hepatic necrosis

in neonates. Despite its having been available for many years, there are no studies demonstrating improved outcomes with the use of THAM. The acute dose in milliliters of 0.3 mol/L solution can be derived by multiplying the decrease in HCO_3^- from normal (in mmol/L) times the body weight in kilograms.. The first 25% to 50% of the dose is given over 5 minutes, and the rest over 1 hour. Alternatively, a steady infusion of no more than 3.5 L/day can be given for several days.

Dichloroacetate has also been used in the treatment of lactic acidosis. This agent stimulates the activity of PDH, increasing the rate of pyruvate oxidation and thereby decreasing lactate levels. A large multicenter trial in humans showed a reduction in serum lactate, an increase in pH, and an increase in the number of patients able to resolve their hyperlactatemia. Despite these favorable changes, no improvement in either hemodynamic parameters or mortality was found.

Various modes of renal replacement therapy have been used in the treatment of lactic acidosis. Standard bicarbonate hemodialysis treats acidosis primarily by diffusion of bicarbonate from the bath into the blood and is thus another form of bicarbonate administration, albeit with several advantages. Hypernatremia and volume overload are not a concern with hemodialysis, as they are with intravenous administration. Also, hemodialysis, in addition to adding bicarbonate, removes lactate. Although the removal of lactate does not increase serum pH, there is some evidence that the lactate ion itself is harmful. However, there have been no randomized, prospective trials demonstrating benefit of dialysis in lactic acidosis, and its use in the absence of other indications cannot be routinely recommended.

Several studies have shown that high-volume hemofiltration using either lactate- or bicarbonate-buffered replacement fluid can rapidly correct metabolic acidosis. These studies have been small, and the degree and type of acidosis have been poorly characterized. In addition, other treatment measures have usually been instituted, making it difficult to draw conclusions about the effectiveness of this treatment. Nevertheless, hemofiltration remains a viable therapeutic option.

Peritoneal dialysis has also been used in the treatment of metabolic acidosis. Although there are case reports of success using this modality, a randomized study comparing lactate-buffered peritoneal dialysis with continuous hemofiltration showed that hemofiltration corrected acidosis more quickly and more effectively than peritoneal dialysis. Whether newer, bicarbonate-buffered peritoneal dialysis solutions would be more efficacious remains to be determined.

Ketoacidosis

Diabetic Ketoacidosis

DKA is another common cause of an AG acidosis. Although DKA may be the initial presentation of diabetes mellitus, patients more commonly have a known diagnosis of diabetes and either have been noncompliant with their insulin regimen or have some other precipitating factor, such as infection. Patients are typically polyuric and polydipsic, but if volume depletion becomes severe enough, polyuria may not be seen. Although DKA is classically seen in type 1 diabetes, it can also occur in patients with type 2 diabetes. DKA results from insulin deficiency and concomitant increase in counter-regulatory hormones such as glucagon, epinephrine, and cortisol. This hormonal milieu leads to an inability of cells to utilize glucose, which causes them to oxidize fatty acids as fuel, producing large amounts of keto acids.

A diagnosis of DKA requires a pH less than 7.35, elevated AG, positive serum ketones of at least 1:2 dilutions, and decreased serum bicarbonate. However, not all patients with DKA meet these criteria. If renal perfusion and the glomerular filtration rate (GFR) are well maintained, ketones (anions) are rapidly excreted by the kidney in place of chloride. With the loss of these anions in the urine, the AG acidosis may be replaced by a mixed AG/hyperchloremic acidosis or even a pure hyperchloremic acidosis. Furthermore, an increase in the NADH/NAD ratio, which frequently occurs during DKA, causes ketones to shift from acetoacetate to β-hydroxybutyrate, which is not detected on the standard nitroprusside test used to identify serum and urinary ketones. If this occurs, serum ketones may appear to be negative or only trace-positive. Finally, vomiting may result in a metabolic alkalosis, which would raise the serum bicarbonate toward the normal range. In this case, the serum AG would almost certainly be elevated, and the astute clinician will not be fooled.

Treatment of Diabetic Ketoacidosis

The treatment of DKA consists of three parts: fluid resuscitation, insulin administration, and correction of potassium deficits. Patients with DKA often have profound deficits of both sodium and free water. Hypovolemia, as demonstrated by hemodynamic compromise, should always be treated first. Patients should rapidly receive 1 to 2 L of 0.9% saline until their blood pressure is stabilized. Thereafter, hypotonic fluids in the form of 0.45% saline should be administered to correct free water deficits while continuing to provide volume. Insulin should be administered only after fluid resuscitation is well underway. If insulin is given precipitously, the rapid uptake of glucose by the cells will cause water to follow because of the fall in extracellular osmolality, potentially resulting in cardiovascular collapse. A regular insulin bolus of 0.1 unit/kg intravenously is given, followed by a continuous infusion of 0.1 unit/kg/hr. If the glucose does not decline by 50 to 100 mg/dL/hr, the infusion should be increased by 50%. The insulin infusion should be continued until the ketosis is resolved, as demonstrated by negative serum ketones, closure of the AG, and near-normalization of the serum pH.

As tissue perfusion improves, β-hydroxybutyrate is converted to acetoacetate, and serum ketones paradoxically increase, but then they should decrease. The closure of the AG, by itself, is unreliable because, as discussed previously, with volume resuscitation the ketones are rapidly excreted and the AG acidosis is replaced by a hyperchloremic acidosis. Serum glucose usually approaches normal before ketosis is resolved.

If the glucose level is less than 250 mg/dL, intravenous fluids should be changed to 5% dextrose in water (D5W) to avoid hypoglycemia while awaiting resolution of ketosis. The insulin infusion can be discontinued after the ketosis has been resolved and the patient is taking food and fluid by mouth. A subcutaneous insulin dose should be given at least 1 hour before stopping the drip, to avoid rebound ketosis.

Most patients with DKA have total-body potassium depletion. Nevertheless, their serum potassium concentration may be normal to high because of a shift of potassium out of the cells caused by the profound insulinopenia. After insulin is restored, extracellular potassium is rapidly taken up by cells, and severe hypokalemia may ensue. Therefore, addition of potassium to the intravenous fluids is recommended, at a concentration of 10 to 20 mEq/L, as soon as the serum potassium level falls below 4.5 mEq/L. Needless to say, this management algorithm requires frequent laboratory tests.

Although bicarbonate therapy has been used in severe DKA, this use is not supported by the literature. In fact, bicarbonate administration, even in patients with pH less than 7.0, has not been shown to be advantageous. In almost all cases, the acidosis rapidly improves with appropriate management without the use of bicarbonate. Therefore, the administration of sodium bicarbonate to patients with DKA cannot be routinely recommended. However, it is important that these patients be monitored in a setting where they can be closely observed and where frequent analyses of their arterial blood gases and electrolytes can be obtained.

Alcoholic Ketoacidosis

Alcoholic ketoacidosis (AKA) usually manifests with an AG acidosis and ketonemia but without significant hyperglycemia. The classic presentation is that of a patient who has been on an alcohol binge, develops nausea and vomiting, and stops eating. The patient typically presents 24 to 48 hours after the cessation of oral intake and may also complain of abdominal pain and shortness of breath. Alcohol levels are low or even unmeasurable by the time AKA develops.

AKA is similar to DKA in that it is a state of insulinopenia and increased counter-regulatory hormones; in fact, the levels of these hormones are similar in both disorders. In AKA, normoglycemia to hypoglycemia is usually observed, despite a hormonal milieu favoring hyperglycemia, because decreased NAD curtails hepatic gluconeogenesis and starvation depletes glycogen stores. However, patients with AKA occasionally present with hyperglycemia, and in those cases distinguishing AKA from DKA can be difficult. AKA almost always produces an AG, but acidemia is less universal. Patients often have concurrent metabolic alkalosis from vomiting or respiratory alkalosis from liver disease. Therefore, patients with AKA may not be acidemic, and they rarely have a simple metabolic acidosis. Because of the increased NADH/NAD ratio, the primary keto acid present is β-hydroxybutyrate, so the serum ketones determination may be reported as negative. This ratio also favors the formation of lactic acid. Finally, electrolyte disorders, including hypokalemia, hypophosphatemia, and hypomagnesemia, are common.

Treatment of Alcoholic Ketoacidosis

Therapy for AKA is straightforward and consists of volume repletion, provision of glucose (except in those patients with hyperglycemia), and correction of any electrolyte abnormalities. Patients are often volume depleted as a result of vomiting combined with poor oral intake. Thiamine must be provided before or concurrently with glucose, to avoid precipitating Wernicke's encephalopathy. Acidosis resolves as insulin increases and counter-regulatory hormones are turned off in response to glucose infusion. The clinician must maintain a high degree of suspicion for this disorder, because the acid-base disturbance may be subtle on routine laboratory analyses, with patients often demonstrating an elevated AG as the only abnormality. Chronic alcoholics often have hypoalbuminemia, which can further obscure the interpretation of the AG. Any patient with nausea and vomiting who has a recent history of alcohol abuse should probably be treated for presumptive AKA until the diagnosis is clearly ruled out.

Starvation Ketosis

During prolonged fasting, insulin levels are suppressed, and levels of glucagon, epinephrine, growth hormone, and cortisol are increased. This hormonal milieu results in increased lipolysis, with release of free fatty acids into the blood and stimulation of hepatic ketogenesis. The concentrations of both β-hydroxybutyrate and acetoacetate increase over the course of several weeks, resulting in a mild AG metabolic acidosis.

Toxins and Drugs

Ethylene Glycol

Ingestion of various toxins can cause severe metabolic acidosis with an increased AG and should always be suspected in these cases. Ethylene glycol is a sweet liquid that is found in antifreeze. Ingestion of 100 mL or more can be fatal. Smaller volumes can be lethal in children; fraudulent mislabeling of a cold syrup of ethylene glycol as glycerol recently led to an epidemic of poisonings in Panama, with numerous fatalities.

Ethylene glycol is metabolized by alcohol dehydrogenase to glycolic acid and subsequently to oxalic acid. This generates NADH, which encourages the formation of lactic acid. The AG acidosis results from the accumulation of the various acid metabolites of ethylene glycol as well as lactic acidosis. Diagnosis can be difficult, because ethylene glycol is not detected on routine toxicology assays. Its ingestion should be suspected in anyone who presents with intoxication, a low blood alcohol content, and a markedly increased AG metabolic acidosis without ketonemia.

The serum osmolar gap may help detect ethylene glycol. Serum osmolar gap is the difference between the calculated serum osmolarity $[([Na^+] \times 2) + (Glucose/18) + (Blood\ urea\ nitrogen/2.8)]$ and the actual serum osmolality as measured by the laboratory. A difference greater than about 10 to 15 mOsm/kg suggests the presence of an unmeasured, osmotically active substance, which in the right clinical setting could be a toxin. However, it is important to understand the limitations of this approach. Some laboratories measure serum osmolality using vapor pressure methodology rather than freezing point depression, and volatile substances such as alcohols may not be detected. Moreover, as the osmotically active alcohol is metabolized into the various acids, the osmolar gap disappears. Therefore the osmolar gap is elevated early after ingestion, without a significant increase in the AG, and as the alcohol is metabolized, the osmolar gap decreases while the AG increases.

Examination of the urine may reveal calcium oxalate crystals, a finding that can be considered pathognomonic. However, the absence of these crystals does not rule out the ingestion of ethylene glycol. Precipitation of calcium oxalate may occasionally cause hypocalcemia. Because fluorescein is added as a colorant to antifreeze, the urine of a patient with antifreeze ingestion may fluoresce under a Wood's lamp.

Methanol

Methanol is an alcohol that is often found in solvents or as an adulterant in alcoholic beverages. Toxicity is caused by ingestion of as little as 30 mL and has also been reported after inhalation. Methanol is metabolized by alcohol dehydrogenase to formaldehyde and then to formic acid, resulting in an elevated AG acidosis. As with ingestions of other alcohols, NAD depletion favors the production of lactate. Methanol is less intoxicating than either ethanol or ethylene glycol. The most characteristic symptom of methanol toxicity is blurry vision. Blindness may occur with optic nerve involvement, and pancreatitis may be seen in up to two thirds of patients. Early after ingestion an osmolar gap may be found, as was described previously. The diagnosis of either ethylene glycol or methanol poisoning can be confirmed by specific toxicologic assays, but treatment should never be delayed while awaiting these results.

Treatment of Toxic Alcohol Ingestions

Treatment of ethylene glycol or methanol toxicity is based on the fact that it is the metabolites of these alcohols that are actually harmful. Both substances are metabolized by alcohol dehydrogenase. Blocking the activity of this enzyme prevents the metabolic acidosis and allows the alcohol to be excreted by the kidneys or removed by dialysis. Because alcohol dehydrogenase has a much higher affinity for ethanol than for either ethylene glycol or methanol, use of ethanol as a competitive inhibitor has been the traditional treatment. Ethanol is supplied as a 10% solution in D5W. A loading dose of 0.8 to 1.0 g/kg body weight, followed by an infusion of 100 mg/kg/hr, should be sufficient to maintain a blood alcohol level of 100 to 150 mg/dL. However, in some patients with marked ethanol tolerance, this rate will need to be doubled.

Fomepizole (4-methylpyrazole), a competitive inhibitor of alcohol dehydrogenase, has now replaced ethanol as the treatment of choice. Fomepizole is a more potent inhibitor of alcohol dehydrogenase than ethanol and does not lead to central nervous system depression. An initial loading dose of 15 mg/kg body weight is followed 12 hours later by 10 mg/kg every 12 hours for four doses, then 15 mg/kg every 12 hours for four more doses. Fomepizole, because of its potency, has begun to call into question the need for dialysis; however, until more studies are available, it is recommended that dialysis be instituted in all patients with suspected ingestions of ethylene glycol or methanol who have end-organ damage (kidney failure or visual impairment) and whose blood pH is less than 7.2.

Both ethylene glycol and methanol are rapidly removed by hemodialysis. Hemodialysis can also help improve the acidosis by providing a source of bicarbonate. It is important to double the rate of any ethanol infusion (or increase the dose of fomepizole) while the patient is undergoing hemodialysis. For either ingestion, gastric lavage with charcoal should be performed if the ingestion occurred within the preceding 2 to 3 hours.

Salicylate Toxicity

The ingestion of salicylates is an important cause of mixed acid-base disturbances, producing both a respiratory alkalosis and a metabolic acidosis. Salicylate is a direct respiratory stimulant. Metabolic acidosis results from the accumulation of both lactic acid and keto acids. Salicylic acid, by itself, accounts for only a small quantity of the acid load. The common presenting sign of salicylate toxicity is tachypnea. The patient may also complain of tinnitus with serum concentrations of salicylic acid of 20 to 45 mg/dL or higher. Other central nervous system manifestations are agitation, seizures, and even coma. Both noncardiogenic pulmonary edema and upper gastrointestinal bleeding may occur. Hypoglycemia occurs in children but is rare in adults. Other symptoms include nausea, vomiting, and hyperpyrexia.

In the setting of salicylate overdose, peak serum concentrations are achieved 4 to 6 hours after ingestion. The severity of the ingestion can be predicted by the Done nomogram, which plots the toxic salicylate level at varying time points after ingestion. This nomogram cannot be used with chronic ingestions or with the ingestion of enteric-coated aspirin. The treatment of salicylate toxicity consists of supportive care, removal of unabsorbed compounds by means of charcoal lavage, administration of bicarbonate, and, if necessary, hemodialysis. Because the dissociation constant (pK) of salicylic acid is 3.0, alkalinization keeps the drug in its polar dissociated form, preventing diffusion into the central nervous system. In addition, because tissue salicylic acid is in equilibrium with the nondissociated compound in the plasma, alkalinization also decreases tissue levels. Concurrent alkalinization of the urine traps salicylate in the tubule, promoting its excretion. Hemodialysis is indicated for all patients with altered mental status, kidney failure that causes a decrease in renal excretion, volume overload that prevents the administration of bicarbonate, or salicylate levels greater than 100 mg/dL.

Kidney Failure

Kidney failure is also a well-recognized cause of metabolic acidosis. With the reduction in nephron mass that occurs in CKD, there is decreased ammoniagenesis in the proximal tubule. Many patients with diminished kidney function also have specific acidification defects in the form of a renal tubular acidosis (RTA). As the GFR declines, the kidney is unable to secrete the daily production of fixed acid. Serum bicarbonate begins to decline when the GFR falls below 40 mL/min/1.73 m².

The acidosis of kidney failure can be associated with either an elevated AG or a normal AG. With mild to moderate reductions in GFR, the anions that comprise the gap are excreted normally; the acidosis reflects decreased ammoniagenesis and is therefore hyperchloremic. As kidney failure worsens, the kidney loses its ability to excrete various anions, and the accumulation of sulfate, phosphate, and other anions produces an elevated AG. Because of better control of phosphorus, more intensive dietary modifications, and earlier initiation of dialysis provided today, even patients who are beginning renal replacement therapy often do not manifest an AG.

Despite a daily net positive acid balance, it is unusual for $[HCO_3^-]$ to fall lower than 15 mmol/L. Why the acidosis of CKD is rarely severe is unclear. Whether this lack of severity is secondary to buffering of the retained protons in bone or to retention of organic anions that are usually lost in the urine but instead are converted to HCO_3^- is controversial. The buffering of protons by bone results in loss of calcium and a negative calcium balance. In addition, chronic acidosis causes protein breakdown, muscle wasting, and a negative nitrogen balance. Maintenance of the acid-base balance close to normal can prevent these consequences.

The metabolic acidosis commonly found in patients with CKD can easily be corrected by oral bicarbonate. Usually, administration of two 650-mg (7.6-mEq) tablets three times a day keeps the serum bicarbonate in the normal range. It is rare that hemodialysis has to be initiated solely for the purpose of correcting the acidosis.

HYPERCHLOREMIC ACIDOSIS

Acidosis associated with a normal AG, called hyperchloremic acidosis (HCMA), has a limited number of causes (**Fig. 8-5**). HCMA can occur in CKD when reduced ammoniagenesis impairs the kidney's ability to excrete the daily acid load. In individuals with normal or near-normal kidney function, cases of HCMA can be divided into those caused by the kidney's failure to reabsorb HCO_3^- or to secrete the daily fixed load of H⁺ (commonly known as RTA) and those in which renal acid-base handling is normal. In contrast to AG acidosis, most cases of HCMA are easily treated with supplemental base.

Renal Causes of Hyperchloremic Metabolic Acidosis

RTA represents a heterogeneous cause of HCMA in which the kidney is unable to maintain acid-base balance despite preservation of normal or near-normal overall kidney function (normal GFR). There is often confusion regarding the

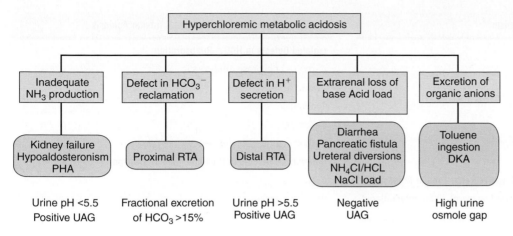

FIGURE 8-5 The etiology of hyperchloremic metabolic acidosis. Shown at the bottom are useful diagnostic tools. AG, anion gap; DKA, diabetic ketoacidosis; PHA, pseudohypoaldosteronism; RTA, renal tubular acidosis; UAG, urine anion gap.

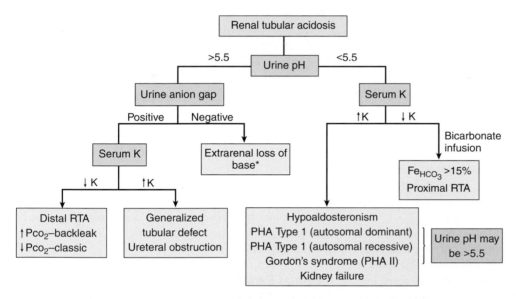

FIGURE 8-6 Evaluation of renal tubular acidosis. By following this algorithm the type of renal defect can be determined. FE_{HCO_3}, fractional excretion of bicarbonate; PHA, pseudohypoaldosteronism; RTA, renal tubular acidosis. *Extrarenal loss of base is not a form of renal tubular acidosis.

various RTAs, because no standard nomenclature exists, numerous diverse transport defects have been identified, and the literature often presents contradictory information. A grasp of the underlying pathophysiology makes the approach to these disorders more comprehensible. The RTAs can be divided into four major categories: (1) primary defects in ammoniagenesis, (2) hypoaldosteronism, (3) disorders of the proximal tubule, and (4) disorders of the distal tubule. The distal tubule defects can be further divided into those associated with hypokalemia and those associated with hyperkalemia (**Fig. 8-6**).

Defective Ammoniagenesis

One of the most common causes of an HCMA is inability of the kidney to generate ammonia because of CKD (see **Fig. 8-4**). By definition, RTA refers to a specific acid excretory defect occurring despite the presence of normal or near-normal kidney function, and it bears emphasis that the HCMA of CKD is not classified as an RTA. As the number of nephrons decreases with development of CKD, there is a proportional decrease in the production of ammonia. As mentioned in the

section on AG acidosis, when the GFR falls to less than 40 mL/min/1.73 m², the kidney is unable to excrete the daily acid load and [HCO_3^-] begins to decline, with a concomitant increase in the serum [Cl^-], producing HCMA. Only when the GFR is lower than 15 to 20 mL/min/1.73 m² does the kidney lose the ability to secrete anions, thus converting this HCMA into an AG acidosis. It needs to be stressed that the acidosis in kidney failure, whether manifested by hyperchloremia or by an AG, is primarily caused by defective ammoniagenesis. Therefore, the UAG will be positive because of the decrease in ammonia excretion, whereas the urine pH will be less than 5.5.

Hypoaldosteronism

Primary or secondary hypoaldosteronism results from common disorders causing hyperkalemia and metabolic acidosis (**Table 8-4**). Hyporeninemic hypoaldosteronism (type IV RTA) is the most frequently encountered variety. This disorder is usually seen in patients with diabetes and mild CKD. The precise cause of hyporeninemia has not been clearly defined. The finding that hypertension is frequently present

TABLE 8-4   Causes of Hypoaldosteronism
Primary Hypoaldosteronism
Addison's disease
Congenital enzyme defects
Drugs
Heparin
Angiotensin-converting enzyme inhibitors
Angiotensin receptor blockers
Hyporeninemic Hypoaldosteronism (Type IV Renal Tubular Acidosis)
Pseudohypoaldosteronism I (Autosomal Dominant)—Mineralocorticoid Resistance

TABLE 8-5   Causes of Proximal Renal Tubular Acidosis
Isolated Defects in HCO_3^- Reabsorption
Carbonic anhydrase inhibitors
Acetazolamide
Topiramate
Sulfamylon
Carbonic anhydrase deficiency
Generalized Defects in Proximal Tubular Transport
Cystinosis
Wilson's disease
Lowe's syndrome
Galactosemia
Multiple myeloma
Light chain disease
Amyloidosis
Vitamin D deficiency
Ifosfamide
Cidofovir
Lead
Aminoglycosides

and that the disorder may be partly reversed with chronic furosemide use suggests that the renin suppression may be secondary to chronic volume overload. Neither has the cause of the hypoaldosteronism been fully explained. Renin lack alone should not cause hypoaldosteronism, because hyperkalemia is a potent stimulus to aldosterone secretion, and anephric individuals still secrete aldosterone. The acidosis is primarily caused by decreased ammoniagenesis as a result of the associated hyperkalemia induced by the aldosterone deficiency. Hypoaldosteronism, by diminishing distal sodium reabsorption, also results in a less negative lumen potential, thus decreasing the rate of H^+ secretion but not the electromotive force of the pump. Because the hydrogen pump is not defective, urine pH is usually less than 5.5.

Patients with type IV RTA are usually asymptomatic, with only minor laboratory abnormalities (mild hyperkalemia and decreased $[HCO_3^-]$). However, whenever renal potassium handling is further perturbed by various stressors, hyperkalemia ensues with a decline in ammoniagenesis. Such stressors include sodium depletion, which decreases delivery of sodium to the distal tubule; high-potassium diet; and use of potassium-sparing diuretics or medications that further decrease renin and aldosterone levels, such as angiotensin-converting enzyme inhibitors, angiotensin receptor blockers, nonsteroidal anti-inflammatory drugs, or heparin. Most patients can be treated by removal of the insult to potassium homeostasis, restriction of potassium intake, and provision of supplemental bicarbonate. Proof that type IV RTA is present requires the demonstration of low renin and aldosterone levels after sodium depletion. Because of practical considerations, these tests are rarely ordered, and most cases are treated empirically.

Autosomal-dominant pseudohypoaldosteronism (PHA) type I is an uncommon disorder caused by a mutation in the renal mineralocorticoid receptor that results in decreased affinity for aldosterone. This genetic disorder manifests in childhood with hyperaldosteronism, hyperkalemia, metabolic acidosis, salt wasting, and hypotension. Autosomal-dominant PHA type I becomes less severe with age. Carbenoxolone (no longer available in the United States) and glycyrrhizic acid (found in true licorice) both inhibit

11-β-hydroxysteroid dehydrogenase, the enzyme in the kidney that converts cortisol (which binds the mineralocorticoid receptor) to cortisone (which does not). They can be used to treat PHA type I by increasing the intrarenal supply of mineralocorticoid.

Proximal Renal Tubular Acidosis

Proximal RTA, often called type II RTA because it was the second type described, is a defect in the ability of the proximal tubule to reclaim filtered HCO_3^- (**Table 8-5**). In type II RTA, the proximal tubule has a diminished threshold (approximately 15 mmol/L instead of the normal 24 mmol/L) for HCO_3^- reabsorption. When the plasma $[HCO_3^-]$ falls below this threshold, complete reabsorption occurs. Proximal RTA can be congenital or acquired, and it may exist as an isolated defect in HCO_3^- reabsorption or as part of a more generalized transport defect known as Fanconi's syndrome, in which there is diminished reabsorption of other solutes across the proximal tubule as well. Patients with proximal RTA and Fanconi's syndrome, in addition to the loss of HCO_3^-, inappropriately excrete amino acids, glucose, phosphorous, and uric acid in their urine.

As would be expected, mutations in the Na^+/H^+ exchanger on the luminal membrane, the Na^+-HCO_3^- cotransporter on the basolateral membrane, and cytosolic carbonic anhydrase have all been implicated in the isolated hereditary and sporadic forms of proximal RTA. Several drugs that block carbonic anhydrase, including the diuretic acetazolamide and the anticonvulsant topiramate, also cause isolated HCO_3^- wasting. Proximal RTA with Fanconi's syndrome is frequently found in patients with cystinosis, Wilson's disease, Lowe's syndrome, multiple myeloma, or light chain disease, among others. A decrease in ATP production, which reduces basolateral Na^+,K^+-ATPase activity, is the presumed cause of this global transport defect. Drugs, particularly the cyclophosphamide analogue, ifosfamide, and cidofovir, which is used in the treatment of cytomegalovirus retinitis, have also been associated with a generalized proximal tubulopathy.

Because distal H^+ excretion is normal, the urine pH during steady state, when the $[HCO_3^-]$ is below the lowered threshold and bicarbonaturia is absent, will be less than 5.5. At the same time, the serum $[HCO_3^-]$ will be between 15 and 18 mEq/L. It is important to recognize that whenever the $[HCO_3^-]$ increases above the reabsorptive threshold, HCO_3^- will appear in the urine and the pH will be greater than 6.5. Although ammoniagenesis is preserved in proximal RTA, direct or indirect measurement of urine NH_4^+ may reveal an inappropriately low excretion. This can occur because HCO_3^-, which escapes proximal reabsorption, serves as a buffer sink for secreted H^+, thus reducing the trapping of NH_4^+. The diagnosis of proximal RTA is established by demonstrating a fractional excretion of HCO_3^- greater than 15% while supplemental bicarbonate is administered in an attempt to increase the serum bicarbonate to normal.

Treatment of proximal RTA is difficult, because administered base is rapidly excreted in the urine. Because extremely large amounts of base (10 to 15 mmol/kg/day) are frequently needed, compliance is limited. The increased delivery of HCO_3^- to the distal nephron induces or exacerbates hypokalemia. It is recommended that frequent doses of a mixture of sodium and potassium salts of bicarbonate and the better-tolerated citrate be used.

Distal Renal Tubular Acidosis

Classic Distal Renal Tubular Acidosis with Hypokalemia

Distal RTA, also known as type I RTA, represents the inability of the distal tubule to acidify the urine (**Table 8-6**). As with proximal RTA, the distal variety can be congenital or acquired. Abnormalities have been identified in both the luminal H^+-ATPase and the basolateral Cl^-/HCO_3^- exchanger (AE1). The acquired form is associated with autoimmune diseases, especially systemic lupus erythematosus and Sjöögren's syndrome; dysproteinemia; and kidney transplant rejection. Immunocytochemical studies have revealed decreased staining of the AE1 in patients with the acquired form of distal RTA. Ifosfamide, which is also associated with a proximal RTA, can also cause a distal defect. Amphotericin, which literally punches holes in membranes forming ion channels, causes a distal RTA by allowing backleak of protons across the luminal membrane. The classic finding in type I RTA is an inappropriately high urine pH (>5.5).

Because H^+ secretion is defective in distal RTA, less NH_4^+ can be trapped in the lumen of the tubule, and the UAG will be positive, reflecting this decrease in NH_4^+ excretion. In addition to an inappropriately high urine pH and a positive UAG, distal RTA can be further characterized by measuring urine PCO_2 during an HCO_3^- infusion. Distal delivery

TABLE 8-6 Causes of Distal Renal Tubular Acidosis with Hypokalemia
Familial
Defective HCO_3^-/Cl^- Exchanger (AE1) (Autosomal Dominant)
Defective H^+-ATPase (autosomal recessive)
Endemic
Thai endemic distal renal tubular acidosis
Drugs
Amphotericin
Toluene
Lithium
Ifosfamide
Foscarnet
Vanadium
Systemic disorder
Sjögren's syndrome
Cryoglobulinemia
Systemic lupus erythematosus
Kidney transplant rejection

of HCO_3^- in the presence of a normal H^+ secretory capacity results in elevated PCO_2 in the urine. If there is a H^+ secretory defect, the urine PCO_2 will not increase. In amphotericin-induced RTA, in which H^+ ion secretion is unaffected, urine PCO_2 increases normally, as would be expected.

Occasionally, it can be difficult to distinguish HCMA induced by diarrhea from a distal RTA. Diarrhea results in HCMA and hypokalemia. Because the hypokalemia increases renal ammoniagenesis, urine pH may be inappropriately elevated. Therefore, on the surface, both forms of acidosis appear similar. However, measurement of the UAG easily distinguishes the markedly elevated urine NH_4^+ and negative AG, found in diarrheal illness, from the low NH_4^+ excretion and positive AG, found with distal RTA. The one caveat is that sodium must be delivered to the distal tubule, as shown by a urine Na^+ greater than 20 mmol/L.

Classic distal RTA is associated with hypokalemia (due to augmented distal K^+ secretion in lieu of H^+ secretion in exchange for Na^+ reabsorption), hypocitraturia (from augmented proximal tubule cell reabsorption), hypercalciuria (from the buffering of H^+ in bone and loss of calcium), and nephrocalcinosis. The treatment of distal RTA consists in simply supplying enough base (2 to 3 mmol/kg/day) to counter the daily fixed production of acid. This can be administered as a mixture of sodium and potassium salts of either bicarbonate or citrate.

Distal Renal Tubular Acidosis with Hyperkalemia

Distal RTA with hyperkalemia can be further divided into two broad general categories: (1) a generalized defect of both distal tubular H^+ and K^+ secretion or (2) a primary defect in Na^+ transport often called a "voltage defect" (**Table 8-7**).

TABLE 8-7 Causes of Distal Renal Tubular Acidosis with Hyperkalemia

Lupus Nephritis

Obstructive Nephropathy

Sickle Cell Anemia

Voltage Defects

Familial

Pseudohypoaldosteronism type I (autosomal recessive)

Pseudohypoaldosteronism type II (autosomal recessive)—Gordon's syndrome

Drugs

Amiloride

Triamterene

Trimethoprim

Pentamidine

Generalized Distal Tubule Defect

Unlike classic distal RTA, a more generalized defect of the distal tubule can occur in which both H^+ and K^+ secretion are impaired. This has been best identified in cases of ureteral obstruction and in patients with interstitial kidney disease resulting from sickle cell anemia or systemic lupus erythematosus. In animals with ureteral obstruction, immunocytochemical staining has revealed loss of the apical H^+-ATPase. Why hyperkalemia occurs is less clear. Because K^+ excretion cannot be augmented by diuretics, a primary defect in K^+ transport is likely. As in classic distal RTA, urine pH is greater than 5.5.

Distal Sodium Transport Defects

Several disorders have been characterized by defective sodium transport in the distal tubule. The reabsorption of Na^+ by the distal tubule generates a lumen-negative potential. This electrical negativity helps promote the secretion of K^+ and H^+. Any drug or disorder that interferes with this lumen-negative potential will diminish both K^+ and H^+ secretion. These are commonly classified as voltage defects. Autosomal-recessive PHA type I is a syndrome in which there is loss of function of the epithelial sodium channel (ENaC) in the distal tubule. Numerous mutations have been described in various subunits of this channel. This disease manifests in childhood with marked hyperkalemia, metabolic acidosis, hyperaldosteronism, and salt wasting. Because the ENaC also exists in other tissues, including lung, colon, and sweat glands, patients with this disorder often have symptoms related to these organs. Treatment consists of providing a high salt intake. Drugs that block ENaC produce a similar metabolic picture; these include the potassium-sparing diuretics, amiloride and triamterene, as well as trimethoprim and pentamidine.

Another well-recognized disorder of distal transport is PHA type II, also known as Gordon's syndrome (see Chapter 66). Individuals with this condition have mild volume overload with suppressed renin and aldosterone, hypertension, hyperkalemia, and metabolic acidosis. Mutations in two members of a family of serine-threonine kinases, WNK1 and WNK4 (*With No K* [K = lysine]) have been shown to be the cause of this syndrome. These kinases appear to have an important role in the regulation of Cl^- transport in numerous tissues. It appears that defects in these kinases result in an increase in the number of neutral NaCl transporters (NCCT) and therefore increase NaCl transport across the distal convoluted tubule. Less sodium is delivered to the more distal tubule segments for reabsorption, which curtails the generation of the lumen-negative potential, resulting in decreased H^+ and K^+ secretion. Supporting this hypothesis is the fact that Gordon's syndrome can be treated with thiazide-type diuretics, which block the NCCT.

The acidosis in all of these sodium transport disorders is secondary to the decreased H^+ secretion caused by an unfavorable electrical gradient in the distal tubule and the decreased ammoniagenesis caused by the hyperkalemia. Whether the urine pH is less than 5.5 depends on how severely H^+ secretion is affected.

Combined Proximal and Distal Renal Tubular Acidosis

An extremely uncommon disorder, which has been called type III RTA, combines proximal and distal RTA. As would be expected, both proximal HCO_3^- reabsorption and distal H^+ secretion are impaired. Mutations in the gene for cytosolic carbonic anhydrase can cause such a defect. As discussed earlier, ifosfamide can also cause a combined defect.

Incomplete Distal Renal Tubular Acidosis

Patients with incomplete distal RTA come to medical attention because of calcium stone disease and nephrocalcinosis. The serum $[HCO_3^-]$ is normal, but urine pH never falls below 5.5, even after acid loading with NH_4Cl or $CaCl_2$. This disorder most likely represents a milder form of distal RTA. Frank metabolic acidosis may become evident when patients are stressed by diarrhea or other conditions that require compensation by augmented renal proton secretion.

Extrarenal Causes of Hyperchloremic Metabolic Acidosis

Extrarenal Bicarbonate Loss

Loss of base during episodes of diarrhea or with overzealous use of laxatives is associated with HCMA (see **Fig. 8-5**). Loss of HCO_3^- can also occur with pancreatic fistula or with a pancreas transplant if drainage of the pancreatic duct is into the bladder. Ureteral diversions using an isolated sigmoid loop were frequently associated with bicarbonate loss because of Cl^-/HCO_3^- exchange in the bowel loop. These ureteral-sigmoidostomies have largely been replaced by ureteral diversions using ileal conduits, which have less surface area and less contact time for loss of HCO_3^- to occur. If these conduits become obstructed, however, HCMA can still develop.

Acid Load

An obvious cause of an HCMA is ingestion or infusion of a chloride salt of an acid. Both NH_4Cl and $CaCl_2$ can result in a metabolic acidosis and can be used as a provocative test to assess urinary acidification. In addition, total parenteral nutrition using hydrochloric acid salts of various amino acids can produce a metabolic acidosis if an insufficient quantity of base (usually acetate) is added to the infusion mixture. Another form of acid load is NaCl. Volume resuscitation with 0.9% NaCl often produces an HCMA. This occurs because of "dilution" of the plasma HCO_3^- by the more acidic saline solution (pH 7.0) and because volume expansion diminishes proximal HCO_3^- reabsorption.

Urinary Loss of Anions

As previously discussed, excretion of organic anions in the urine represents a source of base lost from the body. Although this loss involves the kidney, it cannot be viewed as being caused by an intrinsic kidney defect. Because of the low renal threshold for excretion of keto acids, patients with DKA, if they are able to maintain their intravascular volume or are volume resuscitated, will excrete these anions in place of Cl^-. This results in HCMA.

A similar metabolic disturbance exists after toluene exposure. Toluene is a common solvent found in paint products and glues. Exposure is typically by inhalation, either accidental or intentional. Toluene is rapidly absorbed through the skin and mucous membranes and is metabolized to hippuric acid. Hippurate is quickly excreted by the kidney, leaving behind an HCMA. Although hippurate is not a base, its rapid excretion into the urine conceals the AG origins of this disturbance. Both of these disorders are usually easily discovered on taking an adequate history.

BIBLIOGRAPHY

Alper SL: Genetic diseases of acid-base transporters. Annu Rev Physiol 64:899-923, 2002.

Adrogue HJ, Madias NE: Management of life-threatening acid-base disorders. N Engl J Med 338:26-34. 107–111, 1998.

Bonny O, Rossier B: Disturbances of Na/K balance: Pseudohypoaldosteronism revisited. J Am Soc Nephrol 13:2399-2414, 2002.

Brent J, McMartin K, Phillips S, et al: Fomepizole for the treatment of methanol poisoning. N Engl J Med 344:424-429, 2001.

Carlisle EJ, Donnelly SM, Vasuvattakul S, et al: Glue-sniffing and distal renal tubular acidosis: Sticking to the facts. J Am Soc Nephrol 1:1019-1027, 1991.

Chang CT, Chen YC, Fang JT, Huang CC: Metformin-associated lactic acidosis: Case reports and literature review. J Nephrol 15: 398–394, 2002.

Claessens YE, Cariou A, Monchi M, et al: Detecting life- threatening lactic acidosis related to nucleoside-analog treatment of human immunodeficiency virus-infected patients, and treatment with L-carnitine. Crit Care Med 31:1042-1047, 2003.

Dargan PI, Wallace CI, Jones AL: An evidence based flowchart to guide the management of acute salicylate (aspirin) overdose. Emerg Med J 19:206-209, 2002.

DuBose TD Jr, Mcdonald GA: Renal tubular acidosis. In Dubose TD, Hamm LL Jr (eds): Acid-Base and Electrolyte Disorders: A Companion to Brenner and Rector's The Kidney. Philadelphia, WB Saunders, 2002, pp 189-206.

Figge J, Jabor A, Kazda A: Anion gap and hypoalbuminemia. Crit Care Med 26:1807-1810, 1998.

Fraser AD: Clinical toxicologic implications of ethylene glycol and glycolic acid poisoning. Ther Drug Monit 24:232-238, 2002.

Han J, Kim G-H, Kim J, et al: Secretory-defect distal renal tubular acidosis is associated with transporter defect in H+-ATPase and anion exchanger-1. J Am Soc Nephrol 13:1425-1432, 2002.

Hood VL, Tannen RL: Protection of acid-base balance by pH regulation of acid production. N Engl J Med 339:819-826, 1998.

Igarashi T, Sekine T, Inatomi J, Seki G: Unraveling the molecular pathogenesis of isolated proximal renal tubular acidosis. J Am Soc Nephrol 13:2171-2177, 2002.

Ishihara K, Szerlip HM: Anion gap acidosis. Semin Nephrol 18:83-89, 1998.

Izzedine H, Launay-Vacher V, Isnard-Bagnis C, Derray G: Drug-induced Fanconi's syndrome. Am J Kid Dis 41:292-309, 2003.

Karet FE: Inherited distal renal tubular acidosis. J Am Soc Nephrol 13:2178-2184, 2002.

Kirschbaum B, Sica D, Anderson F: Urine electrolytes and the urine anion and osmolar gaps. J Lab Clin Med 133:597-604, 1999.

Lemann J Jr, Bushinsky DA, Hamm LL: Bone buffering of acid and base in humans. Am J Physiol Renal Physiol 285:F811-F832, 2003.

Levraut J, Grimaud D: Treatment of metabolic acidosis. Curr Opin Crit Care 9:260-265, 2003.

Llushine KA, Harris CR, Holger JS: Methanol ingestion: Prevention of toxic sequelae after massive ingestion. J Emerg Med 24:433-436, 2003.

Mycyk MB, Aks SE: A visual schematic for clarifying the temporal relationship between the anion and osmol gap in toxic alcohol poisoning. Am J Emerg Med 21:333-335, 2003.

Ogedegbe AE, Thomas DL, Diehl AM: Hyperlactataemia syndromes associated with HIV therapy. Lancet Infect Dis 3:329-337, 2003.

Oh M, Carrrol H: Value and determinants of the urine anion gap. Nephron 90:252-255, 2002.

Reynolds HN, Teiken P, Regan ME, et al: Hyperlactatemia, increased osmolar gap, and renal dysfunction during continuous lorazepam infusion. Crit Care Med 28:1631-1634, 2000.

Salpeter SR, Greyber E, Pasternak GA, Salpeter EE: Risk of fatal and nonfatal lactic acidosis with metformin use in type 2 diabetes mellitus: Systematic review and meta-analysis. Arch Intern Med 163:2594-2602, 2003.

Soriano J: Renal tubular acidosis: The clinical entity. J Am Soc Nephrol 13:2160-2170, 2002.

Stacpoole PW: Lactic acidosis and other mitochondrial disorders. Metabolism 46:306-321, 1997.

Uribarri J, Oh MS, Carroll HJ: D-lactic acidosis: A review of clinical presentation, biochemical features, and pathophysiologic mechanisms. Medicine 77:73-82, 1998.

CHAPTER 9

Metabolic Alkalosis

Thomas D. DuBose, Jr.

PATHOGENESIS

The pathogenesis of metabolic alkalosis requires both the generation and the maintenance of this disorder. Generation occurs as a result of net gain of bicarbonate ion (HCO_3^-) or net loss of nonvolatile acid (usually HCl by vomiting) from the extracellular fluid. "New" bicarbonate may be generated as a result of both renal and extrarenal disturbances.

Under normal circumstances, the kidneys have an impressive capacity to excrete HCO_3^-. In the maintenance stage of metabolic alkalosis, the kidneys fail to compensate (by excreting HCO_3^-) because of volume contraction, a low glomerular filtration rate (GFR), or depletion of chloride (Cl^-) or potassium (K^+). Continuation of metabolic alkalosis, therefore, represents a failure of the kidneys to eliminate HCO_3^- in the usual manner. Retention rather than excretion of excess alkali by the kidney is promoted when (1) volume deficiency, Cl^- deficiency, and K^+ deficiency exist in combination with a reduced GFR, or (2) hypokalemia prevails because of autonomous hyperaldosteronism. In the first example, alkalosis is corrected by administration of NaCl and KCl, whereas in the latter example it is necessary to repair the alkalosis by pharmacologic or surgical intervention, not with saline administration.

In assessing a patient with metabolic alkalosis, two questions should be considered: (1) What is the source of alkali gain (or acid loss) that generated the alkalosis? and (2) What renal mechanisms are operating to prevent excretion of excess HCO_3^-, thereby maintaining, rather than correcting, the alkalosis?

DIFFERENTIAL DIAGNOSIS

To establish the cause of metabolic alkalosis (**Table 9-1**), it is necessary to assess the extracellular fluid volume (ECV) status, the recumbent and upright blood pressure, the serum potassium concentration ($[K^+]$), and the renin-angiotensin system. For example, the presence of chronic hypertension and chronic hypokalemia in an alkalotic patient suggests either mineralocorticoid excess or a hypertensive patient receiving diuretics. Low plasma renin activity and urine $[Na^+]$ and $[Cl^-]$ values greater than 20 mEq/L in a patient who is not taking diuretics indicate a primary mineralocorticoid excess syndrome.

The combination of hypokalemia and alkalosis in a normotensive, nonedematous patient can pose a difficult problem. Possible causes to be considered are Bartter's or Gitelman's syndrome, magnesium deficiency, vomiting, exogenous alkali, and diuretic ingestion. Determination of urine electrolytes (especially $[Cl^-]$) and screening of the urine for diuretics may be helpful. When the urine chloride concentration is measured (**Table 9-2**), it should be considered in context with assessment of the ECV status of the patient. A low urine $[Cl^-]$ (i.e., <10 mEq/L) indicates avid Cl^- retention by the kidney and denotes ECV depletion even if the urine Na^+ excretion and urine $[Na^+]$ are high (i.e., >15 mEq/L). A high urine $[Cl^-]$, in the absence of concurrent diuretic use, suggests inappropriate chloruresis resulting from a tubular defect or mineralocorticoid excess. If the urine is alkaline, with an elevated $[Na^+]$ and $[K^+]$ but a urine $[Cl^-]$ lower than 10 mEq/L, the diagnosis is usually either vomiting (overt or surreptitious) or alkali ingestion. If the urine is relatively acid and has low concentrations of Na^+, K^+, and Cl^-, the most likely possibilities are prior vomiting, the posthypercapnic state, or prior diuretic ingestion. If, on the other hand, neither the urine $[Na^+]$, $[K^+]$, nor $[Cl^-]$ is depressed, magnesium deficiency, Bartter's or Gitelman's syndrome, or current diuretic ingestion should be considered. Gitelman's syndrome is distinguished from Bartter's syndrome by the presence of hypocalciuria and, on occasion, hypomagnesemia in the former disorder.

METABOLIC ALKALOSIS DUE TO EXOGENOUS BICARBONATE LOADS

Alkali Administration

Administration of base to individuals with normal kidney function rarely causes alkalosis, because the kidney has a high capacity for HCO_3^- excretion. However, in patients with coexistent hemodynamic disturbances, alkalosis may develop, because the normal capacity to excrete HCO_3^- can be exceeded or there may be enhanced reabsorption of HCO_3^-. Examples include patients receiving oral or intravenous HCO_3^-, acetate loads (parenteral hyperalimentation solutions), citrate loads (transfusions, continuous renal replacement therapy, or infant formula), or antacids plus cation-exchange resins (aluminum hydroxide and sodium polystyrene sulfonate).

Chronic administration of alkali to individuals with normal kidney function results in minimal, if any, alkalosis. In

TABLE 9-1 Causes of Metabolic Alkalosis

Exogenous HCO$_3^-$ Loads	**ECV Expansion, Hypertension, K$^+$ Deficiency, and Hypermineralocorticoidism**
Acute alkali administration	*Associated with high renin*
Milk-alkali syndrome	Renal artery stenosis
Use of crack cocaine in ESRD	Accelerated hypertension
Baking soda pica in pregnancy	Renin-secreting tumor
Bicarbonate precursors (citrate, acetate) in chronic or acute kidney disease	Estrogen therapy
Effective ECV Contraction, Normotension, K$^+$ Deficiency, and Secondary Hyperreninemic Hyperaldosteronism	*Associated with low renin*

Gastrointestinal origin	Primary aldosteronism
	  Adenoma
	  Hyperplasia
	  Carcinoma
	  Glucocorticoid suppressible

Vomiting	
Gastric aspiration	

Congenital chloridorrhea	Adrenal enzymatic defects
	  11β-Hydroxylase deficiency
	  17α-Hydroxylase deficiency

Villous adenoma	

Combined administration of sodium polystyrene sulfonate (Kayexalate) and aluminum hydroxide)	Cushing's syndrome or disease
	  Ectopic corticotropin
	  Adrenal carcinoma
	  Adrenal adenoma
	  Primary pituitary

Cystic fibrosis and volume depletion	
Renal origin	
Diuretics (especially thiazides and loop diuretics)	*Other*
Edematous states	Licorice
Posthypercapnic state	Carbenoxolone
Hypercalcemia–hypoparathyroidism	Chewing tobacco
Recovery from lactic acidosis or ketoacidosis	Lydia Pinkham tablets
Nonreabsorbable anions (e.g., penicillin, carbenicillin)	**Gain-of-Function Mutation of ENaC with ECV Expansion, Hypertension, K$^+$ Deficiency, and Hyporeninemic Hypoaldosteronism**
Mg^{2+} deficiency	Liddle's syndrome
K$^+$ depletion	
Bartter's syndrome (loss-of-function mutation of Cl$^-$ transport in TAL)	
Gitelman's syndrome (loss-of-function mutation in Na$^+$-Cl$^-$ cotransporter)	
Carbohydrate refeeding after starvation	

ECV, extracellular fluid volume; ENaC, epithelial sodium channel; ESRD, end-stage renal disease; TAL, thick ascending limb of the loop of Henle.

patients with acute or chronic kidney functional impairment, overt alkalosis can develop after alkali administration because the capacity to excrete HCO$_3^-$ is exceeded or because coexistent hemodynamic disturbances have caused enhanced HCO$_3^-$ reabsorption.

A dramatic example of acute metabolic alkalosis resulting from alkali ingestion is the association of a pica for baking soda and pregnancy.

Additionally, the use of crack cocaine has been described as a cause of severe alkalosis in patients undergoing hemodialysis. "Free-basing" involves the addition of alkali (NaOH as drain cleaner) to cocaine hydrochloride.

Milk-Alkali Syndrome

A long-standing history of excessive ingestion of milk and antacids is an unusual but historically important cause of metabolic alkalosis. Both hypercalcemia and vitamin D excess

increase renal HCO3$^-$ reabsorption. A critical component of this syndrome is renal insufficiency. Patients with this disorder are prone to develop nephrocalcinosis, renal function impairment, and metabolic alkalosis. Discontinuation of alkali ingestion is usually sufficient to repair the alkalosis, but the kidney disease may be irreversible if nephrocalcinosis is advanced.

METABOLIC ALKALOSIS ASSOCIATED WITH EXTRACELLULAR FLUID VOLUME CONTRACTION, K$^+$ DEPLETION, AND SECONDARY HYPERRENINEMIC HYPERALDOSTERONISM

Gastrointestinal Origin

Gastrointestinal loss of H$^+$, Cl$^-$, Na$^+$, and K$^+$ from vomitus or gastric aspiration results in retention of HCO$_3^-$. The loss of fluid and electrolytes results in contraction of the ECV and stimulation of the renin-angiotensin system. Volume contraction causes a reduction in GFR and an enhanced capacity of the renal tubule to reabsorb HCO_3^-. Excess angiotensin stimulates Na^+/H^+ exchange in the proximal tubule. During active vomiting, there is continued addition of HCO_3^- to plasma in exchange for Cl^-, and the plasma $[HCO_3^-]$ exceeds the reabsorptive capacity of the proximal tubule. Aldosterone and endothelin also stimulate the proton-transporting adenosine triphosphatase (H^+-ATPase) in the distal nephron, so the capacity for distal nephron HCO_3^- absorption is enhanced paradoxically. When the excess $NaHCO_3$ reaches the distal tubule, potassium secretion is enhanced by aldosterone and the delivery of the poorly reabsorbed anion, HCO_3^-. Thus, the predominant cause of the hypokalemia is renal, rather than gastrointestinal, potassium wasting.

Hypokalemia has selective effects on renal bicarbonate absorption and ammonium production that are counterproductive. Hypokalemia dramatically increases the activity of the proton pump (H^+,K^+-ATPase) in the cortical collecting tubule to reabsorb K^+, but at the expense of enhanced net acid excretion and HCO_3^- absorption. Hypokalemia also increases ammonium production independently of acid-base status, which in the face of enhanced H^+ secretion results in increased ammonium excretion and the addition of new bicarbonate to the systemic circulation. Therefore, hypokalemia plays an important role in the seemingly maladaptive response of the kidney to maintain the alkalosis. Because of contraction of the ECV and hypochloremia, Cl^- is avidly conserved by the kidney. This can be recognized clinically by a low urinary chloride concentration (see **Table 9-2**). Correction of the contracted ECV with NaCl and repair of K^+ deficits correct the acid-base disorder.

Congenital Chloridorrhea

Congenital chloridorrhea is a rare autosomal-recessive disorder causes metabolic alkalosis by an extrarenal mechanism and is associated with severe diarrhea, fecal acid loss, and HCO_3^- retention. The disease is the result of mutations in the *SLC26A3* gene that disrupt the ileal and colonic Cl^-/HCO_3^- anion exchange mechanism so that Cl^- cannot be reabsorbed. The parallel Na^+/H^+ ion exchanger remains functional, allowing Na^+ to be reabsorbed and H^+ to be secreted. Therefore, the stool is high in H^+ and Cl^-, causing Na^+ and HCO_3^- retention in the extracellular fluid. The alkalosis is sustained by concomitant ECV contraction, hyperaldosteronism, and K^+ deficiency. Delivery of Cl^- to the distal nephron is low because of volume contraction. As in cystic fibrosis, this low delivery of HCO_3^- results in impaired HCO_3^- secretion by the β-intercalated cell.

Therapy consists of oral supplements of sodium and potassium chloride. Recently, the use of proton pump inhibitors has been advanced as a means of reducing chloride secretion by the parietal cells and thus reducing the diarrhea. The long-term outcome is good with daily supplementation of NaCl and KCl.

TABLE 9-2 Diagnosis of Metabolic Alkalosis

LOW URINARY [CL⁻] (<10 MEQ/L)	HIGH OR NORMAL URINARY [CL⁻] (>15-20 MEQ/L)
Normotensive	**Hypertensive**
Vomiting, nasogastric	Primary aldosteronism
Aspiration	Cushing's syndrome
Diuretics	Renal artery stenosis
Posthypercapnia	Renal failure plus alkali therapy
Bicarbonate treatment of organic acidosis	**Normotensive**
K^+ deficiency	Mg^{2+} deficiency
Hypertensive	Severe K^+ deficiency
Liddle's syndrome	Bartter's syndrome
	Gitelman's syndrome
	Diuretics

Use of Citrate in Continuous Renal Replacement Therapy

If citrate is employed for anticoagulation regionally in patients at high risk for bleeding, or if there is a contraindication to heparin, metabolic alkalosis should be expected. The metabolism of citrate by the liver and skeletal muscle results in net gain of HCO_3^-. Strategies have been advanced to reduce the complications of regional trisodium citrate anticoagulation (hypocalcemia, metabolic alkalosis, use of 0.1 N HCl, and subsequent hyponatremia) by using anticoagulant citrate dextrose formula A.

Villous Adenoma

Metabolic alkalosis has been described in cases of villous adenoma. K^+ depletion probably causes the alkalosis, because colonic secretion is alkaline.

Renal Origin

The generation of metabolic alkalosis through renal mechanisms involves three characteristics to increase distal nephron H^+ secretion and enhance net acid excretion (ammonium excretion): (1) high delivery of Na^+ salts to the distal nephron, (2) excessive elaboration of mineralocorticoids, and (3) K^+ deficiency.

Diuretics

Drugs that induce distal delivery of sodium salts, such as thiazides and loop diuretics (furosemide, bumetanide, torsemide, and ethacrynic acid), diminish ECV without altering total body bicarbonate content. Consequently, the serum $[HCO_3^-]$ increases. The chronic administration of diuretics generates a metabolic alkalosis by increasing distal salt delivery, so that secretion of K^+ and H^+ is stimulated. The alkalosis is maintained by persistence of the contraction of the ECV, secondary hyperaldosteronism, K^+ deficiency, and activation of the H^+,K^+-ATPase, as long as diuretic administration continues. The hypokalemia also enhances ammonium production and excretion.

Repair of the alkalosis is achieved by withholding the diuretic, providing isotonic saline to correct the ECV deficit, and correcting the potassium deficit.

Bartter's Syndrome

Both classic Bartter's syndrome and the antenatal type are inherited as autosomal-recessive disorders and involve impairments in salt absorption in the thick ascending limb of the loop of Henle (TAL); this results in salt wasting, volume depletion, and activation of the renin-angiotensin system. These manifestations are the result of loss-of-function mutations of one of the genes that encode three transporters involved in vectorial NaCl absorption in the TAL. The most prevalent disorder is a mutation of the gene *NKCC2*, which encodes the bumetanide-sensitive Na^+-K^+-$2Cl^-$ cotransporter on the apical membrane. A second mutation has been discovered in the gene *KCNJ1*, which encodes the ATP-sensitive apical K^+ conductance channel (ROMK) that operates in parallel with the Na^+-K^+-$2Cl^-$ cotransporter to recycle K^+. Both defects can be associated with antenatal Bartter's syndrome or with classic Bartter's syndrome. A mutation of the *CLCNKb* gene encoding the voltage-gated basolateral chloride channel (ClC-Kb) is associated only with classic Bartter's syndrome and is milder and rarely associated with nephrocalcinosis. All three defects have the same net effect: loss of Cl^- transport in the TAL.

Antenatal Bartter's syndrome has been observed in consanguineous families in association with sensorineural deafness, a syndrome linked to chromosome 1p31. The responsible gene, *BSND*, encodes a subunit, barttin, that co-localizes with the ClC-Kb channel in the TAL and K^+-secreting epithelial cells in the inner ear. Barttin appears to be necessary for function of the voltage-gated chloride channel. Expression of ClC-Kb is lost when coexpressed with mutant barttins. Therefore, mutations in *BSND* define a fourth category of patients with Bartter's syndrome.

Such defects predictably lead to ECV contraction, hyperreninemic hyperaldosteronism, and increased delivery of Na^+ to the distal nephron, with consequent alkalosis, renal K^+ wasting, and hypokalemia. Secondary overproduction of prostaglandins, juxtaglomerular apparatus hypertrophy, and vascular pressor unresponsiveness then ensue. Most patients have hypercalciuria and normal serum magnesium levels, distinguishing this disorder from Gitelman's syndrome.

Bartter's syndrome is inherited as an autosomal-recessive defect, and, in studies, most patients have been homozygotes or compound heterozygotes for different mutations in one of these four genes. A few patients with the clinical syndrome have no discernible mutation in any of these genes. Plausible explanations include unrecognized mutations in other genes, a dominant-negative effect of a heterozygous mutation, or other mechanisms. Recently, two groups of investigators reported features of Bartter's syndrome in patients with autosomal-dominant hypocalcemia and activating mutations in calcium-sensing receptor, CaSR. Activation of CaSR on the basolateral cell surface of the TAL inhibits function of ROMK. Therefore, mutations in CaSR may represent a fifth gene associated with Bartter's syndrome.

For diagnosis, Bartter's syndrome must be distinguished from surreptitious vomiting, diuretic administration, and laxative abuse. The finding of a low urinary Cl^- concentration is helpful in identifying the vomiting patient (see **Table 9-2**). The urinary Cl^- concentration in a patient with Bartter's syndrome would be expected to be normal or increased, rather than depressed.

The therapy for Bartter's syndrome focuses on repair of the hypokalemia through inhibition of the renin-angiotensin-aldosterone system or the prostaglandin-kinin system, using propranolol, amiloride, spironolactone, prostaglandin inhibitors, and angiotensin-converting enzyme inhibitors, as well as direct repletion of the deficits with potassium and magnesium.

Gitelman's Syndrome

Patients with Gitelman's syndrome resemble the Bartter's syndrome phenotype in that an autosomal-recessive chloride-resistant metabolic alkalosis is associated with hypokalemia, a normal to low blood pressure, volume depletion with secondary hyperreninemic hyperaldosteronism, and juxtaglomerular hyperplasia. However, the consistent presence of hypocalciuria and the frequent presence of hypomagnesemia are useful in distinguishing Gitelman's syndrome from Bartter's syndrome on clinical grounds. These unique features mimic the effects of chronic thiazide diuretic administration. A large number of missense mutations in the gene *SLC12A3*, which encodes the thiazide-sensitive sodium chloride cotransporter in the distal convoluted tubule (NCCT), have been described and account for the clinical features, including the classic finding of hypocalciuria. However, it is not clear why these patients have pronounced hypomagnesemia. A recent study demonstrated that peripheral blood mononuclear cells from patients with Gitelman's syndrome express mutated NCCT messenger RNA (mRNA). In a large consanguineous Bedouin family, missense mutations were noted in *CLCNKb*, but the clinical features overlapped between Gitelman's and Bartter's syndromes.

Compared with Bartter's syndrome, Gitelman's syndrome becomes symptomatic later in life and is associated with milder salt wasting. A large study of adults with proven Gitelman's syndrome and NCCT mutations showed that salt craving, nocturia, cramps, and fatigue were more common than in sex- and age-matched controls. Women experienced exacerbation of symptoms during menses, and many had complicated pregnancies.

Treatment of Gitelman's syndrome, as with Bartter's syndrome, consists of liberal dietary sodium and potassium salts, but with the addition of magnesium supplementation in most patients. Angiotensin-converting enzyme inhibitors have been suggested to be helpful in selected patients but may cause frank hypotension.

Nonreabsorbable Anions and Magnesium Deficiency

Administration of large quantities of nonreabsorbable anions, such as penicillin or carbenicillin, can enhance distal acidification and K^+ secretion by increasing the transepithelial potential difference (negative lumen potential). Mg^{2+} deficiency frequently accompanies hypokalemia, and both electrolyte abnormalities must be corrected to ameliorate the metabolic alkalosis.

Potassium Depletion

Pure K^+ depletion causes metabolic alkalosis, although usually of only modest severity. Hypokalemia independently enhances renal ammonium production, which increases net acid excretion and, thereby, the return of "new" bicarbonate to the systemic circulation. When access to salt and K^+ is restricted, more severe alkalosis develops. Activation of the renal H^+,K^+-ATPase in the collecting duct by chronic hypokalemia probably plays a major role in maintenance of the alkalosis. Specifically, chronic hypokalemia has been shown to markedly increase the abundance of the colonic H^+,K^+-ATPase mRNA and protein in the outer medullary collecting duct.

Alkalosis associated with severe K^+ depletion is resistant to salt administration. Repair of the K^+ deficiency is necessary to correct the alkalosis.

After Treatment of Lactic Acidosis or Ketoacidosis

When an underlying stimulus for the generation of lactic acid or keto acid is removed rapidly, as with repair of circulatory insufficiency or with insulin therapy, the lactate or ketones are metabolized to yield an equivalent amount of HCO_3^-. Other sources of new HCO_3^- are additive to the original amount generated by organic anion metabolism to create a surfeit of HCO_3^-. Such sources include new HCO_3^- added to the blood by the kidneys as a result of enhanced acid excretion during the preexisting period of acidosis and alkali therapy during the treatment phase of the acidosis. Acidosis-induced contraction of the ECV and K^+ deficiency act to sustain the alkalosis.

Posthypercapnia

Prolonged CO_2 retention with chronic respiratory acidosis enhances renal HCO_3^- absorption and the generation of new HCO_3^- (increased net acid excretion). If the partial pressure of carbon dioxide in arterial blood ($Paco_2$) is returned to normal by mechanical ventilation or other means, metabolic alkalosis results from the persistently elevated [HCO_3^-]. Associated ECV contraction does not allow complete repair of the alkalosis by correction of the $Paco_2$ alone, and alkalosis persists until isotonic saline is infused.

METABOLIC ALKALOSIS ASSOCIATED WITH EXTRACELLULAR FLUID VOLUME EXPANSION, HYPERTENSION, AND HYPERALDOSTERONISM

Mineralocorticoid administration or excess production (due to primary aldosteronism of Cushing's syndrome or adrenal cortical enzyme defects) increases net acid excretion and

may result in metabolic alkalosis, which may be worsened by associated K^+ deficiency. ECV expansion from salt retention causes hypertension and antagonizes the reduction in GFR or increases tubule acidification induced by aldosterone and by K^+ deficiency. The kaliuresis persists and causes continued K^+ depletion with polydipsia, inability to concentrate the urine, and polyuria. Increased aldosterone levels may be the result of autonomous primary adrenal overproduction or of secondary aldosterone release due to renal overproduction of renin. In both situations, the normal feedback of ECV on net aldosterone production is disrupted, and hypertension from volume retention can result (see **Table 9-2**).

Liddle's Syndrome

Liddle's syndrome is associated with severe hypertension presenting in childhood, accompanied by hypokalemic metabolic alkalosis. These features resemble those of primary hyperaldosteronism, but the renin and aldosterone levels are suppressed (pseudohyperaldosteronism). Liddle originally described patients with low renin and low aldosterone levels that did not respond to spironolactone. The defect is inherited as an autosomal-dominant form of monogenic hypertension and has been localized to chromosome 16q. The disorder is attributed to an inherited abnormality in the gene that encodes the β or the γ subunit of the renal epithelial Na^+ channel (ENaC) at the apical membrane of principal cells in the cortical collecting duct, leading to constitutive activation of this channel. Either mutation results in deletion of the cytoplasmic tail (C-terminus) of the affected subunit. The C-termini contain a PY amino acid motif that is highly conserved, and essentially all mutations in Liddle's syndrome patients involve disruption or deletion of this motif. Such PY motifs are important in regulating the number of sodium channels in the luminal membrane by binding to the WW domains of the Nedd4-like family of ubiquitin protein ligases. Disruption of the PY motif dramatically increases the surface localization of the ENaC complex, because these channels are not internalized or degraded (Nedd4 pathway) but remain activated on the cell surface. Persistent Na^+ absorption eventuates in volume expansion, hypertension, hypokalemia, and metabolic alkalosis.

Glucocorticoid-Remediable Hyperaldosteronism

Glucocorticoid-remediable hyperaldosteronism is an autosomal-dominant form of hypertension, the features of which resemble those of primary aldosteronism (hypokalemic metabolic alkalosis and volume-dependent hypertension). In this disorder, however, glucocorticoid administration corrects the hypertension as well as the excessive excretion of 18-hydroxysteroid in the urine. This disorder results from unequal crossing over between the two genes located in close proximity on chromosome 8, which is the glucocorticoid-responsive promoter region of the gene encoding the 11-β-hydroxylase (*CYP11B1*), where it is joined to the structural portion of the *CYP11B2* gene encoding aldosterone synthase. The chimeric gene produces excess amounts of aldosterone synthase; this is unresponsive to serum potassium or renin levels but is suppressed by glucocorticoid administration. Although this syndrome is a rare cause of primary aldosteronism, it is important to identify it, because treatment differs, and because the syndrome can be associated with severe hypertension, stroke, and accelerated hypertension during pregnancy.

Cushing's Disease or Syndrome

Abnormally high glucocorticoid production due to adrenal adenoma or carcinoma or to ectopic corticotropin production causes metabolic alkalosis. The alkalosis may be ascribed to coexisting mineralocorticoid (deoxycorticosterone and corticosterone) hypersecretion. Alternatively, glucocorticoids may have the capability of enhancing net acid secretion and NH_4^+ production, which may be caused by occupancy of cellular mineralocorticoid receptors.

Miscellaneous Conditions

Ingestion of licorice or licorice-containing chewing tobacco can cause a typical pattern of mineralocorticoid excess. The glycyrrhizinic acid contained in genuine licorice inhibits 11β-hydroxysteroid dehydrogenase. This enzyme is responsible for converting cortisol to cortisone, an essential step in protecting the mineralocorticoid receptor from cortisol. When the enzyme is inactivated, cortisol is allowed to occupy type I renal mineralocorticoid receptors, mimicking aldosterone. Genetic apparent mineralocorticoid excess (AME) resembles excessive ingestion of licorice, with volume expansion, low renin and aldosterone levels, and a salt-sensitive form of hypertension that may include metabolic alkalosis and hypokalemia. The hypertension responds to thiazides and spironolactone but without abnormal steroid products in the urine. In genetic AME, 11β-hydroxysteroid dehydrogenase is defective, and monogenic hypertension develops.

SYMPTOMS OF METABOLIC ALKALOSIS

Patients with metabolic alkalosis experience changes in central and peripheral nervous system function similar to those of hypocalcemia. Symptoms include mental confusion, obtundation, and a predisposition to seizures, paresthesia, muscular cramping, tetany, aggravation of arrhythmias, and hypoxemia in chronic obstructive pulmonary disease. Related electrolyte abnormalities include hypokalemia and hypophosphatemia.

TREATMENT OF METABOLIC ALKALOSIS

The maintenance of metabolic alkalosis represents a failure of the kidney to excrete bicarbonate efficiently because of chloride or potassium deficiency, continuous

mineralocorticoid elaboration, or both. Treatment is primarily directed at correcting the underlying stimulus for HCO_3^- generation and restoring the ability of the kidney to excrete the excess HCO_3^-. Assistance is gained in the diagnosis and treatment of metabolic alkalosis from directing attention to the urinary chloride, arterial blood pressure, and volume status of the patient (particularly the presence or absence of orthostasis; see **Table 9-1**). Helpful in the history is the presence or absence of vomiting, diuretic use, or alkali therapy.

A high urine chloride level and hypertension suggest that primary mineralocorticoid excess is present. If primary aldosteronism is present, correction of the underlying cause (adenoma, bilateral hyperplasia, Cushing's syndrome) will reverse the alkalosis. Patients with bilateral adrenal hyperplasia may respond to spironolactone. Normotensive patients with a high urine chloride level may have Bartter's or Gitelman's syndrome if diuretic use or vomiting can be excluded. A low urine chloride level and relative hypotension suggest a chloride-responsive metabolic alkalosis such as vomiting or nasogastric suction. Loss of $[H^+]$ by the stomach or kidneys can be mitigated by the use of proton pump inhibitors or the discontinuation of diuretics. The second aspect of treatment is to remove the factors that sustain HCO_3^- reabsorption, such as ECV contraction or K^+ deficiency. Although K^+ deficits should be repaired, NaCl therapy is usually sufficient to reverse the alkalosis if ECV contraction is present, as would be indicated by a low urine $[Cl^-]$.

Patients with congestive heart failure (CHF) or unexplained volume overexpansion represent special challenges in the critical care setting. Patients with a low urine chloride concentration, usually indicative of a "chloride-responsive" form of metabolic alkalosis, may not tolerate normal saline infusion. Renal HCO_3^- loss can be accelerated by administration of the carbonic anhydrase inhibitor acetazolamide (250 mg intravenously) if associated conditions preclude infusion of saline (i.e., elevated pulmonary capillary wedge pressure or evidence of CHF). Acetazolamide is usually effective in patients with adequate kidney function, but can exacerbate urinary K^+ losses and hypokalemia. Dilute hydrochloric acid (0.1N HCl) is also effective but can cause hemolysis and may be difficult to titrate. If it is used, the goal should be to restore the pH, not to normal, but to a level of approximately 7.50. Alternatively, acidification can also be achieved with oral NH_4Cl, which should be avoided in the presence of liver disease. Hemodialysis against a dialysate that is low in $[HCO_3^-]$ and high in $[Cl^-]$ can be effective if kidney function is impaired. Patients receiving continuous renal replacement therapy in the intensive care unit typically develop metabolic alkalosis with high-bicarbonate dialysate or if citrate regional anticoagulation is used. Therapy should include reduction of alkali loads via dialysis by reducing the bicarbonate concentration in the dialysate, or, if citrate is being used, by postfiltration infusion of 0.1 N HCl.

BIBLIOGRAPHY

Birkenhager R, Otto E, Schurmann MJ, et al: Mutation of BSND causes Bartter syndrome with sensorineural deafness and kidney failure. Nat Genet 29:310-314, 2001.

Conn JW, Rovner DR, Cohen EL: Licorice-induced pseudoaldosteronism: Hypertension, hypokalemia, aldosteronopenia, and suppressed plasma renin activity. JAMA 205:492, 1968.

Cruz DN, Shaer AJ, Bia MJ, et al: Gitelman's syndrome revisited: An evaluation of symptoms and health-related quality of life. Kidney Int 59: 719–717, 2001.

Diskin CJ, Stokes TJ, Dansby LM, et al: Recurrent metabolic alkalosis and elevated troponins after crack cocaine use in a hemodialysis patient. *Clin Exp Nephrol* 10:156-158, 2006.

DuBose TD Jr: Disorders of acid-base balance. In Brenner BM (ed): Brenner and Rector's The Kidney, 8th ed. Philadelphia, Saunders, pp 505–546.

Felsenfeld AJ, Levine BS: Milk alkali syndrome and the dynamics of calcium homeostasis. Clin J Am Soc Nephrol 1:641-654, 2006.

Galla JH: Metabolic alkalosis. In DuBose TD, Hamm L (eds): Acid-Base and Electrolyte Disorders: A Companion to Brenner and Rector's The Kidney. Philadelphia, Saunders, 2002, pp 109-128.

Grotegut CA, Dandolu V, Katari S, et al: Baking soda pica: A case of hypokalemic metabolic alkalosis and rhabdomyolysis in pregnancy. Obstet Gynecol 107:484-486, 2006.

Hebert SC, Gullans SR: The molecular basis of inherited hypokalemic alkalosis: Bartter's and Gitelman's syndromes. Am J Physiol 271:F957-F959, 1996.

Hernandez R, Schambelan M, Cogan MG, et al: Dietary NaCl determines severity of potassium depletion-induced metabolic alkalosis. Kidney Int 31:1356, 1987.

Hihnala S, Kujala M, Toppari J, et al: Expression of SLC26A3, CFTR and NHE3 in the human male reproductive tract: Role in male subfertility caused by congenital chloride diarrhea. Mol Hum Reprod 12:107-111, 2006.

Jamison RL, Ross JC, Kempson RL, et al: Surreptitious diuretic ingestion and pseudo-Bartter's syndrome. Am J Med 73:142, 1982.

Kamynina E, Staub O: Concerted action of ENaC, Nedd4-2, and Sgkl in transepithelial Na$^+$ transport. Am J Physiol Renal Physiol 283:F377, 2002.

Lifton RP, Dluhy RG, Powers M, et al: Hereditary hypertension caused by chimaeric gene duplications and ectopic expression of aldosterone synthase. Nat Genet 2:66-74, 1992.

Morgera S, Haase M, Ruckert M, et al: Regional citrate anticoagulation in continuous hemodialysis: Acid-base and electrolyte balance at an increased dose of dialysis. Nephron Clin Pract 101:c211-c219, 2005.

Schroeder ET: Alkalosis resulting from combined administration of a "nonsystemic" antacid and a cation-exchange resin. Gastroenterology 56:868, 1969.

Shimkets RA, Warnock DG, Bositis CM, et al: Liddle's syndrome: Heritable human hypertension caused by mutations in the beta subunit of the epithelial sodium channel. Cell 79:407, 1994.

Zelikovic I, Szargel R, Hawash A, et al: A novel mutation in the chloride channel gene, CLCNKB, as a cause of Gitelman and Bartter syndromes. Kidney Int 63:24-32, 2003.

CHAPTER 10

Respiratory Acidosis and Alkalosis

Nicolaos E. Madias and Horacio J. Adrogué

RESPIRATORY ACIDOSIS

Respiratory acidosis, or primary hypercapnia, is the acid-base disturbance initiated by an increase in carbon dioxide tension of body fluids and in whole-body CO_2 stores. Hypercapnia acidifies body fluids and elicits an adaptive increment in the plasma bicarbonate concentration ($[HCO_3^-]$) that should be viewed as an integral part of the respiratory acidosis. Arterial CO_2 tension (PCO_2) measured at rest and at sea level, is greater than 45 mm Hg in simple respiratory acidosis. Lower values of PCO_2 might still signify the presence of primary hypercapnia in the setting of mixed acid-base disorders (e.g., eucapnia, rather than the expected hypocapnia, in the presence of metabolic acidosis). Another special case of respiratory acidosis is the presence of arterial eucapnia, or even hypocapnia, in association with venous hypercapnia in patients who have an acute severe reduction in cardiac output but relative preservation of respiratory function (i.e., pseudorespiratory alkalosis).

Pathophysiology

Hypercapnia develops whenever CO_2 excretion by the lungs is insufficient to match CO_2 production, thus leading to positive CO_2 balance. Hypercapnia could result from increased CO_2 production, decreased alveolar ventilation, or both. Overproduction of CO_2 is usually matched by increased excretion, so that hypercapnia is prevented. However, patients with marked limitation in pulmonary reserve and those receiving constant mechanical ventilation might experience respiratory acidosis due to increased CO_2 production caused by increased muscle activity (agitation, myoclonus, shivering, seizures), sepsis, fever, or hyperthyroidism. Increments in CO_2 production might also be imposed by the administration of large carbohydrate loads (>2000 kcal/day) to semistarved, critically ill patients or during the decomposition of bicarbonate infused in the course of treating metabolic acidosis. By far, most cases of respiratory acidosis reflect a decrease in alveolar ventilation. Decreased alveolar ventilation can result from a reduction in minute ventilation, an increase in wasted ventilation (increased ratio of dead space volume to tidal volume), or a combination of the two. An increase in wasted ventilation is caused by overventilation of lung regions relative to their perfusion. This situation occurs in emphysema, cystic fibrosis, asthma, pulmonary fibrosis, and other intrinsic diseases, as well as chest wall disorders, including scoliosis.

The major threat to life from CO_2 retention in patients breathing room air is the associated obligatory hypoxemia. When the arterial oxygen tension (PO_2) falls to less than 40 to 50 mm Hg, harmful effects can occur, especially if the fall is rapid. In the absence of supplemental oxygen, patients in respiratory arrest develop critical hypoxemia within a few minutes, long before extreme hypercapnia ensues. Because of the constraints of the alveolar gas equation, it is not possible for PCO_2 to reach values much higher than 80 mm Hg while the level of PO_2 is still compatible with life. Extreme hypercapnia can be seen only during oxygen administration, and, in fact, it is often the result of uncontrolled oxygen therapy.

Secondary Physiologic Response

An immediate increment in plasma $[HCO_3^-]$ owing to titration of nonbicarbonate body buffers occurs in response to acute hypercapnia. This adaptation is complete within 5 to 10 minutes after the increase in PCO_2. On average, plasma $[HCO_3^-]$ increases by about 0.1 mEq/L for each 1 mm Hg acute increment in PCO_2; as a result, the plasma hydrogen ion concentration ($[H^+]$) increases by about 0.75 nEq/L for each 1 mm Hg acute increment in PCO_2. Therefore, the overall limit of adaptation of plasma $[HCO_3^-]$ in acute respiratory acidosis is quite small; even when PCO_2 increases to levels of 80 to 90 mm Hg, the increment in plasma $[HCO_3^-]$ does not exceed 3 to 4 mEq/L. Moderate hypoxemia does not alter the adaptive response to acute respiratory acidosis. On the other hand, preexisting hypobicarbonatemia (from metabolic acidosis or chronic respiratory alkalosis) enhances the magnitude of the bicarbonate response to acute hypercapnia, and such a response is diminished in hyperbicarbonatemic states (from metabolic alkalosis or chronic respiratory acidosis). Other electrolyte changes observed in acute respiratory acidosis include a mild increase in plasma sodium (1 to 4 mEq/L), potassium (0.1 mEq/L for each 0.1 unit decrease in pH), and phosphorus, as well as a small decrease in plasma chloride and lactate concentrations (the latter effect originating from inhibition of the activity of 6-phosphofructokinase and, consequently, glycolysis by intracellular acidosis). A small reduction in the plasma anion gap is also observed, reflecting the decline in plasma lactate and the acidic titration of plasma proteins.

The adaptive increase in plasma $[HCO_3^-]$ observed in the acute phase of hypercapnia is amplified markedly during chronic hypercapnia as a result of generation of new bicarbonate by the kidneys. Both proximal and distal acidification mechanisms contribute to this adaptation, which requires 3 to 5 days for completion. The renal response to chronic hypercapnia includes chloruresis and generation of hypochloremia. On average, plasma $[HCO_3^-]$ increases by about 0.3 mEq/L for each 1 mm Hg chronic increment in P_{CO_2}; as a result, the plasma $[H^+]$ increases by about 0.3 nEq/L for each 1 mm Hg chronic increase in P_{CO_2}. Empiric observations indicate a limit of adaptation of plasma $[HCO_3^-]$ on the order of 45 mEq/L. The renal response to chronic hypercapnia is not altered appreciably by dietary sodium or chloride restriction, moderate potassium depletion, alkali loading, or moderate hypoxemia. It is currently unknown to what extent chronic kidney disease of variable severity limits the renal response to chronic hypercapnia. Obviously, patients with end-stage kidney disease cannot mount a renal response to chronic hypercapnia, so they are more subject to severe acidemia. The degree of acidemia is more pronounced in patients who are receiving hemodialysis rather than peritoneal dialysis, because the former treatment maintains, on average, a lower plasma $[HCO_3^-]$. Recovery from chronic hypercapnia is crippled by a chloride-deficient diet. In this circumstance, despite correction of the level of P_{CO_2}, plasma $[HCO_3^-]$ remains elevated as long as the state of chloride deprivation persists, thus creating the entity of "posthypercapnic metabolic alkalosis." Chronic hypercapnia is not associated with appreciable changes in the anion gap or in plasma concentrations of sodium, potassium, or phosphorus.

Etiology

Respiratory acidosis can develop in patients who have normal or abnormal airways and lungs. **Tables 10-1** and **10-2** present, respectively, causes of acute and chronic respiratory acidosis. This classification takes into consideration the usual mode of onset and duration of the various causes and emphasizes the biphasic time course that characterizes the secondary physiologic response to hypercapnia. Primary hypercapnia can result from disease or malfunction within any element of the regulatory system that controls respiration, including the central and peripheral nervous system, respiratory muscles, thoracic cage, pleural space, airways, and lung parenchyma. Not infrequently, more than one cause contributes to the development of respiratory acidosis in a given patient. Chronic obstructive pulmonary disease (COPD) is the most common cause of chronic hypercapnia.

Clinical Manifestations

Because hypercapnia almost always occurs with some degree of hypoxemia, it is often difficult to determine whether a specific manifestation is the consequence of the elevated P_{CO_2} or the reduced P_{O_2}. Clinical manifestations of respiratory acidosis arising from the central nervous system are collectively known as hypercapnic encephalopathy and include irritability, inability to concentrate, headache, anorexia, mental cloudiness, apathy, confusion, incoherence, combativeness,

TABLE 10-1 Causes of Acute Respiratory Acidosis

NORMAL AIRWAYS AND LUNGS	ABNORMAL AIRWAYS AND LUNGS
Central Nervous System Depression	**Upper Airway Obstruction**
General anesthesia	Coma-induced hypopharyngeal obstruction
Sedative overdosage	Aspiration of foreign body or vomitus
Head trauma	Laryngospasm or angioedema
Cerebrovascular accident	Obstructive sleep apnea
Central sleep apnea	Inadequate laryngeal intubation
Cerebral edema	Laryngeal obstruction postintubation
Brain tumor	**Lower Airway Obstruction**
Encephalitis	Generalized bronchospasm
Neuromuscular Impairment	Severe asthma (status asthmaticus)
High spinal cord injury	Bronchiolitis of infancy and adults
Guillain-Barré syndrome	Disorders involving pulmonary alveoli
Status epilepticus	Severe bilateral pneumonia
Botulism, tetanus	Acute respiratory distress syndrome
Crisis in myasthenia gravis	Severe pulmonary edema
Hypokalemic myopathy	**Pulmonary Perfusion Defect**
Familial hypokalemic periodic paralysis	Cardiac arrest[*]
Drugs or toxic agents (e.g., curare, succinylcholine, aminoglycosides, organophosphorus)	Severe circulatory failure[*]
Ventilatory Restriction	Massive pulmonary thromboembolism
Rib fractures with flail chest	Fat or air embolus
Pneumothorax	
Hemothorax	
Impaired diaphragmatic function (e.g., peritoneal dialysis, ascites)	
IATROGENIC EVENTS	
Misplacement or displacement of airway cannula during anesthesia or mechanical ventilation	
Bronchoscopy-associated hypoventilation or respiratory arrest	
Increased CO_2 production with constant mechanical ventilation (e.g., due to high-carbohydrate diet or sorbent-regenerative hemodialysis)	

[*]May produce "pseudorespiratory alkalosis."
From Madias NE, Adrogué HJ: Respiratory alkalosis and acidosis. In Seldin DW, Giebisch G (eds): The Kidney: Physiology and Pathophysiology. Philadelphia, Lippincott Williams & Wilkins, 2000, pp 2131–2166.

TABLE 10-2 Causes of Chronic Respiratory Acidosis

NORMAL AIRWAYS AND LUNGS	ABNORMAL AIRWAYS AND LUNGS
Central Nervous System Depression	**Upper Airway Obstruction**
Sedative overdosage	Tonsillar and peritonsillar hypertrophy
Methadone/heroin addiction	Paralysis of vocal cords
Primary alveolar hypoventilation (Ondine's curse)	Tumor of the cords or larynx
Obesity-hypoventilation syndrome (pickwickian syndrome)	Airway stenosis after prolonged intubation
Brain tumor	Thymoma, aortic aneurysm
Bulbar poliomyelitis	**Lower Airway Obstruction**
Neuromuscular Impairment	Chronic obstructive lung disease (bronchitis, bronchiolitis, bronchiectasis, emphysema)
Poliomyelitis	**Disorders Involving Pulmonary Alveoli**
Multiple sclerosis	Severe chronic pneumonitis
Muscular dystrophy	Diffuse infiltrative disease (e.g., alveolar proteinosis)
Amyotrophic lateral sclerosis	Interstitial fibrosis
Diaphragmatic paralysis	
Myxedema	
Myopathic disease	
Ventilatory Restriction	
Kyphoscoliosis, spinal arthritis	
Obesity	
Fibrothorax	
Hydrothorax	
Impaired diaphragmatic function	

From Madias NE, Adrogué HJ: Respiratory alkalosis and acidosis. In Seldin DW, Giebisch G (eds): The Kidney: Physiology and Pathophysiology. Philadelphia, Lippincott Williams & Wilkins, 2000, pp 2131–2166.

hallucinations, delirium, and transient psychosis. Progressive narcosis or coma might develop in patients receiving oxygen therapy, especially those with an acute exacerbation of chronic respiratory insufficiency, in whom P_{CO_2} levels of up to 100 mm Hg or even higher can occur. In addition, frank papilledema (pseudotumor cerebri) and motor disturbances, including myoclonic jerks, flapping tremor identical to that observed in liver failure, sustained myoclonus, and seizures may develop. Focal neurologic signs (e.g., muscle paresis, abnormal reflexes) might be observed. The neurologic symptomatology depends on the magnitude of the hypercapnia, the rapidity with which it develops, the severity of the acidemia, and the degree of the accompanying hypoxemia. Severe hypercapnia often is misdiagnosed as a cerebral vascular accident or an intracranial tumor.

The hemodynamic consequences of respiratory acidosis include a direct depressing effect on myocardial contractility. An associated sympathetic surge, sometimes intense, leads to

increases in plasma catecholamines, but during severe acidemia (blood pH lower than about 7.20), receptor responsiveness to catecholamines is markedly blunted. Hypercapnia results in systemic vasodilatation via a direct action on vascular smooth muscle; this effect is most obvious in the cerebral circulation, where blood flow increases in direct relation to the level of P_{CO_2}. By contrast, CO_2 retention can produce vasoconstriction in the pulmonary circulation as well as in the kidneys; in the latter case, the hemodynamic response may be mediated via an enhanced sympathetic activity. Mild to moderate hypercapnia is usually associated with an increased cardiac output, normal or increased blood pressure, warm skin, a bounding pulse, and diaphoresis. However, if hypercapnia is severe or considerable hypoxemia is present, decreases in both cardiac output and blood pressure may be observed. Concomitant therapy with vasoactive medications (e.g., β-adrenergic receptor blockers) or the presence of congestive heart failure may further modify the hemodynamic response. Cardiac arrhythmias, particularly supraventricular tachyarrhythmias not associated with major hemodynamic compromise, are common, especially in patients receiving digitalis as therapy for cor pulmonale. They do not result primarily from the hypercapnia, but rather reflect the associated hypoxemia and sympathetic discharge, concomitant medication, electrolyte abnormalities, and underlying cardiac disease. Retention of salt and water is commonly observed in sustained hypercapnia, especially in the presence of cor pulmonale. In addition to the effects of heart failure on the kidney, multiple other factors may be involved, including the prevailing stimulation of the sympathetic nervous system and the renin-angiotensin-aldosterone axis, increased renal vascular resistance, and elevated levels of antidiuretic hormone and cortisol.

Diagnosis

Whenever hypoventilation is suspected, arterial blood gases should be obtained. If the acid-base profile of the patient reveals hypercapnia in association with acidemia, at least an element of respiratory acidosis must be present. However, hypercapnia can be associated with a normal or an alkaline pH because of the simultaneous presence of additional acid-base disorders (see Chapter 11). Information from the patient's history, physical examination, and ancillary laboratory data should be used for an accurate assessment of the acid-base status.

Therapeutic Principles

Treatment of acute respiratory acidosis should focus on three critical steps: ensuring a patent airway, restoring adequate oxygenation by delivering an oxygen-rich inspired mixture, and securing adequate ventilation in order to repair the abnormal blood gas composition. As noted, acute respiratory acidosis poses its major threat to survival not because of hypercapnia or acidemia, but because of the associated hypoxemia. Achieving a P_{O_2} of 60 mm Hg or higher

TABLE 10-3 Causes of Respiratory Alkalosis

Hypoxemia or Tissue Hypoxia	Subarachnoid Hemorrhage
Decreased inspired O$_2$ tension	Cerebrovascular accident
High altitude	Meningoencephalitis
Bacterial or viral pneumonia	Tumor
Aspiration of food, foreign body, or vomitus	Trauma
Laryngospasm	**Drugs or Hormones**
Drowning	Nikethamide, ethamivan
Cyanotic heart disease	Doxapram
Severe anemia	Xanthines
Left shift deviation of the HbO$_2$ curve	Salicylates
Hypotension*	Catecholamines
Severe circulatory failure*	Angiotensin II
Pulmonary edema	Vasopressor agents
Stimulation of Chest Receptors	Progesterone
Pneumonia	Medroxyprogesterone
Asthma	Dinitrophenol
Pneumothorax	Nicotine
Hemothorax	**Miscellaneous**
Flail chest	Pregnancy
Acute respiratory distress syndrome	Sepsis
Cardiac failure	Hepatic failure
Noncardiogenic pulmonary edema	Mechanical hyperventilation
Pulmonary embolism	Heat exposure
Interstitial lung disease	Recovery from metabolic acidosis
Central Nervous System Stimulation	
Voluntary	
Pain	
Anxiety	
Psychosis	
Fever	

*May produce "pseudorespiratory alkalosis."
HbO$_2$, oxyhemoglobin
From Madias NE, Adrogué HJ: Respiratory alkalosis and acidosis. In Seldin DW, Giebisch G (eds): The Kidney: Physiology and Pathophysiology. Philadelphia, Lippincott Williams & Wilkins, 2000, pp 2131–2166.

Clinical Manifestations

Rapid decrements in Pco$_2$ to half the normal values or lower are typically accompanied by paresthesias of the extremities, chest discomfort, circumoral numbness, lightheadedness, confusion, and, infrequently, tetany or generalized seizures. These manifestations are seldom present in the chronic phase. Acute hypocapnia decreases cerebral blood flow, which in severe cases may reach values less than 50% of normal, resulting in cerebral hypoxia. This hypoperfusion has been implicated in the pathogenesis of the neurologic manifestations of acute respiratory alkalosis along with other

factors, including hypocapnia per se, alkalemia, pH-induced shift of the oxyhemoglobin dissociation curve, and decrements in the levels of ionized calcium and potassium. Some evidence indicates that cerebral blood flow returns to normal in chronic respiratory alkalosis.

Actively hyperventilating patients manifest no appreciable changes in cardiac output or systemic blood pressure. By contrast, acute hypocapnia in the course of passive hyperventilation, as typically observed during mechanical ventilation in patients with a depressed central nervous system or in patients under general anesthesia, frequently results in a major reduction in cardiac output and systemic blood pressure, increased peripheral resistance, and substantial hyperlactatemia. This discrepant response probably reflects the decline in venous return caused by mechanical ventilation in passive hyperventilation and the reflex tachycardia consistently observed in active hyperventilation. Although acute hypocapnia does not lead to cardiac arrhythmias in normal volunteers, it appears that it contributes to the generation of both atrial and ventricular tachyarrhythmias in patients with ischemic heart disease. Chest pain and ischemic ST-T wave changes have been observed in acutely hyperventilating subjects with or without coronary artery disease. Coronary vasospasm and Prinzmetal's angina can be precipitated by acute hypocapnia in susceptible subjects. The pathogenesis of these manifestations has been attributed to the same factors that are incriminated in the neurologic manifestations of acute hypocapnia.

Diagnosis

Careful observation can detect abnormal patterns of breathing in some patients, yet marked hypocapnia may be present without a clinically evident increase in respiratory effort. Therefore, an arterial blood gas analysis should be obtained whenever hyperventilation is suspected. In fact, the diagnosis of respiratory alkalosis, especially the chronic form, is frequently missed; physicians often misinterpret the electrolyte pattern of hyperchloremic hypobicarbonatemia as indicative of a normal anion gap metabolic acidosis. If the acid-base profile of the patient reveals hypocapnia in association with alkalemia, at least an element of respiratory alkalosis must be present. Primary hypocapnia, however, may be associated with a normal or an acidic pH as a result of the concomitant presence of other acid-base disorders. Notably, mild degrees of chronic hypocapnia commonly leave blood pH within the high-normal range. As always, proper evaluation of the acid-base status of the patient requires careful assessment of the history, physical examination, and ancillary laboratory data (see Chapter 11). Once the diagnosis of respiratory alkalosis has been made, a search for its cause should be performed. The diagnosis of respiratory alkalosis can have important clinical implications: It often provides a clue to the presence of an unrecognized, serious disorder (e.g., sepsis) or signals the severity of a known underlying disease.

Therapeutic Principles

Management of respiratory alkalosis must be directed toward correction of the underlying cause, whenever possible. Respiratory alkalosis resulting from severe hypoxemia requires oxygen therapy. The widely held view that hypocapnia, even if severe, poses little risk to health is inaccurate. In fact, transient or permanent damage to the brain, heart, and lungs can result from substantial hypocapnia. In addition, rapid correction of severe hypocapnia can lead to reperfusion injury in the brain and lung. Therefore, severe hypocapnia in hospitalized patients must be prevented whenever possible, and, if it is present, a slow correction is most appropriate.

Rebreathing into a closed system (e.g., a paper bag) may prove helpful for the patient with the anxiety-hyperventilation syndrome, because it interrupting the vicious cycle that can result from the reinforcing effects of the symptoms of hypocapnia. Administration of 250 to 500 mg acetazolamide can be beneficial in the management of signs and symptoms of high-altitude sickness, a syndrome characterized by hypoxemia and respiratory alkalosis. Considering the risks of severe alkalemia, sedation or, in rare cases, skeletal muscle paralysis and mechanical ventilation may be required to temporarily correct marked respiratory alkalosis. Management of pseudorespiratory alkalosis must be directed at optimizing systemic hemodynamics.

BIBLIOGRAPHY

Adrogué HJ, Madias NE: Management of life-threatening acid-base disorders. N Engl J Med 338:26-34;107-111, 1998.

Adrogué HJ, Madias NE. Respiratory Acidosis. In: Gennari FJ, Adrogué HJ, Galla JH, Madias NE(eds). Acid-Base Disorders and their Treatment. Taylor & Francis Group, 597-639, 2005.

Adrogué HJ, Madias NE. Respiratory acidosis, respiratory alkalosis, and mixed disorders. In Feehally J, Floege J, Johnson RJ (eds): Comprehensive Clinical Nephrology, 3rd ed. Philadelphia, Mosby, 2007, pp 167-180.

Adrogué HJ, Rashad MN, Gorin AB, et al: Assessing acid-base status in circulatory failure. Differences between arterial and central venous blood. N Engl J Med 320:1312-1316, 1989.

Amato MB, Barbas CSV, Medeiros DM, et al: Effect of a protective-ventilation strategy on mortality in the acute respiratory distress syndrome. N Engl J Med 338:347-354, 1998.

Arbus GS, Hebert LA, Levesque PR, et al: Characterization and clinical application of the "significance band" for acute respiratory alkalosis. N Engl J Med 280:117-123, 1969.

Brackett NC Jr, Cohen JJ, Schwartz WB: Carbon dioxide titration curve of normal man: Effect of increasing degrees of acute hypercapnia on acid-base equilibrium. N Engl J Med 272:6-12, 1965.

Brackett NC Jr, Wingo CF, Muren O, Solano JT: Acid-base response to chronic hypercapnia in man. N Engl J Med 280: 124-130, 1969.

Dries DJ: Permissive hypercapnia. J Trauma 39:984-989, 1995.

Epstein SK, Singh N: Respiratory acidosis. Respir Care 46:366-383, 2001.

Foster GT, Vaziri ND, Sassoon CSH: Respiratory alkalosis. Respir Care 46:384-391, 2001.

Jardin F, Fellahi J, Beauchet A, et al: Improved prognosis of acute respiratory distress syndrome 15 years on. Intensive Care Med 25:936-941, 1999.

Krapf R, Beeler I, Hertner D, Hulter HN: Chronic respiratory alkalosis: The effect of sustained hyperventilation on renal regulation of acid-base equilibrium. N Engl J Med 324:1394-1401, 1991.

Kollef M: Respiratory failure. In Dale DC, Federman DD (eds): ACP Medicine. New York, WebMD, 2006, pp 2791-2804.

Laffey JG, Kavanagh BP: Hypocapnia. N Engl J Med 347:43-53, 2002.

Madias NE, Adrogué HJ: Respiratory acidosis and alkalosis. In Adrogué HJ (ed): Contemporary Management in Critical Care: Acid-Base and Electrolyte Disorders. New York, Churchill Livingstone, 1991, pp 37-53.

Madias NE, Adrogué HJ: Respiratory alkalosis and acidosis. In Seldin DW, Giebisch G (eds): The Kidney: Physiology and Pathophysiology. Philadelphia, Lippincott Williams & Wilkins, 2000, pp 2131-2166.

Madias NE, Adrogué HJ: Respiratory alkalosis. In DuBose TD, Hamm LL (eds): Acid-Base and Electrolyte Disorders. Philadelphia, WB Saunders, 2002, pp 147-164.

Madias NE, Wolf CJ, Cohen JJ: Regulation of acid-base equilibrium in chronic hypercapnia. Kidney Int 27:538-543, 1985.

Malhotra A: Low-tidal-volume ventilation in the acute respiratory distress syndrome. N Engl J Med 357:1113-1120, 2007.

Tobin MJ: Advances in mechanical ventilation. N Engl J Med 344:1986-1996, 2001.

CHAPTER 11

Approach to Acid-Base Disorders

Ankit W. Mehta and Michael Emmett

Acid-base disorders have major clinical and diagnostic implications. If they generate extreme acidemia or alkalemia, the abnormal pH itself has major pathophysiologic impact. The tertiary structure of proteins is altered by extreme pH conditions, and this may affect the activity of enzymes and ion transport systems. Consequently every metabolic pathway may be affected by acidemia or alkalemia. Extreme acidemia can depress cardiac function, impair the vascular response to catecholamines, generate arteriolar vasodilation, and simultaneously cause venoconstriction. Systemic hypotension and pulmonary edema may result. Insulin resistance, reduced hepatic lactate uptake, and accelerated protein catabolism are also effects of acidemia. Alkalemia can generate cardiac arrhythmias, produce neuromuscular irritability, and generate tissue hypoxemia. Cerebral and myocardial blood flow fall, and respiratory depression occurs. Hypokalemia, a common accompaniment of respiratory and metabolic alkalosis, also contributes to the morbidity of these acid-base disorders.

Although moderate or minor acid-base disorders may not directly affect physiologic function or require treatment, the identification of such disorders may provide extremely important clues to the presence of otherwise unsuspected but serious medical conditions. When an acid-base disorder is identified, elucidation of the underlying cause is often of critical importance. The situation is analogous to the recognition of fever or hypothermia. Very high, or very low, temperatures can themselves be destructive and may require aggressive therapy directed at restoration of a more normal temperature. However, equally important, and most of the time more important, is the effort to elucidate and treat the underlying cause of the abnormal temperature. The recognition of an acid-base disorder must generate a search for its clinical cause or causes.

The acid-base status of the extracellular fluid is carefully regulated to maintain the arterial pH in a narrow range between 7.36 and 7.44 (representing a hydrogen ion concentration, [H$^+$], of 44 to 36 nEq/L). The pH is stabilized by multiple buffer systems in the extracellular fluid, within cells, and in the skeleton. The carbon dioxide tension (PCO_2), which is primarily under neurorespiratory control, and the serum bicarbonate concentration ([HCO$_3^-$]), which is primarily under renal/metabolic regulation, are the most important variables in this complex system of buffers.

There are currently three widely accepted methodologic approaches to the elucidation of simple and mixed acid-base disorders:

1. The *Boston approach*, which utilizes measurements of arterial pH, PCO_2, and [HCO$_3^-$] together with an analysis of the anion gap (AG) and a set of compensation rules.
2. The *Copenhagen approach*, which is based on measurements of arterial pH and PCO_2 and calculation of the so-called base excess (BE).
3. The *Stewart approach*, which utilizes measurements of arterial pH and PCO_2 together with the calculated "strong ion difference" (SID), "total weak acids" and "strong ion gap" (SIG).

Each of these approaches can be effectively used to characterize acid-base disorders; each has its vocal proponents and detractors; and each has unique characteristics that may be particularly helpful under certain conditions. We believe that the Boston approach is the most straightforward, is easiest to understand and use, and is generally acceptable in most clinical circumstances. Therefore, the Boston method has been selected for use in this chapter and throughout this *Primer*.

The Boston approach to the elucidation of acid-base disorders requires the following information:

- Recognition of diagnostic clues provided by the patient's history and physical examination.
- Analysis of the serum [HCO$_3^-$] and arterial pH and PCO_2. Although a blood gas analysis is not always necessary to make a diagnosis, it is usually required for complicated cases.
- Recognition of the predicted compensatory response to simple acid-base disorders.
- Calculation of the AG and consideration of the expected "baseline" AG.
- Analysis of the degree of increase in AG (Δ[AG]) and the degree of decrease in [HCO$_3^-$] (ΔHCO$_3^-$) to determine whether the magnitudes of these respective changes are reciprocal—the so-called Delta/Delta, or ΔAG/ΔHCO$_3^-$.

ACIDEMIA, ALKALEMIA, ACIDOSIS, AND ALKALOSIS

The normal arterial blood pH range is between 7.36 and 7.44 ([H$^+$] between 44 and 36 nEq/L). Acidemia is defined as an arterial pH of less than 7.36 ([H$^+$] >44 nEq/L); it may result from a primary elevation in PCO_2 or a fall in [HCO$_3^-$]. Alkalemia is defined as an arterial pH greater than 7.44

([H$^+$] <36 nEq/L). Alkalemia may result from a primary increase in [HCO$_3$$^-$] or a fall in Pco$_2$.

The relationship between pH, Pco$_2$, and [HCO$_3$$^-$] is described by the familiar Henderson-Hasselbalch equation:

$$pH = 6.1 + \log\left(\frac{\left[HCO_3^-\right]}{0.3 \times Pco_2}\right)$$

Acidosis and alkalosis are pathophysiologic processes that, if unopposed by therapy or complicating disorders, cause, respectively, acidemia and alkalemia.

SIMPLE (SINGLE) ACID-BASE DISTURBANCES AND COMPENSATION

The simple acid-base disorders are divided into primary metabolic and primary respiratory disturbances. Each of these simple, or single, acid-base disorders generates a compensatory response which acts to return the blood pH back toward the normal range. By convention, the Boston approach to acid-base analysis considers the compensatory response to a simple acid-base disorder to be an integral component of that disorder. Hence, there are four primary simple acid-base disturbances (or six, if each respiratory disorder is divided into an acute and a chronic phase):

1. *Metabolic acidosis*: The underlying pathophysiology tends to reduce the serum [HCO$_3$$^-$].* Causes include excess generation of metabolic acids, excessive exogenous acid intake, reduced kidney acid excretion, and exogenous loss of HCO$_3$$^-$ (usually in stool or urine). Metabolic acidosis reduces the arterial plasma pH and generates a hyperventilatory compensatory response that reduces the arterial Pco$_2$ and blunts the degree of acidemia.
2. *Metabolic alkalosis*: The underlying pathophysiology tends to increase the serum [HCO$_3$$^-$]. Causes include exogenous intake of HCO$_3$$^-$ salts (or salts that can be converted to HCO$_3$$^-$) and endogenous generation of HCO$_3$$^-$. Regardless of the origin of the HCO$_3$$^-$, the pathology must also include reduced or impaired renal HCO$_3$$^-$ excretion. Metabolic alkalosis increases the arterial plasma pH and generates a hypoventilatory compensatory response that increases the arterial Pco$_2$ and blunts the degree of alkalemia.
3. *Respiratory acidosis*: The underlying pathophysiology tends to increase the arterial Pco$_2$. The compensatory response is an increase of the plasma [HCO$_3$$^-$] caused by rapid generation from buffers and, over a period of days, renal HCO$_3$$^-$ generation and retention.
4. *Respiratory alkalosis*: The underlying pathophysiology tends to decrease the arterial Pco$_2$. The compensatory response reduces the plasma [HCO$_3$$^-$]. This occurs acutely

as H$^+$ is released from buffers and, over a period of days, as the kidneys excrete HCO$_3$$^-$ and/or retain acid.

The magnitude of each compensatory response is proportional to the severity of the primary disturbance. In general, respiratory responses to primary metabolic acid-base disorders occur rapidly (within 1 hour) and are fully developed within 12 to 36 hours. In contrast, the compensatory metabolic alterations triggered by the primary respiratory disorders require several days before the kidney response is fully developed. Hence, each of the primary respiratory disorders is subdivided into an acute and a chronic phase, to differentiate the expected compensatory response.

The expected degree of compensation for each simple disorder has been determined by studying patients with isolated simple disorders and normal subjects with experimentally induced acid-base disorders. These data have been utilized to create various graphic acid-base nomograms, simple mathematical relationships, and various mnemonic methods for predicting expected compensation ranges. **Figure 11-1** and **Table 11-1** provide some of these "compensation rules". Appropriate compensation should usually exist in all patients with an acid-base disorder; if it is not present, a complex, or mixed, acid-base disorder must be considered.

In general, with one exception, compensatory responses minimize the pH abnormality but do not completely normalize the pH. The exception is chronic respiratory alkalosis, wherein compensation often results in a pH that is in the mid-normal range. With all other disorders, some degree of acidemia or alkalemia remains, even after full compensation. In compensatory responses, the Pco$_2$ always moves in the same direction as the initial [HCO$_3$$^-$] change in metabolic acid-base disorders, and the [HCO$_3$$^-$] always moves in the same direction as the initial Pco$_2$ change in respiratory acid-base disorders (see **Table 11-1**). If the Pco$_2$ and [HCO$_3$$^-$] are abnormal in opposite directions (i.e., one is increased and the other is decreased), then a mixed disturbance must exist.

ANION GAP

The ion profile of normal serum is depicted in **Figure 11-2A**. In any solution, the total cation charge concentration must be equal to the total anion charge concentration (all measured in units of electrical charge concentration, mEq/L). Now consider only the three serum electrolytes that are at the highest concentration; namely, Na$^+$, Cl$^-$, and HCO$_3$$^-$. The cation charge, [Na$^+$], normally exceeds the sum of the anion charges, [Cl$^-$] and [HCO$_3$$^-$]. If the sum of the two cations is subtracted from [Na$^+$], an AG is noted (see **Fig. 11-2B**):

$$AG = \left[Na^+\right] - \left(\left[Cl^-\right] + \left[HCO_3^-\right]\right)$$

This AG is, of course, an arbitrary number that results from the decision to consider only the three "major" serum electrolytes and not some or all of the many other ions that normally exist in serum. Nevertheless, the AG, defined in this fashion, is a very useful diagnostic tool.

The normal value of the AG varies among laboratories because of the wide variety of analyte measurement

---

*Although we refer to serum bicarbonate concentration ([HCO$_3$$^-$]) here, it is often directly measured and reported in the serum electrolyte analysis as total CO$_2$ (tCO$_2$), which includes bicarbonate (HCO$_3$$^-$), carbonic acid (H$_2CO_3$), and dissolved CO$_2$ gas. The latter two components usually account for a very small fraction of the total (roughly 1.2 mEq/L at normal Pco$_2$). Therefore, for clinical purposes, tCO$_2$ is generally equated to the serum [HCO$_3$$^-$].

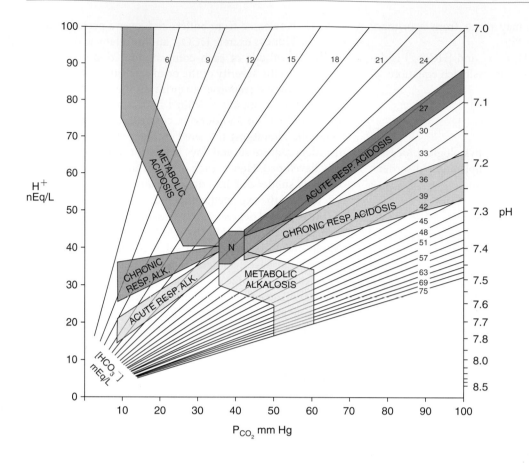

FIGURE 11-1 The acid-base map. Shaded areas represent the 95% confidence limits for zones of adaptation of the simple acid-base disorders. Numbered diagonal lines represent isopleths of plasma bicarbonate concentration ($[HCO_3^-]$). Laboratory values that fall within a marked zone are consistent with the patient's having the diagnosis shown. If the values fall outside a marked zone, a mixed acid-base disturbance is likely. Alk., alkalosis; N, normal range; Resp., respiratory. (Modified and updated from Goldberg M, Green SB, Moss ML, et al: Computer-based instruction and diagnosis of acid-base disorders. JAMA 223:269-275, 1973.)

TABLE 11-1 "Acid-Base Rules": Changes in pH, Pco_2, and $[HCO_3^-]$ and Expected Compensatory Responses in Simple Disturbances

PRIMARY DISORDER	pH	INITIAL CHEMICAL CHANGE	COMPENSATORY RESPONSE	EXPECTED COMPENSATION
Metabolic acidosis	Low	↓ $[HCO_3^-]$	↓ Pco_2	$Pco_2 = (1.5 \times [HCO_3^-]) + 8 \pm 2$ $Pco_2 = [HCO_3^-] + 15$ $Pco_2 = $ decimal digits of pH
Metabolic alkalosis[*]	High	↑ $[HCO_3^-]$	↑ Pco_2	Pco_2 variably increased $Pco_2 = (0.9 \times [HCO_3^-]) + 9$
Respiratory acidosis				$Pco_2 = (0.7 \times [HCO_3^-]) + 20$
Acute	Low	↑ Pco_2	↑ $[HCO_3^-]$	$[HCO_3^-]$ increases 1 mEq/L for every 10 mm Hg increase in Pco_2
Chronic	Low	↑ Pco_2	further ↑ $[HCO_3^-]$	$[HCO_3^-]$ increases 3-4 mEq/L for every 10 mm Hg increase in Pco_2
Respiratory alkalosis				
Acute	High	↓ Pco_2	↓ $[HCO_3^-]$	$[HCO_3^-]$ decreases 2 mEq/L for every 10 mm Hg decrease in Pco_2
Chronic	High	↓ Pco_2	further ↓ $[HCO_3^-]$	$[HCO_3^-]$ decreases 5 mEq/L for every 10 mm Hg decrease in Pco_2

[*]Compensation formulas for metabolic alkalosis have wide confidence limits because the Pco_2 of individuals with this disorder vary greatly at any given $[HCO_3^-]$.
$[HCO_3^-]$, serum bicarbonate concentration; Pco_2, arterial partial pressure of carbon dioxide.

technologies and unique normal ranges for each instrument. In general, the normal AG range is considered to be 8 to 12 mEq/L. The composition of the normal AG is primarily anionic albumin and, to a lesser degree, other proteins, sulfate, phosphate, urate, and various organic acid anions such as lactate. In general, if the concentration of these "unmeasured" anions increases, the AG increases, and, conversely, the AG falls when the concentration of unmeasured anions is reduced. For example, hypoalbuminemia is a common cause

of a reduced AG: The AG falls about 2.5 mEq/L for each 1 g/dL reduction of albumin below its normal range.

Metabolic acidosis disorders can be subdivided according to whether they are associated with an increased or a normal AG. An examination of the AG equation reveals that the only way the $[HCO_3^-]$ can fall while the AG remains normal is for the $[Cl^-]$ to increase relative to the $[Na^+]$. Consequently, all "non-AG" metabolic acidoses must be hyperchloremic metabolic acidoses. This is shown graphically in **Figure 11-3**.

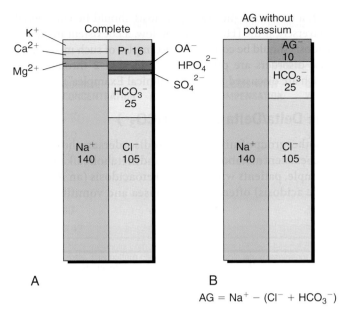

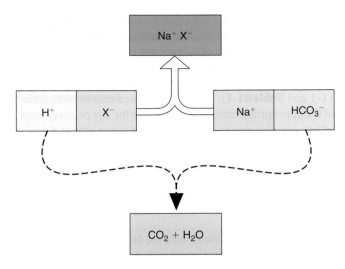

$$AG = Na^+ - (Cl^- + HCO_3^-)$$

FIGURE 11-2 The ionic anatomy of plasma. All units are milliequivalents per liter (mEq/L). **A,** Ion profile of normal serum. **B,** Calculation of the anion gap (AG) using the concentrations of sodium, chloride, and bicarbonate only. OA, organic acid; Pr, Protein.

Most often, an elevated AG indicates the presence of a metabolic acidosis. However, exceptions do exist, and they include

- Dehydration. Loss of water in excess of salts increases the concentration of all electrolytes, including albumin and other unmeasured ions, thereby increasing the AG.
- Rapid infusion, and short-lived accumulation, of metabolizable sodium salts such as lactate, acetate, or citrate. To the extent that these salts are metabolized, they generate $NaHCO_3$, and the AG does not increase; if metabolic conversion is delayed, the AG increases.
- Infusion of nonmetabolizable sodium salts (i.e., salts other than sodium chloride or sodium bicarbonate). For example, anionic antibiotics such as carbenicillin and penicillin G may be infused as sodium (or potassium) salts, and, to the extent that they accumulate, they increase the AG.
- Metabolic alkalosis, causes a small increase in AG (usually <3 to 4 mEq/L) as a result of (1) increased concentration of organic anions, mainly lactate, due to metabolic stimulation of lactate production and (2) increased concentration of albumin, due to extracellular fluid volume contraction
- Laboratory error or measurement artifact of one or more analytes

MIXED ACID-BASE DISTURBANCES

A mixed acid-base disturbance is the simultaneous finding of two or more simple acid-base disturbances in a patient. Mixed acid-base disorders may develop concurrently or sequentially. The disorders may be additive, with each process having a similar directional effect on pH. Alternatively, they may oppose each other, having offsetting effects on pH. Sometimes, three simultaneous acid-base disorders or a triple acid-base disturbance can be identified.

		METABOLIC ACIDOSIS	
	NORMAL	HYPERCHLOREMIC	HIGH AG
Na^+	140	140	140
Cl^-	105	115	105
HCO_3^-	25	15	15
AG	10	10	20
ΔHCO_3^-	0	−10	−10
ΔAG	0	0	+10
Lactate	1	1	11

FIGURE 11-3 If any relatively strong acid, HX (where X^- is an anion), is added to a solution containing $NaHCO_3$, there is decomposition of some HCO_3^- and an equivalent increase in the concentration of X^-. If the HX is HCl, then a hyperchloremic, or normal anion gap (AG), acidosis develops. If the HX is any acid other than HCl, such as lactic acid or a keto acid, then a high AG acidosis develops.

Recognition of mixed acid-base disorders is important for several reasons. First, when these disorders are additive (i.e., metabolic and respiratory acidosis or metabolic and respiratory alkalosis), the pH excursions may become severe, and these extreme conditions are themselves toxic. When offsetting disorders coexist, the pH may be normal or near-normal. Nonetheless, their identification serves as an important diagnostic clue to the underlying pathophysiology. Mixed disorders often suggest specific clinical derangements. For example, the coexistence of AG metabolic acidosis and respiratory alkalosis is typical of salicylate poisoning. Patients with diabetic ketoacidosis often vomit and present with AG metabolic acidosis and metabolic alkalosis.

Inadequate or "Excessive" Compensation

The expected compensatory responses shown in the acid-base nomogram (see **Fig. 11-1**) and described in **Table 11-1** are used to determine whether respiratory compensation for a metabolic disorder, or metabolic compensation for a respiratory disorder, is quantitatively appropriate, inadequate, or excessive. The arterial pH, Pco_2, and $[HCO_3^-]$ values are required for this determination; therefore, a blood gas analysis is necessary for complete characterization of the acid-base disturbance. If a patient with a metabolic acidosis has a Pco_2 that is lower than the expected compensatory response,

TABLE 11-6 Mixed Metabolic Acidosis and Metabolic Alkalosis

| | | | | METABOLIC ALKALOSIS AND METABOLIC ACIDOSIS | |
ION	NORMAL CONCENTRATION	HIGH AG METABOLIC ACIDOSIS WITH APPROPRIATE COMPENSATION	NORMAL AG METABOLIC ACIDOSIS WITH APPROPRIATE COMPENSATION	HIGH AG METABOLIC ACIDOSIS	NORMAL AG METABOLIC ACIDOSIS
Na$^+$	140	140	140	140	140
K$^+$	4.0	5.0	3.8	4.0	4.0
Cl$^-$	105	105	115	95	105
HCO$_3^-$	25	15	15	25	25
AG	10	20	10	20	10
Pco$_2$	40	30	30	40	40
pH	7.42	7.32	7.32	7.42	7.42

AG, anion gap; Pco$_2$, arterial carbon dioxide tension.

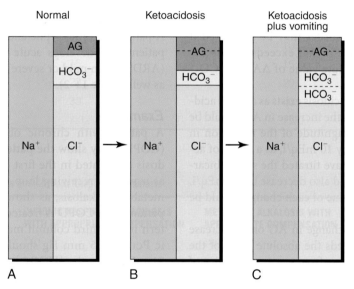

FIGURE 11-4 The effect of ketoacidosis plus vomiting on the ionic profile of blood. **A,** The normal electrolyte pattern. **B,** The development of a typical anion gap (AG) metabolic acidosis. **C,** The superimposed effect of vomiting, which causes proton loss without the loss of any organic acid anions. This results in a decrease in the serum chloride concentration and an increase in the bicarbonate concentration. The latter normalizes the [HCO$_3^-$], but the AG remains large because the keto acids are unchanged by the vomiting.

Example 4

Metabolic alkalosis raises the [HCO$_3^-$], and compensation should increase the Pco$_2$. Respiratory alkalosis decreases the Pco$_2$ and compensation should decrease the [HCO$_3^-$]. If the [HCO$_3^-$] is increased and the Pco$_2$ is decreased, then metabolic alkalosis and respiratory alkalosis coexist (**Table 11-5**). This mixed acid-base disorder is often seen in patients with severe liver disease. Chronic respiratory alkalosis is extremely common as a result of diaphragmatic elevation, arteriovenous shunting, and a deranged hormonal milieu that stimulates ventilation. Nausea and vomiting occur frequently, and nasogastric suction is often employed. Metabolic alkalosis then complicates the chronic respiratory alkalosis. Combined, these disorders can generate extreme alkalemia.

Example 5

The large AG associated with the AG acidoses persists when metabolic alkalosis also develops: The [HCO$_3^-$] increases while the [Cl$^-$] falls, leaving the AG large (**Table 11-6**). Patients with diabetic ketoacidosis have metabolic acidosis with a large AG. With nausea and vomiting, they generate in addition a metabolic alkalosis. Although the final arterial pH is typically acidic, it may sometimes become normal or even overtly alkaline if the alkalosis is more severe than the acidosis. Regardless of the pH, the large AG remains as a clue to the presence of a metabolic acidosis. A similar pattern is seen when uremic patients develop nausea and vomiting. If patients develop hyperchloremic (non-AG) acidosis and metabolic alkalosis, there is no residual AG clue to the presence

TABLE 11-7 Metabolic Acidosis, Metabolic Alkalosis, and Respiratory Alkalosis: A Triple Acid-Base Disturbance

ION	NORMAL CONCENTRATION	METABOLIC ALKALOSIS WITH APPROPRIATE COMPENSATION	HIGH AG METABOLIC ACIDOSIS WITH APPROPRIATE COMPENSATION	MIXED METABOLIC ACIDOSIS AND METABOLIC ALKALOSIS	MIXED METABOLIC ACIDOSIS, METABOLIC ALKALOSIS, AND RESPIRATORY ALKALOSIS
Na^+	140	140	140	140	140
K^+	4.0	3.4	4.5	4.5	4.5
Cl^-	105	93	105	92	92
HCO_3^-	25	34	12	25	25
AG	10	13	23	23	23
Pco_2	40	46	26	40	30
pH	7.42	7.49	7.29	7.42	7.54

AG, anion gap; Pco_2, arterial carbon dioxide tension.

of this mixed disorder; it may be suspected on the basis of the clinical history and physical examination (see next section).

Other Mixed Acid-Base Disorders

The combination of a hyperchloremic metabolic acidosis and metabolic alkalosis is more difficult to diagnose. In these patients, there is no residual AG increase to indicate that an underlying metabolic acidosis exists. Instead, whereas the hyperchloremic acidosis reduces the $[HCO_3^-]$ and increases the $[Cl^-]$, the metabolic alkalosis increases the $[HCO_3^-]$ and decreases the $[Cl^-]$. If the two disorders are of similar intensity, the final $[HCO_3^-]$ and $[Cl^-]$ may be in the normal range, with a normal AG. This mixed disorder can be suspected, however, on the basis of the history, clinical setting, and physical examination. For example, a patient with gastroenteritis who has a history of both watery diarrhea and vomiting may have this mixed acid-base disorder despite a normal pH, Pco_2, $[HCO_3^-]$, AG, and $[Cl^-]$, although marked hypokalemia often develops. If the vomiting improves but the diarrhea continues, overt hyperchloremic metabolic acidosis and acidemia may develop.

Other forms of mixed acid-base disorders are combinations of different metabolic acidosis disorders or, much less commonly, metabolic alkalosis disorders. For example, keto-acidosis not uncommonly coexists with lactic acidosis, and hyperchloremic acidosis caused by diarrhea or type IV renal tubular acidosis may be present together with lactic acidosis or uremic acidosis. Some patients with nausea and vomiting medicate themselves with baking soda and thereby both generate and ingest HCO_3^-.

Mixed respiratory acid-base disorders can also develop and are usually suspected on the basis of the history and clinical setting rather than any specific laboratory results. The patient with COPD who presents with recent pulmonary deterioration due to a mucus plug or pneumonia may

have chronic respiratory acidosis and a superimposed acute respiratory acidosis. A pregnant woman with underlying hyperventilation who ingests an overdose of sedating drugs and develops respiratory depression will have a chronic respiratory alkalosis and a superimposed acute respiratory acidosis.

Triple Acid-Base Disturbances

The most common, and most readily diagnosed, triple acid-base disturbance is the combination of AG metabolic acidosis, metabolic alkalosis, and either respiratory acidosis or respiratory alkalosis. The offsetting effects of the coexistent metabolic acidosis and alkalosis result in a low, normal, or elevated $[HCO_3^-]$. Regardless of the $[HCO_3^-]$, there is a large ΔAG which exceeds the ΔHCO_3^-. This is the clue to the double disorder of metabolic acidosis and metabolic alkalosis. The final $[HCO_3^-]$ which results from these two disorders is the parameter that should determine the degree of respiratory compensation and Pco_2. If the Pco_2 is lower than expected, a third disorder, respiratory alkalosis, exists. If the Pco_2 is higher than expected, the third disorder is respiratory acidosis.

A clinical example is the patient who vomits and develops metabolic alkalosis (**Table 11-7**). The $[HCO_3^-]$ increases to 34 mEq/L. The Pco_2 increases to 46 mm Hg, and the AG increases slightly. If extracellular fluid volume depletion becomes severe, lactic acidosis may ensue. The $[HCO_3^-]$ falls, in this example to 25 mEq/L, and the AG increases to 23 mEq/L. The discrepancy between the normal $[HCO_3^-]$ and the large AG is the clue to the disorder. The normal $[HCO_3^-]$ indicates that the Pco_2 should also be normal. The last column shows an example of a Pco_2 that is too low, indicating that an independent respiratory alkalosis disorder is also present.

The flow charts in **Figures 11-5** and **11-6** show one general approach to the diagnostic workup of a patient with either acidemia or alkalemia.

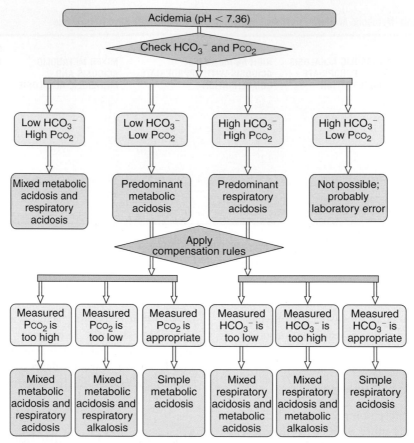

FIGURE 11-5 A flow chart showing one approach to the diagnostic workup of a patient with acidemia.

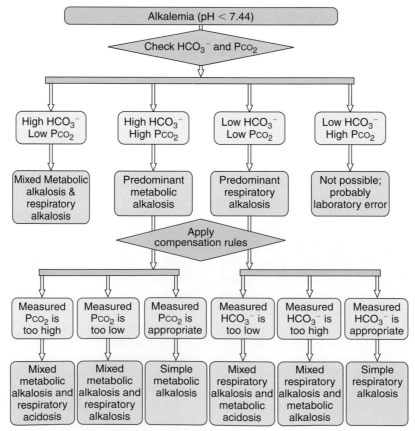

FIGURE 11-6 A flow chart showing one approach to the diagnostic workup of a patient with alkalemia.

BIBLIOGRAPHY

Emmett M, Narins R: Clinical use of the anion gap. Medicine 56: 38-54, 1977.

Emmett M, Seldin DW: Evaluation of acid-base disorders from plasma composition. In Seldin DW, Giebisch G (eds): The Regulation of Acid-Base Balance. New York, Raven Press, 1989, pp 213-263.

Gabow PA, Kaehny WD, Fennessey PV, et al: Diagnostic importance of an increased serum anion gap. N Engl J Med 303:854-858, 1980.

Narins RG, Emmett M: Simple and mixed acid-base disorders: A practical approach. Medicine 59:161-187, 1980.

Palmer BF, Alpern RJ: Metabolic alkalosis. J Am Soc Nephrol 8:1462-1469, 1997.

Rastegar A: Use of the DeltaAG/DeltaHCO$_3^-$ ratio in the diagnosis of mixed acid-base disorders. J Am Soc Nephrol 18:2429-2431, 2007.

CHAPTER 12

Disorders of Potassium Metabolism

Michael Allon

MECHANISMS OF POTASSIUM HOMEOSTASIS

Total body potassium is about 3500 mmol. Approximately 98% of the total is intracellular, primarily in skeletal muscle and to a lesser extent in liver. The remaining 2% (about 70 mmol) is in the extracellular fluid (ECF). Two homeostatic systems help to maintain potassium homeostasis. The first system regulates potassium excretion (kidney and intestine). The second regulates potassium shifts between the extracellular and intracellular fluid (ICF) compartments.

External Potassium Balance

The average American diet contains about 100 mmol of potassium per day. Dietary potassium intake may vary widely from day to day. To stay in potassium balance, it is necessary to increase excretion of K^+ when dietary potassium increases and decrease K^+ excretion when dietary potassium decreases. Normally, the kidneys excrete 90% to 95% of dietary potassium, with the remaining 5% to 10% excreted by the gut. Potassium excretion by the kidney is a relatively slow process: It takes 6 to 12 hours to excrete an acute potassium load.

Renal Handling of Potassium

To understand the physiologic factors that determine renal excretion of potassium, it is critical to review the main features of tubular potassium handling. Plasma K^+ is freely filtered across the glomerular capillary into the proximal tubule. It is subsequently completely reabsorbed by the proximal tubule and loop of Henle. In the distal tubule and the collecting duct, K^+ is secreted into the tubular lumen. For practical purposes, urinary excretion of K^+ can be viewed as a reflection of K^+ secretion into the lumen of the distal tubule and collecting duct. Therefore, any factor that stimulates K^+ secretion increases urinary K^+ excretion; conversely, any factor that inhibits K^+ secretion decreases urinary K^+ excretion.

Physiologic Regulation of Renal Potassium Excretion

Five major physiologic factors stimulate distal K^+ secretion (and thereby increase excretion): aldosterone; high distal sodium delivery; high urine flow rate; high [K^+] in tubular cell; and metabolic alkalosis. Aldosterone directly increases the activity of the sodium-potassium adenosinetriphosphatase (Na^+,K^+-ATPase) in the collecting duct cells, thereby

stimulating secretion of K^+ into the tubular lumen. Medical conditions that impair aldosterone production or secretion (e.g., diabetic nephropathy, chronic interstitial nephritis) and drugs that inhibit aldosterone production or action (e.g., nonsteroidal anti-inflammatory drugs [NSAIDs], angiotensin-converting enzyme [ACE] inhibitors, angiotensin receptor blockers [ARBs], heparin, spironolactone) decrease potassium secretion by the kidney. Conversely, medical conditions associated with increased aldosterone levels (primary aldosteronism, secondary aldosteronism due to diuretics or vomiting) increase potassium excretion by the kidney. Although there is profound secondary hyperaldosteronism in congestive heart failure and cirrhosis, each of these conditions may be associated with hyperkalemia due to decreased delivery of sodium.

Many diuretics increase renal K^+ excretion by a number of mechanisms, including high distal sodium delivery, high urine flow rate, metabolic alkalosis, and hyperaldosteronism due to volume depletion. Poorly controlled diabetes commonly increases urinary K^+ excretion due to osmotic diuresis with high urinary flow rate and high distal delivery of sodium.

Reabsorption of sodium (Na^+) in the collecting duct occurs through selective sodium channels. This creates an electronegative charge within the tubular lumen relative to the tubular epithelial cell, which in turn promotes secretion of cations (K^+ and H^+) into the lumen. Therefore, drugs that block the sodium channel in the collecting duct decrease potassium secretion. Conversely, in Liddle's syndrome, a rare genetic disorder, this sodium channel is constitutively open, resulting in avid sodium reabsorption and excessive potassium secretion.

Adaptation in Renal Failure

In patients with renal failure, the kidney compensates by increasing the efficiency of K^+ excretion. Clearly, there is a limit to renal compensation, and a significant loss of kidney function impairs the ability to excrete K^+, thereby predisposing to a positive potassium balance and a tendency to hyperkalemia. In most patients with chronic renal failure, overt hyperkalemia does not occur until the rate of creatinine clearance falls to less than 10 mL/min. Serum aldosterone levels are elevated in many patients with chronic renal failure. Aldosterone stimulates the activity of both Na^+,K^+-ATPase and H^+,K^+-ATPase, thereby promoting secretion of K^+ in the collecting duct and defending against hyperkalemia. These adaptive mechanisms are less effective in patients with acute renal failure, as compared with chronic renal failure. Moreover, patients with acute renal failure are often hypotensive, resulting in tissue hypoperfusion and release of potassium from ischemic limbs. For these reasons, severe hyperkalemia occurs more frequently in patients with acute, rather than chronic, renal failure.

A subset of patients with chronic renal failure fail to increase aldosterone levels appreciably; as a result, they develop hyperkalemia at moderate levels of renal insufficiency (creatinine clearance <50 mL/min), typically in association with a hyperchloremic, normal anion gap metabolic acidosis (type IV renal tubular acidosis [RTA]). This condition is most commonly associated with diabetic nephropathy and chronic interstitial nephritis. Moreover, administration of drugs that inhibit aldosterone production or secretion (e.g., ACE inhibitors, ARBs, NSAIDs, heparin) may provoke hyperkalemia in patients with mild to moderate chronic renal failure.

Intestinal Potassium Excretion

Like the renal collecting duct, the small intestine and colon secrete K^+. Aldosterone stimulates K^+ excretion by the gut. In normal individuals, intestinal K^+ excretion plays a minor role in potassium homeostasis. However, in patients with significant renal failure, intestinal K^+ secretion is increased threefold to fourfold, contributing significantly to potassium homeostasis. This adaptation is limited, and it is inadequate to compensate for the loss of excretory function in patients with advanced renal failure.

Internal Potassium Balance

Overview

The $[K^+]$ in the ECF is approximately 4 mEq/L, whereas the intracellular $[K^+]$ is about 150 mEq/L. Because of the uneven distribution of K^+ between the fluid compartments, a relatively small net shift of K^+ from the ICF to the ECF compartment produces a marked increase in plasma K^+. Conversely, a relatively small net shift from the extracellular to the ICF compartment produces a marked decrease in plasma K^+. Unlike renal excretion of K^+, which requires several hours, the shift of K^+ between the ECF and ICF compartments (also referred to as *extrarenal potassium disposal*) is extremely rapid, occurring within minutes.

Clearly, in patients with advanced renal failure, whose capacity to excrete K^+ is marginal, extrarenal potassium disposal plays a critical role in the prevention of life-threatening hyperkalemia after potassium-rich meals. The following example illustrates this important principle. Suppose that a 70-kg dialysis patient with a serum $[K^+]$of 4.5 mmol/L eats 1 cup of pinto beans (35 mmol potassium). Initially, the dietary potassium is absorbed into the ECF compartment ($0.2 \times 70 = 14$ L). This amount of dietary potassium will increase the serum $[K^+]$ by 35 mmol ÷ 14 L, or 2.5 mmol/L. In the absence of extrarenal potassium disposal, the patient's serum $[K^+]$ would rise acutely to 7.0 mmol/L, a level frequently associated with serious ventricular arrhythmias. In practice,

the increase in serum $[K^+]$ is much smaller, because of efficient physiologic mechanisms that promote the shift of K^+ into the ICF compartment.

Effects of Insulin and Catecholamines on Extrarenal Potassium Disposal

The two major physiologic factors that stimulate transfer of K^+ from the ECF to the ICF compartment are insulin and epinephrine. The stimulation of extrarenal potassium disposal by insulin and by β_2-adrenergic agonists is mediated by stimulation of the Na^+,K^+-ATPase activity, primarily in skeletal muscle cells. Interference with these two physiologic mechanisms (i.e., insulin deficiency or β_2-adrenergic blockade) predisposes to hyperkalemia. On the other hand, excessive levels of insulin or epinephrine predispose to hypokalemia.

The potassium-lowering effect of insulin is dose-related within the physiologic range of plasma insulin. The potassium-lowering effect of insulin is independent of its effect on plasma glucose. Even the low physiologic levels of insulin that are present during fasting promote extrarenal potassium disposal. In nondiabetic individuals, hyperglycemia stimulates endogenous insulin secretion, thereby decreasing the serum $[K^+]$. In insulin-dependent diabetics, endogenous insulin production is limited, and significant hyperglycemia may occur. Hyperglycemia results in plasma hypertonicity, which promotes the shift of K^+ out of the cells and produces a paradoxic hyperkalemia.

The potassium-lowering action of epinephrine is mediated by β_2-adrenergic stimulation, and is blocked by nonselective β-blockers, but not by selective β_1-adrenergic blockers. α-Adrenergic stimulation promotes shifts of potassium out of the cells and into the ECF compartment, tending to increase serum $[K^+]$. Epinephrine is a mixed α- and β-adrenergic agonist, and its net effect on serum $[K^+]$ reflects the balance between its β-adrenergic (potassium-lowering) and α-adrenergic (potassium-raising) effects. In normal individuals, the β-adrenergic effect of epinephrine predominates, so that the serum $[K^+]$ decreases. In contrast, the α-adrenergic effect of epinephrine on K^+ shifts is much more prominent in patients with severe renal failure; as a result, dialysis patients are refractory to the potassium-lowering effect of epinephrine.

Effect of Acid-Base Disorders on Extrarenal Potassium Disposal

Acid-base disorders produce internal K^+ shifts in a less predictable manner. As a general rule, metabolic alkalosis shifts K^+ into the cells, whereas metabolic acidosis shifts K^+ out of the cells. However, the nature of the metabolic acidosis determines its effect on serum $[K^+]$. Cells are relatively impermeable to chloride (Cl^-). With inorganic acidosis, entry of protons (but not Cl^-) into the cell results in a reciprocal extrusion of K^+ out of the cell to maintain electrical neutrality. In contrast, cells are highly permeable to organic anions. The addition of an organic acid to the ECF results in parallel shifts of protons and organic anions into the cells, with no net change in the electrical balance; as a result, K^+ is not extruded out of the cells. Therefore, a mineral acidosis (i.e., a hyperchloremic, normal anion gap metabolic acidosis) typically results in hyperkalemia, whereas an organic metabolic acidosis (e.g., a lactic acidosis) does not affect the serum $[K^+]$. Bicarbonate administration to individuals with normal renal function decreases serum $[K^+]$, but this effect is largely due to enhanced urinary excretion of K^+. In contrast, bicarbonate administration to dialysis patients (in whom the capacity for urinary K^+ excretion is negligible) does not lower plasma $[K^+]$ acutely. Moreover, bicarbonate administration does not potentiate the potassium-lowering effects of insulin or albuterol in dialysis patients.

LABORATORY TESTS FOR DIFFERENTIAL DIAGNOSIS OF POTASSIUM DISORDERS

Differential Diagnosis of Hypokalemia and Hyperkalemia

The clinical history, review of medications, family history, and physical examination are sufficient in the rapid differential diagnosis of most potassium disorders. In selected patients, the cause of a hypokalemia or hyperkalemia is not apparent, and additional specialized laboratory tests may be useful. Measurements of the fractional excretion of potassium (FE_K) and the transtubular potassium gradient (TTKG) may be useful in distinguishing between renal and nonrenal causes of hyperkalemia and hypokalemia. The general principle underlying these tests is that the kidney compensates for hyperkalemia by increasing K^+ excretion, and it compensates for hypokalemia by decreasing K^+ excretion. If K^+ excretion is inappropriate for the level of serum $[K^+]$, a renal etiology is suggested. The optimal use of FE_K or TTKG in the differential diagnosis requires that these values be obtained before the potassium abnormality (hyperkalemia or hypokalemia) is corrected.

Fractional Excretion of Potassium

FE_K is the percentage of potassium filtered into the proximal tubule that appears in the urine. It represents potassium clearance (Cl_K) corrected for glomerular filtration rate (as represented by the creatinine clearance, Cl_{Cr}):

$$FE_K = Cl_K / Cl_{Cr}$$

Because the clearance of any substance is equal to the volume cleared (V) times the ratio of the urinary to the plasma concentration of the substance, this calculation can be algebraically transformed as follows:

$$FE_K = \frac{(V \times U_K / S_K)}{(V \times U_{Cr} / S_{Cr})} \times 100\%$$

where U_K and U_{Cr} are the concentrations of potassium and creatinine, respectively, in the urine and S_K and S_{Cr} are the corresponding serum concentrations. The V in the numerator and denominator cancel out, giving simplified formula,

$$FE_K = \frac{U_K / S_K}{U_{Cr} / S_{Cr}} \times 100\%$$

For an individual with normal renal function who has an average dietary potassium intake, the FE_K is approximately 10%. If hypokalemia is present due to extrarenal causes (low potassium diet, gastrointestinal losses, potassium shifts into cells), the kidney conserves K^+, and the FE_K is low. In contrast, hypokalemia due to renal K^+ losses is associated with an increased FE_K. Similarly, in the setting of hyperkalemia, a high FE_K suggests an extrarenal cause, whereas a low FE_K is consistent with a renal cause. If a urine creatinine measurement is not available, one can often use U_K alone to differentiate between renal and extrarenal causes of hyperkalemia. Specifically, in a hypokalemic patient, a U_K greater than 20 mEq/L suggests a renal cause, whereas a U_K lower than 20 mEq/L suggests an extrarenal cause.

Transtubular Potassium Gradient

The TTKG is calculated by a formula that estimates the potassium gradient between the urine and the blood in the distal nephron:

$$TTKG = \left[U_K \div (U_{osm} / P_{osm}) \right] \div P_K$$

where U_{osm} and P_{osm} are the urine and plasma osmolalities. The numerator is an estimate of the luminal potassium concentration. The U_{osm}/P_{osm} term is included to correct for the rise in U_K that is due purely to water abstraction and concentration of the urine overall. TTKG values have been derived from empiric measurements in normal individuals under a variety of physiologic conditions. In normal circumstances, the TTKG is between 6 and 8. Hypokalemia with a high TTKG suggests excessive renal potassium losses, whereas hypokalemia with a low TTKG suggests an extrarenal etiology. Similarly, hyperkalemia with a low TTKG suggests a renal cause, whereas hyperkalemia with a high TTKG is consistent with an extrarenal cause.

Limits of Fractional Excretion and Transtubular Gradient in Diagnosis

Several factors limit the utility of FE_K and TTKG in the differential diagnosis of potassium disorders. The FE_K and TTKG are increased when dietary potassium is increased and decreased when dietary potassium is decreased. Furthermore, in patients with chronic renal failure, there is an adaptive increase in K^+ excretion per functioning nephron, such that FE_K and TTKG increase. This means that the "normal" value for a given individual can vary substantially, making it difficult to determine the significance of a high or low FE_K or TTKG.

HYPOKALEMIA

Hypokalemia versus Potassium Deficiency

It is important to distinguish between potassium deficiency and hypokalemia. Potassium deficiency is the state that results from a persistent negative potassium balance (i.e., potassium excretion exceeding potassium intake). Hypokalemia refers to a low plasma [K$^+$]. Hypokalemia can result from potassium deficiency (inadequate potassium intake or excessive potassium losses) or from a net shift of K$^+$ from the ECF to the ICF compartment. A patient may have severe potassium depletion without manifesting hypokalemia.

An important example is a patient who presents with diabetic ketoacidosis. Such patients have typically had severe hyperglycemia with osmotic diuresis for several days, leading to high levels of renal K$^+$ excretion and potassium deficiency. However, as a result of insulin deficiency, there is a concomitant shift of K$^+$ out of the cells into the ECF compartment. At presentation to the hospital, such patients are frequently normokalemic or even hyperkalemic. Once they are treated with exogenous insulin, there is a rapid shift of K$^+$ back into the cells, and within a few hours the patients develop significant hypokalemia. Conversely, patients hospitalized with an acute myocardial infarction commonly have hypokalemia due to stress-induced release of catecholamines and enhanced extrarenal potassium disposal, even though they have a normal external potassium balance.

Clinical Disorders Associated with Hypokalemia

Table 12-1 provides a list of the most common causes of hypokalemia. The kidney can so avidly conserve potassium that hypokalemia due to inadequate potassium intake is a rare event requiring prolonged starvation ("tea and toast diet"). Therefore, hypokalemia is usually caused by excessive K$^+$ losses from the gut or urine or by K$^+$ shifts from the ECF to the ICF compartments. Prolonged vomiting causes potassium losses, in part because of direct loss of potassium present in the gastric juice (approximately 10 mEq/L), but primarily because of renal losses due to secondary aldosteronism from volume depletion. Severe diarrhea, from either disease or laxative abuse, results in significant potassium excretion in the stool.

Excessive renal K$^+$ loss as a cause of hypokalemia is seen with a number of clinical syndromes. Conceptually, it is useful to distinguish between hypokalemia associated with hypertension (see Chapter 66) and hypokalemia associated with a normal blood pressure. If hypokalemia is associated with hypertension, measurements of plasma renin and aldosterone may be helpful in the differential diagnosis. Several physiologic observations are relevant in this regard. Aldosterone, a mineralocorticoid, stimulates Na$^+$ reabsorption and K$^+$ secretion in the collecting duct. The physiologic stimulus for aldosterone secretion is activation of the renin-angiotensin axis. Moreover, aldosterone-induced Na$^+$ retention suppresses the renin-angiotensin axis by negative feedback. Finally, glucocorticoids at high concentrations bind to mineralocorticoid receptors and mimic their physiologic actions. Glucocorticoids are stimulated by corticotropin (ACTH), and they suppress ACTH production by negative feedback.

Primary aldosteronism is caused by autonomous (non–renin-mediated) secretion of aldosterone by the adrenal

TABLE 12-1 **Causes of Hypokalemia**
Inadequate Potassium Intake (Severe Malnutrition)
Extrarenal Potassium Losses
Vomiting
Diarrhea
Hypokalemia Sue to Urinary Potassium Losses
Diuretics (loop diuretics, thiazides, acetazolamide)
Osmotic diuresis (e.g., hyperglycemia)

Hypokalemia with hypertension
  Primary aldosteronism
  Glucocorticoid-remediable aldosteronism
  Malignant hypertension
  Renovascular hypertension
  Renin-secreting tumor
  Essential hypertension with excessive diuretics
  Liddle syndrome
  11β-Hydroxysteroid dehydrogenase deficiency
    Genetic (syndrome of apparent mineralocorticoid excess)
    Drug induced (chewing tobacco, licorice, some French wines)
  Congenital adrenal hyperplasia

Hypokalemia with a normal blood pressure
  Distal renal tubular acidosis (type I)
  Proximal renal tubular acidosis (type II)
  Bartter's syndrome
  Gitelman's syndrome
  Hypomagnesemia (cisplatinum, alcoholism, diuretics)

Hypokalemia Due to Potassium Shifts
Insulin administration
Catecholamine excess (acute stress)
Familial periodic hypokalemic paralysis
Thyrotoxic hypokalemic paralysis

cortex. This results in avid Na$^+$ retention and K$^+$ secretion by the distal nephron. Patients present with volume-dependent hypertension, hypokalemia, and metabolic alkalosis. Biochemical evaluation reveals a high serum aldosterone level and suppressed plasma renin. Abdominal computed tomographic scanning reveals either a unilateral adrenal adenoma or bilateral adrenal hyperplasia. The former is treated surgically, and the latter with spironolactone.

Glucocorticoid-remediable aldosteronism is a rare, autosomal-dominant condition in which there is fusion of the 11β-hydroxylase and aldosterone synthase genes. As a result, aldosterone secretion is stimulated by ACTH, and can be suppressed by an exogenous mineralocorticoid, dexamethasone. Patients with this condition have a very similar clinical presentation to those with primary aldosteronism (i.e., volume-dependent hypertension, hypokalemia, high serum aldosterone, and low serum renin), except that they are younger and have a family history of hypertension.

Patients with *renovascular hypertension, renin-secreting tumors* and severe *malignant hypertension* may also present with severe hypertension and hypokalemia. In contrast to patients with primary aldosteronism, these patient have secondary aldosteronism, demonstrated by high serum renin and aldosterone levels. Of course, patients with essential hypertension may also have hypokalemia and high plasma renin and aldosterone levels if they are treated with loop or thiazide diuretics and are volume depleted.

Patients with *11β-hydroxysteroid dehydrogenase deficiency*, a rare genetic disorder, have a defect in the conversion of cortisol to cortisone in the peripheral tissues. This results in high tissue cortisol levels that activate the mineralocorticoid receptors, producing hypokalemia and hypertension. Such patients have low serum renin and aldosterone levels. Chewing tobacco, certain brands of licorice, and some French red wines contain glycyrrhizic acid, which inhibits 11β-hydroxysteroid dehydrogenase. Ingestion of such foods may produce hypokalemia, volume-dependent hypertension, and low serum renin and aldosterone levels, similar to the clinical presentation of congenital 11β-hydroxysteroid dehydrogenase deficiency.

Patients with *congenital adrenal hyperplasia* have a deficiency of 11β-hydroxylase, an enzyme that is required in the common pathways for mineralocorticoids and glucocorticoids. These patients have low serum renin and aldosterone levels, high levels of deoxycorticosterone acetate (DOCA, a mineralocorticoid), and high levels of androgen. Males have early puberty, and females exhibit virilization, with hirsutism and clitorimegaly. This condition improves with administration of exogenous corticosteroids to suppress ACTH.

Liddle's syndrome is a rare autosomal-dominant disorder caused by a defect of the sodium channel that results in increased Na^+ absorption and K^+ secretion in the collecting duct. Patients present with hypokalemia, hypertension, and volume overload. Their biochemical profile reveals low levels of serum renin and aldosterone. The patients' blood pressure and serum $[K^+]$ improve dramatically with administration of inhibitors of the sodium channel, such as amiloride.

Hypokalemia due to excessive renal K^+ excretion is also seen in a number of clinical conditions in which hypertension is infrequent. Both type I (distal) and type II (proximal) RTA are associated with kaliuresis and hypokalemia, and both conditions manifest with a normal anion gap metabolic acidosis. *Type I RTA* is frequently associated with hypercalciuria and calcium oxalate kidney stones. *Type II RTA* is rare in adults and is often associated with a generalized defect in proximal tubular function, manifesting with glycosuria (with a normal serum glucose concentration), hypophosphatemia with phosphaturia, and a low serum uric acid level with uricosuria.

Bartter's syndrome is a rare familial disease characterized by hypokalemia, metabolic alkalosis, hypercalciuria, normal blood pressure, and high plasma renin and aldosterone levels. It has been associated with a number of mutations that inhibit active Na^+ reabsorption in the thick ascending limb of Henle, including mutations in the Na^+-K^+-2Cl cotransporter (NKCC2), the voltage-gated basolateral chloride channel (ClC-Kb), and the apical K^+ conductance channel (ROMK) (see Chapter 40). Patients act as if they are chronically ingesting loop diuretics; for this reason, they are difficult to distinguish clinically from patients with surreptitious diuretic ingestion. Patients with *Gitelman's syndrome*, a variant of Bartter's syndrome, differ in that they have hypocalciuria and hypomagnesemia. Gitelman's syndrome has been linked to a mutation in the renal thiazide-sensitive Na^+-Cl^- cotransporter (NCCT). These patients act as if they are chronically ingesting thiazide diuretics.

Familial hypokalemic periodic paralysis is a rare, autosomal-dominant disorder in which affected individuals develop periodic episodes of severe muscle weakness in association with profound hypokalemia, caused by rapid shifts of K^+ from the ECF to the ICF compartment. Even when the patient has complete paralysis, however, the diaphragm and bulbar muscles are spared, so that the patient is able to breathe, swallow, talk, and blink. The paralysis resolves within hours after potassium ingestion. Patients are asymptomatic with a normal serum K^+ in between the acute episodes.

Thyrotoxic hypokalemic paralysis is an unusual manifestation of hyperthyroidism, seen primarily in Asian patients. The clinical presentation is similar to that of hypokalemic periodic paralysis, except that the paralytic episodes cease when the hyperthyroidism is corrected.

Drug-Induced Hypokalemia

A number of drugs have the potential to cause hypokalemia, either by stimulating renal K^+ excretion or by blocking extrarenal disposal. Exogenous mineralocorticoids mimic the effects of aldosterone, thereby stimulating distal K^+ secretion. High doses of glucocorticoids possess some mineralocorticoid activity and have a similar effect. Most diuretics, including loop diuretics, thiazide diuretics, and acetazolamide increase renal K^+ excretion. A number of drugs, including alcohol, diuretics, and cisplatinum, cause renal magnesium-wasting and hypomagnesemia. For reasons that are not well understood, hypomagnesemia impairs renal K^+ conservation. Therefore, these patients may have associated hypokalemia that is refractory to potassium supplementation until the magnesium deficit is corrected. (Paradoxically, cyclosporine may produce hypomagnesemia in conjunction with hyperkalemia.)

Drugs that promote extrarenal potassium disposal may also result in hypokalemia. This phenomenon can be seen after the administration of an acute dose of insulin. Similarly, β_2-agonists (either intravenous or nebulized), including albuterol and terbutaline, frequently result in acute hypokalemia.

Clinical Manifestations of Hypokalemia

Hypokalemia may produce electrocardiographic (ECG) abnormalities, including a flattened T wave and a U wave (**Fig. 12-1**). Hypokalemia also appears to increases the risk of ventricular arrhythmias in patients with ischemic heart disease and in patients taking digoxin. Severe hypokalemia is associated with variable degrees of skeletal muscle weakness, even to the point of paralysis. On rare occasions, diaphragmatic paralysis from hypokalemia can lead to respiratory arrest. There may also be decreased motility of smooth muscle, manifesting with ileus or urinary retention. Rarely, severe hypokalemia can result in rhabdomyolysis.

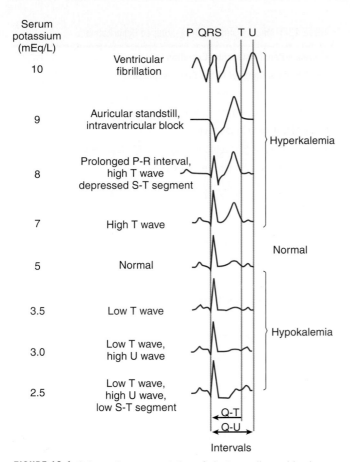

FIGURE 12-1 Schematic representation of electrocardiographic changes and the serum potassium levels at which such changes are typically seen. (From Seldin DW, Giebisch G [eds]: The Regulation of Potassium Balance, New York, Raven, 1989, with permission.)

Severe hypokalemia also interferes with the urinary concentrating mechanism in the distal nephron, resulting in nephrogenic diabetes insipidus. Such patients have a low urine osmolality in the face of high serum osmolality and are refractory to vasopressin.

Treatment of Hypokalemia

The immediate treatment of hypokalemia requires potassium supplementation. This can be given either intravenously or orally. The correlation between serum [K+] and total potassium deficit in hypokalemia patients is poor. A given patient's serum [K+] is a reflection of both the external potassium balance and transcellular potassium shifts. The percentage of administered exogenous potassium that remains in the ECF compartment is variable. Therefore, it is difficult to predict how much potassium replacement a given hypokalemic patient will require. Without adequate monitoring, it is possible to give too much potassium and make the patient hyperkalemic. Therefore, one should give multiple small doses of potassium, with frequent checks of serum [K+] values.

Oral potassium administration is safer than the intravenous route and is less likely to produce an overshoot in the serum [K+]. Each oral dose should not exceed 20 to 40 mEq

of potassium. Intravenous KCl should be reserved for severe, symptomatic hypokalemia (< 3.0 mEq/L) or for patients who cannot ingest oral potassium. Intravenous KCl should not be given any faster than 10 mmol/hr in the absence of continuous ECG monitoring. The serum [K+] should be rechecked every 2 to 3 hours to confirm a clinical response and avoid an overshoot.

Correction of the underlying medical condition may prevent recurrence of hypokalemia after its correction. If the patient has a chronic condition associated with persistent urinary K+ losses, such that hypokalemia is likely to recur, the patient should be encouraged to increase the intake of foods high in potassium (especially fresh fruits, nuts, and legumes). In some patients, chronic oral potassium supplementation may be necessary.

HYPERKALEMIA

Pseudohyperkalemia is a factitious elevation of the serum [K+] caused by in vitro release of potassium from blood cells. It may be seen with in vitro hemolysis, thrombocytosis, or severe leukocytosis. Pseudohyperkalemia due to hemolysis is readily apparent because the serum is pink. Pseudohyperkalemia due to severe thrombocytosis or leukocytosis may be confirmed by drawing simultaneous blood samples in tubes with and without anticoagulant; if the serum [K+] is higher than the plasma [K+], the diagnosis is confirmed.

True hyperkalemia is caused by a positive potassium balance (increased potassium intake or decreased potassium excretion) or an increase in net K+ shift from the ICF to the ECF compartment. **Table 12-2** provides a list of the most common causes of hyperkalemia. In practice, most patients who develop severe hyperkalemia have more than one contributory factor. For example, a patient with moderate renal failure due to diabetic nephropathy may be medicated with an ACE inhibitor and have mild hyperkalemia; however, after indomethacin is started for acute gouty arthritis, the patient rapidly develops severe hyperkalemia.

Drug-Induced Hyperkalemia

A large number of drugs have the potential to cause hyperkalemia, either by inhibiting renal K+ excretion or by blocking extrarenal potassium disposal (**Table 12-3**). Most individuals taking these drugs do not develop hyperkalemia. Patients at risk are those with renal failure, especially if they have a high dietary potassium intake or are on taking additional medication that predisposes to hyperkalemia.

Most diuretics (loop diuretics, thiazide diuretics, acetazolamide) increase urinary K+ excretion and tend to cause hypokalemia. However, potassium-sparing diuretics inhibit urinary K+ excretion and predispose to hyperkalemia by one of two mechanisms. Spironolactone and eplerenone are competitive inhibitors of aldosterone; they bind to the aldosterone receptors in the collecting duct, thereby inhibiting Na+,K+-ATPase activity and indirectly limiting K+ secretion. Interestingly, the immunosuppressant drug, cyclosporine,

TABLE 12-2 Causes of Hyperkalemia

Pseudohyperkalemia

Hemolysis

Thrombocytosis

Severe leukocytosis

Fist clenching

Decreased Renal Excretion

Acute or chronic renal failure

Aldosterone deficiency (e.g., type IV renal tubular acidosis)—
frequently associated with diabetic nephropathy, chronic interstitial
nephritis, or obstructive nephropathy

Adrenal insufficiency (Addison's disease)

Drugs that inhibit potassium excretion (see Table 12-3)

Kidney diseases that impair distal tubule function
Sickle cell anemia
Systemic lupus erythematosus

Abnormal Potassium Distribution

Insulin deficiency

β-Blockers

Metabolic or respiratory acidosis

Familial hyperkalemic periodic paralysis

Abnormal Potassium Release from Cells

Rhabdomyolysis

Tumor lysis syndrome

TABLE 12-3 Mechanisms for Drug-Induced Hyperkalemia

Decrease Renal Potassium Excretion

Block Sodium Channel in the Distal Nephron

Potassium-sparing diuretics: amiloride, triamterene

Antibiotics: trimethoprim, pentamidine

Block Aldosterone Production

ACE inhibitors (e.g., captopril, enalapril, lisinopril, benazepril)

Angiotensin receptor blockers (ARB)

NSAIDs and COX-2 inhibitors

Heparin

Tacrolimus

Block Aldosterone Receptors

Spironolactone

Eplerenone

Block Na^+,K^+-ATPase Activity in the Distal Nephron

Cyclosporine

Inhibit Extrarenal Potassium Disposal

Block $β_2$-adrenergic–mediated extrarenal potassium disposal—
nonselective β-blockers (e.g., propranolol, nadolol, timolol)

Block $Na^+,K+$-ATPase activity in skeletal muscles: digoxin overdose
(not therapeutic doses)

Inhibit insulin release (e.g., somatostatin)

Potassium Release from Injured Cells

Drug-induced rhabdomyolysis (e.g., lovastatin, cocaine)

Drug-induced tumor lysis syndrome (chemotherapy agents in acute
leukemias, high-grade lymphomas)

Depolarizing paralytic agents (e.g., succinylcholine)

Drug-Induced Acute Renal Failure

ACE, angiotensin-converting enzyme; ATPase, adenosine triphosphatase; COX-2,
cyclooxygenase 2; NSAIDs, nonsteroidal anti-inflammatory drugs.

also blocks Na^+,K^+-ATPase activity in the distal nephron. Two other potassium-sparing diuretics, amiloride and triamterene, bind to the sodium channel in the collecting duct. This inhibits Na^+ reabsorption in the distal nephron and thereby limits the establishment of an electrochemical gradient required for K^+ secretion. Two antibiotics, trimethoprim (one of the components of Bactrim) and pentamidine, have also been shown to block the sodium channel in the collecting duct and therefore predispose patients to hyperkalemia. In addition, trimethoprim has been shown to inhibit the collecting tubule H^+,K^+-ATPase.

Because aldosterone plays an important role in enhancing renal K^+ excretion in patients with renal failure, drugs that inhibit aldosterone production (either directly or indirectly) predispose such patients to hyperkalemia. Angiotensin II is a potent stimulator of aldosterone production in the adrenal cortex. Angiotensin converting enzyme (ACE) inhibitors inhibit the production of angiotensin II, thereby decreasing aldosterone levels. Similarly, angiotensin II receptor blockers also inhibit aldosterone production. Prostaglandins directly stimulate renin production, and prostaglandin inhibitors (NSAIDs) inhibit the production of renin, thereby indirectly decreasing aldosterone production. This effect is seen even with "renal-sparing" NSAIDs such as sulindac (a nonselective cyclooxygenase 1 [COX-1] and COX-2 inhibitor). Hyperkalemia may also be caused by selective COX-2 inhibitors. Heparin has been shown to directly inhibit the production of aldosterone in the renal cortex, primarily by decreasing

the number and affinity of angiotensin II receptors in the zona glomerulosa. This effect occurs even with the low doses of subcutaneous heparin used for prophylaxis of venous thrombosis in hospitalized patients (e.g., 5000 units every 12 hours). Tacrolimus, an immunosuppressant drug, may also cause hyperkalemia by inhibiting aldosterone synthesis. Oral contraceptives containing drospirenone (a progestin) inhibit renal K^+ excretion and may provoke hyperkalemia in women with chronic kidney disease.

Given the stimulation of extrarenal potassium disposal by β-adrenergic agonists, it is not surprising that $β_2$-antagonists can predispose to hyperkalemia. This effect is seen primarily with nonselective β-blockers (e.g., propranolol, nadolol), rather than β-selective blockers (e.g., atenolol, metoprolol). There is significant systemic absorption of topical β-blockers, and severe hyperkalemia may rarely be provoked by timolol eye drops. Drugs that inhibit endogenous insulin release, such as somatostatin, have been implicated rarely as a cause of hyperkalemia in patients with renal failure. Presumably, long-acting somatostatin analogues, such as octreotide, would have a similar effect on serum K^+. Digoxin overdose causes inhibition of Na^+,K^+-ATPase activity in skeletal muscle cells and may manifest with hyperkalemia. This effect is rarely seen at therapeutic doses of the drug. Depolarizing paralytic agents used for general anesthesia, such as succinylcholine, can occasionally produce hyperkalemia, by causing K^+ to leak out of the cells.

Finally, drugs can also cause hyperkalemia indirectly by causing the release of intracellular K^+ from injured cells; examples are rhabdomyolysis with lovastatin and cocaine and tumor lysis syndrome when chemotherapy is administered to patients with acute leukemia or high-grade lymphoma. Moreover, drug-induced acute renal failure may be associated with secondary hyperkalemia.

A common clinical dilemma occurs when patients with chronic kidney disease develop hyperkalemia after being started on an ACE inhibitor or ARB. One would like to continue the drug because of its renoprotective benefit. Therapeutic options for this scenario include reducing the dose of ACE inhibitor or ARB, starting or increasing the dose of a loop or thiazide diuretic, discontinuing other medications that promote hyperkalemia, and reinforcing dietary potassium restriction. Fludrocortisone (0.1 to 0.2 mg daily) can be tried in refractory cases, although it may promote peripheral edema and hypertension resulting from avid Na^+ retention.

Fasting Hyperkalemia in Dialysis Patients

Prolonged fasting decreases plasma insulin concentrations, thereby promoting K^+ shifts from the ICF to the ECF compartments. In normal individuals, the excess potassium is excreted in the urine, so that the plasma $[K^+]$ remains constant. In dialysis patients, the potassium entering the ECF compartment during fasting cannot be excreted, and progressive hyperkalemia results. The phenomenon of fasting hyperkalemia may be clinically significant in dialysis patients who are fasted longer than 8 to 12 hours before a surgical or radiologic procedure. Occasionally, such patients develop life-threatening hyperkalemia during a prolonged fast. The hyperkalemia can be prevented by administration of intravenous dextrose (to stimulate endogenous insulin secretion) for the duration of the fast. If the patient is diabetic, insulin must be added to the dextrose infusion to prevent paradoxic hyperkalemia.

Clinical Manifestations of Hyperkalemia

Hyperkalemia may produce progressive ECG abnormalities, including peaked T waves, flattened or absent P waves, widened QRS complexes, and sine waves (see **Fig. 12-1**). The major risk of severe hyperkalemia is the development of life-threatening ventricular arrhythmias. Severe hyperkalemia with ECG changes is a medical emergency.

Severe hyperkalemia, like severe hypokalemia, can cause skeletal muscle weakness, even to the point of paralysis and respiratory failure. Hyperkalemia impairs urinary acidification by decreasing collecting tubule apical H^+,K^+-ATPase, which may result in an RTA (type IV). Hyperkalemia

stimulates endogenous aldosterone secretion. Hyperkalemia stimulates insulin secretion in dogs, but not in humans.

Treatment of Hyperkalemia

Severe hyperkalemia associated with ECG changes (see **Fig. 12-1**) is a life-threatening state requiring emergent intervention. If the patient's ECG is suspicious for hyperkalemia, one should initiate therapy without waiting for the laboratory confirmation. If the patient has renal failure, urgent dialysis is required for removal of potassium from the body. Because of the inevitable delay in initiating dialysis, the following temporizing measures must be initiated promptly.

1. *The first step is to stabilize the myocardium.* Acute administration of intravenous calcium gluconate does not change plasma $[K^+]$ but does transiently improve the ECG. The effect is almost immediate. One should give 10 mL of calcium gluconate over 1 minute. If there is no improvement in the ECG appearance within 3 to 5 minutes, the dose should be repeated.

2. *The second step is to shift potassium* from the ECF to the ICF, so as to rapidly decrease the serum $[K^+]$. This involves the administration of insulin and a β_2-agonist.

   a. *Intravenous insulin* is the fastest way to lower the serum $[K^+]$. The plasma $[K^+]$ starts to decrease within 15 minutes. Intravenous glucose is given concurrently to prevent hypoglycemia. One should give 10 units of regular insulin and 50 mL of 50% dextrose (1 ampoule of D50) as a bolus, followed by a continuous infusion of 5% dextrose at a rate of 100 mL/hr to prevent late hypoglycemia. In diabetic patients, the serum glucose concentration should be ascertained with a Glucometer; if it is greater than 300 mg/dL, the intravenous insulin may be administered alone (i.e., without concomitant 50% dextrose). One should never give dextrose without insulin for the acute treatment of hyperkalemia; in patients with inadequate endogenous insulin production, the resulting hyperglycemia could produce a paradoxic increase in serum K^+.

   b. *β-Agonists:* One should give 20 mg of albuterol (a β_2-agonist) by inhalation over 10 minutes. The onset of action is 30 minutes. Make sure to use the concentrated form (5 mg/mL) of the drug to minimize the volume that needs to be inhaled. The dose required to lower plasma $[K^+]$ is considerably higher than that used to treat asthma, because only a small fraction of nebulized albuterol is absorbed systemically (0.5 mg of intravenous albuterol [not available in the United States] produces a change in plasma $[K^+]$ comparable to that seen after 20 mg of nebulized albuterol. The potassium-lowering effect of albuterol is additive to that of insulin.

   c. *Sodium bicarbonate:* In patients with chronic kidney disease who are not yet undergoing dialysis, bicarbonate administration can lower the serum $[K^+]$ by enhancing renal K^+ excretion. However, bicarbonate administration is of dubious value for treatment of hyperkalemia in patients without residual kidney function. It takes at least 3 to 4 hours for the serum [K⁺] to start to decrease after bicarbonate administration to dialysis patients, so this modality is not useful for the acute management of hyperkalemia. Moreover, bicarbonate administration does not enhance the potassium-lowering effects of insulin or albuterol. Bicarbonate administration is still indicated if the patient has severe metabolic acidosis (serum bicarbonate concentration <10 mmol/L).

3. Once the previous temporizing measures have been performed, further interventions are done to *remove potassium from the body*.
   a. *Diuretics:* These only work if the patient has adequate kidney function.
   b. *Sodium polystyrene sulfonate (Kayexalate):* This resin-exchanger removes K⁺ from the blood into the gut, in exchange for an equal amount of Na⁺. It is relatively slow-acting, requiring 1 to 2 hours before plasma [K⁺] decreases. Each 1 g of resin removes 0.5 to 1.0 mmol of potassium. One should give 50 g in 30 mL sorbitol by mouth, or 50 g in a retention enema; the rectal route is faster and more reliable. One study suggested that a single standard oral dose of resin may not be efficacious in decreasing the serum [K⁺] within 4 hours in normokalemic hemodialysis patients, despite a documented increase in K⁺ excretion by the gut. Whether this modality is effective in hyperkalemic dialysis patients, or when given in multiple doses, remains to be determined. However, given this uncertainty, frequent monitoring of plasma [K⁺] in patients treated with sodium polystyrene sulfonate resin is warranted.
   c. *Hemodialysis:* This is the definitive treatment for patients with advanced renal failure and severe hyperkalemia.

For patients with moderate hyperkalemia, not associated with ECG changes, it is frequently sufficient to discontinue the drugs predisposing to hyperkalemia.

To prevent a recurrence of hyperkalemia once the acute treatment has been provided, the following measures are useful.

1. Counsel the patient to restrict dietary potassium to 40 to 60 mEq/day (**Table 12-4**).
2. Avoid medications that interfere with renal excretion of K⁺, such as potassium-sparing diuretics and NSAIDs. ACE inhibitors and ARBs play a major role in slowing the

TABLE 12-4 Potassium Content of Selected Foods

FOOD	PORTION	POTASSIUM (mg)	POTASSIUM (mEq)
Pinto beans	1 cup	1370	35
Raisins	1 cup	1106	28
Honeydew melon	1/2 melon	939	24
Nuts	1 cup	688	18
Blackeyed peas	1 cup	625	16
Collard greens	1 cup	498	13
Banana	1 medium	440	11
Tomato	1 medium	366	9
Orange	1 large	333	9
Milk	1 cup	351	9
Potato chips	10 chips	226	6

progression of chronic kidney disease. For this reason, when patients taking these medications develop hyperkalemia, one should first attempt to decrease the dietary potassium intake, stop other drugs contributing to hyperkalemia, add a diuretic, or reduce the dose of ACE inhibitor or ARB. Only if all other measures fail to control the hyperkalemia should the ACE inhibitor or ARB be discontinued.

3. Avoid drugs that interfere with K⁺ shifts from the ECF to the ICF compartment (e.g., nonselective β-blockers).
4. When hemodialysis patients are fasted in preparation for surgery or a radiologic procedure, administer intravenous 10% dextrose at 50 mL/hr to prevent hyperkalemia. If the patient is diabetic, add 10 units of regular insulin to each liter of 10% dextrose.
5. In selected patients, chronic medication with loop diuretics can be used to stimulate urinary K⁺ excretion.
6. Specific therapy may be indicated for the underlying cause, if available. For example, patients with adrenal insufficiency require replacement with exogenous glucocorticoids and mineralocorticoids. In patients with hyperkalemic periodic paralysis (see earlier discussion), prophylactic aerosolized albuterol can prevent both exercise-induced hyperkalemia and muscle weakness.

BIBLIOGRAPHY

Allon M: Treatment and prevention of hyperkalemia in end-stage renal disease. Kidney Int 43:1197-1209, 1993.

Allon M: Hyperkalemia in end-stage renal disease: mechanisms and management. J Am Soc Nephrol 6:1134-1142, 1995.

Allon M, Takeshian A, Shanklin N: Effect of insulin-plus-glucose infusion with or without epinephrine on fasting hyperkalemia. Kidney Int 43:212-217, 1993.

DuBose TD: Hyperkalemic hyperchloremic metabolic acidosis: Pathophysiologic insights. Kidney Int 51:591-602, 1997.

Ethier JH, Kamel KS, Magner PO, et al: The transtubular potassium concentration in patients with hyperkalemia and hypokalemia. Am J Kidney Dis 15:309-315, 1990.

Farese RV, Biglieri EG, Shackleton CHL, et al: Licorice-induced hypermineralocorticoidism. N Engl J Med 325:1223-1227, 1991.

Gruy-Kapral C, Emmett M, Santa Ana CA, et al: Effect of single dose resin-cathartic therapy on serum potassium concentration in patients with end-stage renal disease. J Am Soc Nephrol 9:1924-1930, 1998.

Palmer BF: Managing hyperkalemia caused by inhibitors of the renin–angiotensin–aldosterone system. N Engl J Med 351:585-592, 2004.

Krishna GG, Steigerwalt SP, Pikus R, et al: Hypokalemic states. In Narins RG (ed): Clinical Disorders of Fluid and Electrolyte Metabolism. New York, McGraw-Hill, 1994, pp 659-696.

Kurtz I: Molecular pathogenesis of Bartter's and Gitelman's syndromes. Kidney Int 54:1396-1410, 1998.

Lifton RP, Dluhy RG, Powers M, et al: A chimaeric 11 beta-hydroxylase/aldosterone synthase gene causes glucocorticoid-remediable aldosteronism and human hypertension. Nature 355:262-265, 1992.

Salem MM, Rosa RM, Batlle DC: Extrarenal potassium tolerance in chronic renal failure: Implications for the treatment of acute hyperkalemia. Am J Kidney Dis 18:421-440, 1991.

Shimkets RA, Warnock DG, Bositis CM, et al: Liddle's syndrome: Heritable human hypertension caused by mutations in the beta subunit of the epithelial sodium channel. Cell 79:407-414, 1994.

Putcha N, Allon M: Management of hyperkalemia in dialysis patients. Semin Dial 20:431-439, 2007.

Kamel KS, Wei C: Controversial issues in the treatment of hyperkalemia. Nephrol Dial Transplant 18:2215-2218, 2003.

CHAPTER 13

Disorders of Calcium and Phosphorus

Akber Saifullah and Sharon M. Moe

Disorders of mineral metabolism, specifically calcium and phosphorus homeostasis, are common in patients with chronic kidney disease (CKD). The homeostatic regulation of calcium and phosphorus maintains normal serum levels, normal intracellular levels, and optimal mineral content in bone. This regulation occurs in three major target organs (intestine, kidney, and bone) via the complex integration of two hormones (parathyroid hormone [PTH] and vitamin D). There is also increasing evidence for the role of hormones collectively known as "phosphatonins" in the regulation of phosphorus. An understanding of normal physiology is necessary to accurately diagnose and treat disorders of calcium and phosphorus.

NORMAL PHYSIOLOGY

Parathyroid Hormone

PTH is released in response to hypocalcemia (**Fig. 13-1**) and maintains calcium homeostasis by three mechanisms: (1) increasing bone mineral dissolution, thus releasing calcium and phosphorus; (2) increasing renal reabsorption of calcium and excretion of phosphorus; and (3) enhancing the gastrointestinal absorption of both calcium and phosphorus indirectly through its effects on the synthesis of activated vitamin D [$1,25(OH)_2D_3$, or calcitriol]. In healthy subjects, this increase in serum PTH level in response to hypocalcemia effectively restores serum calcium levels and maintains normal serum phosphorus levels.

PTH enhances the synthesis of calcitriol, which in turn decreases PTH secretion at the level of the parathyroid glands, completing a typical endocrine feedback loop. In primary hyperparathyroidism, PTH is secreted autonomously from adenomatous glands without regard to physiologic stimuli. In the initial phase of secondary hyperparathyroidism, PTH is secreted as a normal response, but to abnormal stimuli. Later, after a prolonged period of CKD, the hyperplastic glands become adenomatous and therefore unresponsive to stimuli that would normally suppress PTH secretion. When PTH levels are high enough to produce frank hypercalcemia, tertiary hyperparathyroidism is present. Once in the circulation, PTH binds to PTH receptors that are located throughout the body. Therefore, disorders of PTH excess or insufficiency not only affect serum levels of calcium and phosphorus but also lead to bone, cardiac, skin, neurologic, and other manifestations.

PTH is cleaved from a precursor "pre-pro" hormone to an 84-amino-acid protein in the parathyroid gland, where it is stored with other PTH-protein fragments in secretory granules for release. Once released, the circulating 1-84 amino acid protein has a half-life of 2 to 4 minutes. It is then further cleaved into N-terminal, C-terminal, and mid-region fragments of PTH, which are finally metabolized in the liver and kidney. PTH secretion can be triggered by hypocalcemia, hyperphosphatemia, or calcitriol deficiency. The extracellular concentration of ionized calcium is the most important determinant of minute-to-minute PTH levels. Active secretion of PTH from stored secretory granules in response to hypocalcemia is controlled by the calcium-sensing receptor (CaSR). The CaSR is a member of the G-protein–coupled receptor superfamily, with a 7 membrane-spanning domain. Mutations of the CaSR gene can lead to syndromes of hypercalcemia or hypocalcemia (see Chapter 40). The CaSR is expressed in thyroid C-cells and in the kidney, predominantly in the thick ascending limb of the loop of Henle, where it controls renal excretion of calcium in response to changes in serum calcium concentration.

Over the years, a succession of increasingly sensitive assays have been developed to measure PTH. A major difficulty in accurately measuring PTH is cross-reactivity with inactive, circulating PTH-protein fragments, which may accumulate in CKD. Early assays targeted the C-terminus but were inaccurate in patients with kidney disease because of impaired renal excretion of C-terminal fragments. Subsequent N-terminus assays had similar problems. Accuracy was improved by the development of a two-site antibody test (commonly called "INTACT" assay) to detect full-length (1-84, or active) PTH molecules. In this assay, a capture antibody binds to the N-terminus and a second antibody binds to the C-terminus. However, recent data indicate that this intact assay also detects accumulated C-terminal fragments, commonly termed "7-84." These fragments accumulate in CKD and lead to falsely elevated values in assays of intact PTH. Despite these limitations, the intact PTH assay is currently the most widely used assay in clinical care.

Vitamin D

Vitamin D is called a "vitamin" because it is an essential nutrient that must come from an exogenous source if it cannot be manufactured in humans in sufficient quantity. However, this is a misnomer, because vitamin D can be synthesized

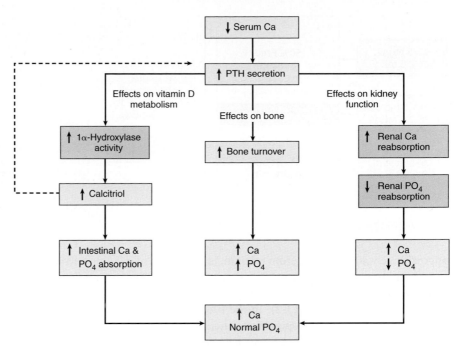

FIGURE 13-1 Normal homeostatic response to hypocalcemia. In the presence of hypocalcemia, secretion of parathyroid hormone (PTH) is increased. PTH acts on three target organs. PTH works at the intestine indirectly by first increasing the 1α-hydroxylase activity in the kidney; this enzyme converts calcidiol to calcitriol, which increases intestinal absorption of both calcium and phosphorus. Calcitriol then negatively feeds back on the parathyroid glands to regulate PTH release *(dotted line)*. In bone, PTH increases bone turnover, resulting in a release of calcium and phosphorus from bone. Lastly, PTH works directly on the kidney to increase renal calcium reabsorption and decrease renal phosphorus reabsorption. The net effect is a rise in serum calcium but no net change in serum phosphorus. The blue boxes indicate homeostatic steps in the kidney that are abnormal in people with chronic kidney disease. Because of diminished kidney mass, conversion of calcidiol to calcitriol and phosphorus excretion are impaired.

in the skin, and it is really a hormone. Vitamin D_2 (ergocalciferol) from plants and vitamin D_3 (cholecalciferol) primarily from oily fish are the main exogenous sources in a Western diet, outside of supplementation in milk. In the skin, 7-dehydrocholesterol is converted to vitamin D_3 in response to sunlight, a process that is inhibited by sunscreen of skin protection factor (SPF) 8 or greater. Once in the blood, vitamins D_2 and D_3 from diet or skin bind to vitamin D–binding protein and are carried to the liver, where they are hydroxylated to yield 25(OH)D, often called calcidiol. Therefore, calcidiol levels in the blood are a direct assessment of the nutritional (dietary) intake of vitamin D. Calcidiol is then converted in the kidney to calcitriol by the action of 1α-hydroxylase (the CYP27B1 isoenzyme of the cytochrome P-450 system). In the kidney, CYP27B activity is affected by almost every hormone involved in calcium homeostasis. Its activity is stimulated by PTH, estrogen, calcitonin, prolactin, growth hormone, low serum calcium, and low serum phosphorus and inhibited by calcitriol.

1,25(OH)$_2$D$_3$ circulates in the bloodstream bound to vitamin D–binding protein. The free form of 1,25(OH)$_2$D$_3$ enters the target cell, where it interacts with its nuclear vitamin D receptor (VDR). This complex then combines with the retinoic acid X receptor to form a heterodimer, which in turn interacts with the vitamin D response element (VDRE) on the target gene. The major functions of 1,25(OH)$_2$D$_3$ are carried out in two target organs: (1) the small intestine, where it regulates the intestinal absorption of calcium and, to a lesser degree, phosphorus; and (2) the parathyroid gland, where it inhibits PTH synthesis at the level of messenger RNA transcription. However, many genes contain the VDRE, the VDR is expressed in multiple organs, and 1α-hydroxylase activity can be detected in extrarenal tissues. These features may mediate autocrine or paracrine effects of vitamin D outside its classic target tissues, including effects on cell

differentiation and proliferation, immune function, and response to infection. Discovery of these nonmineral effects has led to the therapeutic use of vitamin D and congeners in some cancers and skin disorders.

Phosphatonins

The phosphatonins comprise a group of proteins that were identified from the study of several genetic disorders characterized by hypophosphatemia and impaired bone mineralization and from cases of tumor-induced osteomalacia associated with renal phosphate wasting. Fibroblast growth factor 23 (FGF23) is produced by the tumors of such patients; corresponding genetic defects were identified in autosomal dominant hypophosphatemic rickets (ADHR). FGF23 is made by osteocytes, and it directly impedes the conversion of 25(OH)D$_3$ to 1,25(OH)$_2$D$_3$ by inhibition of the 1α-hydroxylase enzyme in the renal tubules. Levels of FGF23 are elevated in patients with CKD, presumably due to net phosphate retention. Another factor, secreted frizzled-related protein 4 (FRP4) also can induce renal phosphate wasting. It is now clear that these factors are important for PTH-independent control of urinary phosphate handling. However, the role of phosphatonins in normal homeostasis of phosphorus is not yet completely clear.

Calcium

Serum calcium levels are tightly controlled within a narrow range, usually 8.5 to 10.5 mg/dL (2.1 to 2.6 mmol/L). However, the serum calcium level is a poor reflection of overall total body calcium, because the intravascular space contains only 0.1% to 0.2% of extracellular calcium, which in turn represents only 1% of total body calcium. The preponderance of total body calcium is stored in bone. Ionized calcium,

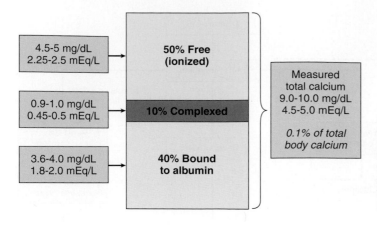

FIGURE 13-2 Distribution of extracellular calcium. Only 0.1% of the total body calcium is in the extracellular space; the other 99.9% is localized in bone. The serum calcium concentration reported by the clinical laboratory is total serum calcium. However, only 50% of this total calcium is the physiologically active ionized component. The 50% bound fraction of serum calcium comprises the 10% of the total calcium that is complexed to anions such as bicarbonate, phosphate, and citrate and the 40% that is bound to albumin.

approximately 40% of total serum calcium, is physiologically active; the remainder of serum calcium, which bound to albumin or anions such as citrate, bicarbonate, and phosphorus, is not active (**Fig. 13-2**). In the presence of hypoalbuminemia, there is a proportionate increase in ionized calcium relative to total calcium, so that measurements of total serum calcium in patients with hypoalbuminemia may underestimate the amount of physiologically active (ionized) calcium. A commonly used formula for estimating ionized calcium from total serum calcium is to add 0.8 mg/dL to the ionized calcium value for every 1 mg decrease in serum albumin below 4 mg/dL. Direct ionized calcium measurements are also widely available now.

Reduced serum levels of ionized calcium stimulate PTH secretion, an effect that helps restore a normal level of ionized calcium (see **Fig. 13-1**). PTH acts to increase bone resorption, increase renal calcium reabsorption, and increase the conversion of $25(OH)D_3$ to $1,25(OH)_2D_3$ in the kidney, thereby stimulating gastrointestinal calcium absorption. In individuals with intact kidneys, net calcium balance varies with age. Children and young adults are usually in a slightly positive net calcium balance, because bone accrual accompanies skeletal growth; after age 25 to 35 years, when bones stop growing, the calcium balance tends to be neutral. Normal individuals are protected against calcium overload by both the suppression of PTH release and the inactivation of $1,25(OH)_2D_3$. Absence of these two hormones leads to increased calciuria and diminished intestinal absorption of calcium.

Calcium absorption across the intestinal epithelium occurs via both a vitamin D–dependent mechanism and a passive, concentration-dependent pathway that is independent of vitamin D. The duodenum is the major site of calcium absorption, although the other segments of the small intestine and the colon also contribute to net calcium absorption. In addition, there is an obligatory secretion of calcium into the gut. Individuals on a calcium-free diet will have a net loss of calcium from the body in stool resulting in a negative calcium balance. In the kidney, the majority (60% to 70%) of calcium is reabsorbed passively in the proximal tubule, driven by a gradient that is generated by reabsorption of sodium and water. In the thick ascending limb, another 20-30% of calcium is reabsorbed via paracellular transport driven by the lumen

positive net charge. The remaining 10% of calcium reabsorption occurs in the distal convoluted tubule, the connecting tubule, and the initial portion of the cortical collecting duct. The final regulation of urinary calcium excretion is carried out in these distal segments.

Calcium enters epithelial cells in the intestine and kidney through specialized channels called transient receptor potential cation channels TRPV5 and TRPV6; it is transported through the cell by a protein called calbindin and then extruded through the basolateral side by the Na^{2+}/Ca^{2+} exchanger (NCX1) or the calcium–adenosine triphosphatase (Ca^{2+}-ATPase) pump (PMCA1b). Genetic defects in these various transporters lead to a variety of rare disorders of calcium homeostasis. Vitamin D actively regulates all of these channels and transporters, and vitamin D deficiency leads to impaired intestinal calcium absorption. At the level of the kidney, vitamin D and PTH work together to control calcium excretion.

Phosphorus

Inorganic phosphorus is critical for numerous normal physiologic functions, including skeletal development, cell membrane phospholipid content and function, cell signaling, platelet aggregation, and energy transfer through mitochondrial metabolism. Normal homeostasis maintains serum concentrations between 2.5 and 4.5 mg/dL (0.81 to 1.45mmol/L). The terms *phosphorus* and *phosphate* are often used interchangeably, but, strictly speaking, "phosphate" refers to the inorganic form that is in equilibrium (pK = 6.8) between HPO_4^{2-} and $H_2PO_4^-$ at physiologic pH in a ratio of about 4:1. For that reason, phosphorus is usually expressed in millimoles (mmol) rather than milliequivalents per liter (mEq/L). However, most laboratories report this inorganic component as "phosphorus," and that is the term we will use in the remainder of this chapter. Levels are highest in infants and decrease throughout growth, reaching adult levels in the late teens.

Total adult body stores of phosphorus are approximately 700 g, of which 85% is contained in bone. Of the remainder, 14% is intracellular, and only 1% is extracellular. Of this extracellular phosphorus, 70% is organic and contained within phospholipids, and 30% is inorganic. Of the latter,

15% is protein bound, and the remaining 85% is either complexed with sodium, magnesium, or calcium or circulating as the free monohydrogen or dihydrogen forms. Only 0.15% of total body phosphorus (15% of extracellular phosphorus) is freely circulating, and this is the portion that is measured. Therefore, as with calcium, serum measurements reflect only a minor fraction of total body phosphorus and do not accurately indicate total body stores in the setting of abnormal homeostasis (e.g., CKD).

The average American diet contains approximately 1000 to 1400 mg phosphorus per day, and the recommended daily allowance (RDA) is 800 mg/day. Approximately two thirds of the ingested phosphorus is excreted in the urine and the remaining third in stool. Many prepackaged, fast food, and dark-colored carbonated beverages (colas but not root beer) contain extra phosphorus as a preservative. Therefore, it is difficult to accurately predict dietary intake based on food type alone. In general, foods high in protein and dairy products contain the most phosphorus, whereas fruits and vegetables contain the least. Between 60% and 70% of dietary phosphorus is absorbed by the gastrointestinal tract, in all intestinal segments. Passive absorption (which is dependent on the luminal phosphorus concentration) occurs via the epithelial brush border sodium-phosphate cotransporter (NPT2b), driven by the sodium gradient created by the energy-using basolateral sodium-potassium ATPase transporter. The NPT2b sits in the terminal web, just below the brush border in "ready-to-use" vesicles that traffic to the brush border in response to acute and chronic changes in phosphorus concentration.

Medications and foods that bind dietary phosphorus (antacids, calcium salts, non–calcium containing phosphate binders) can decrease the net amount of phosphorus absorbed, by decreasing the amount of free phosphate available for absorption.

Calcitriol can upregulate the NPT2b and thereby actively increase phosphorus absorption. Most inorganic phosphorus (phosphate) is freely filtered by the glomerulus. Approximately 70% to 80% of the filtered load is reabsorbed in the proximal tubule, which is the primary site of regulated phosphorus reabsorption in the kidney; the remaining 20% to 30% is reabsorbed in the distal tubule. Hypophosphatemia stimulates 1α-hydroxylase, thereby increasing conversion of calcidiol to calcitriol and in turn increasing intestinal phosphorus absorption. Calcitriol also stimulates renal tubular phosphorus reabsorption, leading to a reduction in urinary phosphorus excretion. In the presence of hyperphosphatemia, there is a rapid increase in urinary excretion of phosphorus, mediated by the serum phosphorus level, PTH, and, most likely, FGF23. Because of the substantial capacity of the kidney to increase urinary phosphorus excretion after dietary ingestion, sustained hyperphosphatemia is not seen clinically without renal impairment. Although the effects are more minor, renal phosphorus excretion is also increased by volume expansion, metabolic acidosis, glucocorticoids, and calcitonin and decreased by growth hormone and thyroid hormone.

Bone

The majority of the total body stores of calcium and phosphorus are located in bone in the form of hydroxyapatite $[Ca_{10}(PO_4)_6(OH)_2]$. Trabecular (cancellous) bone is 15% to 20% calcified. Trabecular bone is located predominately in the epiphyses of the long bones and serves a metabolic function. There is a relatively rapid exchange of calcium between trabecular bone and plasma (days to weeks), as evidenced by a short turnover rate of the radioisotope ^{45}calcium. In contrast, cortical (compact) bone is located in the shafts of long bones and is 80% to 90% calcified. This bone serves primarily a protective and mechanical function and has a calcium turnover rate of months. The nonmineral component of bone consists principally (90%) of highly organized cross-linked fibers of type I collagen; the remainder consists of proteoglycans, and "noncollagen" proteins such as osteopontin, osteocalcin, osteonectin, and alkaline phosphatase. The predominant cell types involved in bone turnover are osteoclasts, the bone-resorbing cells derived from circulating hematopoietic cells, and osteoblasts, the bone-forming cells derived from the marrow. These cells are important in bone remodeling, which occurs in response to hormones, cytokines, and changes in mechanical forces. All of these factors, by inducing bone remodeling, can affect calcium and phosphorus homeostasis.

DISORDERS OF MINERAL METABOLISM
Hypercalcemia

When the level of serum ionized calcium increases above normal, hypercalcemia is present. Ionized calcium is not included in most routine clinical chemistry panels, but it can be estimated from the total serum calcium and serum albumin concentration values using the formula given earlier. In certain circumstances in which the concentration of proteins capable of binding calcium is increased, including paraproteinemia, or if the blood pH is abnormally high or low, direct measurement of serum ionized calcium is more helpful. Ionized calcium represents the biologically active fraction of total serum calcium.

Clinical Manifestations of Hypercalcemia

The severity of symptoms caused by hypercalcemia depends on the degree and rate of rise in serum calcium. Gastrointestinal symptoms such as nausea, vomiting, constipation, abdominal pain, and, rarely, peptic ulcer disease may occur. Neuromuscular involvement includes altered mentation, impaired concentration, fatigue, lethargy, and muscle weakness. Hypercalcemia can impair renal water handling by inducing nephrogenic diabetes insipidus and sodium wasting; the resulting diuresis worsens the hypercalcemia, because volume depletion limits the protective hypercalciuria. Volume depletion may lead to acute renal failure, which further limits calcium excretion and favors a further increase in serum calcium. The hypercalciuria associated with prolonged hypercalcemia can rarely lead to nephrolithiasis and nephrocalcinosis. Cardiovascular effects include hypertension and shortening of the QT interval on the electrocardiogram. Although cardiac arrhythmias are uncommon, hypercalcemia can trigger digitalis toxicity.

Differential Diagnosis of Hypercalcemia

The most common causes of hypercalcemia are malignancy and hyperparathyroidism; in most series, these two diagnoses account for more than 80% of cases. The remaining causes are listed in **Table 13-1**, and a few are discussed in more detail in the following paragraphs.

Malignancy

Malignancy is the most common cause of hypercalcemia. Its presence in cancer patients confers a poor prognosis. Depending on the type of malignancy, hypercalcemia can result from (1) direct invasion of bone by metastatic disease (local osteolytic hypercalcemia, or LOH), (2) production of circulating factors that stimulate osteoclastic resorption of bone, or (3) increased production of calcitriol, which stimulates gastrointestinal absorption of calcium. In LOH, tumor cells within the bone marrow space produce a variety of inflammatory cytokines, collectively termed osteoclast-activating factors, which lead to net bone resorption and hypercalcemia. PTH levels are suppressed in response to the hypercalcemia. This is the usual mechanism seen with hypercalcemia resulting from breast cancer or multiple myeloma. Humoral hypercalcemia of malignancy is caused by secretion of parathyroid hormone–related peptide (PTHrp) by malignant tumor cells. PTHrp bears similarity to PTH only in the initial 8-amino-acid sequence, but this homology permits binding to the PTH receptor, leading to increased bone turnover and hypercalcemia. Specific assays are available to distinguish circulating PTHrp from PTH. Various lymphoid tumors,

most notably Hodgkin's lymphoma, have been shown to synthesize large quantities of calcitriol.

Hyperparathyroidism

The incidence of *primary hyperparathyroidism* has declined dramatically over the last 30 years, but it is still the second most common cause of hypercalcemia. Early diagnosis is possible because of routine measurement of the serum calcium concentration in chemistry panels. In most cases, primary hyperparathyroidism is caused by a benign adenoma of a single parathyroid gland that autonomously secretes PTH. The disorder may be sporadic, familial, or inherited as a component of the constellation of multiple endocrine neoplasia (MEN). The elevation in PTH results in increased intestinal reabsorption of calcium through stimulation of the production of calcitriol, increased osteoclastic bone resorption, and increased renal tubular reabsorption of calcium. However, because of the elevation in serum calcium, the filtered load of calcium exceeds the ability of the kidney to reabsorb calcium, leading to hypercalciuria and potentially to nephrolithiasis.

Secondary hyperparathyroidism is caused by diffuse hyperplasia of all four glands in response to ongoing stimuli such as hypocalcemia or hyperphosphatemia. Hypercalcemia may occur in patients with secondary hyperparathyroidism due to treatments such as calcium-based phosphate binders or calcitriol and its derivatives. Secondary hyperparathyroidism can also cause hypercalcemia via increased bone resorption when the glands become adenomatous and no longer respond to the change in calcium—a stage often called *tertiary hyperparathyroidism*. With a kidney transplant, the PTH continues to be secreted, leading to hypercalcemia.

Lithium may interfere with the CaSR, leading to a "resetting" of the parathyroid gland sensitivity such that higher levels of calcium are needed to decrease PTH. Clinically, these patients may appear to have hyperparathyroidism, but the hypercalcemia resolves when lithium is stopped.

Vitamin D Excess

Toxicity from excessive exogenous intake of native vitamin D supplements (ergocalciferol and cholecalciferol) is rare, because 1α-hydroxylase activity is tightly regulated by calcium levels. In contrast, the excessive administration of calcitriol or of other active vitamin D analogues, such as paricalcitol or doxercalciferol, that bypass the regulation step often leads to hypercalcemia. These drugs are most commonly used in the treatment of secondary hyperparathyroidism in CKD. An endogenous source of excess calcitriol is production by nonkidney tissue (e.g., lymphoma, granuloma). Granulomatous diseases such as sarcoidosis, tuberculosis, and leprosy are thought to cause hypercalcemia via increased production of calcitriol by monocytes and macrophages that possess 1α-hydroxylase activity.

Familial Hypocalciuric Hypercalcemia

Inactivating mutations of the CaSR cause familial hypocalciuric hypercalcemia (FHH), a rare hereditary disease with autosomal dominant transmission. Calcium is unable to

---

TABLE 13-1 Causes of Hypercalcemia

Malignancy
   Local osteolytic hypercalcemia
   Humoral hypercalcemia of malignancy (PTHrp)
   Hematologic malignancies (ectopic calcitriol synthesis)

Hyperparathyroidism

Thyrotoxicosis

Granulomatous diseases

Drug-induced
   Vitamin D
   Thiazide diuretics
   Estrogens and antiestrogens
   Androgens (breast cancer therapy)
   Vitamin A
   Lithium

Immobilization

Total parenteral nutrition

Impaired kidney function (acute renal failure or CKD), usually from medications such as calcium-containing phosphate binders or calcitriol or its analogues)

CKD, chronic kidney disease; PTHrp, parathyroid hormone–related peptide.

activate the mutant receptor, which leads to increased renal reabsorption of calcium into the blood from the tubular fluid and hypocalciuria, usually with urine calcium excretion of less than 100 mg/day. Because this mutation may also affect the receptor at the level of the parathyroid gland, PTH may be slightly elevated out of proportion to the degree of hypercalcemia. Other clues pointing to this diagnosis include a family history of asymptomatic hypercalcemia. Probands are often discovered after parathyroidectomy fails to correct hypercalcemia.

Approach to the Patient with Hypercalcemia

The clinician may approach patients with hypercalcemia by reviewing the list in **Table 13-1**. However, an alternative approach is to formulate a differential diagnosis based on the physiology of calcium homeostasis. As shown in **Figure 13-3**, approaching a patient in this manner allows the clinician to order the appropriate diagnostic studies.

Parathyroid Glands

The normal response to hypercalcemia is suppression of PTH secretion. Interpretation of a PTH level (normal, 10 to 65 pg/mL) must always be done in conjunction with a simultaneously measured calcium level. For example, if the serum calcium level is 11.5 mg/dL and the PTH is 50 pg/mL, the circulating level of PTH is inappropriately high. Despite a PTH in the normal range, these values are suggestive of hyperparathyroidism. Because PTH increases urinary phosphorus excretion, a normal or high-normal PTH level with hypercalcemia and low or low-normal phosphorus level is essentially diagnostic of primary hyperparathyroidism. Radionuclide sestamibi imaging may be helpful in localizing an adenomatous gland. However, there is a high risk of false-negative scans, and an experienced

parathyroid surgeon can usually locate the enlarged gland. Rarely, glands are found in the mediastinum. Parathyroid cancers secrete excess PTH, leading to severe hyperparathyroidism, and marked hypercalcemia may be present.

Bone

Hypercalcemia at the level of the bone occurs either because of enhanced bone turnover (osteoclast activity greater than osteoblast activity, or net bone resorption greater than bone formation) caused by local tumor invasion or as a result of increased secretion of hormonal factors by tumor cells (PTHrp, calcitriol, and excess secretion of PTH). Alternatively, immobilization may lead to release of calcium from the bone, especially in the setting of excess turnover (e.g., Paget's disease). The diagnostic studies for bone-induced hypercalcemia include PTH, PTHrp, urine and serum protein electrophoresis to diagnose multiple myeloma, and an alkaline phosphatase level. The latter is markedly elevated in Paget's disease and other states with high bone turnover.

Intestine

Enhanced intestinal absorption of calcium can occur in conditions that result in elevated circulating levels of calcidiol or calcitriol. This can occur as a result of vitamin D toxicity with very high calcidiol levels, calcitriol therapy in patients with secondary hyperparathyroidism, calcitriol-secreting granulomatous diseases and lymphomas, and hyperparathyroidism, which in turn increases calcitriol synthesis. In addition, excess calcium ingestion, especially with alkali, can lead to hypercalcemia. In the past this was called *milk-alkali syndrome*, named for the combination of therapies used to treat peptic ulcer disease before the advent of histamine 2 blockers. However, it is now rarely

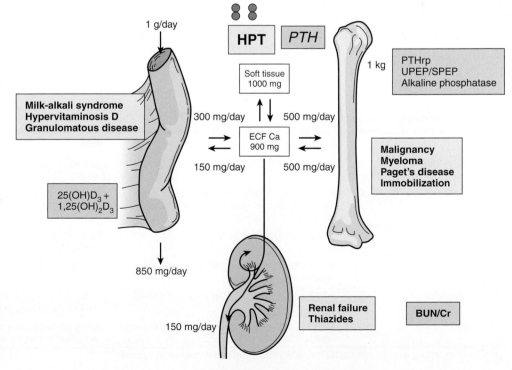

FIGURE 13-3 Approach to patient with hypercalcemia. The normal daily calcium balance is shown, demonstrating the fluxes between the serum compartment and intestine and bone as well as the excretion of calcium. The patient with hypercalcemia must have an abnormality at the parathyroid glands *(top)*, intestine *(left)*, bone *(right)*, or kidney *(bottom)*. The *yellow boxes* represent causes of hypercalcemia that are associated with abnormalities at each of these target organs. The *blue boxes* indicate diagnostic tests that may be abnormal in these disorders. BUN, blood urea nitrogen; Cr, creatinine; ECF, extracellular fluid; HPT, hyperparathyroidism; PTH, parathyroid hormone; PTHrp, parathyroid hormone–related peptide; SPEP, serum protein electrophoresis; UPEP, urine protein electrophoresis.

observed. In order to detect vitamin D toxicity, levels of both calcidiol and calcitriol should be measured. In the setting of exogenous vitamin D intake, calcidiol levels will be high and calcitriol levels normal to high. In the setting of granulomatous production of calcitriol, calcitriol levels will be high; calcidiol levels are nondiagnostic but usually are low-normal.

Kidneys

With volume depletion, serum calcium levels rise, and mild hypercalcemia can result. Thiazide diuretics, by blocking distal tubular sodium reabsorption, enhance the sodium-calcium exchanger, resulting in a reduction in urinary calcium excretion and hypercalcemia. These effects are used to advantage in the treatment of hypercalciuria in patients with nephrolithiasis. In most cases, the rise in calcium in response to thiazide diuretics does not result in frank hypercalcemia. When thiazides induce hypercalcemia, there is often underlying, previously undetected, hyperparathyroidism.

PTH acts at the kidney to increase tubular reabsorption of calcium. Even so, patients with hypercalcemia from hyperparathyroidism tend to have an elevated urine calcium excretion because the filtered load of calcium is so high. In primary hyperparathyroidism, the urinary calcium/creatinine ratio is usually greater than 0.2 (mg/mg), whereas in patients with FHH, the urinary calcium/creatinine ratio is less than 0.01 mg/mg. Ideally, a 24 hour urine collection should be measured, but a spot collection can differentiate primary hyperparathyroidism from FHH.

Treatment of Hypercalcemia

The ultimate goal of therapy is to remedy the underlying cause of hypercalcemia. However, patients who present with acute symptoms of hypercalcemia require immediate treatment to reduce the serum levels of calcium. The safest and most effective treatment in patients with normal cardiac and renal function is intravenous volume expansion with normal saline, which reduces proximal tubular reabsorption of salt, water, and calcium. Most patients with symptomatic hypercalcemia are volume depleted at presentation because of the polyuria and natriuresis induced by hypercalcemia. In more severe cases, very aggressive volume resuscitation, with normal saline boluses followed by continuous administration at 200 to 500 mL/hr, may be required, with close attention to the patient's cardiopulmonary status to avoid volume overload. Once volume expansion is achieved, calcium reabsorption can be further reduced with intravenous loop diuretics, such as furosemide, that block the Na^{2+}-K^+-$2Cl^-$ (NKCC2) cotransporter in the thick ascending limb of the loop of Henle, thereby disrupting the favorable electrochemical gradient for passive (paracellular) calcium reabsorption. It is important to remember that patients must be adequately hydrated before the diuretic is given, to avoid worsening hypovolemia, and therefore accurate assessment of intake and output is critical to optimize this treatment approach.

If these conservative treatments fail to restore normocalcemia, other pharmacologic options should be used (**Table 13-2**). Because the response to these agents is not immediate, their use agents in patients with severe symptoms of hypercalcemia may be appropriate even before the full effect of hydration and furosemide has occurred.

In the United States, two bisphosphonates, pamidronate and zoledronate, are approved for the treatment of malignancy-associated hypercalcemia. These agents block osteoclast-mediated bone resorption by inducing osteoclast apoptosis. Typically, a clinical response is seen within 2 to 4 days, with a nadir in serum calcium within 4 to 7 days. Caution is required, because acute renal failure and osteonecrosis of the jaw are rare side effects of bisphosphonate therapy. Calcitonin has the advantage of rapid reduction of serum calcium, but its use is limited by short duration of action and tachyphylaxis. Glucocorticoids are effective first-line agents, along with saline diuresis, when the hypercalcemia is mediated by elevated circulating levels of calcitriol

TABLE 13-2 Treatments for Hypercalcemia

AGENT	MODE OF ACTION	DOSE
IV hydration with saline	Increases tubular flow and excretion of calcium	Hydration based on patient's cardiovascular and renal status; 200-500 mL/hr
IV furosemide or loop diuretics	Block NKCC2 channel in loop of Henle thus reducing positive electrochemical gradient for calcium reabsorption	20-40 mg after rehydration; dose may need to be adjusted based on kidney function level
IV bisphosphonates	Inhibit osteoclastic activity	Pamidronate, 60-90 mg over 4 hr Zoledronate, 4 mg over 15 min
Calcitonin	Inhibits bone resorption and enhances calcium excretion	4-12 IU IM/SQ every 12 hr
Glucocorticoids	Inhibit conversion of 25(OH)D to 1,25(OH)$_2$D	Hydrocortisone, 200 mg/day IV for 3 days Prednisone, 60 mg PO for 10 days
Cinacalcet	Allosteric activator of CaSR, mimicking increased calcium to reduce PTH	30 mg qd to bid, to a maximum dose of 90 mg bid; give with food to reduce nausea

CaSR, calcium-sensing receptor; NKCC2, Na^{2+}/K^+/$2Cl^{2-}$ cotransporter; PTH, parathyroid hormone.

due to granulomatous disorders or lymphoma. Mild hypercalcemia is usually not symptomatic and may not require aggressive therapy.

The approach to the patient with hyperparathyroidism is more controversial. In primary hyperparathyroidism, intervention may be indicated only if symptoms (nephrolithiasis, lethargy, fatigue) are present. A National Institutes of Health consensus conference recommended that patients undergo surgical removal of the enlarged parathyroid gland if any of the following conditions are satisfied: (1) serum calcium 1.0 mg/dL greater than the laboratory upper limit of normal; (2) urine calcium excretion greater than 400 mg/day; (3) creatinine clearance reduced by 30% or more; (4) dual-energy X-ray absorptiometry (DEXA) T-score of −2.5 present at any major site; and (5) age younger than 50 years. An alternative to surgical parathyroidectomy is the use of cinacalcet, a calcimimetic. This new drug is an allosteric activator of the CaSR. It "mimics" higher levels of calcium, thereby decreasing PTH secretion and serum calcium. For primary hyperparathyroidism, the dose is usually 30 mg twice daily, titrating up to 90 mg twice daily.

Hypocalcemia

With true hypocalcemia, the ionized calcium concentration is low. In patients with hypoalbuminemia, there is a decrease in the total calcium, but not necessarily a decrease in the ionized calcium. In patients with excess citrate (from blood transfusions) or acute administration of bicarbonate, the percentage of calcium that is bound to these negatively charged ions increases; this reduces the free ionized calcium, usually with only a minimal change in total calcium. Acute respiratory alkalosis also lowers the ionized calcium by the same mechanism. A decrease in the hydrogen ion concentration leads to increased protein binding of ionized calcium, as protons dissociate from binding sites on protein, and a decrease in the ionized component. On the other hand, hypoalbuminemia results in a reduction in total serum calcium but does not cause symptomatic hypocalcemia, because there is no true change in the ionized calcium. Because the actual magnitude of any change in these circumstances may be hard to predict, the ionized calcium concentration is best measured directly.

Clinical Manifestations of Hypocalcemia

Most patients with mild hypocalcemia have very few symptoms, but large or abrupt changes in ionized calcium may lead to symptoms. The most specific symptoms are perioral numbness and spasms of the hands and feet. In some patients, progression to tetany or seizures occurs. This increased neuromuscular reactivity can be demonstrated by eliciting Chvostek's sign or Trousseau's sign. Chvostek's sign is tested by tapping on the facial nerve near the temporal mandibular joint and watching for grimacing caused by spasm of the facial muscles. Trousseau's sign is tested by inflating a blood pressure cuff to a pressure greater than the systolic blood pressure for 3 minutes and watching for spasm of the outstretched hand. Of these two signs, Trousseau's is more

specific. If these clinical signs are positive, hypocalcemia should be confirmed by measurement of ionized calcium.

Differential Diagnosis of Hypocalcemia

There are many causes of hypocalcemia. These can be best organized mechanistically.

Vitamin D Deficiency

Vitamin D, once activated to calcitriol, is the primary determinant of intestinal calcium absorption. Individuals may be deficient in vitamin D due to poor absorption from dietary sources (e.g., malabsorption, short bowel, poor nutrition); lack of sun exposure; abnormal conversion of calcidiol to calcitriol in the liver (cirrhosis, some drugs); or decreased renal conversion of calcidiol to calcitriol (CKD). These patients have low levels of vitamin D and an increase in PTH.

Hypoparathyroidism

Deficiency or inactivity of PTH results in hypocalcemia. This may be caused by the inadvertent removal of the parathyroid glands during thyroid surgery or by damage from radiation, congenital defects, or autoimmune disease. These patients have an inappropriately low PTH for their low calcium levels. In the absence of PTH, the only mechanism to increase serum calcium is via intestinal absorption stimulated by the administration of vitamin D (usually in the active form, calcitriol) and oral calcium. Hypomagnesemia may also cause resistance to PTH as well as an impairment in PTH release.

Pseudohypoparathyroidism

The term *pseudohypoparathyroidism* describes a group of disorders that are characterized by hypocalcemia and hypophosphatemia with elevated PTH levels and lack of tissue responsiveness to PTH. The magnesium and calcidiol levels are normal. A PTH infusion test can confirm the tissue resistance. The intravenous administration of PTH normally results in increased urinary cyclic adenosine monophosphate (cAMP) and phosphorus excretion. In patients with pseudohypoparathyroidism, the lack of response is diagnostic. The most common form of pseudohypoparathyroidism is type Ia, Albright's hereditary osteodystrophy, which is also associated with short stature, round facies, obesity, brachydactyly, and other defects.

Tissue Consumption of Calcium

Hypocalcemia may result from the precipitation of calcium into extraskeletal tissue, such as occurs in pancreatitis. In addition, excess bone formation in some malignancies with blastic bone metastases may cause the bone to take up excess calcium acutely. After parathyroidectomy, there is an acute drop in serum calcium and phosphorus because of the "hungry bone syndrome," wherein calcium and phosphorus are rapidly taken up due to the sudden reduction in PTH. This phenomenon is more severe and more protracted in patients with kidney failure who are undergoing parathyroidectomy as a treatment for severe secondary hyperparathyroidism. In acute hyperphosphatemia due to rhabdomyolysis or tumor lysis syndrome, the phosphorus binds to calcium, leading to a fall in ionized calcium. Similarly, the infusion of citrate, a preservative in blood and plasma transfusions, can reduce ionized calcium, as discussed earlier. Lastly, sepsis is also associated with hypocalcemia, although the mechanism is not clear.

Treatment of Hypocalcemia

Intravenous calcium infusions are indicated only in the setting of symptomatic hypocalcemia and should not be given to patients with severe hyperphosphatemia because of the risk of ectopic precipitation of calcium phosphate. Intravenous calcium comes in two forms: calcium gluconate (10-mL vial = 94 mg elemental calcium) and calcium chloride (10-mL vial = 273 mg elemental calcium). The calcium chloride formulation is typically used only during a cardiopulmonary arrest, because its infusion is painful and can cause vein sclerosis. For obvious reasons, care must taken to order the correct formulation of calcium. Importantly, patients who are not symptomatic should be repleted with oral, not intravenous, calcium. The most common oral supplement is calcium carbonate, starting with 1 to 2 g of elemental calcium three times daily (1250 mg calcium carbonate = 500 mg elemental calcium), given separately from meals. The amount of calcium absorbed will be increased if calcitriol (0.25 µg twice daily to start) is given with the calcium. In addition, hypomagnesemia should be treated concomitantly. If appropriate, patients may also be changed from loop diuretics to thiazide diuretics to decrease urinary calcium excretion.

Hyperphosphatemia

Hyperphosphatemia can result from increased intestinal absorption, from cellular release or rapid shifts of phosphorus from the intracellular to the extracellular compartment, or from decreased renal excretion. Persistent hyperphosphatemia (>12 hours) occurs almost exclusively in the setting of impaired kidney function. Increased intestinal absorption is usually caused by either use of phosphate-containing oral purgatives or enemas or by vitamin D overdoses. Increased tissue release of phosphorus is commonly seen in acute tumor lysis syndrome, rhabdomyolysis, hemolysis, hyperthermia, profound catabolic stress, or acute leukemia. These disorders can also lead to acute renal failure, limiting renal phosphate excretion and further exacerbating the hyperphosphatemia. Rarely, thyrotoxicosis or acromegaly leads to hyperphosphatemia. Acute hyperphosphatemia usually does not cause symptoms unless the reciprocal reduction of serum calcium leads to symptoms of hypocalcemia. The treatment of acute hyperphosphatemia includes volume expansion, dialysis, and administration of phosphate binders. In the setting of normal kidney function, or even mild to moderate kidney disease, hyperphosphatemia is usually self-limited because of the capacity of the kidney to excrete a phosphorus load. In CKD, chronic hyperphosphatemia is associated with adverse sequelae including cardiovascular disease. Treatment of hyperphosphatemia related to CKD or end-stage renal disease is discussed in detail in Chapter 58.

TABLE 13-3 Causes of Hypophosphatemia

Decreased Intestinal Absorption
Antacid abuse
Malabsorption and chronic diarrhea
Vitamin D deficiency
Starvation or anorexia
Alcoholism
Increased Urinary Losses
Primary hyperparathyroidism
After renal transplantation
Extracellular fluid volume expansion
Glucosuria (after treatment of DKA)
Post-obstructive or resolving ATN diuresis
Acetazolamide
Fanconi's syndrome
X-linked and vitamin D–dependent rickets
Oncogenic osteomalacia
Redistribution
Respiratory alkalosis
Alcohol withdrawal
Severe burns
Post-feeding syndrome
Leukemic blast crisis
Treatment of hyperglycemia

ATN, acute tubular necrosis; DKA, diabetic ketoacidosis.

Hypophosphatemia

Hypophosphatemia can occur with decreased phosphorus intake (decreased intestinal absorption or increased gastrointestinal losses) or with excess renal wasting due to renal tubular defects or hyperparathyroidism. In addition, low serum phosphorus levels may also occur in the setting of extracellular-to-intracellular shifts. In the case of cellular shifts, total body phosphorus may not be depleted. By convention, hypophosphatemia is often graded as mild (<3.5 mg/dL), moderate (<2.5 mg/dL), or severe (<1.0 mg/dL). Moderate and severe hypophosphatemia usually occur only if there are multiple causes. The causes of hypophosphatemia are listed in **Table 13-3**.

Clinical Manifestations of Hypophosphatemia

Hypophosphatemia is a common finding; it is observed in approximately 3% of all hospitalized patients, 10% of hospitalized alcoholic patients, and 70% of ventilated patients in intensive care. Symptoms usually are seen only in patients with moderate or severe hypophosphatemia and include muscle weakness (and difficulty weaning from the ventilator), hemolysis, impaired platelet and white blood cell function, rhabdomyolysis, and, in rare cases, neurologic disorders. Hypophosphatemia is probably overtreated in the intensive care unit, where the "difficult to wean" patient may be given phosphorus when the low phosphorus levels are actually caused by cellular shifts due to respiratory alkalosis. A careful review of the trend in serum phosphorus with arterial blood pH can help discern which patients need to be treated.

Differential Diagnosis of Hypophosphatemia

The differential diagnosis and treatment approach are based on the cause and site of phosphate loss. Usually, the cause is clinically apparent, but if it is not, the simplest test is to measure 24-hour urine phosphorus excretion. The expected renal response to hypophosphatemia is avid reabsorption. If the urinary excretion is less than 100 mg/24 hr, then the kidney is responding normally to hypophosphatemia, and the cause must be impaired intake, gastrointestinal losses, or extracellular-to-intracellular shifts.

Decreased Oral Intake

The average American diet contains almost two times the RDA of phosphorus. All proteins and dairy products contain phosphorus, and phosphorus is used as a preservative in many processed foods. Decreased intake of phosphorus is usually seen only with generalized poor oral intake, gastrointestinal losses with diarrhea and malabsorption, or alcoholism. Occasionally, patients abuse phosphate-binding antacids.

Redistribution

Approximately 15% of the extraskeletal phosphorus is intracellular, and hypophosphatemia may result from a shift to intracellular stores. In most situations, this shift is not clinically detectable. However, if there is some underlying phosphate depletion, more profound hypophosphatemia may be observed. The most common clinical cause of this form of hypophosphatemia is hyperglycemia with or without ketoacidosis. The glucose-induced osmotic diuresis results in a net deficit of phosphorus, and cellular glucose uptake stimulated by insulin during treatment further causes a shift of the extracellular phosphorus into cells as glycogen stores are repleted. This is usually a transient hypophosphatemia and, in general, should not be treated. In patients who are malnourished, sudden "refeeding" may shift phosphorus into cells. Respiratory, but not metabolic, alkalosis also increases the intracellular flux of phosphorus. Even in normal subjects, severe hyperventilation (to a carbon dioxide tension [PCO_2] of less than 20 mm Hg) may lower serum phosphorus concentrations to less than 1.0 mg/dL. Therefore, in ventilated patients, arterial blood gases may be helpful in differentiating shifts resulting from true phosphorus depletion. Lastly, in hungry bone syndrome after parathyroidectomy (described earlier), there is increased bone uptake of phosphorus and resultant hypophosphatemia.

Increased Urinary Losses

Phosphorus clearance in the kidney is primarily determined by the phosphorus concentration, urinary flow, PTH, and FGF23 and other phosphatonins. Patients who are overly volume expanded have less proximal tubular reabsorption of phosphorus in parallel with reduced proximal salt and water reabsorption. Similarly, patients with glucosuria and post-obstructive diuresis have increased urinary flow and losses. In primary hyperparathyroidism, there is increased urinary phosphorus excretion caused by elevated PTH levels. Both congenital and acquired Fanconi's syndrome are characterized by increased urinary phosphorus excretion due to defects in the proximal tubule, together with renal glucosuria, hypouricemia, aminoaciduria, and, potentially, type 2 renal tubular acidosis. Acquired forms of Fanconi's syndrome may be seen in multiple myeloma and after administration of some chemotherapy drugs (cisplatin, ifosfamide, and 6-mercaptopurine), outdated tetracycline, or the antiretroviral agent tenofovir.

Rickets and Osteomalacia

Hypophosphatemia can lead to impaired bone mineralization. Several genetic disorders are associated with hypophosphatemia and rickets in children, including ADHR and X-linked hypophosphatemic rickets (XLH). These patients have phosphaturia, hypophosphatemia, inappropriately low calcitriol levels, normal to slightly elevated PTH, and normocalcemia. The defective gene in XLH is an endopeptidase called PHEX. In XLH, it has been postulated that PHEX abnormalities may lead to altered FGF23 metabolism, but this remains controversial. In ADHR, FGF23 is mutated; this results in abnormal clearance of the protein, leading to prolonged and inappropriate hypophosphaturia (see also Chapter 40). In tumor-induced osteomalacia, tumors of mesenchymal origin secrete a phosphatonin such as FGF23, matrix extracellular phosphoglycoprotein (MEPE), or FRP4, which upregulates the renal sodium phosphate cotransporter with resultant renal phosphate wasting.

Treatment of Hypophosphatemia

Treatment is usually necessary for patients with moderate to severe hypophosphatemia. Increasing oral intake is the preferred treatment, because acutely administered intravenous phosphate can complex calcium and lead to extraskeletal calcifications. Oral supplementation can be given with skim milk (1000 mg/quart), whole milk (850 mg/quart), Neutra-Phos K capsules (250 mg/capsule; maximum dose, 3 tabs every 6 hours), or Neutra-Phos solution (128 mg/mL). Oral phosphorus may induce or exacerbate diarrhea. Milk is much better tolerated (and cheaper!), and the concomitant administration of vitamin D will enhance its absorption. If necessary, phosphorus may be replaced intravenously as potassium phosphate (3 mmol/mL of phosphorus, 4.4 mEq/mL of potassium) or sodium phosphate (3 mmol/mL of phosphorus, 4.0 mEq/mL of sodium) in a single administration, usually mixed in 50 mL of normal saline.

BIBLIOGRAPHY

Bielesz B: Emerging roles of a phosphatonin in mineral homeostasis and its derangements. Eur J Clin Invest 36(Suppl 2):34-42, 2006.

Bilezikian JP, Silverberg SJ: Clinical practice: Asymptomatic primary hyperparathyroidism. N Engl J Med 350:1746-1751, 2004.

Brunelli SM, Goldfarb S: Hypophosphatemia: Clinical consequences and management. J Am Soc Nephrol 18:1999-2003, 2007.

Clines GA, Guise TA: Hypercalcaemia of malignancy and basic research on mechanisms responsible for osteolytic osteoblastic metastasis to bone. Endocr Relat Cancer 12:549-583, 2005.

D'Amour P: Circulating PTH molecular forms: What we know and what we don't. Kidney Int Suppl 102:S29-S33, 2006.

Friedlander G: Regulation of renal phosphate handling: recent findings. Curr Opin Nephrol Hypertens 5:316-320, 1996.

Imel EA, Econs MJ: Fibroblast growth factor 23: Roles in health and disease. J Am Soc Nephrol 16:2565-2575, 2005.

Jacobs TP, Bilezikian JP: Clinical review: Rare causes of hypercalcemia. J Clin Endocrinol Metab 90:6316-6322, 2005.

Kraft MD, Btaiche IF, Sacks GS: Review of the refeeding syndrome. Nutr Clin Pract 20:625-633, 2005.

Lyman D: Undiagnosed vitamin D deficiency in the hospitalized patient. Am Fam Physcian 71:299-304, 2005.

Rampello E, Fricia T, Malaguarnera M: The management of tumor lysis syndrome. Nat Clin Pract Oncol 3:438-447, 2006.

Ritz E: The clinical management of hyperphosphatemia. J Nephrol 18:221-228, 2005.

Schwartz SR, Futran ND: Hypercalcemic hypocalciuria: A critical differential diagnosis for hyperparathyroidism. Otolaryngol Clin North Am 37:887-896. xi, 2004.

Sedlacek M, Schoolwerth AC, Remillard BD: Electrolyte disturbances in the intensive care unit. Semin Dial 19:496-501, 2006.

Stewart AF: Clinical practice: Hypercalcemia associated with cancer. N Engl J Med 352:373-379, 2005.

Tfelt-Hansen J, Brown EM: The calcium-sensing receptor in normal physiology and pathophysiology: A review. Crit Rev Clin Lab Sci 42:35-70, 2005.

CHAPTER 14

Disorders of Magnesium Homeostasis

Jeffrey S. Berns

MAGNESIUM METABOLISM

The normal adult total body magnesium content is approximately 25 g (about 15 mmol/kg); between 60% and 65% is in bone, with most of the remainder in the intracellular compartment of muscle and other soft tissues. Much of the intracellular magnesium is bound to various cellular constituents such as adenosine triphosphate (ATP), adenosine diphosphate (ADP), proteins, and nucleic acids, or is located within mitochondria, and is only slowly exchangeable with the extracellular fluid (ECF) pool. The free cytosolic concentration is 0.5 to 0.8 mmol/L. Only about 1% of total body magnesium is in the ECF. The normal total plasma magnesium concentration is 1.7 to 2.3 mg/dL (0.71 to 0.96 mmol/L; the atomic weight of magnesium is 24.3, so 1 mmol/L = 2 mEq/L = 2.4 mg/dL). Approximately 30% of magnesium in the ECF is protein bound; the remaining 70% is filterable. This filterable fraction includes free, ionized magnesium (60% to 65% of total plasma magnesium) and magnesium that is complexed to citrate, phosphate, oxalate, and other anions (5% to 10% of total plasma magnesium). Assays to measure ionized, biologically active magnesium in the serum and in red blood cells have been developed but are not yet in routine use.

A typical American adult diet contains about 300 to 400 mg/day of elemental magnesium. Cereal grains, nuts, legumes, green vegetables, and some meats and seafoods, as well as drinking water (especially so-called "hard water"), are significant sources of dietary magnesium.

Normally, about 40% to 50% of dietary magnesium is absorbed in the gastrointestinal tract, primarily in the small intestine. Magnesium is also secreted in the small intestine (approximately 40 mg/day) and reabsorbed in the colon and rectum (approximately 20 mg/day). Absorption of magnesium in the intestine occurs through both passive paracellular absorption and via an active, transcellular pathway mediated by the luminal membrane Mg^{2+}-selective channel, TRPM6 (transient receptor potential channel, subfamily M, member 6). As in the kidney, the mechanism for Mg^{2+} exit from the cell is not certain. There does not appear to be any important hormonal regulation of magnesium absorption in the gastrointestinal tract, although vitamin D may variably increase magnesium absorption.

Renal Handling of Magnesium

Under normal circumstances, 95% to 97% of filtered magnesium is reabsorbed in the kidney, and 3% to 5% appears in the urine. In contrast to most other ions, only about 15% to 25% of the filtered load of magnesium is reabsorbed in the proximal tubule. The cortical thick ascending limb (TAL) of the loop of Henle reabsorbs 60% to 70% of the filtered load via a passive, paracellular process, driven largely by the lumen-positive voltage in this segment. Tight junction proteins called paracellin-1 (claudin-16) and claudin-19 control paracellular permeability to magnesium in the TAL. The medullary TAL does not appear to reabsorb magnesium in humans. Activation of the basolateral membrane extracellular Ca^{2+}/Mg^{2+}-sensing receptor (CaSR), a member of the G protein–coupled receptor superfamily, by either cation reduces magnesium (and calcium) reabsorption in the TAL. This appears to occur via inhibition of intermediate-conductance ROMK apical K^+ channels and the Na^+-K^+-$2Cl^-$ cotransporter, which reduces the transepithelial voltage, and modulation of paracellin-1, which reduces paracellular permeability. Magnesium reabsorption in the distal convoluted tubule (DCT) accounts for 5% to 10% of the filtered load, is active and transcellular, and serves to regulate final urinary magnesium excretion. Cellular uptake is mediated by the luminal membrane Mg^{2+}-selective channel, TRPM6, driven by the transepithelial voltage; exit from the cell is probably mediated by a basolateral membrane Na^+-Mg^{2+} exchanger and/or Mg^{2+}ATPase. It has recently been shown that TRMP6 and cellular Mg^{2+} uptake are activated by epidermal growth factor (EGF) via a basolateral membrane EGF receptor (EGFR). Activation of the CaSR in the DCT also inhibits magnesium reabsorption in this segment, but its physiologic role in magnesium handling is not fully established.

The plasma magnesium concentration is the most important determinant of renal magnesium excretion. Magnesium depletion and hypomagnesemia increase magnesium reabsorption, and hypermagnesemia decreases reabsorption in the TAL and DCT. Hypercalcemia also decreases magnesium reabsorption in these segments. These effects of changes in the plasma concentrations of magnesium and calcium on urinary magnesium excretion are mediated primarily by the basolateral membrane CaSR. Volume contraction increases and volume expansion decreases magnesium reabsorption in the proximal tubule. Unlike calcium and phosphorous, hormonal control of magnesium handling in the kidney appears to be of relatively minor physiologic importance, although complex direct and indirect hormonal influences on urinary magnesium excretion and renal magnesium transport have been described. Experimentally, parathyroid hormone (PTH), calcitonin, $1,25(OH)_2$ vitamin D_3, glucagon, insulin, aldosterone, and vasopressin can be shown to increase magnesium absorption by cells of the TAL and/or the DCT. The effects of aldosterone on renal handling of magnesium are complex. Although aldosterone may increase magnesium absorption in the TAL and DCT, aldosterone-mediated ECF volume expansion reduces magnesium reabsorption in the proximal tubule and can increase urinary magnesium excretion. Loop diuretics decrease magnesium reabsorption in the TAL by reducing the lumen-positive transepithelial voltage that drives paracellular reabsorption in this segment. Acute thiazide diuretic administration and amiloride increase magnesium reabsorption in the DCT by stimulating voltage-sensitive magnesium uptake by DCT cells. The effects of thiazide diuretics on renal magnesium handling are discussed later in this chapter.

HYPOMAGNESEMIA

The plasma magnesium concentration is not a particularly accurate measure of total body magnesium. It is difficult to predict the extent of magnesium deficiency based on the plasma concentration. Intracellular magnesium depletion can be present with low-normal plasma levels.

Causes of Hypomagnesemia

Impaired gastrointestinal tract absorption is a common underlying basis for hypomagnesemia, especially when the small bowel is involved due to disorders associated with malabsorption, chronic diarrhea, steatorrhea, or small intestinal bypass surgery (**Table 14-1**). Because there is some magnesium absorption in the colon, patients with ileostomies can develop hypomagnesemia. Hypomagnesemia with secondary hypocalcemia is a rare autosomal recessive disorder in which intestinal and renal magnesium absorption are impaired as a result of mutations in the gene for TRPM6.

Renal causes of hypomagnesemia are listed in **Table 14-1**. Osmotic and loop diuretics can cause significant urinary magnesium losses and hypomagnesemia. Thiazide diuretics acutely increase magnesium reabsorption in the DCT and do not cause urinary magnesium wasting. With chronic thiazide diuretic use, however, magnesium reabsorption is decreased and magnesium depletion can develop. The mechanisms causing increased urinary magnesium excretion with chronic thiazide use are not fully understood, but recent studies suggest that they may involve primarily downregulation of TRPM6. Experimental studies have also shown reduced magnesium uptake by DCT cells in the presence of hypokalemia and cellular potassium depletion, as may occur with chronic thiazide use. Effects of hyperaldosteronism on the activity of luminal membrane epithelial sodium channels (ENaC) in the DCT, leading to an increase in the lumen-negative transepithelial voltage and reduced reabsorption in this segment, as well as possible indirect effects on paracellin-1 function, have also been postulated. Experimental evidence indicating increased apoptosis of DCT cells with thiazide administration has led to the suggestion that this may reduce

TABLE 14-1 Causes of Hypomagnesemia

Decreased Intake
Chronic alcoholism
Protein-calorie malnutrition
Inadequate magnesium content in total parenteral nutrition or intravenous fluids
Gastrointestinal Losses
Inflammatory bowel disease
Chronic diarrhea
Laxative abuse
Malabsorption
Surgical bowel resection
Inherited hypomagnesemia with secondary hypocalcemia
Renal Losses
Diuretics: osmotic diuretics, loop diuretics, thiazide diuretics (chronic use)
Amphotericin B
Aminoglycosides
Cisplatin
Pentamidine
Cyclosporine, tacrolimus
Foscarnet
Cetuximab
Post-obstructive diuresis or diuretic phase of acute tubular necrosis
Inherited disorders 　Hypomagnesemia with secondary hypocalcemia 　Isolated dominant hypomagnesemia (autosomal dominant renal hypomagnesemia with hypocalciuria) 　Hypomagnesemia with hypercalciuria and nephrocalcinosis 　Autosomal dominant hypocalcemia with hypercalciuria 　Isolated recessive hypomagnesemia 　Gitelman's syndrome 　Bartter's syndrome
Alcohol ingestion
Hypercalcemia
Chronic metabolic acidosis
Miscellaneous
Acute pancreatitis
Hungry bone syndrome
Diabetic ketoacidosis

the overall epithelial cell surface area and thus impair magnesium reabsorption in this segment of the nephron.

Several nephrotoxic drugs, such as amphotericin B, the aminoglycosides, cisplatin, foscarnet, cyclosporine, and tacrolimus, can cause urinary magnesium wasting, in most cases related to impaired magnesium absorption in the TAL and DCT. The magnesium wasting with these drugs can be quite severe, can occur before other evidence of tubular injury or a decline in glomerular filtration rate (GFR) develops, and can persist for months after the drug is stopped.

Urinary magnesium wasting appears to be more common with tacrolimus than with cyclosporine. Cetuximab, a human/mouse chimeric monoclonal antibody that binds to the EGFR and blocks EGF binding, is used for treatment of metastatic colon cancer and causes reversible urinary magnesium wasting and hypomagnesemia. As mentioned earlier, EGF and EGFR are both expressed in the kidney, particularly in the DCT, and appear to be involved in regulation of magnesium handling in this nephron segment.

Urinary magnesium wasting and hypomagnesemia, which can be severe, are seen in most patients with Gitelman's syndrome, which is caused by loss-of-function mutations in the gene that encodes the DCT Na^+-Cl^- cotransporter (NCCT). The pathophysiologic basis for the urinary magnesium wasting in Gitelman's syndrome has not been fully elucidated but is probably multifactorial. Because thiazide diuretics inhibit the DCT NCCT and therefore, in some respects, create a model of Gitelman's syndrome, the mechanisms proposed for urinary magnesium wasting with chronic thiazide administration may also explain the urinary magnesium wasting of this syndrome. An experimental animal model of Gitelman's syndrome in which the NCCT gene has been deleted and urinary magnesium wasting is present may help researchers understand the basis for this disorder. Interestingly, hypokalemia does not develop in these knockout animals, suggesting that, in contrast to chronic thiazide administration, hypokalemia and cellular potassium depletion are not responsible for the urinary magnesium wasting in Gitelman's syndrome.

Urinary magnesium wasting and hypomagnesemia are present in only a minority of patients with Bartter's syndrome and are seen primarily in those with the classic form, which is mediated by mutations in the gene for the TAL basolateral membrane chloride channel (ClC-Kb). Urinary magnesium wasting in these patients is thought to be caused by a reduction in the lumen-positive voltage in the TAL, which reduces the driving force for magnesium reabsorption. It is unclear why urinary magnesium wasting and hypomagnesemia are not seen in most patients with Bartter's syndrome but are typical of Gitelman's syndrome. Because more magnesium is normally reabsorbed in the loop of Henle than in the DCT, urinary magnesium wasting might be expected more commonly with the Bartter's syndrome group of disorders than with Gitelman' syndrome, much as urinary magnesium wasting is more common with loop diuretics than thiazide diuretics. Volume depletion and hyperaldosteronism may attenuate urinary magnesium wasting in patients with Bartter's syndrome, partially explaining why it is less common than otherwise might be expected in these patients. Differences in TRPM abundance or activity may also play a role. A variety of other rare inherited disorders with renal magnesium wasting have been described, some of which result from mutations in the genes for paracellin-1 (familial hypomagnesemia with hypercalciuria/nephrocalcinosis), the CaSR (autosomal dominant hypocalcemia with hypercalciuria), TRPM6 (hypomagnesemia with secondary hypocalcemia), and EGF (isolated recessive hypomagnesemia).

Chronic metabolic acidosis increases urinary loss of magnesium, in association with decreased renal expression of TRPM6. Alcoholics and those on magnesium-deficient diets or parenteral nutrition for prolonged periods can become hypomagnesemic in the absence of abnormal gastrointestinal or kidney function. Addition of 4 to 12 mmol of magnesium per day to the total parenteral nutrition has been recommended to prevent hypomagnesemia. Although urinary magnesium excretion can be reduced to very low levels with magnesium deficiency, hypomagnesemia can still develop because of persistent obligatory losses in urine, stool, and sweat, coupled with the fact that exchange of bone and intracellular magnesium with extracellular magnesium is limited and slow. Alcohol ingestion can cause reversible generalized renal tubular dysfunction with urinary magnesium wasting even in the presence of hypomagnesemia. Hypomagnesemia can occur with acute pancreatitis, probably through the same mechanism that contributes to hypocalcemia in this setting, namely, the precipitation of magnesium (and calcium) in necrotic fat in the pancreatic bed. Hypomagnesemia also appears to be more common among type 2 diabetics than among nondiabetics.

Hypomagnesemia is common among patients in intensive care units, particularly those who have sepsis or who are receiving diuretics. In some studies, patients in intensive care units with hypomagnesemia had higher mortality rates than patients without hypomagnesemia. A beneficial effect of magnesium replacement on outcomes in this setting has not been shown.

In circumstances where the etiology of hypomagnesemia is unclear, a 24-hour urinary magnesium excretion greater than 1 mmol or a calculated fractional excretion of magnesium (FE_{Mg})* greater than 3% suggests inappropriate renal wasting; the FE_{Mg} can decrease to less than 0.5% with magnesium depletion from nonrenal causes.

Clinical Manifestations of Hypomagnesemia

Hypomagnesemia often coexists with hypokalemia and hypocalcemia, which may be caused by the same underlying medical condition (e.g., diuretics, diarrhea). In addition, magnesium depletion enhances renal potassium secretion in the loop of Henle, and possibly in the cortical collecting tubules, through uncertain mechanisms. The hypocalcemia seen with hypomagnesemia is caused by inhibition of PTH secretion and skeletal resistance to the effects of PTH, although inhibition of calcitriol synthesis may also play a role. The hypokalemia and hypocalcemia are often refractory to correction until the hypomagnesemia is corrected.

---

*The FE_{Mg} is calculated from the urinary (U) and plasma (P) concentrations of magnesium (Mg) and creatinine (Cr) as follows:

$$FE_{Mg} = \frac{U_{Mg}/(0.7 \times P_{Mg})}{U_{Cr}/P_{Cr}} \times 100$$

The P_{Mg} is multiplied by 0.7 because approximately 70% of total plasma magnesium is not albumin bound and is thus free to be filtered across the glomerulus.

Neuromuscular manifestations of hypomagnesemia are similar to those of hypocalcemia, including hyperreflexia, carpopedal spasm, tetany, seizures, and positive Chvostek's and Trousseau's signs. These signs can occur in the absence of severe hypocalcemia. Electrocardiographic changes include widening of the QRS complex, prolongation of the QT interval, and peaking of T waves, mimicking changes related to hypokalemia and/or hypocalcemia. Torsades de pointes, premature ventricular beats, ventricular tachycardia, and ventricular fibrillation have also been described with hypomagnesemia and may respond to intravenous administration of magnesium sulfate. Hypomagnesemia also increases the risk of cardiac toxicity from digitalis glycosides. Chronic magnesium deficiency has been variably associated with increased risk for stroke, ischemic coronary artery disease, hypertension, complications of diabetes mellitus, and asthma, albeit through uncertain mechanisms.

Normomagnesemic magnesium depletion should be considered in patients with clinical features consistent with magnesium depletion (e.g., unexplained hypokalemia or hypocalcemia) who are at risk for magnesium depletion. The diagnosis may be suggested by a 24-hour urinary magnesium value of less than 1 mmol, retention of more than 20% of a standardized dose of magnesium (2.4 mg/kg infused over 4 hours) over 24 hours, or response to empiric treatment with magnesium supplementation.

Treatment of Hypomagnesemia

In patients with asymptomatic or chronic hypomagnesemia not responsive to increased dietary magnesium, oral replacement therapy is appropriate (**Table 14-2**). An initial oral dose of 30 to 60 mEq/day in three or four divided doses may be used. Ingestion of magnesium salts can cause diarrhea. Sustained-release preparations are often recommended. For instance, for Slo-Mag, an enteric-coated preparation of magnesium chloride that contains 64 mg (5.3 mEq) of elemental magnesium per tablet, 6 to 12 tablets in divided doses may be taken daily. Although a single 400-mg tablet of magnesium oxide (containing 20 mEq of elemental magnesium) taken two to three times daily may also be adequate, diarrhea with this preparation tends to be more problematic than with sustained-released magnesium chloride. Repletion of body stores usually takes at least several days. Amiloride and the other potassium-sparing diuretics can reduce the renal magnesium wasting caused by other diuretics, aminoglycosides, amphotericin B, Gitelman's syndrome, or other circumstances.

Patients with hypomagnesemia who are unable to take magnesium supplements orally and those with symptomatic or severe hypomagnesemia (<1.0 mEq/L) should receive intravenous magnesium sulfate. In the presence of normal kidney function, as much as 50% of an intravenous magnesium dose administrated over 4 hours will be excreted in the urine even when there is substantial magnesium deficiency. An intravenous dose of magnesium of 1.0 to 1.5 mEq/kg may be given over the first 24 hours, with doses of 0.5 to 1.0 mEq/kg daily thereafter until the plasma magnesium level remains within the normal range. This typically requires several days and as much as 3 to 4 mEq/kg of magnesium. These doses should be reduced commensurate with any reduction in GFR. Intravenous preparations of magnesium sulfate are available in concentrations of 10% to 50%. A common preparation is a 2-mL vial or ampoule of 50% magnesium sulfate (as $MgSO_4 \cdot 7H_2O$) containing 1 g $MgSO_4$ or 8.1 mEq (98.7 mg) of elemental magnesium. Magnesium sulfate can be painful and sclerosing when administered intravenously, so it should be diluted before administration. In emergency situations, 1 to 2 g of $MgSO_4$ (8.1 to 16.2 mEq) may be given intravenously in 50 mL of normal saline or 5% dextrose in water over 5 to 10 minutes. Patients should be monitored during magnesium infusion for hypotension and reduction of deep tendon reflexes. Facial flushing or a feeling of warmth

TABLE 14-2 Preparations for Oral Magnesium Replacement Therapy			
MAGNESIUM SALT	**USUAL TABLET (mg)**	**Mg CONTENT (mg/tablet)**	**Mg CONTENT (mEq/tablet)**
Oxide			
Mg-Ox 400	400	242	20
Uro-Mag	140	84	7
Gluconate*			
Almora, Magtrate, others	500	27	2.3
Chloride			
Slo-Mag (enteric coated)	535	64	5.3
Mag-SR (sustained release)	535	64	5.3
Lactate			
Mag-Tab SR (sustained release)	840	84	7
L-Aspartate HCl			
Maginex (enteric coated)	615	61	5
Maginex DS (enteric coated)	1230	122	10

*Also available in liquid oral formulations.

may indicate an overly rapid rate of infusion. Intramuscular injection of magnesium sulfate is painful and should be used only in the absence of intravenous access.

HYPERMAGNESEMIA

Causes of Hypermagnesemia

Because an increase in the plasma magnesium concentration causes decreased reabsorption in the cortical TAL and increased urinary excretion, hypermagnesemia rarely occurs unless there is a significant degree of kidney functional impairment (GFR <30 mL/min) or a very large load of magnesium is delivered. Even among patients undergoing chronic dialysis, symptomatic hypermagnesemia is rare.

Some of the more common causes of hypermagnesemia are shown in **Table 14-3**. Intentional iatrogenic hypermagnesemia occurs with intravenous magnesium administration for the treatment of severe preeclampsia and eclampsia. Severe hypermagnesemia can also result from excessive use of magnesium-containing enemas, antacids, laxatives, or nutritional supplements or accidental ingestion of Epsom salts. Magnesium-containing enemas and laxatives should be avoided in patients with impaired kidney function. Magnesium-containing antacids should be used very cautiously in such patients.

Uncommon causes of hypermagnesemia include familial hypocalciuric hypercalcemia, which is caused by inactivating mutations in the CaSR gene; theophylline intoxication; lithium ingestion; hyperparathyroidism; adrenal insufficiency; hypothyroidism; milk-alkali syndrome; tumor lysis syndrome; and Dead Sea water ingestion.

Clinical Manifestations of Hypermagnesemia

Clinical sequelae of hypermagnesemia are uncommon with serum concentrations lower than 4.5 to 5.0 mg/dL. Above this level, cutaneous flushing, nausea, vomiting, and mild hypotension may occur. Hyporeflexia typically occurs at magnesium levels of 5 mg/dL and higher. Loss of deep tendon

TABLE 14-3 Principal Causes of Hypermagnesemia
Magnesium Infusion
Therapy for severe preeclampsia and eclampsia
Total parenteral nutrition
Oral Ingestion
Laxatives
Antacids
Epsom salts (magnesium sulfate)
Magnesium-Containing Enemas
Reduced Glomerular Filtration Rate
Acute kidney injury
Chronic kidney disease

reflexes, skeletal muscle weakness, and hypotension, which can be severe, develop with levels of 7 to 10 mg/dL or greater; respiratory muscle paralysis typically occurs at 12 to 15 mg/dL or higher. Electrocardiographic manifestations begin to develop at concentrations of 5 mg/dL and include prolonged PR interval, increased QRS duration, and increased QT interval, along with bradycardia that may progress to complete heart block at levels of 10 to 15 mg/dL or higher and cardiac arrest when levels exceed 15 to 20 mg/dL.

Symptomatic hypocalcemia due to inhibition of PTH secretion can complicate parenteral magnesium therapy for eclampsia. Although hypermagnesemia decreases the anion gap, this appears not to occur with infusion of magnesium sulfate, because retention of the anionic sulfate moiety counterbalances the unmeasured cation.

Treatment of Hypermagnesemia

Hypermagnesemia usually requires no treatment, provided that kidney function is close to normal. Hemodialysis and, to a much lesser extent, peritoneal dialysis can remove excess magnesium. Intravenous calcium (100 to 200 mg over 5 to 10 minutes) can transiently antagonize the cardiac effects of hypermagnesemia.

BIBLIOGRAPHY

Agus ZS: Hypomagnesemia. J Am Soc Nephrol 10:1616-1622, 1999.

Alexander RT, Hoenderop JG, Bindels RJ: Molecular determinants of magnesium homeostasis: insights from human disease. J Am Soc Nephrol. 19:1451-8, 2008.

Chubanov V, Gudermann T, Schlingmann KP: Essential role for TRPM6 in epithelial magnesium transport and body magnesium homeostasis. Pflugers Arch 451:228-234, 2005.

Cole DEC, Quamme GA: Inherited disorders of renal magnesium handling. J Am Soc Nephrol 11:1937-1947, 2000.

Dai L-J, Ritchie G, Kerstan D, et al: Magnesium transport in the renal distal convoluted tubule. Physiology Rev 81:51-84, 2001.

deRouffignac C, Quamme G: Renal magnesium handling and its hormonal control. Physiol Rev 74:305-322, 1994.

Ellison DH: Divalent cation transport by the distal nephron: Insights from Bartter's and Gitelman's syndromes. Am J Physiol Renal Physiol 279:F616-F625, 2000.

Hoenderop JGJ, Bindels RJM: Epithelial Ca^{2+} and Mg^{2+} channels in health and disease. J Am Soc Nephrol 16:15-26, 2005.

Huang CL, Kuo E: Mechanism of hypokalemia in magnesium deficiency. J Am Soc Nephrol 18:2649-52, 2007.

Konrad M, Weber S: Recent advances in molecular genetics of hereditary magnesium-losing disorders. J Am Soc Nephrol 14: 249-260, 2003.

Konrad M, Schlingmann KP, Gudermann T: Insights into the molecular nature of magnesium homeostasis. Am J Physiol Renal Physiol 286:F599-F605, 2004.

Muallem S, Moe OW: When EGF is offside, magnesium is wasted. J Clin Invest 117:2086-2089, 2007.

Naderi AS, Reilly RF Jr: Hereditary etiologies of hypomagnesemia. Nat Clin Pract Nephrol 4:80-9, 2008.

Nijenhuis T, Vallon V, van der Kemp AWCM, et al: Enhanced passive Ca^{2+} reabsorption and reduced Mg^{2+} channel abundance explains thiazide-induced hypocalciuria and hypomagnesemia. J Clin Invest 115:1651-1658, 2005.

Pham P-CT, Pham P-MT, Pham SV, et al: Hypomagnesemia in patients with type 2 diabetes. Clin J Am Soc Nephrol 2:366-373, 2007.

Quamme GA: Renal magnesium handling: New insights in understanding old problems. Kidney Int 52:1180-1195, 1997.

Reikes S, Gonzalez EA, Martin KJ: Abnormal calcium and magnesium metabolism. In DuBose TD Jr, Hamm LL (eds): Acid-Base and Electrolyte Disorders. Philadelphia, Saunders, 2002, pp 453-487.

Ricci J, Oster JR, Gutierrez R, et al: Influence of magnesium-sulfate-induced hypermagnesemia on the anion gap: Role of hypersulfatemia. Am J Nephrol 10:409-411, 1990.

Simon DB, Lu Y, Choate KA, et al: Paracellin-1, a renal tight junction protein is required for paracellular Mg^{2+} resorption. Science 285:103-106, 1999.

Tong GM, Rude RK: Magnesium deficiency in critical illness. J Intensive Care Med 20:3-17, 2005.

Whang R, Whang DD, Ryan MP: Refractory potassium depletion: A consequence of magnesium deficiency. Arch Intern Med 152:40-45, 1992.

CHAPTER 15

Edema and the Clinical Use of Diuretics

David H. Ellison

Edema is usually a manifestation of expanded extracellular fluid volume (ECFV) resulting from heart failure, hepatic cirrhosis, nephrotic syndrome, or impaired kidney function; it can also result from local factors or lymphatic obstruction. The ECFV commonly expands when the kidneys retain NaCl in excess of dietary NaCl intake. Primary increases in renal NaCl reabsorption typically lead to hypertension but not edema, because the elevated blood pressure normalizes NaCl excretion (pressure natriuresis) before edema develops. In contrast, if NaCl is retained because the *effective* arterial blood volume is reduced, as in patients with heart failure or cirrhosis, or if it is retained in the setting of fluid redistribution, as in patients with nephrotic syndrome, edema results. Regardless of its cause, the best treatments for generalized edema include dietary NaCl restriction and treatment of the primary disorder. Despite these interventions, or if they are impossible, ECFV frequently remains expanded unacceptably, and, for this reason, diuretics are prescribed.

The term *diuretic* defines a substance that increases urine production (from the Greek *dia*, "thoroughly," and *ourein*, "urine"). Until recently, all of the diuretics used clinically increased salt excretion primarily. Recently, the first of a new class of diuretics that increase water excretion without increasing salt excretion was approved for use in the United States. Thus, diuretics now comprise both natriuretics (including all of the older diuretics) and aquaretics (the vasopressin receptor–blocking drugs). Natriuretic diuretics are powerful drugs that, if used carefully, can play an important role in the treatment of symptomatic edema. The prompt, dramatic, and sustained symptomatic improvement that occurs when such diuretics are administered intravenously to a patient with acute pulmonary edema remains one of the most gratifying responses in clinical medicine. Furthermore, careful diuretic use remains essential for the chronic treatment of most edematous patients, making diuretics among the most frequently prescribed drugs. Aquaretics represent a new option for the treatment of hyponatremia; they may also become an important part of the therapeutic armamentarium, but current experience is limited.

In addition to their use for edema, diuretic drugs are indicated for a wide variety of nonedematous disorders. Specific details of diuretic treatment of hypertension, acute renal failure, nephrolithiasis, and hyponatremia are discussed in other chapters of this *Primer*. This chapter focuses on renal mechanisms of diuretic action and diuretic treatment of edema.

THE PHYSIOLOGIC BASIS OF DIURETIC ACTION

The amount of filtered Na^+ is equal to the plasma sodium concentration ($[Na^+]$) times the glomerular filtration rate (GFR). The amount of NaCl excreted by the kidneys is the difference between filtered Na^+ and the quantity reabsorbed by the renal tubules. Assuming a normal GFR (approximately 150 L/day) and a normal plasma $[Na^+]$ (approximately 150 mM), about 23 moles of Na^+ are filtered each day (equivalent to about 3 pounds of table salt). When individuals are in salt balance and urinary NaCl excretion equals dietary NaCl intake (typically 100 to 300 mEq of Na^+ per day), more than 99% of the filtered Na^+ is reabsorbed. All of the natriuretic drugs in clinical use act primarily on the renal tubules to inhibit Na^+ reabsorption and increase fractional Na^+ excretion.

A simple and clinically useful classification of diuretic drugs is based on the nature of the induced diuresis (Na^+ or water) and on the sites and mechanisms of action along the nephron (**Table 15-1**). All active NaCl reabsorption by renal epithelial cells is driven by the sodium-potassium adenosine triphosphatase (Na^+,K^+-ATPase) pump, which is expressed at the basolateral membrane (the blood side) of epithelial cells along the nephron. This pump uses metabolic energy

TABLE 15-1 Physiologic Classification of Diuretic Drugs*

Natriuretics

Proximal Diuretics

Carbonic anhydrase inhibitors: acetazolamide

Loop Diuretics

NKCC2 inhibitors: furosemide, bumetanide, torsemide, ethacrynic acid

DCT Diuretics

NCC inhibitors: hydrochlorothiazide, metolazone, chlorthalidone, indapamide†, many others

Distal K+-Sparing Diuretics

ENaC inhibitors: amiloride, triamterene

Aldosterone antagonists: spironolactone, eplerenone

Aquaretics

Vasopressin receptor blockers: conivaptan

*Classification based on site and mechanism of action.
†Indapamide and metolazone may have other actions as well.
DCT, distal convoluted tubule; ENaC, epithelial sodium channel; NCC, Na^+-Cl^- cotransporter; NKCC2, Na^+-K^+-$2Cl^-$ cotransporter.

(derived from hydrolysis of ATP) to extrude Na^+ from the cell into the interstitium and blood and to move K^+ into the cell. The action of the Na^+,K^+-ATPase keeps the cellular Na^+ concentration low and the cellular K^+ concentration high. Because the exchange of Na^+ for K^+ exchange occurs at a 3:2 ratio, the action of the Na^+,K^+-ATPase also contributes to making the cell interior electrically negative with respect to the extracellular fluid (the high intracellular $[K^+]$ being the other factor). The low cellular $[Na^+]$ and the cell-negative voltage create a driving force for Na^+ ions to enter the cell across the luminal membrane from tubule fluid. Although Na^+,K^+-ATPase pumps are present at the basolateral cell membranes of almost every epithelial cell, each nephron segment possesses unique apical mechanisms that permit Na^+ to move across the luminal membrane; these specific transport pathways form the molecular basis of most natriuretic action. Together, active Na^+ extrusion from the basolateral membrane and passive Na^+ entry across the luminal membrane permit vectorial Na^+ transport in the absorptive direction. Aquaretic diuretics, in contrast, block the action of arginine vasopressin (AVP), the antidiuretic hormone of humans, at basolateral receptors in the collecting ducts of the kidney.

NATRIURETICS
Proximal Tubule Diuretics

Approximately two thirds of the water and Na^+ that is filtered is reabsorbed along the proximal tubule. Sodium can enter proximal tubule cells together with other solutes such as glucose, amino acids, and phosphate, using the electrochemical gradient that favors Na^+ entry to drive the coupled solute into the cell. Additionally, Na^+ can enter the cell in exchange for H^+, indirectly coupling bicarbonate and chloride reabsorption to Na^+ absorption (see later discussion). Because the epithelium is electrically "leaky" (i.e., highly permeable to ions), large transepithelial ion gradients do not develop, and solute absorption along this segment is isosmotic.

The exchange of Na^+ for H^+ across the lumen of the proximal tubule is mediated largely by a Na^+/H^+ exchanger (NHE3, gene symbol *SLC9A3*) (**Fig. 15-1**). Protons that are extruded across the luminal membrane of proximal cells titrate bicarbonate (HCO_3^-) that has been filtered by the glomeruli. This forms carbonic acid (H_2CO_3), which dehydrates to CO_2 and H_2O, a reaction catalyzed by the carbonic anhydrase in the brush border of proximal tubule cells. By these mechanisms, $NaHCO_3$ is functionally reabsorbed across the luminal membrane into the cell. For transepithelial $NaHCO_3$ reabsorption to continue at steady state, Na^+ and HCO_3^- must leave the cell across the basolateral membrane. Sodium leaves via the Na^+,K^+-ATPase pump. Bicarbonate, with Na^+, leaves via a $NaHCO_3$ transport pathway. A second pool of carbonic anhydrase, located within proximal tubule cells, generates H^+ ions for extrusion across the apical membrane and HCO_3^- ions that exit across the basolateral membrane.

Carbonic anhydrase inhibitors interfere with enzyme activity both inside the cell and within the brush border. Their action in the brush border inhibits Na^+/H^+ exchange by slowing the rate at which carbonic acid dehydrates: Carbonic acid accumulates in tubule fluid, acidifying it. Their action

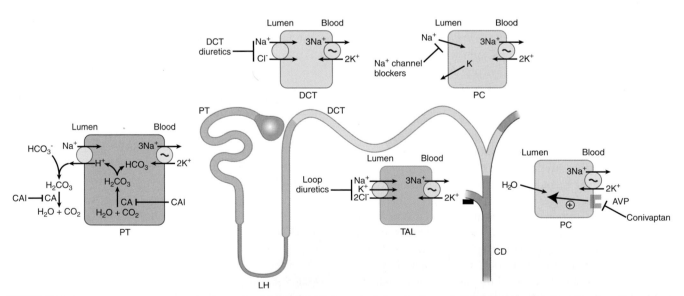

FIGURE 15-1 Predominant sites and mechanisms of action of clinically important diuretic drugs. Patterns identify sites of action along the nephron and corresponding cell types. The proximal tubule (PT, purple segment) is represented by a typical PT cell, shown in purple. The loop of Henle (LH) includes a thick ascending limb (TAL, green segment), and a typical TAL cell is shown in green. The distal convoluted tubule (DCT, blue segment) is represented by a typical DCT cell in blue. The collecting duct (CD, yellow and orange segments) includes principal cells (PC), shown in yellow. Note that, for clarity, two principal cells are shown. Both water and salt pathways are present in the same cells. Both intracellular and luminal actions of carbonic anhydrase inhibitors (CAI) in suppressing carbonic anhydrase (CA) are important in their ability to reduce Na^+ reabsorption by the renal proximal tubule. Note that Na^+ channel blockers probably act along the last half of the DCT and in the connecting tubule as well as in the CD. Spironolactone and eplerenone (not shown) are competitive aldosterone antagonists and act primarily in the cortical collecting tubule. Aquaretics, such as conivaptan, inhibit water reabsorption by principal cells by blocking the action of arginine vasopressin (AVP) on V_2 receptors. These receptors stimulate insertion of aquaporin 2 water channels in the apical membrane.

inside the cell inhibits HCO_3^- production, thereby interfering with basolateral base exit. The net result of carbonic anhydrase inhibition is impaired Na^+, and HCO_3^- reabsorption. This inhibits water reabsorption, which is driven by solute movement. Further, the usual increase in luminal $[Cl^-]$ caused by water removal from the tubule lumen is reduced, leading to impaired Cl^- reabsorption, as well. When administered acutely, these drugs provoke a moderate alkaline diuresis. When administered chronically, their natriuretic potency is relatively weak, because compensatory processes develop. Several mechanisms underlie this adaptation. First, when $NaHCO_3$ reabsorption along the proximal tubule is inhibited, much of the solute and fluid that escapes reabsorption by the proximal tubule can be reabsorbed by more distal nephron segments. Second, inhibition of solute reabsorption along the proximal tubule increases solute delivery to the macula densa. This activates the tubuloglomerular feedback mechanism, which suppresses GFR and decreases the filtration of Na^+, HCO_3^-, and Cl^-. Finally, alkaline diuresis induces metabolic acidosis; when the serum $[HCO_3^-]$ declines, less HCO_3^- is filtered, and the carbonic anhydrase–dependent component of Na^+ reabsorption declines.

Because carbonic anhydrase inhibitors are relatively weak diuretics in chronic use, and because they often result in metabolic acidosis, their use as natriuretic drugs is limited. However, they are commonly employed to treat open-angle glaucoma, where they reduce the formation of aqueous humor by as much as 50%. Furthermore, they can be used to prevent acute mountain sickness and to treat metabolic alkalosis at times when the Cl^- needed to correct it cannot be administered because of ECFV expansion. This is especially useful in patients whose respiratory drive is compromised by metabolic alkalosis; careful use of carbonic anhydrase inhibitors may correct the alkalosis and improve the respiratory drive. Carbonic anhydrase inhibitors may also be used in combination with other classes of diuretics to induce diuresis in otherwise resistant cases (see "Resistance to Diuretics").

Loop Diuretics

Approximately 25% of filtered NaCl is reabsorbed along the loop of Henle. Transcellular NaCl reabsorption along the medullary and cortical thick ascending limb (TAL) is driven by Na^+,K^+-ATPase at the basolateral membrane. An electroneutral pathway at the luminal membrane (NKCC2, gene symbol *SLC12A1*) carries 1 Na^+, 1 K^+, and 2 Cl^- from tubule fluid into the cell, driven by the electrochemical gradient for Na^+ (see **Fig. 15-1**). Much of the K^+ that is taken up via this pathway recycles across the luminal membrane through K^+ channels (ROMK, gene symbol *KCNJ1*). The Na^+-K^+-$2Cl^-$ pathway, therefore, generates net NaCl reabsorption and (because of the K^+ recycling) a voltage across the wall of the tubule that is oriented such that the lumen is positive relative to the extracellular fluid.

Loop diuretics such as furosemide, bumetanide, and torsemide inhibit the action of the NKCC2 directly. These diuretics are anions that circulate bound to protein; because of the extensive protein binding, very little diuretic reaches tubule fluid via glomerular filtration. Instead, loop diuretics are secreted into the lumen of the proximal tubule by an organic anion transport pathway. Mice deficient in the first isoform of organic anion transporter (OAT1) show resistance to furosemide, owing to impaired renal clearance. Once secreted, loop diuretics travel downstream to the TAL, where they bind directly to the Na^+-K^+-$2Cl^-$ transporter and inhibit its action. Although the mechanism by which ethacrynic acid inhibits NaCl reabsorption is not as clear, its net effect on transport along the TAL is qualitatively similar. Loop diuretics are potent ("high-ceiling") drugs that promote the excretion of Na^+ and Cl^-, together with K^+. Although they inhibit K^+ reabsorption along the TAL, their effects on K^+ excretion reflect predominantly their tendency to increase K^+ secretion along the distal nephron (see "Complications of Diuretic Treatment"). Loop diuretics increase excretion of Ca^{2+} and Mg^{2+} by reducing the magnitude of the lumen-positive voltage in the TAL. This tends to impair Ca^{2+} and Mg^{2+} reabsorption, which is driven across the paracellular pathway by the lumen-positive voltage.

Loop diuretics impair the ability of the kidney to elaborate urine that is either very concentrated or very dilute. The NKCC2 removes Na^+ and Cl^- from the lumen as fluid courses up the TAL. Because this segment of the nephron is impermeable to water, solute removal dilutes the tubule fluid. By blocking the predominant solute removal pathway, loop diuretics inhibit free water generation. The action of the NKCC2 also provides the so-called single effect that is responsible for countercurrent multiplication. Solute removal from the TAL contributes to generation of a high solute concentration in the medullary interstitium, which drives water reabsorption from the medullary collecting tubule, under the control of AVP. By blocking NKCC2, loop diuretics inhibit the kidney's ability to generate concentrated urine; this is one reason these diuretics can be useful in treating the syndrome of inappropriate antidiuretic hormone secretion (SIADH).

Loop diuretics have important hemodynamic effects, both within the kidney and systemically. They increase secretion of vasodilatory prostaglandins and often reduce cardiac preload when administered acutely. Loop diuretics also strongly stimulate renin release. Diuretic-stimulated renin release results both from a reduction in pressure in the afferent arteriole, owing to ECFV depletion, and from direct interference with NaCl entry across the apical membrane of macula densa cells. This second mechanism explains why loop diuretics stimulate renin secretion in an ECFV-independent manner. The tendency to stimulate renin (and ensuing production of angiotensin II and aldosterone) can have negative consequences. In some situations, loop diuretics can elicit a vasoconstrictor response that may impair cardiac performance acutely; this anomalous response results from enhanced renin secretion and may be blocked by angiotensin-converting enzyme (ACE) inhibitors. Loop diuretics tend to maintain or increase the GFR, even in the face of ECFV depletion, because they block the tubuloglomerular feedback mechanism and because diuretic-induced prostaglandin secretion dilates the afferent arterioles.

Distal Convoluted Tubule Diuretics (Thiazides and Others)

The distal tubule, the nephron segment just beyond the loop of Henle, reabsorbs 5% to 10% of the filtered NaCl. The Na^+ concentration in distal convoluted tubule (DCT) cells is maintained at a low level by Na^+,K^+-ATPase. Na^+ and Cl^- enter the cell across the luminal membrane via an electroneutral Na^+-Cl^- cotransport pathway that is molecularly and functionally distinct from the pathway in the TAL (NCC, gene symbol *SLC12A3*; see **Fig. 15-1**). Although DCT diuretics are commonly called "thiazides" (benzothiadiazines), many such drugs (e.g., chlorthalidone) are not true thiazides; the more general term that defines them by their site of action is preferred. DCT diuretics are anions that, like the loop diuretics, circulate in the bloodstream bound to protein and are secreted into the lumen of the proximal tubule by the organic anion transport pathway described earlier. They are carried downstream to the distal tubule, where they bind to the NCC protein and inhibit its action. Because the distal tubule is relatively water impermeable, NaCl reabsorption along the DCT contributes to urinary dilution. DCT diuretics therefore impair urinary diluting capacity, but they have no effect on urinary concentrating ability. Most DCT diuretics, with the possible exception of metolazone, become less effective when the GFR declines below 40 mL/min, although this is not true if the DCT diuretic is used together with a loop diuretic.

DCT diuretics increase Mg^{2+} excretion modestly but, in contrast to loop diuretics, inhibit urinary Ca^{2+} excretion. Two mechanisms have been invoked to explain the effects of DCT diuretics on Ca^{2+} excretion. First, DCT diuretics stimulate Ca^{2+} reabsorption along the proximal tubule because they contract ECFV and increase proximal Na^+ reabsorption (Ca^{2+} transport varies in parallel with Na^{2+} transport along the proximal tubule). Second, DCT diuretics stimulate Ca^{2+} reabsorption along the distal tubule through their action on the NCC. When the entry pathway is blocked, intracellular concentrations of Na^+ and Cl^- decline. Low intracellular $[Cl^-]$ make the cell interior more electrically negative with respect to the extracellular fluid, because Cl^- tends to diffuse into the cell from the interstitium. This opens voltage-activated calcium channels in the luminal membrane (probably the transient receptor potential cation channel, TRPV5). The cellular negativity, coupled with a decrease in cellular $[Na^+]$, also stimulates $3Na^+/Ca^{2+}$ exchange at the basolateral cell membrane, which is an electrogenic process. It is now clear that effects of DCT diuretics along *both* the proximal tubule (owing to ECFV depletion) and the distal tubule (owing to effects on transepithelial Ca^{2+} transport) contribute to the ability of DCT diuretics to reduce Ca^{2+} excretion. These effects form the basis for the use of DCT diuretics to reduce the recurrence of calcium nephrolithiasis.

Distal Potassium-Sparing Diuretics

Sodium reabsorption by the aldosterone-sensitive distal nephron (ASDN), amounts to only 3% to 5% of the filtered Na^+ load, but it is physiologically important because it is tightly regulated. The ASDN is now believed to comprise a short segment of the DCT, the connecting tubule, and the cortical collecting duct. As in the other tubule segments, the Na^+,K^+-ATPase keeps the $[Na^+]$ inside cells below the electrochemical equilibrium, generating a driving force for Na^+ entry across the apical membrane. Unlike more proximal segments, however, Na^+ transport along the ASDN is primarily electrogenic (current-generating), because Na^+ enters across the luminal membrane through epithelial sodium ion channels (ENaC) that carry an electrical charge. As Na^+ moves out of the lumen, it generates a voltage across the tubule wall that is oriented with the lumen negative, relative to blood. This lumen-negative voltage helps to drive K^+ movement in the secretory direction via separate K^+ channels (primarily ROMK). Although Na^+ and K^+ do not traverse the same channel, transport rates are electrically linked, and modulation of the transport of one of these cations indirectly affects the transport of the other.

Two major groups of natriuretics act predominantly along the ASDN. Sodium channel blockers, such as triamterene and amiloride, act from the lumen to inhibit Na^+ movement through ENaC. Because these drugs impair Na^+ movement, the transepithelial voltage declines, inhibiting K^+ secretion secondarily. This effect accounts for their K^+-sparing action. It should be emphasized that, although amiloride inhibits renal Na^+/H^+ exchange in the proximal tubule, the proximal effect probably does not contribute to its diuretic action in humans, because the concentrations of amiloride achieved in the lumen of the proximal tubule during oral administration are insufficient to interfere with Na^+/H^+ exchange.

The second class of natriuretics that act along the ASDN is the aldosterone antagonists, represented by spironolactone and eplerenone. Aldosterone, a mineralocorticoid hormone secreted by the adrenal gland in response to angiotensin II or serum K^+, stimulates Na^+ reabsorption and K^+ secretion along the late DCT (the DCT2), the connecting tubule, and the cortical collecting duct. This process increases the magnitude of the lumen-negative transepithelial voltage. Spironolactone and eplerenone are competitive antagonists of the mineralocorticoid receptor that cause mild natriuresis and K^+ retention. Spironolactone stimulates estrogen receptors, leading to troubling side effects, especially gynecomastia. Eplerenone binds more specifically to mineralocorticoid receptors than spironolactone does, and it has a lower incidence of estrogenic side effects.

Distal K^+-sparing diuretics are relatively modest in potency, at least when given acutely, partly because they inhibit distal Na^+ reabsorption incompletely. (In contrast, inherited diseases of aldosterone action or ENaC activity are associated with profound salt wasting.) They are sometimes used as sole agents in situations in which excessive aldosterone secretion plays a central pathogenic role or, more commonly, in combination with other diuretics to reduce K^+ excretion. Further, in patients with hypertension caused by adrenocortical hyperplasia, adequate blood pressure control can often be obtained with oral spironolactone or amiloride. Recently, indications for use of distal K^+-sparing diuretics have increased, stimulated largely by suggestions that extrarenal actions of aldosterone may contribute to the pathogenesis of heart failure and vascular disease. Aldosterone antagonists are now recommended for patients with moderate to severe systolic heart failure, because they can prolong life, but complications, including hyperkalemia and kidney failure, can occur.

Osmotic Diuretics

Unlike other classes of natriuretics, osmotic diuretics do not interfere directly with specific transport proteins or receptors; rather, they act as osmotic particles in tubule fluid. Water reabsorption throughout the nephron is driven by the osmotic gradients that are generated by solute transport. When an agent such as mannitol is administered, it is filtered but very poorly reabsorbed. Because the mannitol is retained in the tubule lumen, the osmolality of tubule fluid remains higher than normal, inhibiting fluid reabsorption. NaCl reabsorption is also inhibited, in this case because solute reabsorption dilutes tubule fluid, predisposing to NaCl backflux. Thus, these drugs tend to increase the excretion not only of water but also of Na^+, K^+, Cl^-, HCO_3^-, and other solutes. The urinary osmolality during osmotic diuresis tends to approach that of plasma, regardless of the state of hydration. Osmotic diuretics increase renal blood flow and wash out the medullary solute gradient, effects that contribute to the diuretic-induced impairment in urinary concentrating capacity.

Osmotic diuretics have been used in an attempt to prevent acute renal failure after cardiopulmonary bypass, rhabdomyolysis, or radiocontrast exposure. Mannitol is frequently employed to reduce cerebral edema, first by osmotic fluid removal from the brain and then by promoting diuresis. Although data in the settings of cardiopulmonary bypass and rhabdomyolysis are inconclusive, a controlled study of patients exposed to radiocontrast agents indicated that hydration with half-normal saline was as effective or more effective than mannitol in reducing the incidence of acute renal failure; therefore, mannitol should not be used to reduce the risk of contrast-mediated acute renal failure.

AQUARETICS

Vasopressin Receptor Antagonists

AVP (also called antidiuretic hormone, or ADH) regulates water excretion by the kidney in a process that is largely, although incompletely, separate from the regulation of NaCl excretion. Circulating AVP binds to two major receptor subtypes, V_1 and V_2. V_1 receptors are expressed in many cell types, including vascular smooth muscle (V_{1a}) and adenohypophysis (V_{1b}). V_2 receptors are expressed in vascular endothelium and in the kidney, where they are localized to principal cells of the connecting tubule and the cortical and medullary collecting duct. In the kidney, binding of AVP to V_2 receptors leads to insertion of aquaporin 2 water channels into the apical membrane of epithelial cells along the distal nephron and, consequently, increased water reabsorption. Many clinical disorders such as cirrhosis, congestive heart failure, and SIADH are associated with high levels of AVP that prevent appropriate water excretion, resulting in hyponatremia.

A nonpeptide combined $V_{1a}R/V_2R$ vasopressin receptor antagonist (conivaptan) is now available for clinical use in the United States in an intravenous preparation; it is indicated to treat euvolemic and hypervolemic hyponatremia. Additional information concerning conivaptan's safety profile, appropriate clinical use, and therapeutic role will certainly become available during the next several years, and it is likely that oral aquaretic drugs will be available shortly.

ADAPTATION TO DIURETIC DRUGS

When a loop diuretic drug is administered acutely, excretion of Na^+ and fluid increases transiently. This natriuresis is followed by a period of positive NaCl balance, termed post-diuretic NaCl retention (**Fig. 15-2**). The net effect of the diuretic on ECFV during a 24-hour period is equal to the sum of NaCl losses during diuretic action (excretion > intake) and NaCl retention during periods when the drug concentration is low (intake > excretion). Factors that influence the relation between natriuresis and post-diuretic NaCl retention include the dietary NaCl intake, the dose of diuretic, its half-life, and the frequency with which it is administered. When loop diuretics are administered once daily to patients ingesting a high-NaCl diet, post-diuretic NaCl retention often compensates entirely for NaCl losses during the period of drug action; no net Na^+ losses ensue, despite the effective natriuresis (see **Fig. 15-2**). When NaCl intake is restricted, Na^+ avidity during the post-diuretic period cannot overcome the initial NaCl losses, Na^+ is lost from the body, and ECFV declines. This relationship between dietary NaCl intake and the net effect of diuretics accounts for the central role of dietary NaCl restriction in effective diuretic therapy.

Even when diuretic treatment does induce negative NaCl and fluid balance initially, NaCl balance is restored after several days to weeks because other adaptive mechanisms come into play, limiting the magnitude of the diuretic response; this is known as the "braking phenomenon" (see **Fig. 15-2**). Several mechanisms contribute to adaptation during chronic diuretic treatment. Contraction of the ECFV, at least relative to pretreatment levels, may stimulate secretion of renin, aldosterone, and ADH, which mediate renal NaCl and fluid retention. Contraction of the ECFV may increase the activity of renal nerves, which stimulate renal NaCl retention via direct effects on renal tubules. Contraction of the ECFV may also reduce renal perfusion pressure and the GFR. In addition to adaptations that depend on changes in ECFV, specific intrarenal effects of diuretics may also contribute to adaptation. Loop diuretics inhibit solute reabsorption along

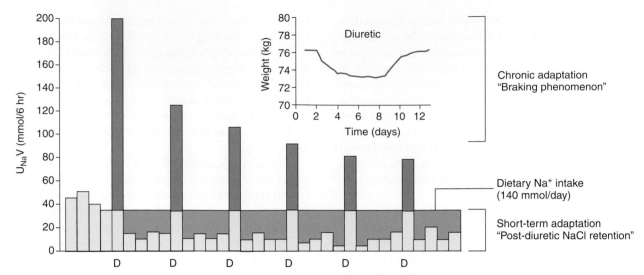

FIGURE 15-2 Effects of a loop diuretic on urinary sodium excretion. Each bar represents 6 hours. Purple bars indicate periods during which urinary Na+ excretion ($U_{Na}V$) exceeds dietary intake. Blue areas indicate periods of post-diuretic NaCl retention, during which dietary Na+ intake exceeds urinary Na+ excretion. Changes in the magnitude of the natriuretic response over several days (D) are indicative of diuretic "braking." Horizontal black line indicates dietary Na+ intake per 24-hour period. Inset shows effect of diuretics on weight (and extracellular fluid volume) during several days of diuretic administration. (Data redrawn from Wilcox CS, Mitch WE, Kelly RA, et al: Response of the kidney to furosemide: I. Effects of salt intake and renal compensation. J Lab Clin Med 102:450-458, 1983.)

the TAL, thereby increasing solute delivery to, and solute reabsorption from, the distal nephron. When solute delivery to the distal tubule is increased chronically (as during long-term diuretic therapy), distal tubule cells undergo substantial hypertrophy, with increases in the abundance and activity of transport proteins. These changes are associated with increases in NaCl transport capacity, which participates in returning the patient to NaCl balance. Such adaptations must occur; if not, ECFV would continue to decline beyond desired levels. However, if such adaptations occur before acceptable levels of ECFV (the desired response to diuretics) are achieved, they contribute importantly to diuretic resistance, as discussed later. Diuretic adaptations occur whenever the drugs are administered chronically, but it is only when the ECFV remains unacceptably expanded that the adaptations are viewed as dysfunctional.

It should be emphasized that the goal of diuretic treatment of edema is not simply to increase urinary NaCl or fluid excretion. Instead, the goal is to reduce ECFV to a clinically acceptable level and to maintain that volume chronically. To achieve this goal, urinary NaCl excretion must increase initially (see **Fig. 15-2**), but excretion rates of NaCl and fluid always return to pretreatment levels once steady state occurs. Therefore, during successful diuretic treatment of edema, when the patient's weight has stabilized, urinary NaCl excretion matches dietary intake; it is not increased above normal values.

COMPLICATIONS OF DIURETIC TREATMENT

The most common complications of diuretic treatment result directly from the effects of these drugs on renal fluid and electrolyte excretion. They include ECFV depletion, hyponatremia, hypokalemia, and, for distal K+-sparing diuretics,

hyperkalemia. Although both DCT and loop diuretics predispose to hypokalemia, the incidence and the implications of diuretic-induced hypokalemia depend on the indication for treatment, the class of drug, the dose, the dietary Na+ and K+ intake, and the duration of treatment. In the treatment of essential hypertension, mild hypokalemia occurs more frequently with DCT diuretics, such as hydrochlorothiazide and chlorthalidone, than with loop diuretics; this side effect is clearly dose related. Luckily, DCT diuretics are effective antihypertensive drugs at doses that cause only mild K+ wasting; for this reason, lower doses of DCT diuretics (12.5 to 25 mg of hydrochlorothiazide or chlorthalidone) are now recommended to treat hypertension than were commonly used in the past. In the Antihypertensive and Lipid-Lowering Treatment to Prevent Heart Attack Trial (ALLHAT), serum K+ concentrations lower than 3.5 mEq/L occurred in 12.7% of patients receiving chlorthalidone (12.5 or 25 mg/day) at 2 years and in 8.5% at 4 years. Debate continues about the need to treat mild hypokalemia during DCT diuretic therapy, but marked hypokalemia should alert the clinician that increased renin or aldosterone secretion may be present and that the presence of primary hyperaldosteronism or renovascular disease should be considered.

Loop diuretics are prescribed most commonly to treat heart failure. Cardiac dysfunction activates the renin-angiotensin-aldosterone axis, which predisposes to hypokalemia, especially when diuretic drugs are superimposed. Furthermore, many patients with systolic dysfunction or with atrial fibrillation receive digitalis glycosides, which predispose to hypokalemic arrhythmias. Several studies have indicated that the risk of ventricular arrhythmias increases as serum [K+] declines, so hypokalemia is often treated more aggressively in this patient population. In one study, serum [K+] of less than 3.5 mEq/L was observed in 25% of patients treated with K^+-losing diuretics, such as loop diuretics. Changes in clinical practice during the past 15 years, including the increasing use of ACE inhibitors, aldosterone antagonists, and β-adrenergic blocking drugs, has increased the risk of hyperkalemia in patients with heart failure (see later discussion).

Several mechanisms contribute to the tendency of loop and DCT diuretics to cause hypokalemia. First, both classes of diuretics increase fluid flow through the distal nephron, the site at which K^+ secretion determines urinary K^+ excretion rates. High fluid flow rates stimulate K^+ secretion directly by reducing luminal K^+ concentrations; yet, a second class of secretory K^+ channels has recently been identified in the distal nephron. These maxi K^+ channels appear to respond directly to increases in tubule flow rate. Second, both loop and DCT diuretics stimulate aldosterone secretion, which further increases K^+ secretion along the distal nephron; in several studies, the net effect of diuretics on K^+ balance correlated best with elevations in serum aldosterone concentration. Finally, both DCT and loop diuretics predispose to hypomagnesemia, which contributes to the development of hypokalemia, perhaps by opening secretory K^+ channels in the distal nephron. Hypokalemia has several adverse consequences. These include ventricular arrhythmias, especially during the administration of digitalis glycosides or when hypomagnesemia is present. Hypokalemia may also contribute to glucose intolerance, a known complication of DCT diuretic use.

Methods to prevent or treat hypokalemia during diuretic therapy include (1) using the lowest effective diuretic dose (especially for hypertension), (2) supplementing dietary K^+ and, if that is insufficient, prescribing KCl orally, (3) preventing hypomagnesemia, and (4) using distal K^+-sparing diuretics together with loop or DCT diuretics. Serum $[Na^+]$ and $[K^+]$ should be monitored in every patient who is treated with diuretics, and patients should be encouraged to consume a diet that is rich in K^+ and low in Na^+. Many physicians prescribe potassium supplements to patients whose serum $[K^+]$ falls to less than 3.5 mmol/L, although others have suggested that $[K^+]$ levels between 3.0 and 3.5 mmol/L do not require treatment. Certainly, in patients who are at risk for complications of hypokalemia, such as patients receiving digitalis glycosides and those with hepatic cirrhosis, serum $[K^+]$ should be maintained at greater than 3.5 mmol/L. Of note, adding a distal K^+-sparing diuretic not only corrects hypokalemia in many patients but may also prevent hypomagnesemia, which is suggested to act synergistically with hypokalemia to predispose to ventricular arrhythmias.

DCT diuretics and, less commonly, loop diuretics also predispose to glucose intolerance, hyperlipidemia, and hyperuricemia, when administered chronically. Although the mechanisms by which these complications develop are not completely clear, hypokalemia and ECFV contraction may contribute. Serum concentrations of glucose, lipids, and uric acid should be monitored in patients receiving chronic diuretic treatment, and hypokalemia should be treated as described earlier.

Hyperkalemia is a complication of distal K^+-sparing diuretics. Hyperkalemia occurs most commonly in patients with CKD and in those taking ACE inhibitors, angiotensin receptor blockers, or β-blockers concomitantly. The use of spironolactone to treat heart failure may be contributing to a rise in potentially life-threatening hyperkalemia, when it (or, presumably, eplerenone) is used to treat patients with heart failure who have a concomitant decrease in kidney function. It must be noted that all clinical trials of spironolactone to treat heart failure have excluded patients with significant degrees of renal dysfunction and that bioactive metabolites of spironolactone have long half-lives, making the development of associated hyperkalemia more difficult to treat. Triamterene metabolism is impaired in patients with cirrhosis, and this drug precipitates hyperkalemia in this group of patients.

Mild metabolic alkalosis occurs frequently during treatment with loop and DCT diuretics. These drugs promote urinary losses of NaCl (leaving HCO_3^- behind). Further, they increase aldosterone secretion, which stimulates H^+ secretion directly. Metabolic alkalosis can exacerbate hepatic encephalopathy and can inhibit respiratory drive. Severe metabolic alkalosis is often a manifestation of aggressive therapy. Loop diuretics or combination diuretic therapy (see later discussion) may also lead to excessive ECFV depletion and vascular collapse.

Hyponatremia may develop during treatment with loop diuretics, but this complication is much more common with DCT diuretics (thiazides and their congeners). Some patients treated with DCT diuretics develop severe and potentially life-threatening hyponatremia, often several days to weeks after initiation of diuretic therapy. This complication is much more common in women and the elderly and can be life-threatening. The mechanisms underlying this response are incompletely understood, but they include the inhibition by DCT diuretics of urinary diluting capacity, the development of potassium deficiency, and central stimulation of thirst.

Toxic side effects of diuretics are drug or group specific. Allergic interstitial nephritis is an idiosyncratic reaction to diuretics that may precipitate skin rash and acute renal failure. Ototoxicity is a toxic effect of loop diuretics that occurs most commonly when high doses are administered rapidly (e.g., furosemide IV >15 mg/min) to patients with renal insufficiency. Triamterene can cause renal stones and may precipitate acute renal failure when administered with nonsteroidal anti-inflammatory drugs (NSAIDs). Spironolactone causes gynecomastia, especially in patients with cirrhosis of the liver.

DIURETIC TREATMENT OF EDEMA

Edema is a manifestation of disordered NaCl homeostasis. The NaCl retention often reflects a physiologic response to inadequate effective arterial blood volume, as occurs in heart failure or cirrhosis. In other situations, NaCl retention may reflect an abnormal renal response, resulting from damage to the kidney, as occurs with reduced kidney function or nephrotic syndrome. In either case, therapeutic maneuvers should be aimed first at correcting the primary disorder. Often, however, such maneuvers are not available or do not contract the ECFV adequately, and more direct methods of effecting NaCl removal are needed.

Before initiating treatment with diuretic drugs, it is important to institute a low-NaCl diet. ECFV varies directly with NaCl intake, in both normal and edematous individuals. For patients with mild ECFV expansion, a "no added salt" diet may be appropriate (4 g Na$^+$/day); for more severe edema, a low-Na$^+$ diet (2 g Na$^+$/day) should be prescribed. Even if dietary restriction alone is unsuccessful and diuretic drugs are administered, the dietary Na$^+$ intake must be restricted to less than 4 g/day for diuretics to be effective. A second important consideration before initiating diuretic therapy is to improve the general management by discontinuing, if possible, drugs that predispose to NaCl retention or interfere with diuretic efficacy. NSAIDs promote renal NaCl retention directly and interfere with the efficacy of loop and DCT diuretics. Many vasodilators promote edema; minoxidil frequently causes significant ECFV expansion; and nifedipine promotes edema despite intrinsic natriuretic properties, through local vasodilation. The thiazolidinediones, drugs frequently used to treat diabetes, commonly expand the ECFV and can induce symptomatic heart failure.

Once the decision to initiate diuretic therapy has been made, the initial choice of drug and dosage depends on the underlying cause of edema and its severity. Hypertension often responds to very low doses of a DCT diuretic (12.5 mg/day of chlorthalidone, for example), doses that tend to cause few side effects. Cirrhotic edema and ascites may respond to spironolactone alone (50 to 300 mg daily), but the most effective choice is to combine furosemide and spironolactone, beginning with a dose of 40 mg furosemide and 100 mg spironolactone. This ratio should be maintained as the dosage is increased to treat more resistant edema, because it is effective and maintains normokalemia. Moderate edema associated with heart failure may respond to a DCT diuretic such as chlorthalidone, in doses of 25 to 50 mg/day, but when edema from heart failure, cirrhosis, or nephrotic syndrome is more than mild, when kidney function is impaired, or in the presence of pulmonary congestion or severe symptoms, loop diuretics are the drugs of choice. As mentioned earlier, the addition of a small dose of spironolactone (25 to 50 mg/day) or eplerenone to traditional therapies for heart failure can reduce mortality in patients with left ventricular dysfunction; because this use of mineralocorticoid antagonists is indicated primarily to prolong life, rather than to reduce symptoms of ECFV overload, it will not be discussed at length in this chapter.

Loop diuretics have the highest natriuretic potency, are active at all levels of renal function, and act rapidly, even after oral administration. The drugs have steep dose-response relationships: As the dose is increased, there is little response until a critical threshold is reached, above which diuretic effectiveness increases rapidly to a maximum (**Fig. 15-3**). If a loop diuretic is administered in a dose that exceeds the threshold, most patients

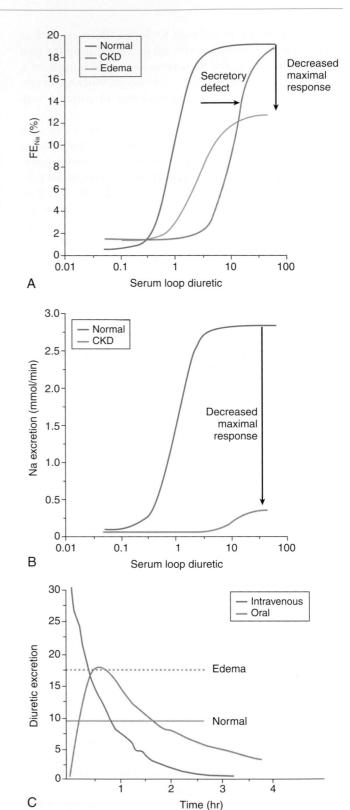

FIGURE 15-3 A, Comparison of effects of chronic kidney disease (CKD) and edematous conditions (edema) on the loop diuretic dose response, expressed as the fractional Na$^+$ excretion (FE$_{Na}$). Diuretic delivery via secretion into the lumen is impaired by CKD (pharmacokinetic effect), whereas the response to delivered drug is diminished with edema (pharmacodynamic effect). **B,** Effect of CKD on the absolute response to a loop diuretic. Compare with panel **A. C,** Pharmacokinetics of intravenous and oral loop diuretics. The diuretic thresholds for normal and edematous individuals are shown as horizontal lines. Note that, whereas a normal individual responds to either intravenous or oral diuretic, some edematous individuals achieve therapeutic levels only after intravenous treatment.

experience an increase in urine output that is noticeable during the several hours after diuretic ingestion. To be effective, each dose of loop diuretic must exceed this threshold. When initiating oral diuretic therapy, a target is set for weight loss, and a low dose of loop diuretic (20 mg furosemide or its equivalent) is begun once or twice daily. If urine output rises during the 4 to 6 hours after diuretic ingestion (the patient can usually report a noticeable increase in urine volume), the same dose is continued on a daily basis (unless weight loss exceeds the target value). If urine output does not rise, the patient may double the dose on the following day (to 40 mg once or twice daily). If there is no response, the dose can be doubled each day until a response is obtained or until the maximum safe dose is achieved (usually about 120 mg furosemide per dose, unless the patient has decreased kidney function). In normal individuals, 40 mg of furosemide orally produces maximal diuresis, but in patients with edema or reduced kidney function, larger doses are frequently necessary (see **Fig. 15-3**).

If kidney function is reduced, the loop diuretic dose-response curve shifts to the right. If the fractional Na^+ excretion is plotted, the maximal effectiveness of loop diuretics appears unchanged. However, the maximal effectiveness is markedly reduced in CKD if effectiveness is expressed as absolute Na^+ excretion, the more physiologically relevant parameter (see **Fig. 15-3**). Even in renal failure, however, there is little to be gained by increasing beyond 240 mg furosemide or 8 mg bumetanide per dose, because these doses reach the plateau of the dose-response curve. Some clinicians have reported that much higher doses of loop diuretics can be effective. **Figure 15-3C** shows that very high doses of loop diuretics can enhance natriuresis, because serum diuretic levels are maintained above the threshold for a longer period. This prolonged duration, however, comes at the price of potential toxicity (mostly ototoxicity). Most clinicians believe that more frequent but moderate doses are just as effective and better tolerated. Adding an afternoon dose of a loop diuretic is often useful or even necessary for therapeutic success; but each dose must exceed the diuretic threshold to be effective.

Often, the dose that elicits an increase in urine output can be continued indefinitely, because adaptive mechanisms, such as those discussed earlier, bring the patient back into NaCl balance once ECFV has been reduced. Sometimes, however, patients may be maintained with lower doses than were necessary to elicit diuresis initially, once control of the ECFV is achieved.

DIURETIC RESISTANCE: CAUSES AND TREATMENT

Control of ECFV expansion can be attained in most edematous patients using the approach outlined here. In some circumstances, however, moderate or high doses of loop diuretics do not reduce ECFV to the desired level, even when used appropriately. Such patients are often deemed resistant

to diuretic therapy. The level of ECFV that is acceptable to the patient and to the physician depends on many factors, including the severity of the underlying disease, patient preference, and comorbid illness. If ECFV is expanded beyond acceptable limits, a systematic approach to diuretic resistance usually leads to a treatment regimen that is safe and effective (**Fig. 15-4**).

One of the most common causes of apparent resistance to diuretic drugs is dietary indiscretion; as discussed previously, dietary NaCl excess abrogates the effect of most diuretic regimens. The influence of dietary NaCl intake is most pronounced for the loop diuretics, because their half-lives are relatively short. If the patient's weight is stable but edema remains troubling, dietary compliance can be assessed by measuring the amount of Na^+ excreted during 24 hours. One should always measure creatinine excretion at the same time, to validate the completeness of the collection. A urinary Na^+ excretion rate greater than 100 to 120 mmol/day (equivalent to 2.3 to 2.8 g Na^+ per day) indicates both that the patient is ingesting too much NaCl and that true diuretic resistance is not present. Daily Na^+ excretion rates greater than 120 mmol will lead to ECFV loss if the patient ingests less than 2 g of Na^+ daily. Of course, dietary compliance cannot always be assured, and more intensive regimens (discussed later) may provide effective diuresis for patients who continue to ingest too much NaCl.

Gastrointestinal absorption of many diuretics is variable. The gastrointestinal absorption of furosemide (both Lasix and the unbranded generic) varies by as much as 60% from day to day in a single individual and averages only 50% to 60%. Gastrointestinal absorption may be slowed further by edema of the gut, such as occurs in some patients with heart failure. In contrast, the bioavailability of torsemide and bumetanide exceeds 80%, and some studies suggest that this may provide more reliable diuresis. If diuresis is urgent, loop diuretics are frequently administered intravenously to ensure bioavailability and consistent effect; once clinical improvement occurs, diuretic absorption through the gastrointestinal tract may improve, and oral therapy may once again become effective.

Impaired renal diuretic clearance may also contribute to resistance. Once a loop or DCT diuretic drug has been absorbed into the bloodstream, it reaches the kidney tubular lumen via the organic anion secretory pathway located in the proximal tubule. This pathway also interacts with NSAIDs, probenecid, and endogenous anions that accumulate when kidney function is reduced. With administration of NSAIDs, or with reduced kidney function, diuretic secretion into the lumen of the proximal tubule is inhibited, and less diuretic reaches its active site for any given serum concentration. To overcome the inhibition, higher serum levels (higher doses) are needed. This is one reason that high doses of diuretic drugs are required to elicit diuresis in patients with reduced kidney function. Of note, although the ratio of equipotent doses of furosemide to bumetanide is 40:1 in patients with normal renal function, it is only 20:1 in patients with renal functional impairment, because the renal clearance of

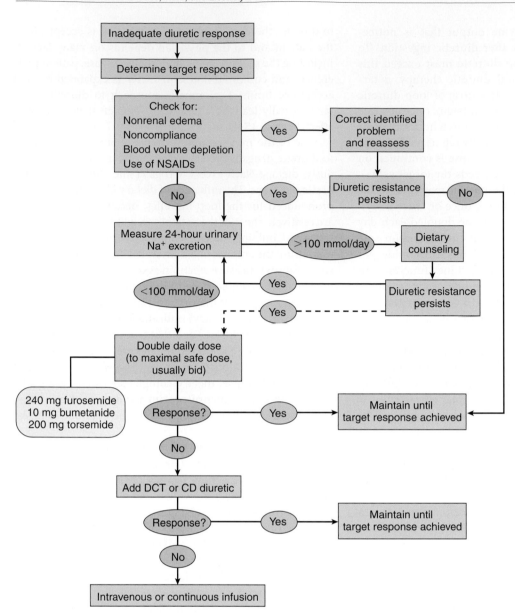

FIGURE 15-4 Algorithm for diuretic resistance. Regimens for combination therapy are given in the text. Maximal recommended single doses are provided in the yellow box. Note that higher doses have been used to treat patients with acute renal failure. Higher doses may provide additional natriuresis because of prolonged actions, but at the expense of increased side effects. CD, collecting duct; DCT, distal convoluted tubule; NSAIDS, nonsteroidal anti-inflammatory drugs. (Modified with permission from Wilcox CS: Diuretics. In Brenner B [ed.]: Brenner and Rector's The Kidney, 5th ed. Philadelphia, WB Saunders, 1996.)

furosemide is reduced (leading to relatively higher serum levels and relatively higher potency), whereas the clearance of bumetanide is maintained. In general, when switching from intravenous to oral furosemide, the starting oral dose should be twice the intravenous dose (because of the limited bioavailability). When switching from intravenous to oral torsemide or bumetanide, the conversion is 1 to 1, because bioavailability is higher. In each case, however, it is necessary to confirm that an effective oral dose has been selected by making sure that a detectable diuresis follows each drug dose.

Diuretic resistance is common in patients with the nephrotic syndrome. Several causes have been postulated, including increased diuretic volume of distribution (resulting from hypoalbuminemia) and drug binding to filtered protein in tubule fluid. Hypoalbuminemia itself may also predispose to renal vasoconstriction and may inhibit diuretic secretion into kidney tubules directly. Yet,

it appears that increased volume of distribution in the setting of mild to moderate hypoalbuminemia is not the key mediator of resistance for most patients. In these situations, increasing the diuretic dose or changing from oral to intravenous therapy often suffices. The use of albumin with loop diuretics has been extremely controversial. Several controlled studies showed modest improvements in natriuresis when albumin was infused with furosemide, compared with furosemide alone, in patients with nephrotic syndrome, but the effects appeared to be relatively modest. A systematic review noted that results in the literature have been conflicting but suggested that the totality of the evidence supports the use of albumin with furosemide in selected patients who are severely hypoalbuminemic and for whom aggressive traditional approaches have failed. In this setting, albumin may be cost-effective when mixed together with furosemide (in a ratio of 5 mg furosemide per 1 g of albumin).

Experiments in animal models suggested that diuretics bind to filtered albumin within kidney tubules of nephrotic patients. In several experimental model systems, this was shown to inhibit diuretic action. A more recent clinical study, however, indicated that urinary protein binding does not contribute significantly to the diuretic resistance of nephrotic patients, and several recent studies indicate that changes in diuretic delivery to kidney tubules are also not primary contributors to diuretic resistance. Therefore, the main cause of diuretic resistance in nephrotic syndrome is the strong primary stimulus to NaCl retention. High doses of loop diuretics, often used in combination with DCT diuretics, may be necessary to achieve diuresis in this patient population.

Hemodynamic factors frequently contribute to diuretic resistance. For patients with low cardiac output, dopamine (2 to 4 µg/kg/min) may increase renal plasma flow and increase urine flow (dopamine may also increase urine flow in patients with acute renal failure), but the effects of "renal dose" dopamine are controversial and poorly documented (see Chapter 37). The effects of drugs used to reduce cardiac afterload on renal NaCl excretion are complex. When treatment with ACE inhibitors or nitroprusside increases cardiac output effectively, it may stimulate natriuresis and reduce edema. On the other hand, when aggressive therapy with these agents reduces blood pressure beyond a critical threshold (which may be surprisingly high in patients with severe vascular disease), it may lead to NaCl retention and even acute renal failure. Permitting the mean arterial pressure to rise by a few millimeters of mercury can often be effective in this setting, at least acutely. Relative hypotension is problematic during concomitant administration of NSAIDs, when bilateral renal artery stenosis is present, and during very aggressive diuretic therapy. Renal vasoconstrictors, such as NSAIDs and adrenergic agonists, have many effects, including reduction of GFR, that lead to diuretic resistance. They should always be avoided in the diuretic-resistant patient.

One approach to diuretic resistance in patients with systolic dysfunction who are hospitalized is to use intravenous nesiritide (B-type natriuretic peptide). In addition to increasing urinary excretion of Na^+, Cl^-, and water, this agent reduces pulmonary capillary wedge pressure and systemic vascular resistance and increases cardiac output. Unlike the loop diuretics, nesiritide suppresses the renin-angiotensin-aldosterone axis. Nevertheless, enthusiasm for use of nesiritide has waned because of concerns about renal toxicity and other morbidity.

Not uncommonly, simple approaches to diuretic resistance fail. Several strategies can be used to control of ECFV in such patients (see **Fig. 15-4**). First, it is often necessary to increase the frequency of loop diuretic administration, especially if post-diuretic NaCl retention is contributing importantly to NaCl retention. Recall, however, that each dose must be greater than the diuretic threshold to be effective (see **Fig. 15-3**). Patients are often able to notice a distinct increase in urine output within several hours after each dose of diuretic if the dose is in the appropriate range. Second,

another class of diuretic may be added to a regimen that includes a loop diuretic. This strategy produces true synergism: The combination of agents is more effective than the sum of the responses to each agent alone. DCT diuretics are the class of drug most commonly combined with loop diuretics, although diuretic synergism also occurs when loop diuretics are combined with carbonic anhydrase inhibitors. The addition of acetazolamide to a loop diuretic is especially useful for patients in whom metabolic alkalosis is exacerbating hypoventilation, in the setting of volume overload. DCT diuretics may act synergistically with loop diuretics for several reasons. Loop diuretics increase NaCl delivery to the distal tubule, a site at which NaCl transport depends on the luminal NaCl concentration. Loop diuretics, therefore, stimulate NaCl reabsorption along the nephron segment that is sensitive to DCT diuretics. Adding a DCT diuretic inhibits NaCl transport along the stimulated segment, thereby eliciting a larger effect than would a DCT diuretic given alone. Further, when loop diuretics are administered chronically, cells in the distal tubule become hypertrophic, increasing their ability to reabsorb NaCl. DCT diuretics inhibit the increased NaCl reabsorption that accompanies hypertrophy of the distal nephron and therefore counteract the effects of hypertrophy. Finally, DCT diuretics have longer half-lives than loop diuretics. For this reason, they can prevent or attenuate NaCl retention during the periods when loop diuretic action wanes, thereby increasing their net effect. Therefore, at least three mechanisms contribute to the ability of DCT diuretics to act synergistically with loop-acting drugs.

When two diuretics are combined, the DCT diuretic is often administered before the loop diuretic (1 hour is reasonable), to ensure that NaCl transport in the distal nephron is blocked by the time the tubule is flooded with solute. If an intravenous DCT diuretic is required, chlorothiazide (500 to 1000 mg) may be employed. Metolazone is the DCT diuretic most frequently combined with loop diuretics, because its half-life is relatively long (as formulated in Zaroxolyn) and because it has been reported to be effective even when renal failure is present. However, other thiazide and thiazide-like diuretics are probably equally effective, even when renal failure is present. The dramatic effectiveness of combination diuretic therapy is accompanied by complications in a significant number of patients. Massive fluid and electrolyte losses have led to circulatory collapse during combination therapy, and patients must be monitored carefully. The lowest effective dose of DCT diuretic should be added to the loop diuretic regimen. Patients can frequently be treated with combination therapy for only a few days and then placed back on a single-drug regimen. If continuous combination therapy is needed, low doses of DCT diuretic (2.5 mg metolazone or 25 mg hydrochlorothiazide), administered only 2 or 3 times per week, may be sufficient.

For hospitalized patients who are resistant to diuretic therapy, a different approach is to infuse loop diuretics continuously (**Table 15-2**; see **Fig. 15-4**). Continuous diuretic infusions have several advantages over bolus diuretic administration. First, because they avoid peaks and

TABLE 15-2 Continuous Diuretic Infusion

DIURETIC	LOADING DOSE (mg)	Continuous Dose (mg/hr)		
		GFR <25 mL/min	GFR 25-75 mL/min	GFR >75 mL/min
Furosemide	40	20-40	10-20	10
Torsemide	20	10-20	5-10	5
Bumetanide	1	1-2	0.5-1	0.5

GFR: glomerular filtration rate.
Data from Brater DC: Diuretic therapy. N Engl J Med 339:387-395, 1998.

troughs of diuretic concentration, continuous infusions prevent periods of positive NaCl balance (post-diuretic NaCl retention) from occurring. Second, continuous infusions are more efficient than bolus therapy (the amount of NaCl excreted per milligram of drug administered is greater). Third, some patients who are resistant to large doses of diuretics given by bolus respond to continuous infusion. Fourth, diuretic response can be titrated. In the intensive care unit, where obligate fluid administration must be balanced by fluid excretion, excellent control of NaCl and water excretion can be obtained. Finally, complications associated with high doses of loop diuretics, such as ototoxicity, appear to be less common when large doses are administered as continuous infusions. Total daily furosemide doses exceeding 1 g have been tolerated well when administered over 24 hours, but a more cautious dosing regimen is provided in **Table 15-2**. A Cochrane database review concluded that, whereas studies in general suggested efficacy and safety with this approach, definitive conclusions regarding the merits of bolus versus

continuous loop diuretic use could not be reached at the time of the review.

In some patients with ECFV expansion and resistant edema, ultrafiltration may be employed. Recent studies suggest that such approaches are effective and safe in selected individuals with heart failure. Whether they prove more effective than aggressive treatment with diuretics and inotropes remains unclear, but, like large-volume paracentesis, they may provide more rapid symptomatic improvement in selected patients.

Most patients who are deemed resistant to diuretics respond to the approaches described here. Side effects of diuretic therapy, such as increases in serum creatinine concentration, often limit the ability to reduce ECFV, rather than a lack of efficacy. Obtaining effective control of ECFV without provoking complications requires a thorough understanding of diuretic physiology and a commitment to use diuretics rationally and carefully. When used in this manner, they remain among the most powerful drugs in clinical medicine.

BIBLIOGRAPHY

Brater DC, Diuretic therapy. N Engl J Med 339:387-395, 1998.

Costanzo MR, Guglin ME, Saltzberg MT, et al; Investigators UT: Ultrafiltration versus intravenous diuretics for patients hospitalized for acute decompensated heart failure [see comment]. J Am Coll Cardiol 49:675-683, 2007.

Ellison DH: Diuretic therapy and resistance in congestive heart failure. Cardiology 96:132-143, 2001.

Ellison DH, Wilcox CS: Diuretics. In Brenner BM (ed): Brenner and Rector's The Kidney, 8th ed., vol 2. Philadelphia, WB Saunders, 2008, pp 1646-1678.

Eraly SA, Vallon V, Vaughn DA, et al: Decreased renal organic anion secretion and plasma accumulation of endogenous organic anions in OAT1 knock-out mice. J Biol Chem 281:5072-5083, 2006.

Faris R, Flather MD, Purcell H, et al: Diuretics for heart failure. Cochrane Database Syst Rev (1):CD003838, 2006.

Greenberg A: Diuretic complications. Am J Med Sci 319:10-24, 2000.

Howard PA, Dunn MI: Severe heart failure in the elderly: Potential benefits of high-dose and continuous infusion diuretics. Drugs Aging 19:249-256, 2002.

Karalliedde J, Buckingham RE: Thiazolidinediones and their fluid-related adverse effects: Facts, fiction and putative management strategies. Drug Saf 30:741-753, 2007.

Rosner MH, Gupta R, Ellison DH, Okusa MD: Management of cirrhotic ascites: Physiologic basis of diuretic action. Eur J Intern Med 17:8-19, 2006.

Sackner-Bernstein JD, Kowalski M, Fox M, Aaronson K: Short-term risk of death after treatment with nesiritide for decompensated heart failure: A pooled analysis of randomized controlled trials. JAMA 293:1900-1905, 2005.

Salvador DR, Rey NR, Ramos GC, Punzalan FE: Continuous infusion versus bolus injection of loop diuretics in congestive heart failure. Cochrane Database Syst Rev(3): CD003178, 2005.

Wilcox CS: New insights into diuretic use in patients with chronic renal disease. J Am Soc Nephrol 13:798-805, 2002.

Glomerular Diseases

CHAPTER 16

Glomerular Clinicopathologic Syndromes

J. Charles Jennette and Ronald J. Falk

Injury to glomeruli results in a multiplicity of signs and symptoms of disease, including proteinuria caused by altered permeability of capillary walls, hematuria caused by rupture of capillary walls, azotemia caused by impaired filtration of nitrogenous wastes, oliguria or anuria caused by reduced urine production, edema caused by salt and water retention, and hypertension caused by fluid retention and disturbed renal homeostasis of blood pressure. The nature and severity of disease in a given patient is dictated by the nature and severity of glomerular injury.

Specific glomerular diseases tend to produce characteristic syndromes of kidney dysfunction, but different glomerular diseases can produce the same syndrome (**Tables 16-1** and **16-2**). The diagnosis of a glomerular disease requires recognition of one of these syndromes followed by collection of data to determine which specific glomerular disease is present. Alternatively, if reaching a specific diagnosis is not possible or not necessary, the physician should at least narrow the differential diagnosis to a likely candidate disease.

Evaluation of pathologic features identified in a kidney biopsy specimen is often required for a definitive diagnosis. The pathologic features of various glomerular diseases are described in the corresponding chapters of this *Primer*. **Figure 16-1** depicts some of the clinical and pathologic features used to resolve the differential diagnosis in patients with antibody-mediated glomerulonephritis, **Figures 16-2** through **16-5** illustrate the distinctive ultrastructural features of some of the major categories of glomerular disease, and **Figure 16-6** illustrates some of the major patterns of immune deposition identified by immunofluorescence microscopy.

ASYMPTOMATIC HEMATURIA AND RECURRENT GROSS HEMATURIA

Hematuria is usually defined as greater than 3 red blood cells per high-power field observed by microscopic examination of a centrifuged urine sediment (see Chapters 3 and 4). Hematuria is asymptomatic when the patient is unaware of its presence and it is not accompanied by clinical manifestations of nephritis or nephrotic syndrome (i.e., without azotemia, oliguria, edema, or hypertension). Asymptomatic microscopic hematuria occurs in 5% to 10% of the general population. Recurrent gross hematuria may be superimposed on asymptomatic microscopic hematuria, or it may occur in isolation. The patient observes urine discoloration, which often is described as tea-colored or cola-colored.

Most hematuria is not of glomerular origin. Glomerular diseases cause less than 10% of hematuria in patients who do not have proteinuria; almost 80% is caused by bladder, prostate, or urethral disease. Hypercalciuria and hyperuricosuria also can cause asymptomatic hematuria, especially in children.

Microscopic examination of the urine can help determine whether hematuria is of glomerular or nonglomerular origin. Chemical (e.g., osmotic) and physical damage to red blood cells as they pass through the nephron causes structural changes that are not present in red blood cells that have passed directly into the urine from a gross parenchymal injury in the kidney (e.g., a neoplasm or infection) or from a lesion in the urinary tract (e.g., renal pelvis traumatized by stones or an inflamed bladder). Dysmorphic red blood cells that have transited the urinary tract from the glomeruli usually have lost their biconcave configuration and hemoglobin, and they often have multiple membrane blebs, sometimes producing acanthocytes and "Mickey Mouse" cells. The presence of red blood cell casts and substantial proteinuria (>2 g/24 hr) also supports a glomerular origin for hematuria.

Published kidney biopsy series conducted in patients with asymptomatic hematuria show differences in the frequencies of identified underlying glomerular lesions. Differences in the nature of the population analyzed (e.g., military recruits versus patients undergoing routine physical examination) and differences in pathologic analysis (e.g., failure of earlier studies to recognize thin basement membrane nephropathy) account for the observed disparities. The data presented in **Table 16-3** are derived from patients with hematuria who underwent diagnostic kidney biopsy. The data in the first column equate with asymptomatic hematuria and are similar to findings in other recent series. In these patients with hematuria, less than 1 g/24 hr proteinuria, and serum creatinine less than 1.5 mg/dL, the three major findings were no pathologic abnormality (30%), thin basement membrane nephropathy (26%), and immunoglobulin A (IgA) nephropathy (28%). Whereas thin basement membrane nephropathy virtually always manifests as asymptomatic hematuria or recurrent gross hematuria, IgA nephropathy can manifest as any of the syndromes listed in **Table 16-1**.

Alport's syndrome is a hereditary disease caused by a defect in the genes that code for basement membrane type IV collagen (see Chapter 44). Approximately 85% of patients have a mutation in the X-chromosomal $\alpha 5$ gene and 15% in the autosomal $\alpha 3$ and $\alpha 4$ genes. In affected men, Alport's

TABLE 16-1 Clinical Manifestations of Glomerular Diseases and Representative Diseases that Cause Them*

Asymptomatic Proteinuria

Focal segmental glomerulosclerosis

Mesangioproliferative GN

Nephrotic Syndrome

Minimal change glomerulopathy

Membranous glomerulopathy

Idiopathic (primary)

Secondary (e.g., lupus)

Focal segmental glomerulosclerosis

Mesangioproliferative GN

Type I membranoproliferative GN

Type II membranoproliferative GN

Fibrillary GN

Diabetic glomerulosclerosis

Amyloidosis

Light chain deposition disease

Asymptomatic Microscopic Hematuria

Thin basement membrane nephropathy

IgA nephropathy

Mesangioproliferative GN

Alport's syndrome

Recurrent Gross Hematuria

Thin basement membrane nephropathy

IgA nephropathy

Alport's syndrome

Acute Nephritis

Acute postinfectious GN

Poststreptococcal GN

Poststaphylococcal GN

Focal or Diffuse Proliferative GN

IgA nephropathy

Lupus nephritis

Type I Membranoproliferative GN

Type II Membranoproliferative GN

Fibrillary GN

Rapidly Progressive Nephritis

Crescentic GN

Anti-GBM GN

Immune complex GN

ANCA GN

Pulmonary-Renal Vasculitic Syndrome

Goodpasture's (anti-GBM) syndrome

Immune complex vasculitis

Lupus

ANCA Vasculitis

Microscopic polyangiitis

Wegener's granulomatosis

Churg-Strauss syndrome

Chronic Kidney Disease

Chronic sclerosing GN

ANCA, antineutrophil cytoplasmic antibody; GBM, glomerular basement membrane; GN, glomerulonephritis; IgA, immunoglobulin A.

*The same manifestations can be caused by different diseases, and the same disease can manifest in different ways.

TABLE 16-2 Tendencies of Glomerular Diseases to Manifest Nephrotic and Nephritic Features*

DISEASE	NEPHROTIC FEATURES	NEPHRITIC FEATURES
Minimal change glomerulopathy	++++	—
Membranous glomerulopathy	++++	+
Diabetic glomerulosclerosis	++++	+
Amyloidosis	++++	+
Focal segmental glomerulosclerosis	+++	++
Fibrillary glomerulonephritis	+++	++
Mesangioproliferative glomerulopathy†	++	++
Membranoproliferative glomerulonephritis‡	++	+++
Proliferative glomerulonephritis†	++	+++
Acute postinfectious glomerulonephritis§	+	++++
Crescentic glomerulonephritis#	+	++++

*Most diseases can manifest both nephrotic and nephritic features, but there usually is a tendency for one to predominate. Number of plus signs indicates strength of tendency.

†Mesangioproliferative and proliferative glomerulonephritis (focal or diffuse) are structural manifestations of a number of glomerulonephritides, including immunoglobulin A nephropathy and lupus nephritis.

‡Both type I (mesangiocapillary) and type II (dense deposit disease).

§Often a structural manifestation of acute poststreptococcal glomerulonephritis.

#Can be immune complex mediated, anti–glomerular basement membrane antibody mediated, or associated with antineutrophil cytoplasmic antibodies.

Modified from Jennette JC, Mandal AK: The nephrotic syndrome. In Mandal AK, Jennette JC (eds): Diagnosis and Management of Renal Disease and Hypertension. Durham, NC, Carolina Academic Press, 1994.

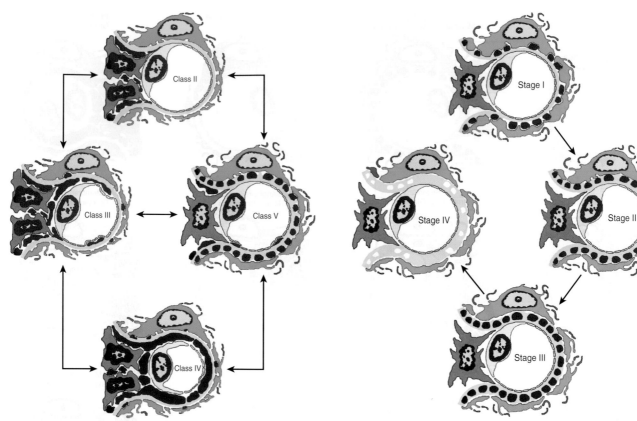

FIGURE 16-4 Ultrastructural features of the major classes of lupus nephritis. The sequestration of immune deposits within the mesangium in class II (mesangioproliferative) lupus glomerulonephritis causes only mesangial hyperplasia and mild renal dysfunction. Substantial amounts of subendothelial immune deposits, which are adjacent to the inflammatory mediator systems of the blood, cause focal (class III) or diffuse (class IV) proliferative lupus glomerulonephritis with overt nephritic signs and symptoms. Localization of immune deposits predominantly in the subepithelial zone causes membranous (class V) lupus glomerulonephritis, which usually manifests predominantly as the nephrotic syndrome. (Courtesy of J. Charles Jennette, MD)

FIGURE 16-5 Ultrastructural stages in the progression of membranous glomerulopathy. Stage I has subepithelial electron-dense immune complex deposits without adjacent projections of basement membrane material. Stage II has adjacent glomerular basement membrane (GBM) projections that eventually surround the electron-dense immune deposits in stage III. Stage IV has a markedly thickened GBM with electron-lucent zones replacing the electron-dense deposits. (Courtesy of J. Charles Jennette, MD)

[ISN/RPS] class I minimal mesangial and class II mesangioproliferative lupus glomerulonephritis) are induced by predominantly mesangial localization of immune complexes, which usually causes only mild nephritis or asymptomatic hematuria and proteinuria. Localization of substantial amounts of nephritogenic immune complexes in the subendothelial zones of glomerular capillaries where they are adjacent to the inflammatory mediator systems in the blood induces overt glomerular inflammation (focal or diffuse proliferative lupus glomerulonephritis, class III or IV lupus nephritis) and usually causes severe clinical manifestations of nephritis. Qualitative and quantitative characteristics of the pathogenic immune complexes that result in localization predominantly in subepithelial zones where they are not in contact with the inflammatory mediator systems in the blood induces membranous lupus glomerulonephritis (class V lupus nephritis). This variant usually causes the nephrotic syndrome rather than nephritis. As the nephritogenic immune response in a given patient changes over time, sometimes modified by treatment, transitions may occur between the various lupus nephritis phenotypes.

The structurally most severe form of active glomerulonephritis is crescentic glomerulonephritis, which usually manifests clinically as rapidly progressive glomerulonephritis. In patients with new-onset kidney disease who have a nephritic sediment and a serum creatinine concentration greater than 3 mg/dL, glomerulonephritis with crescents is the most common finding in kidney biopsy specimens (see **Table 16-3**). Crescents are proliferations of cells within Bowman's capsule that include both mononuclear phagocytes and glomerular epithelial cells. Crescent formation is a response to glomerular rupture and therefore is a marker of severe glomerular injury. Crescents do not indicate the cause of glomerular injury, however, because many different pathogenic mechanisms can cause crescent formation. There is no consensus on how many glomeruli should have crescents in order to use the term *crescentic glomerulonephritis* in the diagnosis. Most pathologists use the term if more than 50% of glomeruli have crescents, but the percentage of glomeruli with crescents should be specified in the diagnosis

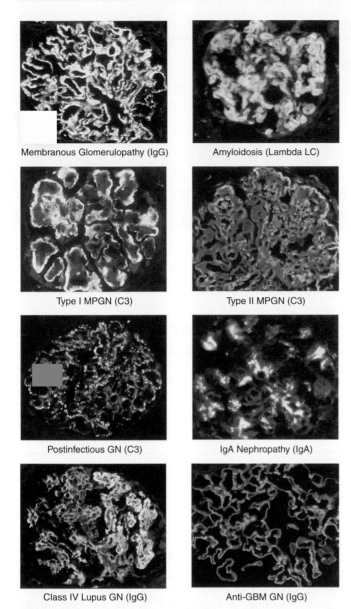

Membranous Glomerulopathy (IgG)

Amyloidosis (Lambda LC)

Type I MPGN (C3)

Type II MPGN (C3)

Postinfectious GN (C3)

IgA Nephropathy (IgA)

Class IV Lupus GN (IgG)

Anti-GBM GN (IgG)

FIGURE 16-6 Immunofluorescence microscopy staining patterns for membranous glomerulopathy. Note the global granular capillary wall staining for immunoglobulin G (IgG). In AL amyloidosis, note the irregular fluffy staining for light chains (LC). In type I membranoproliferative glomerulonephritis (MPGN), note the peripheral granular to bandlike staining for C3. In type II MPGN, note the bandlike capillary wall and coarsely granular mesangial staining for C3. In acute postinfectious glomerulonephritis (GN), note the coarsely granular capillary wall staining for C3. In IgA nephropathy, note the mesangial staining for IgA. In class IV lupus GN, note the segmentally variable capillary wall and mesangial staining for IgG. In anti–glomerular basement membrane (anti-GBM) GN, note the linear GBM staining for IgG.

even if it is less than 50% (e.g., IgA nephropathy with focal proliferative glomerulonephritis and 25% crescents). Within a specific pathogenic category of glomerulonephritis (e.g., anti-GBM disease, ANCA disease, lupus glomerulonephritis, IgA nephropathy, poststreptococcal glomerulonephritis), the higher the fraction of glomeruli with crescents, the worse the prognosis. Among pathogenetically different forms of glomerulonephritis, however, the pathogenic category may be more important in predicting outcome than the presence

of crescents. For example, a patient with poststreptococcal glomerulonephritis with 50% crescents has a much better prognosis for kidney survival, even without immunosuppressive treatment, than a patient with anti-GBM glomerulonephritis or ANCA glomerulonephritis with 25% crescents.

This importance of pathogenic category in predicting the natural history of glomerulonephritis indicates that the pathologic classification of glomerulonephritis by light microscopy into the morphologic categories shown in **Figure 16-7** is not adequate for optimal management. In addition to determining the morphologic severity of glomerular inflammation, the pathogenic or immunopathologic category of disease must be determined. If a kidney biopsy is performed, this is usually done by immunohistology and electron microscopy (see **Figs. 16-1** through **16-6**). Immunohistology reveals the presence or absence of immunoglobulins and complement components. The distribution (e.g., capillary wall, mesangium), pattern (e.g., granular, linear), and composition (e.g., IgA-dominant, IgG-dominant, IgM-dominant) of immunoglobulin are useful for determining specific types of glomerulonephritis; this is discussed in detail in later chapters that address specific types of glomerular disease.

Table 16-4 gives the frequencies of the major pathologic categories of glomerulonephritis in patients with crescents who have undergone kidney biopsy. The immune complex category comprises a variety of diseases, including lupus nephritis, IgA nephropathy, and poststreptococcal glomerulonephritis. Note that most patients with greater than 50% crescents have little or no immunohistologic evidence for immune complex or anti-GBM antibody localization within glomeruli; that is, they have pauci-immune glomerulonephritis. More than 80% of these patients with pauci-immune crescentic glomerulonephritis have circulating ANCAs. Therefore, ANCA glomerulonephritis is the most common form of crescentic glomerulonephritis, especially in older adults.

Because both the structural severity (such as the morphologic stages shown in **Fig. 16-7**) and the immunopathologic category of disease (such as the categories given in **Figs. 16-1** through **16-6**) are important in predicting the course of disease in a patient with glomerulonephritis, the most useful diagnostic terms should include information about both. Examples are "focal proliferative IgA nephropathy," "diffuse proliferative lupus glomerulonephritis," and "crescentic anti-GBM glomerulonephritis."

Many types of glomerulonephritis are immune-mediated inflammatory diseases and are treated with corticosteroids, cytotoxic drugs, or other anti-inflammatory and immunosuppressive agents. The aggressiveness of the treatment, of course, should match the aggressiveness of the disease. For example, active class IV lupus nephritis warrants immunosuppressive treatment, whereas class I or class II lupus nephritis does not.

The two most aggressive forms of glomerulonephritis are anti-GBM crescentic glomerulonephritis and ANCA crescentic glomerulonephritis. The most important factor in improving renal outcome is early diagnosis and treatment. Once extensive sclerosis of glomeruli and advanced chronic

TABLE 16-3 Renal Disease in Patients with Hematuria Undergoing Kidney Biopsy*

DISEASE	PROT <1 g/24 hr, Cr <1.5 mg/dL	PROT 1-3 g/24 hr	Cr 1.5-3.0 mg/dL	Cr >3 mg/dL
No abnormality	30%	2%	1%	0%
Thin BM nephropathy	26%	4%	3%	0%
IgA nephropathy	28%	24%	14%	8%
GN without crescents[†]	9%	26%	37%	23%
GN with crescents[†]	2%	24%	21%	44%
Other kidney disease[‡]	5%	20%	24%	25%
Total	100% (n = 43)	100% (n = 123)	100% (n = 179)	100% (n = 255)

BM, basement membrane; Cr, serum creatinine; GN, glomerulonephritis; IgA, immunoglobulin A; Prot, proteinuria.

*An analysis of kidney biopsy specimens evaluated by the University of North Carolina Nephropathology Laboratory. Patients with systemic lupus erythematosus were excluded from the analysis.

[†]Proliferative or necrotizing GN other than IgA nephropathy or lupus nephritis.

[‡]Includes causes for the nephrotic syndrome, such as membranous glomerulopathy and focal segmental glomerulosclerosis.

Adapted from Caldas MLR, Jennette JC, Falk RJ, Wilkman AS: NC Glomerular Disease Collaborative Network: What is found by renal biopsy in patients with hematuria? Lab Invest 62:15A, 1990.

TABLE 16-4 Frequency of Pathologic Categories of Crescentic Glomerulonephritis in Consecutive Native Kidney Biopsy Specimens, by Age of Patient*

AGE (yr)	PAUCI-IMMUNE	IMMUNE COMPLEX	ANTI-GBM	OTHER[†]
All (n = 632)	60%	24%	15%	1%
1-20 (n = 73)	42%	45%	125	0%
21-60 (n = 303)	48%	35%	15%	3%
61-100 (n = 256)	79%	65%	15%	0%

*Crescentic glomerulonephritis was defined as glomerular disease with 50% or more crescents.

[†]The "other" category includes all other glomerular diseases, such as thrombotic microangiopathy, diabetic glomerulosclerosis, and monoclonal immunoglobulin deposition disease.

Modified from Jennette JC: Rapidly progressive and crescentic glomerulonephritis. Kidney Int 63:1164-1172, 2003.

tubulointerstitial injury have developed, significant response to treatment is unlikely. Both diseases are treated with immunosuppressive regimens, such as pulse methylprednisolone and intravenous or oral cyclophosphamide. Plasmapheresis is usually added to the regimen for anti-GBM disease and for ANCA disease with pulmonary hemorrhage or severe renal failure. Immunosuppressive treatment usually can be terminated after 4 to 5 months in patients with anti-GBM glomerulonephritis with little risk for recurrence (see Chapter 21). The initial induction of remission for ANCA glomerulonephritis often is performed for 6 to 12 months, and even then there is a risk of approximately 25% for recurrence that will require additional immunosuppression (see Chapter 23).

GLOMERULONEPHRITIS ASSOCIATED WITH SYSTEMIC DISEASES

Some patients with acute or rapidly progressive glomerulonephritis have a pathogenetically related systemic disease. These forms of glomerulonephritis with known systemic disease causes may be referred to as *secondary glomerulonephritides.* Immune complex–mediated glomerulonephritis that is induced by infection may involve an antecedent or a concurrent infection, such as streptococcal pharyngitis or

pyoderma preceding acute poststreptococcal glomerulonephritis or hepatitis C infection concurrent with type I membranoproliferative glomerulonephritis (MPGN). As noted earlier, glomerulonephritis with any of the morphologic expressions shown in **Figure 16-7**, as well as membranous glomerulopathy, can be caused by systemic lupus erythematosus (see **Fig. 16-4**).

Because glomeruli are vessels, glomerulonephritis is a frequent manifestation of systemic small-vessel vasculitides, such as Henoch-Schönlein purpura, cryoglobulinemic vasculitis, microscopic polyangiitis, Wegener's granulomatosis, or Churg-Strauss syndrome (see Chapter 23). Henoch-Schönlein purpura is caused by vascular localization of IgA-dominant immune complexes, which manifests as IgA nephropathy in the glomeruli. Cryoglobulinemic vasculitis is caused by cryoglobulin deposition in vessels and often is associated with hepatitis C infection. In glomeruli, cryoglobulinemia usually causes type I MPGN, but other phenotypes of proliferative and even membranous glomerulonephritis may develop. In microscopic polyangiitis, Wegener's granulomatosis, and Churg-Strauss syndrome, there is typically a paucity of immune deposits in vessel walls, usually, but not always, accompanied by circulating ANCAs. Glomerulonephritis associated with and probably caused by ANCAs is characterized pathologically by fibrinoid necrosis and crescent formation

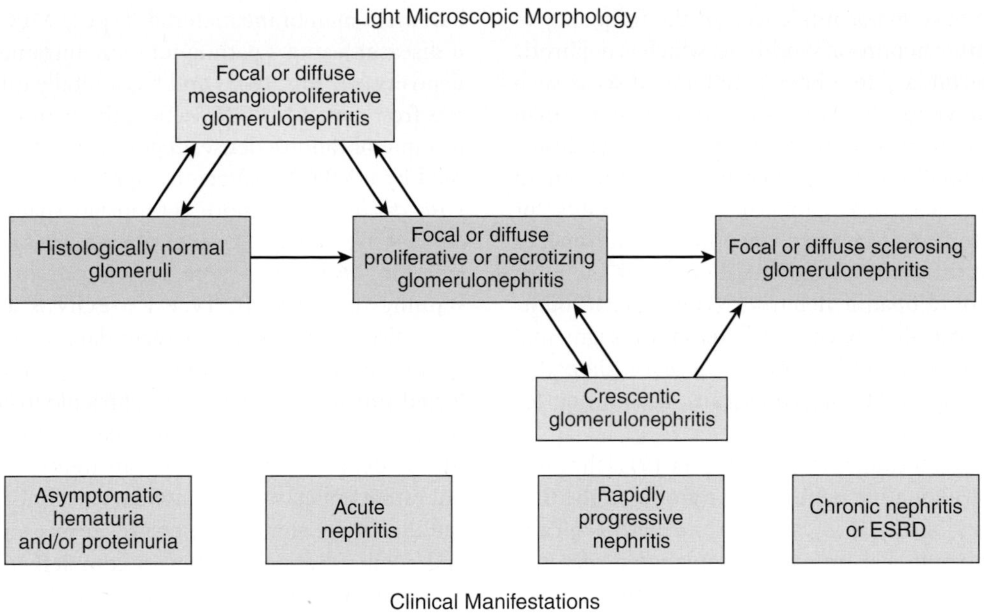

Light Microscopic Morphology

Clinical Manifestations

FIGURE 16-7 Morphologic stages of glomerulonephritis (*top*) aligned with the usual clinical manifestations (*bottom*). Certain glomerular diseases, such as anti–glomerular basement membrane (anti-GBM) and antineutrophil cytoplasmic antibody (ANCA) glomerulonephritis, usually exhibit crescentic glomerulonephritis with rapid decline in kidney function if not promptly treated. Others, such as lupus nephritis, have a predilection for causing focal or diffuse proliferative glomerulonephritis with variable rates of progression depending on the activity of the glomerular lesions. Immunoglobulin A (IgA) nephropathy tends to begin as mild mesangioproliferative lesions but may progress to more severe proliferative lesions. Poststreptococcal glomerulonephritis typically develops an active acute proliferative glomerulonephritis initially but then resolves through a mesangioproliferative phase to normal. Still others, such as IgM mesangial nephropathy, rarely progress past the mesangioproliferative phase. ESRD, end-stage renal disease. (From Jennette JC, Mandal AK: Syndrome of glomerulonephritis. In Mandal AK, Jennette JC [eds]: Diagnosis and Management of Renal Disease and Hypertension, 2nd ed. Durham, NC, Carolina Academic Press, 1994, with permission.)

and often manifests as a rapidly progressive decline in kidney function. Patients with vasculitis-associated glomerulonephritis typically have clinical manifestations of vascular inflammation in multiple organs, such as skin purpura caused by dermal venulitis, hemoptysis caused by alveolar capillary hemorrhage, abdominal pain caused by gut vasculitis, and peripheral neuropathy (mononeuritis multiplex) caused by vasculitis in the small epineural arteries of peripheral nerves.

A distinctive and severe clinical presentation for glomerulonephritis is pulmonary-renal vasculitic syndrome, in which rapidly progressive glomerulonephritis is combined with pulmonary hemorrhage. **Table 16-1** lists the most common causes for pulmonary-renal vasculitic syndrome. Histologic and immunohistologic examination of involved vessels, including glomeruli in kidney biopsy specimens, is useful in making a definitive diagnosis (see **Fig. 16-1**). Serologic analysis for anti-GBM antibodies, ANCA, and markers for immune complex disease (e.g., antinuclear antibodies, cryoglobulins, anti-hepatitis C and B antibodies, complement levels) also may indicate the appropriate diagnosis (see **Fig. 16-1**). ANCA small-vessel vasculitis is the most frequent cause for pulmonary-renal vasculitic syndrome.

ASYMPTOMATIC PROTEINURIA AND NEPHROTIC SYNDROME

When proteinuria is severe, it causes the nephrotic syndrome. Less severe proteinuria, or severe proteinuria of short duration, may be asymptomatic. The nephrotic syndrome is characterized by massive proteinuria (>3 g/24 hr per 1.73 m^2), hypoproteinemia (especially hypoalbuminemia), edema, hyperlipidemia, and lipiduria. The most specific microscopic urinalysis finding is the presence of oval fat bodies (see Chapter 3). These are sloughed tubular epithelial cells that have reabsorbed some of the excess lipids and lipoproteins in the urine.

Severe nephrotic syndrome predisposes to thrombosis secondary to loss of hemostasis control proteins (e.g., antithrombin III, protein S, protein C), infection secondary to loss of immunoglobulins, and, possibly, accelerated atherosclerosis because of the hyperlipidemia. Volume depletion and inactivity may increase the risk for venous thrombosis in nephrotic patients. In nephrotic patients with frequent bacterial infections, administration of intravenous gamma globulin may be required.

Any type of glomerular disease can cause proteinuria. In fact, proteinuria is a sensitive indicator of glomerular damage. However, not all proteinuria is of glomerular origin. For example, tubular damage can cause proteinuria, but rarely of more than 2 g/24 hr.

As noted in **Table 16-2**, some glomerular diseases are more likely to manifest as nephrotic syndrome than others, although virtually any form of glomerular disease may be the cause. The two primary kidney diseases that most often manifest as nephrotic syndrome are minimal change glomerulopathy and membranous glomerulopathy; the two secondary forms of kidney disease that most often manifest as nephrotic syndrome are diabetic glomerulosclerosis and amyloidosis.

Age and race have major influences on the frequency of causes for idiopathic nephrotic syndrome, which is nephrotic syndrome not secondary to a known systemic disease such as diabetes or amyloidosis. Among children younger than 10 years of age, about 80% of idiopathic nephrotic syndrome is caused by minimal change glomerulopathy. Throughout adulthood, minimal change glomerulopathy accounts for only about 10% to 15% of idiopathic nephrotic syndrome. In Caucasian adults, membranous glomerulopathy is the most common cause for idiopathic nephrotic syndrome, accounting for approximately 40% of cases, whereas focal segmental glomerulosclerosis is the most common cause for idiopathic nephrotic syndrome in African Americans, accounting for more than 50% of cases.

Membranous glomerulopathy (see Chapter 19) is the most frequent cause of idiopathic nephrotic syndrome in the fifth and sixth decades of life. It is characterized pathologically by numerous subepithelial immune complex deposits (see **Figs. 16-2**, **16-5**, and **16-6**). The glomerular lesion evolves over time, with progressive accumulation of basement membrane material around the capillary wall immune complexes (see **Fig. 16-5**) and eventual development of chronic tubulointerstitial injury in those patients with progressive disease. If the Heymann nephritis animal model is analogous to human disease, idiopathic (primary) membranous glomerulopathy may be caused by autoantibodies specific for antigens on visceral epithelial cells, which would allow immune complex formation in the subepithelial zone but not in the subendothelial zone or the mesangium of glomeruli. On the other hand, in addition to the numerous subepithelial immune deposits, membranous glomerulopathy secondary to immune complexes composed of antigens and antibodies in the systemic circulation often exhibits immune complex deposits in the mesangium and may have small subendothelial deposits (see **Fig. 16-2**). Therefore, the ultrastructural identification of mesangial or subendothelial deposits should raise the level of suspicion for secondary membranous glomerulopathy, such as membranous glomerulopathy caused by a systemic autoimmune disease (e.g., lupus, mixed connective tissue disease, autoimmune thyroiditis), infection (e.g., hepatitis B or C, syphilis), or neoplasm (e.g., lung or gut carcinoma). In very young and very old patients, the likelihood of secondary membranous glomerulopathy is greater, although still uncommon. Membranous glomerulopathy occurring in young patients raises the possibility of systemic lupus erythematosus or hepatitis B infection, and in very old patients it raises the possibility of occult carcinoma.

Both type I and type II MPGN typically manifest with mixed nephrotic and nephritic features, sometimes accompanied by hypocomplementemia and C3 nephritic factor, which is an autoantibody against the C3 convertase of the alternative complement activation pathway. Both types often exhibit glomerular capillary wall thickening and hypercellularity by light microscopy. Type I MPGN (mesangiocapillary glomerulonephritis) is characterized ultrastructurally by subendothelial immune complex deposits that stimulate subendothelial mesangial interposition and replication of basement membrane material. Type II MPGN (dense deposit disease) features pathognomonic intramembranous dense deposits (see **Fig. 16-3**) and has a totally different pathogenesis from type I MPGN. In fact, the pathognomonic feature, intramembranous dense deposits, is not always accompanied by a MPGN pattern by light microscopy, so *dense deposit disease* is the more appropriate diagnostic term. Both MPGN types have extensive glomerular staining for C3 (see **Fig. 16-6**), with type I having more immunoglobulin staining than type II. Type I MPGN is an immune complex disease that may be secondary to cryoglobulinemia, neoplasms, or chronic infections (e.g., hepatitis C or B; infected prostheses, such as a ventriculoatrial shunt; chronic bacterial endocarditis; chronic mastoiditis). Type II MPGN (dense deposit disease) is not an immune complex disease but rather appears to be secondary to abnormal activation of the alternative complement pathway by a variety of inherited and acquired abnormalities in complement regulation. For example, rare patients have inherited defects in the complement control protein factor H.

When taken as a group, the various forms of proliferative glomerulonephritis account for a substantial proportion of patients who have nephrotic-range proteinuria. Patients with proliferative glomerulonephritis and marked proteinuria usually also have features of nephritis, especially hematuria. Included in this group are patients with lupus nephritis and IgA nephropathy who have nephrotic-range proteinuria. In the United States, approximately 15% of adults with unexplained nephrotic-range proteinuria are unexpectedly found to have IgA nephropathy by renal biopsy.

Amyloidosis as a cause for the nephrotic syndrome is most frequently seen in older adults. Overall, approximately 10% of adults with unexplained nephrotic syndrome are found to have amyloidosis at the time of renal biopsy. Currently in the United States, amyloid causing the nephrotic syndrome is approximately 75% AL amyloid rather than AA amyloid. Approximately 75% of AL amyloid is composed of λ rather than κ light chain. Patients with κ light chain paraproteins and the nephrotic syndrome are more likely to have light chain deposition disease (i.e., nodular sclerosis without amyloid fibrils) rather than amyloidosis (see Chapter 27). Amyloid composition can be determined by immunofluorescence microscopy (see **Fig. 16-6**). In less developed areas of the world, where chronic infections are more prevalent, AA amyloidosis is more frequent than AL amyloidosis.

CHRONIC GLOMERULONEPHRITIS AND END-STAGE RENAL DISEASE

Most glomerular disease, with the possible exceptions of uncomplicated minimal change glomerulopathy and thin basement membrane nephropathy, can progress to chronic glomerular sclerosis with progressively declining kidney function and, eventually, to ESRD. Chronic glomerular disease is the third leading cause of ESRD in the United States, after diabetic and hypertensive kidney disease. Clinicopathologic studies of glomerular diseases have revealed marked differences in their natural histories. Some diseases, such as anti-GBM and ANCA crescentic glomerulonephritis, have a high risk for rapid progression to ESRD unless treated. Other diseases, such as IgA nephropathy and focal segmental glomerulosclerosis, have more indolent but persistent courses, with ESRD eventually ensuing in a significant number of patients. Some forms of glomerulonephritis, such as acute poststreptococcal glomerulonephritis, may initially manifest a rather severe nephritis but usually resolve completely with little risk for progression to ESRD. And some diseases are unpredictable, such as membranous glomerulopathy, which may remit spontaneously, produce persistent nephrosis for decades without a decline in kidney function, or progress over several years to ESRD.

Chronic glomerulonephritis is characterized pathologically by varying degrees of glomerular scarring that is always accompanied by cortical tubular atrophy, interstitial fibrosis, interstitial infiltration by chronic inflammatory cells, and arteriosclerosis. As the glomerular, interstitial, and vascular sclerosis worsen, they eventually reach a point at which histologic evaluation of the kidney tissue cannot reveal the initial cause for the kidney injury, and a pathologic diagnosis of ESRD is all that can be concluded.

Clinically, chronic glomerulonephritis that is progressing to ESRD eventually results in uremia that must be managed by dialysis or kidney transplantation. As the term implies, patients with uremia have accumulation of nitrogenous wastes (urea, uric acid, creatinine) in the blood. Other clinical manifestations of uremia include nausea and vomiting, hiccups, anorexia, pruritus, lethargy, pericarditis, myopathies, neuropathies, and encephalopathy.

KIDNEY BIOPSY: INDICATIONS AND METHODS

In a patient with kidney disease, a kidney biopsy provides tissue that can be used to determine the diagnosis, indicate the cause, predict the prognosis, direct treatment, and collect data for research, although not all potential applications are accomplished by every kidney biopsy.

Kidney biopsy is indicated in a patient with kidney disease when all three of the following conditions are met: (1) the cause cannot be determined or adequately predicted by less invasive diagnostic procedures; (2) the signs and symptoms suggest parenchymal disease that can be diagnosed by pathologic evaluation; and (3) the differential diagnosis includes diseases that have different treatments, different prognoses, or both. Situations in which a kidney biopsy serves an important diagnostic function include nephrotic syndrome in adults, steroid-resistant nephrotic syndrome in children, glomerulonephritis in adults other than clearcut acute poststreptococcal glomerulonephritis, and acute renal failure of unknown cause. In some kidney diseases for which the diagnosis is relatively definite based on clinical data, a kidney biopsy may be of value not only for confirming the diagnosis but also for assessing the activity, chronicity, and severity of injury (e.g., in patients with

suspected lupus glomerulonephritis). Although the diagnosis is strongly supported by positive serologic results in patients with anti-GBM and ANCA glomerulonephritis, the extremely toxic treatment that is used for these diseases warrants the additional level of confirmation that a kidney biopsy provides; and a kidney biopsy also provides information about the severity and potential reversibility of the glomerular damage. **Table 16-5** demonstrates the types of native kidney disease that have prompted kidney biopsy among the nephrologists who refer specimens to the University of North Carolina Nephropathology Laboratory. Approximately 80% of these biopsies were performed by nephrologists in community practice. Diseases that typically cause nephrotic syndrome (e.g., membranous glomerulopathy, focal segmental glomerulosclerosis) were most frequently the impetus for biopsy, followed by diseases that cause nephritis (e.g., lupus nephritis, IgA nephropathy).

Contraindications to percutaneous kidney biopsy include an uncooperative patient, solitary kidney, hemorrhagic diathesis, uncontrolled severe hypertension, severe anemia or dehydration, cystic kidney, hydronephrosis, multiple renal arterial aneurysms, acute pyelonephritis or perinephric abscess, renal neoplasm, and ESRD. Transjugular kidney biopsy and open kidney biopsy are advocated by some as safer procedures in patients with these risk factors.

Clinically significant complications of kidney biopsy are relatively infrequent but must be kept in mind when determining the risk/benefit ratio of the procedure. Small perirenal hematomas that can be seen on imaging studies (e.g., ultrasonography) are relatively common if sought carefully. Gross hematuria occurs in fewer than 10% of patients, arteriovenous fistula in fewer than 1%, hemorrhage requiring surgery in fewer than 1%, and death in fewer than 0.1%.

Current percutaneous needle biopsy procedures usually employ localization of the kidney by real-time ultrasound guidance, determination of kidney location and depth by ultrasonography immediately before biopsy, or computed tomography–guided localization of the kidney. Many varieties of biopsy needles have been used over the years, most of which are effective in experienced hands. Currently, most kidney biopsies are performed with spring-loaded disposable gun devices. Extensive experience and multiple published studies indicate that the use of larger biopsy needles (e.g., 15 and 16 gauge) provides more useful tissue with no more morbidity than smaller needles (e.g., 18 gauge), which are more likely to provide inadequate tissue for diagnosis and especially for prognosis. Therefore, 15- and 16-gauge needle provide a better cost/benefit ratio for the patient.

Light microscopy alone is not adequate for the diagnosis of native kidney diseases, although it may be adequate for assessing the basis for kidney allograft dysfunction during the first few weeks after transplantation. All native kidney biopsy samples should be processed for at least light microscopy and immunofluorescence microscopy. Most renal pathologists advocate performing electron microscopy on all native kidney biopsy specimens; however, some fix tissue for

Minimal Change Nephrotic Syndrome

Howard Trachtman

Minimal change nephrotic syndrome (MCNS) is a victim of poor nomenclature. By focusing solely on the benign microscopic appearance, one is easily lured into a false sense of security based on the mistaken impression that MCNS is not a genuine disease. Nothing could be further from the truth, because MCNS represents a fascinating instance of organ dysfunction caused by a variable interaction between intrinsic structural defects and immunologic disturbances. Moreover, MCNS can be the cause of significant short-term morbidity and can follow a chronic relapsing course with long-term adverse consequences. Finally, both first-line treatments and secondary therapeutic options for more difficult cases can lead to serious toxicity. Therefore, although the long-term prognosis is excellent, optimal management of MCNS requires clinical acumen to balance the risks of untreated disease activity against the hazards of available pharmacologic choices. This chapter reviews the definition, incidence, presentation, and treatment options for MCNS, highlighting key differences between pediatric and adult patients, with the goal of providing a rational basis for the management of this disorder.

DEFINITION

As a cause of nephrotic syndrome, MCNS is characterized by the presence of edema, selective proteinuria, hypoalbuminemia, hypercholesterolemia, and a normal glomerular filtration rate. It is defined as a distinct and separate medical entity by its histologic appearance when kidney tissue is available for examination, or operationally if empiric treatment is offered. If a renal biopsy is performed, the histopathology reveals a normal-looking kidney without cellular proliferation, immune deposits, tubulointerstitial changes, or alterations in the glomerular basement membrane (GBM). The only abnormality is diffuse effacement and fusion of epithelial cell foot processes.

In current pediatric practice, if there is a high degree of confidence that a patient has MCNS, then a renal biopsy is not routinely done and the disease is defined by its response to a standard course of oral corticosteroids. There is a general consensus among pediatric nephrologists that 4 to 6 weeks of daily prednisone followed by 4 to 6 weeks of alternate-day therapy constitutes adequate treatment to define steroid responsiveness and a diagnosis of MCNS. The situation is different in adult patients. MCNS is not the leading cause of nephrotic syndrome in adults, and a biopsy is almost always required to define the cause of idiopathic nephrotic syndrome. Therefore, the diagnosis of MCNS in an adult is established by biopsy. Moreover, in adults, the renal pathology frequently is associated with atherosclerotic disease, especially in the setting of acute renal failure. The definition of a standard course of oral corticosteroids is not universally accepted in adults, and more extended periods of steroid therapy are often required to confirm steroid resistance. Therefore, the definition of MCNS based on response to steroids is adequate in children but clearly not in adults.

The interplay between these two methods of defining MCNS varies based on factors such as the age of the patient and the circumstances of each clinical practice. It is important to recognize that there is no specific blood or urine test or histologic finding that consistently distinguishes MCNS from other causes of idiopathic or secondary nephrotic syndrome. In routine practice, the diagnosis is made by negative inference—that is, the absence of features of any other cause of new-onset nephrotic syndrome with steroid responsiveness.

INCIDENCE

MCNS is one of the causes of primary or idiopathic nephrotic syndrome, to be distinguished from the secondary causes of nephrotic syndrome, such as diabetic nephropathy or amyloidosis. Overall, the incidence of primary or idiopathic nephrotic syndrome, including MCNS and its variants, focal segmental glomerulosclerosis (FSGS), membranous nephropathy, and membranoproliferative glomerulonephritis, is approximately 3 to 5 cases per 100,000 population per year in children and adults. The contribution of MCNS to this general category varies greatly with the age of the patient. In prepubertal patients, MCNS accounts for almost 90% of all cases of idiopathic nephrotic syndrome. In adults, the percentage of cases attributable to MCNS falls to 20% to 40%, depending on the patient sample. Adolescence represents a transition between the two ends of the spectrum, although the findings in adolescents, overall, more closely resemble those in adults than those in school-age children.

PATHOPHYSIOLOGY

Nephrotic-range proteinuria occurs because of defective glomerular barrier function and can arise from an altered charge density or from increased effective pore size in the filtration

differences in their natural histories. Some diseases, such as anti-GBM and ANCA crescentic glomerulonephritis, have a high risk for rapid progression to ESRD unless treated. Other diseases, such as IgA nephropathy and focal segmental glomerulosclerosis, have more indolent but persistent courses, with ESRD eventually ensuing in a significant number of patients. Some forms of glomerulonephritis, such as acute poststreptococcal glomerulonephritis, may initially manifest a rather severe nephritis but usually resolve completely with little risk for progression to ESRD. And some diseases are unpredictable, such as membranous glomerulopathy, which may remit spontaneously, produce persistent nephrosis for decades without a decline in kidney function, or progress over several years to ESRD.

Chronic glomerulonephritis is characterized pathologically by varying degrees of glomerular scarring that is always accompanied by cortical tubular atrophy, interstitial fibrosis, interstitial infiltration by chronic inflammatory cells, and arteriosclerosis. As the glomerular, interstitial, and vascular sclerosis worsen, they eventually reach a point at which histologic evaluation of the kidney tissue cannot reveal the initial cause for the kidney injury, and a pathologic diagnosis of ESRD is all that can be concluded.

Clinically, chronic glomerulonephritis that is progressing to ESRD eventually results in uremia that must be managed by dialysis or kidney transplantation. As the term implies, patients with uremia have accumulation of nitrogenous wastes (urea, uric acid, creatinine) in the blood. Other clinical manifestations of uremia include nausea and vomiting, hiccups, anorexia, pruritus, lethargy, pericarditis, myopathies, neuropathies, and encephalopathy.

KIDNEY BIOPSY: INDICATIONS AND METHODS

In a patient with kidney disease, a kidney biopsy provides tissue that can be used to determine the diagnosis, indicate the cause, predict the prognosis, direct treatment, and collect data for research, although not all potential applications are accomplished by every kidney biopsy.

Kidney biopsy is indicated in a patient with kidney disease when all three of the following conditions are met: (1) the cause cannot be determined or adequately predicted by less invasive diagnostic procedures; (2) the signs and symptoms suggest parenchymal disease that can be diagnosed by pathologic evaluation; and (3) the differential diagnosis includes diseases that have different treatments, different prognoses, or both. Situations in which a kidney biopsy serves an important diagnostic function include nephrotic syndrome in adults, steroid-resistant nephrotic syndrome in children, glomerulonephritis in adults other than clearcut acute poststreptococcal glomerulonephritis, and acute renal failure of unknown cause. In some kidney diseases for which the diagnosis is relatively definite based on clinical data, a kidney biopsy may be of value not only for confirming the diagnosis but also for assessing the activity, chronicity, and severity of injury (e.g., in patients with

suspected lupus glomerulonephritis). Although the diagnosis is strongly supported by positive serologic results in patients with anti-GBM and ANCA glomerulonephritis, the extremely toxic treatment that is used for these diseases warrants the additional level of confirmation that a kidney biopsy provides; and a kidney biopsy also provides information about the severity and potential reversibility of the glomerular damage. **Table 16-5** demonstrates the types of native kidney disease that have prompted kidney biopsy among the nephrologists who refer specimens to the University of North Carolina Nephropathology Laboratory. Approximately 80% of these biopsies were performed by nephrologists in community practice. Diseases that typically cause nephrotic syndrome (e.g., membranous glomerulopathy, focal segmental glomerulosclerosis) were most frequently the impetus for biopsy, followed by diseases that cause nephritis (e.g., lupus nephritis, IgA nephropathy).

Contraindications to percutaneous kidney biopsy include an uncooperative patient, solitary kidney, hemorrhagic diathesis, uncontrolled severe hypertension, severe anemia or dehydration, cystic kidney, hydronephrosis, multiple renal arterial aneurysms, acute pyelonephritis or perinephric abscess, renal neoplasm, and ESRD. Transjugular kidney biopsy and open kidney biopsy are advocated by some as safer procedures in patients with these risk factors.

Clinically significant complications of kidney biopsy are relatively infrequent but must be kept in mind when determining the risk/benefit ratio of the procedure. Small perirenal hematomas that can be seen on imaging studies (e.g., ultrasonography) are relatively common if sought carefully. Gross hematuria occurs in fewer than 10% of patients, arteriovenous fistula in fewer than 1%, hemorrhage requiring surgery in fewer than 1%, and death in fewer than 0.1%.

Current percutaneous needle biopsy procedures usually employ localization of the kidney by real-time ultrasound guidance, determination of kidney location and depth by ultrasonography immediately before biopsy, or computed tomography–guided localization of the kidney. Many varieties of biopsy needles have been used over the years, most of which are effective in experienced hands. Currently, most kidney biopsies are performed with spring-loaded disposable gun devices. Extensive experience and multiple published studies indicate that the use of larger biopsy needles (e.g., 15 and 16 gauge) provides more useful tissue with no more morbidity than smaller needles (e.g., 18 gauge), which are more likely to provide inadequate tissue for diagnosis and especially for prognosis. Therefore, 15- and 16-gauge needle provide a better cost/benefit ratio for the patient.

Light microscopy alone is not adequate for the diagnosis of native kidney diseases, although it may be adequate for assessing the basis for kidney allograft dysfunction during the first few weeks after transplantation. All native kidney biopsy samples should be processed for at least light microscopy and immunofluorescence microscopy. Most renal pathologists advocate performing electron microscopy on all native kidney biopsy specimens; however, some fix tissue for

TABLE 16-5 Frequency of Diagnoses among 7257 Kidney Biopsy Samples Evaluated in the University of North Carolina Nephropathology Laboratory*

Diseases that Often Cause Nephrotic Syndrome (42%)	3067	**Diseases that Often Cause Hematuria and Nephritis (29%)**	2109
Idiopathic membranous glomerulopathy	847	Lupus nephritis (all classes)	636
Focal segmental glomerulosclerosis (FSGS)	768	Immunoglobulin A nephropathy	538
Minimal change glomerulopathy	398	Other immune complex proliferative GN	375
Diabetic glomerulosclerosis	246	Pauci-immune/ANCA GN	301
Type I membranoproliferative GN	190	Acute diffuse proliferative (postinfectious) GN	86
Mesangioproliferative GN	145	Thin basement membrane nephropathy	82
Amyloidosis	108	Anti-GBM GN	56
C1q nephropathy	99	Alport's syndrome	35
Collapsing variant of FSGS	87	**Diseases that Often Cause Chronic Kidney Disease (8%)**	583
Glomerular tip lesion variant of FSGS	65	Arterionephrosclerosis	229
Fibrillary GN	59	Chronic sclerosing GN	166
Light chain deposition disease	26	End-stage renal disease	114
Type II membranoproliferative GN	14	Chronic tubulointerstitial nephritis	74
Preeclampsia/eclampsia	6	**Miscellaneous Other Diseases (3%)**	199
Immunotactoid glomerulopathy	6	**No Pathologic Lesion Identified (2%)**	141
Collagenofibrotic glomerulopathy	3	**Adequate Tissue with Nonspecific Abnormalities (5%)**	370
Diseases that Often Cause Acute Renal Failure† (5%)	371	**Inadequate Tissue for Definitive Diagnosis (6%)**	417
Thrombotic microangiopathy (all types)	126		
Acute tubulointerstitial nephritis	101		
Acute tubular necrosis	69		
Atheroembolization	34		
Light chain cast nephropathy	31		
Cortical necrosis	10		

ANCA, antineutrophil cytoplasmic antibody; GBM, glomerular basement membrane; GN, glomerulonephritis.

*Specimens with nonspecific abnormalities (e.g., interstitial fibrosis, tubular atrophy, glomerular scarring, arteriosclerosis), specimens with no identifiable pathologic abnormality (e.g., in a patient with asymptomatic hematuria), and some specimens with inadequate tissue for definitive diagnosis (e.g., a very small specimen with only a few glomeruli but with negative immunofluorescence microscopy) may nevertheless provide useful clinical information, especially with respect to ruling out diseases that were in the differential diagnosis.
†Other than glomerulonephritis.

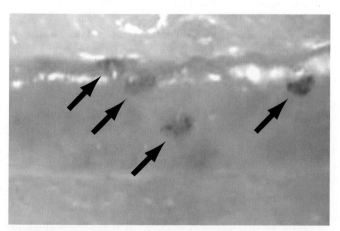

FIGURE 16-8 Photograph of a fresh 15-gauge needle renal biopsy showing red blushes (*arrows*) corresponding to glomeruli in the renal cortex.

electron microscopy but perform the procedure only if the other microscopic findings suggest that it will be useful.

The needle biopsy core sample should be examined with a magnifying glass or a dissecting microscope to confirm that kidney tissue is present and to determine whether it is cortex or medulla. When gently prodded and pulled with forceps, adipose tissue is mushy and strings out, skeletal muscle tissue falls apart into little clumps, and kidney tissue maintains a cylindrical shape. At 15× or higher magnification, adipose tissue looks like clusters of tiny fat droplets (i.e., adipose cells), skeletal muscle is red-brown with irregular bundles of fibers, and kidney tissue is pale pink to tan. Glomeruli in the renal cortex appear as reddish blushes or hemispheres projecting from the surface of the core (**Fig. 16-8**). Straight red striations produced by the vasa recta are markers for the medulla. If there is extensive glomerular hematuria, the convoluted tubules in the cortex appear as red corkscrews. Once the tissue landmarks are identified, portions of tissue should be separated for processing for light, immunofluorescence, and electron microscopy.

In our experience with kidney biopsy specimens sent to us from more than 200 different nephrologists per year, most of whom are in community practice, approximately 6% of kidney biopsy specimens are inadequate for a definitive diagnosis (see **Table 16-5**). The most common inadequacy is kidney tissue with too little or no cortex. This can be remedied by beginning the sampling procedure with the biopsy needle just barely penetrating the outer cortex. Obviously, if the biopsy needle is inserted too deeply into or through the cortex, the specimen will contain only medulla. Even specimens that are considered inadequate for a definitive diagnosis may provide useful information. For example, in a patient with nephrotic syndrome, a kidney biopsy specimen that has no glomeruli for light or electron microscopy may have one glomerulus that stains negative for immunoglobulins and complement by immunofluorescence microscopy, which rules out any form of immune complex glomerulonephritis (e.g., membranous glomerulopathy) and focuses the differential diagnosis on minimal change glomerulopathy versus focal segmental glomerulosclerosis.

BIBLIOGRAPHY

Appel GB: Renal biopsy: The clinician's viewpoint. In Silva FG, D'Agati VD, Nadasdy T (eds): Renal Biopsy Interpretation. New York, Churchill Livingstone, 1996, pp 21-29.

Bolton WK: Goodpasture's syndrome. Kidney Int 50:1753-1766, 1996.

Cameron JS: Nephrotic syndrome in the elderly. Semin Nephrol 16:319-329, 1996.

D'Agati VD, Fogo AB, Bruijn JA, et al: Pathologic classification of focal segmental glomerulosclerosis: A working proposal. Am J Kidney Dis 43:368-382, 2004.

Eddy AA, Symons JM: Nephrotic syndrome in childhood. Lancet 362:629-639, 2003.

Feneberg R, Schaefer F, Zieger B, et al: Percutaneous renal biopsy in children: A 27-year experience. Nephron 79:438-446, 1998.

Glassock RJ: Diagnosis and natural course of membranous nephropathy. Semin Nephrol 23:324-332, 2003.

Glassock RJ, Cohen AH: The primary glomerulopathies. Dis Mon 42:329-383, 1996.

Haas M, Meehan SM, Karrison TG, Spargo BH: Changing etiologies of unexplained adult nephrotic syndrome: A comparison of renal biopsy findings from 1976-1979 and 1995-1997. Am J Kidney Dis 30:621-631, 1997.

Haas M, Spargo BH, Wit EJ, Meehan SM: Etiologies and outcome of acute renal insufficiency in older adults: A renal biopsy study of 259 cases. Am J Kidney Dis 35:433-447, 2000.

Jennette JC: Rapidly progressive and crescentic glomerulonephritis. Kidney Int 63:1164-1172, 2003.

Jennette JC, Olson JL, Schwartz MM, Silva FG: Primer on the pathologic diagnosis of renal disease. In Jennette JC, Olson JL, Schwartz MM, Silva FG (eds): Heptinstall's Pathology of the Kidney. 6th ed., Philadelphia, Lippincott Williams & Wilkins, 2007, pp 100-126.

Jouet P, Meyrier A, Mai F, et al: Transjugular renal biopsy in the treatment of patients with cirrhosis and renal abnormalities. Hepatology 24:1143-1147, 1996.

Mariani AJ, Mariani MC, Macchioni C, et al: The significance of adult hematuria: 1,000 Hematuria evaluations including a risk-benefit and cost-effectiveness analysis. J Urol 141:350-355, 1989.

Niles JL, Bottinger EP, Saurina GR, et al: The syndrome of lung hemorrhage and nephritis is usually an ANCA-associated condition. Arch Intern Med 156:440-445, 1996.

Schena FP: Survey of the Italian Registry of Renal Biopsies: Frequency of the renal diseases for 7 consecutive years. The Italian Group of Renal Immunopathology. Nephrology Dial Transplant 12:418-426, 1997.

Smith RJ, Alexander J, Barlow PN, et al: New approaches to the treatment of dense deposit disease. J Am Soc Nephrol 18:2447-56, 2007.

van der Loop FT, Monnens LA, Schroder CH, et al: Identification of COL4A5 defects in Alport's syndrome by immunohistochemistry of skin. Kidney Int 55:1217-1224, 1999.

Walker PD, Cavallo T, Bonsib SM; Ad Hoc Committee on Renal Biopsy Guidelines of the Renal Pathology Society: Practice guidelines for the renal biopsy. Mod Pathol 17:1555-1563, 2004.

Weening JJ, D'Agati VD, Schwartz MM, et al: The classification of glomerulonephritis in systemic lupus erythematosus revisited. Kidney Int 65:521-530, 2004.

Minimal Change Nephrotic Syndrome

Howard Trachtman

Minimal change nephrotic syndrome (MCNS) is a victim of poor nomenclature. By focusing solely on the benign microscopic appearance, one is easily lured into a false sense of security based on the mistaken impression that MCNS is not a genuine disease. Nothing could be further from the truth, because MCNS represents a fascinating instance of organ dysfunction caused by a variable interaction between intrinsic structural defects and immunologic disturbances. Moreover, MCNS can be the cause of significant short-term morbidity and can follow a chronic relapsing course with long-term adverse consequences. Finally, both first-line treatments and secondary therapeutic options for more difficult cases can lead to serious toxicity. Therefore, although the long-term prognosis is excellent, optimal management of MCNS requires clinical acumen to balance the risks of untreated disease activity against the hazards of available pharmacologic choices. This chapter reviews the definition, incidence, presentation, and treatment options for MCNS, highlighting key differences between pediatric and adult patients, with the goal of providing a rational basis for the management of this disorder.

DEFINITION

As a cause of nephrotic syndrome, MCNS is characterized by the presence of edema, selective proteinuria, hypoalbuminemia, hypercholesterolemia, and a normal glomerular filtration rate. It is defined as a distinct and separate medical entity by its histologic appearance when kidney tissue is available for examination, or operationally if empiric treatment is offered. If a renal biopsy is performed, the histopathology reveals a normal-looking kidney without cellular proliferation, immune deposits, tubulointerstitial changes, or alterations in the glomerular basement membrane (GBM). The only abnormality is diffuse effacement and fusion of epithelial cell foot processes.

In current pediatric practice, if there is a high degree of confidence that a patient has MCNS, then a renal biopsy is not routinely done and the disease is defined by its response to a standard course of oral corticosteroids. There is a general consensus among pediatric nephrologists that 4 to 6 weeks of daily prednisone followed by 4 to 6 weeks of alternate-day therapy constitutes adequate treatment to define steroid responsiveness and a diagnosis of MCNS. The situation is different in adult patients. MCNS is not the leading cause of nephrotic syndrome in adults, and a biopsy is almost always required to define the cause of idiopathic nephrotic syndrome. Therefore, the diagnosis of MCNS in an adult is established by biopsy. Moreover, in adults, the renal pathology frequently is associated with atherosclerotic disease, especially in the setting of acute renal failure. The definition of a standard course of oral corticosteroids is not universally accepted in adults, and more extended periods of steroid therapy are often required to confirm steroid resistance. Therefore, the definition of MCNS based on response to steroids is adequate in children but clearly not in adults.

The interplay between these two methods of defining MCNS varies based on factors such as the age of the patient and the circumstances of each clinical practice. It is important to recognize that there is no specific blood or urine test or histologic finding that consistently distinguishes MCNS from other causes of idiopathic or secondary nephrotic syndrome. In routine practice, the diagnosis is made by negative inference—that is, the absence of features of any other cause of new-onset nephrotic syndrome with steroid responsiveness.

INCIDENCE

MCNS is one of the causes of primary or idiopathic nephrotic syndrome, to be distinguished from the secondary causes of nephrotic syndrome, such as diabetic nephropathy or amyloidosis. Overall, the incidence of primary or idiopathic nephrotic syndrome, including MCNS and its variants, focal segmental glomerulosclerosis (FSGS), membranous nephropathy, and membranoproliferative glomerulonephritis, is approximately 3 to 5 cases per 100,000 population per year in children and adults. The contribution of MCNS to this general category varies greatly with the age of the patient. In prepubertal patients, MCNS accounts for almost 90% of all cases of idiopathic nephrotic syndrome. In adults, the percentage of cases attributable to MCNS falls to 20% to 40%, depending on the patient sample. Adolescence represents a transition between the two ends of the spectrum, although the findings in adolescents, overall, more closely resemble those in adults than those in school-age children.

PATHOPHYSIOLOGY

Nephrotic-range proteinuria occurs because of defective glomerular barrier function and can arise from an altered charge density or from increased effective pore size in the filtration

unit. MCNS is unique in that it reflects predominantly a decrease in the negative charge present in endothelial cells, the GBM, and podocytes, which causes selective proteinuria. The reduction in negative charge appears to be a diffuse abnormality that is manifested in capillaries throughout the body, with leakage of albumin in the peripheral circulation and accumulation of interstitial fluid. The cause of the diminished negative charge density probably is related to immune-mediated defects that inhibit sulfate incorporation into the GBM, rather than a genetic mutation in a podocyte protein. In addition, immunoeffector cells may elaborate soluble molecules, such as vascular endothelial growth factor, that directly increase GBM permeability to protein. A linkage between abnormal T-cell function and MCNS was initially proposed more than 30 years ago by Shalhoub, and many studies since then have documented altered subtype distribution and activity of lymphocytes in children with MCNS. A recent study in which albuminuria and podocyte foot process effacement were induced by injection of CD34-positive stem cells isolated from patients with MCNS or FSGS into immunodeficient (NOD/SCID) mice underscored the pivotal role of the immune system in the pathogenesis of MCNS.

Although MCNS can occur in a familial pattern with both vertical and horizontal transmission, it has not been linked to mutations in any of the well-recognized proteins associated with FSGS, such as podocin, Wilms' tumor 1 (WT-1), the transient receptor potential cation channel 6 (TRPC6), or α-actinin 4. However, there have been observations linking frequently relapsing childhood MCNS to allelic heterogeneity in the gene for nephrin, a key component of the slit diaphragm and a major genetic locus for congenital nephrotic syndrome. Further work is needed to ascertain the frequency and impact of genetic abnormalities in podocyte-related proteins in MCNS.

CLINICAL PRESENTATION

The most common presentation of MCNS is edema. The clinical presentation of MCNS in adult patients is a distinguishing feature of this form of nephrotic syndrome, with rapidly developing edema that can be pedal in distribution but can also manifest as anasarca. In children, edema can occur anywhere in the body, including the periorbital region, scrotum, or abdomen. It is essential to exclude other nonrenal causes of edema, such as congestive heart failure, cirrhosis, protein-losing enteropathy, and malabsorption. Less frequent presenting complaints include infections such as cellulitis secondary to localized fluid accumulation and skin breakdown or bacterial peritonitis in patients with ascites. Thromboembolic events, including renal vein thrombosis and pulmonary emboli, are much more common in adult patients. Another clinical presentation can be acute renal failure associated with sudden development of proteinuria in the setting of substantial vascular disease. As a cause of primary nephrotic syndrome, MCNS is not associated with systemic manifestations such as fever, rash, or joint pains. Therefore, the physical examination is usually normal except for the edema.

DIAGNOSTIC EVALUATION

The diagnostic evaluation of patients with new-onset nephrotic syndrome when MCNS is suspected should include the following: (1) complete serum biochemical profile with creatinine, albumin, and cholesterol concentrations; (2) complete blood count; (3) quantitation of urinary protein excretion; and (4) serum C3 level. For quantitation of urinary protein excretion, determination of the protein/creatinine ratio (both measured in milligrams per deciliter) in an early-morning urine sample has been validated as a reliable method in pediatric patients. Normal urinary protein excretion is characterized by a ratio lower than 0.2, and nephrotic-range proteinuria is at least 10-fold higher than normal (i.e., >2). In adults, proteinuria may also be quantitated as the amount of protein in a 24-hour urine collection, with a cutoff level of 3 g, or as a protein/creatinine ratio greater than 3.

Mild azotemia may be present in up to 20% of cases. Overt acute renal failure secondary to severe intravascular volume depletion or renal edema and tubular obstruction can occur in both adults and children, although the complication is much less common in pediatric patients. The urinalysis, which should preferably be performed by the physician, may show hematuria in 20% to 30% of cases on dipstick testing. Microscopic examination of the urine may reveal waxy casts and oval fat bodies. All other diagnostic tests, such as serologic markers of systemic lupus erythematosus, hepatitis B or C, or human immunodeficiency virus infection, should be geared to the individual clinical circumstance.

In general, the diagnosis of MCNS can be confirmed in pediatric patients by the patient's responsiveness to a standard course of corticosteroids (see "Initial Treatment"). Therefore, in cases of new-onset nephrotic syndrome in pediatric patients, a kidney biopsy is warranted only if the clinical and laboratory evidence (i.e., age <6 months or older than adolescence, unexpected systemic manifestations, or a low serum C3 level) suggests that the patient does *not* have MCNS. In adult patients, a diagnosis of MCNS cannot be conclusively established based on responsiveness to steroids, and MCNS is much less frequently the cause of new-onset nephrotic syndrome in adults than children. Because of these issues, a kidney biopsy is warranted in the workup of adults with new-onset nephrotic syndrome. Some nephrologists perform a kidney biopsy only in adults who are steroid resistant and base this practice on decision analysis.

INITIAL TREATMENT

Corticosteroids represent the time-honored initial therapy for presumed MCNS. Prednisone is the usual drug that is prescribed, and the standard dose is 60 mg/m^2 or 2 mg/kg daily for 4 to 6 weeks, followed by 40 mg/m^2 or 1 mg/kg every other day for 4 to 6 weeks. Seventy percent of pediatric patients achieve remission after 10 to 14 days of treatment, and most will no longer have proteinuria after 4 weeks of therapy. The time to response is longer in adults, especially those given alternate-day steroids from the onset of treatment, who may require 4 to 6 months to manifest a response to the initial course of therapy.

There are conflicting data in the literature as to whether lengthening the course of the initial treatment from 8 to 12 weeks delays the time to first relapse and reduces overall exposure to steroids. Efficacy may vary depending on the patient population, and the details of treatment should be guided by the experience at each center. In adult patients, it is common to prescribe more modest doses at the outset (e.g., 40 mg), on an alternate-day regimen for a more prolonged period (often up to 6 months), to achieve remission without the toxicity associated with daily administration of the drug. Lower doses and alternate-day treatment schedules are less likely to induce remission in patients with MCNS.

Relapse therapy involves similar doses but usually for a shorter period. Various modifications in corticosteroid dosing have been tried to prevent relapses and minimize side effects, such as use of extended tapering schedules, complete avoidance of every-other-day administration, and prolonged low-dose hydrocortisone to prevent adrenal insufficiency. Different formulations of steroids (e.g., deflazacort) have also been tried, with mixed results. Adults do not tolerate relapsing disease as well as children, as a consequence of the intrinsic morbidity of MCNS and the toxicity related to repeated exposures to corticosteroids. Therefore, these patients are often candidates for prompt implementation of immunosuppressive therapy.

SHORT-TERM COURSE

MCNS is usually a chronic relapsing disease (**Fig. 17-1**). Fewer than 10% of patients will remain completely free of relapses after the initial episode. The rest can be divided into three categories. One third will have infrequent relapses that are easily managed by intermittent administration of courses of corticosteroids. Another third will have frequent relapses, defined as two or more relapses in a 6-month period.

However, they too are successfully managed with intermittent administration of courses of corticosteroids and do not manifest significant steroid-induced side effects. The final third comprises frequently relapsing patients and those with steroid dependence, defined as relapse occurring on alternate-day steroid treatment or within 2 weeks after discontinuing corticosteroids. It has proved difficult to predict the short-term prognosis (i.e., up to 2 years after disease onset) in individual patients. Those children who go into remission during the first week of corticosteroid treatment and who have no hematuria are more likely to be infrequent relapsers, defined as fewer than two relapses in 6 months or fewer than three in 1 year. The presence of small involuted glomeruli that can be distinguished from other causes of global glomerulosclerosis by the presence of vital podocytes and parietal epithelial cells may be a marker of frequently relapsing MCNS in children.

The last category of patients usually experience steroid toxicity and are candidates for the second-line treatments outlined later. Key steroid-induced side effects in children are impaired linear growth, obesity, behavioral changes, and cosmetic changes. Besides these clinical effects, children with MCNS also experience an altered quality of life and psychosocial adjustment that is linked both to illness-related variables and alterations in the family climate. In adults, additional evidence of steroid toxicity includes cataracts and altered bone density. Hypertension and hyperlipidemia occur across the age spectrum. It is this third category of patients who will require referral to a nephrologist for ongoing management and care.

LONG-TERM TREATMENT
Immunosuppressive Therapy

Second-line therapy is used for patients who relapse frequently or who are steroid dependent and manifest steroid side effects as a consequence of repeated exposure to the drug (**Table 17-1**). The first class of drugs used in these circumstances was

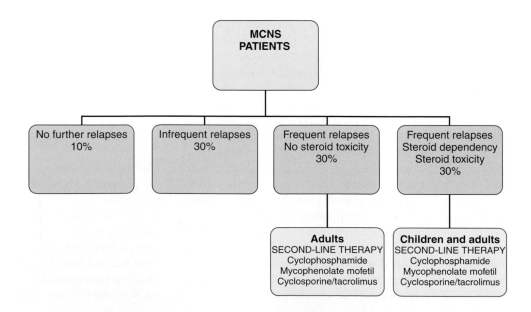

FIGURE 17-1 Minimal change nephrotic syndrome: short-term natural history.

alkylating agents such as cyclophosphamide or chlorambucil. They usually achieve a prolonged remission of at least 1 year in 70% of patients. Most patients require at least 12 weeks of therapy, and patients should be carefully monitored for side effects including leukopenia, infection, hemorrhagic cystitis (cyclophosphamide), gonadal toxicity, and malignancy. However, more than 25% of patients with MCNS who were treated with cyclophosphamide were not in sustained remission after puberty and required prolonged immunosuppressive treatment. Therefore, because of the serious toxicity associated with the alkylating agents and the guarded long-term effect, there has been greater reliance on alternative medications for frequently relapsing or steroid-dependent patients with MCNS.

Antimetabolites such as azathioprine or mycophenolate mofetil can reduce the relapse rate by approximately 50%, although they are not as effective as alkylating agents in inducing a permanent remission. They are useful because they have a more favorable side effect profile, can be administered for an extended period, and require less intensive monitoring.

Finally, a third option is a calcineurin inhibitor such as cyclosporine or tacrolimus. These agents can induce a prolonged remission in 80% to 90% of patients while the patient is taking the drug. However, they can cause undesirable cosmetic changes (hair growth and gingival hyperplasia), hepatotoxicity, hypertension, and nephrotoxicity. Therefore, patients taking calcineurin inhibitors for longer than 1 year may require periodic blood tests and serial kidney biopsies to ensure that irreversible renal injury does not occur.

The decision to recommend one of these medications in an effort to alleviate the adverse consequences of steroids must be weighed on an individual basis, taking into account the patient's age, gender, and likely compliance with treatment. Consideration should be given to the severity of the side effects, the likelihood of reversal of the complication, and the odds that the MCNS will spontaneously resolve. Although a number of other immunomodulatory agents have been tried in the past for patients with MCNS, the data have been collected in relatively small studies that hinder broad generalizations about efficacy. In addition, drugs such as levamisole are often not available in the United States for use in patients with MCNS. This underscores the need to develop newer agents that can be used to control proteinuria in patients with MCNS, especially in children with steroid toxicity and in adults with relapsing disease.

Supportive Care

After the initial diagnosis, patients with MCNS are usually monitored with daily dipstick testing for proteinuria. In most patients, relapses are detected by the onset of proteinuria for 3 or 4 consecutive days before edema ensues. Moreover, because proteinuria resolves rapidly in response to corticosteroid therapy, significant edema is not usually present. However, in those patients who develop edema before a relapse is recognized or who respond slowly to prednisone, edema can be controlled by prescribing a low-salt diet (2 g sodium per day) and oral diuretics. Options include loop diuretics such as furosemide (1 to 2 mg/kg/dose given once or twice daily) or a thiazide diuretic. The duration of action of the drugs may be diminished secondary to hypoalbuminemia and enhanced clearance, but this rarely is clinically significant, because the medications are only needed for 1 to 2 weeks, until proteinuria resolves. Children who have frequent relapses and persistent edema are at risk for bacterial peritonitis and can be given prophylactic penicillin. Immunization with the pneumococcal vaccine is also helpful under these circumstances; however, if feasible, the timing of vaccine administration should be delayed for at least 2 weeks after administration of prednisone, to ensure maximal immunologic response.

TABLE 17-1 Minimal Change Nephrotic Syndrome: Second-Line Treatments

DRUG	DOSE	EFFICACY	SIDE EFFECTS
Alkylating Agents			
Cyclophosphamide	*Children and adults:* 2-3 mg/kg/day × 8-12 wk*	Prolonged remission (>1 yr) in 70%	Leukopenia, hemorrhagic cystitis, alopecia, seizures, gonadal toxicity, malignancy
Chlorambucil	*Children and adults:* 0.15 mg/kg/day × 8-12 wk*		
Antimetabolites			
Mycophenolate mofetil	*Children:* 24-36 mg/kg/day OR 600 mg/m^2/dose bid *Adults:* 1-1.5 g bid	50% reduction in overall relapse rate	Gastrointestinal complaints, leucopenia, elevated liver enzymes
Calcineurin Inhibitors			
Cyclosporine	*Children and adults:* 4-6 mg/kg/day†	80-90% of patients achieve complete remission on treatment	Gingival hyperplasia (cyclosporine), tremor, elevated liver enzymes, nephrotoxicity
Tacrolimus	*Children and adults:* 0.05-0.3 mg/kg/day†		

*It is recommended that the duration of therapy be extended to 12 wk in patients with steroid-dependent disease.

†Target trough levels for cyclosporine and tacrolimus are 100-200 ng/ml and 4-8 ng/ml, respectively. Children may require more frequent dosing to maintain a therapeutic drug level.

PROGNOSIS

The prognosis for patients with MCNS is excellent; according to the literature, the disease eventually resolves without further relapses in more than 95% of patients. However, this presumed benign course is based on scarce data about patients followed into adulthood. A recent study of 42 adult patients (median age, 28 years) who were monitored for a median of 22 years after the diagnosis of MCNS demonstrated that 33% were still relapsing in adulthood. Pediatric patients who had a relapsing course and/or required immunosuppressive medications were more likely to have persistent disease in adulthood. Moreover, although final height was normal, almost half of the adult patients with relapsing MCNS had excess weight gain and osteoporosis.

Whether MCNS has any long-term effect on the incidence or age at onset of cardiovascular disease in adults remains unclear. Clinical outcomes in patients enrolled in large health maintenance organizations have indicated that nephrotic syndrome is associated with an increased incidence of atherosclerotic disease. The relative risk in patients with MCNS versus more refractory forms of idiopathic nephrotic syndrome requires further study. Based on the persistence beyond childhood of relapsing disease and the development of serious side effects, transition from a pediatric to an internal medicine nephrologist is warranted for patients who have relapsing MCNS or a history of prolonged steroid or immunosuppressive drug use for MCNS as they reach adulthood.

The overwhelming majority of children with MCNS have no evidence of a decline in kidney function. Recognizing that the diagnosis of FSGS can be difficult to establish if a kidney biopsy specimen does not include the few abnormal glomeruli at the corticomedullary junction, it is conceivable that the rare cases of presumed MCNS with a poor outcome and progression of chronic kidney disease may represent unidentified FSGS.

CONCLUSION

In summary, although MCNS is not a common illness, it causes short-term morbidity related to edema and infection. Initial treatment with corticosteroids results in remission of proteinuria in almost all patients. However, 90% of patients experience a frequently relapsing or steroid-dependent course with steroid toxicity. These patients are candidates for treatment with second-line drugs such as cyclophosphamide, mycophenolate mofetil, or tacrolimus. The choice of drug varies from center to center and reflects local experience and preferences of the individual physician. The long-term outcome is for preservation of the glomerular filtration rate. The disease can persist into adulthood and can lead to chronic sequelae such as bone demineralization, atherosclerosis, and obesity. Therefore, long-term follow-up is warranted in those patients who continue to relapse and require immunosuppressive medication. Further research is needed to better define the cause of MCNS (i.e., the immunologic basis and the role of podocyte protein abnormalities) in order to develop more effective treatments that can promote long-term remission without the side effects associated with current therapeutic options.

BIBLIOGRAPHY

Bazzi C, Petrini C, Rizza V, et al: A modern approach to selectivity of proteinuria and tubulointerstitial damage in nephrotic syndrome. Kidney Int 58:1732-1741, 2000.

Chesney RW: The changing face of childhood nephrotic syndrome. Kidney Int 66:1294-1302, 2004.

Constantinescu AR, Shah HB, Foote EF, Weiss LS: Predicting first-year relapses in children with nephrotic syndrome. Pediatrics 105:492-495, 2000.

Dijkman HBPM, Wetzels JFM, Gemnick JH, et al: Glomerular involution in children with frequently relapsing minimal change nephrotic syndrome: An unrecognized form of glomerulosclerosis? Kidney Int 71:44-52, 2007.

Fakhouri F, Bocqueret N, Taupin P, et al: Children with steroid-sensitive nephrotic syndrome come of age: Long-term outcome. J Pediatr 147:202-207, 2005.

Hlatky M: Is renal biopsy necessary in adults with nephrotic syndrome? Lancet 310:1264-1268, 1982.

Kitamura A, Tsukaguchi H, Hiramoto R, et al: A familial childhood-onset relapsing nephrotic syndrome. Kidney Int 71:946-951, 2007.

Knebelmann B, Broyer M, Grunfeld JP, Niaudet P: Steroid-sensitive nephrotic syndrome: From childhood to adulthood. Am J Kidney Dis 41:550-557, 2003.

Kyriels HA, Levtchenko EN, Wetzels JF: Long-term outcome after cyclophosphamide treatment in children with steroid-dependent and frequently relapsing minimal change nephrotic syndrome. Am J Kidney Dis 49:592-597, 2007.

Orth SR, Ritz E: The nephrotic syndrome. N Engl J Med 338:1202-1211, 1998.

Ruth EM, Landolt MA, Neuhaus TJ, Kemper MJ: Health-related quality of life and psychosocial adjustment in steroid-sensitive nephrotic syndrome. J Pediatr 145:778-783, 2004.

Sellier-Leclerc AKL, Duval A, Riveron S, et al: A humanized mouse model of idiopathic nephrotic syndrome suggests a pathogenic role for immature cells. J Am Soc Nephrol 18:2732-2739, 2007.

Stadermann MB, Lilien MR, van de Kar NCAJ, et al: Is biopsy required prior to cyclophosphamide in steroid-sensitive nephrotic syndrome? Clin Nephrol 60:315-317, 2003.

CHAPTER 18

Focal Segmental Glomerulosclerosis

Nidhi Aggarwal and Gerald B. Appel

Focal segmental glomerulosclerosis (FSGS) is a clinicopathologic syndrome associated with glomerular injury that may be either idiopathic or secondary to one of a number of other disorders (**Table 18-1**). The most common manifestation is proteinuria, which ranges from asymptomatic to nephrotic levels. FSGS accounts for 7% to 20% of cases of idiopathic nephrotic syndrome in children but as many as 35% of cases in adults. FSGS is the most common pattern of idiopathic nephrotic syndrome among African Americans, and in some series it is the most common pattern among all races. Recent U.S. studies have documented an increased incidence of FSGS in biopsies of adults, especially among nephrotic patients. This is true even in Caucasian populations. Untreated idiopathic FSGS frequently progresses to end-stage renal disease (ESRD). Among patients who do not experience a remission of the nephrotic syndrome, only 20% to 40% have kidney survival at 10 years. Patients with partial or complete remissions of nephrotic-range proteinuria have 10-year kidney survival rates of 65% to 90%. However, the ideal type and duration of immunosuppressive therapy as well as adjunctive therapy for idiopathic FSGS remain controversial.

PATHOLOGY

The histopathologic diagnosis of FSGS is characterized by areas of glomerular scarring in some glomeruli (focal lesions) in some parts of the glomerular tufts (segmental lesions) (**Fig. 18-1**). The diagnosis of "idiopathic" FSGS on renal biopsy requires the absence of lesions of other types of focal glomerulonephritis that could heal as focal sclerosing lesions and the absence of immune complex deposition by electron microscopy (EM). Immunoglobulin M (IgM) and C3 localized by immunofluorescence microscopy to the areas of segmental sclerosis are not infrequently seen, but they are believed to result from entrapment of immunoglobulin and complement components rather than from true immune complex deposition. The remainder of the glomerular tuft and the glomeruli unaffected by glomerulosclerosis typically have some degree of foot process effacement noted by EM, but they do not have evidence of immune complex deposition. Although biopsies taken early in the course, when renal function is still normal, show few glomeruli with segmental sclerosing lesions and almost no global sclerosis, there is still extensive foot process effacement in patients with large amounts of proteinuria. At a later stage, as renal function deteriorates, many glomeruli will show segmental or global sclerosis. Some investigators believe that the segmental sclerosing lesions are initially present in the juxtamedullary glomeruli and spread outward with time to involve the rest of the renal cortex. Interstitial fibrosis is also a common finding in biopsies with significant glomerulosclerosis.

Several morphologic variants of FSGS have recently been precisely defined (**Table 18-2**). These include a "tip" lesion, a perihilar lesion, a cellular variant, and a collapsing variant. If none of these features is present, the biopsy is classified as FSGS-NOS (not otherwise specified). Some variants

TABLE 18-1 Causes of Focal Segmental Glomerulosclerosis (FSGS)

Primary (Idiopathic) FSGS

Secondary FSGS

Genetic—mutations in podocin, α-actinin 4, WT-1, CD2AP, TRPC6, mitochondrial cytopathies

Viral related—human immunodeficiency virus, parvovirus B19

Medication- or drug-related—heroin, interferon-alfa, lithium, pamidronate

Associated with reduced nephron mass and hyperfiltration—oligomeganephronia, unilateral renal agenesis, renal dysplasia, reflux nephropathy, secondary to surgical or traumatic ablation, chronic allograft nephropathy, other causes of nephron loss

Other—obesity-related, hypertensive, atheroembolic, cyanotic congenital heart disease, sickle cell disease, Hodgkin's disease, non-Hodgkin's lymphoma

CD2AP, CD2-associated protein; TRPC6, the transient receptor potential cation channel 6; WT-1, Wilms' tumor 1.

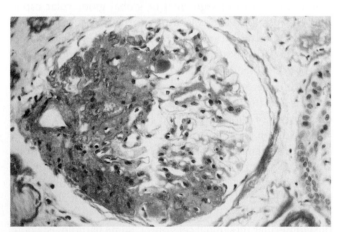

FIGURE 18-1 Glomerulus from a patient with focal segmental glomerulosclerosis, showing perihilar sclerosis with adhesion to Bowman's capsule (periodic acid–Schiff stain, original magnification ×300). (Courtesy of Dr. J. C. Jennette.)

TABLE 18-2 **Proposed Morphologic Classification of Focal Segmental Glomerulosclerosis (FSGS)**

FSGS-NOS—at least one glomerulus with segmental increase in matrix obliterating capillary lumina (excludes other variants)

Perihilar Variant—at least one glomerulus with perihilar hyalinosis

Cellular Variant—at least one glomerulus with segmental endocapillary hypercellularity occluding lumina with or without foam cells and karyorrhexis

Tip Variant—at least one segmental, either cellular or sclerosing lesion involving the outer 25% of the glomerulus next to the origin of the proximal tubule

Collapsing Variant—at least one glomerulus with segmental or global collapse and overlying podocyte hyperplasia.

NOS, not otherwise specified.

Modified from D'Agati VD, Fogo AB, Bruijn AJ, Jennette JC: Pathologic classification of focal segmental glomerulosclerosis: A working proposal. Am J Kidney Dis. 43:368-382, 2004.

have clearly been associated with a unique presentation and course. Others, although appearing different histologically, remain to be defined by distinct clinical features or response to therapy at this time. The glomerular "tip" lesion is characterized by the presence of at least one glomerulus with a segmental lesion with swelling, vacuolation, and proliferation of epithelial cells and later sclerosis and hyalinosis in the segment of the glomerulus adjacent to the origin of the proximal tubule. The remainder of the glomerulus has changes that are similar by light microscopy and EM to those seen in minimal change nephrotic syndrome (MCNS). This pattern is associated with a relatively good response to treatment and a better renal survival than classic FSGS.

The perihilar variant has at least one glomerulus with perihilar hyalinosis with or without sclerosis. The cellular variant has at least one glomerulus with segmental endocapillary hypercellularity occluding the lumina of the glomerular capillaries and does not appear to have unique clinical features or a unique course from other patterns of FSGS. Another variant of FSGS is associated with at least one glomerulus showing segmental or global glomerular capillary collapse and sclerosis with overlying visceral epithelial cell hypertrophy and hyperplasia similar to that seen in glomerulopathy associated with human immunodeficiency virus (HIV) infection. This so called "collapsing" variant of glomerulosclerosis is more common in African Americans and has a distinctive and more ominous clinical course than other forms of idiopathic FSGS.

In addition, there are a number of lesions often considered as variants of either MCNS or FSGS, including IgM nephropathy (a picture of minimal change by light microscopy but with positivity for IgM on immunofluorescence microscopy and with EM mesangial dense deposits), C1q nephropathy, and diffuse mesangial hypercellularity (mild proliferation of the glomerular mesangial cells only). Some pathologists note on the biopsy report any changes suggestive of secondary forms of FSGS, such as glomerulomegaly or less complete effacement of the visceral epithelial foot processes.

PATHOGENESIS

It has become clear that FSGS, once thought to be a uniform entity, is a syndrome with multiple causes, including disorders associated with genetic mutations, with an enhanced glomerular permeability, or with increased intracapillary glomerular pressure or glomerular hyperfiltration. In all of these conditions, the resultant phenotype is the focal sclerosing lesion. The pathogenesis of idiopathic FSGS, by definition, is unknown. Some patients who initially appear on biopsy to have minimal change disease are found to have FSGS on repeat biopsy. Whether this represents missed segmental lesions that were present on the initial biopsy in only a few glomeruli or the fact that minimal change disease and FSGS are really part of a continuum of disease is unknown.

Several genetic mutations produce the FSGS phenotype. All are related to defects in proteins involved in podocyte signaling or the structural apparatus of the slit diaphragm. Mutations in the podocyte gene *NPHS1* encode for defects in nephrin, and those in *NPHS2* encode for defects in podocin, both of which are proteins found at the slit diaphragm. Caucasian patients with podocin defects have autosomal recessive steroid-resistant FSGS. Defects in the actinin 4 gene lead to actinin 4 protein abnormalities of the podocytes, associated with steroid-resistant autosomal dominant FSGS. Mutations in *CD2AP* lead to abnormalities in the scaffolding protein, CD2-associated protein (CD2AP), which is involved in the regulation of actin cytoskeleton. Mutation of the transient receptor potential cation channel 6 (TRPC6) causes an increase of intracellular calcium in the podocytes and affects critical interactions with the podocyte structural proteins.

In idiopathic FSGS, a genetic predisposition may lead to susceptibility for a "second hit" phenomenon when the immune system is stimulated by viral or other insults. A number of animal models of FSGS have been created and are helping clarify the pathogenesis of the lesions in human FSGS. Although some studies have noted an association between FSGS and prior infection with parvovirus or other viruses, the data are far from consistent.

The plasma of some FSGS patients contains a circulating permeability factor which, in vitro, promotes the permeability of glomeruli to albumin. The presence of this permeability factor, which is not an immunoglobulin and has been defined as a small, hydrophobic glycoprotein, has been used to predict the rapid development of recurrent proteinuria in the allograft of some FSGS patients who reach ESRD and undergo transplantation. Moreover, some patients with recurrent FSGS in the allograft respond to plasmapheresis or use of a protein absorption column with a reduction in proteinuria, suggesting that the removal of this factor may reverse the disease.

The proteinuria in FSGS is often less selective than in minimal change disease, implying leakage of larger macromolecules through "larger pores" in the glomerular basement membrane. Drug-induced minimal change lesions in some animal models (e.g., puromycin nephrosis, doxorubicin nephrosis) can develop into a picture of FSGS with nonselective proteinuria. In these models, the nonselective proteinuria correlates with lifting off of the visceral epithelial foot processes from the glomerular basement membrane.

The pathogenesis of the glomerular sclerosing lesions and their progressive nature is unclear. Podocytes in several forms of FSGS display a dysregulated phenotype, with dedifferentiation and apoptosis. In collapsing FSGS, podocytes lose their highly differentiated cytoarchitecture. Humans with idiopathic FSGS often have, initially, a high glomerular filtration rate (GFR) and evidence of hyperfiltration, suggesting that hyperfiltration and increased intracapillary glomerular pressure may be mediators of FSGS. Likewise, in secondary FSGS, maladaptive hemodynamic alterations may be present in patients with reduced nephron numbers. Such patients with glomerulomegaly also have a high incidence of proteinuria, hyperfiltration, and FSGS. Secondary FSGS without increased glomerular capillary pressure or glomerulomegaly may relate to hyperlipidemia or alterations in intraglomerular coagulation.

It is likely that the pattern of FSGS seen on biopsy represents a common pathway for a number of distinct entities with different pathogenetic mechanisms and clinical courses.

CLINICAL FEATURES

Most patients with idiopathic FSGS present with proteinuria ranging from asymptomatic levels (10% to 30% of patients) to the full nephrotic syndrome. Children with asymptomatic proteinuria are most commonly detected by routine pediatric checkups and camp or sports physical examinations. In adults, asymptomatic detection occurs at military induction examinations, routine gynecologic or obstetric checkups, and insurance or employment physical examinations. Patients with the nephrotic syndrome usually present with edema.

Hypertension is found in 30% to 50% of children and adults with FSGS. Microscopic hematuria is found in 25% to 75% of these patients, and a decreased GFR is noted at presentation in 20% to 30%. Daily urinary protein excretion ranges from less than 1 g to between 20 and 30 g. Proteinuria is typically nonselective; that is, the urine contains not only albumin but also higher-molecular-weight proteins as well. Nevertheless, albumin still is the largest component of the urine protein. Complement levels and other serologic tests are normal. Occasionally, a patient has glycosuria, aminoaciduria, phosphaturia, or a concentrating defect indicating tubular damage as well as glomerular injury.

DIAGNOSIS

The diagnosis of FSGS requires a renal biopsy. Early on, only a minority of the glomeruli will have segmental sclerosing lesions. Even these lesions may show a predilection for the juxtamedullary region of the kidney, so the renal biopsy may look identical to that of MCNS. Likewise, a small sample of glomeruli in a biopsy in an older adult may show some glomeruli identical to minimal change disease and one or two globally sclerotic glomeruli. These may be the result of

FSGS or merely the obsolescent glomeruli that are found in the kidneys of older patients. The finding of tubulointerstitial damage in a biopsy otherwise described as minimal change disease also suggests the possibility of unobserved FSGS. Clinically, patients thought to have MCNS with a poor response to corticosteroids or other immunosuppressive agents are likely to have FSGS. The biopsy may also provide clues to a secondary form of FSGS. In HIV-associated nephropathy, there is often a collapsing variant of glomerulosclerosis with global rather than segmental involvement, and tubuloreticular inclusions are commonly found on EM. In patients with remnant kidneys and other forms of hyperfiltration-induced FSGS, there is often less effacement of the foot processes than in idiopathic FSGS, correlating with the lesser degrees of proteinuria.

COURSE AND THERAPY

Although variable, the course of untreated primary FSGS is usually one of progressive proteinuria and declining GFR. Patients with asymptomatic proteinuria typically develop the nephrotic syndrome over time. Only a small minority of patients (5% to 10%) experience a spontaneous remission of proteinuria and/or the nephrotic syndrome. Unfortunately, many children and adults have a similar course. Most develop ESRD 5 to 20 years after initial presentation. Several clinical and histologic features have been associated with a more rapid progression to renal failure in idiopathic FSGS, including African American race, higher serum creatinine and heavier proteinuria at biopsy, the collapsing pattern of FSGS, and more tubulointerstitial damage at biopsy (**Table 18-3**). On the other hand, patients with the "tip" lesion have a more favorable prognosis. During the course of treatment of FSGS, a partial or complete remission of the nephrotic syndrome at any time conveys a better prognosis.

Idiopathic FSGS may recur in a transplanted kidney, with severe proteinuria and the nephrotic syndrome, either immediately after transplantation or years later. Pediatric patients and those patients who present with a more rapid course to renal failure in their native kidneys are two groups at greater risk for recurrence in the allograft. Those with prior loss of an

TABLE 18-3	Risk Factors for Progressive Renal Disease in Focal Segmental Glomerulosclerosis (FSGS)
Clinical Features at Time of Biopsy	
Nephrotic-range proteinuria or massive proteinuria	
Elevated serum creatinine	
Black race	
Certain genetic mutations (e.g., podocin mutation in children)	
Histopathologic Features at Time of Biopsy	
Collapsing variant	
Tubulointerstitial fibrosis	
Clinical Features during the Course of the FSGS	
Failure to achieve partial or complete remission	

allograft due to recurrent FSGS are at highest risk for recurrence. Plasmapheresis has been used successfully to induce remissions of the proteinuria associated with recurrence, but the results are more favorable in children than in adults.

The treatment of FSGS is controversial, and there have been few randomized, controlled trials. Patients with a sustained remission of their nephrotic syndrome are unlikely to progress to ESRD, whereas those with unremitting nephrotic syndrome are likely to have progression. In early studies, only 10% to 30% of patients responded to corticosteroids or to other immunosuppressive agents with a remission of proteinuria, and most responders subsequently relapsed. Therefore, many American nephrologists considered FSGS to be unresponsive to therapy and did not advocate immunosuppressive treatment.

A seminal Canadian study in 1987 noted that 44% of children responded with a remission of proteinuria. The response rate for treated adults was similar (39%), but most adults did not receive any therapy. Other studies using corticosteroids and other immunosuppressive agents in FSGS have confirmed initial response rates of 25% to 60 %. Among pediatric patients, 20% to 25% experience a complete remission with a short course of corticosteroids, and up to 50% have remission with more intensive therapy. Among adults, an Italian study using much longer courses of prednisone, cyclophosphamide, and/or azathioprine found that 60% of FSGS patients had a complete remission of the nephrotic syndrome with excellent long-term renal survival. Subsequent trials in children and adults using either steroids alone or long-term immunosuppression with corticosteroids and cytotoxic agents also found high complete and partial remission rates of proteinuria and low rates of progression to renal failure. The median duration of steroid treatment to achieve complete remission is 3 to 4 months, with most patients responding by 6 months. Therefore, initial therapy should include at least 6 months of daily or alternate-day corticosteroids before steroid resistance is diagnosed. The dose of steroids is usually tapered after the first 6 to 8 weeks of therapy.

Several trials have used low-dose cyclosporine (4 to 6 mg/kg/day for 2 to 6 months) to treat steroid-resistant FSGS, with complete plus partial remission rates of 60% to 70%, compared with 17% to 33% in the placebo groups. The largest study, The North American Collaborative Study of Cyclosporine in Nephrotic Syndrome, reported 12% complete remission and more than 70% complete and/or partial remission with use of cyclosporine in steroid-resistant FSGS. Even patients who have been unresponsive to cytotoxic agents may respond to this therapy. Although there is a potential for increased renal damage from the cyclosporine itself, this blinded randomized trial showed better long-term preservation of renal function in the group receiving cyclosporine compared with placebo. Cyclophosphamide, often considered in the past as the second-line agent of choice after treatment failure with steroids, leads to a remission in fewer than 20% of adults. Therefore, many clinicians prefer to use cyclosporine or newer, less toxic alternative immunosuppressives.

Tacrolimus has also demonstrated high rates of complete and partial remission in patients with steroid-resistant or steroid-dependent nephrotic syndrome, in studies with smaller numbers of FSGS patients. However, calcineurin inhibitors should be avoided in patients with significant vascular or interstitial disease on renal biopsy and in those who have an estimated GFR of less than 40 mL/min/1.73 m^2, because of potential nephrotoxicity.

Several uncontrolled studies have documented successful treatment of steroid-resistant FSGS with mycophenolate, producing significant decreases in proteinuria without adversely affecting renal function. A current large, well-designed National Institutes of Health trial is comparing mycophenolate plus dexamethasone with cyclosporine alone for steroid-resistant FSGS.

Sirolimus has proved to have mixed results in steroid-resistant FSGS. Because this drug has been associated with new-onset de novo FSGS in kidney allografts, its current usage in FSGS should certainly be considered experimental.

In a study involving five pediatric patients with steroid-resistant nephrotic syndrome, rituximab led to complete remission in three patients and partial remission in two. Resolution of proteinuria with rituximab has also been seen in other FSGS patients. However, further studies are required to determine the efficacy and safety of this medication. Plasmapheresis, which has been successful in treating some patients with recurrent FSGS in a renal allograft, has not proved useful in patients with disease in their native kidneys.

At the present, the ideal regimen to treat idiopathic FSGS is unknown (**Table 18-4**). Many clinicians would not use immunosuppressives to treat patients who have subnephrotic

---

TABLE 18-4 Therapeutic Options in Focal Segmental Glomerulosclerosis (FSGS)

Immunosuppressive Therapy for Idiopathic FSGS

First-line therapy: corticosteroids (daily or every other day with taper for at least 6 mo)

Second-line therapy (or in those with increased risks from steroids (e.g., diabetes, obesity): cyclosporine, tacrolimus, mycophenolate, or cyclophosphamide

Experimental therapies: rituximab, sirolimus, plasmapheresis

For Secondary FSGS—Treatment Directed at the Underlying Etiology

Nephropathy associated with HIV infection: highly active antiretroviral therapy

Nephropathy associated with heroin use: discontinue use

Nephropathy related to use of pamidronate: discontinue the medication

Nephropathy related to obesity: weight loss

Nonimmunosuppressive Therapy for Both Idiopathic and Secondary Forms

Optimal blood pressure control (<130/80 mm Hg)

Use of ACE inhibitors or angiotensin receptor blockers

Optimal lipid control with the use of statins

Low-protein diet

ACE, angiotensin-converting enzyme; HIV, human immunodeficiency virus.

levels of proteinuria and show little damage on their renal biopsies. Almost all would just use angiotensin-converting enzyme inhibitors and/or angiotensin receptor blockers to reduce proteinuria. For patients at increased risk of renal failure, such as those with nephrotic-range proteinuria, elevated serum creatinine levels, and interstitial scarring on biopsy, most clinicians would treat with a prolonged course (at least 6 months) of daily or every-other-day corticosteroids (starting with 60 mg of prednisone daily or 120 mg every other day and tapering to lower doses after 6 to 8 weeks) or other immunosuppressive medication in the hope of inducing a remission of the nephrotic syndrome and preventing eventual ESRD. Many would avoid use of steroids entirely in patients who are morbidly obese or diabetic and instead turn directly to other immunosuppressive medications. Likewise, in patients with the collapsing variant, vigorous therapy with combination regimens including a calcineurin inhibitor are frequently used.

For patients with secondary forms of FSGS, treatment of the primary disorder, although rarely possible, is the first step in management. Some patients with FSGS secondary to obesity or heroin nephropathy have had remissions of proteinuria after weight reduction or cessation of drug use, respectively. Use of blockers of the renin-angiotensin system and other nonspecific methods to reduce proteinuria and the manifestations of the nephrotic syndrome may also be beneficial. Immunosuppressive medications have not yet been proven to be clearly effective in any form of secondary FSGS. In those patients with either primary idiopathic or secondary forms of the FSGS who remain nephrotic, control of fluid retention and edema can be managed with salt restriction and diuretics. In addition, attention should be given to control of hypertension to optimal levels (<130/80 mm Hg), to control of hyperlipidemia with diet and statins, and perhaps to prevention of hyperfiltration by avoidance of high-protein diets.

BIBLIOGRAPHY

Appel GB, Pollak M, D'Agati VD: Focal segmental gomerulosclerosis. In Johnson R, Floege J, Feehaly J (eds): Comprehensive Clinical Nephrology. Philadelphia, Mosby Elsevier, 2007, pp 217-230.

Appel GB, Waldman M, Radhakrishnan J: New approaches to the treatment of glomerular disease. Kidney Int 70:S45-S50, 2006.

Barisoni L, Kriz W, Mundel P, et al: The dysregulated podocyte phenotype: A novel concept in the pathogenesis of collapsing idiopathic FSGS and HIV associated nephropathy. J Am Soc Nephrol 10:51-61, 1999.

Cattran D, Appel GB, Hebert L, et al: A randomized trial of cyclosporine in patients with steroid resistant FSGS. Kidney Int 56:2220-2226, 1999.

Cattran DC, Wang MM, Appel G, et al: Mycophenolate mofetil in the treatment of focal segmental glomerulosclerosis. Clin Nephrol 62:405-411, 2004.

Choi MJ, Eustace JA, Gimenez LF, et al: Mycophenolate mofetil treatment for primary glomerular disease. Kidney Int 61:1098-1114, 2002.

Chun MJ, Korbet SM, Schwatz MM, Lewis EJ: FSGS in nephrotic adults: Presentation, prognosis, and response to therapy of the histologic variants. J Am Soc Nephrol 15:2169-2177, 2004.

D'Agati VD, Fogo AB, Bruijn AJ, Jennette JC: Pathologic classification of focal segmental glomerulosclerosis: A working proposal. Am J Kidney Dis. 43:368-382, 2004.

Duncan N, Dhaygude A, Owen J, et al: Treatment of focal and segmental glomerulosclerosis in adults with tacrolimus monotherapy. Nephrol Dial Transplant 19:3062, 2004.

Haas M, Spargo BH, Coventry S: Increasing incidence of FSGS among adult nephropathies: A 20-year renal biopsy study. Am J Kidney Dis 26:740-750, 1995.

Heering P, Braun N, Mullejans R, et al: Cyclosporin A and chlorambucil in the treatment of idiopathic focal segmental glomerulosclerosis. Am J Kidney Dis 43:10-18, 2004.

Kambham N, Markowitz GS, Valeri AM, et al: Obesity related glomerulomegaly: An emerging epidemic. Kidney Int 59:1498-1509, 2001.

Korbet SM: Treatment of primary focal and segmental glomerulosclerosis. Kidney Int 62:2301-2310, 2002.

Matalon A, Markowitz GS, Joseph RE, et al: Plasmapheresis treatment of recurrent FSGS in adult transplant recipients. Clin Nephrol 56:271-278, 2001.

Pei Y, Cattran D, Delmore T, et al: Evidence suggesting undertreatment of adults with idiopathic FSGS. Am J Med 82:938-944, 1987.

Pollak M: Inherited podocytopathies: FSGS and nephrotic syndrome from a genetic viewpoint. J Am Soc Nephrol 13:3016-3023, 2002.

Savin VJ, McCarthy ET, Sharma M: Permeability factors in FSGS. Semin Nephrol 23:147-161, 2003.

Schwimer JA, Markowitz GS, Valeri A, Appel GB: Collapsing glomerulopathy. Semin Nephrol 23:209-219, 2003.

Stokes MB, Markowitz GS, Lin J, et al: Glomerular tip lesion: A distinct entity within the minimal change disease/FSGS spectrum. Kidney Int 65:1690-1702, 2004.

Swaminathan S, Leung N, Lager DJ, et al. Changing Incidence of Glomerular Disease in Olmstead County, Minnesota: a 30 yr renal biopsy study. Clin J Am Soc Nephrol 2006; 1:483-7.

Thomas DB, Franceschini N, Hogan SL, et al: Clinical and pathologic characteristics of focal segmental glomerulosclerosis pathologic variants. Kidney Int 69:920-926, 2006.

Troyanov S, Wall CA, Miller JA, et al: for the Toronto Glomerulonephritis Registry Group: Focal and segmental glomerulosclerosis: Definition and relevance of a partial remission. J Am Soc Nephrol 16:1061-1068, 2005.

Valeri A, Barisoni L, Appel GB, et al: Idiopathic collapsing FSGS: A clinicopathologic study. Kidney Int 50:1734-1746, 1996.

Weins A, Kenlan P, Herbert S, et al: Mutational and biological analysis of alpha-actinin-4 in focal segmental glomeruloslcerosis. J Am Soc Nephrol 16:3694-3701, 2005.

Winn MP, Conlon PJ, Lynn KL, et al: A mutation in the TRPC6 cation channel causes familial FSGS. Science 308:1801-1804, 2005.

CHAPTER 19

Membranous Nephropathy

Daniel C. Cattran

Membranous nephropathy remains the most common histologic entity associated with adult-onset nephrotic syndrome. This histologic pattern is more properly called "glomerular nephropathy" than "glomerulonephritis," because there is rarely any inflammatory response in the glomeruli or interstitium (i.e., no nephritis). In most industrialized countries, the etiology is unknown in 70% to 80% of patients with membranous glomerular nephropathy (MGN), and the disorder is termed *idiopathic*. In the other 20% to 30% of cases, a defined cause can be identified, and the disease is categorized as *secondary*.

The list of known causes in **Table 19-1** is not complete but gives an indication of the variety of disorders that have been seen in association with this histologic pattern. In some, such as hepatitis B or thyroiditis, the specific antigen has been identified as part of the immune complex within the deposits in the glomeruli. In others, the association is less well defined, but the designation remains because treatment of the underlying condition or removal of the putative agent results in disappearance of the clinical and histologic features of the disease.

The renal manifestations of both the primary and secondary types of MGN are similar by clinical, laboratory, and histologic features; therefore, a careful history, with attention to potential secondary causes, must be obtained. Ongoing vigilance is also necessary, because the causative agent may not be obvious for months or even years after presentation. This histologic pattern is rare in children, and, if it is found, careful and repeated screenings for immunologically mediated disorders such as systemic lupus erythematosus are necessary. In the older patient, neoplasms become the most common cause of secondary MGN.

There are also marked geographic differences in etiology. In Europe and North America, by far the most common etiologic designation is idiopathic, but infectious agents account for a higher percentage of cases in other geographic areas. In Africa, for instance, malaria is a common cause; and in East Asia, hepatitis B.

CLINICAL FEATURES

MGN manifests in 60% to 70% of cases with features associated with the nephrotic syndrome, including edema, heavy proteinuria, hypoalbuminemia, and hypercholesterolemia. The other 30% to 40% of cases manifest with asymptomatic proteinuria, usually in the subnephrotic range (≤3.5 g/day). This is commonly found on urine testing done as part of a routine physical examination or as an insurance policy requirement. The majority of patients present with a normal glomerular filtration rate (i.e., a normal serum creatinine and creatinine clearance), but about 10% have diminished kidney function. The urine sediment is often bland, but 30% to 40% of patients have microhematuria, and 10% to 20% have granular casts. Hypertension is uncommon at presentation, occurring in only 10% to 20% of cases.

The clinical features associated with nephrotic-range proteinuria in MGN can be severe. The patient almost always has ankle swelling, but ascites, pleural effusions, and, rarely, pericardial effusions may be present. This pattern is particularly common in the elderly, and, unless a urinalysis is performed, these symptoms may be incorrectly labeled as signs of primary cardiac failure. Complications of this disorder include thromboembolic events and hyperlipidemia. Renal vein thrombosis has been found in 10% to 30% of cases at some time during the course of this disorder, and subsequent embolic events have been reported in up to 30% of patients. Secondary hyperlipidemia is also common and is characterized by increases in both total cholesterol and low-density lipoprotein (LDL) cholesterol, often with a decrease in high-density lipoproteins (HDL). This is a profile known to be associated with accelerated atherogenesis.

PATHOLOGY

In early idiopathic MGN, the glomeruli appear normal by light microscopy. Increasing size and number of immune complexes in the subepithelial space produce a thickening as

TABLE 19-1 Secondary Causes of Membranous Nephropathy

CAUSE	EXAMPLES
Neoplasm	Carcinomas (especially solid organ tumors of the lung, colon, breast, and kidney), leukemia, lymphoma (non-Hodgkin's)
Infections	Malaria, hepatitis B and C, secondary or congenital syphilis, leprosy
Drugs	Penicillamine, gold
Immunologic	Systemic lupus erythematosus, mixed connective tissue disease, thyroiditis, dermatitis herpetiformis
After renal transplantation	Recurrent disease, de novo membranous nephropathy
Miscellaneous	Sickle cell anemia

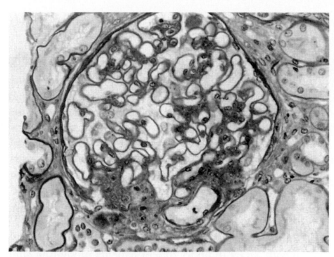

FIGURE 19-1 Glomerulus from a patient with membranous nephropathy. The capillary walls are diffusely thickened, and there is no increase in mesangial cells or matrix (periodic acid–Schiff stain, original magnification ×250).

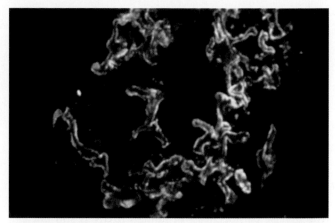

FIGURE 19-3 Glomerulus with diffuse granular capillary wall staining with anti–immunoglobulin G antibody (immunofluorescence microscopy, original magnification ×250).

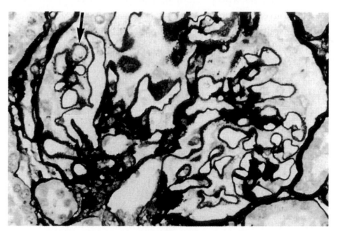

FIGURE 19-2 Classic spike pattern along glomerular basement membrane (GBM) as it grows around deposits (*arrow* at upper left) (periodic acid–Schiff stain, original magnification ×400).

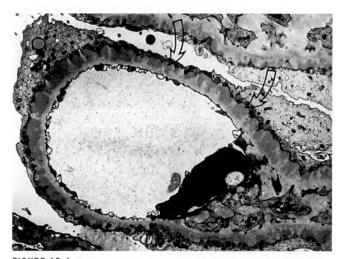

FIGURE 19-4 Electron photomicrograph of capillary loop with multiple electron-dense deposits along the subepithelial side of the GBM (*open arrows*) (original magnification ×7500).

well as a rigid appearance of the normally lacy-looking glomerular basement membrane (GBM) on light microscopy (**Fig. 19-1**). Over time, new GBM is formed around the immune complexes (deposits do not stain), producing the spikes along the epithelial side of the GBM that are particularly well visualized with the use of silver methenamine stains (**Fig. 19-2**). In contrast, on immunofluorescence microscopy, these immune complexes do stain, most commonly with anti–human immunoglobulin G (anti-IgG) and complement (**Fig. 19-3**). This produces a beaded appearance along the GBM (capillary wall) that is pathognomonic of MGN on immunofluorescence. In the most extreme cases, this beading can become so dense that careful examination is required to distinguish it from a linear pattern.

On electron microscopy, these deposits are initially formed in the subepithelial space (**Fig. 19-4**). A classification system has been developed based on the specific location of deposits on electron microscopic examination: in stage I, the deposits are located only on the surface of the

GBM in the subepithelial location, without evidence of new GBM formation; in stage II, the deposits are partially surrounded by new GBM; in stage III, they are surrounded and incorporated into the GBM; and in stage IV, the capillary walls are diffusely thickened, but rarefaction (lucent) zones are seen in intramembranous areas previously occupied by deposits. However, the clinical and laboratory correlations with these stages are poor. In some individual cases of MGN, the electron microscopic pattern appears as if there had been waves of complex deposition, with all of the preceding stages present in the same glomerulus; in other cases, the deposits appear as if there had been a continuous production of complexes, with the deposits growing in size over time, producing lesions that are all at a similar stage and that may extend from the surface of the subepithelial space and penetrate all the way through the GBM.

Although a specific cause cannot usually be determined by standard pathology, hints that may suggest a specific underlying cause can sometimes be seen. In a patient with systemic lupus erythematosus, for instance, more-mesangial cell proliferation and mesangial matrix formation may be present, and on immunofluorescent staining all of the immunoglobulins, rather than just IgG, may be seen along the capillary wall. In rare cases, a cause can be confirmed by the use of a specific antibody directed against the suspected causative agent. Such an example would be finding the carcinoembryonic antigen in the glomeruli of a patient with bowel cancer through use of the appropriate antibody.

PATHOGENESIS

The precise pathogenesis of human MGN is still unclear. In experimental animal models, lesions identical to human MGN have been produced by a variety of techniques using known antigens. However, the identification of the causative antigen in the majority of human cases has remained elusive. A recent report cast new light on the pathobiology of the disease. Several families were described in which a neonate was found to be nephrotic at birth and renal biopsies confirmed the classic MGN lesion. Subsequent evaluation showed mutations in neutral endopeptidase (NEP, an antigen normally found in the podocyte of the human glomerulus) of the mother. With pregnancy, the mother had formed antibodies to NEP, generated from exposure of the maternal circulation to the NEP antigen of the fetus. These anti-NEP antibodies crossed the placental barrier to the fetus and led to the in situ formation of immune complex in the subepithelial space of the glomeruli in the kidney of the fetus, with resultant damage to the GBM and the clinical findings of the nephrotic syndrome in the newborn.

The complexing of antigen and antibody in the subepithelial space is unique, because the binding occurs on the urinary side of the GBM. The subsequent activation of complement and cytokine factors is modified, because the site of the deposit is remote from the activators that are normally present in the circulation. The reduced response produces a lesion that looks benign on light microscopy (i.e., no inflammatory cells in the glomeruli or interstitium). The detection and the amount of the terminal complement membrane attack complex (C5b-9) in the urine (because complement deposition and activation occurs in the urinary space after the immune complex has been formed) has been reported to mirror both kidney survival and treatment efficacy. This has not been confirmed in prospective studies in humans, perhaps because of more recent data supporting tubular cell interactions with complement that produce the same terminal components even in non–MGN-related proteinuric kidney disease.

It is possible that there are susceptibility genes and genes associated with the more progressive variants, but these are probably polygenic traits, and the balance of hereditary factors versus environmental ones remains largely undetermined in this disorder.

DIAGNOSIS

MGN is a diagnosis based on histology. The idiopathic designation is made by exclusion. Secondary MGN is usually diagnosed by a careful history and physical and laboratory examinations aided by features identified on pathology. In the developed nations, most cases in the 20- to 55-year-old age range are idiopathic. In all patients that have clinical features suggestive of a secondary cause, however, investigations should include the appropriate screening tests, such as a complement profile and assays for antinuclear antibodies, rheumatoid factor, hepatitis B surface antigen and hepatitis C antibody, thyroid antibodies, and cryoglobulins.

Although idiopathic MGN remains the most common cause in all age groups, malignancy has been found in association with MGN in up to 20% of patients presenting after the age of 60 years. More recent epidemiologic data suggest that the standardized incidence ratio of malignancy in MGN is in the range of 2 to 3 in all age groups, independent of gender. Patients who present with MGN in this age category should have a focused history and physical examination, with the clinician looking for an occult tumor. Laboratory tests should include a chest radiograph (or better, a computed tomographic study of the thorax), examination for occult blood in the stools (or better, a colonoscopy), perhaps a mammogram in women, and a prostate-specific antigen assay in men. The precise cost/benefit ratio for this additional screening in the absence of symptoms remains unknown.

TREATMENT OF SECONDARY MEMBRANOUS GLOMERULAR NEPHROPATHY

In the secondary types of MGN, attention should be focused on removal of the putative agent or treatment of the underlying cause. If this can be done successfully, both the histopathology and the clinical manifestations will largely resolve with time.

NATURAL HISTORY AND TREATMENT GOALS OF IDIOPATHIC MEMBRANOUS GLOMERULAR NEPHROPATHY

The natural history of idiopathic MGN has been documented in several studies and must be understood before specific treatment is considered. Spontaneous complete remissions of proteinuria occur in 20% to 30% of patients with idiopathic MGN, and progressive kidney failure develops in 20% to 40% of cases, but only over 5 to 15 years of observation. In the remaining patients, mild to severe proteinuria persists. A summary review of 11 large studies demonstrated a 10-year kidney survival rate of 65% to 85%, and a more recent pooled analysis of 32 reports indicated a 15-year kidney survival rate of 60%. Complicating the understanding of the natural history is the fact that idiopathic MGN often follows a spontaneous remitting and relapsing course. Spontaneous complete remission rates have been reported in 20% to 30%

of long-term (>10 years) follow-up studies, with 20% to 50% of these cases having at least one relapse. A complete remission and a lower relapse rate are more common in patients with persistent low-grade (subnephrotic) proteinuria and in female patients. In contrast, male gender, age greater than 50 years, high levels of proteinuria (>6 g/day), abnormal kidney function at presentation, and tubulointerstitial disease (including focal and segmental lesions on biopsy) have all been associated with a lower renal survival rate.

Predicting Outcome

A semiquantitative method of predicting outcome has been developed and validated. It uses the clinical parameters of proteinuria and creatinine clearance estimates over fixed periods of time. In its simplest form, it demonstrated greatly improved overall accuracy in predicting outcome, compared with nephrotic-range proteinuria at presentation, when proteinuria values over 6-month time frames were monitored. If the proteinuria was 4 g/day or greater, the overall accuracy of the model was 71%; if 6 g/day or greater, 79%; and if 8 g/day, 84%. If the patient had a below-normal creatinine clearance estimation at the beginning of the period or deteriorating function during the 6 months of observation, the odds of progressing were higher. The advantages of the algorithm are that it requires only standard measurements of kidney function and that its nature is dynamic; that is, the risk can be calculated by measuring creatinine clearance and 24-hour urine protein estimates, and it can be calculated repeatedly over the period of follow-up. The issues of age, gender, degree of sclerosis, and hypertension are relevant but are not necessary in this model, because they do not add to its predictive ability.

A different approach to quantitation of outcome has been developed. It uses urinary excretion rates of large-molecular-weight proteins (e.g., IgG) that may reflect glomerular injury and can be combined with measurements of the urinary excretion rates of small-weight proteins (e.g., β_2-microglobulin) that may reflect damaged tubular cells. Excretion rates of these protein species above certain levels have also been reported to predict both treatment responsiveness and kidney survival

It is in light of this natural history background that current therapies must be evaluated. One helpful framework is to establish "risk of progression" categories based on the algorithm relating initial creatinine clearance, quantity of proteinuria, and change in function over 6 months to outcome. The following categories may be established:

1. Patients with low risk for progression have normal serum creatinine and creatinine clearance estimates and proteinuria of less than 4 g/day over 6 months of observation.
2. Medium-risk patients have normal or near-normal creatinine and creatinine clearance estimates and persistent proteinuria over 6 months of between 4 and 8 g/day.
3. High-risk patients include those with high-grade proteinuria (≥8 g/day) that is persistent over 3 to 6 months and/or creatinine clearance estimates declining during this observation period.

4. Alternatively, the finding of a urinary IgG excretion rate greater than 250 mg/24 hr and/or a urinary β_2-microglobulin clearance rate greater than 0.5 µg/min is associated with a higher likelihood of progressive MGN disease.

By examination of the laboratory data obtained at entry into the major clinical trials that are available, patients can be segregate into these risk categories. The treatment benefits in preventing progression compared to the risks associated with treatment are then easier to assess. This is important, because most of the current immunosuppressive routines have potentially significant adverse effects, and these, rather than the symptoms of the disease, are often the overriding concern of both physicians and patients dealing with this disease.

Response Goals

The appropriate target for treatment in MGN has been debated for some time. Obviously, the best outcome would be a permanent state of complete remission (<0.15 g/day proteinuria), but with current approaches this happens in only 30% to 50% of cases, even when spontaneous remissions are combined with those that occur in response to specific drug treatment. However, there is now good evidence that an appropriate and valid target is the achievement of a state of partial remission (<3.5 g/day and a 50% reduction from peak proteinuria). Achieving a partial remission is associated with both a very significant slowing in the rate of kidney disease progression and a doubling of renal survival at 10 years, compared with patients who do not have a remission.

TREATMENT OF IDIOPATHIC MEMBRANOUS GLOMERULAR NEPHROPATHY

Treatment can be considered in four broad categories:
1. Nonspecific, nonimmunosuppressive therapy focused on reducing proteinuria and perhaps secondarily slowing the progression rate of the kidney disease
2. Immunosuppressive therapy aimed at slowing or stopping the immune-mediated component of the disease
3. Treatment of the effects of the disease on other systems
4. Treatment aimed at reducing the complications of the immunosuppressive drugs

Specific Immunosuppressive Treatments

Patients with a Low Risk for Progression

The prognosis of patients with a low risk for progression based on their level of proteinuria and function (i.e., asymptomatic proteinuria ≤4 g/day with normal kidney function) is excellent. In a series of more than 300 cases from three distinct geographic regions that were followed for more than 5 years, fewer than 8% of patients went on to develop a decrease in kidney function. Normalization of the blood pressure and reduction of protein excretion through the use of agents such as angiotensin-converting enzyme (ACE) inhibitors and/or angiotensin receptor blockers (ARBs) should be used. Because the percentage of patients who progress is not zero, long-term follow-up should include regular measurements of blood pressure and kidney function, including protein excretion. Immunosuppressive therapy is not recommended as long as patients remain in this low-risk category. Approximately 50% of patients who present with non-nephrotic proteinuria in MGN eventually progress to nephrotic-range proteinuria. In most cases (70%), this progression occurs during the first year after biopsy has confirmed the diagnosis

Patients with a Medium Risk for Progression

There is evidence for a benefit of treatment when corticosteroids are combined with a cytotoxic agent. In a series of randomized trials from Italy, significant increases in both partial and complete remission in proteinuria and long-term improved kidney survival at 10 years were seen after an initial 6-month course of corticosteroids and chlorambucil. Therapy consisted of 1 g of intravenous methylprednisolone on the first 3 days of months 1, 3, and 5, followed by 27 days of oral methylprednisolone at 0.4 mg/kg/day, alternating in months 2, 4, and 6 with chlorambucil at 0.2 mg/kg/day. This therapeutic regimen was compared by the same authors to no specific treatment, to methylprednisolone alone, and to cyclophosphamide substituted for chlorambucil. In their first study comparing chlorambucil/prednisone versus no treatment, 40% of untreated patients reached end-stage renal disease after 10 years, compared with only 8% of treated patients. Proteinuria also improved with this regimen: the non-nephrotic state was maintained during 58% of the follow-up time in the treatment group, compared with 22% of the time in the control group. When this regimen was compared with methylprednisolone alone, there was a significant initial benefit in the patients receiving the combination therapy, but this difference was not significant by the end of 4 years of follow-up. The original regimen was remarkably safe, with only 4 of 42 treated patients stopping therapy. All adverse events were reversed after stopping the drugs.

When 2.5 mg/kg/day oral cyclophosphamide was substituted for chlorambucil and compared with the original regimen, similar results in terms of complete and partial remission rates of proteinuria were observed. However, a substantial relapse rate of approximately 30% was seen within 2 years in both groups, regardless of whether they were treated with chlorambucil or cyclophosphamide. Fewer patients had to discontinue cyclophosphamide (5%) compared with the chlorambucil (14%). Kidney function was equally well preserved in both groups for up to 3 years. Similar improvement in long-term results using this same regimen was recently reported from a randomized, controlled trial in India. Other regimens using longer-term cyclophosphamide (1 year) together with lower-dose prednisone have also demonstrated an improved outcome, although in these studies the patients were compared with historical controls and not in a prospective, randomized, controlled trial. These results are in contrast to those of other uncontrolled studies, in which cyclophosphamide alone was used; in those studies,

the frequency of remission was found to be similar to that in untreated patients. Mycophenolate mofetil, a newer immunosuppressive agent that has proved effective in reducing rejection in the field of solid organ transplantation but is associated with less toxicity than cyclophosphamide, has also been used in treatment trials of patients with MGN. Initial results have been similar to those observed with cyclophosphamide therapy but with a significantly higher relapse rate (70% by 3 years after treatment).

A different regimen using the immunosuppressive agent cyclosporine showed results similar to those of the cytotoxic/steroid regimen in terms of improving proteinuria in the group of patients with medium risk for progression. Those patients who remained nephrotic after a minimum of 6 months of observation and were unresponsive to a course of high-dose prednisone were given 6 months of cyclosporine (3 to 5 mg/kg/day) plus low-dose prednisone (maximum of 10 mg/day) and compared with a group receiving placebo plus prednisone. Complete or partial remission of proteinuria was seen in 70% of the cyclosporine group, compared with 24% of the control group. There was no difference in kidney survival, but the follow-up period was relatively short at 2 years. Relapses were common, with a rate similar to that seen in the Italian cytotoxic trials—approximately 35% within 2 years after discontinuation of the drug. A recent study using more prolonged cyclosporine treatment at a dose of 2 to 4 mg/kg/day showed a much lower relapse rate of approximately 20% within the 2-year period following a 50% reduction in the cyclosporine dosage (maintaining the cyclosporine therapy in the range of 1.5 mg/kg/day). More recently a 12-month randomized, controlled trial using monotherapy with tacrolimus (a different calcineurin inhibitor) confirmed the benefit of this class of agents, producing a partial or complete remission in proteinuria in 75% to 80% of the treated group as well as a significant slowing in the progression rate of the kidney disease compared to a control group.

Corticosteroids such as prednisone alone have been shown to be ineffective in inducing remission of proteinuria in all controlled trials conducted to date and in preventing progression in all but one study. Although the follow-up periods were limited to less than 4 years and the dose and duration of corticosteroid treatment varied, it is generally held that these drugs alone should not be used in the treatment of idiopathic MGN. This view was supported by a meta-analysis of studies using corticosteroids alone in MGN. A recent report (although not a controlled trial) in patients from Japan did show a benefit for prednisone therapy alone, suggesting that there may be a specific racial effect to this class of drugs in the treatment of MGN.

Newer therapeutic options have included year-long injections of synthetic adrenocorticotrophic hormone (ACTH). There have been two small but controlled trials with this agent showing short-term benefits similar to the results seen with the cytotoxic/steroid regimen, with relatively minor adverse effects. These results need to be confirmed but do seem to suggest that this regimen could be used as an alternative to the options previously described. The mechanism underlying this benefit is currently unknown. Another exciting potential alternative agent is rituximab, the chimeric monoclonal antibody to B cells carrying the CD20 epitope. In two small pilot trials, the use of this drug as monotherapy resulted in a complete or partial remission of proteinuria in approximately 66% of the patients by the end of 1 year of follow-up. Moreover, in the later of these pilot studies, the patients were a selected cohort that had been resistant to many of the other treatment options.

Patients with a High Risk for Progression

The group of MGN patients with a high risk for progression includes those with worsening kidney function and/or persistent high-grade proteinuria. The percentage of patients with idiopathic MGN in this category is small, and randomized, controlled trials focused on this subgroup are rare. In most cases, if an improvement in proteinuria with conservative therapy is not seen within the first 3 months, an earlier start to immunosuppressive therapy is often warranted. In terms of randomized, controlled trials, only the use of cyclosporine in patients with documented renal disease progression has been reported. In that trial, 17 of 64 patients in the conservative, pretreatment phase of the study fulfilled the entry criterion of an absolute reduction in kidney function (10 mL/min reduction in creatinine clearance). These patients were randomized to receive either cyclosporine or placebo for 1 year. Cyclosporine produced a substantial improvement in proteinuria, compared with placebo, that was sustained for up to 2 years in 50% of cases. The rate of progression, as measured by the slope of the change in creatinine clearance, was significantly slowed compared with the predrug period (>60% during cyclosporine treatment), but there was no improvement in the placebo group. This drug has substantial nephrotoxic potential, and monitoring for nephrotoxic and other adverse events must be part of any treatment routine that includes this class of agent.

The use of cytotoxic drugs in this category of patients has been limited. One such study reported the treatment of a small group of patients who had progressive deterioration in kidney function with prednisone, 1 mg/kg tapering over 6 months to 0.5 mg/kg every other day, plus chlorambucil, 0.15 mg/kg for 14 weeks, and found a significant improvement in both proteinuria and kidney survival at 8 years, compared with an historical control group with similar presenting characteristics. Recent reports have compared more prolonged cytotoxic therapy (i.e., 1 year of cyclophosphamide plus prednisone—see details in the discussion of treatment for medium-risk patients) and found that even repeated courses (up to three) benefited these patients in terms of reducing proteinuria and slowing the rate of renal disease progression. Obviously, the risks associated with prolonged and repeated exposure to this potent cytotoxic agent, particularly in relation to the increasing incidence of cancer as drug exposure increases, must be considered. In contrast, in a randomized trial in patients with idiopathic MGN who had documented progression, treatment by pulse cyclophosphamide combined with pulse methylprednisolone and oral

prednisone failed to show any significant benefit when compared with prednisone alone.

Although the algorithm for the management of the high-risk patient (**Fig. 19-5**) lists the option of switching to the regimen cytotoxics plus prednisone if there is a failure to respond to cyclosporine, it must be realized that both options are powerful immunosuppressive regimens and carry significant risks of infection. In addition, if renal impairment is significant, the dose of cyclophosphamide must be adjusted downward to avoid the risk of significant bone marrow toxicity. The decision to treat this group is not to be undertaken without careful consideration of the risks to the patient, and often a second opinion is warranted before initiating this therapy.

Three small, uncontrolled studies from several years ago used a modification of the Italian regimen (prednisone alternating monthly with chlorambucil) in patients with MGN and progressively deteriorating kidney function. Among a total of 34 patients, approximately 50% showed sustained improvement in kidney function, but the rate of adverse effects was high even with the appropriate reduction in dosage of chlorambucil. Two smaller, nonrandomized trials also showed a benefit to long-term oral cyclophosphamide with and without prednisone therapy. However, prolonged cytotoxic therapy did result in significant problems, and these results have limited the use of this treatment regimen.

Monotherapy with steroids in high-risk patients has not been tested. A subgroup analysis of patients with abnormal

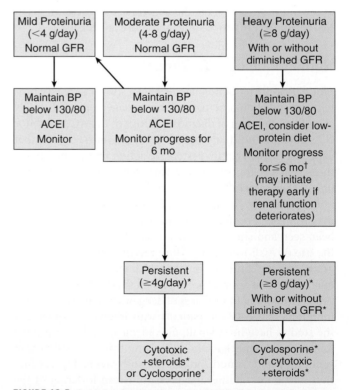

FIGURE 19-5 Guideline for the treatment of idiopathic membranous nephropathy. Patients may change from one category to another during the course of follow-up. Asterisks indicate risk-reduction strategies. ACEI, angiotensin-converting enzyme inhibitor; BP, blood pressure (mm Hg); GFR, glomerular filtration rate.

kidney function at the time of diagnosis from one of the corticosteroid-alone trials found no difference in the rate of deterioration over 4 years of follow-up between the prednisone-treated group and the control group. One small, uncontrolled trial using pulse methylprednisolone for 5 days followed by a tapering dose of prednisone did show initial stabilization in 15 patients of their chronic kidney disease. By the time of follow-up, however, 2 patients had died and 5 had gone on to end-stage renal disease, suggesting only a transient benefit. These data support the view that corticosteroids alone are not effective in slowing the progression rate in patients with a high risk of progression.

Specific treatment as well as therapy directed toward secondary effects of the disease may need to be started before the end of the intended monitoring time in these patients, especially if there is associated deterioration in filtration function (i.e., an increase in serum creatinine) persistant high grade (>8g/day) proteinuria.

Other Treatments

A large number of other therapies have been tried in this disorder. The reported studies have been small or uncontrolled, or the series have included patients in a variety of risk categories. Some have been focused on treating the downstream inflammatory effects of the disease (e.g., with eculizumab and a C5b-9 inhibitor), others on the possible benefits of antioxidant therapy (e.g., probucol) or the potential role of antifibrotic agents (e.g., pentoxifylline). There is insufficient evidence at the moment to support the general use of these agents in MGN. Studies are proceeding, and more are needed.

Nonimmunologic Treatments

Blood pressure reduction has also been shown to reduce proteinuria and should be part of the management of all MGN cases from the time of diagnosis. Drugs of the ACE inhibitor class have produced improvement in proteinuria beyond that expected by their antihypertensive action alone, and, unless there is a specific contraindication, they should be the first line of therapy in all cases, even when the blood pressure is not significantly elevated. Similar results from ARBs in the management of proteinuria in diabetic nephropathy have also been seen and should be considered if problems arise with the use of ACE inhibitors. More recently, studies have suggested that the combination of an ACE inhibitor with an ARB may be the best approach. Some data suggest there is a renal protective benefit to this class of drug or combination of ACE inhibitors and ARBs in patients with idiopathic MGN, but the studies have been small, uncontrolled, and with limited follow-up. The mechanism underlying this potential benefit is not fully understood, but it is not solely related to a reduction in the intraglomerular pressure (from lowering of the systemic blood pressure). The effect on progression has also been examined using these conservative measures. Stabilization of function may occur, because the decrease in protein trafficking across the tubular cell results in reduced interstitial

toxicity. Patients with idiopathic MGN have been included in these studies, but not in sufficient numbers to allow a determination as to whether a specific benefit in this particular type of glomerular disease occurs with these agents.

Other nonspecific measures to reduce proteinuria and perhaps slow the rate of kidney disease progression have been studied. Although dietary protein restriction has never been associated with a complete remission of the nephrotic syndrome, it does have its biggest impact in reducing proteinuria and in slowing progression in patients with the highest grades of proteinuria. Certainly many patients with idiopathic MGN fulfill this criterion. However, overdoing the dietary protein restriction risks malnutrition, and it is important to monitor this closely and compensate for the high urinary protein losses by additions to the diet.

Treatment of the Secondary Effects of the Disease

In addition to the efforts to reduce proteinuria and prevent kidney failure, attention must be directed to the associated hyperlipidemia and the increased risks for thromboembolism in patients with idiopathic MGN. Patients with the nephrotic syndrome have elevated serum cholesterol and triglycerides, with normal or low levels of HDL and increased LDL. This hyperlipidemia probably plays a role in the increased risk for cardiovascular disease in patients with prolonged high-grade proteinuria. Although no trial has been conducted to determine whether cholesterol lowering reduces the risk for cardiovascular disease in such patients, most clinicians apply evidence from nonrenal patients to advocate the use of statins in patients with idiopathic MGN and persistent high-grade proteinuria. A recent meta-analysis did show a small benefit in regard to proteinuria with the use of statins, although no beneficial effect on glomerular filtration rate in these proteinuric conditions could be determined. The addition of ezetimibe, the inhibitor of cholesterol absorption from the gut, is certainly possible for patients whose LDL remains high despite statin therapy or for those in whom statins cannot be used because of adverse effects.

Studies of the risk for thrombotic disease in idiopathic MGN have shown a wide variation in prevalence. This is partly related to the rigor of screening (all patients versus selection of high-risk patients) and partly to the detection methods used. In a recent review, deep venous thrombosis was reported in 11% of patients with idiopathic MGN, clinically significant pulmonary emboli in 11%, and renal vein thrombosis in 35%. Certainly, if this incidence of thromboembolic events is viewed in the light of data from patients receiving long-term anticoagulants for nonrenal indications, the benefits would appear to outweigh the risks. However, other studies have reported a lower incidence rate and a higher-than-average risk with long-term anticoagulant therapy, given the hypoalbuminemic state of these patients. No consensus has emerged as to whether prophylactic anticoagulation should be used in this disease. A majority of physicians use this therapy as primary prevention only in high-risk cases or reserve its use until after documentation of a thromboembolic event. A positive family history, a previous thrombotic event before the patient was known to have MGN, and a prolonged serum albumin level lower than 2.0 g/dL are indicators that should prompt earlier use of prophylactic anticoagulation. The precise mechanism of this hypercoagulable state is unclear, although a variety of factors do converge that heighten the thrombotic risk, including a local decrease in perfusion pressure in the renal vein (from the lowered oncotic pressure), loss of clotting factors in the urine, increased hepatic production of clotting factors, and perhaps even a genetic predisposition to clot.

Treatment Prophylaxis

Many large studies in the kidney transplantation field and in postmenopausal women have indicated that agents such as bisphosphonates reduce bone loss during long-term use of corticosteroids. Certainly, the use of such agents in patients with idiopathic MGN should be considered if the course of therapy includes prolonged prednisone treatment.

Trimethoprim-sulfamethoxazole has reduced the incidence of *Pneumocystis carinii* pneumonia (PCP) in patients receiving prolonged immunosuppressive therapy in both the transplantation field and in certain autoimmune diseases. Its use when the patients with idiopathic MGN are exposed to prolonged glucocorticoid treatment, cytotoxic agents, or calcineurin inhibitors seems prudent.

MANAGEMENT PLAN

Figure 19-5 gives a graphic display of a treatment framework for patients with idiopathic MGN. In addition, the following general rules should be applied.
1. Establish whether the disease is primary or secondary, and take appropriate actions for known causes.
2. For patients with idiopathic MGN, monitor kidney function over a 6-month period (3 months for patients at high risk) and establish a "risk for progression" score.
3. If persistent nephrotic-range proteinuria or deterioration in kidney function occurs despite maximum conservative therapy, introduce treatment for the secondary effects of the disease, including a lipid-lowering agent and possibly anticoagulants.
4. Introduce risk-reduction strategies such as bisphosphonates if long-term corticosteroids are used and trimethoprim-sulfamethoxazole if long-term immunosuppressive drugs are used.
5. The first choice as specific therapy for patients with a medium risk for progression is chlorambucil or cyclophosphamide plus prednisone for 6 months, or cyclosporine combined with low-dose prednisone for 6 to 12 months.
6. Specific therapy for high-risk patients should be cyclosporine for 6 to 12 months. If this fails, a short course of chlorambucil combined with up to 6 months of prednisone should be considered.
7. If both regimens fail and the clinical status warrants further attempts at treatment, consider one of the newer treatments, such as ACTH therapy or rituximab.
8. A significant proportion of patients who achieve either partial or complete remission experience relapse. Retreatment with the previously successful regimen (or with one of the other proven routines if toxicity is a major concern) should be undertaken. The case should not be labeled a treatment failure, because even a partial remission is associated with significantly improved kidney survival.

BIBLIOGRAPHY

Alexopoulos E, Papagianni A, Tsamelashvili M, et al: Induction and long-term treatment with cyclosporine in membranous nephropathy with the nephrotic syndrome. Nephrol Dial Transplant 21:3127-3132, 2006.

Adachi JD, Benson WG, Brown J, et al: Intermittent etidronate therapy to prevent corticosteroid induced osteoporosis. N Engl J Med 337:382-387, 1997.

Bjorneklett R, Viksc BE, Svarstad E, et al: Long-term risk of cancer in membranous nephropathy patients. Am J Kidney Dis 50: 396-403, 2007.

Branten AJ, du Buf-Vereijken PW, Klasen IS, et al: Urinary excretion of beta 2 microglobulin and IgG predict prognosis in idiopathic membranous nephropathy: A validation study. J Am Soc Nephrol 16:169-174, 2005.

Branten AJ, du Buf-Vereijken, Vervloet M, Wetzels JF: Mycophenolate mofetil in idiopathic membranous nephropathy: A clinical trial with comparison to a historical control group treated with cyclophosphamide. Am J Kidney Dis 50:248-256, 2007.

Branten AJ, Reichert LJ, Koene RA, et al: Oral cyclophosphamide versus chlorambucil in the treatment of patients with membranous nephropathy and renal insufficiency. Q J Med 91:359-366, 1998.

Cattran DC, Appel GB, Hebert LA, et al: Cyclosporine in patients with steroid resistant membranous nephropathy: A randomized trial. Kidney Int 59:1484-1490, 2001.

Cattran DC, Greenwood C, Ritchie S, et al: A controlled trial of cyclosporine in patients with progressive membranous nephropathy. Canadian Glomerulonephritis Study Group. Kidney Int 47:1130-1135, 1995.

Cattran DC, Pei Y, Greenwood CM, et al: Validation of a predictive model of idiopathic membranous nephropathy: Its clinical and research implications. Kidney Int 51:901-907, 1997.

Debiec H, Guigonis V, Mougenot B, et al: Antenatal membranous glomerulonephritis due to anti-neutral endopeptidase antibodies. N Engl J Med 346:2053-2060, 2002.

Fervenza FC, Cosio FG, Ericsson SB, et al: Rituximab treatment of idiopathic membranous nephropathy. Kidney Int 73:117-125, 2007.

The GISEN Group: Randomized placebo-controlled trial of the effect of ramipril on decline in glomerular filtration rate and risk of terminal renal failure in proteinuric, non-diabetic nephropathy. (Gruppo Italiano di Studi Epidemiologici in Nefrologia). Lancet 349:1857-1863, 1997.

Honkanen E, Tornroth T, Gronhagen-Riska C: Natural history, clinical course and morphological evolution of membranous nephropathy. Nephrol Dial Transplant 7(Suppl 1):35-41, 1992.

Jha V, Ganguli A, Saha TK, et al: A randomized, controlled trial of steroids and cyclophosphamide in adults with nephrotic syndrome caused by idiopathic membranous nephropathy. J Am Soc Nephol 18:1899-1904, 2007.

Laluck BJ Jr, Cattran DC: Prognosis after a complete remission in adult patients with idiopathic membranous nephropathy. Am J Kidney Dis 33:1026-1032, 1999.

Nicholas TL, Radhakrishnan J, Appel GB: Hyperlipidemia and thrombotic complications in patients with membranous nephropathy. Semin Nephrol 23:406-411, 2003.

Praga M, Barrio V, Juarez GF, et al: Tacrolimus mono therapy in membranous nephropathy: A randomized controlled trial. Kidney Int 71:924-930, 2007.

Ponticelli C, Passerini P, Salvadori M, et al: A randomized pilot trial comparing methylprednisolone plus a cytotoxic agent versus synthetic adrenocorticotrophic hormone in idiopathic membranous nephropathy. Am J Kidney Dis 47:233-240, 2006.

Ponticelli C, Zucchelli P, Passerini P, et al: A 10-year follow-up of a randomized study with methylprednisolone and chlorambucil in membranous nephropathy. Kidney Int 48:1600-1604, 1995.

Rabelink TJ, Zwaginga JJ, Koomans HA, et al: Thrombosis and hemostasis in renal disease. Kidney Int 46:287-296, 1994.

Ruggenenti P, Chiurchiu C, Brusegan V, et al: Rituximab in idiopathic membranous nephropathy: A one-year prospective study. J Am Soc Nephrol 14:1851-1857, 2003.

Schieppati A, Mosconi L, Perna A, et al: Prognosis of untreated patients with idiopathic membranous. N Engl J Med 329:85-89, 1993.

Torres A, Dominguez-Gil B, Carreno A, et al: Conservative versus immunosuppressive treatment of patients with idiopathic membranous nephropathy. Kidney Int 61:219-227, 2002.

Troyanov S, Roasio L, Pandes M, et al: Renal pathology in idiopathic membranous nephropathy: A new perspective. Kidney Int 69:1641-1648, 2006.

Troyanov S, Wall CA, Miller JA, et al: Idiopathic membranous nephropathy: Definition and relevance of a partial remission. Kidney Int 66:1199-1205, 2004.

Wheeler DC, Bernard DB: Lipid abnormalities in the nephrotic syndrome: Causes, consequences, and treatment. Am J Kidney Dis 23:331-346, 1994.

CHAPTER 20

Immunoglobulin A Nephropathy and Related Disorders

Ronald J. Hogg

Immunoglobulin A (IgA) nephropathy, or IgAN, is defined by the presence of IgA deposits in glomerular mesangial areas, sometimes accompanied by IgA deposits in other areas of the glomeruli, in the absence of coexisting diseases such as systemic lupus erythematosus. These deposits may be accompanied by other immunoreactants, but the IgA must be dominant or codominant. The condition was first described by Professor Jean Berger and his colleagues in the late 1960s. The original description of the condition indicated that it was relatively mild. However, it is now known that the renal histologic abnormalities in patients with IgAN range from virtually normal to severe proliferative glomerulonephritis. The clinical course may indeed be mild, or it may lead to end-stage renal disease. In the later stages of disease, glomerulosclerosis may predominate. The condition was originally called Berger's disease, but this term has been replaced by the descriptive name, IgAN.

RENAL BIOPSY FINDINGS

Light Microscopy

In most cases, there is focal or diffuse mesangial hypercellularity that may vary from mild to severe (**Fig. 20-1**). Mesangial hypercellularity is accompanied by an increase in mesangial matrix that may be more evident than the increase in cellularity.

Endocapillary lesions may be proliferative or sclerosing. In some biopsies, the histology may even resemble that of focal segmental glomerulosclerosis. Extracapillary hypercellularity is often associated with a more aggressive clinical course. Crescentic glomerulonephritis, in which more than 50% of the glomeruli contain crescents, is observed in approximately 5% of cases. In mild cases, the tubulointerstitium appears normal, whereas in patients with progressive disease, tubular injury often results in fibroproliferative changes and infiltration of inflammatory cells. More severe cases may exhibit significant interstitial fibrosis and tubular atrophy.

Immunohistology

The presence of IgA in the glomeruli may be demonstrated either by immunofluorescence of unstained frozen sections or by immunoperoxidase staining of paraffin sections. C3 is usually present in addition to IgA, but C1q is typically absent. IgG and IgM are seen in approximately 50% of biopsies, although they are usually less dominant than IgA (**Fig. 20-2**).

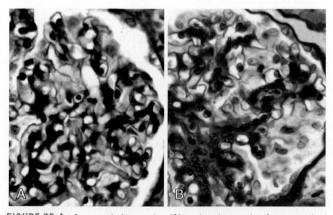

FIGURE 20-1 A normal glomerulus (**A**) and a glomerulus from a patient with immunoglobulin A nephropathy (**B**). Note that the glomerulus in **B** has increased mesangial hypercellularity and increased mesangial matrix (periodic acid–Schiff stain).

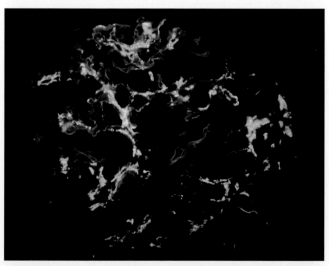

FIGURE 20-2 Immunofluorescence microscopy demonstrating mesangial immunoglobulin A (IgA) in a glomerulus from a patient with IgA nephropathy.

Electron Microscopy

IgA deposits are usually seen only in mesangial areas (**Fig. 20-3**). However, capillary wall deposits may also be seen in approximately 30% of biopsies. These are usually subendothelial. In rare cases, there may be extensive subendothelial deposits associated with endocapillary lesions, leading to a membranoproliferative pattern.

Clinicopathologic Correlations

The severity of the histologic lesions in patients with IgAN usually mirrors the clinical features. The presence of glomerulosclerosis, fibrous crescents, interstitial fibrosis, or tubular atrophy, as individual or combined lesions, provides the most reliable histologic indicator of a poor outcome. It is also important to distinguish between chronic, irreversible lesions and active, potentially reversible lesions that may respond to therapy.

ETIOLOGY

The etiology of IgAN remains unclear. The development of gross hematuria immediately after an episode of upper respiratory infection led to the view that IgAN is a complication of such infections. Although some authors have implicated specific microorganisms as causative agents, no individual viral or bacterial organism has been consistently associated with the development of IgAN. It has also been suggested that IgAN may be caused by hypersensitivity to food antigens, because there are some reports showing its association with gluten-sensitive enteropathy. However, there is no evidence of hypersensitivity to food antigens in most patients with IgAN. At this time, there is consensus that IgAN usually develops as a consequence of an aberrant IgA immune response to a variety of different antigens, whether this be an infecting organism or a food antigen.

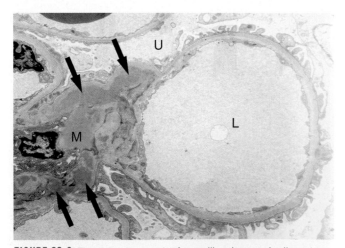

FIGURE 20-3 Electron micrograph of a capillary loop and adjacent mesangium from a patient with immunoglobulin A nephropathy, demonstrating mesangial electron-dense deposits (*arrows*). L, capillary lumen; M, mesangium; U, urinary space.

PATHOGENESIS

The initiating event in the pathogenesis of IgAN appears to be mesangial deposition of IgA. Although codeposition of IgG and C3 complement is often identified in IgAN biopsies, the presence or absence of these immunoreactants does not correlate with the severity of disease activity or risk of clinical progression.

Production of Immunoglobulin A

In humans, IgA is produced in two forms, IgA1 and IgA2, and is secreted from mucosal surfaces, with very little reaching the systemic circulation. Both IgA1 and IgA2 are produced at different mucosal sites. Increased levels of circulating IgA in immune complexes have been documented in some patients with IgAN during exacerbations of disease. However, attempts to correlate the levels of these complexes with disease activity have not produced consistent findings. Some patients with IgAN have been noted to have abnormalities in IgA production, but it is known that an increased plasma level of IgA per se is not sufficient to produce mesangial IgA deposition. Therefore, patients with IgAN must have circulating IgA molecules with abnormal characteristics that lead to mesangial deposition.

Abnormal Galactosylation of IgA1 Molecules

There is now increasing evidence that the molecular abnormality in IgAN patients involves a defect in galactosylation of the IgA1 hinge region. Altered sialylation of IgA1 has also been described in some patients. The initial reports of abnormal galactosylation of IgA1 *O*-glycans were confined to studies of serum IgA, but recent studies have shown the same *O*-galactosylation abnormalities in IgA eluted from glomeruli of patients with IgAN. A similar abnormality in galactosylation in these patients has been demonstrated for IgA1 produced in vitro by their tonsillar lymphocytes. Abnormally galactosylated IgA has also been reported in the urine of patients with IgAN, but not in patients with other forms of glomerular disease.

Clearance of Immunoglobulin A

Another possible contributor to increased levels of IgA in the circulation and likelihood of IgA deposition in glomeruli is defective clearance of IgA immune complexes. Recent studies have confirmed that there may be reduced catabolism of IgA by leucocytes in IgAN. Mesangial IgA accumulation occurs in IgAN either because the rate of deposition exceeds the glomerular IgA clearance capacity or because the deposited IgA is in some way resistant to mesangial clearance. However, it is also known that IgA deposition is not irreversible, because mesangial IgA deposits resolve when a kidney from a renal transplant donor with unrecognized, subclinical IgAN is transplanted into a recipient who developed kidney failure from some other cause.

The Glomerular Response to Immunoglobulin A

IgAN is not usually associated with marked cellular infiltration into the glomeruli, suggesting that most of the glomerular injury is mediated by an expansion of resident glomerular cells. This occurs predominantly through IgA-induced activation of mesangial cells. It is known that mesangial cells are capable of binding with IgA and that this confers on the cells a pro-inflammatory phenotype. Recent studies have also shown increased binding of IgA immune complexes to human mesangial cells, in particular the complexes that contain undergalactosylated IgA1. This increased binding is associated with mesangial proliferation, apoptosis, and increased synthesis of extracellular matrix components. IgA immune complexes and mesangial IgA1 can activate complement to enhance the inflammatory cascade and potentiate glomerular injury in IgAN. However, the contribution of this complement activation to progressive glomerular injury is not known.

EPIDEMIOLOGY

IgAN is the most common form of glomerulonephritis in some parts of the world, including many countries in Asia, where it accounts for up to 40% of patients who undergo a kidney biopsy, but it is relatively uncommon in some other populations. Although it is possible that genetic or environmental differences may be largely responsible for these variances, ascertainment bias probably also plays a significant role. The threshold for performing a biopsy varies with local practice, and the adoption of national mandates for urinary screening programs in many areas of Southeast Asia may also be important, because this policy has resulted in the detection of more patients with covert clinical presentations.

Genetics

Over the past 3 decades, many families with several members who have biopsy-proven IgAN have been described. More recent studies have shown that some patients with IgAN and asymptomatic blood relatives may share an abnormality in glycosylation of the *O*-linked hinge-region glycans in the IgA1 molecule, as discussed earlier, whereas individuals who married into these families, and who therefore had a similar environment, do not exhibit this glycosylation defect. Familial aggregation of IgAN was first reported in two families 30 years ago and has been the subject of great interest in recent years. In the some parts of Europe, up to 10% of patients with IgAN have a family history of renal disease. In a large Italian study, more than 20% of asymptomatic relatives of patients with IgAN were found to have abnormal urinalyses.

The largest studies of the genetic predisposition to the development of IgAN in the United States were carried out in eastern Kentucky. In these studies, it was found that 53 (55%) of 96 IgAN patients who lived in eastern or central Kentucky had at least one relative with IgAN. Similar findings were later reported from Australia and Italy.

Taken as a whole, these reports suggest that familial IgAN is quite common, although often not diagnosed. Using hematuria as the criterion for disease in relatives of IgAN patients, familial disease may be responsible for 10% to 15% of all cases in northern Italy and eastern Kentucky. The low incidence of clinical expression of disease among close relatives probably reflects the need for multiple susceptibility genes for full expression of disease.

CLINICAL FEATURES

Patients with IgAN present with widely differing clinical findings. The original descriptions of the disease emphasized the synpharyngitic presentation—an episode of gross hematuria coincident with or immediately following an upper respiratory tract infection. This is still recognized as the most frequent mode of presentation in children and young adults in the Western hemisphere, but a small number of patients show clinical signs of the nephritic or nephrotic syndrome. Many others, especially adult patients with IgAN, are asymptomatic. This more covert mode of presentation is also been common among children in the Eastern hemisphere, where children are often referred for nephrology evaluation after they are found to have urinary abnormalities during school screening. This applies especially to children in Japan, Korea, Taiwan and Singapore where school screening has been in place for many years. It should be noted, however, that 60% of the patients who are diagnosed with IgAN after they are discovered to have microscopic hematuria subsequently develop gross hematuria on at least one occasion.

Clinical Course and Prognosis

The clinical course of patients with IgAN is heterogeneous and often unpredictable. A small percentage of patients have a benign course that may be associated with spontaneous resolution of their urinary abnormalities, although most have persistent microscopic hematuria. In patients who do not have proteinuria or hypertension, the prognosis is usually good, and such patients are usually managed conservatively.

Many prognostic markers for progressive disease in patients with IgAN have been published over the past 25 years. Persistent proteinuria, hypertension, and impairment in the glomerular filtration rate (GFR) are the principal clinical features of progressive disease. The approach to therapy in individual patients should take into account their relative risk of progressive disease based on both clinical features and biopsy findings. Many asymptomatic patients with IgAN are not biopsied before presenting with hypertension and advanced renal failure; such patients are usually not diagnosed in time for therapy to be effective. It is important to note that the prognosis for patients with

Mycophenolate Mofetil

Recent trials of mycophenolate mofetil (MMF) in patients with severe IgAN have produced mixed results, with two studies showing benefit and two others showing no benefit. The relatively small size, short duration, and mixed results of the studies so far available justifies further evaluation, and other studies are awaited. Until then, there is insufficient evidence to recommend MMF therapy for the treatment of progressive IgAN.

Stepwise Approach to Treatment of Immunoglobulin A Nephropathy

This remains a controversial area, but, based on published data, many authors recommend that therapy with corticosteroids or immunosuppressives should be considered only in patients who have persistent risk factors for progressive disease (e.g., sustained proteinuria) despite achieving a target blood pressure of 125/75 mm Hg with full RAS blockade. Based on recent clinical trials, it appears that relatively few patients fulfill these criteria. It is evident from the previous discussion that the efficacies of corticosteroids, cyclophosphamide, and MMF have not been adequately evaluated by large-scale randomized, controlled trials in the context of such a standard.

HENOCH-SCHÖNLEIN PURPURA NEPHRITIS

Clinical Features and Presentation

Henoch-Schönlein purpura (HSP) is a small-vessel vasculitis associated with IgA-dominant immune deposits in the skin, gut, and kidney. It most often manifests in the first decade of life but can occur at any age. The geographic distribution of HSP is similar to that of primary IgAN; the syndrome is common in Southeast Asia and some parts of Europe but is less common in North America and Africa. Approximately two thirds of patients have a triggering event, most often an infection or an allergic reaction to one of several common drugs or vaccinations. Patients with HSP usually develop a purpuric rash that is symmetrically distributed over the extensor surfaces of the lower limbs and forearms and over the sides and buttocks. Skin biopsies show the lesions to be a leukocytoclastic vasculitis of dermal vessels with IgA deposits in the vascular walls.

Gastrointestinal symptoms and transient arthralgias due to oligoarticular synovitis are reported in 50% to 70% of all patients. In contrast, the prevalence of renal involvement during the course of HSP ranges from 20% to 60%. Isolated microscopic hematuria is the most common renal manifestation of the disease. It usually resolves within a few months of onset, but in a small percentage of children (<10% in most series), the hematuria persists. Proteinuria often develops in these patients, with nephrotic-range levels occurring in 2% to 5%. In long-term follow-up, progression to end-stage renal disease is observed in about 2% to 3% of the children with initial signs of renal involvement. It is important to note that, in long-term follow-up studies of patients with this condition, late progression was observed after 25 years in up to 25% of children, mostly in those with nephritic and/or nephrotic presentations. However, such progression may also occur in rare instances in patients with apparent full recovery 2 years after onset.

Risk Factors for Progression

Proteinuria during follow-up is the only clinical variable that has been shown to be predictive of progression to renal failure in patients with HSP nephropathy. The presence and degree of chronic and irreversible renal sclerotic lesions is the histopathologic lesion that represents the most significant risk factor for progression.

Treatment

Patients with mild HSP nephropathy do not require treatment, provided that monitoring of their urine protein levels and blood pressure is carried out to ensure that they do not develop increasing levels of proteinuria or hypertension. Retrospective studies have failed to demonstrate any benefit of prednisone for children with established HSP nephropathy. A few children with progressive HSP nephropathy may present with features of the nephrotic syndrome or persisting nephritic syndrome. In such cases, more aggressive treatment has been advocated, and methylprednisolone pulses (1 g/1.73 m^2 in three pulses on alternate days) followed by oral prednisone for 3 months has provided a significant benefit. The most encouraging results with such therapy have been reported in patients with epithelial crescents involving more than 50% of glomeruli or with nephrotic syndrome—patients who without treatment often develop progressive renal failure. However, there are no controlled clinical trials that have evaluated this type of approach.

BIBLIOGRAPHY

Ballardie FW: Quantitative appraisal of treatment options for IgA nephropathy. J Am Soc Nephrol 18:2806-2809, 2007.

Ballardie FW, Roberts ISD: Controlled prospective trial of prednisolone and cytotoxics in progressive IgA nephropathy. J Am Soc Nephrol 13:142-148, 2002.

Barratt J, Feehally J: Treatment of IgA Nephropathy. Kidney Int 69:1934, 2006.

Barratt J, Feehally J, Smith AC: Pathogenesis of IgA nephropathy. Semin Nephrol 24:197-217, 2004.

Barratt J, Smith AC, Feehally J: The pathogenic role of IgA1 O-linked glycosylation in the pathogenesis of IgA nephropathy [review]. Nephrology (Carlton) 12:275-284, 2007.

Bartosik LP, Lajoie G, Sugar L, Cattran DC: Predicting progression in IgA nephropathy. Am J Kidney Dis 38:728-735, 2001.

Coppo R, D'Amico G: Factors predicting progression of IgA nephropathies. J Nephrol 18:503-512, 2005.

D'Amico G: Natural history of idiopathic IgA nephropathy and factors predictive of disease outcome. Semin Nephrol 24:179-196, 2004.

Donadio JV, Bergstralh EJ, Grande JP, Rademcher DM: Proteinuria patterns and their association with subsequent end-stage renal disease in IgA nephropathy. Nephrol Dial Transplant 17: 1197-1203, 2002.

Haas M: Histological subclassification of IgA nephropathy: A clinicopathologic study of 244 cases. Am J Kidney Dis 29:829-842, 1997.

Hogg RJ, Lee J, Nardelli N, et al: Placebo-controlled clinical trial evaluating omega-3 fatty acids and alternate day prednisone in patients with IgA nephropathy. Clin J Am Soc Nephrol 1:467-474, 2006.

Izzi C, Sanna-Cherchi S, Prati E, et al: Familial aggregation of primary glomerulonephritis in an Italian population isolate: Valtrompia study. Kidney Int 69:1033-1040, 2006.

Kanno Y, Okada H, Saruta T, Suzuki H: Blood pressure reduction associated with preservation of renal function in hypertensive patients with IgA nephropathy: A 3-year follow-up. Clin Nephrol 54:360-365, 2000.

Kawasaki Y, Suzuki J, Sakai N, et al: Clinical and pathological features of children with Henoch-Schönlein purpura nephritis: Risk factors associated with poor prognosis. Clin Nephrol 60:153-160, 2003.

Mestecky J, Suzuki H, Yanagihara T, et al: IgA nephropathy: Current views of immune complex formation. Contrib Nephrol 157:56-63, 2007.

Monteiro RC: Pathogenic role of IgA receptors in IgA nephropathy. Contrib Nephrol 157:64-69, 2007.

Obara W, Iida A, Suzuki Y, et al: Association of single-nucleotide polymorphisms in the polymeric immunoglobulin receptor gene with immunoglobulin A nephropathy (IgAN) in Japanese patients. J Hum Genet 48:293-299, 2003.

Pillebout E, Thervet E, Hill G, et al: Henoch-Schönlein purpura in adults: Outcome and prognostic factors. J Am Soc Nephrol 13:1271-1278, 2002.

Samuels JA, Strippoli GF, Craig JC, et al: Immunosuppressive treatments for immunoglobulin A nephropathy: A meta-analysis of randomized controlled trials. Nephrology (Carlton) 9:177-185, 2004.

Tomana M, Novak J, Julian BA, et al: Circulating immune complexes in IgA nephropathy consist of IgA1 with galactose-deficient hinge region and antiglycan antibodies. J Clin Invest 104:73-81, 1999.

Tumlin JA, Hennigar RA: Clinical presentation, natural history, and treatment of crescentic proliferative IgA nephropathy. Semin Nephrol 24:256-268, 2004.

Tumlin JA, Madaio MP, Hennigar R: Idiopathic IgA nephropathy: Pathogenesis, histopathology, and therapeutic options. Clin J Am Soc Nephrol 2:1054-1061, 2004.

Wakai K, Kawarmura T, Endoh M, et al: A scoring system to predict renal outcome in IgA nephropathy: From a nationwide prospective study. Nephrol Dial Transplant 21:2800-2808, 2006.

Wyatt RJ, Hogg RJ: Evidence-based assessment of treatment options for children with IgA nephropathies. Pediatr Nephrol 16:156-167, 2001.

CHAPTER 21

Goodpasture's Syndrome and Other Anti–Glomerular Basement Membrane Disease

Alan D. Salama and Charles D. Pusey

The term *Goodpasture's syndrome* was first used by Stanton and Tange in 1957 in their report of nine patients with pulmonary renal syndrome; it referred back to the original patient described by Goodpasture in 1919. It was not until the 1960s that the development of immunofluorescence techniques led to the detection of immunoglobulin deposited along the glomerular basement membrane (GBM) in this condition. Today the term *Goodpasture's syndrome* is often used to describe the combination of rapidly progressive glomerulonephritis (RPGN), pulmonary hemorrhage, and anti-GBM antibodies. However, some researchers use *Goodpasture's syndrome* to refer to those patients with the characteristic clinical features from any cause and *Goodpasture's disease* to describe those who in addition have anti-GBM antibodies. The term *anti-GBM disease* is also widely used to describe any patient with the typical autoantibodies, regardless of clinical features.

CLINICAL FEATURES

There is a bimodal age distribution, with peak incidences in the third and sixth decades of life, and a slight preponderance toward males. Most patients present with RPGN and lung hemorrhage, although about one third present with isolated glomerulonephritis. Rarely, patients present with isolated lung hemorrhage without renal failure, although many of them have hematuria and proteinuria. General malaise, fatigue, and weight loss are the most common systemic features and may relate to anemia.

Pulmonary Disease

Pulmonary hemorrhage occurs in about two thirds of patients and is more common in young men. It may precede the development of kidney disease. Patients often complain of breathlessness and cough, which may be accompanied by minor or massive hemoptysis. Hemoptysis can be triggered by cigarette smoking, inhaled toxins, sepsis, or fluid overload. Clinical signs include tachypnea, respiratory crackles, and eventually cyanosis, but these are often indistinguishable from the signs of pulmonary edema or infection. Radiographic features are nonspecific but usually involve patchy or diffuse alveolar shadowing in the central lung fields (**Fig. 21-1**). The most sensitive test is an elevation in the carbon monoxide diffusion capacity of the lungs, which is caused by the presence of hemoglobin in the alveolar spaces. Bronchoscopy may reveal diffuse hemorrhage, but it is perhaps of more importance in excluding infection. Despite the common presentation of pulmonary hemorrhage, long-term pulmonary sequelae are uncommon in treated patients.

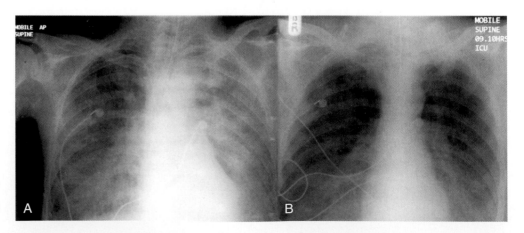

FIGURE 21-1 Chest radiographs of a patient with Goodpasture's disease. **A,** Alveolar hemorrhage. **B,** Resolution after 4 days of treatment.

Renal Disease

Patients may present with isolated hematuria or mild renal functional impairment, but they most commonly present with acute renal failure due to RPGN. The clinical features are not distinguishable from those of any other cause of RPGN, although systemic features (other than lung hemorrhage) are uncommon, unlike RPGN associated with systemic vasculitis. Urine microscopy reveals numerous erythrocytes of glomerular origin, red cell casts, and mild to moderate proteinuria (nephrotic-range proteinuria is rare). Hypertension and oliguria are late features. Renal ultrasonography usually reveals normal-sized kidneys and is helpful in excluding other kidney disorders.

PATHOLOGY

Light microscopy of the kidney biopsy specimen usually reveals a diffuse crescentic glomerulonephritis, with most of the crescents at the same stage of evolution (**Fig. 21-2**). Often, segmental necrosis of glomeruli and some cellular proliferation are present. Blood vessels are usually normal, but vasculitis has been reported rarely. There is usually a prominent interstitial cellular infiltrate. The immunohistology is characteristic, with linear deposits of immunoglobulin G (IgG), sometimes accompanied by IgA or IgM, and complement C3 along the GBM (**Fig. 21-3**). Less intense linear staining with IgG may occasionally be seen in patients with diabetes, systemic lupus erythematosus, myeloma, or transplanted kidney. Lung histology findings are rarely obtained, because transbronchial biopsy does not provide adequate specimens. Open-lung biopsy can reveal alveoli full of red cells, hemosiderin-laden macrophages, and fibrin. Immunofluorescence is technically difficult but may reveal linear deposits of IgG along the alveolar basement membrane.

DIFFERENTIAL DIAGNOSIS

It is important to distinguish anti-GBM disease from other causes of pulmonary renal syndrome and RPGN, because treatment and prognosis are different. Primary systemic vasculitis associated with antineutrophil cytoplasmic antibodies (ANCA) is the most common cause of pulmonary renal syndrome and is the main consideration in the differential diagnosis. Occasionally, patients have both anti-GBM antibodies and ANCA. Other conditions to consider include systemic lupus erythematosus, cryoglobulinemia, Henoch-Schönlein purpura, and various causes of pulmonary renal syndrome (**Table 21-1**). The diagnosis of anti-GBM disease can be made by kidney biopsy or by the detection of circulating anti-GBM antibodies. Various enzyme-linked immunosorbent assays (ELISA) are available for serologic testing; although their specificity is generally equivalent, they may vary in their sensitivity. A screen for other relevant antibodies (e.g., ANCA, anti-DNA antibodies) is usually performed at the same time. Rarely, anti-GBM disease can occur in the absence of detectable circulating anti-GBM antibodies but with positive immunohistology on renal biopsy. These cases have similar antibody properties on biosensor analysis but are not detected on standard ELISA tests. The vast majority of patients' anti-GBM antibodies react with the noncollagenous domain of the α3 chain of type IV collagen, although rare reports of reactivity to other collagen chains have been published. Anti-GBM antibodies appear to correlate with disease activity, and their removal via plasmapheresis is associated with clinical improvement.

ASSOCIATED DISEASES

Anti-GBM disease is rarely associated with other autoimmune disorders, except for systemic vasculitis. Up to 30% of patients have been shown to have ANCA, most commonly perinuclear ANCA (P-ANCA) specific for myeloperoxidase. Conversely, relatively few patients with ANCA-associated vasculitis also have anti-GBM antibodies (5% to 10%). A number of recent series have demonstrated that these "double-positive" patients have a renal prognosis that initially resembles that of patients with isolated anti-GBM disease, in that they are unlikely to recover kidney function once on dialysis. In contrast to patients with anti-GBM disease, however, relapse in the double-positive group is

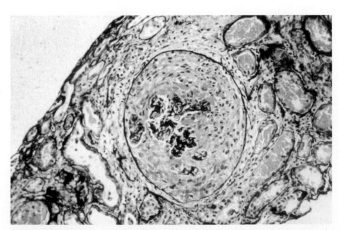

FIGURE 21-2 Renal biopsy from a patient with Goodpasture's disease showing acute crescentic glomerulonephritis (silver stain).

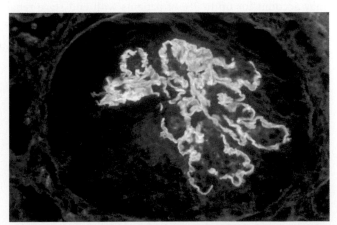

FIGURE 21-3 Renal biopsy from a patient with Goodpasture's disease. Immunofluorescence microscopy shows linear deposition of immunoglobulin G along the glomerular basement membrane.

TABLE 21-1 Causes of Pulmonary Renal Syndrome

More Common Causes
Microscopic polyangiitis
Wegener's granulomatosis
Goodpasture's disease
Systemic lupus erythematosus
Less Common Causes
Churg-Strauss syndrome
Henoch-Schönlein purpura
Hemolytic uremic syndrome
Behçet's disease
Essential mixed cryoglobulinemia
Rheumatoid vasculitis
Penicillamine therapy

more common and resembles that in the ANCA-positive patients. Several patients with membranous nephropathy have been reported to develop anti-GBM disease. It has also been reported to occur after lithotripsy and after urinary tract obstruction. Anti-GBM disease may develop in the transplanted kidney in patients with Alport's syndrome. Patients with X-linked Alport's syndrome inherit a defect in the α5 chain of type IV collagen but also lack the α3 chain, which contains the Goodpasture antigen. Transplantation of a normal kidney therefore exposes the immune system to an antigen to which tolerance has not developed, and an immune response is provoked. The antibodies may be against either the α5 or the α3 chain. Although many patients show antibody deposition along the GBM of the allograft, only a minority develop severe glomerulonephritis.

EPIDEMIOLOGY

Limited epidemiologic studies have suggested that anti-GBM disease has an incidence of 0.5 to 1 case per million population per year. It is found in up to 2% of kidney biopsies and may account for up to 7% of patients with end-stage renal failure. It is predominantly a disease of whites and is less common in those of African or Asian origin.

Genetic Predisposition

Goodpasture's disease has been reported in siblings and in two sets of identical twins. However, discordant twins with the disease have also been documented. As in other autoimmune diseases, there are associations with the major histocompatibility complex. There is a strong association with human leukocyte antigen (HLA) DR2, which is carried by about 85% of patients with Goodpasture's disease. Molecular analysis of HLA class II alleles has confirmed the positive association with DRB1*1501 and DRB1*1502, as well as weaker associations with DRB1*04 and DRB1*03. There are negative associations with DRB1*07 and DRB1*01, suggesting that these are protective alleles. Because of linkage disequilibrium, there are also positive associations with the DQ genes DQA1*01 and DQB1*06.

Environmental Factors

There are several case reports documenting exposure to hydrocarbons before the onset of clinical disease. There are also case-control studies showing a higher incidence of anti-GBM antibodies (usually borderline levels) in those exposed to inhaled industrial hydrocarbons. Cigarette smoking undoubtedly precipitates pulmonary hemorrhage, but it is of uncertain relevance to the etiology. Several clusters of cases have been reported, and there are suggestions of associations with viral infection. However, no clear association with any specific infectious agent has been proved.

PATHOGENESIS

There is good evidence that anti-GBM disease is caused by the development of autoimmunity to a component of the GBM known as the Goodpasture antigen. The GBM is formed from a network of type IV collagen molecules, of which the α1 and α2 chains are widespread in vascular basement membranes, whereas the α3, α4, and α5 chains are restricted to the GBM and certain other specialized basement membranes. The Goodpasture antigen is present in the noncollagenous 1 (NC1) domain of the α3 chain of type IV collagen [α3(IV)NC1]. The main antibody epitope is localized to the amino terminus of the molecule, and the epitope is usually sequestered, suggesting that tolerance is broken after exposure of the cryptic epitope to the immune system. This hypothesis is further supported by the development of anti-GBM disease after renal insults such as lithotripsy and membranous glomerulonephritis. Such epitopes may also be generated after the action of reactive oxygen species on GBM. The antigen is also found in basement membranes of the alveoli, choroid plexus, cochlea, and eye.

Autoimmunity

In Goodpasture's disease, the presence of anti-GBM antibodies is closely linked to the development of clinical features. There is a broad correlation between anti-GBM antibody levels at presentation and severity of disease, and the disease recurs immediately in kidney transplants if the recipient still has circulating antibodies. Importantly, the transfer of anti-GBM antibodies from patients to squirrel monkeys has confirmed that the antibodies are directly pathogenic. However, T cells are also involved in pathogenesis, both by providing help for autoreactive B cells and probably by contributing to cell-mediated glomerular injury. In certain rodent models GBM-specific T cells are capable of mediating disease with minimal antibody responses, demonstrating that either cellular or humoral immunity may predominate in particular individuals and

TABLE 21-2 Initial Treatment of Goodpasture's Disease

Plasma exchange	Daily 4-L exchange for 5% human albumin solution. Use 300-600 mL fresh plasma within 3 days after invasive procedure (e.g., biopsy) or in patients with pulmonary hemorrhage. Continue for 14 days or until antibody levels are fully suppressed. Withhold if platelet count is $<70 \times 10^9$/mL, fibrinogen <1 g/L or hemoglobin is <9 g/dL. Watch for coagulopathy, hypocalcemia, and hypokalemia.
Cyclophosphamide	Daily oral dosing at 2-3 mg/kg/day (round down to nearest 50 mg; use 2 mg/kg/day in patients >55 years). Stop if white cell count is less than 4×10^9/mL, and restart at lower dose when count increases to $>4 \times 10^9$/mL.
Prednisone	Daily oral dosing at 1 mg/kg/day (maximum, 60 mg). Reduce dose weekly to 20 mg by week 6, and then more slowly. There is no evidence of benefit of IV methylprednisolone, and it may increase infection risk (possibly use if plasma exchange not available).
Prophylactic treatments	Use oral nystatin and amphotericin (or fluconazole) for oropharyngeal fungal infection. Use histamine 2 blocker or proton-pump inhibitor for steroid-promoted gastric ulceration. Use low-dose cotrimoxazole for *Pneumocystis jiroveci* pneumonia (PCP).

lead to the same final result. A population of regulatory T cells can be detected in patients who have recovered from the disease, and this regulatory mechanism may account for the rarity of recurrence.

TREATMENT

Untreated anti-GBM disease is usually rapidly fatal, and kidney function does not recover. However, the introduction in the 1970s of treatment with plasma exchange, cyclophosphamide, and corticosteroids (together with dialysis when required) now allows the great majority of patients to survive. The rationale behind this treatment regimen is that plasma exchange rapidly removes circulating anti-GBM antibodies, while cyclophosphamide prevents further antibody synthesis. There has been only one small trial of plasma exchange compared with drug treatment alone, and it suggested a trend toward improved outcome. However, the widely reported improvement in mortality and in kidney function after introduction of the treatment regimen described previously has led to its widespread use. The protocol we currently use is shown in **Table 21-2**. Some patients have been treated with intravenous methylprednisolone, but there is no convincing evidence that it confers a benefit, and it may be associated with a greater risk for infection. Cyclosporine, mycophenolate mofetil, and the anti-CD20 monoclonal antibody (rituximab) have occasionally been used in patients unresponsive to other therapy, but their role is not yet clear and they cannot be recommended as first-line therapy. In general, long-term treatment is not necessary, and patients can stop cyclophosphamide after 3 months. Some authors then change to azathioprine, but there is little evidence that this is necessary. Steroids may be tailed off after about 6 months.

PROGNOSIS

Most patients now survive the acute disease, although pulmonary hemorrhage and infection remain important causes of death. In recent series, 1-year patient survival was 75% to 90%, but only about 40% of survivors recovered independent kidney function. The serum creatinine concentration usually starts to decrease within 1 or 2 weeks after the initiation of treatment, and most patients with a creatinine level of less than 6.8 mg/dL at presentation recover kidney function. However, it has been reported that those who have a creatinine level greater than 6.8 mg/dL, or who are oliguric, rarely recover kidney function. A single-center study of 71 treated patients did show that almost all of the patients with a creatinine level of less than 5.7 mg/dL recovered kidney function, as did most of those with a level of greater than 5.7 mg/dL, but not those on dialysis. As in previous studies, very few patients recovered kidney function once on dialysis. Crescent scores of greater than 50% are usually, but not always, associated with a poor renal prognosis. Patients presenting with dialysis-dependent renal failure may therefore not benefit from immunosuppression, unless they also have pulmonary hemorrhage. This is in marked contrast to the outcome in patients with ANCA-associated RPGN, in whom the majority should recover kidney function, even if presenting with a creatinine level of greater than 6.8 mg/dL or on dialysis.

Exacerbations of pulmonary hemorrhage and worsening kidney function may occur early in the disease, in the presence of anti-GBM antibodies, and are often triggered by infection. True late recurrence after anti-GBM antibodies have become undetectable is rare. Kidney transplantation may be performed once anti-GBM antibodies are undetectable, but we usually delay this, on an empiric basis, until at least 6 months after the disappearance of antibodies.

BIBLIOGRAPHY

Borza DB: Autoepitopes and alloepitopes of type IV collagen: Role in the molecular pathogenesis of anti-GBM antibody glomerulonephritis. Nephron Exp Nephrol 106:e37-e43, 2007.

Herody M, Bobrie G, Gouarin C, et al: Anti-GBM disease: Predictive value of clinical, histological and serological data. Clin Nephrol 40:249-255, 1993.

Johnson JP, Moore JJ, Austin HJ, et al: Therapy of anti-glomerular basement membrane antibody disease: Analysis of prognostic significance of clinical, pathological and treatment factors. Medicine (Baltimore) 64:219-227, 1985.

Lerner RA, Glassock RJ, Dixon FJ: The role of anti-glomerular basement membrane antibodies in the pathogenesis of human glomerulonephritis. J Exp Med 126:989-1004, 1967.

Levy JB, Hammad T, Coulthart A, et al: Clinical features and outcome of patients with both ANCA and anti-GBM antibodies. Kidney Int 66:1535-1540, 2004.

Levy JB, Turner AN, Rees AJ, Pusey CD: Long-term outcome of anti-glomerular basement membrane antibody disease treated with plasma exchange and immunosuppression. Ann Intern Med 134:1033-1942, 2001.

Lockwood CM, Rees AJ, Pearson TA, et al: Immunosuppression and plasma exchange in the treatment of Goodpasture's syndrome. Lancet 1:711-715, 1976.

Merkel F, Pullig O, Marx M, et al: Course and prognosis of anti-basement membrane antibody mediated disease: A report of 35 cases. Nephrol Dial Transplant 9:372-376, 1994.

Phelps RG, Rees AJ: The HLA complex in Goodpasture's disease: A model for analyzing susceptibility to autoimmunity. Kidney Int 56:1638-1653, 1999.

Pusey CD: Anti-glomerular basement membrane (anti-GBM) disease. Kidney Int 64:1535-1550, 2003.

Rutgers A, Slot M, van Paassen P, et al: Coexistence of anti-glomerular basement membrane antibodies and myeloperoxidase-ANCAs in crescentic glomerulonephritis. Am J Kidney Dis 46:253-62, 2005.

Salama AD, Chaudhry AN, Holthaus KA, et al: Regulation by CD25+ lymphocytes of autoantigen-specific T-cell responses in Goodpasture's (anti-GBM) disease. Kidney Int. 64:1685-1694, 2003.

Salama AD, Dougan T, Levy JB, et al: Goodpasture's disease in the absence of circulating anti-glomerular basement membrane antibodies as detected by standard techniques. Am J Kidney Dis 39:1162-1167, 2002.

Salama AD, Pusey CD: Immunology of anti-glomerular basement membrane disease. Curr Opin Nephrol Hypertens 11:279-286, 2002.

Saus J, Wieslander J, Langeveld JPM, et al: Identification of the Goodpasture antigen as the $\alpha 3$(IV) chain of collagen IV. J Biol Chem 263:13374-13380, 1988.

Sinico RA, Radice A, Corace C, et al: Anti-glomerular basement membrane antibodies in the diagnosis of Goodpasture syndrome: A comparison of different assays. Nephrol Dial Transplant 21:397-401, 2006.

Turner N, Mason PJ, Brown R, et al: Molecular cloning of the human Goodpasture antigen demonstrates it to be the alpha 3 chain of type IV collagen. J Clin Invest 89:592-601, 1992.

Wilson CB, Dixon FJ: Anti-glomerular basement membrane antibody-induced glomerulonephritis. Kidney Int 3:74-89, 1973.

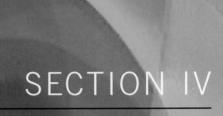

The Kidney in Systemic Disease

CHAPTER 22

Postinfectious Glomerulonephritis

Alain Meyrier

Infection remains a common cause of proliferative glomerulonephritis (GN). Kidney biopsies demonstrate that the same agent may induce more than one histologic type of GN and that a given glomerular lesion may be the consequence of a wide array of pathogens. Thirty years ago, this chapter would have been almost entirely devoted to acute poststreptococcal glomerulonephritis (PSGN). However, the epidemiology of postinfectious GN has considerably evolved in the Western world. In fact, what is now true in industrialized countries is not entirely applicable to all parts of the world, and PSGN remains a significant public health problem in Latin America, in Africa, and most probably in Eastern Europe. Any proliferative GN for which the cause is unclear should prompt consideration of an infectious origin, even if this is not readily suggested by the clinical context.

CLINICAL APPROACH

The clinical presentation of postinfectious GN spans a large spectrum. A bacterial cause should be considered in any patient with the acute nephritic syndrome, acute or rapidly progressive GN, or nephrotic syndrome with progressively declining renal function. An infectious cause is readily suggested when any of these glomerular syndromes follows or accompanies evident bacterial infection. However, the infection may be covert, or it may be overlooked in the patient's history. These considerations justify wide indications for renal biopsy, because it may be the renal pathologist who alerts the clinician to the presence of a possible infectious cause. One such example is a biopsy done in the course of a febrile episode that discloses glomerular lesions strongly suggestive of infective endocarditis.

Acute Nephritic Syndrome

The typical clinical presentation of acute GN, irrespective of the offending organism, is the acute nephritic syndrome. *Streptococcus* and *Staphylococcus* are the most common agents. However, this syndrome is not pathognomonic of postinfectious GN and may be observed in immunoglobulin A (IgA) nephropathy, Henoch-Schönlein purpura, idiopathic membranoproliferative GN (MPGN), and, occasionally, crescentic pauci-immune GN, among others.

The illness is characterized by rapid onset of edema, hypertension, and oliguria, with heavy proteinuria, microscopic or macroscopic hematuria, and low urinary sodium, as well as a concentrated urine. In contrast to nephrotic syndrome, volume expansion involves both the intravascular and the interstitial compartments. Therefore, hypertension, cardiac enlargement, and pulmonary edema may be present. The clinical presentation in children can be fulminant, with abdominal pain, acute cerebral edema, and seizures. In the elderly, volume overload may lead to a presentation with acute pulmonary edema. Renal function ranges from normal to oliguric acute renal failure.

In contrast to IgA nephropathy, in which macroscopic hematuria follows soon after an upper respiratory tract infection (synpharyngitic hematuria), in postpharyngitic forms of postinfectious GN, the episode of bloody urine is delayed by 10 to 20 days after infection (see Chapter 20).

Acute or Rapidly Progressive Renal Functional Impairment

Postinfectious GN can manifest as rapidly progressive or even acute renal functional impairment that is not necessarily correlated with the type of the glomerular lesions. Some cases with purely proliferative and exudative GN may be oliguric at onset but resolve completely. However, severely impaired renal function may also indicate the presence of extracapillary proliferation. A kidney biopsy is almost always required in this setting, both to establish the diagnosis and to guide therapy.

Nephrotic Syndrome and Progressive Renal Functional Impairment

The presence of hypertension, abundant proteinuria, microscopic hematuria and, usually, edema points to a chronic form of glomerular disease. Usually, the date of onset is not known, except when the initial infectious focus is identified, as in shunt nephritis (discussed later), or there has been a clearly identified clinical episode. The membranoproliferative variant of postinfectious GN usually leads to chronic kidney disease and eventually to end-stage renal disease (ESRD). Chronic GN with nephrotic proteinuria is an indication for kidney biopsy.

PATHOLOGY

The glomerular lesions found in postinfectious GN fall into three patterns: acute endocapillary exudative GN, endocapillary plus extracapillary (crescentic) GN, and MPGN.

Acute Endocapillary Exudative Glomerulonephritis

Acute endocapillary exudative glomerulonephritis is the classic appearance of acute PSGN. However, no routine markers are available for histologic identification of the offending microorganism, and the lesions are the same in acute GN resulting from infection with *Staphylococcus*, other bacteria, and viruses. Many pediatricians would defer a biopsy when the clinical picture is typical. This approach is certainly arguable in adults.

Cell Proliferation

By light microscopy, diffuse hypercellularity involves all glomeruli, so that the diagnosis can be made on a renal sample comprising just a few or only a single glomerulus. The glomerular tufts are greatly enlarged, with minimal urinary space remaining and few open capillaries (**Fig. 22-1**). Hypercellularity results both from proliferation of resident glomerular cells (mainly mesangial) and from the influx of polymorphonuclear leukocytes, monocyte-macrophages, and plasma cells. The term *exudative* refers to the presence of abundant polymorphonuclear cells, some of which may be eosinophils. It is possible, although unusual, to find small focal regions of necrosis with fibrin in some glomeruli. Overall, cell proliferation may range from massive infiltration obstructing virtually all capillary lumina to mild inflammation with a moderate increase in mesangial cellularity and greater than normal numbers of polymorphonuclear leukocytes (i.e., ≥5 per glomerulus).

Glomerular Basement Membrane Changes

The most characteristic change in acute GN is the postinfectious subepithelial hump. It is usually easily detected on silver staining (**Fig. 22-2**) and appears as a triangular or oval structure on the outer aspect of the glomerular basement membrane (GBM) that is overlain by a continuous layer of podocyte cytoplasm. The rest of the GBM is normal. Humps are not absolutely pathognomonic of postinfectious GN, but light microscopy and immunofluorescence easily eliminate other causes such as Henoch-Schönlein and MPGN. Humps are especially prominent within the first weeks of disease. In most cases, the typical silver-stain and immunofluorescence appearance make electron microscopy unnecessary. However, light microscopy may yield ambiguous findings. Electron microscopy is then of diagnostic value, because it shows distinct subepithelial and intramembranous deposits indicative of a postinfectious glomerular injury (**Fig. 22-3**).

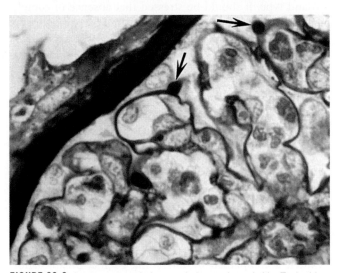

FIGURE 22-2 Acute poststaphylococcal glomerulonephritis. Typical humps are visible on the outer aspect of the glomerular basement membranes (*arrows*) (silver methenamine stain).

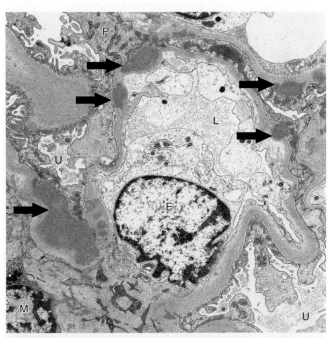

FIGURE 22-3 Transmission electron micrograph showing a capillary loop from a patient with acute poststreptococcal glomerulonephritis, demonstrating scattered subepithelial electron-dense deposits, called humps (*arrows*). E, endothelial cell nucleus; L, polymorphonuclear leukocyte; M, mesangial cell nucleus; P, podocyte cytoplasm; U, urinary space. (Courtesy of Dr. J. Charles Jennette.)

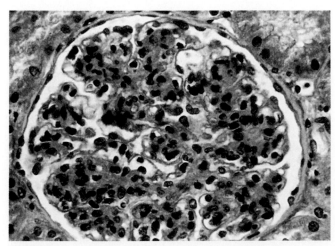

FIGURE 22-1 Acute glomerulonephritis. Marked endocapillary proliferation is seen. Few capillary lumens remain open (Masson's trichrome stain).

Immunofluorescence

Specific antisera disclose granular IgG and complement C3 deposits along the capillary wall and within the mesangium (**Fig. 22-4**). Humps appear brightly fluorescent. Two immunofluorescence patterns have been described. The "garland" type mainly follows the outline of capillary walls, and immunofluorescence shows numerous humps. This type is often associated with heavy proteinuria. The "starry sky" pattern consists of coarser deposits with mesangial predominance and fewer humps. Proteinuria is less abundant than in the garland type. It should be stressed that absence of complement components on immunofluorescence preparations casts strong doubt on the infectious origin of a glomerulopathy.

Endocapillary Plus Extracapillary (Crescentic) Glomerulonephritis

The classic picture of GN associated with systemic bacterial infection consists of focal GN with cellular and necrotic lesions in some of the glomerular tuft lobules. This pattern was described a century ago as "embolic" GN in the course of subacute bacterial endocarditis. However, the most common picture complicating endocarditis and other forms of septicemia, as well as visceral abscesses with negative blood cultures, consists of endocapillary plus extracapillary proliferation (**Fig. 22-5**). Crescent formation is an ominous finding and is often accompanied by interstitial edema, inflammation, and tubular atrophy. Crescents appear as layers of inflammatory cells comprising parietal (Bowman's capsule) cells and macrophages. Necrosis is characterized by the presence of fibrin. The size and distribution of crescents vary from one glomerulus to another. Circumferential crescents anticipate glomerular obsolescence. The spared lobules show the same proliferative changes as described previously. Immunofluorescence shows IgG and C3 deposits, as well as fibrin within crescents.

Membranoproliferative Glomerulonephritis

That MPGN may be the consequence of infection has been demonstrated in the case of shunt nephritis. The lesions include mesangial proliferation, exudative polymorphonuclear cell infiltration, and characteristic GBM changes. The latter changes consist of double contours that result from the interposition of mesangial cells beneath the basement membrane, which elaborates an additional layer of silver-stained mesangial matrix (**Fig. 22-6**). Humps and abundant C3 deposits are strongly suggestive of a postinfectious origin of this type of glomerulopathy and help to differentiate it from the more common idiopathic variety.

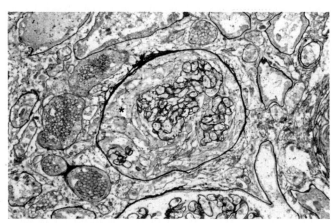

FIGURE 22-5 Crescentic glomerulonephritis complicating a case of slow bacterial endocarditis in an elderly patient with urinary tract infection due to *Enterococcus faecalis*. A circumferential crescent (*asterisk*) surrounds the remaining glomerular tuft (silver methenamine stain).

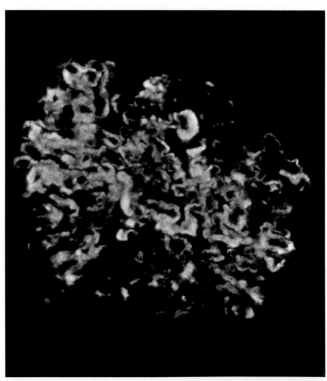

FIGURE 22-4 Acute poststreptococcal glomerulonephritis. Immunofluorescence with an anti-C3 antiserum discloses widespread "garland"-type C3 labeling, mostly along the glomerular basement membranes.

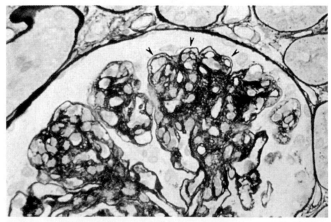

FIGURE 22-6 Membranoproliferative glomerulonephritis in a 50-year-old man with a lifelong history of acne. Typical glomerular basement membrane double contours (*arrowheads*) are visible (silver methenamine stain).

ETIOLOGY AND EPIDEMIOLOGY

Acute Postinfectious Glomerulonephritis

Acute PSGN due to nephritogenic strains of *Streptococcus pyogenes*, group A, remains common in tropical and subtropical regions. It affects mostly children and otherwise healthy adults, including the elderly. The illness can be epidemic. The nephropathy is characterized by rapid onset of the acute nephritic syndrome 10 to 20 days after a pharyngeal or cutaneous infection. The offending microorganism is not always identified, but serologic markers usually confirm that the etiologic agent is *Streptococcus*. The complement profile is characterized by hypocomplementemia with activation of both the classic and the alternative pathways and depressed C3 and C4 levels, followed by normalization within approximately 6 weeks.

Spontaneous recovery is the rule. Proteinuria wanes over weeks. Microscopic hematuria can last a few months before disappearing. Acute PSGN is in most cases a benign disease. However, in some cases, acute GN with an initial histologic appearance of acute exudative GN may progress without remission to crescentic GN. Persistently low complement levels weeks and months after the initial episode, along with heavy proteinuria and hematuria and rising serum creatinine levels, indicate that the disease is not following its usual self-limited course and is progressing to chronic GN. Such progression is an incentive to carry out repeat renal biopsy.

Regarding long-term prognosis, publications dating back as much as 3 decades have indicated that, in the long run, after a protracted period of apparent cure, some patients experience hypertension and renal vascular lesions and can progress to ESRD. However, it is difficult to determine the actual long-term outcome of acute GN, because, in many early publications, biopsies were not performed. The reported rate of recovery varied from 28% to 100%. The course appears to be more benign in children than in adults. Studies carried out during epidemics have determined that the renal disease is clinically silent in a substantial number of affected children, with GN detectable only on screening urinalyses, which demonstrate proteinuria and microscopic hematuria. How many of these clinically silent cases might later eventuate in chronic GN is an unsettled issue. This ascertainment bias may account for the impression that the disease is less severe in children. It has never been clearly established whether cases that are clinically mild and detected only by screening have a better long-term prognosis than the sporadic adult cases that come to attention because renal involvement is more severe.

A systematic retrospective electron microscopic screening of 1012 consecutive renal biopsy specimens performed at Johns Hopkins University School of Medicine found evidence of resolving or largely healed postinfectious GN in 57 of 543 cases in which a diagnosis of a secondary immune complex–related glomerular disease (e.g. cryoglobulinemia, fibrillary GN, lupus nephritis) had been ruled out. These 57 cases included 26 cases with an established diagnosis of postinfectious GN. The others were considered to show "incidental" postinfectious GN based on electron microscopic

TABLE 22-1 Infectious Agents Associated with Glomerulonephritis	
BACTERIA	**VIRUSES**
Streptococcus	Hepatitis B
Staphylococcus	Hepatitis C
Pneumococcus	Echovirus
Enterobacteriaceae	Adenovirus
Salmonella typhi	Coxsackievirus
Meningococcus	Cytomegalovirus
Treponema pallidum	Epstein-Barr virus
Brucella	Enteroviruses
Leptospira	Measles
Yersinia	Mumps
Rickettsia	Varicella
Legionella	Rubella

criteria typical of an infectious etiology. Such findings seem to indicate that clinically silent or overlooked postinfectious GN is, in fact, frequent, especially among diabetics (40% of the 57 biopsies in this study).

Acute GN can occur after infection with a host of microorganisms. Acute GN complicating staphylococcal infection is virtually indistinguishable from acute PSGN, or from acute GN caused by most of the other etiologic agents listed in **Table 22-1**. In the Western world, the incidence of classic acute PSGN has steadily declined in recent decades, and it has become rare in children. On the other hand, microorganisms other than *Streptococcus* are increasingly recognized as etiologic agents for acute GN. Therefore, the overall incidence of postinfectious GN has remained the same, but with a different distribution of glomerular lesions. In adults, an immunocompromised background is emerging as a predisposing factor, especially in alcoholic, cirrhotic, and diabetic patients. However, individuals with human immunodeficiency virus (HIV) carriage, those with acquired immunodeficiency syndrome (AIDS), and those receiving immunosuppressive medications do not seem to be at increased risk for acute GN.

Postinfectious Glomerulonephritis with Rapid or Subacute Development

As noted previously, the typical endocapillary exudative acute GN does not always resolve spontaneously. However, an unfavorable course is now mainly, although not exclusively, restricted to patients whose renal involvement consists of endocapillary plus extracapillary (crescentic) GN. This variety of postinfectious GN is not new; crescentic GN occurring after septicemia (e.g., infectious endocarditis) has been known for almost a century. Nevertheless, its relative frequency, at least in industrialized countries, has grown in as that of acute PSGN has diminished. Its mode of onset and clinical features are more varied than those of acute PSGN. The onset may be heralded by acute nephritic syndrome or rapidly progressive renal functional impairment; alternatively, the disorder may not be detected until chronic kidney disease has developed. The initial focus of infection is not always easy to identify. Most cutaneous, dental, and visceral infections can be complicated by endocapillary and extracapillary GN. Several simultaneous candidate foci may be found in a given patient, growing both gram-positive and gram-negative organisms. In contrast to acute PSGN, extrarenal manifestations, especially purpura, may be present. In a febrile patient with GN and purpura, a search for endocarditis by ultrasound examination and repeated blood cultures is mandatory. In our experience, low serum complement levels were found in only 24% of 25 patients with crescentic GN, probably indicating that the acute initial phase of the disease had occurred at a remote time in the past.

Risk factors for this form of postinfectious GN include alcoholism, drug addiction, malnutrition, and low socioeconomic level, because of poor dental and cutaneous hygiene and delayed access to medical care. The prognosis depends on the severity of infection, the immunologic status and age of the host, and the findings on kidney biopsy. The extent of crescentic proliferation on a biopsy (i.e., encompassing a sufficient number of glomeruli) is the best predictor of development to ESRD. Early recognition and eradication of the infectious foci by antibiotic treatment and, if necessary, by visceral or dental surgery, is probably the best means of preventing progression of kidney disease.

Postinfectious Membranoproliferative Glomerulonephritis

MPGN was long considered to be idiopathic in most cases. However, some forms were evidently postinfectious, such as shunt nephritis. Ventriculoatrial shunting was devised 4 decades ago to relieve hydrocephalus, mostly in children. It consists of a silicon catheter and a valve connecting the cerebral ventricle to the right atrium. This prosthetic material can become colonized with *Staphylococcus epidermidis* or, more rarely, other organisms; about 160 cases have been published. The disease is characterized by fever, arthralgias, wasting, purpura, and severe anemia. Laboratory findings are suggestive of immune complex disease, with low serum complement levels, complement-driven hemolytic anemia, antinuclear antibodies, rheumatoid factor, and cryoglobulins. Renal signs and symptoms consist of proteinuria, microhematuria, and renal insufficiency that can be rapidly progressive. Kidney biopsy usually discloses type I MPGN, often with numerous endocapillary polymorphonuclear cells and abundant C3 deposits. Endocapillary and extracapillary GN has also been observed. Removal of the shunt and antibiotic treatment may be followed by stabilization and even regression of the glomerular lesions, a demonstration that type I MPGN is not invariably irreversible. Nevertheless, only half of the patients experience a complete remission.

Several observations are consistent with the theory that some cases of "idiopathic" MPGN also are of infectious origin. These include the presence of C3 by immunofluorescence

and epidemiologic studies demonstrating the striking simultaneous decrease in incidence of both acute GN and MPGN in western Europe.

PATHOGENESIS
The Offending Microorganisms

A host of microorganisms, including microbes, viruses, and parasites, can be responsible for postinfectious GN. For historical reasons, the most consistent data deal with streptococci. It has been established that only certain strains of group A streptococci lead to acute GN, especially Lancefield type 12, although not all strains of type 12 are nephritogenic. The main sites of streptococcal infection are the throat, especially in the winter and early spring, and the skin, in the late summer and early fall. A tropical or subtropical climate favors skin infection, whereas in temperate climates, a pharyngeal origin is more common. In highly populated areas with low socioeconomic status, PSGN is often epidemic. Studies from both the United States and western Europe have documented a decline in the incidence of acute PSGN in recent decades in urban areas, contrasting with a stable incidence in rural areas. The same has been observed in the Shanghai area in China. In fact, the sharply declining incidence of acute PSGN (as well as acute rheumatic fever) in industrialized countries contrasts with a continuing high incidence in the tropical regions of Africa, Latin America, and the Caribbean. Its prevalence remains high in the countries of Mediterranean Africa, which have a dry climate but a low per capita income.

Is this declining incidence just the consequence of better socioeconomic conditions? A French government-sponsored study that focused on eradication of rheumatic heart disease employing the systematic free distribution of oral phenoxymethylpenicillin in the French Caribbean was immediately followed by a dramatic decrease in the annual incidence of both rheumatic fever and acute GN. Therefore, the weight of the evidence is that early eradication of *S. pyogenes* group A infection is effective in preventing acute GN. The same is probably true for staphylococcal and other etiologic agents.

The Complex Issue of Postinfectious Glomerular Inflammation

Acute postinfectious GN is an immunologic disease. A good clinical argument for this contention is the latent interval between clinical signs of infection and the onset of GN, at least when the onset of infection can be identified. This interval is usually easy to determine in acute GN, but less readily discerned in endocapillary and extracapillary forms, and rarely apparent in cases of MPGN.

Overall, all forms of proliferative GN appear to follow a triphasic course: (1) induction, which is dependent on an antigen; (2) transduction, characterized by immunoglobulin deposits; and (3), mediation. This last phase involves a host of cytokines that originate from monocytes and macrophages, glomerular mesangial cells, platelets, and endothelial cells, including the C5a and C3a complement fractions, and interferon-γ as well as interleukin 2 (IL-2). Activation of these mediators leads to generation of IL-1, tumor necrosis factor-α, platelet-derived growth factor, and transforming growth factor-β. The role of the complement membrane attack complex (C5b-9) in inducing release of arachidonic acid, free oxygen radicals, and IL-1 is probably important. The initial event might be deposition of circulating immune complexes, including a bacterial component, or fixation of bacterial antigens with in situ immune complex formation.

In human disease, the nephritogenic bacterial antigens are seldom identified within the glomeruli, except in some studies dealing with streptococcal or staphylococcal infections. In this respect, it is noteworthy that hepatitis B viral epitopes have been identified within the glomeruli of carriers of hepatitis B surface antigen (HBsAg) with various types of GN. Nephritis-associated plasmin receptor, a group A streptococcal antigen identified as a glyceraldehyde phosphate dehydrogenase (GAPDH), as well as the cationic cysteine proteinase exotoxin B (SPE B), have been detected in the glomeruli of patients with acute GN following group A streptococcal infection. An antibody response to the SPE B was present. It is likely that these antigens, and especially SPE B, have a pathogenic role in patients with acute PSGN. However, considering the diversity of microorganisms and viruses capable of inducing postinfectious GN, identification of specific antigens appears to be a formidable task.

Whatever the triggering mechanism, the usual course of poststreptococcal and poststaphylococcal endocapillary exudative acute GN is that of a self-limited disease. This is not the case for crescentic GN. Crescent formation in various conditions seems to be related to segmental destruction of the GBM by polymorphonuclear and macrophagic enzymes. Through these gaps, immune cells, plasma, fibrin, and inflammatory mediators gain access to Bowman's space and induce an intense proliferative reaction of Bowman's capsule parietal epithelial cells. Podocytes detached from the outer aspect of the GBM may participate in crescent formation. The natural history of untreated crescentic GN is evolution to fibrosis and glomerular obsolescence. It is not readily apparent why other forms of postinfectious GN produce the chronic form of MPGN. The fact that the incidence of acute PSGN and that of MPGN have diminished in parallel suggests that, at least in some cases, the latter might be a mode of progression of an initial occult streptococcal glomerular injury.

PROGNOSTIC INDICATORS AND OUTCOME

Prognostic indicators stem from both the patient's background and the severity of the infectious focus, as well as from features of the glomerulopathy. Patients with poor general health due to malnutrition or cirrhosis are more likely to have an unfavorable course. Patients with septicemia and those with such sites of infection as visceral abscesses, empyema, meningitis, or endocarditis are more likely to die from the primary disorder than from the consequences of their

glomerulopathy. Risk of death is significantly higher in older patients and in those with purpura. Initial presentation with nephrotic syndrome or a serum creatinine concentration greater than 2.7 mg/dL and the presence of crescents and interstitial fibrosis on renal biopsy usually herald irreversible renal damage. Two factors at presentation apparently predict a favorable prognosis: the upper respiratory tract as the initial site of infection and pure endocapillary proliferation with an immunofluorescence "starry sky" pattern. Proteinuria of less than 1.5 g/day is well correlated with recovery in patients with pure endocapillary proliferation, whereas nephrotic syndrome at presentation is often followed by persistent chronic GN. Persistently low serum complement levels are associated with an adverse outcome.

TREATMENT

In the cases of pure endocapillary GN from 3 decades ago, the course was considered to be almost uniformly favorable. More recent experience indicates that the location of the infectious focus is much more varied than simply throat and skin, and it is often still present at the time of kidney biopsy. If a repeat kidney biopsy is performed months or even years after the initial one, it discloses ongoing inflammatory lesions in patients whose infection persists, whereas in those in whom infection had been eradicated, the glomerular lesions are mainly inactive and fibrous. This reinforces the need to eradicate any persistent infection with appropriate antibiotic therapy and, if necessary, a surgical or dental procedure.

Definitive treatment recommendations for the crescentic form of postinfectious GN are not available. Anecdotal experience with glomerular complications of endocarditis suggests that corticosteroid therapy, cyclophosphamide, or plasmapheresis has a favorable effect on kidney function. Such observations are uncontrolled. However, they suggest that the prognosis of postinfectious crescentic GN is not necessarily disastrous if an aggressive anti-inflammatory and possibly immunosuppressive regimen is used after eradication of infection has been achieved.

Postinfectious GN is a public health problem with significant cost implications. In this respect, early and easy access to medical and dental care, control of drug addiction, and the same prophylactic measures that have proved effective in preventing bacterial endocarditis should be implemented to reduce the incidence of the kidney disease.

Glomerulonephritis Related to Viral Infection

Viral infections can be complicated by various types of glomerulopathies, both proliferative and nonproliferative. This confirms the notion that the same agent can induce different histologic types of glomerular diseases.

Hepatitis B Virus–Related Glomerulopathies

The main type of hepatitis B virus (HBV)-related glomerulopathy is membranous glomerulopathy (MGN). It is endemic in Asia and usually affects children infected via maternal-fetal transmission. In the United States, it is found primarily in immigrant children from endemic areas and in adult drug addicts. The second most common form of GN reported with HBV infection is MPGN. The clinical picture consists of nephrotic syndrome. A history of recent acute hepatitis is usually found in adults. The patients carry HBsAg, hepatitis B core antigen (HBcAg), and hepatitis B early antigen (HbeAg). Hypocomplementemia and circulating immune complexes are frequently identified. Viral antigens can be revealed in the glomeruli by immunohistochemistry. Electron microscopy shows virus-like particles incorporated into the GBM. Some forms of HBV infection are accompanied by vasculitis in the form of polyarteritis nodosa. Vasculitic lesions may be found in renal arteries. The natural history of HBV-MGN in children is usually characterized by spontaneous clinical remission, with only rare progression to ESRD. Corticosteroid treatment is contraindicated. Specific antiviral therapy is indicated for the liver disease, because it has the potential to eventuate in cirrhosis and hepatocellular carcinoma. Drug treatment is based on lamivudine or interferon alfa, or both, but there is no general agreement on the superiority of single versus combined therapy. There are no publications on the specific effect of viral load reduction on HBV-related glomerulopathy.

Hepatitis C Virus–Related Glomerulopathies

That HCV infection is related to cryoglobulinemia and renal disease was recognized in 1993. Athralgias, peripheral neuropathy, and purpura are common and indicate that the cryoglobulinemia induces a generalized vasculitis. The patients may have elevated serum aminotransferase levels, but this laboratory indication of liver involvement waxes and wanes and may be negative at times. The glomerulopathy is characterized by moderate to nephrotic proteinuria and impaired kidney function. In rare cases, the kidney biopsy shows MGN. Typically, it discloses a particular form of MPGN comprising diffuse thickening of the glomerular capillary walls and double contours but also massive glomerular infiltration by activated macrophages and eosinophilic thrombi in some capillary loops that are characteristic of cryoglobulinemia. Immunofluorescence shows glomerular subepithelial and mesangial deposition of large amounts of IgG, IgM, and C3, especially on the thrombi. On electron microscopy, large subendothelial deposits are present. Virus-like particles along with HCV RNA were identified by electron microscopy in the renal tissue in half of a series of patients with HCV and glomerulopathy. Cryoglobulins (i.e. immune complexes that precipitate in vitro at 4° C) are present in the serum.

The classification of cryoglobulins distinguishes three subsets. All are immune complexes. Type I is found in monoclonal gammopathies and consists of M component alone. Type II comprises a monoclonal immunoglobulin (typically IgM or IgA) with rheumatoid factor activity that binds to and precipitates with polyclonal immunoglobulins. Type III consists of polyclonal immunoglobulin. Types II and III occur in HCV-related glomerulopathy.

Type II cryoglobulins (essentially IgG) are found in 75% of HCV-related cases. The remainder have type III (polyclonal IgM/IgG) cryoglobulins. They contain HCV RNA with concentrations 1000-fold higher than in the serum, as well as IgG anti-HCV antibodies to the nucleocapsid core antigen (c22-3). Circulating IgM rheumatoid factors are usually present. The complement components C4 and C1q are usually low.

Treatment pursues two goals: reduce the viral load and treat the glomerular inflammation by immunosuppressive therapy. However, immunosuppressive therapy may induce a flare-up in viral replication and aggravate liver injury.

Anti–hepatitis C Virus Therapy

Trials using ribavirin monotherapy have been credited with a beneficial effect on the viral load and on the glomerulopathy in immunocompetent patients. Ribavirin plasma concentrations must be monitored, aiming at a trough level of 10 to 15 mmol/L. However, this dosage adjustment does not always prevents the occurrence of hemolytic anemia, especially in patients with renal insufficiency. Interferon alfa may suppress viremia and simultaneously ameliorate the course of the glomerulopathy. The combination of standard interferon alfa and ribavirin may be more effective than interferon alfa alone in preventing the frequent viral and renal relapses that occur after conclusion of a treatment course. Recent data seem to indicate that pegylated interferon is more effective than standard interferon alfa to promote HCV RNA clearance.

Immunosuppressive Therapy

Regarding treatment of the glomerulopathy, previous uncontrolled studies employed plasmapheresis, methylprednisolone pulses, and cyclophosphamide aimed at suppressing cryoglobulin production and concentration and thereby diminishing the deposition of cryoglobulins in the glomeruli. They provided encouraging results, because they seemed to control the acute phase of the disease. However, immunodepression induced flare-ups of HCV RNA concentration and could aggravate the HCV-related liver disease.

Recently, rituximab, an anti-CD20 monoclonal antibody that targets this B-cell subset, has been tried in the treatment of HCV-related GN. In a few trials conducted in a limited number of patients, some patients responded with rapid disappearance of proteinuria and hematuria, whereas others did not respond. Tolerability was better than that of cyclophosphamide. However, in the case of transplanted HCV-infected patients, the rate of infectious complications was high. Prospective studies using rituximab followed by antiviral therapy, to assess the value of this new treatment option, are still lacking.

Glomerulonephritis Associated with Other Viruses

Numerous publications report anecdotal cases of virus-associated GN. They are listed in **Table 22-1**. In children, viral glomerulopathies may be accompanied with the hemolytic uremic syndrome.

Nephrotic focal segmental glomerulosclerosis (FSGS), especially with the histologic appearance of "collapsing glomerulopathy," is a typical picture of HIV-associated nephropathy. Recent observations indicate that parvovirus B19 and simian virus SV40 may also injure the glomerular podocytes. In this respect, some forms of FSGS can also be listed among glomerulopathies of viral origin (FSGS and HIV-associated renal disease are covered in Chapters 18 and 29, respectively).

BIBLIOGRAPHY

Bach JF, Chalons S, Forier E, et al: Ten-year educational programme aimed at rheumatic fever in two French Caribbean Islands. Lancet 347:644-648, 1996.

Batsford S, Mezzano S, Mihatsch M, et al: Is the nephritogenic antigen in post-streptococcal glomerulonephritis pyrogenic exotoxin B (SPE B) or GAPDH? Kidney Int 68:1120-1129, 2006.

Daimon S, Mizuno Y, Fujii S, et al: Infective endocarditis-induced crescentic glomerulonephritis dramatically improved by plasmapheresis. Am J Kidney Dis 32:309-313, 1998.

Haas M: Incidental healed postinfectious glomerulonephritis: A study of 1012 renal biopsy specimens examined by electron microscopy. Hum Pathol 34:3-10, 2003.

Haffner D, Schindera F, Aschoff A, et al: The clinical spectrum of shunt nephritis. Nephrol Dial Transplant 12:1143-1148, 1997.

Kamar N, Rostaing L, Alric C: Treatment of hepatitis C virus-related glomerulonephritis. Kidney Int 69:436-439, 2006.

Lai KN, Ho RTH, Tam JS, et al: Detection of hepatitis B virus DNA and RNA in kidneys of HBV-related glomerulonephritis. Kidney Int 50:1965-1977, 1996.

Lesavre P, Davison AM: Infection related glomerulonephritis. In Davison AM, Cameron JS, Grünfeld JP, et al (eds): Oxford Textbook of Clinical Nephrology, vol 1, 3rd ed. Oxford, Oxford University Press, 2005, pp 601-623.

Montseny JJ, Meyrier A, Kleinknecht D, Callard P: The current spectrum of infectious glomerulonephritis: Experience with 76 patients and review of the literature. Medicine 74:63-73, 1995.

Rocatello D, Fornasieri A, Ghiachino O, et al: Multicenter study on hepatitis C virus-related cryoglobulinemic glomerulonephritis. Am J Kidney Dis 49:69-82, 2007.

Roy SI, Stapleton FB: Changing perspectives in children hospitalized with poststreptococcal acute glomerulonephritis. Pediatr Nephrol 4:585-589, 1990.

Sabry AA, Sobh MA, Irving WL, et al: A comprehensive study of the association between hepatitis C virus and glomerulopathy. Nephrol Dial Transplant 17:239-245, 2002.

Silva FG: Acute postinfectious glomerulonephritis and glomerulonephritis complicating persistent bacterial infection. In Jennette JC, Olson JL, Schwartz MM, Silva FG (eds): Heptinstall's Pathology of the Kidney. 5th ed. Philadelphia, Lippincott-Raven, 1998, pp 389-453.

CHAPTER 23

Kidney Involvement in Systemic Vasculitis

J. Charles Jennette and Ronald J. Falk

The kidneys are affected by many forms of system vasculitis (**Fig. 23-1**), which cause a wide variety of sometimes confusing clinical manifestations. Large-vessel vasculitides, such as giant cell arteritis and Takayasu's arteritis, can narrow the abdominal aorta or renal arteries, resulting in renal ischemia and renovascular hypertension. Vasculitides of the medium-sized vessels, such as polyarteritis nodosa and Kawasaki's disease, also can reduce flow through the renal artery and may affect intrarenal arteries, resulting in infarction and hemorrhage. Small-vessel vasculitides, such as microscopic polyangiitis, Wegener's granulomatosis, Henoch-Schönlein purpura, and cryoglobulinemic vasculitis, frequently involve the kidneys and especially the glomerular capillaries, resulting in glomerulonephritis.

PATHOLOGY

As depicted in **Figure 23-1** and described in **Table 23-1**, different types of systemic vasculitis affect different vessels within the kidney. In addition, each type of vasculitis has different histologic and immunohistologic features.

Giant cell arteritis and Takayasu's arteritis predominantly affect the aorta and its major branches. Takayasu's arteritis is an important cause of renovascular hypertension, especially in young patients. Giant cell arteritis only rarely causes clinically significant kidney disease, although asymptomatic pathologic involvement is common. Giant cell arteritis often involves the extracranial branches of the carotid arteries, including the temporal artery. Some patients, however, do not have temporal artery involvement, and patients with other types of vasculitis (e.g., microscopic polyangiitis, Wegener's granulomatosis) may have temporal artery involvement. Therefore, temporal artery disease is neither a required nor a sufficient pathologic feature of giant cell arteritis.

Histologically, both giant cell arteritis and Takayasu's arteritis are characterized by focal chronic inflammation that frequently has a granulomatous appearance, often, but not always, with multinucleated giant cells. With chronicity, the inflammatory injury evolves into fibrosis and frequently results in vascular narrowing, which is the basis for renovascular hypertension when a renal artery is involved.

Polyarteritis nodosa and Kawasaki's disease affect medium-sized arteries (i.e., main visceral arteries) such as the mesenteric, hepatic, coronary, and main renal arteries. These diseases also may involve small arteries, such as arteries within the parenchyma of skeletal muscle, liver, heart, pancreas, spleen, and kidney (e.g., interlobar and arcuate arteries). By the definitions in **Table 23-1**, polyarteritis nodosa and Kawasaki's disease affect arteries exclusively, and not capillaries or venules. Therefore, they do not cause glomerulonephritis. The presence of arteritis with glomerulonephritis indicates some form of small-vessel vasculitis rather than a medium-vessel vasculitis.

Histologically, the acute arterial injury of Kawasaki's disease and polyarteritis nodosa is characterized by focal artery wall necrosis and infiltration of inflammatory cells. The acute injury of polyarteritis nodosa typically includes conspicuous fibrinoid necrosis, which is absent or less apparent in Kawasaki's disease. Fibrinoid necrosis results from plasma coagulation factors' spilling into the necrotic areas, where they are activated to form fibrin. Early in the acute injury of polyarteritis nodosa, neutrophils predominate, but within a few days mononuclear leukocytes are most numerous. Thrombosis may occur at the site of inflammation, resulting in infarction. Focal necrotizing injury to vessels erodes into the vessel wall and adjacent tissue, producing an inflammatory aneurysm, which may rupture and cause hemorrhage. Thrombosis of the inflamed arteries causes downstream ischemia and infarction.

Although small-vessel vasculitides may affect medium-sized arteries, these disorders favor small vessels such as arterioles, venules (e.g., in the dermis), and capillaries (e.g., in glomeruli and pulmonary alveoli) (see **Fig. 23-1**). As described in **Table 23-1**, there are a variety of clinically and pathogenetically distinct forms of small-vessel vasculitis that have in common focal necrotizing inflammation of small vessels. In the acute phase, this injury is characterized histologically by segmental fibrinoid necrosis and leukocyte infiltration (**Fig. 23-2**), sometimes with secondary thrombosis. The neutrophils often undergo karyorrhexis (leukocytoclasia). With chronicity, mononuclear leukocytes become predominant and fibrosis develops.

The various forms of small-vessel vasculitis differ from one another with respect to the presence or absence of distinctive features, as summarized in **Table 23-1** and **Figure 23-1**. For example, Wegener's granulomatosis is characterized by necrotizing granulomatous inflammation, Churg-Strauss syndrome by blood eosinophilia and asthma, Henoch-Schönlein purpura by immunoglobulin A (IgA)-dominant vascular immune deposits, and cryoglobulinemic vasculitis by circulating cryoglobulins.

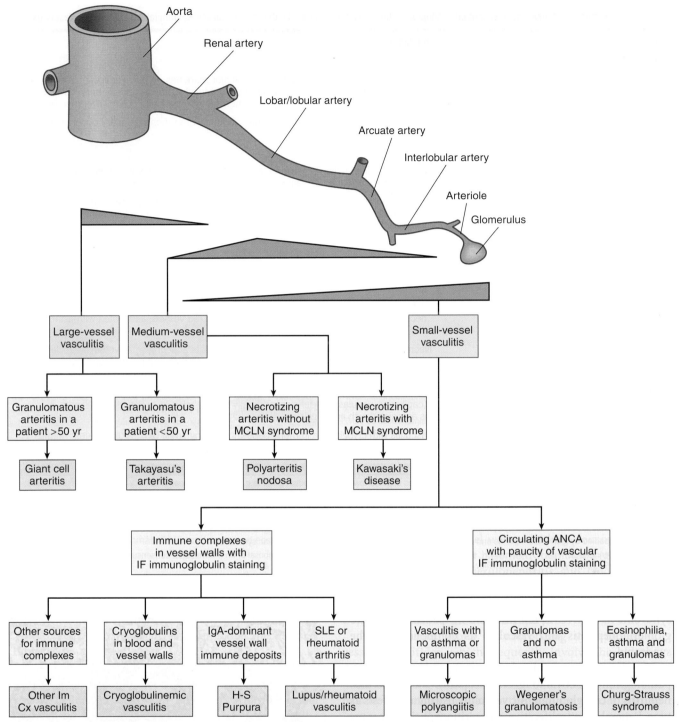

FIGURE 23-1 Predominant distribution of renal vascular involvement by systemic vasculitides and the diagnostic clinical and pathologic features that distinguish among them. The width of the blue triangles indicates the predilection of small-, medium-, and large-vessel vasculitides for various portions of the renal vasculature. Note that medium-sized renal arteries can be affected by large-, medium-, or small-vessel vasculitides, but arterioles and glomeruli are affected by small-vessel vasculitides alone, based on the definitions in **Table 23-1**. ANCA, antineutroophil cytoplasmic antibodies; H-S, Henoch-Schönlein; IF, immunofluorescence; IgA, immunoglobulin A; Im Cx, immune complex; MCLN, mucocutaneous lymph node syndrome; SLE, systemic lupus erythematosus.

The glomerular lesions of microscopic polyangiitis, Wegener's granulomatosis, and Churg-Strauss syndrome are identical pathologically and are characterized by segmental fibrinoid necrosis, crescent formation (**Fig. 23-3**), and a paucity of glomerular staining for immunoglobulin (i.e., pauci-immune glomerulonephritis). Leukocytoclastic angiitis of medullary vasa recta (**Fig. 23-4**) also occurs in the antineutrophil cytoplasmic antibody (ANCA) vasculitides and rarely is severe enough to cause papillary necrosis. More than 85% of patients with active untreated microscopic polyangiitis or Wegener's granulomatosis have circulating ANCAs. Fewer than half of patients with Churg-Strauss

neutrophil staining are observed that discriminate between the two major subtypes of ANCAs: cytoplasmic-staining (C-ANCA) and perinuclear-staining (P-ANCA). With the use of specific immunochemical assays such as enzyme-linked immunosorbent assays (ELISAs), most C-ANCAs are found to be specific for a neutrophil and monocyte proteinase called proteinase 3 (PR3-ANCA), and most P-ANCAs are specific for myeloperoxidase (MPO-ANCA).

The leading hypothesis about the pathogenesis of ANCA-associated vasculitides proposes that ANCAs react with cytoplasmic antigens (PR3 and MPO) that are present at the surface of cytokine-stimulated leukocytes, causing the leukocytes to adhere to vessel walls, degranulate, and generate toxic oxygen metabolites. The interaction of ANCAs with neutrophils involves Fc receptor engagement, perhaps by immune complexes formed between ANCAs and ANCA antigens in the microenvironment surrounding the leukocyte. ANCA binding to ANCA antigens on the surface of neutrophils also may be involved in neutrophil activation. ANCA antigens also may become planted in vessel walls or even produced by endothelial cells, thus providing a nidus for in situ immune complex formation in vessel walls. If such in situ formation is present, it must be at a level that cannot be detected by immunofluorescence microscopy, because ANCA vasculitides are characteristically pauci-immune. The most compelling experimental evidence that ANCAs cause vasculitis is the observation that circulating antibodies specific for MPO cause pauci-immune crescentic glomerulonephritis and small-vessel vasculitis in mice and rats. The most convincing clinical observation that supports the pathogenicity of ANCA is one reported occurrence of transplacental transfer of MPO-ANCA IgG that apparently caused glomerulonephritis and pulmonary capillaritis in a newborn.

CLINICAL FEATURES

The diagnosis and management of systemic vasculitis can be very challenging. The clinical features are extremely varied and are dictated by the category of vasculitis, the type of vessel involved, the organ system distribution of vascular injury, and the stage of disease. Regardless of the type of vasculitis, most patients have accompanying constitutional features of inflammatory disease, such as fever, arthralgias, myalgias, and weight loss. These probably are caused by increased circulating levels of proinflammatory cytokines.

Giant cell arteritis and Takayasu's arteritis typically manifest with evidence for ischemia in tissues supplied by involved arteries. Patients with Takayasu's arteritis often develop claudication (especially in the upper extremities), absent pulses, and bruits. Approximately 40% of patients with Takayasu's arteritis develop renovascular hypertension, a feature that only rarely complicates giant cell arteritis. Giant cell arteritis can affect virtually any organ in the body, but signs and symptoms of involvement of arteries in the head and neck are the most common clinical manifestations. Superficial arteries (e.g., the temporal artery) may be swollen and tender.

Arterial narrowing causes ischemic manifestations in affected tissues (e.g., headache, jaw claudication, loss of vision). About half of the patients with giant cell arteritis have polymyalgia rheumatica, which is characterized by aching and stiffness in the neck, shoulder girdle, or pelvic girdle.

Medium-vessel vasculitides, such as polyarteritis nodosa and Kawasaki's disease, often manifest with clinical evidence for infarction in multiple organs, such as abdominal pain with occult blood in the stool and skeletal muscle and cardiac pain with elevated serum muscle enzymes. Laboratory evaluation often demonstrates clinically silent organ damage, such as liver injury with elevated liver function tests and pancreatic injury with elevated serum amylase.

Polyarteritis nodosa frequently causes multiple renal infarcts and aneurysms. Unlike microscopic polyangiitis, polyarteritis nodosa typically does not cause severe impairments in kidney function. Rupture of arterial aneurysms with massive retroperitoneal or intraperitoneal hemorrhage is a life-threatening complication of polyarteritis nodosa.

Kawasaki's disease almost always occurs in children younger than 6 years of age and has a predilection for coronary, axillary, and iliac arteries. Kawasaki's disease is accompanied by the mucocutaneous lymph node syndrome that includes fever, nonpurulent lymphadenopathy, and mucosal and cutaneous inflammation. Although the renal arteries frequently are affected pathologically, clinically significant renal involvement is rare in patients with Kawasaki's disease.

Patients with small-vessel vasculitides often present with evidence of inflammation in vessels in multiple organs, but initially there may be involvement of only one organ, followed later by development of disease in other organs. Hematuria, proteinuria, and impaired kidney function caused by glomerulonephritis are frequent clinical features of all forms of small-vessel vasculitis listed in **Table 23-1**. Other manifestations include purpura caused by leukocytoclastic angiitis in dermal venules and arterioles, abdominal pain and occult blood in the stool from mucosal and bowel wall infarcts, mononeuritis multiplex from arteritis in peripheral nerves, necrotizing sinusitis from upper respiratory tract mucosal angiitis, and pulmonary hemorrhage from alveolar capillaritis.

In addition to these features, which are shared by patients with any type of small vessel vasculitis, patients with Wegener's granulomatosis or Churg-Strauss syndrome have distinctive clinical features that set them apart. Patients with Wegener's granulomatosis have necrotizing granulomatous inflammation, most often in the upper or lower respiratory tract, and rarely in other tissues (e.g., skin, orbit). In the lungs, this inflammation produces irregular nodular lesions that can be observed by radiography. These lesions may cavitate and hemorrhage. However, massive pulmonary hemorrhage in patients with Wegener's granulomatosis is usually caused by capillaritis rather than granulomatous inflammation. By definition, patients with Churg-Strauss syndrome have blood eosinophilia and a history of asthma. They also develop eosinophil-rich tissue inflammation, especially in the lungs and gut.

TABLE 23-3 Approximate Frequency of PR3-ANCA or MPO-ANCA in Pauci-Immune Small-Vessel Vasculitis

ANTIBODY	MICROSCOPIC POLYANGIITIS	WEGENER'S GRAULOMATOSIS	CHURG-STRAUSS SYNDROME	RENAL-LIMITED VASCULITIS
PR3-ANCA	40%	75%	5%	25%
MPO-ANCA	50%	20%	40%	65%
ANCA-negative	10%	5%	55%	10%

MPO-ANCA, myeloperoxidase antineutrophil cytoplasmic antibody; PR3-ANCA, proteinase 3 antineutrophil cytoplasmic antibody.

DIAGNOSIS

Multisystem disease in a patient with constitutional signs and symptoms of inflammation, such as fever, arthralgias, myalgias, and weight loss, should raise suspicion of systemic vasculitis. Data that will assist in resolving the differential diagnosis include the age of the patient, organ distribution of injury, concurrent syndromes (e.g., mucocutaneous lymph node syndrome in Kawasaki's disease, polymyalgia rheumatica in giant cell arteritis, asthma in Churg-Strauss syndrome), type of vessel involved (e.g., large artery, visceral artery, small vessel other than an artery), lesion histology (e.g., granulomatous, necrotizing), lesion immunohistology (e.g., immune deposits, pauci-immune), and serologic data (e.g., cryoglobulins, hepatitis C antibodies, hypocomplementemia, antinuclear antibodies, ANCAs) (see **Fig. 23-1**).

Signs and symptoms of tissue ischemia along with angiography demonstrating irregularity, stenosis, occlusion, or, less commonly, aneurysms of large and medium-sized arteries should suggest giant cell arteritis or Takayasu's arteritis. A useful discriminator between giant cell arteritis and Takayasu's arteritis is age. The former disorder is rare in individuals younger than 50 years of age, and the latter is rare in patients older than 50 years. The presence of polymyalgia rheumatica is a clinical marker for giant cell arteritis.

Polyarteritis nodosa and Kawasaki's disease cause visceral ischemia, particularly in the heart, kidneys, liver, spleen, and gut. Arteritis in skeletal muscle and subcutaneous tissues causes tender erythematous nodules that can be identified on physical examination. Angiographic demonstration of aneurysms in medium-sized arteries (e.g., renal arteries) indicates that some type of vasculitis is present, but it is not disease specific, because giant cell arteritis, Takayasu's arteritis, polyarteritis nodosa, Kawasaki's disease, Wegener's granulomatosis, microscopic polyarteritis, and Churg-Strauss syndrome all can produce arterial aneurysms. Kawasaki's disease almost always occurs in children younger than 6 years of age and is by definition accompanied by the mucocutaneous lymph node syndrome.

A small-vessel vasculitis should be suspected if there is evidence for inflammation of vessels smaller than arteries, such as glomerular capillaries (hematuria and proteinuria), dermal venules (palpable purpura), or alveolar capillaries (hemoptysis). To discriminate among the small-vessel vasculitides, evaluation of serologic data, vessel immunohistology, or concurrent nonvasculitic disease (e.g., asthma, eosinophilia, lupus, hepatitis) is required (see **Fig. 23-1**).

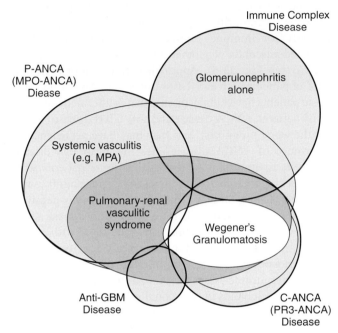

FIGURE 23-5 Relationship of vasculitic clinicopathologic syndromes to immunopathologic categories of vascular injury in patients with crescentic glomerulonephritis. The circles represent the major immunopathologic categories of vascular inflammation that affect the kidneys, and the shaded ovals represent the clinicopathologic expressions of the vascular inflammation. Note that clinical syndromes can be caused by more than one immunopathologic process; for example, pulmonary-renal vasculitic syndrome can be caused by anti-GBM antibodies (i.e., Goodpasture's syndrome), immune complex localization (e.g., lupus erythematosus), or ANCA-associated disease (e.g., MPA, Wegener's granulomatosis). ANCA, antineutrophil cytoplasmic antibody; GBM, glomerular basement membrane; MPA, microscopic polyangiitis. (From Jennette JC: Anti-neutrophil cytoplasmic autoantibody-associated disease: A pathologist's perspective. Am J Kidney Dis 18:164-170, 1991, with permission.)

Evaluation of vessels in biopsy specimens, such as glomerular capillaries in kidney biopsies, alveolar capillaries in lung biopsies, or dermal venules in skin biopsies, can be helpful, especially if immunohistology is performed. The pauci-immune vasculitides lack immune deposits, anti-GBM disease produces linear immunoglobulin deposits, and immune complex vasculitides have granular immune deposits, such as the IgA-dominant deposits of Henoch-Schönlein purpura.

Serology, especially ANCA analysis, is useful in differentiating among the small-vessel vasculitides. Wegener's granulomatosis, microscopic polyangiitis, and, to a lesser extent, Churg-Strauss syndrome are associated with ANCAs (**Table 23-3**). As depicted in **Figure 23-5** and listed in **Table 23-3**, most patients with active untreated Wegener's granulomatosis have C-ANCA (PR3-ANCA). A minority of patients have P-ANCA (MPO-ANCA). Therefore, C-ANCA is not completely specific for Wegener's granulomatosis, because some patients with C-ANCA have systemic small-vessel vasculitis without granulomatous inflammation (i.e., microscopic polyangiitis), and others have pauci-immune necrotizing and crescentic glomerulonephritis alone. Patients with Churg-Strauss syndrome have the lowest frequency of ANCAs and the lowest frequency of renal involvement by glomerulonephritis. A minority of patients with immunopathologic evidence for immune complex–mediated or anti-GBM–mediated vasculitis or glomerulonephritis have concurrent ANCA (see **Fig. 23-5**). Approximately one fourth to one third of patients with anti-GBM disease are ANCA positive. These patients have kidney disease that is intermediate in severity between ANCA disease and anti-GBM disease (which has the worst prognosis), and they may have persistence or recurrence of ANCA disease after the anti-GBM disease remits. It is important to realize that some patients with Wegener's granulomatosis, microscopic polyangiitis, and especially Churg-Strauss syndrome are ANCA-negative. In some patients, ANCA titers correlate with disease activity. However, in many patients, especially those with MPO-ANCA, ANCA titers do not mirror disease activity.

Diagnostic serologic tests for immune complex–mediated vasculitides include assays for circulating immune complexes (e.g., cryoglobulins in cryoglobulinemic vasculitis), assays for antibodies known to participate in immune complex formation or to mark the presence of a disease that generates immune complexes (e.g., antibodies to hepatitis B or C, streptococci, DNA), and assays for consumption or activation of humoral inflammatory mediator system components (e.g., assays for reduced complement components or for activated membrane attack complex).

THERAPY AND OUTCOME

All of the vasculitides discussed in this chapter respond to anti-inflammatory or immunosuppressive therapy. The aggressiveness of treatment should match the aggressiveness of the disease.

Takayasu's arteritis and giant cell arteritis usually respond well to high-dose corticosteroid treatment (e.g., prednisone, 1 mg/kg body weight per day) during the acute phase of the disease, followed by tapering and low-dose maintenance for several months to 1 year depending on disease activity. Patients with severe disease or steroid toxicity benefit from other immunosuppressive agents, including methotrexate, cyclophosphamide, or azathioprine. If present, renovascular hypertension should be controlled. After the inflammatory phase has passed and the sclerotic phase has developed, reconstructive vascular surgery may be required to improve flow to ischemic tissues, especially in patients with Takayasu's arteritis.

Some patients with polyarteritis nodosa have a persistent viral infection, especially hepatitis B virus infection. These patients are usually ANCA negative. In these cases, antiviral therapy with or without plasma exchange is recommended. In patients with no evidence for infection, management usually consists of corticosteroids with or without cytotoxic drugs.

Corticosteroid treatment is not recommended for Kawasaki's disease, because it may worsen the coronary artery disease, which is the most life-threatening feature of Kawasaki's disease. The preferred treatment is a combination of aspirin and high-dose intravenous gamma globulins. This controls the inflammatory manifestations of the disease (e.g., the mucocutaneous lymph node syndrome), prevents thrombosis of injured arteries, and retards the frequency of coronary artery involvement. With appropriate treatment, more than 90% of patients with Kawasaki's disease have complete resolution of the disease.

Most patients with Henoch-Schönlein purpura have mild, self-limited disease that requires only supportive care (see Chapter 20). Arthralgias are relieved by nonsteroidal anti-inflammatory drugs. Corticosteroid treatment is beneficial for patients who have severe abdominal pain caused by intestinal vasculitis. The treatment of severe glomerulonephritis in patients with Henoch-Schönlein purpura is controversial. There is anecdotal evidence indicating that aggressive crescent glomerulonephritis should be treated with high-dose corticosteroids, cytotoxic agents, or plasmapheresis, but this has not been documented in controlled trials. Data from a large pediatric population suggest that corticosteroid treatment may decrease the risk for development of kidney involvement in those patients with severe abdominal pain and rash.

Cryoglobulinemic vasculitis caused by hepatitis C infection may respond to interferon-alfa in combination with antiviral therapy (e.g., ribavirin). The relative response to treatment varies according to the study population. As many as 25% to 50% of patients have either partial or complete response to therapy.

High-dose corticosteroids (e.g., pulse methylprednisolone) and cytotoxic agents (e.g., cyclophosphamide) are the treatments of choice for necrotizing and crescentic glomerulonephritis associated with microscopic polyangiitis, Wegener's granulomatosis, or the Churg-Strauss syndrome or for renal-limited vascular inflammation. Patients with pulmonary-renal vasculitic syndromes in whom hemoptysis is a major clinical feature require emergent therapy with plasma exchange. Adjunctive plasma exchange also improves renal survival in patients with severe renal disease at the time of diagnosis.

Induction therapy includes pulse methylprednisolone at a dose of 7 mg/kg/day for 3 days, followed by daily oral prednisone or plasmapheresis therapy for 7 to 14 days in addition to daily oral prednisone. Prednisone treatment is typically converted to alternate-day treatment during the second month of therapy. Corticosteroid treatment is terminated by the fourth or fifth month after diagnosis. There are a number of cyclophosphamide protocols, including intravenous or oral cyclophosphamide, that induce remission in almost 90% of patients. The optimal duration of cyclophosphamide treatment has not been defined. Once the patient is in remission, treatment may be switched to maintenance therapy that includes azathioprine or mycophenolate mofetil. Some patients may not require any kind of immunosuppressive therapy once they are in remission after 6 to 12 months of overall therapy.

As many as 75% to 85% of ANCA-vasculitic patients enter remission with aggressive immunosuppressive therapy, but approximately 20% to 40% have a relapse within 2 years. Relapses typically occur in the same organ system as the primary disease, although relapses may occur in another organ system as well. Depending on the severity of the relapse, patients may be treated either with another course of corticosteroids and cyclophosphamide or with less toxic therapy, including mycophenolate mofetil, glucocorticoids, or azathioprine.

BIBLIOGRAPHY

Alric L, Plaisier E, Thebault S, et al: Influence of antiviral therapy in hepatitis C virus-associated cryoglobulinemic MPGN. Am J Kidney Dis 43:617-623, 2004.

de Lind van Wijngaarden RA, Hauer HA, Wolterbeek R, et al: Chances of renal recovery for dialysis-dependent ANCA-associated glomerulonephritis. J Am Soc Nephrol 18:2189-2197, 2007.

Guillevin L, Durand-Gasselin B, Cevallos R, et al: Microscopic polyangiitis: Clinical and laboratory findings in eighty-five patients. Arthritis Rheum 42:421-430, 1999.

Guillevin L, Lhote F, Gherardi R: The spectrum and treatment of virus-associated vasculitides. Curr Opin Rheumatol 9:31-36, 1997.

Hogan SL, Falk RJ, Chin H, et al: Predictors of relapse and treatment resistance in antineutrophil cytoplasmic antibody-associated small-vessel vasculitis. Ann Intern Med 143:621-631, 2005.

Jayne D, Rasmussen N, Andrassy K, et al: A randomized trial of maintenance therapy for vasculitis associated with antineutrophil cytoplasmic autoantibodies. N Engl J Med 349:36-44, 2003.

Jayne DR, Gaskin G, Rasmussen N, et al: Randomized trial of plasma exchange or high-dosage methylprednisolone as adjunctive therapy for severe renal vasculitis. J Am Soc Nephrol 18:2180-2188, 2007.

Jennette JC, Falk RJ: Small vessel vasculitis. N Engl J Med 337:1512-1523, 1997.

Jennette JC, Falk RJ, Andrassy K, et al: Nomenclature of systemic vasculitides: Proposal of an international consensus conference. Arthritis Rheum 37:187-192, 1994.

Jennette JC, Thomas DB: Pauci-immune and antineutrophil cytoplasmic autoantibody glomerulonephritis and vasculitis. In Jennette JC, Olson JL, Schwartz MM, Silva FG (eds): Heptinstall's Pathology of the Kidney. 6th ed. Philadelphia, Lippincott Williams & Wilkins, 2007, pp 643-674.

Jennette JC, Thomas DB, Falk RJ: Microscopic polyangiitis (microscopic polyarteritis). Semin Diagn Pathol 18:3-13, 2001.

Jennette JC, Xiao H, Falk RJ: The pathogenesis of vascular inflammation by antineutrophil cytoplasmic antibodies. J Am Soc Nephrol 17:1235-1242, 2006.

Kaku Y, Nohara K, Honda S: Renal involvement in Henoch-Schönlein purpura: A multivariate analysis of prognostic factors. Kidney Int 53:1755-1759, 1998.

Kamesh L, Harper L, Savage CO: ANCA-positive vasculitis. J Am Soc Nephrol 13:1953-1960, 2002.

Klemmer PJ, Chalermskulrat W, Reif MS, et al: Plasmapheresis therapy for diffuse alveolar hemorrhage in patients with small-vessel vasculitis. Am J Kidney Dis 42:1149-1153, 2003.

Langford CA, Balow JE: New insights into the immunopathogenesis and treatment of small vessel vasculitis of the kidney. Curr Opin Nephrol Hypertens 12:267-272, 2003.

Morgan MD, Harper L, Williams J, Savage C: Anti-neutrophil cytoplasm-associated glomerulonephritis. J Am Soc Nephrol 17:1224-1234, 2006.

Nachman PH, Hogan SL, Jennette JC, Falk RJ: Treatment response and relapse in ANCA-associated microscopic polyangiitis and glomerulonephritis. J Am Soc Nephrol 7:23-32, 1996.

Rieu P, Noel LH: Henoch-Schönlein nephritis in children and adults: Morphological features and clinicopathological correlations. Ann Intern Med 150:151-159, 1999.

Rossi P, Bertani T, Baio P, et al: Hepatitis C virus-related cryoglobulinemic glomerulonephritis: Long-term remission after antiviral therapy. Kidney Int 63:2236-2241, 2003.

CHAPTER 24

Renal Manifestations of Systemic Lupus Erythematosus

James E. Balow

Systemic lupus erythematosus (SLE) is a complex systemic autoimmune disease that exhibits a protean array of clinical manifestations and laboratory test abnormalities. The basis for development of autoimmunity in SLE is incompletely understood, but there is strong and rapidly emerging evidence from genome-wide association studies for genetic susceptibility factors. The current paradigm for SLE pathogenesis posits that environmental factors, such as sunlight, drugs, or infections, provoke excessive apoptosis and release of nuclear antigens from endogenous host cells. Constellations of gene variants that affect antigen presentation, interferon biology, and lymphocyte activation create a fertile environment for the excessive nuclear antigens to drive autoimmune responses and create pathogenic circulating immune complexes.

Autoantibodies to a range of constitutive nuclear antigens are cardinal elements in the definition of SLE. Of these, anti-DNA antibodies and related immune complexes appear to be the most nephritogenic. There is evidence from experimental murine models and from human subjects with SLE that genetic variants of receptors for immunoglobulin Fc receptor–mediated immune complex clearance are also susceptibility factors. The classic paradigm for lupus nephritis involves deposition of preformed circulating immune complexes, initially in the mesangial interstices with eventual spillover into the subendothelial space, which initiates progressive stages of inflammation as well as mesangial and endocapillary proliferative disease. An alternative model suggests that circulating nuclear remnants resulting from excessive apoptotic cellular breakdown are bound to glomerular capillary sites, with subsequent binding of autoantibodies to the "planted" antigens and local formation of immune complex aggregates.

Observations in the Heymann nephritis animal model of membranous nephropathy and in rare congenital forms of human membranous nephropathy indicate that autoantibodies are capable of reacting with constitutive (nonnuclear) antigens of the glomerular podocytes. This in situ production and accumulation of immune complexes along the external (subepithelial) aspect of the glomerular capillary has not been definitively proven to be operant in human lupus membranous nephropathy.

Autoimmunity based on direct cell-mediated injury to various components of the nephron has been proposed, based primarily on the high frequency of mononuclear cell infiltration in various forms of lupus nephritis. Despite the common presence of infiltrating lymphoid cells, there is no direct proof of a pathogenic mechanism (analogous to the nephron damage of cell-mediated renal allograft rejection) in human lupus nephritis.

RENAL INVOLVEMENT IN SUBSETS OF PATIENTS WITH SYSTEMIC LUPUS ERYTHEMATOSUS

Characteristic patterns of inflammation of skin, joints, and kidneys, along with antinuclear antibodies, are the usual basis for diagnosis of SLE. However, there is a broad range of SLE phenotypes, and subsets of patients with unique natural histories of disease tend to be associated with different subspecialty practices. Frequencies of renal involvement differ among the various subsets of patients. For example, a minority of SLE patients whose predominant clinical problems are of a dermatologic, neurologic, or hematologic nature appears to have clinically significant lupus nephritis, whereas the majority of SLE patients with predominantly rheumatic manifestations have clinical and/or pathologic evidence of renal involvement. Ideally, the diagnosis of SLE should be based on the presence of four or more criteria defined by the American College of Rheumatology, but it should be emphasized that these criteria are intended to standardize eligibility criteria for inclusion of subjects in SLE research studies, rather than to establish diagnostic criteria for SLE in clinical practice.

SYMPTOMS AND SIGNS OF LUPUS NEPHRITIS

Glomerulonephritis is uncommonly the sentinel manifestation of SLE. An exception to this principle is membranous lupus nephritis, wherein up to one quarter of patients present with no extrarenal manifestations, and diagnosis of SLE may emerge only during extended follow-up.

The key challenge for diagnosticians is to detect clinically significant lupus nephritis before the appearance of overt symptoms. Patients with a likely or proven diagnosis of SLE should be carefully questioned about what they may ordinarily consider to be trivial changes in urine color, nocturia, and foam-producing urination, each of which may mark the onset of occult lupus nephritis. Hypertension is more frequent in patients with diffuse proliferative lupus nephritis, compared with focal proliferative or membranous lupus nephritis. Edema, which is proportional to the degree of nephrotic syndrome, is common in lupus membranous and diffuse proliferative nephropathy but rare in milder mesangial or focal proliferative forms of lupus nephritis.

LABORATORY FINDINGS

As one of the major components of the American College of Rheumatology Criteria for Classification for Systemic Lupus Erythematosus, the renal criteria include the presence of (1) persistent proteinuria greater than 0.5 g/day or (2) cellular casts, including red cell, hemoglobin, granular, tubular, or mixed casts. Evidence of hematuria, proteinuria, or pathologic urine sediment on screening urinalysis usually portends the presence of lupus nephritis. However, the astute clinician should be mindful that false-negative urinalyses are disappointingly common in high-throughput clinical laboratories. Errors in identifying abnormalities of urine sediment such as dysmorphic erythrocytes and cellular casts are common. As an offset, it is judicious to "flag" urinalyses from patients with SLE for special scrutiny by laboratory personnel; alternatively, the clinician may consider personally examining the urine sediment in high-risk cases.

Proteinuria is traditionally quantified by 24-hour urine collection. However, a spot urine protein-to-creatinine ratio (the value of which approximates the number of grams per day of proteinuria) is becoming widely accepted as the more convenient alternative for patients, particularly for monitoring changes in proteinuria over time. This method has the cost and convenience advantage of affording more data from which to interpret meaningful and reproducible changes in proteinuria.

Serologic testing includes antinuclear, anti-DNA, and anti-phospholipid antibodies, which are useful for diagnosis of SLE and its complications. The clotting diathesis conferred by the anti-phospholipid syndrome may compound the thromboembolic risk of persistent nephrotic syndrome. Elevated anti-DNA titers and depressed levels of C3 and C4 complement levels correlate with active proliferative lupus nephritis; changes in these levels tend to be more useful than their absolute levels for monitoring activity of nephritis during follow-up.

RENAL BIOPSY

Renal biopsy is primarily valuable for staging the type and severity of lupus nephritis. The classification scheme has recently been revised and updated (**Table 24-1**). **Figures 24-1** and **24-2** depict representative pathology findings of biopsies from patients with lupus nephritis.

Characteristic clinical features of patients with the various classes of pathology can be summarized as follows:

- Class I, Minimal mesangial lupus glomerulonephritis (LGN)—normal urine or microscopic hematuria

- Class II, Mesangial proliferative LGN—microscopic hematuria and/or low-grade proteinuria
- Class III, Focal proliferative LGN—nephritic urine sediment and subnephrotic proteinuria
- Class IV, Diffuse proliferative LGN—nephritic and nephrotic syndromes, hypertension, azotemia
- Class V, Membranous LGN—nephrotic syndrome
- Class VI, Sclerosing disease—hypertension and reduced kidney function

Microvascular thromboses of glomerular capillaries and of extraglomerular vessels occur in a small minority of cases of lupus nephritis. The sensitivity and specificity of anti-phospholipid antibodies for these vasculopathies are low. Lupus patients with high titers of anti-phospholipid antibodies have modestly increased risk of arterial and venous thromboses, clinically manifested as strokes, thrombophlebitis, pulmonary emboli, renal vein thromboses, placental infarcts, and fetal loss.

Discordances among clinicopathologic findings are common over time, and repeat renal biopsy may be needed to stage (or potentially reclassify) the renal disease. Knowledge of the findings of renal biopsy pathology strongly influences therapeutic decisions in lupus nephritis. Institution of intensive therapy, particularly cytotoxic drugs, has been shown to occur earlier when clinicians have the benefit of renal pathology data.

TABLE 24-1 International Society of Nephrology—Renal Pathology Society, 2004 Classification of Lupus Glomerulonephritis

DESIGNATION	DESCRIPTION
Class I: Minimal mesangial LGN	Near-normal glomeruli by LM; mesangial deposits are present by IF and/or EM
Class II: Mesangial proliferative LGN	Mesangial hypercellularity and matrix expansion, with mesangial deposits by IF and EM
Class III: Focal LGN	<50% of glomeruli display active or inactive segmental (<50% of the tuft) or global (>50% of the tuft) endocapillary proliferation or sclerosis; predominantly mesangial and subendothelial deposits are present on IF and EM
Class IV: Diffuse LGN	>50% of glomeruli have endocapillary or extracapillary glomerulonephritis; predominantly mesangial and subendothelial deposits are present on IF and EM; two subsets are defined
Class IV-S: Segmental diffuse LGN	>50% of affected glomeruli have segmental lesions
Class IV-G: Global diffuse LGN	>50% of affected glomeruli have global lesions
Class V: Membranous LGN	Capillary loop thickening in association with predominantly subepithelial deposits by IF and EM
Class VI: Advanced sclerosis	>90% of glomeruli are obsolescent, with substantial activity in remaining glomeruli

EM, electron microscopy; IF, immunofluorescence; LGN, lupus glomerulonephritis; LM, light microscopy

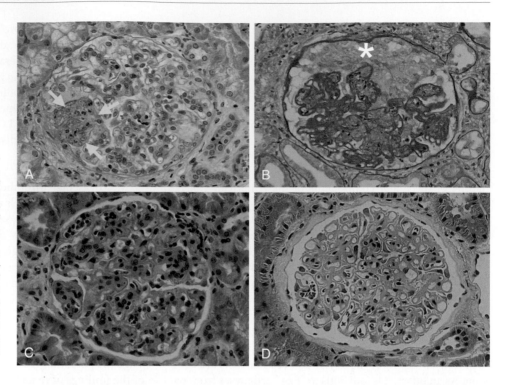

FIGURE 24-1 Light microscopic changes in lupus glomerulonephritis (LGN). **A,** Segmental proliferative LGN. The glomerulus shows a discrete segmental lesion with karyorrhexis and necrosis *(gold arrows)*; the remaining capillary loops are patent with only mild mesangial expansion (hematoxylin and eosin stain). **B,** Global proliferative LGN with an extracapillary cellular crescent *(asterisk)*; the integrity of the glomerular tuft is compromised by proliferation and thickening of the capillary loops (hematoxylin and eosin stain). **C,** Pure global proliferative LGN (hematoxylin and eosin stain). **D,** Membranous LGN; capillary loops are uniformly thickened (hematoxylin and eosin stain).

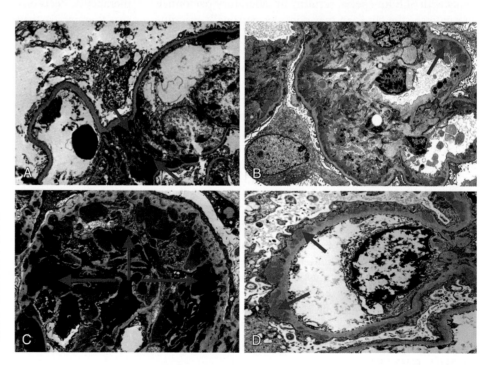

FIGURE 24-2 Ultrastructural changes in lupus glomerulonephritis (LGN). **A,** Mesangial proliferative LGN; electron-dense deposits corresponding to immune complexes are concentrated in mesangial region *(red arrows)*. **B** and **C,** Continuum of subendothelial and intraluminal electron-dense deposits characteristic of proliferative forms of LGN *(red arrows)*. **D,** Subepithelial electron-dense deposits characteristic of membranous LGN *(red arrows)*.

COMPLICATIONS

The complications of lupus nephritis result from the pathophysiology intrinsic to the glomerular disease, including hypertension, nephritic and nephrotic syndromes, and renal failure, as well as from side effects of treatment. Although clinicians treating lupus nephritis have traditionally focused on therapeutic interventions to reduce the risks of renal failure, there is emerging appreciation that treatment may be required to interdict the cardiovascular and thromboembolic complications engendered by protracted nephrotic syndrome. Indeed, evidence supports the notion that achieving even partial remission of proteinuria (to the subnephrotic level) has a salutary effect on patient and renal survival. Beyond standard immunosuppressive therapies, implementation of the full armamentarium of renal protection strategies, particularly angiotensin antagonists and lipid-lowering statin drugs, is warranted in the management of lupus nephritis.

TREATMENT

The natural history of SLE is known most precisely from studies of murine models, in which death from progressive lupus nephritis regularly occurs unless the disease is arrested by effective immunosuppressive regimens. A comparably ominous natural history of human lupus nephritis is occasionally demonstrated by severe damage and renal failure in patients who lack access to modern medical therapies. It is gratifying that numerous therapeutic advances have dramatically improved the prognosis of lupus nephritis over the past few decades.

Optimal care of patients with lupus nephritis usually requires the integrated expertise of both nephrologists and rheumatologists. Most patients with SLE require some dosage of corticosteroids, antimalarial agents, and nonsteroidal anti-inflammatory drugs for control of their commonly debilitating extrarenal disease, which is best evaluated and managed by rheumatologists. Conversely, delineation of the more arcane aspects of renal disease and integration of the results of renal biopsy are best evaluated and managed by nephrologists. Conjointly staffed clinics offer the best environment for effective communication and comprehensive care of patients with SLE and lupus nephritis.

Immunosuppressive drug options for management of lupus nephritis are summarized in **Table 24-2**. Evidence-based clinical recommendations derived from completed controlled clinical trials are limited, and consensus in developing clinical practice guidelines has not been achieved. Results of ongoing multicentered clinical trials are expected to help prioritize the current therapeutic options for treatment of the various forms of lupus nephritis within the next few years.

Corticosteroids

Patients with new-onset class III, IV, or V lupus nephritis warrant a limited therapeutic trial of high-dose corticosteroids. If full remission of nephritis is not achieved within 6 to 8 weeks, treatment with adjunctive cytotoxic drug therapy (cyclophosphamide or mycophenolate mofetil) should be instuted, as described later. Based on current evidence, those patients with more than one quarter of their glomeruli affected by fibrinoid necrosis or cellular crescents on renal biopsy should be directly initiated on therapy with combined pulse methylprednisolone and pulse cyclophosphamide for a period of 6 months or longer.

Cyclophosphamide

Results of early treatment of murine lupus nephritis and meta-analyses of human trials indicate that cyclophosphamide is among the most effective immunosuppressive drugs for lupus nephritis. Side effects of daily cyclophosphamide are formidable, particularly beyond 3 months, and, for this reason, prescription of daily therapy has become limited. The therapeutic index of cyclophosphamide is improved by administration of intermittent pulse therapy, which has become widely accepted as the standard approach to administration of cyclophosphamide therapy. This acceptance arose from observations in several long-term clinical trials reported from the U.S. National Institutes of Health. The composite

TABLE 24-2 Immunosuppressive Drug Options and Guidelines for Administration in Lupus Nephritis

DRUG	GUIDELINES
Corticosteroids	
Prednisone	Start with 1 mg/kg/day for approximately 6-8 wk; taper to approximately 0.25 mg/kg/day over next 6-8 wk; strive for low-dose alternate-day maintenance therapy; patients with membranous lupus nephritis are often initiated on treatment with comparable doses of alternate-day prednisone.
Pulse methylprednisolone	Start with three daily intravenous pulses, 1 g each; continue with single monthly pulses for 6 mo or longer in patients with severe lupus nephritis (usually in conjunction with pulse cyclophosphamide).
Cyclophosphamide	
Pulse cyclophosphamide	If estimated GFR is >30 mL/min, start single monthly doses of 0.75 g/m² BSA administered intravenously over 1 hr; if GFR is <30 mL/min, the starting dose is 0.5 g/m² BSA; adjust subsequent doses to a maximum of 1.0 g/m² BSA according to WBC nadir count (not less than 1500/μL) at days 10 and 14 after treatment. All cyclophosphamide pulse treatments should include bladder protection by administration of oral or intravenous mesna, forced fluids to achieve diuresis >150 mL/hr, and frequent voiding for 24 hr; consider preemptive antiemetic treatment with dexamethasone 10 mg single dose plus ondansetron or granisetron before cyclophosphamide infusions; pulse regimens usually continue monthly for 6 mo, with conversion to maintenance therapy with azathioprine, mycophenolate, or cyclosporine.
Daily oral cyclophosphamide	Start with 2 mg/kg/day (as a single morning dose); taper dose as necessary to keep WBC >4000/μL; duration of therapy is usually <3 mo; after 3 mo, consider transition to maintenance therapy with azathioprine, mycophenolate, or cyclosporine.
Azathioprine	Start at 2 mg/kg/day as maintenance therapy after substantial improvement of nephritis (usually after 3-6 mo of induction therapy).
Mycophenolate Mofetil	Start at 0.5 g bid, escalating weekly to target of 1.0 g tid according to gastrointestinal tolerance.
Cyclosporine	Start at 5 mg/kg/day, adjusting dose downward according to side effects, particularly azotemia and hyperkalemia.

BSA, body surface area; GFR, glomerular filtration rate; WBC, white blood cell.

CHAPTER 25

Pathogenesis and Pathophysiology of Diabetic Nephropathy

Maria Luiza Caramori and Michael Mauer

Diabetic nephropathy is the single most common cause of end-stage renal disease (ESRD) in adults. In the United States, almost half of patients entering ESRD programs in 2005 were diabetic, and most of them (≥80%) had type 2 diabetes. The annual cost of caring for these patients, in the United States alone, exceeds $10 billion. The mortality rate of patients with diabetic nephropathy is high, and a marked increase in cardiovascular risk accounts for more than half of the increased mortality among these patients. Once overt diabetic nephropathy (proteinuria) is present, ESRD can be postponed, but in most instances not prevented, by effective antihypertensive treatment and careful glycemic control. Therefore, in the last decades, there has been intensive research into early pathophysiologic mechanisms of diabetic renal injury, predictors of diabetic nephropathy risk, and early intervention strategies.

EPIDEMIOLOGY

About 0.5% of the population in the United States and Central Europe has type 1 diabetes. The prevalence is higher in the northern Scandinavian countries and lower in southern Europe and Japan. Diabetic nephropathy will develop in 25% to 35% of these patients, with a peak in the incidence after 20 years of diabetes. Type 2 diabetes is about nine times more prevalent than type 1 diabetes, accounting in part for the greater contribution of type 2 diabetic patients to ESRD incidence. Studies in type 2 diabetic patients from Western Europe and in Pima Indians from Arizona showed rates of progression to nephropathy similar to those of type 1 diabetic patients. The risk of developing ESRD is much higher in black than in white American patients with type 2 diabetes. Glycemic control, systemic blood pressure levels, and genetic factors seem to be very important in determining diabetic nephropathy risk. Other factors such as lipid levels, smoking habits, and vitamin D intake may also have a role in modulating this risk.

Vitamin D has a role beyond the regulation of calcium metabolism. There is evidence that the vitamin D system is also involved in regulation of the immune system, cell growth, and differentiation. Vitamin D binds to its nuclear receptor, and later to the vitamin D response element of target genes, to regulate gene transcription. It has been demonstrated that the vitamin D system has a negative in vivo regulatory effect on the intrarenal renin-angiotensin system. Vitamin D metabolites can also suppress activation of transforming growth factor-β (TGF-β). These effects suggest a potential role for vitamin D in diabetic nephropathy. Vitamin D levels were shown to be lower in type 2 diabetic patients than in controls, and they were also lower in microalbuminuric and proteinuric compared with normoalbuminuric type 2 diabetic patients (**Table 25-1**). Of note, vitamin D replacement reduced proteinuria in about half of diabetic patients with stage 3 or 4 chronic kidney disease in a placebo-controlled trial.

NATURAL COURSE OF DIABETIC NEPHROPATHY

For simplicity, the course of renal involvement in type 1 diabetes can be divided in five stages (**Table 25-2**). Stage I, present at diagnosis, is that of renal hypertrophy-hyperfunction. At this stage, patients at risk and not at risk of diabetic nephropathy cannot be clearly separated. Although some studies suggest that the presence of a glomerular filtration rate (GFR) above the normal range (glomerular hyperfiltration) is an important risk factor, this remains controversial. In an inception cohort study of adult-onset type 1 diabetic subjects, a greater albumin excretion rate within the normal range, male gender, higher mean blood pressure and hemoglobin A1c, and shorter stature were independent predictors of development of microalbuminuria over 18 years of follow-up. Genetic factors associated with predisposition to or protection from diabetic nephropathy could, in the future, add to prediction of risk during this period.

Stage II is defined by the presence of detectable glomerular lesions in patients with normal albumin excretion rates and normal blood pressure levels. Normoalbuminuric patients with more severe glomerular lesions might be at increased risk of progression, as described later. Also, 24-hour blood pressure monitoring may reveal failure of the normal nocturnal blood pressure decline (i.e., night/day ratios >0.9 and non-dipping) as an early diabetic nephropathy indicator that often precedes the development of persistent microalbuminuria.

Microalbuminuria, typically occurring after 5 or more years of diabetes, defines stage III. Microalbuminuria may be present earlier, particularly during adolescence and in patients with poor glycemic control and high-normal blood pressure

TABLE 25-1 Categories of Urinary Albumin Excretion

CATEGORY	TIMED COLLECTION (μg/min)	24-hr COLLECTION (mg/24 hr)	SPOT COLLECTION (μg/mg creatinine)
Normoalbuminuria	<20	<30	<30
Microalbuminuria	20-200	30-300	30-300
Proteinuria	>200	>300	>300

levels. Compared with normoalbuminuric patients, patients with persistent microalbuminuria have threefold to fourfold greater risk of progression to proteinuria and ESRD. Current studies indicate that between 20% and 45% of microalbuminuric type 1 diabetic patients will progress to proteinuria after about 10 years of follow-up, whereas 20% to 25% will return to normoalbuminuric levels and the rest will remain microalbuminuric. At this stage, glomerular lesions are generally more severe than in the previous stages, and blood pressure tends to be increasing, often into the hypertensive range. Other laboratory abnormalities, such as increased levels of cholesterol, triglycerides, fibrinogen, Von Willebrand's factor, and prorenin, can be detected in some patients. Diabetic retinopathy, lower extremity amputation, coronary heart disease, and stroke are also more frequent in this group. GFR is usually normal and stable or slowly declining.

Stage IV occurs after 10 to 20 years of diabetes and is characterized by the presence of dipstick-positive proteinuria. Hypertension is present in about 75% of these patients, and reduced GFR and dyslipidemia are also common. Retinopathy and peripheral and autonomic neuropathy are present in most patients. In addition, the risk for cardiovascular events is extremely high, and asymptomatic myocardial ischemia is frequent. Without therapeutic interventions, GFR declines by about 1.2 mL/min/month in proteinuric type 1 diabetic patients.

Progression to ESRD (stage V) occurs 5 to 15 years after the development of proteinuria.

In type 2 diabetic patients, microalbuminuria may reflect a state of generalized endothelial dysfunction in addition to, or rather than, renal damage per se, and type 2 diabetic patients can have proteinuria at diagnosis, at least in part because the diagnosis of type 2 diabetes is often delayed. GFR decline is more variable in this group of patients, and those with a faster GFR decline usually have more advanced, typical diabetic glomerulopathy lesions and worse metabolic control. In these patients, the duration of diabetes is usually not precisely known, and they can have been diabetic for 5 to 10 years before diagnosis. Therefore, at diagnosis, about 20% of type 2 diabetic patients have retinopathy, 10% have nephropathy, 70% have hypertension, and 60% have dyslipidemia. Nevertheless, in Pima Indians studies in which the onset of type 2 diabetes was dated more precisely, the clinical course of diabetic kidney disease was similar to that of type 1 diabetic patients.

It is important to keep in mind that these categories are general and that progression is highly variable and often not linear. The expression and natural history of these overlapping

TABLE 25-2 Stages of Diabetic Nephropathy

DIABETES DURATION (yr)	STAGE	MANIFESTATIONS
0 to 3-5	I	Renal hypertrophy Increased GFR
3-5 or more	II	Basement membrane thickening Mesangial expansion
7-15 or more	III	Microalbuminuria Elevated blood pressure
15-20 or more	IV	Proteinuria Hypertension Decreased GFR
After 15-25	V	ESRD

ESRD, end-stage renal disease; GFR, glomerular filtration rate.

stages may be influenced by complex genetic, environmental, and treatment interactions, which may greatly affect progression and outcome. Therefore, the scheme presented here can serve as a useful general guide but not as an accurate predictor of the course in individual patients.

PATHOGENESIS

Although important modulating factors may exist, diabetic nephropathy is secondary to the long-term metabolic aberrations found in diabetes. Exposure to elevated glucose levels is necessary for the expression of this disorder. Studies in type 1 and type 2 diabetes have found that improved glycemic control can reduce the risk of diabetic nephropathy. Moreover, the development of the earliest diabetic renal lesions can be slowed or prevented by strict glycemic control, as was demonstrated in a randomized trial in type 1 diabetic kidney transplant recipients. Also, intensive insulin treatment decreased the progression rates of glomerular lesions in a controlled trial in microalbuminuric type 1 diabetic patients. Finally, regression of established diabetic glomerular lesions was demonstrated in the native kidneys of type 1 diabetic patients with prolonged normalization of glycemic levels after successful pancreas transplantation. These studies strongly suggest that hyperglycemia is necessary not only for diabetic nephropathy lesions to develop but also to sustain established lesions. Removal of hyperglycemia allows expression of reparative mechanisms which ultimately result in healing of the original diabetic glomerular injury.

Hemodynamic mechanisms may be also involved in the pathogenesis of diabetic nephropathy. Glomerular hyperfiltration could directly promote extracellular matrix (ECM) accumulation, by mechanisms such as increased expression of TGF-β, modeled in vitro by the mechanical stretching of mesangial cells. Glomerular hyperfiltration could also be a marker of other processes, such as increased activity of the renin-angiotensin, TGF-β, and protein kinase C (PKC) systems. However, patients with other causes of hyperfiltration, such as uninephrectomy, do not develop diabetic lesions. Therefore, glomerular hyperfiltration alone cannot fully explain the genesis of the early lesions of diabetic nephropathy. Clinical observations suggest that hemodynamic factors may be more important in modulating the rate of progression of already well-established diabetic lesions. It is worth noting that the presence of reduced GFR in normoalbuminuric patients with type 1 diabetes has been associated with presence of more severe glomerular lesions, and these patients may be at increased risk of progression to overt diabetic nephropathy. Systemic blood pressure levels are implicated in progression and, as noted earlier, lack of normal nocturnal blood pressure dipping may be implicated in the genesis of diabetic nephropathy. Intensive blood pressure control has been associated with decreased rates of progression from normoalbuminuria to microalbuminuria and from microalbuminuria to proteinuria in both normotensive and hypertensive type 2 diabetic patients.

Genetic predisposition to or protection from diabetic nephropathy appears to be the most important determinant of diabetic nephropathy risk in both type 1 and type 2 diabetics. Differences in the prevalence of microalbuminuria, proteinuria, and ESRD in different patient populations (e.g., marked excess of diabetic nephropathy among black type 2 diabetic patients) support this view. Moreover, only about half of patients with decades of poor glycemic control will develop diabetic nephropathy, whereas some patients will do so despite relatively good control, findings consistent with genetically modulated susceptibility or resistance factors. Genetic predisposition to diabetic nephropathy has been suggested by studies in type 1 and type 2 siblings concordant for diabetes. These studies show extremely high concordance in diabetic nephropathy risk. Moreover, there is a strong correlation for the severity and patterns of glomerular lesions in type 1 diabetic sibling pairs. Predisposition to hypertension and cardiovascular disease has also been linked to increased diabetic nephropathy risk. Diabetic patients with advanced nephropathy had higher mean arterial blood pressures during adolescence. Prediabetic blood pressure levels predicted albumin excretion rate after diabetes onset in type 2 diabetic Pima Indians. Diabetic patients with a family history of hypertension or cardiovascular disease also have higher risk of diabetic nephropathy; thus, the pathogenesis of diabetic nephropathy is linked to factors that also favor the development of atherosclerosis. Other data also suggest that albumin excretion rate and blood pressure are heritable and linked in Caucasian families with type 2 diabetes.

There are ongoing searches for genetic loci related to diabetic nephropathy susceptibility, through both genome screening and candidate gene approaches. Neither approach has yet yielded definitive results, but indications are that multiple genes associated with risk and with protection may be involved. Genome-wide scans revealed linkage to a locus on chromosome 3q in Caucasian, Turkish, and Russian type 1 diabetic patients. Several loci have been implicated in increased susceptibility to diabetic nephropathy in type 2 diabetic patients, including regions on chromosomes 3, 7, 9, 18, and 20. Genetic polymorphisms affecting background vascular risk in the general population, such as polymorphisms of genes related to the renin-angiotensin system, have been evaluated in many studies in diabetic patients. A polymorphism in the gene that encodes the angiotensin-converting enzyme (ACE), consisting of insertion or deletion (I/D) of a 287-base-pair sequence, has been associated with diabetic nephropathy, but this may be related more to disease progression than to development. Positive results have been also found for polymorphisms in other genes related to hemodynamic factors, such as angiotensinogen and angiotensin II type 1 receptor genes.

The Pittsburgh Epidemiology of Diabetes Complications Study found that the estimated glucose disposal rate strongly predicted diabetic nephropathy in type 1 diabetic patients, and polymorphisms in genes related to insulin resistance, such as the genes for ectonucleotide pyrophosphatase/phosphodiesterase-1 (*ENPP1*, previously known as PC-1), peroxisome proliferator-activated receptor-γ2 (*PPARG2*), glucose transporter 1, apolipoprotein E, and lipoprotein lipase (HindIII) have been associated with diabetic nephropathy risk. The frequency of Q carriers of K121Q polymorphism in *ENPP1* was higher among proteinuric and ESRD type 1 diabetic patients than among those with normoalbuminuria. Similarly, the *ENPP1* Q121 variant and the ACE DD genotype were associated with a faster GFR decline in microalbuminuric and proteinuric type 1 diabetic patients. Type 2 diabetic carriers of the Ala12 allele of *PPARG2* had lower albumin excretion rates than noncarriers. Also, the Ala allele was more frequent in normoalbuminuric type 2 diabetic patients than in those with diabetic nephropathy, suggesting that the presence of the Ala allele may confer protection.

There is increasing interest in monocyte-macrophage renal infiltration in diabetic nephropathy. The chemokine receptor 5 (CCR5) promoter 59029 A-positive genotype (G/A or A/A) and the leukocyte-endothelial adhesion molecule 1 (LECAM-1) P213 genotype were associated with increased diabetic nephropathy risk in Japanese patients. Also, a leucine repeat of the carnosinase gene (*CNDP1*) gene was associated with diabetic nephropathy risk in type 2 diabetic patients. Variations in the superoxide dismutase 1 gene (*SOD1*) have recently been associated with the development and progression of diabetic nephropathy in type 1 diabetic patients enrolled in the longitudinal Diabetes Control and Complications Trial (DCCT)/Epidemiology of Diabetes Interventions and Complications (EDIC) study. Of interest, *SOD1* variations were not reflected in differences in either SOD1 messenger RNA (mRNA) expression or activity in lymphoblast cell lines.

PATHOPHYSIOLOGY

The renal lesions of diabetic nephropathy appear to be mainly related to ECM accumulation, which occurs in the glomerular basement membrane (GBM) and in the tubular basement membrane (TBM) and is the principal cause of mesangial expansion and a contributor to interstitium expansion late in the disease. This accumulation is secondary to an imbalance between ECM synthesis and degradation. Many regulatory mechanisms have been proposed to explain the linkage between a high ambient glucose concentration and ECM accumulation.

Increased levels of growth factors, particularly TGF-β, can be associated with increased production of ECM molecules. TGF-β can also downregulate the synthesis of ECM-degrading enzymes and upregulate inhibitors of these enzymes. Angiotensin II can also stimulate ECM synthesis through TGF-β activity. High glucose can directly activate PKC, stimulating ECM production through the cyclic adenosine monophosphate (cAMP) pathway. A link between PKC activation and stimulation of TGF-β action may exist, but TGF-β action is not directly mediated by PKC signaling.

It has been suggested that the accumulation of glycosylation products (generated by nonenzymatic reactions between reducing sugars, such as glucose, and free amino groups, lipids, or nucleic acids) may contribute to the development of diabetic complications. Increased advanced glycation end-products (AGE) can stimulate the synthesis of various growth factors, including insulin-like growth factor I and TGF-β. Binding of AGE proteins to AGE receptors on cell surfaces induces increased intracellular oxidative stress in vitro, characterized by increased nuclear factor kappa-B (NF-κB). These glycosylation products may influence ECM dynamics or change ECM molecules to render them less degradable. In diabetic patients, oxidative or nonoxidative products of glycated proteins or lipids could accumulate in the vascular wall and induce release of cytokines and growth factors, contributing to vascular injury. Further studies of the role of glycation in the pathogenesis of diabetic nephropathy are warranted. However, the fact that glycation is an nonenzymatic process that is dependent on the duration and magnitude of glycemia currently leaves unexplained why only about half of patients with very poor glycemic control develop clinical diabetic nephropathy. Hypothetically, genetic variability in cellular responses to AGE could explain these variabilities in risk.

Aldose reductase, the enzyme that catalyzes the reduction of glucose to sorbitol in the polyol pathway, has been associated with diabetic nephropathy and other microvascular complications of diabetes. Increased activity of aldose reductase leads to accumulation of sorbitol, which is further converted to fructose by the sorbitol dehydrogenase enzyme, using nonreduced nicotinamide adenine dinucleotide (NAD^+) as substrate. The ratio of NAD^+ to the reduced form (NADH) decreases, and the conversion of glyceraldehyde-3-phosphate to 1,3-bisphosphoglycerate is blocked, leaving more substrate (glyceraldehyde-3-phosphate) for the

synthesis of α-glycerol phosphate, a diacylglycerol precursor. Diacylglycerol is a PKC activator that could regulate ECM synthesis and removal. Also, increased activity of aldose reductase consumes reduced NAD phosphate (NADPH), leading to decreased or depleted glutathione. Glutathione is an antioxidant coenzyme used by glutathione peroxidase to reduce peroxide or superoxide, yielding oxidized glutathione. Glutathione can also detoxify carbonyl compounds.

There is also rapidly growing evidence that oxidative stress is increased in diabetes and is related to diabetic nephropathy. Skin fibroblasts from type 1 diabetic patients with diabetic nephropathy, when exposed to a high glucose condition in vitro, do not show the expected increase in activity and mRNA expression for the antioxidant enzymes, catalase and glutathione peroxidase. Also, siblings concordant for type 1 diabetes and glomerular lesions are concordant for catalase skin fibroblast mRNA expression levels. These findings suggest that increased oxidative stress in type 1 diabetic patients with diabetic nephropathy is associated with a decreased response of antioxidant enzymes to high glucose concentrations. Studies have demonstrated increased oxidative stress in families of type 1 diabetic patients, suggesting that an abnormal redox state could precede diabetes onset. Interestingly, erythrocyte glutathione content is correlated to Na^+/H^+ exchanger (NHE) activity, linking oxidative stress to an ion transport system associated with hypertension and with diabetic nephropathy risk.

There is an association between oxidative stress, altered nitric oxide (NO) production and action, and endothelial dysfunction. Endothelium-derived NO is a potent vasodilator that also has antiatherogenic properties, including decreased platelet and leukocyte adhesion to the endothelium and inhibition of smooth muscle cell migration. Exposure to high glucose concentrations increases expression of the endothelial NO synthase (eNOS) gene and NO release, with a concomitant increase in superoxide production. Superoxide inactivates and reacts with NO to form peroxynitrite, a potent oxidant, leading to endothelial dysfunction. Normalization of NO-mediated vasorelaxation in high glucose conditions by superoxide dismutase, a scavenger that transforms superoxide anion into hydrogen peroxide, further adds to this association. Increased oxidative stress has been linked to alterations in other key downstream pathways, including PKC and NF-κB activation, AGE formation, and increased flux through the aldose reductase and hexosamine pathways.

Glomerular mononuclear cell infiltration may also be associated with diabetic nephropathy. Monocyte chemoattractant protein 1 (MCP-1) recruits monocytes and lymphocytes to the glomerulus. High levels of glucose lead to increased expression of human mesangial cell MCP-1 mRNA and downregulation of MCP-1 receptor mRNA expression. Plasma and urinary MCP-1 levels and fluorescent products of lipid peroxidation and malondialdehyde content are higher in microalbuminuric and macroalbuminuric type 1 and type 2 diabetic patients than in normoalbuminuric diabetic subjects or controls. Plasma levels of intercellular adhesion molecule 1 (ICAM-1), a glomerular leukocyte recruitment mediator, were also higher in microalbuminuric or macro-albuminuric than in normoalbuminuric type 2 diabetic patients or controls.

Insulin resistance, associated with obesity, blood pressure elevation, and disturbed lipid metabolism, may also be a risk factor for diabetic nephropathy. As described earlier, insulin sensitivity was found to be the strongest predictor of overt nephropathy in type 1 diabetic patients, and polymorphisms in genes related to insulin resistance have been associated with diabetic nephropathy in type 1 and type 2 diabetes. Other mechanisms possibly associated with diabetic nephropathy include abnormalities of the endothelin and prostaglandin pathways and decreased glycosaminoglycan content in basement membranes.

Thus, the various hypotheses overlap and intersect. Polyol pathway-induced redox changes or hyperglycemia-induced formation of reactive oxygen species could potentially account for most of the other biochemical abnormalities. These mechanisms could also be influenced by genetic determinants of susceptibility or resistance to hyperglycemic damage.

PATHOLOGY

Type 1 Diabetes

In type 1 diabetics, glomerular lesions are absent at onset but can be demonstrated after diabetes has been present for a few years. The same is true when a normal kidney is transplanted into a diabetic patient. The changes in kidney structure caused by diabetes are specific, creating a pattern not seen in any other disease. The severity of these diabetic lesions is related to the functional disturbances of the clinical renal

disease and also to diabetes duration, degree of glycemic control, and genetic factors. However, the relationship between duration of type 1 diabetes and extent of glomerular pathology is not precise. This is consonant with the marked variability in susceptibility to this disorder, such that some patients may be in renal failure after having diabetes for 15 years whereas others escape complications despite having type 1 diabetes for many decades.

Light Microscopy

The earliest renal structural change in type 1 diabetes, renal hypertrophy, is not reflected in any specific light microscopic changes. In many patients, glomerular structure remains normal or near-normal even after decades of diabetes. Others develop progressive diffuse mesangial expansion seen mainly as increased periodic acid–Schiff (PAS)-positive ECM mesangial material (**Fig. 25-1**). In about 40% to 50% of patients developing proteinuria, there are areas of extreme mesangial expansion called Kimmelstiel-Wilson nodules or nodular mesangial expansion. Mesangial cell nuclei in these nodules are palisaded around masses of mesangial matrix material with compression of surrounding capillary lumina. Nodules are thought to result from earlier glomerular capillary microaneurysm formation. Note that about half of patients with severe diabetic nephropathy do not have these nodular lesions. Therefore, although Kimmelstiel-Wilson nodules are diagnostic of diabetic nephropathy, they are not necessary for severe renal dysfunction to develop.

Early changes often include arteriolar hyalinosis lesions involving replacement of the smooth muscle cells of afferent and efferent arterioles with PAS-positive waxy, homogenous material (see **Fig. 25-1**). The severity of these lesions is directly related to the frequency of global glomerulosclerosis,

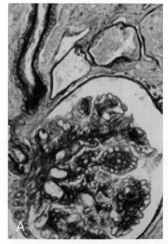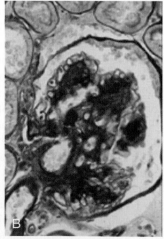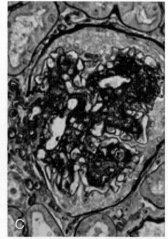

FIGURE 25-1 Light microscopy photographs of glomeruli in sequential kidney biopsies performed at baseline and after 5 and 10 years of follow-up in a patient with long-standing normoalbuminuric type 1 diabetes with progressive mesangial expansion and renal function deterioration. **A,** Note the diffuse and nodular mesangial expansion and arteriolar hyalinosis in this glomerulus from a patient who was normotensive and normoalbuminuric at the time of this baseline biopsy, 21 years after diabetes onset [periodic acid–Schiff [PAS] stain, original magnification ×400). **B,** Five-year follow-up biopsy showing worsening of the diffuse and nodular mesangial expansion and arteriolar hyalinosis in this now microalbuminuric patient with declining glomerular filtration rate (GFR) (PAS stain, ×400). **C,** Ten-year follow-up biopsy showing more advanced diabetic glomerulopathy in this now proteinuric patient with further reduced GFR. Note also the multiple small glomerular (probably efferent) arterioles in the hilar region of this glomerulus (PAS stain, ×400) and in the glomerulus shown in **A.**

perhaps as the result of glomerular ischemia. GBM and TBM thickening may also be detected by light microscopy, although they are often more easily seen by electron microscopy. In addition, atubular glomeruli and glomerulotubular junction abnormalities are present in proteinuric type 1 diabetic patients and may be important in the progressive loss of GFR in diabetic nephropathy. Finally, usually quite late in the disease, tubular atrophy and interstitial fibrosis occur, as in most chronic renal disorders.

Light microscopy changes seen with nephropathies such as amyloidosis might resemble those of diabetes, but the mesangial expansion is not fibrillar as it is in diabetic nephropathy, and the vascular hyalinosis is absent. Moreover, clinical and laboratory features and immunofluorescence and electron microscopy studies can easily differentiate these entities.

Immunofluorescence

Diabetes is characterized by linear GBM, TBM, and Bowman's capsule increased staining, especially for immunoglobulin G (mainly IgG4) and albumin. This staining is removed only by strong acid conditions, consistent with strong ionic binding. The intensity of staining is not related to the severity of the underlying lesions. Care is needed to avoid confusing these findings with anti–basement membrane antibody disorders.

Electron Microscopy

With the use of morphometric techniques, the first measurable nephropathy change observed is thickening of the GBM, which can be detected as early as 1.5 to 2.5 years after onset of type 1 diabetes (**Fig. 25-2**). TBM thickening can also be detected, and it parallels GBM thickening. Increase in the relative area of the mesangium becomes measurable by 4 to 5 years. The fraction of the volume of the glomerulus that is mesangium increases from about 0.2 in the normal state to about 0.4 when proteinuria begins and between 0.6 and 0.8 in those patients whose GFR has been reduced to approximately 40% to 50% of normal. Immunohistochemical studies indicate that these changes in mesangium, GBM, and TBM represent expansion of the intrinsic ECM components at these sites, most likely including types IV and VI collagen, laminin, and fibronectin.

Qualitative and quantitative changes in the renal interstitium are observed in patients with various renal diseases. Interstitial fibrosis is characterized by an increase in ECM proteins and cellularity. Preliminary studies suggest that the pathogenesis of interstitial changes in diabetic nephropathy is different from that of the mesangial matrix, GBM, and TBM changes. Initial observations indicate that, for all but the later stages of the disease, GBM, TBM, and mesangial matrix changes represent the accumulation of basement membrane ECM material, whereas interstitial expansion, early on, is largely due to cellular alterations. Only later, when GFR is already compromised, is interstitial expansion associated with increased interstitium fibrillar collagen and peritubular capillary loss.

Detailed electron microscopy studies revealed that the fraction of GBM covered by intact, nondetached foot processes was decreased in proteinuric patients compared with control subjects and normoalbuminuric or microalbuminuric type 1 diabetic patients. Moreover, the fraction of the glomerular capillary luminal surface covered by fenestrated endothelium was reduced in normoalbuminuric, microalbuminuric, and proteinuric type 1 diabetics compared with controls.

Type 2 Diabetes

Glomerular structure in type 2 diabetes is less well studied, but seems to be more heterogeneous than in type 1. Between one-third and one-half of type 2 patients with clinical features of diabetic nephropathy have typical changes of diabetic nephropathy, including diffuse and nodular mesangial expansion and arteriolar hyalinosis (**Fig. 25-3**). Other patients, despite microalbuminuria or even proteinuria, have no or only mild diabetic glomerulopathy. Some patients have disproportionately severe tubular and interstitial abnormalities and/or vascular lesions and/or an increased number of globally sclerosed glomeruli. Microalbuminuric type 2 diabetic patients, as a group, more frequently have morphometric glomerular structural measures in the normal range on electron microscopy and less severe lesions than microalbuminuric or proteinuric type 1 diabetic patients. Many of these observations have been confirmed in Japanese patients with type 2 diabetes. On the other hand, Pima Indian type 2 diabetic patients, who are known to be at very high risk of ESRD, appear to have lesions more typical of those seen in type 1 diabetic patients.

It is currently unclear why some studies show more structural heterogeneity in type 2 than in type 1 diabetes while others do not. Whether this is a result of differences in patient populations or to other yet unknown variables remains to be determined. However, this is an important question, since the rate of progression towards ESRD in type 2 diabetes appears to be related, at least in part, to the severity of the classic changes of diabetic glomerulopathy. There are reports that type 2 diabetic patients have an increased incidence of nondiabetic lesions, such as proliferative glomerulonephritis and membranous nephropathy, but this is most likely because biopsies were done in atypical cases. When biopsies are performed for research purposes, the incidence of other definable renal diseases is very low (<5%).

STRUCTURAL-FUNCTIONAL RELATIONSHIPS IN DIABETIC NEPHROPATHY

The progression rates vary greatly among individuals. Type 1 diabetic patients with proteinuria who are biopsied for research purposes rather than for diagnosis of atypical clinical characteristics always have advanced glomerular lesions, and usually vascular, tubular, and interstitial lesions as well. Microalbuminuric research patients usually have well-established lesions, but these vary from mild to levels of

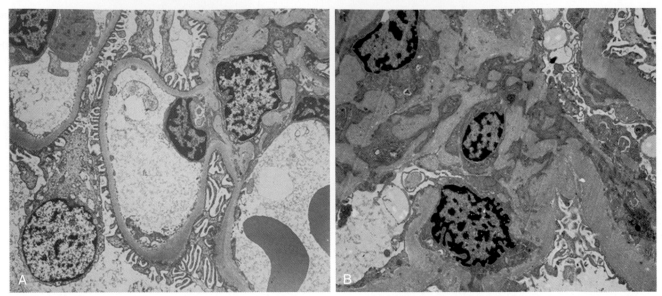

FIGURE 25-2 Electron microscopy photographs of mesangial area in a normal control subject **(A)** and in a patient with type 1 diabetes **(B)** (original magnification ×3900). Note the increase in mesangial matrix and cell content, the glomerular basement membrane thickening, and the decrease in the capillary luminal space in the diabetic patient **(B)**.

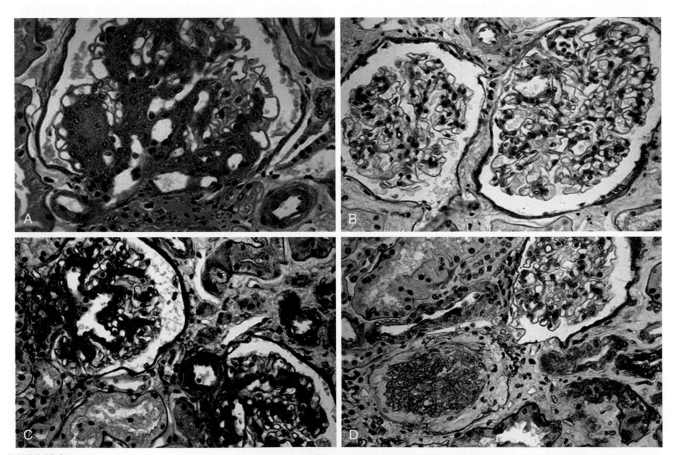

FIGURE 25-3 Light microscopy photographs of glomeruli from type 1 **(A)** and type 2 **(B through D)** diabetic patients. **A,** Diffuse and nodular mesangial expansion and arteriolar hyalinosis in a glomerulus from a microalbuminuric type 1 diabetic patient (periodic acid–Schiff [PAS] stain, original magnification ×400). **B,** Normal or near-normal renal structure in a glomerulus from a microalbuminuric type 2 diabetic patient (PAS stain, ×400). **C,** Changes "typical" of diabetic nephropathology (glomerular, tubulointerstitial, and arteriolar changes occurring in parallel) in a renal biopsy specimen from a microalbuminuric type 2 diabetic patient (PAS stain, ×400). **D,** "Atypical" patterns of injury, with absent or only mild diabetic glomerular changes associated with disproportionately severe tubulointerstitial changes. Note also a glomerulus undergoing glomerular sclerosis (PAS stain, ×400). (**B** through **D,** courtesy of Dr. Paola Fioretto.)

pathology bordering on those regularly seen in proteinuric patients. There is considerable overlap in glomerular structure between long-standing normoalbuinuric and microalbuminuric patients, because normoalbuminuric patients with long-standing type 1 diabetes can have quite advanced renal lesions. On the other hand, many long-standing normoalbuminuric diabetic patients have structural measurements within the normal range.

Expansion of the mesangium, mainly resulting from ECM accumulation, is believed ultimately to reduce or obliterate the glomerular capillary luminal space, decreasing the glomerular filtration surface and the GFR. The fraction of the glomerulus occupied by mesangium is a good correlate of GFR in type 1 diabetic patients, and it is also related to albumin excretion rate and hypertension. The total peripheral GBM filtration surface per glomerulus is directly correlated with GFR and inversely correlated with the degree of mesangial expansion. GBM thickness is also directly related to the albumin excretion rate; however, in sequential biopsy studies, increasing albuminuria was related to increasing mesangial expansion and not to other structural changes. Percentage of global glomerulosclerosis and interstitial expansion are also correlated with the clinical manifestations of diabetic nephropathy (proteinuria, hypertension, and declining GFR). In addition, foot processes width is inversely correlated with GFR in type 1 diabetes and directly correlated with albumin excretion rate in both type 1 and type 2 diabetes. Progressive tubular atrophy, interstitial fibrosis, renal glomerular arteriolar hyalinosis, arteriosclerosis, and glomerulosclerosis are also important components of diabetic nephropathy that may contribute to the reduction in GFR. Finally, atherosclerosis of the larger vessels, perhaps especially in type 2 diabetes, may lead to ischemic renal tissue damage.

In type 1 diabetic patients, glomerular, tubular, interstitial, and vascular lesions tend to progress more or less in parallel, whereas in type 2 diabetic patients this often is not the case. Preliminary observations suggest that long-standing normoalbuminuric type 1 diabetic patients who progress to diabetic nephropathy have more advanced glomerular lesions than those patients who remain normoalbuminuric after long-term follow-up, but these findings are unconfirmed. Current evidence suggests that type 2 diabetic microalbuminuric patients with typical diabetic glomerulopathy have a higher risk of progressive GFR loss than those with lesser degrees of glomerular changes.

A remarkably high frequency of glomerular tubular junction abnormalities can be observed in proteinuric type 1 diabetic patients. Most of these abnormalities are associated with tuft adhesions to Bowman's capsule at or near the glomerular tubular junction (tip lesions). The frequency and severity of these lesions, as well as the presence of completely atubular glomeruli, greatly increase understanding of the structural basis of GFR loss in this disease.

NOVEL THERAPEUTIC STRATEGIES

Better understanding of the processes involved in the pathogenesis of diabetic nephropathy may lead to the development of new therapeutic strategies for its prevention, arrest, or reversal. Conversely, responses to novel therapies could inform understanding of the pathogenesis. These novel strategies might include AGE inhibitors and cross-link breakers, PKC inhibitors, and oxidative stress inhibitors.

Treatment with an inhibitor of glycated albumin formation reduced albumin excretion, prevented GFR decline, reduced mesangial matrix accumulation and normalized cortical mRNA expression of $\alpha 1(IV)$ collagen in *db/db* mice. Pyridoxamine, an intermediate of vitamin B_6 metabolism, improved renal dysfunction in diabetic rats; however, phase II trials in proteinuric type 1 and type 2 diabetic patients showed mixed results. Treatment with the glycation end-product cross-link breaker alagebrium (ALT-711) reduced albumin excretion, blood pressure, renal lesions, cardiac dysfunction, and atherosclerosis in experimental diabetes. Treatment with a PKCβ inhibitor, ruboxistaurin (LY 333531) normalized GFR, decreased albumin excretion, and ameliorated glomerular lesions in diabetic rodents. Treatment with ruboxistaurin for 1 year also prevented GFR decline and reduced the albumin excretion rate in proteinuric type 1 diabetic patients. These findings need to be confirmed in larger prospective trials.

High doses of thiamine and benfotiamine retarded the development of microalbuminuria in experimental diabetic nephropathy. This was associated with decreased activation of PKC and decreased protein glycation and oxidative stress. Sulodexide, a drug that might be capable of repleting glomerular capillary wall change sites, was associated with albuminuria reduction in microalbuminuric and proteinuric type 1 and type 2 diabetic patients. Recently, 12 weeks of osiglitazone, a thiazolidinedione insulin sensitizer, was shown to reduce urinary albumin excretion in normoalbuminuric and microalbuminuric type 2 diabetic patients. This may be a class effect, because proteinuric type 2 diabetic patients receiving pioglitazone in addition to losartan for 12 months had significantly lower albumin excretion rates than patients receiving losartan alone. Histone deacetylase inhibitors also demonstrated antifibrotic and renoprotective effects in animal models of diabetic nephropathy, possibly through modulation of oxidative stress mechanisms. In a 6-month, double-blind, placebo-controlled pilot study, raloxifene, a selective estrogen receptor modulator, slightly decreased the ratio of albumin to creatinine in microalbuminuric and proteinuric postmenopausal women with type 2 diabetes.

In summary, the effects of a number of novel therapies related to the mechanisms of diabetic nephropathy are currently been evaluated in experimental and human diabetic nephropathy, and some of these agents will probably be available for clinical use in the near future.

BIBLIOGRAPHY

Babaei-Jadidi R, Karachalias N, Ahmed N, et al: Prevention of incipient diabetic nephropathy by high-dose thiamine and benfotiamine. Diabetes 52:2110-2120, 2003.

Bangstad HJ, Osterby R, Dahl-Jørgensen K, et al: Improvement of blood glucose control in IDDM patients retards the progression of morphological changes in early diabetic nephropathy. Diabetologia 37:483-490, 1994.

Baynes JW, Thorpe SR: Role of oxidative stress in diabetic complications: A new perspective on an old paradigm. Diabetes 48:1-9, 1999.

Bolton WK, Cattran DC, Williams ME, et al: Randomized trial of an inhibitor of formation of advanced glycation end products in diabetic nephropathy. Am J Nephrol 24:32-40, 2004.

Bennet PH, Haffner S, Kasiske BL, et al: Screening and management of microalbuminuria in patients with diabetes mellitus: Recommendations to the Scientific Advisory Board of the National Kidney Foundation from an ad hoc committee of the Council on Diabetes Mellitus of the National Kidney Foundation. Am J Kidney Dis 25:107-112, 1995.

Bilous RW, Mauer SM, Viberti GC: Genetic aspects of diabetic nephropathy. In Morgan SH, Grünfeld J-P (eds): Inherited Disorders of the Kidney: Investigation and Management. Oxford, Oxford University Press, 1998, pp 427-448.

Caramori ML, Canani LH, Costa LA, et al: The human peroxisome proliferator activated receptor γ2 (PPARγ2) Pro12Ala polymorphism is associated with decreased risk of diabetic nephropathy in patients with type 2 diabetes. Diabetes 52: 3010-3013, 2003.

Caramori ML, Fioretto P, Mauer M: Low glomerular filtration rate in normoalbuminuric type 1 diabetic patients: An indicator of more advanced glomerular lesions. Diabetes 52:1036-1040, 2003.

Caramori ML, Kim Y, Huang C, et al: Cellular basis of diabetic nephropathy: 1. Study design and structural-functional relationships in patients with long-standing type 1 diabetes. Diabetes 51:506-513, 2002.

Coughlan MT, Forbes JM, Cooper ME: Role of the AGE crosslink breaker, alagebrium, as a renoprotective agent in diabetes. Kidney Int Suppl 106:S54-S60, 2007.

The Diabetes Control and Complications Trial Research Group: Effect of intensive therapy on the development and progression of diabetic nephropathy in the Diabetes Control and Complications Trial. Kidney Int 47:1703-1720, 1995.

Fioretto P, Mauer M, Brocco E, et al: Patterns of renal injury in NIDDM patients with microalbuminuria. Diabetologia 39: 1569-1576, 1996.

Fioretto P, Steffes MW, Mauer SM: Glomerular structure in nonproteinuric insulin-dependent diabetic patients with various levels of albuminuria. Diabetes 43:1358-1364, 1994.

Forbes JM, Thallas V, Thomas MC, et al: The breakdown of preexisting advanced glycation end products is associated with reduced renal fibrosis in experimental diabetes. FASEB J 17: 1762-1764, 2003.

Hadjadj S, Gourdy P, Zaoui P, et al: Effect of raloxifene—a selective oestrogen receptor modulator—on kidney function in post-menopausal women with type 2 diabetes: Results from a randomized, placebo-controlled pilot trial. Diabetes Med 24:906-910, 2007.

Hansson L, Zanchetti A, Carruthers SG, et al: Effects of intensive blood-pressure lowering and low-dose aspirin in patients with hypertension: Principal results of the Hypertension Optimal Treatment (HOT) randomised trial. Lancet 351:1755-1762, 1998.

Hovind P, Tarnow L, Rossing P, et al: Predictors for the development of microalbuminuria and macroalbuminuria in patients with type 1 diabetes: Inception cohort study. BMJ 328:1105, 2004.

Huang C, Kim Y, Caramori ML, et al: Cellular basis of diabetic nephropathy: II. The transforming growth factor-beta system and diabetic nephropathy lesions in type 1 diabetes. Diabetes 51:3577-3581, 2002.

Jin HM, Pan Y: Renoprotection provided by losartan in combination with pioglitazone is superior to renoprotection provided by losartan alone in patients with type 2 diabetic nephropathy. Kidney Blood Press Res 30:203-211, 2007.

Katz A, Caramori ML, Sisson-Ross S, et al: An increase in the cell component of the cortical interstitium antedates interstitial fibrosis in type 1 diabetic patients. Kidney Int 61:2058-2066, 2002.

Kelly DJ, Zhang Y, Hepper C, et al: Protein kinase C beta inhibition attenuates the progression of experimental diabetic nephropathy in the presence of continued hypertension. Diabetes 52: 512-518, 2003.

Kiritoshi S, Nishikawa T, Sonoda K, et al: Reactive oxygen species from mitochondria induce cyclooxygenase-2 gene expression in human mesangial cells: Potential role in diabetic nephropathy. Diabetes 52:2570-2577, 2003.

Krolewski AS: Genetics of diabetic nephropathy: Evidence for major and minor gene effects. Kidney Int 55:1582-1596, 1999.

Lee HB, Noh H, Seo JY, et al: Histone deacetylase inhibitors: A novel class of therapeutic agents in diabetic nephropathy. Kidney Int Suppl 106:S61-S66, 2007.

Lewis EJ, Hunsicker LG, Bain RP, et al: The effects of angiotensin-converting-enzyme inhibition on diabetic nephropathy. The Collaborative Study Group. N Engl J Med 329:1456-1462, 1993.

Lurbe E, Redon J, Kesani A, et al: Increase in nocturnal blood pressure and progression to microalbuminuria in type 1 diabetes. N Engl J Med 347:797-805, 2002.

Mauer M, Mogensen CE, Friedman EA: Diabetic nephropathy. In Schrier RW, Gottschalk CW (eds): Diseases of the Kidney. Boston, Little, Brown, 1996, pp 2019-2061.

Mauer SM, Steffes MW, Ellis EN, et al: Structural-functional relationships in diabetic nephropathy. J Clin Invest 74:1143-1155, 1984.

Meltzer S, Leiter L, Daneman D, et al: 1998 Clinical practice guidelines for the management of diabetes in Canada. Canadian Diabetes Association. Can Med Assoc J 159(Suppl 8):S1-S29, 1998.

Mogensen CE: Microalbuminuria, blood pressure and diabetic renal disease: Origin and development of ideas. Diabetologia 42:263-285, 1999.

Nishikawa T, Edelstein D, Brownlee M: The missing link: A single unifying mechanism for diabetic complications. Kidney Int 77:S26-30, 2000.

Orchard TJ, Chang YF, Ferrell RE, et al: Nephropathy in type 1 diabetes: A manifestation of insulin resistance and multiple genetic susceptibilities? Further evidence from the Pittsburgh Epidemiology of Diabetes Complication Study. Kidney Int 62:963-970, 2002.

Østerby R: Glomerular structural changes in type 1 (insulin-dependent) diabetes mellitus: Causes, consequences, and prevention. Diabetologia 35:803-812, 1992.

Ruggenenti P, Fassi A, Ilieva AP, et al: Preventing microalbuminuria in type 2 diabetes. N Engl J Med 351:1941-1951, 2004.

Tuttle KR, Bakris GL, Toto RD, et al: The effect of ruboxistaurin on nephropathy in type 2 diabetes. Diabetes Care 28:2686-2690, 2005.

United Kingdom Prospective Diabetes Study Group: Intensive blood-glucose control with sulphonylureas or insulin compared with conventional treatment and risk of complications in patients with type 2 diabetes (UKPDS 33). Lancet 352:837-853, 1998.

United Kingdom Prospective Diabetes Study Group: Tight blood pressure control and risk of macrovascular and microvascular complications in type 2 diabetes: UKPDS 38. BMJ 317:703-713, 1998.

United States Renal Data System. 2007 Annual Data Report. Available at http://www.usrds.org (accessed July 15, 2008).

Williams ME, Bolton WK, Khalifah RG, et al: Effects of pyridoxamine in combined phase 2 studies of patients with type 1 and type 2 diabetes and overt nephropathy. Am J Nephrol 27:605-14, 2007.

CHAPTER 26

Management of Diabetic Nephropathy

Fuad N. Ziyadeh

SUMMARY OF CLINICAL FEATURES

Up to 35% of all patients with either type 1 or type 2 diabetes eventually develop nephropathy after 25 to 30 years of diabetes. Almost 45% of patients starting chronic dialysis in the United States have diabetic nephropathy as the cause of their end-stage renal disease (ESRD). The point incidence of ESRD due to diabetes has been flattening in recent years, perhaps reflecting improved medical care. However, according to the U.S. Renal Data System's 2007 Annual Data Report (available at http://www.usrds.org), the point prevalence of ESRD due to diabetes is projected to increase by more than 50% between 2005 and 2020 in the United States, largely reflecting the growing population of individuals with type 2 diabetes mellitus.

Five clinical stages characterize the progression of diabetic nephropathy. Staging is based on the values of the glomerular filtration rate (GFR), the urinary albumin excretion (UAE), and systemic blood pressure (**Table 26-1**). The stages are best delineated in the setting of type 1 diabetes: these patients are often young and typically do not have other coexisting systemic diseases (e.g., essential hypertension), and the onset of diabetes is more easily pinpointed. In these patients, microalbuminuria due to diabetic nephropathy rarely develops before 10 years from diabetes onset, and it develops at a rate of 2% to 3% per year. The incidence of microalbuminuria over a lifetime of diabetes is approximately 50%. About one third of individuals with microalbuminuria will progress to proteinuria, at a rate of 2% to 3% per year, and almost all proteinuric patients will eventually develop ESRD. Interestingly, recent studies in type 1 diabetic patients suggest that approximately one third of patients with microalbuminuria will revert to normal UAE, and only one third will progress to proteinuria. Such studies indicate that the appearance of overt nephropathy is perhaps being delayed.

The natural history for patients with type 2 diabetes is not as easily characterized, because 5% to 20% of these patients have some degree of albuminuria at the time of recognition of diabetes. In contrast to type 1 diabetics, patients with type 2 diabetes commonly have hypertension at presentation. Nevertheless, several studies in white type 2 diabetic patients have demonstrated rates of development of microalbuminuria and proteinuria that are approximately comparable to those in type 1 patients. In nonwhite populations, cross-sectional studies indicated a prevalence of microalbuminuria of 30% to 60%, and longitudinal studies of Pima Indians, a native American tribe with an alarmingly high incidence of early-onset type 2 diabetes, have revealed a rate of progression from normal UAE to microalbuminuria of approximately 4% per year. Because of increased cardiovascular mortality, many type 2 diabetic patients die before they progress to ESRD. The patient with diabetes who has microalbuminuria or proteinuria has a twofold to fourfold increased risk for morbidity and mortality from cardiovascular disease. Even with chronic dialysis, the cardiac death rate of diabetic patients is approximately 50% higher than that of nondiabetic patients, reaching 120 deaths per 1000 patients after 1 year of dialysis.

The discrete structural lesions in the renal parenchyma and vasculature typically become more severe with advancing stages and roughly track the functional changes in GFR, UAE, and blood pressure, but the diagnosis of diabetic nephropathy is often made on clinical grounds, without the need for kidney biopsy except in atypical presentations. The earliest renal manifestations in type 1 diabetes are nephromegaly and glomerular hypertrophy, which are accompanied by afferent arteriolar vasodilation, renal hyperperfusion, and glomerular hyperfiltration (stage I). Microscopically, there is thickening of the glomerular and tubular basement

TABLE 26-1 Clinical Stages of Diabetic Nephropathy				
STAGE	**GFR**	**UAE (mg/day)**	**BLOOD PRESSURE**	**YEARS AFTER DIAGNOSIS**
I. Hyperfiltration	Supernormal	<30	Normal	0
II. Microalbuminuria	High-normal to normal	30-300	Rising	5-15
III. Proteinuria	Normal to decreasing	>300	Elevated	10-20
IV. Progressive nephropathy	Decreasing	Increasing	Elevated	15-25
V. ESRD	<15 mL/min	Massive	Elevated	20-30

ESRD, end-stage renal disease; GFR, glomerular filtration rate; UAE, urinary albumin excretion.

membranes, which appears even if the patient is not destined to develop established diabetic nephropathy. During stage II, there is a significant degree of mesangial matrix expansion, with further thickening of the glomerular and tubular basement membranes. Podocyte loss due to detachment and/or apoptosis may also manifest at this early stage and is a pivotal, irreversible lesion that heralds excess protein leakage and progressive glomerulosclerosis. In stage III and beyond, the glomeruli typically demonstrate diffuse or nodular glomerulosclerosis, and further podocyte loss, slit diaphragm abnormalities, and focal areas of foot process effacement are present. Variable degrees of mesangiolysis and microaneurysm formation also appear. Arteriolar hyalinosis develops in both the afferent and efferent arterioles, and there is a variable degree of tubulointerstitial fibrosis. Diabetic vasculopathy can lead to papillary necrosis given the sparse blood flow to the hyperconcentrated regions of the medulla/papilla and the flow-dependence on vasodilatory prostanoids. Ischemic necrosis of the papilla may occur especially if there are predisposing factors for oxidative stress such as vasoconstriction, pyelonephritis, or frequent use of analgesics or nonsteroidal anti-inflammatory agents. Papillary necrosis can often be an incidental finding on imaging studies, and it can be associated with flank pain, hematuria, urinary tract infection, and obstruction due to sloughed papillae.

SCREENING

The Diabetes Control and Complications Trial (DCCT) and the Stockholm Diabetes Intervention Study (SDIS) in type 1 diabetes, and the United Kingdom Prospective Diabetes Study (UKPDS) and the Kumamoto Study in type 2 diabetes, have all shown that the onset and progression of nephropathy can be delayed by interventions, provided they are instituted early in the course of disease. For this reason, screening is of paramount importance. It is recommended that a urinalysis be performed annually, starting at approximately 5 years after the onset of type 1 diabetes or at the time of recognition of type 2 diabetes. In the absence of overt proteinuria, a test for microalbuminuria should be conducted. Conveniently, this is done by measuring the albumin-to-creatinine ratio on a random urine sample. A 24-hour urine collection is also useful for measuring total protein excretion and creatinine clearance. It is important to note that a transient increase in UAE can be caused by uncontrolled hyperglycemia or hypertension, fever, urinary tract infection, congestive heart failure, or physical exertion. Therefore, persistent microalbuminuria should be confirmed by two more urine samples over the following 3 to 6 months.

Once a patient develops proteinuria, it is important to rule out causes other than diabetes. This is particularly important in type 1 patients who have had the diagnosis of diabetes for less than 5 years or longer than 30 years or who do not exhibit concomitant signs of diabetic retinopathy. In these cases, the patient should be evaluated for conditions such as viral hepatitis B or C, human immunodeficiency virus infection, lupus nephritis, multiple myeloma, amyloidosis, or use of nonsteroidal anti-inflammatory drugs. In many of these cases, there may be a nephritic urine sediment with either red blood cells or casts. Some studies have suggested that patients with type 2 diabetes are at increased risk for development of primary glomerulopathies, compared with the general population. If the presence of glomerular disease other than diabetic nephropathy is suspected, a kidney biopsy may be required for confirmation. However, a kidney biopsy is neither required nor advised in what appear to be typical cases of diabetic nephropathy. Finally, in addition to causing chronic kidney disease (CKD), diabetes can affect the urinary system, causing neurogenic bladder, pyelonephritis, and papillary necrosis. Renal ultrasonography should be performed to rule out obstruction from any cause, including sloughed papillae.

MEDICAL MANAGEMENT

Treatment of diabetic nephropathy is based on the clinical stage of the disease process. In this section, therapeutic options are discussed for the following categories: prevention of diabetic nephropathy, treatment of established nephropathy, and management options for renal replacement therapy (RRT). Both renal and cardiovascular morbidity and mortality are increased markedly in patients with type 2 diabetes. The level of albumin excretion is predictive of renal and cardiovascular outcome. Therefore, in addition to the classic risk factors and markers such as glucose, blood pressure, blood lipid profile, and lifestyle (smoking, overweight), novel risk markers are identified, and among them is the magnitude of UAE.

Prevention of Diabetic Nephropathy

Both the DCCT and the SDIS in type 1 diabetes and the UKPDS in type 2 diabetes showed the benefit of intensive glucose control in the prevention of microvascular complications (i.e., the development of retinopathy or microalbuminuria). Tight glucose control has also been shown to reduce the degree of nephromegaly and glomerular hyperfiltration in type 1 diabetes. In the DCCT, intensive control of blood glucose with multiple daily insulin injections (glycated hemoglobin [HbA1c] <7%) reduced the occurrence of microalbuminuria (defined in that study as a UAE ≥40 mg/day) by 39% in the primary and secondary cohorts combined (patients with and without baseline retinopathy). Nevertheless, 16% of patients treated to an average blood glucose concentration of 155 mg/dL progressed from normoalbuminuria to microalbuminuria over an average period of 9 years of follow-up. Therefore, there appear to be additional risk factors for the development of microalbuminuria other than chronic hyperglycemia. In neither the DCCT nor the UKPDS study was a threshold for HbA1c delineated, below which further reduction in nephropathy risk was not gained. So, for prevention of nephropathy, the lowest possible HbA1c for the individual patient is the target.

better blood pressure control and lower rates of UAE in patients with diabetic nephropathy. The renoprotective effect of the novel antihypertensive class of renin inhibitors has yet to be determined in randomized clinical trials in patients with proteinuric diabetic kidney disease.

There is an increased risk for hyperkalemia with any agent that intercepts the RAS system, especially with combination therapy and the addition of aldosterone blockers. Serum potassium and creatinine should be monitored closely, starting within 1 week after the initiation of therapy and periodically thereafter. The use of loop diuretics, sodium bicarbonate, or, occasionally, sodium polystyrene sulfonate (Kayexalate) may be effective in controlling the hyperkalemia during therapy. Patients should be instructed to avoid foods that have a high content of potassium (e.g., bananas, oranges, dried fruits, nuts, potatoes, chocolate) and to limit their total intake of potassium to less than 2000 mg/day. Interventions other than blood pressure medications used to delay progression of CKD include dietary sodium restriction to 2000 mg/day or less, limited alcohol consumption (no more than two drinks per day for men and one drink per day for women), control of hyperlipidemia, cessation of smoking, and dietary protein restriction.

Glycemic Control

Attempts at sustained reductions in hyperglycemia continue to be of therapeutic importance in type 1 and type 2 diabetic patients with either incipient or overt nephropathy. In the DCCT, intensive control of blood glucose reduced the occurrence of macroalbuminuria by 54% in the primary and secondary cohorts combined (with and without baseline retinopathy). Also, tight glucose control has been shown to stabilize or even decrease UAE in patients with microalbuminuria, but this effect may take a few years to be clinically evident. Observational studies in type 1 diabetic patients with reduced GFR showed that worse glycemic control was associated with a faster rate of GFR decline even if blood pressure was fairly well controlled. In a prospective, multiyear, observational study of 227 patients with type 2 diabetes and overt nephropathy, one of the determinants of the rate of decline in GFR, as measured by chromium 52–labeled ethylenediamine tetra-acetic acid (^{51}Cr-EDTA), was a higher baseline HbA1c (along with systolic blood pressure and albuminuria).

Caution should be exercised in the management of hyperglycemia when the patient has significant CKD. Because insulin is degraded by the kidney, dose reduction may be needed to prevent hypoglycemia. Reduction in the doses of oral hypoglycemic agents may also be necessary, especially some sulfonylurea compounds that are metabolized by the kidney. The insulin-sensitizing agent metformin is contra-indicated in the presence of kidney dysfunction, defined as a serum creatinine concentration greater than 1.5 mg/dL in males or greater than 1.4 mg/dL in females or a creatinine clearance rate of less than 60 mL/min, because of the risk for life-threatening lactic acidosis. Metformin should also be discontinued before surgery or administration of contrast media. Thiazolidinediones, such as rosiglitazone or pioglitazone, may aggravate edema and congestive heart failure. Caution should be exercised with the use of thiazolidinediones, because no data are available on their long-term cardiovascular safety and efficacy in patients with CKD.

Dietary Protein Restriction

A meta-analysis of five clinical trials in type 1 diabetic patients with nephropathy concluded that dietary protein restriction (to approximately 0.6 g/kg/day of high–biologic value protein with adequate calorie intake) has a significant long-term beneficial effect in slowing the rate of decline in GFR and lowering the UAE without demonstrable evidence of malnutrition. Currently, the ADA recommends 0.8 g/kg/day of protein restriction for diabetic patients with increased UAE, which is a manageable and safe recommendation for most patients with challenging dietary prescriptions related to their diabetes and CKD. Dietary counseling by a nutritionist is desirable for patients with advanced CKD in order to avoid protein-calorie malnutrition before RRT, which has been shown to be a strong predictor for subsequent increased morbidity and mortality during maintenance dialysis. Dietary counselors can also advise on issues of salt, potassium, and phosphate restriction and can advise patients on the choice of carbohydrates and fats.

Lipid Management

The treatment of hyperlipidemia is known to be important in the prevention of atherosclerosis. There is some circumstantial evidence that treatment of hyperlipidemia with statins may protect against the development of glomerulosclerosis, as reflected by decreased UAE and improved serum creatinine levels. There are a number of proposed mechanisms for this finding, including beneficial effects on nitric oxide and endothelin-1 as well as suppression of glucose-mediated upregulation of TGF-β. The current treatment goals set by the ADA are a low-density lipoprotein cholesterol level of less than 100 mg/dL, triglycerides less than 150 mg/dL, and high-density lipoprotein greater than 40 mg/dL. A multi-pronged approach of intensive combined therapy, aimed at lowering HbA1c, blood pressure, serum cholesterol, and body mass index, as well as a program for anemia management, increased physical activity, and smoking cessation, can lead to a significant decrease in cardiovascular events and slowing of progressive nephropathy, not to mention a greater sense of well-being.

Treatment of End-Stage Renal Disease in Diabetes

Once a diabetic patient approaches ESRD, various options for RRT should be offered: peritoneal dialysis, hemodialysis, or kidney transplantation. Survival with either modality of dialysis is generally worse for patients with diabetes compared with nondiabetic patients. Survival is also inversely related to age, presumably reflecting a greater burden of cardiovascular disease in older patients. In fact, more than 70% of deaths in the diabetic ESRD population are attributed to a cardiovascular cause. In patients undergoing hemodialysis, a preexisting severely compromised cardiovascular condition, vascular access problems, diabetic foot disease, interdialytic weight gain, and intradialytic hypotension explain most of the less favorable outcomes in terms of morbidity and mortality as compared with nondiabetic patients. In diabetic CKD patients undergoing hemodialysis, poor glycemic control is also an independent predictor of prognosis. In the United States, approximately 80% of diabetic patients with ESRD are treated with hemodialysis, and more than 80% of these patients receive their treatments in specialized centers.

The choice of dialysis modality in diabetic patients should be similar in consideration to that for any patient with ESRD. However, there are some special considerations in patients with diabetes. Some patients with autonomic neuropathy have frequent episodes of hypotension associated with large fluid shifts during hemodialysis; these may be avoided with the more gradual fluid shifts of peritoneal dialysis. On the other hand, patients with diabetes who are undergoing peritoneal dialysis are at risk for absorption of the dextrose present in the dialysate and may have worsened blood glucose control and hypertriglyceridemia and increased insulin requirements as well as weight gain. Older diabetic patients may have severe peripheral vascular disease, limiting the success of vascular access for hemodialysis. Similarly, peripheral vascular disease may make the peritoneum less than optimal for fluid and electrolyte exchange. Diabetic patients tend to be more prone to development of infectious complications; however, this would put them at greater risk for complications from both peritonitis and vascular access infections. After adjusting for appropriate comorbidities and potential confounders, some observational studies showed that the mortality rate of older diabetic patients is higher with peritoneal dialysis than with hemodialysis. More patients undergoing peritoneal dialysis, compared with hemodialysis, switched the type of dialysis over time, and the reason for switching was often a consequence of the technique. In both forms of dialysis, diabetic patients tend to be more sensitive than other ESRD patients to the symptoms of underdialysis. The newer options of nocturnal hemodialysis or short daily hemodialysis might provide better outcomes for these patients, but data are lacking. Also, for the young diabetic patient who cannot get a kidney transplant, there are suggestions that initiating RRT with peritoneal dialysis and continuing it for 1 to 2 years, before switching to maintenance hemodialysis as residual renal function declines, may afford better overall survival.

For those diabetic patients who are eligible, survival is much improved with renal transplantation compared with dialysis. Two-year survival may be up to four times better with receipt of a kidney transplant compared with staying on dialysis. It could be argued that there is a selection bias for survival after transplantation, because younger and healthier patients are more likely to receive transplants. However, studies looking at the survival of patients who received transplants compared with matched controls of similar health who were awaiting a transplant showed a survival benefit for the patients who underwent transplantation. Although statistics vary by center, the 5-year patient survival rate after transplantation is approximately 70%. Although these survival data are worse than for nondiabetic patients undergoing transplantation, they are better than those for dialysis patients with diabetes, in whom the 5-year survival rate is usually less than 35%. As for patients with other forms of kidney disease, kidney allografts from living donors survive significantly longer than those from deceased donors.

Recurrence of lesions of diabetic nephropathy develops in almost all solitary kidney allografts (i.e., without pancreas or islet cell transplantation). Within 2 years after solitary kidney transplantation, glomerular ultrastructural changes can be seen on biopsy, pointing to the importance of glycemic control in the development of nephropathy. However, graft failure due to recurrent disease is rare, because most patients die before their allografts fail from recurrent diabetic nephropathy.

Pancreas transplantation can be the preferred option for relatively young patients with type 1 diabetes whose blood glucose is especially difficult to control or who have hypoglycemic unawareness but are otherwise in reasonably good health. If the patient also has early nephropathy (microalbuminuria) but well-preserved kidney function, pancreas transplantation alone (PTA) may be considered. Based on the sequential morbidities of the surgery and long-term immunosuppression, the ADA recommends that PTA be considered only in patients who exhibit the following: frequent, acute, and severe metabolic complications requiring medical attention (e.g., recurrent hypoglycemic unawareness); incapacitating clinical and emotional problems with exogenous insulin therapy; and medical failure of exogenous insulin to prevent acute complications.

If the patient has advanced CKD and is approaching dialysis or is already on dialysis, a simultaneous pancreas-kidney (SPK) transplantation is a good alternative. For this procedure, the patient receives the pancreas and the kidney from the same deceased donor (or, rarely, from different donors) during the same operation. The goal of pancreatic transplantation is to restore euglycemia and thereby attempt to prevent or improve secondary complications of diabetes, including CKD. Sustained euglycemia improves the renal lesions of diabetes in the native kidney (in PTA) and also prevents their appearance in the kidney allograft (in SPK transplantation). At the present time, it is not clear whether SPK transplantation confers an additive patient survival advantage over kidney transplantation alone. However, benefits of chronic euglycemia after pancreas transplantation may include stabilization of peripheral neuropathy, improved life expectancy in patients with autonomic insufficiency, improved fertility and pregnancy outcomes, and improved quality of life.

Another option is for the patient to receive a kidney allograft, preferably from a living donor, followed at a later time by transplantation of a pancreas from a deceased donor; this is known as pancreas-after-kidney (PAK) transplantation. There are no prospective, controlled trials comparing outcomes of these various transplantation approaches.

Observational surveys show that 1-year pancreas graft survival is about 85% in SPK transplantation and about 75% in PAK transplantation. This difference most likely reflect the fact that there is not an easily measured, sensitive marker for early pancreatic rejection, whereas an elevation in the serum creatinine concentration provides an advantage to timely diagnosis and treatment of kidney allograft rejection. In general, minimizing or avoiding the need for dialysis altogether is associated with the best survival rates after transplantation. For this reason and because kidney transplantation alone has a dramatic impact on patient longevity, living donor kidney transplantation is recommended for all patients with type 1 diabetes who have a suitable donor, even if they are potential candidates for pancreatic transplantation. Moreover, kidney graft survival rates are generally superior with live-donor compared with deceased-donor kidney transplants. In this scenario, live-donor recipients may then be eligible for subsequent PAK transplantation.

In the workup for transplantation, full cardiovascular assessment is essential, with stress testing, echocardiography, and angiography as indicated in an individual patient. Coronary angioplasty or even bypass surgery may be required before transplantation.

Transplantation of isolated islets using the Edmonton approach can be an option for the treatment of type 1 diabetes mellitus. However, the promising short-term benefits in many diabetic patients are not associated with sustained long-term efficacy. A North American registry reported complete insulin independence in more than 55% of patients 1 year after transplantation, but this state was not sustained permanently, because only 10% of patients remained insulin-free after 5 years. Larger series from multicenter trials are needed to appreciate the full impact of this novel treatment. Moreover, the greatest hurdle for islet cell transplantation is organ shortage because of the need for two donor pancreata per recipient.

BIBLIOGRAPHY

Adler AI, Stratton IM, Neil HA, et al: Association of systolic blood pressure with macrovascular and microvascular complications of type 2 diabetes (UKPDS 36): Prospective observational study. BMJ 321:412-419, 2000.

American Diabetes Association: Nutrition Recommendations and Interventions for Diabetes: A position statement of the American Diabetes Association. Diabetes Care 30(Suppl 1):S48-S65, 2007.

American Diabetes Association: Standards of medical care in diabetes—2007. Diabetes Care 30(Ssuppl 1):S4-S41, 2007.

Barnett AH, Bain SC, Bouter P, et al: Diabetics Exposed to Telmisartan and Enalapril Study Group: Angiotensin-receptor blockade versus converting-enzyme inhibition in type 2 diabetes and nephropathy. N Engl J Med 351:1952-1961, 2004.

Brenner BM, Cooper ME, de Zeeuw D, et al: Effects of losartan on renal and cardiovascular outcomes in patients with type 2 diabetes and nephropathy. N Engl J Med 345:861-869, 2001.

Buse JB, Ginsberg HN, Bakris GL, et al: Primary prevention of cardiovascular diseases in people with diabetes mellitus: A scientific statement from the American Heart Association and the American Diabetes Association. Circulation 115:114-126, 2007.

Diabetes Control and Complications (DCCT) Research Group: Effect of intensive therapy on the development and progression of diabetic nephropathy in the Diabetes Control and Complications Trial. Kidney Int 47:1703-1720, 1995.

Hamilton RA: Angiotensin-converting enzyme inhibitors and type 2 diabetic nephropathy: A meta-analysis. Pharmacotherapy 23:909-915, 2003.

Hansen HP, Tauber-Lassen E, Jensen BR, et al: Effect of dietary protein restriction on prognosis in patients with diabetic nephropathy. Kidney Int 62:220-228, 2002.

Lewis EJ, Hunsicker LG, Bain RP, et al: The effect of angiotensin-converting enzyme inhibition on diabetic nephropathy. N Engl J Med 329:1456-1462, 1993.

Lewis EJ, Hunsicker LG, Clarke WR, et al: Renoprotective effect of the angiotensin-receptor antagonist irbesartan in patients with nephropathy due to type 2 diabetes. N Engl J Med 345:851-860, 2001.

MacKinnon M, Shurraw S, Akbari A, et al: Combination therapy with an angiotensin receptor blocker and an ACE inhibitor in proteinuric renal disease: A systematic review of the efficacy and safety data. Am J Kidney Dis 48:8-20, 2006.

Ming CS, Chen ZH: Progress in pancreas transplantation and combined pancreas-kidney transplantation. Hepatobiliary Pancreat Dis Int 6:17-23, 2007.

Mogyorosi A, Ziyadeh FN: Diabetic nephropathy. In Massry SG, Glassock RJ (eds): Textbook of Nephrology. 4th ed., Philadelphia, Lippincott, Williams & Wilkins, 2001, pp 874-895.

Molitch ME: Management of dyslipidemias in patients with diabetes and chronic kidney disease. Clin J Am Soc Nephrol 1:1090-1099, 2006.

Parving HH, Lehnert H, Bröchner-Mortensen J, et al: The effect of irbesartan on the development of diabetic nephropathy in patients with type 2 diabetes. N Engl J Med 345:870-878, 2001.

Rossing K, Christensen PK, Hovind P, et al: Progression of nephropathy in type 2 diabetic patients. Kidney Int 66:1596-1605, 2004.

Rossing K, Schjoedt KJ, Smidt UM, et al: Beneficial effects of adding spironolactone to recommended antihypertensive treatment in diabetic nephropathy: A randomized, double-masked, crossover study. Diabetes Care 28:2106-2112, 2005.

Shahab I, Khanna R, Nolph KD: Peritoneal dialysis or hemodialysis? A dilemma for the nephrologist. Adv Perit Dial 22:180-185, 2006.

Strippoli GF, Craig M, Schena FP, Craig JC: Antihypertensive agents for primary prevention of diabetic nephropathy. J Am Soc Nephrol 16:3081-3091, 2005.

Venstrom JM, McBride MA, Rother KI, et al: Survival after pancreas transplantation in patients with diabetes and preserved kidney function. JAMA 290:2817-2823, 2003.

Witkowski P, Zakai SB, Rana A, et al: Pancreatic islet transplantation: What has been achieved since Edmonton break-through. Ann Transplant 11:5-13, 2006.

Wolf G, Chen S, Ziyadeh FN: From the periphery of the glomerular capillary wall toward the center of disease: Podocyte injury comes of age in diabetic nephropathy. Diabetes 54:1626-1634, 2005.

Wolf G, Ritz E: Combination therapy with ACE inhibitors and angiotensin II receptor blockers to halt progression of chronic renal disease: Pathophysiology and indications. Kidney Int 67:799-812, 2005.

Wolf G, Sharma K, Ziyadeh FN: Pathophysiology and pathogenesis of diabetic nephropathy. In Alpern RJ, Hebert SC (eds): Seldin & Giebisch's The Kidney. 4th ed., Philadelphia, Elsevier/Academic Press, 2007, pp 2215-2233.

The Writing Team for the Diabetes Control and Complications Trial/Epidemiology of Diabetes Interventions and Complications Research Group: Sustained effect of intensive treatment of type 1 diabetes mellitus on development and progression of diabetic nephropathy. The Epidemiology of Diabetes Interventions and Complications (EDIC) study. JAMA 290:2159-2167, 2003.

Ziyadeh FN: Mediators of diabetic renal disease: The case for TGF-beta as the major mediator. J Am Soc Nephrol 15(Suppl 1): S55-S57, 2004.

Ziyadeh FN, Hoffman BB, Han DC, et al: Long-term prevention of renal insufficiency, excess matrix gene expression, and glomerular mesangial matrix expansion by treatment with monoclonal antitransforming growth factor-beta antibody in *db/db* diabetic mice. Proc Natl Acad Sci U S A 97:8015-8020, 2000.

CHAPTER 27

Dysproteinemias and Amyloidosis

Paul W. Sanders

Paraproteinemic renal diseases are typically the result of deposition of immunoglobulin fragments (heavy chains and light chains) in specific parts of the nephron (**Fig. 27-1**). They can be divided generally into those diseases that manifest primarily as glomerular or as tubulointerstitial injury (**Table 27-1**). The category of glomerular diseases includes AL-type amyloidosis (amyloid composed of light chains), AH-type amyloidosis (amyloid composed of heavy chains), monoclonal light-chain and light- and heavy-chain deposition disease (collectively termed MLCDD in this review), monoclonal heavy-chain deposition disease, immunotactoid glomerulopathy, glomerulonephritis associated with monoclonal immunoglobulin deposition, and glomerulonephritis associated with type I cryoglobulinemia. In this review, AL-type amyloidosis, MLCDD, fibrillary glomerulonephritis, and immunotactoid glomerulopathy are discussed. Patterns of tubular injury include a proximal tubulopathy and cast nephropathy (also known as "myeloma kidney"). In addition to these paraproteinemic renal lesions, this chapter includes a discussion of Waldenström macroglobulinemia.

Aside from some notable exceptions, such as AH-type amyloidosis and heavy-chain deposition disease, immunoglobulin light-chain deposition is directly responsible for most of the various renal pathologic alterations in paraproteinemia. The type of renal lesion induced by light chains depends on the physicochemical properties of these proteins.

IMMUNOGLOBULIN LIGHT-CHAIN METABOLISM AND CLINICAL DETECTION

The original description of immunoglobulin light chains was attributed to Dr. Henry Bence Jones, who published his findings in 1847. He was the first to characterize these unique proteins, which bear his name. More than a century later, Berggård and Peterson demonstrated that Bence Jones proteins were immunoglobulin light chains.

Plasma cells synthesize light chains that become part of the immunoglobulin molecule (see **Fig. 27-1**). A slight excess production of light, compared to heavy, chains appears to be required for efficient immunoglobulin synthesis but results in release of free light chains into the circulation. Once in the bloodstream, light chains are handled similarly to other low-molecular-weight proteins, which are usually removed from the circulation by glomerular filtration. Unlike albumin, monomers (molecular weight, approximately 22 kDa) and dimers (approximately 44 kDa) are readily filtered through the glomerulus and reabsorbed by the proximal tubule. Endocytosis of light chains into the proximal

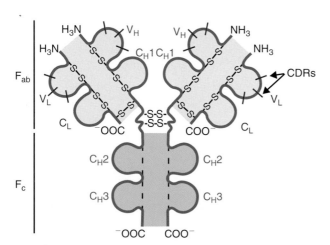

FIGURE 27-1 Diagram of the immunoglobulin G molecule, which consists of two heavy chains and two light chains that are stabilized by intermolecular and intramolecular disulfide bonds (-S-S-). Light chains consist of two domains that are termed constant (C_L) and variable (V_L) regions. Within the V_L domain are the complementarity-determining regions (CDRs, indicated by *short red lines*) that are primarily responsible for variations in the amino acid sequences among light chains. Heavy chains also consist of a variable domain (V_H) and three constant domains (C_H1, C_H2, C_H3). F_{ab} and Fc are the fragments generated by papain cleavage. Amino termini are labeled H_3N and NH_3; carboxyl termini, ^-OOC and COO^-.

TABLE 27-1 Monoclonal Light Chain–Related Renal Lesions
Glomerulopathies
Monoclonal light-chain and light- and heavy-chain deposition disease (MLCDD)
AL-type amyloidosis
Cryoglobulinemia
Tubulointerstitial Lesions
Cast nephropathy ("myeloma kidney")
Fanconi's syndrome
Proximal tubule injury (acute tubular necrosis)
Tubulointerstitial nephritis (rare)
Vascular Lesions
Asymptomatic Bence Jones Proteinuria
Hyperviscosity Syndrome
Neoplastic Cell Infiltration (Rare)

tubule occurs through a single class of heterodimeric, multiligand receptors that are composed of megalin and cubilin. After endocytosis, lysosomal enzymes hydrolyze the proteins, and the amino acid components are returned to the circulation. The uptake and catabolism of these proteins are very efficient and readily handle the approximate 500 mg of free light chains that are produced daily by the normal lymphoid system. In the setting of a monoclonal gammopathy, however, production of monoclonal light chains increases. Binding of light chains to the megalin-cubilin complex can become saturated, allowing light chains to be delivered to the distal nephron and to appear in the urine.

Light chains are modular proteins that possess two independent globular regions, termed constant (C_L) and variable (V_L) domains (see **Fig. 27-1**). Light chains can be isotyped as kappa (κ) or lambda (λ), based on sequence variations in the constant region of the protein. Within the globular V_L domain are four framework regions consisting of beta sheets that develop a hydrophobic core. The framework regions separate three hypervariable segments that are known as complementarity determining regions (CDR1, CDR2, and CDR3) (see **Fig. 27-1**). The CDRs tend to form loop structures and constitute part of the antigen-binding site of the immunoglobulin; the CDR domains represent those regions of sequence variability in the light chain. Diversity among the CDR regions occurs because the V_L domain is synthesized by rearrangement of multiple gene segments. Therefore, although they possess similar structures and biochemical properties, no two light chains are identical, but there are enough sequence similarities among light chains to permit categorizing them into subgroups. There are four κ and ten λ subgroups, although of the λ subgroups, most patients (94%) with multiple myeloma express λI, λII, λIII, or λV. Free light chains, particularly the λ isotype, often homodimerize before secretion into the circulation.

The multiple renal lesions from monoclonal light-chain deposition affect virtually every compartment of the kidney (see **Table 27-1**) and may be explained by sequence variations, particularly in the V_L domain of the offending monoclonal light chain. The light chains that are responsible for monoclonal light-chain deposition disease (MLCDD) are frequently members of the κIV subfamily and appear to possess unusual hydrophobic amino acid residues in CDR1. In AL-type amyloidosis, sequence variations in the V_L domain of the precursor light chain confer the propensity to polymerize to form amyloid. A classic renal presentation of multiple myeloma is Fanconi's syndrome, which is produced almost exclusively by members of the κI subfamily. Unusual nonpolar residues in the CDR1 region and absence of accessible side chains in the CDR3 loop of the variable domain of κI light chains result in homotypic crystallization of the light chain. In cast nephropathy, the secondary structure of CDR3 is a critical determinant of cast formation. In summary, sequence variations in the V_L domain appear to determine the type of renal lesion that occurs with monoclonal light-chain deposition.

Light chains were originally detected using turbidimetric and heat tests. Because these tests lack sensitivity, they are no longer in use. The qualitative urine dipstick test for protein also has a low sensitivity for detection of light chains. Although some Bence Jones proteins react with the chemical impregnated onto the strip, other light chains cannot be detected; the net charge of the protein may be an important determinant of this interaction. Because of the relative insensitivity of routine serum protein electrophoresis and urinary protein electrophoresis for light chains, these tests are not recommended as screening tools in the diagnostic evaluation of the underlying etiology of renal disease. Highly sensitive and reliable immunoassays are available to detect the presence of monoclonal light chains in the urine and serum and are adequate tests for screening when both are used together. If a clone of plasma cells exists, significant amounts of monoclonal light chains appear in the circulation and in the urine. In healthy adults, the urinary concentration of polyclonal light-chain proteins is about 2.5 µg/mL. Causes of monoclonal light-chain proteinuria, a hallmark of plasma cell dyscrasias, are listed (**Table 27-2**). Urinary light chain concentration is generally between 0.020 and 0.5 mg/mL in patients with monoclonal gammopathy of undetermined significance (MGUS) and is often much higher (range, 0.02 to 11.8 mg/mL) in patients with multiple myeloma or Waldenström macroglobulinemia. Immunofixation electrophoresis is very sensitive and detects monoclonal light chains and immunoglobulins even in very low concentrations, but it is a qualitative assay that may be limited by interobserver variation.

Quantification of serum free κ and λ light chains is available and is also very useful, because most of the renal lesions in paraproteinemias are caused by light chain overproduction; the presence of excess heavy chains or intact immunoglobulins is much less common. Because an excess of light chains, compared to heavy chains, is synthesized and released into the circulation, this sensitive assay detects small amounts of serum free light chains in healthy individuals. This assay can also distinguish polyclonal from monoclonal light chains and further quantifies the level of free light chains in the serum. Quantification of serum light chain levels may be of use clinically to monitor chemotherapy as well as to assess risk for development of renal failure, because baseline serum free monoclonal light chain levels greater than 75 mg/dL correlate with depressed renal function (serum creatinine

TABLE 27-2 Causes of Monoclonal Light-Chain Proteinuria

Multiple myeloma

AL-type amyloidosis

Monoclonal light-chain deposition disease

Waldenström macroglobulinemia

Monoclonal gammopathy of undetermined significance

POEMS syndrome (rare)

Heavy (µ) chain disease (rare)

Lymphoproliferative disease (rare)

POEMS, polyneuropathy, organomegaly, endocrinopathy, M protein, and skin changes.

concentration, 2 mg/dL) and more aggressive myeloma. Perhaps the best combination of screening tests for plasma cell dyscrasias during the evaluation of renal disease comprises immunofixation electrophoresis of serum and urine and quantification of serum free κ and λ light chains.

GLOMERULAR LESIONS OF PLASMA CELL DYSCRASIAS

AL-Type Amyloidosis

Twenty different types of the amyloid family of proteins have been identified. They are named according to the precursor protein that polymerizes to produce amyloid. AL-type amyloidosis, which is also known as *primary amyloidosis,* represents a plasma cell dyscrasia that is characterized by organ dysfunction related to deposition of amyloid and, usually, only a mild increase in monoclonal plasma cells in the bone marrow. However, about 20% of patients with AL-type amyloidosis have overt multiple myeloma or other lymphoproliferative disorder. In AL-type amyloidosis, the amyloid deposits are composed of immunoglobulin light chains.

AA-type amyloidosis, or secondary amyloidosis, is a different disease process that occurs in the course of chronic inflammatory conditions, such as rheumatoid arthritis or connective tissue diseases, and familial Mediterranean fever. The amyloid precursor protein in secondary amyloidosis is serum amyloid A protein, which is an acute phase reactant. The treatment of AA-type amyloidosis is completely different from that of AL-type amyloidosis and includes measures to decrease inflammation and treatment with eprodisate, an agent that is thought to interfere with amyloid deposition and was found to be useful in a recent clinical trial. The identification of the type of amyloid protein is an essential first step in the management of this disorder.

AL-type amyloidosis is a systemic disease that typically involves multiple organs (**Table 27-3**). Cardiac infiltration frequently produces congestive heart failure and is a common presenting manifestation of primary amyloidosis. Infiltration of the lungs and gastrointestinal tract is also common but usually produces few clinical manifestations. Dysesthesias, orthostatic hypotension, diarrhea, and bladder dysfunction due to peripheral and autonomic neuropathies can occur. Amyloid deposition can also produce an arthropathy that resembles rheumatoid arthritis, a bleeding diathesis, and a variety of skin manifestations including purpura. Kidney involvement is common in primary amyloidosis.

Pathology

Glomerular lesions are the dominant renal features of AL-type amyloidosis. They are characterized by the presence of mesangial nodules and progressive effacement of glomerular capillaries (**Fig. 27-2**). In the early stage, amyloid deposits are usually found in the mesangium and are not associated with an increase in mesangial cellularity. Deposits may also be seen along the subepithelial space of capillary loops in more advanced stages. Immunohistochemistry demonstrates that the deposits consist of light chains, although the sensitivity of this test is not high. Amyloid has characteristic tinctorial properties and stains with Congo red, which produces an apple-green birefringence when the tissue section is examined under polarized light, and with thioflavins T and S. On electron microscopy, the deposits are characteristic randomly oriented, nonbranching fibrils 7 to 10 nm in diameter. In some cases of early amyloidosis, glomeruli may appear normal on light microscopy. Careful examination, however, can identify scattered monotypic light chains on immunofluorescence microscopy. Ultrastructural examination with immunoelectron microscopy to reveal the fibrils of AL-amyloid may be required to establish the diagnosis early in the course of renal involvement. As the disease advances, mesangial deposits progressively enlarge to form nodules of amyloid protein that compress the filtering surfaces of the glomeruli and cause renal failure. Epithelial proliferation and crescent formation are rare in AL-type amyloidosis.

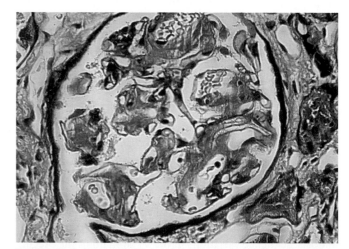

FIGURE 27-2 Glomerulus from a patient with AL-type amyloidosis, showing segmentally variable accumulation of amorphous acidophilic material that is effacing portions of the glomerular architecture (periodic acid–Schiff–hematoxylin [PASH] stain, original magnification ×40).

TABLE 27-3 **Relative Frequency of Organ Infiltration by Light Chains in MLCDD and in AL-Type Amyloidosis***

TYPE OF DYSCRASIA	ISOTYPE	Organ Involvement					
		RENAL	CARDIAC	LIVER	NEUROLOGIC	GI	PULMONARY
MLCDD	κ > λ	++++	+++	+++	+	Rare	Rare
AL-amyloid	λ > κ	+++	+++	+	+	+++	++++

GI, gastrointestinal; MLCDD, monoclonal light-chain and light- and heavy-chain deposition disease.

*Plus signs indicate increasing frequency, from +, uncommon but can occur during the course of the disease, to ++++, extremely common in the course of the disease.

Clinical Features

Proteinuria and renal insufficiency are the two major renal manifestations of AL-type amyloidosis. Proteinuria ranges from asymptomatic non-nephrotic proteinuria to nephrotic syndrome. Isolated microscopic hematuria and nephritic syndrome are not common in AL-type amyloidosis. More than 90% of patients have monoclonal light chains in either urine or blood, but occasionally even sensitive assays will not detect a circulating monoclonal light chain in patients with documented renal involvement from AL-amyloid. Renal insufficiency is present in 58% to 70% of patients at the time of diagnosis. Ultrastructural and immunohistochemical examination of biopsy specimens from an affected organ establish the diagnosis, although tissue diagnosis of AL-type amyloidosis can also be difficult, because commercially available antibodies may not detect the presence of the light chain in the tissue. Scintigraphy using iodine 123–labeled serum amyloid P component, which binds to amyloid, can assess the degree of organ involvement resulting from amyloid infiltration, but this test is not widely available.

Pathogenesis

The pathogenesis of AL-type amyloidosis is incompletely understood. Internalization and processing of light chains by mesangial cells produces amyloid in vitro. The finding that N-terminal sequences of light-chain fragments in amyloid are identical to the sequence of soluble light chains suggests that proteolytic cleavage of light chains may play a role in causing amyloid. Presumably, intracellular oxidation or proteolysis of light chains allows formation of amyloid, which is then extruded into the extracellular space. With continued production of amyloid, the mesangium expands, compressing the filtering surface of the glomeruli and producing progressive renal failure. Not all light chains are amyloidogenic. Members of the λ family are more commonly associated with AL-type amyloidosis, and sequence variations in the V_L domain appear to confer the propensity to polymerize to form amyloid.

Treatment and Prognosis

Patients with both multiple myeloma and AL-type amyloidosis should be managed with treatment regimens that target the myeloma. For those patients who have AL-type amyloidosis but lack the criteria for multiple myeloma, the initial approach to management should be to ensure that the patient has AL-type amyloidosis and not amyloidosis related to a nonlymphoid precursor protein, because the approaches to treatment are quite different.

Since a randomized trial suggested improved survival in patients who received chemotherapy, more aggressive anti–plasma cell therapies have been undertaken in AL-type amyloidosis, including high-dose chemotherapy with autologous peripheral stem cell transplantation (HDT/SCT). Although renal dysfunction may not be an exclusion criteria, treatment-related mortality with HDT/SCT is increased in higher-risk subjects, so more conservative approaches

should be considered for patients with age 80 years or older, decompensated congestive heart failure, left ventricular ejection fraction less than 0.40, systolic blood pressure less than 90 mm Hg, oxygen saturation less than 95% on room air, or significant overall functional impairment. Patients who have evidence of multiorgan system dysfunction, particularly cardiac disease, and are considered ineligible for HDT/SCT have an expected median survival time of only 4 months. In contrast, one study reported a median survival time of 4.6 years in 312 patients who underwent HDT/SCT. Almost half achieved a complete hematologic response, which portended improved long-term survival. Whereas carefully selected patients with AL-type amyloidosis can respond favorably to HDT/SCT, in a randomized clinical trial comparing HDT/SCT with chemotherapy that included melphalan and high-dose dexamethasone, the outcome was not superior with transplantation. Patients with AL-type amyloidosis usually die from organ decompensation due to amyloid infiltration and not from tumor burden, and an important observation is that survival and organ dysfunction can improve with successful reduction in the monoclonal plasma cell population and reduction of light chain production.

Other chemotherapeutic regimens may be of benefit in AL-type amyloidosis and are being considered, particularly given the potential toxicity of chronic treatment with alkylating agents. The recent success of thalidomide as an alternative treatment of multiple myeloma has prompted treatment of AL-type amyloidosis with this agent in an uncontrolled fashion, although thalidomide is not well tolerated in these patients, and dosage reductions are often required. Lenalidomide, an analogue of thalidomide, is also a potentially attractive therapy in AL-type amyloidosis. Randomized, controlled trials are needed to determine the efficacy of these pharmacologic agents in the treatment of AL-type amyloidosis.

Monoclonal Light-Chain Deposition Disease

MLCDD is a systemic disease that typically manifests initially with isolated renal injury related to a glomerular lesion associated with nonamyloid electron-dense granular deposits of monoclonal light chains with or without heavy chains. Isolated deposition of monoclonal heavy chains, termed heavy-chain deposition disease, is extremely rare. MLCDD may accompany other clinical features of multiple myeloma or another lymphoproliferative disorder, or it may be the sole manifestation of a plasma cell dyscrasia.

Pathology

Nodular glomerulopathy with distortion of the glomerular architecture by amorphous eosinophilic material is the most common pathologic finding observed with light microscopy (**Fig. 27-3**). These nodules, which are composed of light chains and extracellular matrix proteins, begin in the mesangium. The appearance is reminiscent of diabetic nephropathy. Less commonly, other glomerular morphologic changes

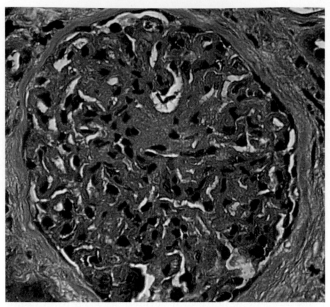

FIGURE 27-3 Glomerulus from a patient with monoclonal κ light-chain deposition disease, showing expansion of the mesangium, related to matrix protein deposition, and associated compression of capillary lumens (hematoxylin and eosin stain, original magnification ×40).

TABLE 27-4 Standard Therapy for Cast Nephropathy
Chemotherapy to decrease light chain production
Increase free water intake to 2-3 L/day as tolerated
Treat hypercalcemia aggressively
Avoid exposure to diuretics, radiocontrast agents, and nonsteroidal anti-inflammatory agents

besides nodular glomerulopathy can be seen in MLCDD. Immunofluorescence microscopy demonstrates the presence of monotypic light chains in the glomeruli. Under electron microscopy, deposits of light-chain proteins are present in a subendothelial position along the glomerular capillary wall, along the outer aspect of tubular basement membranes, and in the mesangium.

There are significant differences between amyloidosis and MLCDD. For amyloid deposition to occur, amyloid P glycoprotein must also be present. The amyloid P component is not part of the amyloid fibrils, but binds them. This glycoprotein is a constituent of normal human glomerular basement membrane and elastic fibrils. In contrast to AL-type amyloid, in MLCDD the light-chain deposits are punctate, granular, and electron dense and are identified in the mesangium or the subendothelial space or both; amyloid P component is absent. Unlike amyloid, the granular light chain deposits of MLCDD do not stain with Congo red or thioflavin T and S. Another difference between these lesions is the tendency for κ light chains to compose the granular deposits of MLCDD, whereas usually λ light chains constitute AL-amyloid. Both diseases can involve organs other than the kidney (**Table 27-4**). Amyloidosis more commonly involves the gastrointestinal tract and lungs, whereas deposits of MLCDD infiltrate the liver more frequently than amyloidosis does.

Clinical Features

The typical clinical presentation is reminiscent of a rapidly progressive glomerulonephritis. The major findings in MLCDD include proteinuria, sometimes in the nephrotic range; microscopic hematuria; and decreased kidney function. Albumin and monoclonal free light chains are the dominant proteins in the urine. The presence of albuminuria and other findings of nephrotic syndrome are important clues to the presence of glomerular injury and not cast nephropathy. The amount of excreted light chain is usually less than that found in cast nephropathy and can very be difficult to detect in some patients. A progressive decline in kidney function in untreated patients is common. Because renal manifestations generally predominate and are often the sole presenting features, it is not uncommon for nephrologists to diagnose the plasma cell dyscrasia. Renal biopsy is necessary to establish the diagnosis. Dysfunction of other organs, especially liver and heart, can develop and is related to deposition of light chains in those organs. Although extrarenal manifestations of overt multiple myeloma can manifest at presentation or over time, a majority (approximately 74%) of patients with MLCDD do not develop myeloma or other malignant lymphoproliferative disease.

Pathogenesis

MLCDD represents a prototypical model of progressive kidney disease that has a pathogenesis related to glomerulosclerosis from increased production of transforming growth factor-β (TGF-β). The response to light-chain deposition includes expansion of the mesangium by extracellular matrix proteins to form nodules and, eventually, glomerular sclerosis. Experimental studies have shown that mesangial cells exposed to light chains obtained from patients with biopsy-proven MLCDD produce TGF-β, which serves as an autacoid to stimulate these same cells to produce matrix proteins, including type IV collagen, laminin, and fibronectin. Thus, TGF-β plays a central role in glomerular sclerosis from MLCDD. As is true for AL-type amyloidosis, not all light chains can produce MLCDD. Many of offending light chains are κ chains, particularly the κIV subfamily, and they appear to possess unusual hydrophobic amino acid residues in the V_L domain.

Whereas deposition of light chain is the prominent feature of these glomerular lesions, heavy chains, along with light chains, can be identified in the deposits. In those specimens, the punctate, electron-dense deposits appear larger and more extensive than deposits that contain only light chains, but it is unclear whether the clinical course of these patients differs from the course of those with isolated light-chain deposition without heavy-chain components. The management is similar.

Treatment and Prognosis

For patients with both multiple myeloma and MLCDD, therapy is directed at the myeloma. The treatment of MLCDD without an associated lymphoproliferative disorder is difficult, because guidance from randomized, controlled trials is unavailable. However, patients appear to benefit from the same therapeutic approach as that given for multiple myeloma. The serum creatinine concentration at presentation appears to be an important predictor of subsequent outcome, so intervention should occur early in the course of the disease.

Therapy with melphalan and prednisone improves renal prognosis, but the long-term toxicity of melphalan makes this approach less attractive. More aggressive anti–plasma cell therapy in the form of HDT/SCT has been used in MLCDD. In the small numbers of patients who underwent HDT/SCT, the procedure-related death rate was low and, when a complete hematologic response was observed, improvement in affected organ function with histologic evidence of regression of the light-chain deposits occurred.

The high incidence of progressive kidney disease in MLCDD has prompted treatment with renal transplantation, but the disease will recur in the allograft if the underlying plasma cell dyscrasia is not addressed. The study with the largest collection of patients (seven) concluded that recurrence of MCLDD in the renal allograft was common and significantly reduced long-term graft survival; these findings emphasize the need to control monoclonal light-chain production before renal transplantation in MLCDD.

Fibrillary Glomerulonephritis and Immunotactoid Glomerulopathy

Fibrillary glomerulonephritis is a rare disorder that is characterized ultrastructurally by the presence of amyloid-like, randomly arranged, fibrillary deposits in the capillary wall (**Fig. 27-4**). Unlike amyloid, these fibrils are thicker (18 to 22 nm), and Congo red and thioflavin T stains are negative. Immunofluorescence microscopy typically reveals immunoglobulin G (usually IgG4) and complement C3. Most patients with fibrillary glomerulonephritis do not have a plasma cell dyscrasia; occasionally, however, a plasma cell dyscrasia is present, so screening is advisable. Tests for cryoglobulins and hepatitis C virus infection should be performed. Patients typically manifest nephrotic syndrome and varying degrees of renal failure; progression to end-stage renal failure is the rule. No standard treatment for the idiopathic variety is currently available.

Immunotactoid, or microtubular, glomerulopathy is even more uncommon than fibrillary glomerulonephritis and is usually associated with a plasma cell dyscrasia or other lymphoproliferative disorder. The deposits in this lesion contain thick (>30 nm), organized, microtubular structures that are located in the mesangium and along capillary walls. Cryoglobulinemia, which is covered in Chapter 22, should be considered in the differential diagnosis and ruled out clinically. Treatment of the underlying plasma cell dyscrasia is indicated for this rare disorder.

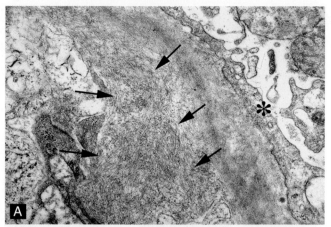

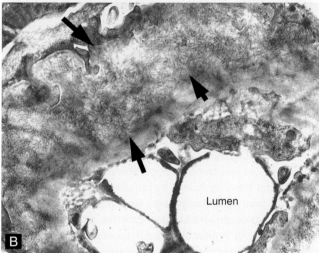

FIGURE 27-4 A, Electron micrograph of a glomerulus from a patient with AL-type amyloidosis. Note the randomly arranged, relatively straight fibrils with an approximate diameter of 7 to 10 nm *(arrows)*. A useful distinction from fibrillary glomerulonephritis (**B**) is that amyloid fibrils stain with Congo red or thioflavin T. Note fusion of the foot processes *(asterisk)* of the adjacent epithelial cell. **B,** Electron micrograph of a glomerulus from a patient with fibrillary glomerulonephritis. The same random arrangement of nonbranching fibrils *(arrows)* is seen. Careful examination demonstrates that the fibrils are larger (approximately 20 nm in diameter). The overall ultrastructural appearance resembles amyloid except that the fibrils are approximately twice as thick. (**A,** Courtesy of Dr. J. Charles Jennette; **B,** courtesy of Dr. William Cook.)

TUBULOINTERSTITIAL LESIONS OF PLASMA CELL DYSCRASIAS

Cast Nephropathy

Pathology

Cast nephropathy is an inflammatory tubulointerstitial renal lesion. Characteristically, multiple intraluminal proteinaceous casts are identified mainly in the distal portion of the nephrons (**Fig. 27-5**). The casts are usually acellular, homogeneous, and eosinophilic, with multiple fracture lines. Immunofluorescence and immunoelectron microscopy confirm that the casts contain light chains and Tamm-Horsfall glycoprotein. Persistence of the casts produces the giant cell inflammation and tubular atrophy that typify myeloma kidney. Glomeruli are usually normal in appearance.

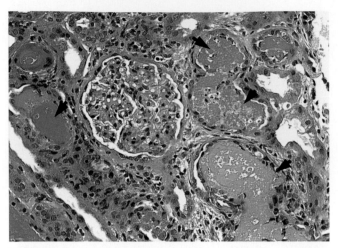

FIGURE 27-5 Renal biopsy tissue from a patient with cast nephropathy. The findings include tubules filled with cast material *(arrows)* and presence of multinucleated giant cells. Glomeruli are typically normal in appearance (hematoxylin and eosin stain, original magnification ×20).

Clinical Features

Renal failure from this lesion may manifest acutely or as a chronic progressive disease, and it may develop at any stage of myeloma. Diagnosis of multiple myeloma is usually evident when chronic bone pain, pathologic fractures, and hypercalcemia are complicated by proteinuria and renal failure. However, many patients present to nephrologists primarily with findings of impaired kidney function or undefined proteinuria; further evaluation then discloses a malignant process. Cast nephropathy should be considered if proteinuria (often >3 g/day) is found, particularly without concomitant hypoalbuminemia or albuminuria, in a patient who is in the fourth decade of life or older. Hypertension is not a common consequence of cast nephropathy. Diagnosis of myeloma may be confirmed by finding monoclonal immunoglobulins or light chains in the serum and urine and by bone marrow examination, although typical intraluminal cast formation on kidney biopsy is virtually pathognomonic. Almost all patients with cast nephropathy have detectable monoclonal light chains in the urine or blood.

Pathogenesis

Intravenous infusion of nephrotoxic human light chains in rats elevates proximal tubule pressure and simultaneously decreases the single-nephron glomerular filtration rate; intraluminal protein casts can be identified in these kidneys. Myeloma casts contain Tamm-Horsfall glycoprotein and occur initially in the distal nephron, which provides an optimal environment for precipitation of light chains. Casts occur primarily because light chains coaggregate with Tamm-Horsfall glycoprotein. This glycoprotein, which is synthesized exclusively by cells of the thick ascending limb of the loop of Henle, comprises the major fraction of total urinary protein in healthy individuals and is the predominant constituent of urinary casts. Cast-forming Bence Jones proteins bind to the same site on the peptide backbone of Tamm-Horsfall glycoprotein; binding results in coaggregation of these proteins

and subsequent occlusion of the tubule lumen by the precipitated protein complexes. Intranephronal obstruction and renal failure ensue. Light chains that bind to Tamm-Horsfall glycoprotein are potentially nephrotoxic. The CDR3 domain of the light chain determines binding affinity.

Coaggregation of Tamm-Horsfall glycoprotein with light chains also depends on the ionic environment and the physicochemical properties of the light chain; not all patients with myeloma develop cast nephropathy, even when the urinary excretion of light chains is very high. Increasing concentrations of sodium chloride or calcium, but not magnesium, facilitate coaggregation. The loop diuretic, furosemide, augments coaggregation and accelerates intraluminal obstruction in vivo in the rat. Finally, the lower tubule fluid flow rates of the distal nephron allow more time for light chains to interact with Tamm-Horsfall glycoprotein and subsequently to obstruct the tubular lumen. Conditions that further reduce flow rates, such as volume depletion, can accelerate tubule obstruction or convert nontoxic light chains into cast-forming proteins. Volume depletion and hypercalcemia are recognized factors that promote acute renal failure due to cast nephropathy.

Treatment and Prognosis

The principles used to guide therapy in cast nephropathy include decreasing the concentration of circulating light chains and preventing coaggregation of light chains with Tamm-Horsfall glycoprotein (see **Table 27-4**). Prompt and effective chemotherapy should start on diagnosis of multiple myeloma, which is present in virtually all patients with cast nephropathy. The traditional treatment with alkylating agents and steroids has been replaced by HDT/SCT, particularly in younger patients. An advantage with a more aggressive approach is the potential for rapid reductions in the levels of circulating monoclonal light chain. Several randomized trials showed that patients who received HDT/SCT had improved overall survival rates, compared with patients who received conventional chemotherapy. Therapy is often initiated with a combination of vincristine, doxorubicin, and dexamethasone (VAD) before HDT/SCT, because VAD can produce a rapid reduction in the plasma cell clone. Often, only two courses of treatment are necessary to determine whether a patient will respond to this chemotherapy. For this reason, VAD may be particularly beneficial in the setting of reduced kidney function related to deposition of light chains, and the physician can rapidly determine the efficacy of such an approach. Chronic treatment with alkylating agents is typically avoided before HDT/SCT, because these drugs may impede peripheral stem cell harvest and are associated with myelodysplasia and acute myelogenous leukemia.

Other therapeutic approaches have been attempted but presently lack randomized, controlled trials to support their use. For example, patients with advanced renal failure and refractory myeloma have been treated successfully with bortezomib and thalidomide, which may replace VAD in induction chemotherapeutic regimens and may even obviate the need for HDT/SCT. Nonmyeloablative allogeneic stem-cell transplantation, so-called mini-allograft therapy, may also provide beneficial results in myeloma without the attendant complications such as severe graft-versus-host disease.

The role of plasmapheresis in cast nephropathy remains controversial. One randomized trial suggested benefit, but two others failed to confirm a survival advantage for the use of plasmapheresis. The most recent of these suggested no clinical benefit from plasma exchange for patients with acute renal failure, although there were limitations to this study. Renal biopsy was not a prerequisite for entry into the study, and, in perhaps one third of the patients with myeloma and acute renal failure, the etiology was not cast nephropathy but was related instead to obstruction (nephrolithiasis, papillary necrosis, amyloid deposition in the ureters), hypercalcemia, or hyperviscosity syndrome, in addition to other causes seen in the general population, such as drug-related renal injury and contrast nephropathy. Even though a significant number of patients participated in the trial, the study may have been underpowered to detect differences between the groups, in part because of the entry criteria that did not require documentation of cast nephropathy as the cause of the acute renal failure. Serum free light chains were not quantified either before or after the plasma exchange. Despite these limitations, a significant issue related to plasma exchange therapy is the relatively inefficient removal of circulating light chains, and other techniques for rapid reduction in serum light chain concentrations may become available in the near future. Until additional data are provided, it is probably prudent not to recommend plasmapheresis for most patients with acute renal failure, although there may be a subset of patients who respond favorably to plasmapheresis. If plasma exchange is performed, demonstration of the efficacy of treatment by quantification of changes in serum free light chain levels should be performed. Finally, hyperviscosity syndrome remains an indication for plasma exchange.

Prevention of the aggregation of light chains with Tamm-Horsfall glycoprotein is a cornerstone of therapy. Volume repletion, normalization of electrolytes, and avoidance of complicating factors such as loop diuretics and nonsteroidal anti-inflammatory agents are helpful in preserving and improving renal function. Although not all patients with light-chain proteinuria develop acute renal failure after exposure to radiocontrast agents, it is difficult to predict who is at risk for this complication, so caution is suggested in the use of radiocontrast agents for all patients with multiple myeloma. Fluid intake up to 3 L/day in the form of electrolyte-free fluids should be encouraged, although the serum sodium concentration should be monitored periodically. Alkalinization of the urine with oral sodium bicarbonate (or citrate) to keep the urine pH higher than 7 may also be therapeutic but may be mitigated by the requisite sodium loading, which favors coaggregation of these proteins. It should also be avoided in patients who have symptomatic extracellular fluid volume overload.

Hypercalcemia occurs during the course of the disease in more than 25% of patients with multiple myeloma.

In addition to being directly nephrotoxic, hypercalcemia enhances the nephrotoxicity of light chains. Treatment of volume contraction with the infusion of saline often corrects mild hypercalcemia. Loop diuretics also increase calcium excretion, but furosemide, because it may facilitate nephrotoxicity from light chains, should not be administered until the patient is clinically euvolemic. Glucocorticoid therapy (e.g., methylprednisolone) is helpful for acute management of the multiple myeloma as well as the hypercalcemia. Bisphosphonates (e.g., pamidronate, zoledronic acid) are used to treat moderate hypercalcemia (serum calcium >3.25 mmol/L or 13 mg/dL) that is unresponsive to other measures. Bisphosphonates lower serum calcium by interfering with osteoclast-mediated bone resorption. Although the hypercalcemia of myeloma responds to bisphosphonates, these agents can be nephrotoxic and should be administered only to euvolemic patients. Renal function should be monitored closely during therapy. Treatment with pamidronate or zoledronic acid allows outpatient management of mild hypercalcemia. Besides controlling hypercalcemia, bisphosphonates appear to inhibit the growth of plasma cells and have been used to treat multiple myeloma, particularly in patients with osseous lesions and bone pain.

Renal replacement therapy in the form of hemodialysis or peritoneal dialysis is generally recommended for patients with renal failure resulting from monoclonal light chain–related renal diseases. Recovery of renal function sufficient to survive without dialysis occurs in as many as 5% of patients with multiple myeloma, although in some patients this requires months to achieve, probably because the traditional chemotherapeutic regimens slowly reduce circulating levels of light chains. Despite the susceptibility to infection in multiple myeloma, the peritonitis rate for continuous ambulatory peritoneal dialysis (one episode every 14.4 months) is not unacceptably high. Neither peritoneal dialysis nor hemodialysis appears to provide a superior survival advantage in patients with myeloma. Renal transplantation has also been successfully performed in selected patients with multiple myeloma in remission. Because the light chain is the underlying cause of cast nephropathy, tests that ensure absence of circulating free light chains are useful in the evaluation of candidacy for renal transplantation.

Other Tubulointerstitial Renal Lesions

Unlike most endogenous low-molecular-weight proteins, light chains have a propensity to produce tubular damage. Proximal tubule injury and tubulointerstitial nephritis can occur. A classic renal presentation of multiple myeloma is Fanconi's syndrome, which is characterized by a renal tubular acidosis type II and defective sodium-coupled cotransport processes, producing aminoaciduria, glycosuria, and phosphaturia. Renal biopsy typically shows crystals of light-chain protein within the epithelium of the proximal tubule. Fanconi's syndrome may precede overt multiple myeloma. Plasma cell dyscrasia should therefore be considered in the differential diagnosis when this syndrome occurs in adults.

Although there is growing concern that proteinuria in general may be nephrotoxic, multiple studies have shown that light chains can injure the proximal tubule epithelium directly. Damage to the proximal tubule epithelium by light chains can produce clinical manifestations of acute renal failure. A major mechanism of damage to the proximal epithelium is related to accumulation of toxic light chains in the endolysosome system. Endocytosis of monoclonal light chains into proximal tubular cells activates nuclear factor kappaB (NF-κB), which in turn promotes expression of cytokines and chemokines, such as monocyte chemotactic factor-1 (MCP-1), that participate in tubulointerstitial inflammation and scarring. Light chains appear to produce hydrogen peroxide and generate sufficient intracellular oxidant stress to promote the production of MCP-1.

WALDENSTRÖM MACROGLOBULINEMIA

Waldenström macroglobulinemia comprises about 5% of monoclonal gammopathies and is characterized by the presence of a monoclonal B-cell malignancy consisting of lymphocytoid plasma cells. This condition clinically behaves more like lymphoma, although the malignant cell secretes IgM (macroglobulin), which usually produces most of the clinical symptoms. Lytic bone lesions are uncommon, but hepatosplenomegaly and lymphadenopathy are frequently identified. IgM is a very large molecule that is not excreted and accumulates in the plasma to produce hyperviscosity syndrome, which consists of neurologic symptoms (headaches, stupor, deafness, dizziness), visual impairment (due to hemorrhages and edema), bleeding diathesis (related to IgM-complexing clotting factors and to platelet dysfunction), renal failure, and symptoms of hypervolemia. Renal function impairment is usually mild but occurs in about 30% of patients. Hyperviscosity syndrome and precipitation of IgM in the lumen of glomerular capillaries are the most common causes of impaired kidney function. About 10% to 15% of patients develop AL-type amyloidosis, but cast nephropathy is rare.

Because of the typically advanced age at presentation (sixth to seventh decade) and the slowly progressive course, the major therapeutic goal is relief of symptoms. All patients with monoclonal IgM levels greater than 3 g/dL should have serum viscosity determined. Plasmapheresis is indicated in symptomatic patients and should be continued until symptoms resolve and serum viscosity normalizes. Severe renal failure requiring renal replacement therapy is uncommon. The course of the disease can vary, but it is often protracted. Factors that portend a worse outcome include age greater than 65 years and organomegaly. Patients lacking these risk factors have a median survival time of 10.6 years, whereas those patients with either of these risk factors have a reduced chance for survival (median, 4.2 years). Symptomatic patients are usually treated with an alkylating agent. Newer treatments of Waldenström macroglobulinemia are on the horizon but await more extensive clinical trials to confirm their efficacy.

BIBLIOGRAPHY

Barlogie B, Shaughnessy J, Tricot G, et al: Treatment of multiple myeloma. Blood 103:20-32, 2004.

Child JA, Morgan GJ, Davies FE, et al: High-dose chemotherapy with hematopoietic stem-cell rescue for multiple myeloma. N Engl J Med 348:1875-1883, 2003.

Clark WF, Stewart AK, Rock GA, et al: Plasma exchange when myeloma presents as acute renal failure: A randomized, controlled trial. Ann Intern Med 143:777-784, 2005.

Dember LM, Hawkins PN, Bouke PC, et al: Eprodisate for the treatment of renal disease in AA amyloidosis. N Engl J Med 356:2349-2360, 2007.

Deret S, Denoroy L, Lamarine M, et al: Kappa light chain-associated Fanconi's syndrome: Molecular analysis of monoclonal immunoglobulin light chains from patients with and without intracellular crystals. Protein Eng 12:363-369, 1999.

Dispenzieri A, Kyle RA, Lacy MQ, et al: Superior survival in primary systemic amyloidosis patients undergoing peripheral blood stem cell transplantation: A case-control study. Blood 103:3960-3963, 2004.

Gertz MA, Lacy MQ, Dispenzieri A: Immunoglobulin light chain amyloidosis and the kidney. Kidney Int 61:1-9, 2002.

Ghobrial IM, Fonseca R, Gertz MA, et al: Prognostic model for disease-specific and overall mortality in newly diagnosed symptomatic patients with Waldenstrom macroglobulinaemia. Br J Haematol 133:158-64, 2006.

Jaccard A, Moreau P, Leblond V, et al: High-dose melphalan versus melphalan plus dexamethasone for AL amyloidosis. N Engl J Med 357:1083-1093, 2007.

Lachmann HJ, Booth DR, Booth SE, et al: Misdiagnosis of hereditary amyloidosis as AL (primary) amyloidosis. N Engl J Med 346:1786-1791, 2002.

Leung N, Lager DJ, Gertz MA, et al: Long-term outcome of renal transplantation in light-chain deposition disease. Am J Kidney Dis 43:147-153, 2004.

Madore F: Does plasmapheresis have a role in the management of myeloma cast nephropathy. Nat Clin Pract Nephrol 2:406-407, 2006.

Rocca A, Khamlichi AA, Aucouturier P, et al: Primary structure of a variable region of the V kappa I subgroup (ISE) in light chain deposition disease. Clin Exp Immunol 91:506-509, 1993.

Rosenstock JL, Markowitz GS, Valeri AM, et al: Fibrillary and immunotactoid glomerulonephritis: Distinct entities with different clinical and pathologic features. Kidney Int 63:1450-1461, 2003.

Royer B, Arnulf B, Martinez F, et al: High dose chemotherapy in light chain or light and heavy chain deposition disease. Kidney Int 65:642-648, 2004.

Sanchorawala V, Wright DG, Rosenzweig M, et al: Lenalidomide and dexamethasone in the treatment of AL amyloidosis: Results of a phase 2 trial. Blood 109:492-496, 2007.

Skinner M, Sanchorawala V, Seldin DC, et al: High-dose melphalan and autologous stem-cell transplantation in patients with AL Amyloidosis: An 8-year study. Ann Intern Med 140:85-93, 2004.

Tagouri YM, Sanders PW, Pickens MM, et al: In vitro AL-amyloid formation by rat and human mesangial cells. Lab Invest 74:290-302, 1996.

van Rhee F, Bolejack V, Hollmig K, et al: High serum free-light chain levels and their rapid reduction in response to therapy define an aggressive multiple myeloma subtype with poor prognosis. Blood 110:827-832, 2007.

Wang, P-X, PW Sanders: Immunoglobulin light chains generate hydrogen peroxide. J Am Soc Nephrol 18:1239-1245, 2007.

Weichman K, Dember LM, Prokaeva T, et al: Clinical and molecular characteristics of patients with non-amyloid light chain deposition disorders, and outcome following treatment with high-dose melphalan and autologous stem cell transplantation. Bone Marrow Transplant 38:339-343, 2006.

Ying W-Z, Sanders PW: Mapping the binding domain of immunoglobulin light chains for Tamm-Horsfall protein. Am J Pathol 158:1859-1866, 2001.

Zhu L, Herrera GA, Murphy-Ullrich JE, et al: Pathogenesis of glomerulosclerosis in light chain deposition disease: Role for transforming growth factor-β. Am J Pathol 147:375-385, 1995.

CHAPTER 28

Thrombotic Microangiopathies

Sharon Adler and Cynthia C. Nast

The thrombotic microangiopathies are a group of diverse disorders that are classified together based on common morphologic features in the kidney. **Table 28-1** lists some of the more common underlying causes. This review focuses on four of the most common: thrombotic thrombocytopenic purpura (TTP), hemolytic uremic syndrome (HUS), the anti-phospholipid syndrome (APLS), and scleroderma renal crisis.

PATHOLOGY

Figure 28-1 demonstrates the characteristic features of the thrombotic microangiopathies. The histopathologic changes are characterized by fibrin accumulation in the lumina and walls of arteries, arterioles, and glomerular capillaries. By light microscopy, fibrin and platelet thrombi are present in many or few capillaries of variable numbers of glomeruli. As the disease progresses, glomeruli may have a lobular appearance with capillary wall double contours, or they may be ischemic, characterized by wrinkled and partially collapsed capillaries (see **Fig. 28-1A** and **B**). Arterioles and, to a lesser extent, arteries are thrombosed and contain fibrin in the walls, which also show muscular hypertrophy and mucoid intimal thickening, resulting in luminal narrowing (see **Fig. 28-1C** and **D**). Areas of infarcted renal parenchyma are found in patients with cortical necrosis. Immunofluorescence reveals fibrin in glomerular capillaries and in vascular walls and lumina. Ultrastructurally, glomerular capillary walls have wide subendothelial zones containing flocculent electron-lucent and -dense material representing altered fibrin, which may contain trapped erythrocytes (see **Fig. 28-1E** and **F**). There may be a new layer of basement membrane material beneath the widened subendothelial zone, accounting for the double-contour appearance of capillaries. Endothelial cells are swollen, capillary lumina are narrowed, and occasionally capillaries contain tactoids of fibrin. In ischemic glomeruli, capillary basement membranes are wrinkled. There are no electron-dense (immune complex) deposits.

All thrombotic microangiopathic renal lesions are morphologically similar, although subtle differences have been described. Some have suggested that biopsy specimens from patients with HUS may show more fibrin and erythrocytes within the thrombi. In contrast, TTP thrombi are composed of more platelets with little fibrin, and immunohistochemistry has demonstrated von Willebrand's factor (vWF),

probably the large multimer form. Patients with HUS also may be more likely to have cortical necrosis than those with TTP. However, the pathologic findings are not sufficiently different to allow a specific diagnosis based on histology for most processes causing thrombotic microangiopathy, apart from scleroderma (see later discussion). The distinction among the thrombotic microangiopathies requires clinical assessment.

THROMBOTIC THROMBOCYTOPENIC PURPURA

Pathogenesis

TTP was once thought to be a disorder that was pathogenetically linked to HUS but differed somewhat in involvement of end organs or severity. However, a more thorough

TABLE 28-1 Causes of Thrombotic Microangiopathy

INFECTIOUS CAUSES	MEDICATIONS
Enteric pathogens	Interferon-alfa
Escherichia coli O157:H7	Aprotinin
Shigella species	Bleomycin
Salmonella species	Cisplatinum
Campylobacter jejuni	Clopidogrel
Yersinia	Cocaine
Human immunodeficiency virus	Cyclosporine
Mycoplasma pneumoniae	Cytosine arabinoside
Legionella infection	Doxycycline
Streptococcus pneumoniae	Daunorubicin
Coxsackie A and B virus	Gemcitabine
Histoplasmosis	Interferon
Brucellosis	Mitomycin C
Bartonella	Sunitinib
Systemic Diseases	Tacrolimus
Systemic lupus erythematosus	Ticlopidine
Malignant hypertension	Vinblastine
Neoplasms	**Miscellaneous Causes**
Thrombotic thrombocytopenic purpura	Vaccinations
Hemolytic uremic syndrome	Radiation
Antiphospholipid syndrome	Transplantation
Scleroderma	

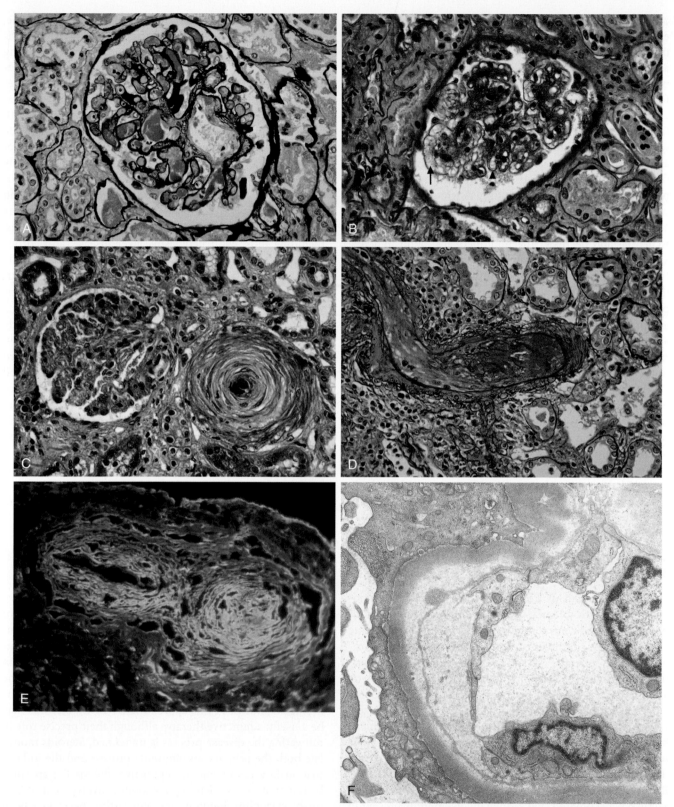

FIGURE 28-1 Kidney biopsy findings in thrombotic microangiopathy. **A,** Glomerulus showing many capillary lumina occluded by fibrin thrombi (periodic acid–methenamine silver stain, original magnification ×20). **B,** Glomerulus with a membranoproliferative glomerulonephritis type I pattern of injury including capillary wall double contours *(arrowheads)* and a capillary microaneurysm *(arrow)* overlying an area of mesangiolysis (periodic acid–Schiff stain, original magnification ×20). **C,** Ischemic glomerulus with wrinkled and partially collapsed capillary walls, lying adjacent to an arteriole. The arteriole has typical "onion skin" thickening of the wall and a fibrin thrombus (Masson's trichrome stain, original magnification ×10). **D,** An interlobular artery with mucoid intimal thickening, fibrin in the wall and lumen, and swollen endothelial cells (periodic acid–methenamine silver stain, original magnification ×10). **E,** Immunofluorescence for fibrin showing positive staining in the wall and lumen of an artery similar to **D** (original magnification ×10). **F,** Electron micrograph of a capillary wall from an involved glomerulus. There is a wide subendothelial lucent zone containing flocculent material; the endothelial cell is swollen; and podocyte foot processes are effaced (original magnification ×6000).

understanding of the pathogenetic mechanisms of these entities underscores the notion that TTP and HUS are distinct conditions. TTP is a complex syndrome, and most cases are characterized by diminished activity of vWF-cleaving protein, resulting either from an inherited mutation or from the presence of inactivating autoantibodies. This vWF-cleaving protein is the 13th member of a family of zinc metalloproteases termed "*A Disintegrin And Metalloprotease with ThromboSpondin type 1 repeat*," commonly known as ADAMTS-13. Decreased ADAMTS-13 activity results in defective vWF cleavage and results in abnormally large and numerous circulating vWF multimers which bind to extracellular matrix and platelets, induce platelet aggregation and activation, and lead to intravascular platelet thrombi, organ ischemia, and necrosis. The multimers are found in active TTP but not in states of remission, and they distinguish TTP from other causes of hemolysis, thrombosis, or thrombocytopenia. Mutations of the ADAMTS-13 gene are observed in patients with familial and recurrent forms of TTP, whereas autoantibodies to ADAMTS-13 cause most cases of acute sporadic TTP. Studies suggest that ADAMTS-13 deficiency may require additional genetic or environmental factors for initiation of acquired and familial TTP.

Diminished ADAMTS-13 activity distinguishes patients with TTP from those with HUS, in that patients with TTP tend to have less than 5% of the functional ADAMTS-13 activity observed in healthy controls. Inhibition of a less severe nature may be seen in other disorders, including HUS. In animal models, inhibition or genetic elimination of vascular endothelial growth factor (VEGF) induces thrombotic microangiopathy. Medications that inhibit VEGF rarely have been reported to induce TTP in patients.

Clinical Presentation and Laboratory Manifestations

The classic pentad of TTP consists of fever, microangiopathic hemolytic anemia, thrombocytopenic purpura, kidney disease, and central nervous system symptoms ranging from lethargy, somnolence, and confusion to focal neurologic signs, seizures, or coma. The neurologic symptoms often dominate the overall clinical picture. The hemolytic anemia is characterized by the presence of numerous circulating fragmented erythrocytes in the form of schistocytes and helmet cells, which are presumably produced by shear stress injury as blood flows through vessels narrowed by platelet thrombi. Associated high levels of lactate dehydrogenase correlate with the severity of the disease. Renal signs and symptoms are common but often mild. Some have estimated that kidney involvement is present in as many as 88% of patients. Manifestations include microscopic (rarely gross) hematuria, mild to moderate proteinuria, and azotemia. Acute renal failure occurs in up to 10% of patients and is usually not severe; the need for dialysis is uncommon.

The disorder may occur either as an acquired acute disease or in a chronic relapsing form. The acquired forms may be triggered by certain medications, of which quinine, mitomycin-C, calcineurin inhibitors, pamidronate, and ticlopidine are the most common. Antibodies to vWF-cleaving protein have been identified in patients with ticlopidine-associated TTP, but a systematic search for antibodies associated with other medication-related TTPs has not been reported. TTP rarely has been reported in association with clopidogrel therapy. Acquired TTP also may complicate collagen-vascular disorders such as systemic lupus erythematosus (SLE). Neoplasms and infections (most notably human immunodeficiency virus infection) have been associated with TTP. For many patients with acquired TTP, no underlying cause is established. ADAMTS-13 activity may be modestly low in patients with some of these conditions, including those with neoplasms, liver disease, and chronic inflammatory conditions. However, antibodies to the ADAMTS-13 vWF-cleaving protein are not always identified, suggesting that there are other potential mechanisms whereby its function may be disturbed.

Most often, TTP in adults does not recur, particularly if an underlying causative factor can be eliminated. However, in 11% to 36% of patients, recurrences are experienced at irregular intervals. The chronic relapsing form, caused by mutations in the gene for ADAMTS-13 on chromosome 9q34, is rare. Patients usually present in childhood, although, for unknown reasons, some may present later in life. This disorder is sometimes called Upshaw-Schulman syndrome.

vWF activity may be measured by a test that is readily available from commercial clinical laboratories. Very low levels of activity (e.g., <5% of normal) are most consistent with a diagnosis of TTP, but moderately low levels, and occasionally even severely low levels, also have been reported in other thrombocytopenic disorders.

Therapy

Infusion of plasma or cryosupernatant (cryoprecipitate-poor plasma) is the mainstay of therapy and provides missing enzyme activity. However, plasma exchange may provide synergism by removing any circulating vWF-cleaving protein inhibitor (e.g., in the acquired form) and by facilitating the infusion of large amounts of fresh-frozen plasma (FFP) (the average course of FFP is approximately 21 L). Steroids may be a useful adjunctive therapy, although their precise role in mitigating the disease process is undefined. Steroids modulate both the primary autoimmune process and the inflammation in areas of injury. Supportive dialysis therapy may be required in cases with severe kidney involvement. Rituximab, cyclophosphamide, and vincristine have also been used with some success in a few patients with refractory TTP. Splenectomy and platelet inhibitors are of unproven value but are occasionally used in desperation for cases refractory to standard therapy. Platelet infusions and aspirin are contraindicated. Response to therapy is best monitored by monitoring with serial platelet counts and serum levels of lactate dehydrogenase.

Course and Prognosis

If TTP is left untreated, the mortality rate approaches 90%. With the advent of plasma infusion, with or without plasma exchange therapy, 60% to 90% of patients now survive. Most patients who go into remission have an excellent long-term prognosis. A subset of patients develop chronic TTP or have TTP as the result of an inherited mutation and require long-term treatment, including repetitive infusions of plasma or cryosupernatant for acute exacerbations.

HEMOLYTIC UREMIC SYNDROME

Pathogenesis

As previously noted, HUS and TTP were once thought to be different clinical expressions of a single disease process, with HUS predominantly presenting features of hemolytic anemia and kidney disease. However, more recent biochemical and genetic information regarding defective ADAMTS-13 in TTP but not in HUS challenged that assumption, and these disorders are now believed to be distinct.

HUS has two major clinical presentations: a diarrheal form (previously termed D⁺HUS and now called *typical HUS*) and a nondiarrheal form (previously termed D⁻HUS and now called *atypical HUS*). In typical HUS, it is postulated that a Shiga-like toxin binds to colonic epithelium and induces elaboration of chemokines and cytokines, resulting in influx of polymorphonuclear cells (PMNs) and abrogation of barrier function; this permits the Shiga-like toxin to enter the circulation in a free form or bound to PMNs. Circulating toxin then binds to the glycolipid Gb3 membrane receptor on glomerular and renal arteriolar endothelial cells and platelets, resulting in endothelial death by suppression of protein synthesis with associated inflammation, thrombosis, and acute renal failure.

The pathogenesis of atypical HUS is not fully understood, although progress has been made, and this topic recently has been reviewed. In circumstances associated with medication use, neoplasms, infections, pregnancy, or collagen-vascular disease, presumably a change in the coagulation cascade or in the endothelial cell membrane creates a prothrombotic environment. Deficiency in the antithrombotic prostacyclin prostaglandin I_2 has been implicated in some cases of HUS. In addition, atypical HUS rarely may manifest as a familial disease associated with impaired regulation of complement activation. Mutations of at least three genes with complement regulatory functions have been implicated in the development of the familial form of atypical HUS; they include genetic deficiency or loss of activity of complement factor H, complement factor I, or membrane cofactor protein (MCP, or CD46). In individuals with reduced levels of factor H, there is an autosomal recessive mode of inheritance associated with low C3 levels and earlier onset of disease. Autosomal dominant inheritance is related to abnormal function of factor H with normal serum levels; patients have normal complement levels and later onset of HUS. This latter form

also is associated more often with a number of underlying factors or events (discussed later) that may initiate complement activation.

In all forms of familial HUS, there is dysregulation of complement activation and complement consumption. Complement factors H and I stabilize the C3 convertase of the alternative pathway. Similarly, complement factors H and I, and MCP cleave and inactivate surface-bound C3b and C4b. When these complement regulatory proteins are mutated or are nonfunctional due to the presence of antibodies, complement activity proceeds in an unregulated fashion at the cell surface, resulting in endothelial cell injury and stimulating platelet aggregation, thereby initiating or exacerbating HUS.

Clinical Presentation and Laboratory Manifestations

HUS manifests as a classic triad consisting of microangiopathic hemolytic anemia, thrombocytopenia, and kidney disease, with peak incidence in the summer. The signs and symptoms tend to overlap with those of TTP, but in HUS the hematologic and especially the renal features predominate.

Typical HUS is associated with infection with organisms that produce a Shiga-like toxin (predominantly *Escherichia coli* O157:H7) or other enteric infections (*Shigella, Salmonella, Campylobacter,* or *Yersinia*). Epidemics associated with ingestion of undercooked hamburger or raw vegetables contaminated with *E. coli* occur sporadically. Multiple cases in young children have occurred after contact with animal feces at a state fair or other petting zoo. Diarrhea ranges from watery to hemorrhagic. The atypical form is associated with a number of underlying clinical predisposing factors, which are detailed in **Table 28-1**. The other systemic manifestations of the typical and atypical forms are similar. The classic features of microangiopathic hemolytic anemia and kidney dysfunction frequently manifest as acute renal failure in adults, but less commonly in children. Leukocytosis and fever are seen frequently. Other systemic manifestations include fluid and electrolyte disturbances, severe hypertension, cerebral edema and seizures, congestive heart failure, pulmonary edema, and cardiac arrhythmias.

The genetic variants of the atypical form are very uncommon, numbering less than 100 (complement factor I and MCP) to a few hundred (complement factor H) so far reported in the literature. Most are autosomal recessive with variable penetrance, and the initial presentation has been reported at ages from infancy through adulthood. Some clinical features are common to all genotypes, such as hypertension and acute renal failure. Neurologic complications are observed in all three genotypes, but at a lower frequency than in TTP. Although recurrences may suggest repetitive exposure to an environmental trigger, consideration of the presence of a genetic mutation should be seriously considered. The factor H activity assay is widely available in commercial laboratories, facilitating diagnosis, although variability among assays can complicate matters.

Therapy

Therapy is supportive for patients with the nongenetic forms of atypical HUS. There is no proven value for treatment with antibiotics, anticoagulants, fibrinolytics, intravenous immunoglobulin, plasma infusion, plasmapheresis, prostacyclin infusion, or antiplatelet agents. For individuals with genetic forms of HUS, a trial of plasma infusion is advised, but the response may not be as rewarding as it is in TTP, especially for patients with MCP mutations. Plasma infusion is contraindicated for patients with HUS caused by *Streptococcus pneumoniae*.

Course and Prognosis

A poor outcome has been associated with marked leukocytosis, older age at onset, presence of atypical HUS, pregnancy, *Shigella* or pneumococcal infection, anuria, persistent proteinuria, hypertension, or cortical necrosis. Thrombotic microangiopathy occurred in 29% of patients undergoing renal transplantation for HUS, compared to 0.8% of patients with renal failure from other causes. Recurrence is less likely in the transplanted kidney of patients with the MCP mutation than in patients with mutations of factors H or I.

ANTI-PHOSPHOLIPID SYNDROME

Pathogenesis

APLS is induced by the actions of a family of autoantibodies with broad reactivity to phospholipid epitopes or to the phospholipid-binding protein β_2-glycoprotein 1 (β_2GP1), which result in thrombotic microangiopathy. It now appears that most autoimmune anticardiolipin antibodies are directed against the phospholipid-binding protein rather than phospholipids themselves, and that the complex of antigen and antibody against β_2GP1 is necessary to activate endothelium and produce a pro-inflammatory and procoagulant phenotype. The syndrome may be present as a primary disorder or as a secondary disorder, the latter usually in association with SLE. Numerous mechanisms have been proposed to account for the hypercoagulable state. Activation of endothelial cells, with upregulation of adhesion molecules, activation of nuclear factor kappaB (NF-κB), the elaboration of cytokines, and alterations in the balance of prothrombotic thromboxane and anticoagulant prostacyclins, has been postulated. Oxidant-mediated endothelial injury may play a role, with autoantibodies to oxidized low-density lipoprotein (LDL) occurring along with anticardiolipin antibodies. In fact, some anticardiolipin antibodies cross-react with oxidized LDL. Finally, anti-phospholipid antibodies may interfere with the function of phospholipid-binding proteins involved in the regulation of coagulation. Candidates for such interference include β_2GP1, prothrombin, protein C, and tissue factor, with β_2GP1 and prothrombin the main targets of anti-phospholipid antibodies.

Clinical and Laboratory Manifestations

The Sapporo classification was adopted in 1999 and requires at least one laboratory and one clinical manifestation. However, the criteria for classification of the APLS were updated in 2006, and the impact of these changes currently is under study.

Diagnostic laboratory studies fall into three categories: lupus anticoagulants, anticardiolipin antibodies, and antibodies to phospholipid-binding proteins. Lupus anticoagulants are identified by abnormalities in coagulation assays. These include prolonged prothrombin time or partial thromboplastin time, particularly if the latter is not normalized when patient plasma is mixed with normal plasma (i.e., indicating the presence of an antibody-mediated clotting inhibition rather than a factor deficiency); abnormal Russell viper venom test results; and abnormalities in the kaolin cephalin clotting time or in the thromboplastin inhibition test. Anticardiolipin antibodies are identified by immunoassays that measure pathologic reactivity to anionic phospholipids, including the anticardiolipin antibody or anti-phospholipid antibody, or by a false-positive Venereal Disease Research Laboratory (VDRL) test result. Finally, antibodies to the phospholipid-binding protein β_2GP1 are frequent and are included in the most recent classification. The anticardiolipin antibody, lupus anticoagulant, or anti-β_2GP1 antibody must be detected twice, at least 12 weeks apart. Approximately 1% to 5% of healthy individuals have circulating anticardiolipin antibodies. It is unclear how many of these results are false-positives and how many occur in individuals who will eventually develop a clinical syndrome. The presence of these antibodies and anticoagulants is associated with venous thromboses, spontaneous abortion, premature myocardial infarction, and cerebrovascular accidents. Among patients with SLE, it has been estimated that 12% to 30% have anticardiolipin antibodies, and 15% to 34% have evidence of a lupus anticoagulant. As many as 50% to 70% of these individuals may have an associated clinical event over the course of 20 years of follow-up.

The clinical diagnostic criteria include a vascular occlusion involving veins, arteries, or capillaries in any organ or pregnancy complications including at least three spontaneous abortions before the 10th gestational week, death of a normal fetus after 10 weeks, or prematurity of a normal fetus (earlier than 34 weeks). The APLS may involve numerous organs, including the central nervous system, kidney, endocrine organs, gastrointestinal tract, lungs, skin, and cerebrovascular and cardiovascular systems. Thrombocytopenia is frequent.

Kidney manifestations in the APLS were recognized relatively recently and are usually mild, although there are exceptions. Kidney involvement is noted in fewer than 25% of patients with the anticardiolipin syndrome. The kidney manifestations are protean and include microscopic hematuria, proteinuria, rarely acute renal failure, mild to malignant hypertension, cortical necrosis, thrombotic microangiopathy, progressive chronic kidney disease sometimes culminating in end-stage renal disease, and thrombosis of kidney allografts. Reports of these manifestations include case reports and small series, and their actual frequencies are not known. Whether the superimposition of the APLS on a classic form of lupus nephritis worsens the prognosis remains conjectural.

The syndrome may occur in a "catastrophic" form, defined by involvement of at least three organ systems contemporaneously. The kidney is the most frequently affected organ and is involved in 78% of cases. This is accompanied by hypertension, which is often malignant. Dialysis is required in 25% of those with kidney involvement. Other end-organ involvement includes pulmonary (66%), central nervous system (56%), cardiac (50%), and dermatologic (50%). Disseminated intravascular coagulation is uncommon.

Therapy

The mainstay of therapy is anticoagulation. Therapy with warfarin is recommended for the primary syndrome and for those with SLE. Low rates of recurrent thrombosis have been reported in patients in whom the International Normalized Ratio (INR) was kept in the range of 2 to 3. In addition to anticoagulation, therapy should include avoidance of prothrombotic drugs such as calcineurin inhibitors, oral contraceptives, hydralazine, procainamide, and chlorpromazine. Aspirin should be prescribed for women with prior pregnancy complications. The role of hydroxychloroquine or chloroquine to prevent thrombosis in patients with SLE is controversial. Although reports are not evidence based, glucocorticosteroids, plasmapheresis, and intravenous immunoglobulin have been implemented as salvage therapy in patients with severe or multiple organ involvement.

Course and Prognosis

The APLS requires long-term anticoagulation. The mortality rate for patients with the catastrophic syndrome is high, approximating 50%.

SCLERODERMA RENAL CRISIS

Pathology

The renal parenchymal changes in scleroderma are similar to those in other forms of thrombotic microangiopathy, but there are subtle features more often associated with scleroderma. The involved vessels more often are the arcuate and interlobular arteries, with abnormalities of arterioles being less common. Arteries are thickened, with loose edematous and mucinous intimal fibrosis and swollen endothelial cells, without inflammation. There often is a concentric appearance to proliferating intimal cells that produces an "onion skin" effect in the artery walls. In more chronic disease, this pattern may be observed as a result of reduplication of the internal elastic lamina. Muscular hypertrophy is variable, and there may be fibrosis of the adventitia of arteries. Glomeruli

display varying degrees of ischemia with capillary wall wrinkling and other features of thrombotic microangiopathy, although capillary thrombi are comparatively rare. The juxtaglomerular apparatus often is expanded. The immunofluorescence and electron microscopic changes are similar to those of the other thrombotic microangiopathies.

Pathogenesis

The pathogenesis of scleroderma is complex and not fully understood, involving both genetic and environmental factors. Exposure to infectious agents, chemicals, and physical agents has been proposed as a predisposing event, but no findings are conclusive. Scleroderma is a lesion of fibrosis and vascular injury, encompassing abnormalities of the microvasculature, cell- and humoral-mediated immune alterations, and aberrant production and accumulation of extracellular matrix. It is possible that this heterogeneous disorder may involve different pathogenetic mechanisms operative in different affected individuals.

Vascular dysfunction most likely is initiated by endothelial injury, which appears to be the primary process in scleroderma renal crisis. Causes of the damage to endothelium may include effects of antiendothelial antibodies, with upregulation of growth factors and cytokines, decrease in intrinsic complement regulatory proteins, proteolytic activities in serum, and cell-mediated immunity. Endothelial injury results in altered permeability and vascular intimal edema, myointimal proliferation with increased extracellular matrix production, platelet activation with aggregation and adhesion, and fibrin deposition. The subsequent vascular narrowing and reduced renal perfusion increase renin production, exacerbating hypertension. A reduction in number and differentiation of bone marrow–derived endothelial progenitor (CD34-positive) cells has been observed and may impair vascular healing. There is no firm evidence that cold temperatures, cardiac dysfunction, pregnancy, or specific drugs such as nonsteroidal anti-inflammatory drugs or calcium channel blockers induce this process, although the administration of high steroid doses over time has been linked to scleroderma renal crisis.

A plethora of autoantibodies is associated with scleroderma, and there appears to be some specificity linked to the pattern of clinical disease presentation. Anti-RNA polymerase III and anti-Th/To ribonucleoprotein are identified frequently in patients who develop scleroderma renal crisis. It is not known whether these phenotype-specific antibodies have a pathogenetic role or are merely markers of disease. Abnormal immune response may influence the onset or progression of scleroderma via several mechanisms. Antibody binding can change the sites of antigen proteolysis or promote the uptake of complexed proteins, which can spread the immune response to different antigenic components (epitope spreading), enhancing the immune reaction. It is plausible that autoantibodies are directly pathogenic; 25% to 85% of patients with scleroderma have antiendothelial cell antibodies, which could induce injury, resulting in vascular damage as described previously. Affected tissues often are infiltrated with T cells and macrophages, possibly in response to environmental stimuli, and an imbalance of T-cell cytokines has been observed, with predominance of Th2 factors likely contributing to fibrosis. In addition, altered B cells may upregulate complement receptor signaling, further inducing target cell injury and augmenting T-cell effector responses.

In patients with scleroderma, fibroblasts overproduce extracellular matrix components, but it is not known whether this is an abnormal response to injury or a dysregulation of the relevant gene expression. Fibroblasts in scleroderma patients express increased levels of transforming growth factor-β (TGF-β) receptors and become persistently activated by small amounts of TGF-β. When there is immune activation due to one or more inciting events, fibroblasts undergo altered signaling and produce excessive amounts of extracellular matrix material, which accumulates in the target organs. Fibroblast stimulation appears to be a final pathway, regardless of the upstream pathogenetic mechanisms involved.

Clinical and Laboratory Manifestations

Kidney disease was not noted as a major cause of morbidity and mortality in systemic sclerosis until 1952. Classic scleroderma renal crisis, defined by the presence of new-onset, often severe hypertension or rapidly progressive acute renal failure in a patient with systemic sclerosis, occurs in approximately 10% of patients. Patients with diffuse systemic sclerosis carry the greatest risk, with up to 25% developing this complication. In contrast, patients with the CREST syndrome (*Calcinosis*, *Raynaud's* phenomenon, *Esophagitis*, *Sclerodactyly*, and *Telangiectasias*) and limited or localized systemic sclerosis are much less likely to develop renal crisis (approximately 1%). Increased risk for developing renal crisis is associated with the presence of diffuse disease, especially rapid skin thickening on the trunk or proximal limbs; anti-topoisomerase III as opposed to anti-centromere antibodies; African-American ethnicity; male gender; onset of scleroderma within the prior 5 years, especially the prior 1 year; fatigue, weight loss, and polyarthritis; carpal tunnel syndrome; edema; and tendon friction rubs. Nevertheless, patients with minimal signs of scleroderma have on occasion been reported to develop renal crisis.

The hypertension and increased plasma renin levels characteristic of the disease emerge abruptly, and there are cases in which these were clearly normal within days of an acute presentation. Microscopic hematuria, proteinuria, and diminished glomerular filtration rate frequently accompany accelerated or malignant hypertension at presentation, but they are not helpful in predicting the onset of renal crisis. Striking blood pressure elevation is the most common presenting manifestation, occurring in 90% of patients. The diastolic blood pressure exceeds 120 mm Hg in 30%. In the minority of patients with normal blood pressure levels, a significant increment for that individual within the normal range often is observed. In the latter setting, microangiopathic hemolytic anemia and thrombocytopenia are clinical clues to the presence of scleroderma renal crisis. The occasional occurrence of scleroderma, acute renal failure, hemolytic anemia, and thrombocytopenia in the absence of severe hypertension suggests that thrombotic microangiopathy may occur in scleroderma via a mechanism independent of or in addition to malignant hypertension.

Extrarenal manifestations occasionally precede the onset of renal crisis, including pericardial effusions, congestive heart failure, ventricular arrhythmias, microangiopathic hemolytic anemia, and thrombocytopenia. Seizures occur rarely with renal crisis.

Plasma renin levels are invariably high in these patients, but whether this is the cause of the hypertension and renal ischemia or a reflection of it has not been resolved. In an era of angiotensin-converting enzyme (ACE) inhibitor therapy, which causes increased renin levels, monitoring of this parameter does not have any clinical utility. Other laboratory features on presentation include non-nephrotic proteinuria, dysmorphic (usually microscopic) hematuria, and an elevated serum creatinine concentration. Microangiopathic hemolytic anemia occurs in 43% of patients. Thrombocytopenia occurs, but the platelet count rarely falls below 50,000/mm^3.

Mild hypertension, proteinuria, microhematuria, and azotemia may be noted in as many as 50% to 60% of patients with systemic sclerosis who do not have renal crisis, and up to 80% may have kidney disease if abnormalities on kidney biopsy are included in the definition. However, causes of these processes other than systemic sclerosis usually are identifiable. Causes include use of D-penicillamine, severe congestive heart failure, prerenal azotemia, and use of nonsteroidal anti-inflammatory drugs. Membranous nephropathy and perinuclear-staining antineutrophil cytoplasmic antibody (P-ANCA)-positive pauci-immune crescentic glomerulonephritis occasionally have been reported in patients with systemic sclerosis.

Therapy

The use of ACE inhibitors is the mainstay of treatment for patients with renal crisis. Inasmuch as they are effective both in patients with hypertension and in the occasional patient without hypertension, their mechanism of action most likely reaches beyond blood pressure control. If ACE inhibitors alone cannot adequately control hypertension, other antihypertensives should be prescribed to achieve a goal blood pressure of 125/75 mm Hg. In the treatment of renal crisis, the ACE inhibitor should not be stopped because of concerns that it might be diminishing renal perfusion pressure and exacerbating the decline in kidney function. Anecdotal case reports suggest that combining ACE inhibitors with angiotensin receptor blockers may worsen the renal outcome.

Course and Prognosis

Scleroderma renal crisis was once almost universally fatal at 1 year, but patients receiving treatment with ACE inhibitors can anticipate a 5-year survival rate of 65%. Late initiation of ACE inhibitor therapy (e.g., after serum creatinine levels exceed 3 mg/dL) is associated with worse prognosis, as is inadequate blood pressure control. For those who progress to require dialysis, continued ACE inhibitor therapy is recommended, because approximately 50% of patients recover sufficient kidney function over 3 to 18 months to discontinue

dialysis. Patients with renal crisis undergoing dialysis had somewhat poorer graft survival and patient survival than in the general dialysis population. Few patients have undergone transplantation, but recurrence in an allograft from an identical twin has been reported.

BIBLIOGRAPHY

Andreoli SP, Trachtman H, Acheson DWK, et al: Hemolytic uremic syndrome: Epidemiology, pathophysiology, and therapy. Pediatr Nephrol 17:293-298, 2002.

Chizzolini C: Update on pathophysiology of scleroderma with special reference to immunoinflammatory events. Ann Med 39:42-53, 2007.

Crowther MA, Ginsberg JS, Julian J, et al: A comparison of two intensities of warfarin for the prevention of recurrent thrombosis in patients with the antiphospholipid antibody syndrome. N Engl J Med 349:1133-1138, 2003.

Fischer M, Rauch J, Levine JS: The antiphospholipid syndrome. Sem Nephrol 27:35-46, 2007.

Fogo A: Atlas of renal pathology: Thrombotic microangiopathy. Am J Kidney Dis 34:E7, 1999.

Giannakopoulos B, Passam F, Rahgozar S, Krilis SA: Current concepts on the pathogenesis of the antiphospholipid syndrome. Blood 109:422-430, 2007.

Harris ML, Rosen A: Autoimmunity in scleroderma: Pathogenetic role and clinical significance of autoantibodies. Curr Opin Rheumatol 15:778-784, 2003.

Hosler GA, Cusumano AM, Hutchins GM: Thrombotic thrombocytopenic purpura and hemolytic uremic syndrome are distinct pathologic entities. Arch Pathol Lab Med 127:834-839, 2003.

Jimenez SA, Derk CT: Following the molecular pathways toward an understanding of the pathogenesis of systemic sclerosis. Ann Intern Med 140:37-50, 2004.

Levine JS, Branch DW, Rauch J: The antiphospholipid syndrome. N Engl J Med 346:752-763, 2002.

Miyakis S, Lockshin MD, Atsumi T, et al: International consensus statement on an update of the classification criteria for definite antiphospholipid syndrome. J Thromb Haemost 4:295-306, 2006.

Moake JL: Mechanisms of disease: Thrombotic microangiopathies. N Engl J Med 347:589-600, 2002.

Noris M, Remuzzi G: Hemolytic uremic syndrome. J Am Soc Nephrol 16:1035-1050, 2005.

Remuzzi G, Galbusera M, Noris M, et al, and the Italian Registry of Recurrent and Familial HUS/TTP: Von Willebrand factor cleaving protease (ADAMTS13) is deficient in recurrent and familial thrombotic thrombocytopenic purpura and hemolytic uremic syndrome. Blood 100:778-785, 2002.

Rock GA, Shumack KH, Buskard NA, et al, and the Canadian Apheresis Group: Comparison of plasma exchange with plasma infusion in the treatment of thrombotic thrombocytopenic purpura. N Engl J Med 325:393-397, 1991.

Ruggenenti P, Noris M, Remuzzi G: Thrombotic microangiopathy, hemolytic uremic syndrome, and thrombotic thrombocytopenic purpura. Kidney Int 60:831-846, 2001.

Steen VD: Scleroderma renal crisis. Rheum Dis Clin North Am 29:315-333, 2003.

Takehara K: Pathogenesis of systemic sclerosis. J Rheumatol 30:755-759, 2003.

Tsai H-M: Von Willebrand factor, ADAMTS13, and thrombotic thrombocytopenic purpura. J Mol Med 80:639-647, 2002.

Tsai H-M: Advances in the pathogenesis, diagnosis and treatment of thrombotic thrombocytopenic purpura. J Am Soc Nephrol 14:1072-1081, 2003.

Tsai HM: The molecular biology of thrombotic microangiopathy. Kidney Int 70:16-23, 2006.

Tsai H-M: Current concepts in thrombotic thrombocytopenic purpura. Annu Rev Med 57:419-436, 2006.

Zakarija A, Bennett C: Drug-induced thrombotic microangiopathy. Semin Thromb Hemost 31:681-690, 2005.

CHAPTER 29

Kidney Disorders in Human Immunodeficiency Virus Infection

Christina M. Wyatt, Marianne Monahan, and Paul E. Klotman

Kidney disease occurs frequently in the course of human immunodeficiency virus (HIV) infection, and it has become a leading contributor to morbidity and mortality in patients with HIV and acquired immunodeficiency syndrome (AIDS) in the era of highly active antiretroviral therapy (HAART). The kidney disorders associated with HIV infection can be divided into several categories: fluid and electrolyte disorders, acid-base disorders, acute kidney injury, and chronic kidney disease (CKD), including HIV-associated nephropathy (HIVAN) and immune-mediated glomerular disease (**Table 29-1**). Many of these disorders are similar to those seen in the HIV-negative population. Others, such as HIVAN, are attributable to HIV infection itself, or are the side effects of medications used in the treatment of HIV infection or AIDS-related illnesses. Many of these complications are preventable or treatable, making early recognition and intervention essential.

FLUID AND ELECTROLYTE DISORDERS

Sodium

Electrolyte and acid-base abnormalities are common in patients with HIV infection, although the distribution of electrolyte and acid-base disorders has changed since the introduction of HAART. Hyponatremia was the most common fluid and electrolyte disorder observed in hospitalized AIDS patients before the HAART era. Although data are limited, hyponatremia appears to be less common in HIV populations with access to HAART. Most cases can be attributed to volume depletion resulting from diarrhea, emesis, poor oral intake, or increased insensible losses due to fever or pulmonary disease. Other causes of low serum sodium include the syndrome of inappropriate antidiuretic hormone secretion (SIADH), adrenal insufficiency, and renal sodium wasting caused by nephrotoxic medications such as amphotericin and pentamidine. Common drug-related toxicities are listed in **Table 29-2**.

Hypernatremia, though less common, can be observed in HIV or AIDS. Hypernatremia also occurs in the setting of volume depletion, and it may be associated with acquired nephrogenic diabetes insipidus from medications such as amphotericin or foscarnet.

Potassium

Hypokalemia, like hyponatremia, may occur in the setting of volume depletion secondary to gastrointestinal losses. Amphotericin nephrotoxicity can also manifest with hypokalemia, often associated with magnesium depletion. Hypokalemia has also been observed as a complication of the antiviral nucleotide analogues adefovir and tenofovir.

Hyperkalemia may occur in patients with HIV or AIDS. As in seronegative patients with hyperkalemia, increased serum potassium levels may be a result of impaired kidney function, adrenal insufficiency, and acidosis. Medications used in the treatment of *Pneumocystis* pneumonia have been shown to increase blood potassium levels through direct mechanisms. The effect of trimethoprim on the distal nephron is similar to that of the potassium-sparing diuretics; it inhibits sodium reabsorption via the epithelial sodium channel (ENaC) of the collecting duct and thereby limits potassium secretion. Pentamidine has been shown to act on the distal tubule in a similar manner, but it may also increase serum potassium indirectly by decreasing the glomerular filtration rate.

Calcium, Phosphorus, and Magnesium

Abnormal serum calcium levels may be observed in both hospitalized AIDS patients and ambulatory HAART-treated patients. In some cases, low serum calcium may reflect hypoalbuminemia rather than true hypocalcemia. Medications including foscarnet, pentamidine, and didanosine have also been implicated in hypocalcemia. Severe, symptomatic hypocalcemia manifested by paraesthesias and Trousseau's or Chvostek's signs has been reported in patients treated concurrently with pentamidine and foscarnet. Increased serum calcium levels may be seen in patients with granulomatous disease or disseminated cytomegalovirus infection.

Hypophosphatemia is commonly observed in HAART-treated patients with HIV; it occurred in 17% of patients in one European cohort. Hypophosphatemia may occur as a complication of treatment with the nucleotide analogues cidofovir, adefovir, and tenofovir, and it may be accompanied by other signs of tubular toxicity. Isolated hypophosphatemia is also common in HAART-treated HIV patients who are not

TABLE 29-1 Common Kidney Disorders in Patients with HIV Infection

Fluid-Electrolyte and Acid-Base Disturbances

Hyponatremia and hypernatremia

Hypokalemia and hyperkalemia

Hypocalcemia and hypercalcemia

Hypophosphatemia and hyperphosphatemia

Hypomagnesemia

SIADH

Nephrogenic diabetes insipidus

Fanconi's syndrome

Renal tubular acidosis

Lactic acidosis

Acute Kidney Injury*

Prerenal acute renal failure

Acute tubular necrosis

Interstitial nephritis

    Allergic processes

    Infectious processes

Crystalluria/obstructive uropathy

HUS/TTP

Glomerular Syndromes

HIV-associated nephropathy

HIV-related immune complex disease

Hepatitis virus–related glomerular disease

    Membranoproliferative glomerulonephritis

    Membranous glomerulopathy

Minimal change disease

Postinfectious glomerulonephritis

Comorbid diabetic or hypertensive disease

HIV, human immunodeficiency virus; HUS/TTP, hemolytic uremic syndrome/thrombotic thrombocytopenic purpura; SIADH, syndrome of inappropriate antidiuretic hormone secretion.

*Some of the diagnoses classified as acute kidney injury may also manifest as chronic kidney disease, in particular interstitial nephritis, crystalluria/obstruction, or HUS/TTP.

TABLE 29-2 Drug-Induced Nephrotoxicity in Patients with HIV-1 Infection

DRUG	TOXICITY
Acyclovir	Acute tubular necrosis
	Crystalluria/obstructive nephropathy
Adefovir	Proximal tubular damage
Aminoglycosides	Acute tubular necrosis
	Renal tubular acidosis
Amphotericin	Acute tubular necrosis
	Hypokalemia or hyperkalemia
	Hypomagnesemia
	Renal tubular acidosis
Atazanavir	Nephrolithiasis
Cidofovir	Proximal tubular damage
Foscarnet	Hypocalcemia or hypercalcemia
	Hypophosphatemia or hyperphosphatemia
	Hypomagnesemia
	Nephrogenic diabetes insipidus
Indinavir	Crystalluria/obstructive nephropathy
	Nephrolithiasis
	Acute and chronic renal failure
NSAIDs	Acute tubular necrosis
	Interstitial nephritis
Pentamidine	Acute tubular necrosis
	Hyperkalemia
	Hypocalcemia
Rifampin	Allergic interstitial nephritis
Sulfadiazine	Crystalluria/obstructive nephropathy
	Allergic interstitial nephritis
Tenofovir	Proximal tubular damage
	Acute renal failure
	Decreased GFR

GFR, glomerular filtration rate; HIV, human immunodeficiency virus; NSAIDs, nonsteroidal anti-inflammatory drugs.

receiving nucleotide analogues, although the mechanisms are unknown. Vitamin D deficiency is also common and may further complicate calcium and phosphorus metabolism.

Renal magnesium wasting, resulting in hypomagnesemia, may occur as a complication of treatment with either pentamidine or amphotericin. Drug-induced tubular injury is the proposed mechanism.

ACID-BASE DISORDERS

Low serum bicarbonate levels are common in HAART-treated patients, occurring in almost 14% of patients in a large European cohort. Non–anion gap metabolic acidosis due to bicarbonate loss in the stool may result from acute or chronic diarrhea in AIDS patients with increased susceptibility to opportunistic enteric pathogens. Lactic acidosis is most often associated with sepsis in patients with HIV; however a type B

lactic acidosis may occur with exposure to the nucleoside reverse transcriptase inhibitors (NRTIs), in particular didanosine and stavudine. The presumed mechanism is inhibition of DNA γ-polymerase resulting in mitochondrial dysfunction in liver and skeletal muscle cells, with resultant overproduction of lactic acid.

Other medications have also been implicated in acid-base disturbances. Renal tubular acidosis may complicate treatment with gentamicin, amphotericin B, or the nucleotide analogues. A series of patients who developed unexplained renal tubular acidosis while receiving high-dose trimethoprim-sulfamethoxazole has also been reported.

Pulmonary infections and sepsis can induce respiratory alkalosis due to hyperventilation. Respiratory acidosis may also occur later in the course of pulmonary infections because of respiratory muscle fatigue.

Proximal Tubular Injury

Urinary bicarbonate losses may occur as a result of proximal tubular injury in patients with HIV infection. Tubular toxicity is the dose-limiting side effect of cidofovir and adefovir, two nucleotide analogues with potent antiviral activity. The mechanism of toxicity is unknown but probably involves accumulation in proximal tubular epithelial cells after uptake by the human organic anion transporters hOAT1 and hOAT3.

In clinical trials of cidofovir for the treatment of cytomegalovirus retinitis, approximately 5% to 7% of patients developed signs of proximal tubular damage, including elevated serum creatinine, glycosuria, and urinary bicarbonate wasting. Cidofovir toxicity can be reduced by coadministration of probenecid, which decreases tubular cell uptake. The related nucleotide analogue, adefovir, has activity against both HIV and hepatitis B. In clinical trials of adefovir for HIV, Fanconi's syndrome developed in up to 30% of patients undergoing treatment for longer than 6 months at doses of 30 mg or higher. Manifestations included bicarbonate wasting, hypophosphatemia, glycosuria, aminoaciduria, and hypokalemia, which resolved with discontinuation of the drug. At the 10-mg dose approved for the treatment of chronic hepatitis B infection, adefovir has not been associated with significant nephrotoxicity.

The nucleotide reverse transcriptase inhibitor tenofovir is less cytotoxic in vitro and did not demonstrate significant nephrotoxicity in clinical trials for the treatment of HIV. Since the approval of tenofovir, proximal tubular toxicity and acute renal failure have been reported, and several cohort studies have observed small reductions in glomerular filtration rate among tenofovir-treated patients. Longitudinal data from the tenofovir expanded access program demonstrated some degree of nephrotoxicity in approximately 2% of treated patients. Tubular toxicity is usually reversible with early recognition and discontinuation of tenofovir, although the long-term effects of continued therapy in the setting of mildly decreased glomerular filtration rate are not known. Risk factors for tenofovir toxicity are not well established; however, patients with unrecognized kidney dysfunction are likely to be at the highest risk.

ACUTE KIDNEY INJURY

Patients with HIV infection or AIDS are at increased risk for acute renal failure; the causes are similar to those identified in patients without HIV. Approximately half of the episodes of acute renal failure observed in an ambulatory HAART-treated population were attributed to infection, manifested as either prerenal acute renal failure or acute tubular necrosis. Almost one third of the cases were medication related, manifesting as acute tubular necrosis, interstitial nephritis, obstructive nephropathy, or prerenal acute renal failure. Ten percent of cases were associated with end-stage liver disease, which is an increasingly common complication of HIV-hepatitis virus coinfection.

Prerenal acute renal failure may occur in the setting of volume depletion, sepsis, heart failure, or cirrhosis. Volume depletion may result from vomiting, diarrhea, fever, or poor oral intake in both hospitalized and ambulatory patients. Prolonged or severe hypoperfusion may result in acute tubular necrosis.

Acute interstitial nephritis may be caused by infection or by a hypersensitivity drug reaction. Infectious agents associated with interstitial nephritis include cytomegalovirus, candida, tuberculosis, and histoplasmosis. Medications used to treat AIDS-related illness that are commonly associated with acute interstitial nephritis include β-lactams, quinolones, sulfonamides, rifampin, and nonsteroidal anti-inflammatory drugs. Treatment requires discontinuation of the medication.

Thrombotic microangiopathy, manifesting as hemolytic uremic syndrome or thrombotic thrombocytopenic purpura (HUS/TTP), is increasingly rare in the HAART era. The clinical manifestations and pathologic findings of HIV-related HUS/TTP are similar to those of the idiopathic forms. Although HIV-related thrombotic microangiopathy most commonly manifests as acute kidney injury, it may also persist or present as progressive CKD. Treatment with plasmapheresis and fresh-frozen plasma replacement may be effective but has not been studied in the HAART era.

Postrenal causes of acute renal failure should be considered in patients with HIV infection or AIDS. Crystal-induced obstructive nephropathy may occur in patients who are receiving sulfadiazine, intravenous acyclovir, or indinavir. Treatment consists of discontinuation of the drug and vigorous hydration. The protease inhibitor indinavir is associated with asymptomatic crystalluria in up to 20% of patients, with symptoms of dysuria and renal colic occurring in approximately 8%. Atazanavir has also been associated with an increased risk of nephrolithiasis, and other protease inhibitors have been implicated in isolated cases.

In addition to the antiretroviral agents discussed previously, many HIV patients are enrolled in clinical trials with investigational medications. A high index of suspicion for medication toxicity should be maintained and explored whenever one is evaluating acute renal failure in a patient with HIV infection.

CHRONIC KIDNEY DISEASE

With the aging of the HAART-treated population, CKD and end-stage renal disease (ESRD) are becoming increasingly common. HIV-related CKD is significantly more common among blacks, and growing racial disparities in new HIV diagnoses have made kidney disease a major concern for the HIV community. Whereas CKD is rare among HAART-treated European patients, urban U.S. clinic populations may have prevalence rates of 15% or higher. The potential public health implications for sub-Saharan Africa are staggering and will become increasingly relevant as HAART becomes available in high-prevalence regions. Common causes of CKD in patients with HIV include HIVAN and other

HIV-related kidney diseases, as well as kidney disease secondary to comorbid diabetes and hypertension.

Management of Chronic Kidney Disease and End-Stage Renal Disease

Regardless of etiology, management of CKD in HIV-positive patients is similar to that in HIV-negative patients. Unique considerations are reviewed in guidelines published by the Infectious Diseases Society of America, with a particular focus on appropriate medication dose adjustment.

Treatment options for the HIV patient with ESRD include hemodialysis and peritoneal dialysis, as well as kidney transplantation in carefully selected patients. Survival of HIV-positive dialysis patients has significantly improved as a result of HAART. Transmission of HIV in hemodialysis units is very unlikely if standard blood precaution practice guidelines (Universal Precautions) are followed, and the Centers for Disease Control does not recommend special machines or isolation procedures for HIV-positive patients undergoing hemodialysis.

Studies to evaluate kidney transplantation in patients infected with HIV are still underway, with promising results. Eligible patients should have undetectable viral burden on a stable HAART regimen, no evidence of neoplasms or opportunistic infections, and CD4 counts greater than 200 cells/μL. One-year patient survival rates are similar to unmatched survival data from the United Network for Organ Sharing database. Median CD4 counts have remained stable, and the risk of opportunistic infections is similar to that in the general transplant population. Acute rejection rates are increased in HIV-positive kidney transplant recipients. Although the mechanism of increased acute rejection is unknown, challenges in achieving and maintaining therapeutic immunosuppressive drug levels may contribute. Significant drug interactions between immunosuppressive agents and HAART require close monitoring and communication between transplant teams and HIV providers.

Human Immunodeficiency Virus–Associated Nephropathy

HIVAN is a disease with unique clinical, pathologic, and epidemiologic features, including a strong predilection for patients of African descent. HIVAN was first described in the early 1980s and is now a leading cause of ESRD in African Americans. The salient features of HIVAN are listed in **Table 29-3** and discussed in this section. Other glomerular diseases associated with HIV infection are less strongly associated with black race and are discussed separately.

Presentation

The diagnosis of HIVAN is remarkably restricted to black patients; in the United States, almost 90% of cases occur in African Americans, and the remaining 10% of patients are almost exclusively of mixed-heritage or Hispanic. Patients with HIVAN usually present with azotemia and proteinuria.

TABLE 29-3 Clinical Presentation of HIV-Associated Nephropathy

Epidemiology	Affects blacks disproportionately
	Natural history improved with HAART
Presentation	Proteinuria
	Rapid progression
	Normal or large, echogenic kidneys
	CD4 count usually <200 cells/μL
Pathology	Collapsing FSGS
	Microcystic dilatation of tubules
	Interstitial inflammation
Pathogenesis	Direct HIV infection of the kidney
	Host genetic factors
Treatment	HAART
	ACE inhibitor or ARB
	Corticosteroids in selected cases

ACE, angiotensin-converting enzyme; ARB, angiotensin receptor blocker; FSGS, focal segmental glomerulosclerosis; HAART, highly active antiretroviral therapy; HIV, human immunodeficiency virus.

On renal sonography, the kidneys are typically normal or slightly increased in size and are often described as echogenic. HIVAN was initially believed to be a late complication of HIV infection, because it appeared in patients with low CD4 counts and a history of opportunistic infections. In a series of 114 patients with biopsy-proven HIVAN, all but 6 had CD4 counts of less than 200 cells/μL. However, there have been case reports of HIVAN occurring in the setting of acute HIV seroconversion, indicating that HIVAN may develop at any time in the course of HIV infection.

Pathology

The histopathologic features of HIVAN include focal segmental glomerular sclerosis (FSGS) in combination with microcystic distortion of the tubulointerstitium (**Fig. 29-1**). Collapsing glomerulosclerosis is a common variant in patients with HIVAN (**Fig. 29-2A and B**), although this form of FSGS has also been described in seronegative patients. Microcysts are often filled with proteinaceous casts, and in some patients there is modest interstitial infiltration by lymphocytes, plasma cells, and monocytes. Immunofluorescence is usually nonspecific. Electron microscopic examination may reveal tubuloreticular inclusions, although this finding is rare in the HAART era. Biopsy confirmation of HIVAN is extremely important. Even when HIVAN is suspected, approximately 40% of patients are found to have another diagnosis on pathologic examination.

Pathogenesis

Much has been learned about the cellular mechanisms responsible for the development of HIVAN. Evidence from both clinical and animal studies supports a direct role for HIV infection of tubular and glomerular epithelial cells. Transgenic mice expressing a replication-defective HIV construct developed proteinuria, reduced kidney function, and

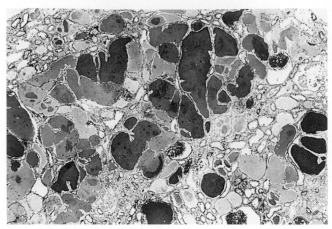

FIGURE 29-1 Kidney biopsy sample of a patient with human immuno-deficiency virus–associated nephropathy (HIVAN). The classic features of HIVAN are present in this specimen, with microcystic tubular dilatation, proteinaceous casts, modest interstitial infiltrate, and collapsing glomerulosclerosis (periodic acid–Schiff stain, original magnification ×50). (Courtesy of Dr. Vivette D'Agati.)

histologic disease almost identical to HIVAN. Reciprocal transplantation studies using this mouse model demonstrated that HIVAN develops only in kidneys expressing the transgene. Moreover, HIV RNA and DNA have been detected in podocytes and renal tubular epithelial cells of patients with HIVAN. The mechanism by which HIV enters kidney epithelial cells is unknown. Recent studies indicate that these epithelial cells are able to support a productive viral life cycle, making the kidney a potential reservoir for HIV.

Kidney biopsy samples of patients with HIVAN demonstrate increased epithelial cell proliferation and apoptosis. Proliferation of tubular epithelial cells probably contributes to microcyst formation and may explain why kidneys are normal or large in size. Increased proliferation of podocytes is an important component of the collapsing FSGS found in HIVAN.

The racial predilection of HIVAN for black patients indicates that host factors are important determinants of response to epithelial cell infection. In an effort to determine the influence of genetic background on HIVAN pathogenesis, the HIV transgenic mouse model of HIVAN has been manipulated to identify genetic loci that are associated with the development of kidney disease. This approach may elucidate novel candidate genes that are important for the development of HIVAN.

Treatment

Approaches to the treatment of HIVAN are directed at slowing progression to ESRD and treating the underlying HIV infection. Small studies have suggested that ACE (angiotensin-converting enzyme) inhibitors or immune modulators, including prednisone and cyclosporine, may be efficacious in slowing the progression of HIVAN to ESRD. Studies demonstrating efficacy of ACE inhibitors were not randomized and lacked proper controls, but therapy with ACE inhibitors is currently considered to be standard care based on the favorable risk profile. In addition, angiotensin

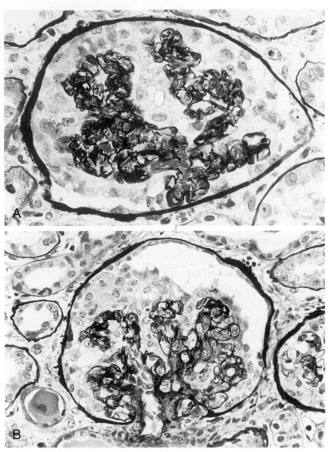

FIGURE 29-2 Focal segmental glomerulosclerosis of the collapsing variant. Both focal (**A**) and global (**B**) collapse can be seen in association with HIV infection (Jones's methenamine silver stain; original magnification ×500 in **A**, ×325 in **B**).

receptor blockers (ARBs) may be beneficial, in light of evidence from studies of other proteinuric glomerular diseases. Use of ACE inhibitors and ARBs should not detract from an aggressive antiretroviral strategy.

The use of immunosuppression in the treatment of late-stage HIVAN has also been explored in small studies. Treatment with prednisone at 60 mg/day for up to 11 weeks reduced serum creatinine and lowered proteinuria in one small, prospective study. Long-term outcome, however, was not substantially different from historical controls, and serious opportunistic infections occurred. Cyclosporine has been used in a small number of HIV-positive children with FSGS; in some, the nephrotic syndrome resolved.

Although there have been no randomized controlled clinical trials to evaluate HAART for the treatment of HIVAN, case series and retrospective studies suggest that the rate of progression of HIVAN to ESRD has been slowed by the introduction of antiretroviral therapy. Data provided by the United States Renal Data System provide further evidence that HAART has improved the natural history of HIVAN. During the first half of the 1990s, the incidence of ESRD due to HIVAN rose rapidly, increasing by more than 550%. Incidence rates dropped slightly from 1995 to 1996 and then reached a plateau. The plateau in incidence of HIVAN coincided with the introduction of HAART. In addition, there are several case reports of patients with biopsy-proven HIVAN who experienced clinical and histologic improvement in their kidney disease after initiating HAART.

Other Forms of Glomerular Disease Associated with HIV Infection

Although FSGS secondary to HIVAN is the most common glomerular lesion seen in HIV-positive patients, biopsy series have revealed a wide spectrum of lesions in these patients, including membranoproliferative glomerulonephritis, minimal change disease, membranous glomerulopathy, IgA nephropathy, amyloidosis, and a variety of parenchymal infections. Coinfection with hepatitis B or C virus is common in HIV-positive patients, especially those with a history of intravenous drug use. Because hepatitis B and C are also associated with immune-mediated kidney disease independent of HIV infection, the specific etiology of the kidney disease should be addressed in an individual patient. The importance of HIV in the pathogenesis of other HIV-related kidney diseases remains unclear.

BIBLIOGRAPHY

Ahuja TS, Grady J, Khan S: Changing trends in the survival of dialysis patients with human immunodeficiency virus in the United States. J Am Soc Nephrol 13:1889-1993, 2002.

Bagnis CI, Du Montcel ST, Fonfrede M, et al: Changing electrolyte and acido-basic profile in HIV-infected patients in the HAART era. Nephron Physiol 103:131-138, 2006.

Burns GC, Paul SK, Toth IR, Sivak SL: Effect of angiotensin converting enzyme inhibition in HIV-associated nephropathy. J Am Soc Nephrol 8:1140-1146, 1997.

Cozzolino M, Vidal M, Arcidiacono MV, et al: HIV-protease inhibitors impair vitamin D bioactivation to 1,25-dihydroxyvitamin D. AIDS 17:513-520, 2003.

D'Agati V, Appel GB: Renal pathology of human immunodeficiency virus infection. Semin Nephrol 18:406-421, 1998.

Franceschini N, Napravnik S, Eron JJ Jr, et al: Incidence and etiology of acute renal failure among ambulatory HIV-infected patients. Kidney Int 67:1526-1531, 2005.

Fine DM, Perazella MA, Lucas GM, Atta MG: Kidney biopsy in HIV: Beyond HIV-associated nephropathy. Am J Kidney Dis 51:504-514, 2008.

Gerntholtz TE, Goetsch SJ, Katz I: HIV-related nephropathy: A South African perspective. Kidney Int 69:1885-1891, 2006.

Gharavi AG, Ahmad T, Wong RD, et al: Mapping a locus for susceptibility to HIV-1-associated nephropathy to mouse chromosome 3. Proc Natl Acad Sci U S A 101:2488-2493, 2004.

Gupta SK, Eustace JA, Winston JA, et al: Guidelines for the management of chronic kidney disease in HIV-infected patients: Recommendations of the HIV Medicine Association of the Infectious Diseases Society of America. Clin Infect Dis 40:1559-1585, 2005.

Rao TK, Filippone EJ, Nicastri AD, et al: Associated focal and segmental glomerulosclerosis in the acquired immunodeficiency syndrome. N Engl J Med 310:669-673, 1984.

Roland ME, Adey D, Carlson LL, et al: Kidney and liver transplantation in HIV-infected patients: Case presentations and review. AIDS Patient Care and STDs 17:501-507, 2003.

Stock PG, Roland ME, Carlson L, et al: Kidney and liver transplantation in human immunodeficiency virus-infected patients: A pilot safety and efficacy study. Transplantation 76:370-375, 2003.

Stokes MB, Chawla H, Brody RI, et al: Immune complex glomerulonephritis in patients coinfected with human immunodeficiency virus and hepatitis C virus. Am J Kidney Dis 29:514-525, 1997.

Szczech LA, Gupta SK, Habash R, et al: The clinical epidemiology and course of the spectrum of renal diseases associated with HIV infection. Kidney Int 66:1145-1152, 2004.

Winston J, Klotman ME, Klotman PE: HIV-associated nephropathy is a late, not early, manifestation of HIV-1 infection. Kidney Int 55:1036-1040, 1999.

Wyatt CM, Arons RR, Klotman PK, Klotman MK: Acute renal failure in hospitalized patients with HIV: Risk factors and impact on in-hospital mortality. AIDS 20:561-565, 2006.

Wyatt CM, Klotman PE: Antiretroviral therapy and the kidney: Balancing benefit and risk in patients with human immunodeficiency virus infection. Expert Opin Drug Saf 5:275-287, 2006.

Wyatt CM, Winston JA, Malvestutto C, et al: Chronic kidney disease in HIV infection: An urban epidemic. AIDS 21:2101-2103, 2007.

CHAPTER 30

Kidney Function in Congestive Heart Failure

Eberhard Ritz

Congestive heart failure (CHF) is a leading cause of morbidity and mortality, affecting mainly the elderly and the survivors of myocardial infarction. Despite the considerable progress made in the clinical management of CHF, its prognosis continues to be worse than in many common cancers. A close link exists between heart function and kidney function. Baseline renal function and, particularly, worsening of renal function are potent predictors of adverse outcome. Whereas evaluation of renal function is usually based on measurements of serum creatinine, cystatin C is a more sensitive indicator of glomerular filtration rate (GFR) and is linearly associated with the incidence of heart failure.

In a prospective, single-center study, worsening of renal function was an independent predictor of death or rehospitalization apart from a history of chronic kidney disease, low left ventricular ejection fraction, and daily furosemide dose. The short-term statistics show a graded relationship between mortality and the acute decrease in renal function, including even small changes, as was found in a recent analysis and confirmed in a systematic meta-analysis.

HETEROGENEITY OF THE SYNDROME "CONGESTIVE HEART FAILURE"

Heart failure is a clinical syndrome that may result from any structural or functional cardiac disorder that impairs the ability of the ventricle to fill or to eject blood. The main cardiac manifestations are dyspnea and fatigue, limited exercise tolerance, and fluid retention, leading to pulmonary and peripheral edema.

The clinical presentation of CHF is quite heterogeneous. It has recently become clear that not all CHF is created equal. It is advantageous to subclassify this syndrome into two major categories: (1) acute cardiac failure from cardiovascular causes, mainly hypertension, and (2) acute decompensated heart failure (ADHF) due to primary cardiac causes. The former is a more rapidly progressive disorder characterized by high blood pressure and severe acute dyspnea and is commonly encountered in emergency settings. The linkage of hypertension to acute heart failure with pulmonary edema is supported by the observation of higher blood pressure and, frequently, a marked blood pressure increase in patients with this condition, associated with increased vascular resistance and superimposed on reduced and deteriorating cardiac contractility. Combined ventricular and arterial stiffening

beyond that associated with aging has been demonstrated in patients with CHF and preserved ejection fraction, and this may explain the beneficial effect of vasodilators.

ADHF resulting from primary cardiac causes is a syndrome of more slowly worsening symptoms and signs, with infrequent pulmonary edema but with increased jugular venous pressure, hepatomegaly, peripheral edema, and poor peripheral perfusion. These are mostly patients with a primary cardiac cause (e.g., postmyocardial infarction), and the symptoms are often triggered by factors such as ingestion of anti-inflammatory agents, negative inotropic agents, concomitant infection, or acute ventricular contractility deficit.

The underlying pathophysiology presumably differs in this second form, and it may be necessary to revise past paradigms. The classic view was that fluid accumulation was a crucial step in the development of symptomatic CHF. More recent studies with consistent invasive and noninvasive monitoring showed that fluid accumulation does not play a pivotal role. An increase in pulmonary pressure was found days to weeks before weight gain was first observed, and such weight gain usually did not exceed 2 kg. In a prospective cohort of patients with chronic CHF, no difference in weight gain was found between those who developed acute heart failure and those who did not. This has led to the concept that the underlying mechanism may be fluid redistribution rather than fluid accumulation. Redistribution appears to be caused by a reduction in the capacitance of large veins and an increase in arterial resistance. The former leads to increased venous return and increased preload, the latter to increased resistance and increased afterload.

A strong argument for the presence of fluid redistribution is the documented superiority of high-dose nitrates with low-dose diuretics, compared to low-dose nitrates with high-dose diuretics. Conversely, a discrepancy is found between weight loss and symptom improvement or outcome. In the Initiation Management Predischarge Assessment of Carvedilol Therapy in Heart Failure (IMPACT-HF) Registry, the degree of weight loss during admission for CHF was not associated with the improvement in fatigue, paroxysmal nocturnal dyspnea, or dyspnea at rest. This agrees with the observation in the Endovascular Valve Edge-to-Edge REpair STudy (EVEREST) trials, in which administration of the aquaretic tolvaptan led to a reduction in weight but failed to produce a clinically significantly improvement in the patient's short-term symptoms or to affect long-term outcome.

PATHOPHYSIOLOGY

Role of Effective Arterial Volume

The kidney receives information triggered by cardiac dysfunction and responds with functional alterations resulting in salt retention and volume expansion. According to this view, initially adaptive mechanisms become ultimately maladaptive by increasing the preload and afterload, thereby compromising cardiac function. When hypovolemia is sensed in the arterial system, the response includes activation of the sympathetic nervous system and the renin-angiotensin-aldosterone system (RAS). The trigger for the response is thought to be arterial underfilling; this stimulates the baroreceptors, which perceive a decrease in the effective arterial volume even when extracellular volume is expanded. The resulting counterregulation of salt and fluid retention is useful in acute hemorrhage but less useful as a compensatory effort in chronic reduction of effective arterial volume (**Fig. 30-1**).

In the kidney, initially plasma flow is reduced, but GFR is unchanged, or at least proportionately less reduced, so that the filtration fraction increases. This response is ultimately maladaptive and explains why in CHF many signs and symptoms are not directly related to impaired cardiac performance but actually result from the maladaptive renal counterregulatory mechanisms.

Neuroendocrine Activation

Sympathetic Activation

Arterial underfilling as a result of cardiac pump failure is sensed by arterial baroreceptors in the large vessels. Their activation results in increased sympathetic tone, which raises cardiac output via increased heart rate and cardiac

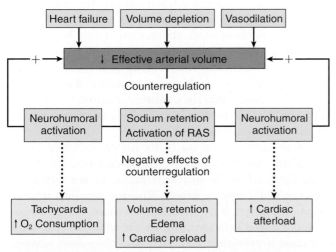

FIGURE 30-1 Cardiorenal volume regulation. Counterregulatory adaptive mechanisms may have negative, maladaptive effects. Heart failure or any other decrease in effective arterial volume activates several counterregulatory cardiorenal mechanisms to increase the effective arterial volume by stimulating renal sodium and volume retention and by increasing vascular resistance. In heart failure, the chronic activation of these counterregulatory mechanisms has a multiplicity of negative effects, which characterize the clinical syndrome of congestive heart failure. RAS, renin-angiotensin-aldosterone system.

contractility. Concomitant venoconstriction increases venous return and cardiac filling, thus augmenting preload. The resulting increase in cardiac work and oxygen consumption is unfavorable. In the kidney, sympathetic activation causes renal vasoconstriction and stimulation of the RAS. In the past, it was thought that, in contrast to the "bad" catecholamines adrenaline and noradrenaline, dopamine was a "good" catecholamine with beneficial effects on the kidney; however, studies of patients in acute renal failure showed no benefit and potential harm from dopamine.

Activation of the Renin-Angiotensin-Aldosterone System

Via β-adrenergic mechanisms, sympathetic activation stimulates the release of renin from the juxtaglomerular apparatus. Angiotensin II is produced and contributes to vasoconstriction in the systemic circulation and in the kidney. Principal effects of angiotensin II generated either systemically or locally within the kidney include the following:

- Direct stimulation of sodium reabsorption in the proximal tubule
- Preferential constriction of the efferent more than the afferent glomerular arteriole, thereby raising intraglomerular pressure and maintaining GFR despite decreased renal blood flow. (In the initial stages, this is a beneficial effect that maintains renal function.)
- Powerful dipsogenic stimulation
- Upregulation of synthesis and secretion of aldosterone in the zona glomerulosa of the adrenal cortex. (Aldosterone is a major player in the cardiac complications of CHF, as evidenced by the dramatic beneficial effect of mineralocorticoid receptor blockade by spironolactone or eplerenone.)

Antidiuretic Hormone

The sensing of arterial underfilling by baroreceptors stimulates the secretion of antidiuretic hormone, also called arginine vasopressin (AVP), from the posterior pituitary. The release of AVP is, under normal circumstances, regulated by hypothalamic osmoreceptors. In CHF, overriding the osmotic control, AVP is secreted despite normal or even low serum osmolality, a phenomenon termed nonosmotic stimulation of AVP release. In the kidney, AVP stimulates V_2 vasopressin receptors in the collecting duct, increasing the synthesis and translocation of the water channel aquaporin 2, and thereby facilitating tubular water absorption. This provides the rationale for the use of aquaretic AVP inhibitors (see later discussion). Like angiotensin II, AVP is also a potent dipsogen.

Natriuretic Peptides

Under physiologic conditions, natriuresis occurs when salt is ingested. Sodium balance is restored as a result of tubular glomerular feedback and the action of natriuretic peptides on distal tubular segments. Atrial natriuretic peptide (ANP) is secreted by the atrium in response to increased wall stretch resulting from volume expansion. Brain natriuretic peptide (BNP) is secreted from the ventricular wall. Apart from reducing sodium reabsorption in the renal collecting duct, and thus promoting natriuresis, these factors also cause glomerular afferent arteriolar vasodilatation and efferent arteriolar vasoconstriction, raising GFR. In addition, they cause systemic vasodilatation, which attenuates the effect of increased effective arterial volume, thus antagonizing vasoconstricting and sodium-retaining mechanisms.

In CHF, plasma ANP and BNP are increased (as a result both of increased secretion and, potentially, reduced elimination). Their concentrations, particularly that of the N-terminal pro-BNP, predict adverse outcome.

The acute beneficial effects of natriuretic peptides have led to efforts to produce analogues with better pharmacokinetic properties. However, randomized, double-blind, placebo-controlled clinical trials failed to show the expected beneficial effect (e.g., with nesiritide).

ACUTE KIDNEY FAILURE IN CONGESTIVE HEART FAILURE

Although the mechanisms described earlier preferentially reduce renal plasma flow more than glomerular filtration by increasing the filtration fraction, GFR frequently decreases. This is mainly a reflection of the intensity of the compensatory counterregulatory mechanisms, and it explains why low GFR, and particularly a decrease in GFR, is correlated with poor outcome. It follows from the above description of the pathophysiologic mechanisms that are in effect that interference with vasodilating prostaglandins by nonsteroidal anti-inflammatory agents, or interference with the RAS by angiotensin converting enzyme (ACE) inhibitors or angiotensin receptor blockers (ARBs) may produce acute deterioration of kidney function.

Low GFR is presumably not only a marker but also a culprit. Even in subjects without CHF, reduced GFR is a powerful predictor of cardiovascular events and mortality in the general population, and particularly in cardiac patients.

HYPONATREMIA IN CONGESTIVE HEART FAILURE

Hyponatremia is mainly caused by nonosmotic release of AVP, but it may be modified by factors such as solute and fluid delivery to the diluting segment in the nephron and by the function of the diluting sites (i.e., the ascending limb of the loop of Henle and the distal convoluted tubule and collecting duct). Solute delivery may be reduced in response to decreased effective circulating volume and the resulting augmentation of proximal tubular reabsorption. Furthermore, loop diuretics and diuretics acting on the distal convoluted tubule may interfere with the action of the diluting sites. Development of hyponatremia is associated with poor outcome, but whether it is only a marker or is directly responsible for poor outcome is unclear. Whether the high AVP levels responsible for hyponatremia are deleterious is also unknown. In the EVEREST trial, long-term treatment of ADHF patients with tolvaptan, a selective blocker of the vasopressin V_2 receptor responsible for water retention but not of the V_{1a} receptor responsible for AVP's pressor effect, did not improve survival.

MANAGEMENT OF CONGESTIVE HEART FAILURE

The American College of Cardiology/American Heart Association guidelines state that symptomatic left ventricular dysfunction should be routinely managed with a combination of drugs, including (unless otherwise contraindicated) a diuretic, an ACE inhibitor, a β-adrenergic blocker, and, usually, digitalis, although its use is still controversial.

A number of new agents for the treatment of acute heart failure syndromes are available, but a recent systematic review concluded that no new agent has demonstrated a clear benefit in terms of long-term clinical outcomes compared with placebo or conventional therapies.

Management of renal malfunction in the patient with CHF has two main goals: to control the development of edema, and to interfere with neurohormonal activation.

Diuretics

Presence of edema in the patient with CHF may point to sodium and volume overload as a result of positive sodium balance, although redistribution may play an important role (see earlier discussion). Positive sodium balance results from either increased sodium load (in the diet or in the intravenous fluid prescription) or decreased natriuresis, or a combination of both.

The recommended dietary intake of salt (NaCl) in the general population is 6 g/day (2.4 g sodium), and this should be reduced in patients with CHF, who should be counseled to follow a diet limited to 2 g sodium per day. A potential source of increased sodium supply is sodium-containing intravenous fluids or medications. Care should be taken to avoid the gratuitous inclusion of sodium in the intravenous fluid prescription. Additional benefits from sodium restriction include reduction of thirst and limitation of urinary potassium loss during diuretic treatment, because the reduced delivery of Na^+ to the distal renal tubule lowers the rate of Na^+-K^+ exchange at that site.

Sodium restriction alone is not usually sufficient to reduce edema, and most patients require diuretics. Those that act on the distal tubule, such as *thiazides*, are not very effective as monotherapy, especially if intense proximal tubular sodium reabsorption (as occurs in advanced CHF) reduces the sodium load delivered to their site of action. Thiazides may cause hypokalemia and, particularly in elderly women, hyponatremia. In mild heart failure, edema may respond to thiazide diuretic monotherapy.

Potassium-sparing agents acting further downstream than thiazides (e.g., amiloride, triamterene) are also weak natriuretic agents as monotherapy. Spironolactone or eplerenone have similar tubular actions, but their main benefit accrues from blocking the action of aldosterone on nonepithelial tissues, particularly the heart. The addition of a potassium-sparing agent reduces diuretic-induced hypokalemia, but close monitoring of the patient is necessary. Potassium-sparing agents are more effective than potassium supplements, but one must be aware of the potential risk for life-threatening hyperkalemia, especially in patients with reduced kidney function or RAS blockade. The risk of hyperkalemia is accentuated by a high-potassium diet, potassium supplements, and potassium-containing salt substitutes but reduced by the concomitant administration of kaliuretic loop diuretics.

Loop diuretics are the most effective agents available for the treatment of volume overload. Their site of action is the Na^+-K^+-$2Cl^-$ transporter in the thick ascending limb of Henle's loop, which accounts for reabsorption of approximately 20% of the filtered sodium load. A note of caution is indicated, however, because in several studies the dose of loop diuretics was correlated with weight loss but also with higher mortality, particularly at daily doses exceeding 300 mg of furosemide. It is unclear whether this simply reflects more severe CHF and diuretic resistance or whether diuretics play an adverse pathogenetic role, perhaps because they stimulate renin release. The effect of the loop diuretic can be amplified by sequential nephron blockade—that is, a combination of the loop diuretic with a diuretic (e.g., a thiazide) acting downstream from Henle's loop. With the exception of torsemide, loop diuretics such as furosemide have relatively short half-lives, so that several doses per day or continuous intravenous infusion is necessary, the latter particularly in the intensive care unit. See Chapter 15 for an extensive discussion of the use of diuretics in resistant edema.

Bed rest has traditionally been an ancillary therapeutic measure, but except in advanced cases, current guidelines recommend even moderate physical exercise. Nevertheless, when bed rest is necessary, it must be kept in mind that aggressive mobilization of edema by diuretics increases the risk of venous thromboembolic events during bed rest. Compression stockings and, if appropriate, prophylactic anticoagulation should be considered.

Angiotensin-Converting Enzyme Inhibition and Aldosterone Antagonism

ACE inhibitors form a mainstay of therapy in patients with symptomatic left ventricular systolic dysfunction—apart from the fact that they can prevent heart failure in patients with high-risk cardiovascular profiles. Benefit from the use of ACE inhibitors in patients with heart failure and preserved ejection fraction has not been consistently demonstrated. It has been suggested that attempts should be made to titrate the dosage of ACE inhibitors, if tolerated, to the target doses that have been used in clinical trials. There is good evidence for benefit from ARBs and mineralocorticoid receptor blockers

in this indication. The recommendations of the Seventh Report of the Joint National Committee on Detection, Evaluation and Treatment of High Blood Pressure (JNC VII) for initial treatment of hypertension recognize CHF as a compelling indication for selection of an ACE inhibitor or ARB.

Management of Anemia

Low hemoglobin in hospitalized CHF patients is associated with higher morbidity and mortality, but it is not an independent risk factor for mortality in patients with CHF after adjustment for increased N-terminal pro-BNP and decreased kidney function. Ongoing studies are examining the efficacy of raising hemoglobin with erythropoietin, but one randomized, controlled, double-blind study failed to show a beneficial effect on exercise tolerance, functional status, plasma BNP, or hospitalization rate. It has been hypothesized that erythropoietin may provide benefit through cardioprotective actions in addition to raising hemoglobin.

Treatment of Hyponatremia

Hyponatremia is a frequent complication of severe CHF and a predictor of poor outcome. AVP acts on two receptors, V_2 and V_1. The V_2 receptor mediates its hydro-osmotic effect and the V_1 receptor its pressor effect. These receptors are specifically inhibited by the novel aquaretics. Recently, both selective V_2 antagonists (tolvaptan, lixivaptan, satavaptan) and a combined V_{1a}/V_2 receptor antagonist (conivaptan) were studied in clinical trials, and the latter is now approved by the U.S. Food and Drug Administration for treatment of hyponatremia in euvolemic and hypervolemic (CHF) patients. Clinical trials showed that tolvaptan was well tolerated, reduced body weight, reduced edema, and normalized serum sodium in hyponatremic patients; no significant effect on left ventricular volumes was seen in well-treated, stable CHF patients, however. As noted earlier, the large-scale EVEREST trial failed to document an effect on long-term mortality or heart failure–related morbidity despite favorable acute effects and improved short-term prognosis in smaller studies.

Mechanical Pumped Blood Ultrafiltration, Peritoneal Dialysis, and Continuous Ambulatory Peritoneal Dialysis

The complex and expensive treatment termed extracorporeal ultrafiltration has recently raised considerable interest, and several small studies with short follow-up have suggested benefit in refractory cases. The procedure has not yet gained widespread use. In contrast, prolonged peritoneal ultrafiltration (peritoneal dialysis) has been quite effective in large observational series, with good outcomes.

BIBLIOGRAPHY

Coca SG, Peixoto AJ, Garg AX, et al: The prognostic importance of a small acute decrement in kidney function in hospitalized patients: A systematic review and meta-analysis. Am J Kidney Dis 50:712-720, 2007.

Cotter G, Metra M, Milo-Cotter O, et al: Fluid overload in acute heart failure: Re-distribution and other mechanisms beyond fluid accumulation. Eur J Heart Fail 10:165-169, 2008.

Cotter G, Metzkor E, Kaluski E, et al: Randomised trial of high-dose isosorbide dinitrate plus low-dose furosemide versus high-dose furosemide plus low-dose isosorbide dinitrate in severe pulmonary oedema. Lancet 351:389-393, 1998.

Damman K, Navis G, Voors AA, et al: Worsening renal function and prognosis in heart failure: Systematic review and meta-analysis. J Card Fail 13:599-608, 2007.

De Luca L, Mebazaa A, Filippatos G, et al: Overview of emerging pharmacologic agents for acute heart failure syndromes. Eur J Heart Fail 10:201-213, 2008.

Gheorghiade M, Konstam MA, Burnett JC Jr, et al: Short-term clinical effects of tolvaptan, an oral vasopressin antagonist, in patients hospitalized for heart failure: The EVEREST Clinical Status Trials. JAMA 297:1332-1343, 2007.

Gheorghiade M, Niazi I, Ouyang J, et al: Vasopressin V2-receptor blockade with tolvaptan in patients with chronic heart failure: Results from a double-blind, randomized trial. Circulation 107:2690-2696, 2003.

Hasselblad V, Gattis Stough W, Shah MR, et al: Relation between dose of loop diuretics and outcomes in a heart failure population: Results of the ESCAPE trial. Eur J Heart Fail 9:1064-1069, 2007.

Hunt SA, Abraham WT, Chin MH, et al: ACC/AHA 2005 Guideline Update for the Diagnosis and Management of Chronic Heart Failure in the Adult: A report of the American College of Cardiology/American Heart Association Task Force on Practice Guidelines (Writing Committee to Update the 2001 Guidelines for the Evaluation and Management of Heart Failure). Developed in collaboration with the American College of Chest Physicians and the International Society for Heart and Lung Transplantation; endorsed by the Heart Rhythm Society. Circulation 112:e154-e235, 2005.

Hunt SA, Baker DW, Chin MH, et al: ACC/AHA Guidelines for the Evaluation and Management of Chronic Heart Failure in the Adult: Executive Summary. A Report of the American College of Cardiology/American Heart Association Task Force on Practice Guidelines (Committee to Revise the 1995 Guidelines for the Evaluation and Management of Heart Failure): Developed in Collaboration with the International Society for Heart and Lung Transplantation; Endorsed by the Heart Failure Society of America. Circulation 104:2996-3007, 2001.

Kawaguchi M, Hay I, Fetics B, Kass DA: Combined ventricular systolic and arterial stiffening in patients with heart failure and preserved ejection fraction: Implications for systolic and diastolic reserve limitations. Circulation 10:714-720, 2003.

Kazory A, Ross EA: Contemporary trends in the pharmacological and extracorporeal management of heart failure: A nephrologic perspective. Circulation 117:975-983, 2008.

Konstam MA, Gheorghiade M, Burnett JC Jr, et al: Effects of oral tolvaptan in patients hospitalized for worsening heart failure: The EVEREST Outcome Trial. JAMA 297:1319-1331, 2007.

Metra M, Nodari S, Parrinello G, et al: Worsening renal function in patients hospitalised for acute heart failure: Clinical implications and prognostic significance. Eur J Heart Fail 10:188-195, 2008.

Moran A, Katz R, Smith NL, et al: Cystatin C concentration as a predictor of systolic and diastolic heart failure. J Card Fail 14:19-26, 2008.

O'Connor CM, Stough WG, Gallup DS, et al: Demographics, clinical characteristics, and outcomes of patients hospitalized for decompensated heart failure: Observations from the IMPACT-HF registry. J Card Fail 11:200-205, 2005.

Petretta M, Scopacasa F, Fontanella L, et al: Prognostic value of reduced kidney function and anemia in patients with chronic heart failure. J Cardiovasc Med (Hagerstown) 8:909-916, 2007.

Ponikowski P, Anker SD, Szachniewicz J, et al: Effect of darbepoetin alfa on exercise tolerance in anemic patients with symptomatic chronic heart failure: A randomized, double-blind, placebo-controlled trial. J Am Coll Cardiol 49:753-762, 2007.

Prevention, detection, evaluation, and treatment of high blood pressure (JNC 7), Hypertension 42:1206, 2003.

Schrier RW, Fassett RG: Pathogenesis of sodium and water retention in cardiac failure. Ren Fail 20:773-781, 1998.

Udelson JE, McGrew FA, Flores E, et al: Multicenter, randomized, double-blind, placebo-controlled study on the effect of oral tolvaptan on left ventricular dilation and function in patients with heart failure and systolic dysfunction. J Am Coll Cardiol 49:2151-2159, 2007.

van Kimmenade RR, Januzzi JL Jr, Baggish AL, et al: Amino-terminal pro-brain natriuretic peptide, renal function, and outcomes in acute heart failure: Redefining the cardiorenal interaction? J Am Coll Cardiol 48:1621-1627, 2006.

Verma A, Anavekar NS, Meris A, et al: The relationship between renal function and cardiac structure, function, and prognosis after myocardial infarction: The VALIANT Echo Study. J Am Coll Cardiol 50:1238-1245, 2007.

Westenbrink BD, Voors AA, Ruifrok WP, et al: Therapeutic potential of erythropoietin in cardiovascular disease: Erythropoiesis and beyond. Curr Heart Fail Rep 4:127-133, 2007.

Witteles RM, Kao D, Christopherson D, et al: Impact of nesiritide on renal function in patients with acute decompensated heart failure and pre-existing renal dysfunction: A randomized, double-blind, placebo-controlled clinical trial. J Am Coll Cardiol 50:1835-1840, 2007.

CHAPTER 31

Renal Function in Liver Disease

Vicente Arroyo, Javier Fernández, and Wladimiro Jiménez

PATHOGENESIS

The *peripheral arterial vasodilation hypothesis* of renal sodium and water retention and the *forward theory of ascites formation* are the most accepted mechanisms of kidney dysfunction and ascites formation in cirrhosis and constitute the rationale on which modern treatment of this condition is based. The peripheral arterial vasodilation hypothesis, as formulated initially, holds that the primary event of renal sodium and water retention in cirrhosis is splanchnic arterial vasodilation caused by a massive release of local vasodilators (i.e., nitric oxide) secondary to portal hypertension. In the initial phases of the disease, compensation occurs through the development of a hyperdynamic circulation (high plasma volume, cardiac index, and heart rate). As the disease progresses and splanchnic arterial vasodilation increases, however, this compensatory mechanism is insufficient to maintain circulatory homeostasis. Arterial pressure decreases, leading to stimulation of baroreceptors; homeostatic activation of the sympathetic nervous system (SNS) and the renin-angiotensin-aldosterone system (RAS) and production of antidiuretic hormone (ADH, or vasopressin); and renal sodium and water retention.

The forward theory of ascites formation follows from the peripheral arterial vasodilation hypothesis and holds that arterial vasodilation in the splanchnic circulation induces the formation of ascites by simultaneously impairing the systemic circulation, leading to sodium and water retention, and the splanchnic microcirculation, where the forward increase in capillary pressure and permeability from the greatly increased inflow of blood at high pressure into the splanchnic capillaries leads to leakage of fluid into the abdominal cavity.

During the last few years, evidence has been presented indicating that the pathogenesis of circulatory dysfunction in cirrhosis is more complex than that just described, in which the main mechanism of the impairment in circulatory function in cirrhosis is the worsening of splanchnic arterial vasodilation that occurs in parallel with the progression of the disease. Recent studies indicate that there is also a progressive decrease in cardiac function caused by an impairment in both cardiac inotropic and chronotropic functions. The net effect of these abnormalities is a reduction in cardiac output and a decrease or disappearance of the hyperdynamic circulation. The peripheral arterial vasodilation hypothesis should therefore be reformulated. Progression of circulatory dysfunction; stimulation of the RAS, the SNS, and ADH production; and impairment of renal function in cirrhosis are caused by both an increase in splanchnic arterial vasodilation and a primary impairment in cardiac function.

The mechanism of cardiac dysfunction in cirrhosis is not well established, but it is probably multifactorial. There is a cirrhotic cardiomyopathy characterized by impaired diastolic function. On the other hand, the cardiac output increases significantly in cirrhosis after volume expansion or after the insertion of a transjugular intrahepatic shunt, which increases venous return. Together these findings suggest a role for decreased cardiac preload. Finally, during the course of cirrhosis, there is a progressive overactivity of the SNS in the absence of an increase in heart rate. The acute activation of the SNS during the course of a severe bacterial infection or hypovolemia (i.e., after large-volume paracentesis) in cirrhosis also fails to increase the heart rate. All of these mechanisms may account for the progressive decrease in cardiac output observed in patients with advanced cirrhosis.

A second major change in understanding of the pathogenesis of renal dysfunction and ascites in cirrhosis relates to hepatorenal syndrome (HRS). Traditionally, type 1 and type 2 HRS were considered to be different expressions of an identical disorder. New evidence suggests that they are completely different syndromes. Type 2 HRS represents genuine functional renal failure. It is the extreme expression of the impairment in circulatory function that slowly but spontaneously develops in patients with decompensated cirrhosis. In contrast, type 1 HRS is acute renal failure caused by the rapid deterioration of circulatory function that occurs in close temporal association with a precipitating event, commonly severe infection. Acute impairment in the function of other organs, including liver, brain, heart, and adrenal glands, is typically also present.

NATURAL COURSE OF KIDNEY DYSFUNCTION IN CIRRHOSIS

A reduction in the ability to excrete sodium and free water and a decrease in renal perfusion and glomerular filtration rate (GFR) are the main kidney function abnormalities in cirrhosis. Their course is usually progressive, except that, in alcoholic cirrhotics, kidney function may improve after alcohol withdrawal. The main consequence of the reduced ability to excrete sodium in cirrhosis is the development of sodium retention and ascites. This occurs when renal sodium excretion decreases to less than the sodium intake.

This represents a marked impairment in renal sodium handling. The kidney's ability to excrete free water is reduced in most patients with cirrhosis and ascites. Dilutional hyponatremia (arbitrarily defined as a serum sodium concentration of <130 mEq/L) develops when electrolyte-free water clearance is severely reduced. Finally, the main consequence of the impaired renal perfusion and GFR is type 2 HRS, which is defined as a GFR of less than 40 mL/min (or a serum creatinine concentration of >1.5 mg/dL) in the absence of any other potential cause of kidney dysfunction. Sodium retention, dilutional hyponatremia, and HRS appear at different times during the evolution of the disease. Therefore, the clinical course of cirrhosis can be divided into phases according to the onset of each of these complications.

Phase 1: Impaired Renal Sodium Metabolism in Compensated Cirrhosis

Chronologically, the first kidney function abnormality that occurs in cirrhosis is impairment of renal sodium handling, which can already be detected before the development of ascites, when the disease is still compensated. At this phase of the disease, patients have portal hypertension, increased cardiac output, reduced peripheral vascular resistance, normal or reduced mean arterial pressure, and normal renal perfusion, GFR and free water clearance. They remain able to excrete the sodium ingested with the diet. However, subtle abnormalities in renal sodium excretion are present. For example, these patients have a reduced natriuretic response to the acute administration of sodium chloride (i.e., infusion of saline solution) and may not be able to escape from the sodium-retaining effect of mineralocorticoids. Abnormal natriuretic responses to changes in posture are another relevant feature at this phase of the disease. Urinary sodium excretion is reduced in the upright and increased in the supine posture, compared with normal subjects.

Phase 2: Renal Sodium Retention Without Activation of the Renin-Angiotensin-Aldosterone System and Sympathetic Nervous System

As the disease progresses, patients become unable to excrete their regular sodium intake. Sodium is then retained together with water, and the fluid accumulates in the abdominal cavity as ascites. Urinary sodium excretion, although reduced, is usually higher than 10 mEq/day, and in some cases it is greater than 50 to 90 mEq/day; therefore, reduction of the sodium content of the diet alone may be sufficient to effect a negative sodium balance and loss of ascites. Renal perfusion, GFR, the ability to excrete free water, plasma renin activity, and the plasma concentrations of norepinephrine and ADH are normal. Sodium retention is therefore unrelated to any abnormality of the RAS or SNS, the two most important regulators of renal sodium excretion so far identified. The plasma levels of atrial natriuretic peptide, brain natriuretic peptide, and natriuretic hormone are increased in these patients, indicating that sodium retention is not caused by a reduced synthesis of endogenous natriuretic peptides. It has been suggested that circulatory dysfunction at this phase, although greater than in compensated cirrhosis without ascites, is not intense enough to stimulate the RAS and the SNS but does activate a still unknown, extremely sensitive, sodium-retaining mechanism (renal or extrarenal). There has been no study comparing the systemic hemodynamics in patients with portal hypertension and compensated cirrhosis with those in patients at this phase of the disease. However, two studies in the latter group of patients clearly showed the presence of a hyperdynamic circulation with high cardiac output, low peripheral vascular resistance, and hypervolemia.

Phase 3: Stimulation of the Endogenous Vasoconstrictor Systems with Preserved Renal Perfusion and Glomerular Filtration Rate

When sodium retention is intense (urinary sodium excretion <10 mEq/day), the plasma renin activity and the plasma concentrations of aldosterone and norepinephrine are invariably increased. Aldosterone increases sodium reabsorption in the distal and collecting tubules. In contrast, renal SNS activity stimulates sodium reabsorption in the proximal tubule and loop of Henle. Therefore, sodium retention in patients in this phase is caused by increased sodium reabsorption throughout the nephron.

The plasma volume and peripheral vascular resistance do not differ from those observed in the previous phase. These features are compatible with a progression of splanchnic arterial vasodilation compensated by vasoconstriction in extrasplanchnic organs secondary to the increased activity of the SNS and RAS. In fact, renal, cerebral, and muscle blood flow in cirrhosis correlates inversely with plasma renin activity and the concentration of norepinephrine. The most interesting feature is that cardiac output in patients at phase 3, although higher than in normal subjects, is lower than in patients at phase 2, indicating that progression of circulatory dysfunction is caused not only by an increase in splanchnic arterial vasodilation but also by a decrease in cardiac output. Arterial pressure at this phase of the disease is critically dependent on increased activity of the RAS and SNS and ADH production, and the administration of drugs that interfere with these systems (angiotensin receptor blockers, angiotensin-converting enzyme inhibitors, clonidine, and vasopressin V_{1a} receptor antagonists) may precipitate arterial hypotension.

Although angiotensin II, norepinephrine, and vasopressin are powerful renal vasoconstrictors, renal perfusion and GFR are normal or only moderately reduced, because the effects of these hormones on the renal circulation are antagonized by intrarenal vasodilator mechanisms, particularly prostaglandins and nitric oxide. Cirrhosis is the human condition in which renal perfusion and GFR are most dependent on the renal production of prostaglandins, and severely impaired kidney function may occur at this phase if renal prostaglandins are inhibited with the use of nonsteroidal anti-inflammatory drugs.

The ability to excrete free water is reduced at this phase of the disease because of the high circulating plasma levels of ADH. However, only a few patients have significant hyponatremia, because the effect of ADH is partially inhibited by an increased renal production of prostaglandin E_2.

Phase 4: Development of Type 2 Hepatorenal Syndrome

Type 2 HRS is a functional impairment that develops secondary to intense renal hypoperfusion. It is characterized by a moderate and steady decrease in kidney function (serum creatinine between 1.5 and 2.5 mg/dL) in the absence of other potential causes of renal failure. The International Ascites Club considers that the serum creatinine concentration should be higher than 1.5 mg/dL or the GFR lower than 40 mL/min for the diagnosis of HRS to be made. However, many patients with a GFR lower than 40 mL/min have a normal serum creatinine concentration. Therefore, the frequency of type 2 HRS is underestimated when serum creatinine alone is used in the clinical evaluation.

Type 2 HRS develops in very advanced phases of cirrhosis in the setting of a significant deterioration of circulatory function. Patients with type 2 HRS have very high plasma levels of renin, norepinephrine, and ADH, as well as significant arterial hypotension. The arterial vascular resistance in these patients is increased not only in the kidneys but also in the brain, muscle, and skin, indicating a generalized arterial vasoconstriction attempting to compensate for intense splanchnic arterial vasodilation. Type 2 HRS is probably caused by the extreme overactivity of the endogenous vasoconstrictor systems, which overcomes the intrarenal vasodilatory mechanisms. The cardiac output in patients with type 2 HRS is lower than in patients who have ascites but a normal serum creatinine concentration. A significant number of these patients have a normal cardiac output, indicating the disappearance of the hyperdynamic circulation. The progression of circulatory dysfunction causing type 2 HRS is therefore related to both an increase in the degree of arterial vasodilation and a decrease in cardiac output.

The degree of sodium retention is intense in patients with type 2 HRS. The mechanism is a reduction in filtered sodium and a marked increase in sodium reabsorption in the proximal tubule. The delivery of sodium to the distal nephron, the site of action of diuretics, is very low. Therefore, most of these patients do not respond to diuretics and have refractory ascites. Free water clearance is also markedly reduced, and most patients have significant hyponatremia. The prognosis of patients with type 2 HRS is poor, with a mortality rate of 50% at 6 months after the onset of impaired kidney function.

Phase 5: Development of Type 1 Hepatorenal Syndrome

Type 1 HRS is characterized by a rapidly progressive decline in kidney function, defined as a doubling of the serum creatinine concentration reaching a level greater than 2.5 mg/dL in less than 2 weeks. Although type 1 HRS may arise spontaneously, it frequently occurs in close chronologic relationship with a precipitating factor such as a severe bacterial infection, acute hepatitis (ischemic, alcoholic, toxic, viral) superimposed on cirrhosis, a major surgical procedure, or massive gastrointestinal hemorrhage. Severe bacterial infections, mainly spontaneous bacterial peritonitis (SBP), are the most common precipitating event. Patients with type 2 HRS are predisposed to develop type 1 HRS, although it may also develop in patients with normal serum creatinine concentrations. However, most of these latter patients have high plasma levels of renin and norepinephrine and, frequently, dilutional hyponatremia, indicating that type 1 HRS occurs after a precipitating event in patients who already have severe circulatory dysfunction. The prognosis of patients with type 1 HRS is extremely poor, with 80% of patients dying less than 2 weeks after the onset of HRS. Patients succumb from progressive circulatory, hepatic, and renal failure, along with encephalopathy.

Type 1 HRS has been closely examined in SBP, because 30% of patients with SBP develop this type of renal failure. The two most important predictors of type 1 HRS development in SBP are an increased serum creatinine concentration before the infection and an intense intra-abdominal inflammatory response, as suggested by high concentrations of polymorphonuclear leukocytes and cytokines (tumor necrosis factor-α and interleukin-6) in the ascitic fluid at infection diagnosis.

Type 1 HRS after SBP occurs in the setting of an acute and severe deterioration of circulatory function, as indicated by a significant decrease in arterial pressure and a marked increase in the plasma levels of renin and norepinephrine. Two recent studies assessed systemic hemodynamics and kidney function in patients with and without SBP before and after the development of type 1 HRS. These studies suggested that the impairment in circulatory function in patients with HRS is far more complex than initially considered. In addition to an accentuation of the arterial vasodilation, a significant decrease in cardiac output compared with values obtained at infection diagnosis was observed. In some cases, resting cardiac output decreased to values below normal (5 L/min). Whether this decrease in heart function is caused by cirrhotic or sepsis-related cardiomyopathy, or by a decreased cardiac preload resulting from central hypovolemia, or both, is currently unknown. The demonstration that use of albumin to expand the plasma volume of patients with SBP at infection diagnosis reduces the incidence of type 1 HRS by more than 60% and decreases hospital mortality is consistent with the second hypothesis. Cardiac chronotropic function is severely impaired in these patients, because there is no increase in heart rate despite a significant reduction in arterial pressure and a marked increase in plasma norepinephrine concentration and SNS activity.

The development of HRS in patients with SBP is associated not only with a deterioration of circulatory and kidney functions but also with an acute impairment in hepatic function leading to hepatic encephalopathy. It has been shown that there is an increase in intrahepatic vascular resistance, a reduction in liver blood flow, and an increase in portal pressure gradient that correlate closely with an increase in renin and norepinephrine. Finally, adrenal function is also markedly impaired in these patients, and treatment with hydrocortisone in cirrhotic patients with severe sepsis and renal failure is associated with improved survival. Type 1 HRS is therefore a complex syndrome that includes acute deterioration of cardiovascular, liver, renal, cerebral, and adrenal functions. It is a multiorgan failure of circulatory origin.

MANAGEMENT OF KIDNEY DYSFUNCTION AND ASCITES IN CIRRHOSIS

Low-Sodium Diet

Mobilization of ascites occurs when a negative sodium balance is achieved. In 10% of patients, those with normal plasma aldosterone and norepinephrine concentrations and relatively high urinary sodium excretion, this can be obtained simply by reducing the sodium intake to between 60 and 90 mEq/day. (A greater reduction in sodium intake interferes with nutrition and is not advisable.) In most cases, however, urinary sodium excretion is very low, and a negative sodium balance cannot be achieved without diuretics. Even in these cases, sodium restriction is important, because it reduces diuretic requirements. Sodium restriction is essential in patients who respond poorly to diuretics. A frequent cause of apparently refractory ascites is inadequate sodium restriction. This should be suspected if ascites does not decrease despite a good natriuretic response to diuretics (see Chapter 15).

Diuretics

Furosemide and spironolactone are the diuretics most commonly used in the treatment of ascites in cirrhosis. In contrast to healthy subjects, in whom furosemide is more potent than spironolactone, in cirrhotic patients with ascites the reverse is true. Cirrhotic patients with ascites and marked hyperaldosteronism (50% of the patients with ascites) do not respond to furosemide. In contrast, most cirrhotic patients with ascites respond to spironolactone. Patients with a normal or slightly increased plasma aldosterone concentration respond to low doses of spironolactone (100 to 150 mg/day), but as much as 300 to 400 mg/day may be required in patients with marked hyperaldosteronism. The mechanism of the resistance to furosemide in patients with hyperaldosteronism is pharmacodynamic. With reduced GFR and avid proximal sodium reabsorption, delivery of sodium to the loop of Henle, where furosemide acts, is reduced. In addition, most of the sodium that is not reabsorbed in the loop because of the action of furosemide is subsequently reabsorbed in the distal nephron due to stimulation by aldosterone. Therefore, spironolactone is the preferred drug for the management of cirrhosis and ascites. The simultaneous administration of furosemide and spironolactone increases the natriuretic effect

of both agents and reduces the incidence of hypokalemia or hyperkalemia that may be observed when these drugs are given alone. There is general agreement that patients not responding to 400 mg/day of spironolactone and 160 mg/day of furosemide will not respond to higher diuretic dosage.

Diuretic treatment in cirrhosis is not free of complications, particularly in patients who require high diuretic doses. Approximately 20% of patients develop significant renal functional impairment (increase in blood urea and serum creatinine concentrations), which is usually moderate and always reversible after diuretic withdrawal. Hyponatremia secondary to a decrease in the renal ability to excrete free water also occurs in approximately 20% of these patients. The most severe complication related to diuretic treatment is hepatic encephalopathy, which occurs in approximately 25% of patients who are hospitalized with tense ascites requiring a high diuretic dosage.

The term *refractory ascites* is applied when ascites cannot be mobilized, when its early recurrence after therapeutic paracentesis cannot be prevented due to lack of response to sodium restriction and maximal diuretic treatment (diuretic-resistant ascites), or when diuretic-induced complications preclude the use of an effective diuretic dosage (diuretic-intractable ascites). Refractory ascites is an infrequent condition, occurring in fewer than 10% of patients hospitalized with tense ascites. Most of these patients have type 2 HRS (serum creatinine concentration >1.5 mg/dL) or less severe but still significant decreases of GFR (serum creatinine between 1.2 and 1.5 mg/dL). It has been estimated that a serum creatinine concentration greater than 1.2 mg/dL reflects a decrease in GFR of more than 50%. Impaired access of diuretics to the renal tubules (due to reduced renal perfusion) and reduced delivery of sodium to the loop of Henle and distal nephron (secondary to the low GFR and increased sodium reabsorption in the proximal tubule) are the mechanisms of diuretic-resistant ascites. Insufficient sodium restriction or treatment with nonsteroidal anti-inflammatory drugs should be excluded before the diagnosis of diuretic-resistant ascites is made.

Arterial Vasoconstrictors

It is well known that plasma volume expansion alone (e.g., after the insertion of a LeVeen shunt) does not improve kidney function in patients with HRS, despite a significant suppression of plasma renin activity and norepinephrine concentration. Also, the administration of vasoconstrictors alone does not produce clinically significant increases in GFR in these patients. In contrast, simultaneous treatment using intravenous albumin as a plasma expander along with vasoconstrictors for 7 to 14 days in patients with type 1 HRS is associated with an increase in arterial pressure, a suppression of plasma renin activity and norepinephrine concentration to normal levels, a marked increase in GFR, and a normalization of serum sodium and serum creatinine concentrations in a significant number of patients. Type 1 HRS usually does not recur after discontinuation of therapy.

These data are consistent with the hypothesis that type 1 HRS is related to both an accentuation of arterial vasodilation, which is corrected by the vasoconstrictor, and decreased cardiac output related to central hypovolemia, which is corrected by the administration of albumin. Very few patients develop side effects related to treatment. The probability of survival after normalization of serum creatinine increases, and a significant proportion of patients may survive to liver transplantation. Terlipressin (0.5 to 2.0 mg every 4 hours) has been the most frequently used vasoconstrictor for the treatment of type 1 HRS. It is a vasopressin agonist not available for use in the United States. The α-adrenergic agonists noradrenaline and midodrine, at doses that increase arterial pressure by more than 10 mm Hg, are also effective. An initial dose of albumin of 1 g per kilogram of body weight, followed by 20 to 40 g/day over 7 to 14 days, is the schedule for volume expansion recommended by some investigators.

Although serum creatinine is normalized in many patients with type 1 HRS responding to treatment with vasoconstrictors and albumin, GFR remains very low (it increases from values of <10 mL/min to between 30 and 50 mL/min), suggesting that treatment with vasoconstrictors and albumin is effective for correcting the type 1 HRS component of the syndrome but not the reduced GFR that was present before the development of type 1 HRS in most patients. Two features further support this contention. First, and contrary to what occurs with type 1 HRS, type 2 HRS frequently recurs soon after discontinuation of therapy with vasoconstrictors and albumin. Second, sequential treatment with vasoconstrictors and albumin followed by the insertion of a transjugular intrahepatic shunt normalizes serum creatinine and GFR in most patients with type 1 HRS.

V$_2$ Vasopressin Antagonists

Dilutional hyponatremia is the most common abnormality of serum electrolytes in patients with cirrhosis and ascites. Traditionally, hyponatremia was considered a minor problem in cirrhosis, because it is usually asymptomatic, even in patients with markedly reduced serum sodium concentration. The presence of hyponatremia does not contraindicate diuretic treatment in patients with cirrhosis and ascites. In fact, many cirrhotics with ascites and hyponatremia respond to diuretics without a further reduction in serum sodium. Recent studies, however, suggest that hyponatremia may be more relevant than previously thought. Its presence is associated with a very poor prognosis. The probability of hepatic encephalopathy is significantly higher in patients with hyponatremia than in those with comparable deterioration of hepatic function without hyponatremia. Finally, the incidence of severe neurologic events after liver transplantation in patients with dilutional hyponatremia, probably related to the rapid correction of extracellular osmolality during the operation, is relatively high. Therefore, treatment of hyponatremia could be beneficial in patients with decompensated cirrhosis.

Dilutional hyponatremia in cirrhosis is related to a severe impairment in the ability of the kidney to excrete free water.

ADH hypersecretion plays a major role in the pathogenesis of this abnormality. Other mechanisms involved in the impairment of water retention in cirrhosis are impaired renal production of prostaglandin E$_2$, a powerful antagonist of the tubular effect of ADH, and reduced sodium and water delivery to the ascending limb of the loop of Henle and the distal convoluted tubule, where urinary dilution occur. Treatment of dilutional hyponatremia in cirrhosis with ascites should, therefore, be directed toward reducing total body water. The administration of sodium may produce a transient increase in serum sodium, but at the expense of increasing the rate of ascites formation.

A number of vasopressin receptor antagonists are under development (see Chapter 6). The main clinical experience, including several randomized, controlled trials in patients with hyponatremia, is with the selective vasopressin V$_2$ receptor antagonists, tolvaptan and lixivaptan, and with the nonselective vasopressin V$_{1a}$/V$_2$ receptor antagonist, conivaptan. These drugs produced a rapid and marked increase in urine volume with a reduction in urine osmolality and an increase in serum osmolality and serum sodium concentration. A significant clinical effect (increase in serum sodium concentration to >135 mEq/L or >5 mEq/L) was obtained within a few days in 60% of patients with hyponatremia. However, in a substantial proportion of patients (40% in some studies), hyponatremia was refractory to the effect of these aquaretic drugs. At present, only conivaptan is available in the United States. Its use in cirrhosis requires further study, because it blocks not only the V$_2$ receptor responsible for water retention but also the V$_{1a}$ receptor responsible for vasoconstriction in the splanchnic and other vascular beds. The available studies suggest that selective V$_2$ receptor antagonists, when they are released, can be safely used in patients with cirrhosis.

Therapeutic Paracentesis

Paracentesis is a rapid, effective, and safe treatment of ascites in cirrhosis. It is considered the treatment of choice for tense ascites. The mobilization of ascites by paracentesis is associated with a deterioration of circulatory function, as manifested by a marked increase in plasma renin activity and aldosterone concentration, in 60% to 70% of the patients. This impairment in circulatory function results from accentuation of the arterial vasodilation already present in these patients. The incidence of this complication is reduced to 30% to 40% if paracentesis is accompanied by plasma volume expansion with synthetic plasma volume expanders (dextran 70 or polygeline), and to only 18 % if it is accompanied by plasma volume expansion with albumin (8 g per liter of ascitic fluid removed).

The prevalence of circulatory dysfunction after paracentesis also depends on the amount of ascitic fluid removed. In patients receiving synthetic plasma expanders, circulatory dysfunction occurred in 18%, 30%, and 54% of patients who had removal of less than 5 L, between 5 and 9 L, and more than 9 L of ascitic fluid, respectively. The corresponding

Acute Kidney Injury

CHAPTER 32

Pathophysiology of Acute Kidney Injury

Lakshman Gunaratnam and Joseph V. Bonventre

The term *acute renal failure* (ARF) has traditionally described a syndrome whose key feature is the rapid decline in the glomerular filtration rate (GFR) that occurs over a period of hours to weeks. The syndrome can be defined by one or more factors: an increase in blood urea nitrogen or serum creatinine concentration, a decrease in urine output or the requirement for renal replacement therapy. Many more quantitative definitions have been used over the years, such as a 25% or 50% increase in the creatinine level if the patient has a normal baseline creatinine value or an increase of 1 to 2 mg/dL if the baseline creatinine value is abnormal or renal replacement therapy is needed.

Varying definitions have led to difficulty in comparing studies in the literature. Recently, the Acute Kidney Injury Network (AKIN) recommended that the term *acute kidney injury* (AKI) replace the term ARF to include the entire spectrum of ARF, recognizing that an acute decline in kidney function is often secondary to an injury that causes functional or structural changes in the kidneys and that the injury can have important consequences for the patient even if it does not lead to organ failure and a requirement for renal replacement therapy. The AKIN defined AKI as "an abrupt (within 48 hours) reduction in kidney function, currently defined as an absolute increase in serum creatinine level of more than or equal to 0.3 mg/dL (26.4 µmol/L), a percentage increase in serum creatinine of more than or equal to 50% (1.5-fold from baseline), or a reduction in urine output (documented oliguria of less than 0.5 mL/kg/hr for more than 6 hours)." We therefore use the term AKI instead of ARF to describe this syndrome in the clinical setting, although many clinicians will continue to use the term ARF.

In considering the pathophysiology of ARF or AKI, it is important to recognize that the serum creatinine level is a very insensitive biomarker for AKI, because its increase is delayed and the level is affected by several factors other than the GFR, which it is used to estimate. Identification of early, sensitive, and specific biomarkers of acute injury, similar to troponin in cardiology, should enable clinicians to recognize earlier periods during AKI when the concentration of serum creatinine has not yet been affected. Studies are underway to determine whether estimating the GFR by using creatinine or injury biomarkers can better predict outcome or the need for therapeutic intervention in human AKI.

Historically, AKI has been classified based on its causes—prenal, intrinsic renal, or postrenal—to simplify the approach to a differential diagnosis. Prerenal AKI, which is common, is a physiologic response to renal hypoperfusion without tubular injury. A functional change in the GFR can result from depletion of the intravascular volume, caused by bleeding, low serum protein level and oncotic pressure, or capillary leak; congestive heart failure, reduced cardiac output; or liver disease, associated with splanchnic vasoconstriction and third spacing of total body water. The integrity of the renal parenchyma is not disrupted in prerenal AKI, and glomerular filtration is restored on re-establishment of more normal renal perfusion. Postrenal causes of AKI include the various forms of obstruction of urinary outflow (e.g., prostatic hypertrophy). Intrinsic renal or intrarenal AKI is associated with conditions that affect the renal parenchyma (glomeruli, tubules, interstitium, or vasculature). Ischemia, nephrotoxin exposure, and sepsis are among the most common causes of intrarenal AKI. Other causes of intrinsic AKI are discussed in various chapters of this *Primer*. The clinical approach to differentiating prerenal azotemia, intrinsic causes, and obstruction in AKI is discussed in Chapter 33.

The term *acute tubular necrosis* (ATN) frequently is used to refer to AKI resulting from severe or prolonged hypoperfusion or toxic injury. This is a controversial term because it is a pathologic description, not a clinical one. The term should not be applied to a patient unless there is physical evidence of tubular cell necrosis such as casts in the urine or biopsy proof. Prerenal azotemia and ATN are at opposite ends of the spectrum of manifestations of renal hypoperfusion.

Ischemic or toxic AKI often follows predictable stages: an initiation phase, characterized by steady increments in serum creatinine levels and reduced urinary volumes; a maintenance phase, in which the GFR is stable at a reduced level and the urinary volume may vary; and a recovery phase, in which the serum creatinine level falls and tubule function is restored. The initiation phase can be further subdivided into initiation and extension periods, because the injury may not occur all at once, but instead may be stuttering. All cases of AKI, however, do not follow such a well-defined sequence of events, nor do they all result in oliguria.

This chapter focuses on ischemic and toxic AKI, because understanding of the pathophysiologic mechanisms in AKI is largely derived from animal models and human studies aimed at examining these disease entities. In the following sections, we discuss five characteristics of the pathophysiology of AKI: (1) imbalance between vasoconstrictive and vasodilatory factors, (2) inflammation, (3) tubular dysfunction and intratubular obstruction, (4) cell death by necrosis or apoptosis, and (5) repair and regeneration.

PATHOGENESIS

The pathogenesis of AKI often can be traced to a mismatch at the level of the nephron between oxygen or nutrient delivery and energy demand or to direct toxicity to the tubular cell or vascular endothelium. Relative oxygen deprivation often is not generalized, because certain regions of the kidney are differentially susceptible to injury due to variations in blood flow or oxygen demand. Because of the complexity of vascular and tubular relationships in the kidney, localized tubular injury can have amplified functional consequences. **Figure 32-1** summarizes the complex interplay of vascular and tubular processes that ultimately lead to organ dysfunction.

Vascular Factors

Although a transient reduction in renal blood flow has been observed upon reflow in animals after renal ischemia, many cases of profound changes in the GFR in humans are not believed to be related to large generalized reductions in renal blood flow. In toxic AKI, there is little perturbation of renal hemodynamics, but there can be significant organ

dysfunction and pathology. The contribution of intrarenal vasoconstriction to the pathophysiology of AKI has become increasingly recognized. Potent vasoconstrictors have been identified in the ischemic kidney, including endothelin 1, angiotensin II, thromboxane A_2, prostaglandin H_2, leukotrienes C_4 and D_4, and adenosine, and there is increased sympathetic nerve stimulation. Results of several studies indicate that blockade of endothelin receptors before an ischemic insult protects the rat kidney from injury. Angiotensin receptor blockade, however, is widely implicated in the induction of ischemic injury through paralysis of postglomerular arterioles. Successful diminution of postinjury vasoconstriction in animal models with improved functional response has not, however, translated into practical therapies for humans. [Renal vasoconstriction in the face of global vasodilation in sepsis-associated AKI is hypothesized to be a physiologic protective mechanism to maintain perfusion pressure to other vital organs such as the brain and heart].

AKI is also characterized by decreased responsiveness of the resistance vessels to vasodilators such as acetylcholine, bradykinin, and nitric oxide and decreased production of certain of the vasodilators. The postischemic kidney endures further injury from perturbations to blood flow within the renal parenchyma due to vascular congestion and hypoperfusion to the outer medulla. Intrarenal hypoperfusion often persists even after blood flow improves after reperfusion. Excess production of vasoconstrictors such as endothelin and reduced abundance of vasodilators such as nitric oxide is believed to explain this phenomenon. During early periods of vasoconstriction, there is relative preservation of tubular

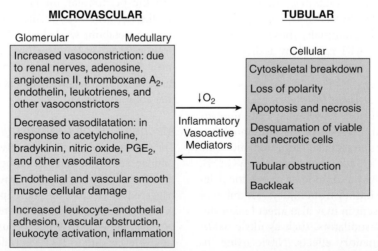

FIGURE 32-1 The pathophysiology of acute kidney injury may be divided into a microvascular component and a tubular component. With acute kidney injury, there is enhanced vasoconstriction in response to a number of agents, and there is decreased vasodilatation in response to agents that are present in the postischemic kidney. With increased endothelial and vascular smooth muscle cellular damage, there is enhanced leukocyte-endothelial adhesion, leading to activation of the coagulation system, vascular obstruction, leukocyte activation, and potentiation of inflammation. At the level of the tubule epithelial cell, there is cytoskeletal breakdown and loss of polarity, followed by apoptosis and necrosis (see **Fig. 32-2**), intratubular obstruction, and backleak of glomerular filtrate through a denuded basement membrane. Tubule cells generate inflammatory vasoactive mediators, which can enhance vascular compromise. In a positive-feedback process, vascular compromise results in decreased oxygen delivery to the tubules, which generates vasoactive inflammatory mediators that enhance the vasoconstriction and the endothelial-leukocyte interactions. PGE_2, prostaglandin E_2.

integrity, but as the reduction in blood flow persists further, it exacerbates tissue hypoxia and contributes to cellular injury in the outer medullary tubules. Reduced blood flow to the outer medulla can have particularly detrimental effects on the tubular cells in that region of the kidney, because the outer medulla is normally relatively hypoxic due to the countercurrent exchange properties of the vasa recta.

Inflammation

Inflammation is an important component of human AKI. For instance, ischemia and reperfusion cause renal synthesis of pro-inflammatory cytokines, infiltration of the kidney by leukocytes (neutrophils, macrophages, B cells, T cells), activation of the complement system, and upregulation of vascular adhesion molecules. Although it is incompletely understood, inflammation contributes in an important way to both the reduction in local blood flow within the kidney and the direct tubular injury that leads to reduced kidney function.

The innate and adaptive immune responses are fundamental contributors to the pathobiology of ischemic injury. The innate component is responsible for the early response to infection or injury and is foreign antigen independent. Toll-like receptors, which are important for the detection of exogenous microbial products and development of antigen-dependent adaptive immunity, recognize host material released during injury and play a central role in activation of the innate immune system.

Anti-inflammatory influences may come into play to decrease the injury associated with ischemia and reperfusion or toxins. Resolvins and protectins are two newly identified families of naturally occurring omega-3 fatty acid docosahexaenoic acid metabolites. They are produced in animals in response to ischemia and reperfusion injury; when administered to animals, these compounds can reduce the severity of AKI caused by ischemia and reperfusion.

Leukocyte-Endothelial Interactions

With ischemia and reperfusion, endothelial cells upregulate integrins, selectins, and members of the immunoglobulin superfamily, including intercellular adhesion molecule 1 (ICAM-1) and vascular cell adhesion molecule (VCAM). In animal studies, anti–ICAM-1 antibodies or genetic deletion of *ICAM1* protects the kidney from injury. A number of vasoactive compounds present in may also affect leukocyte-endothelial interactions. Vasodilators, such as nitric oxide, also can have anti-inflammatory effects. Nitric oxide inhibits adhesion of neutrophils to endothelial cells exposed to tumor necrosis factor-α (TNF-α). Enhanced leukocyte-endothelial interactions can result in cell–cell adhesion, which can physically impede blood flow. These interactions also activate leukocytes and endothelial cells and contribute to the generation of local factors that promote vasoconstriction, especially in the presence of other vasoactive mediators. These factors all contribute to compromised

local blood flow and impaired tubule cell metabolism and, if severe enough, cell death. Because of the anatomic relationships of vessels and tubules in the outer medulla, these leukocyte-endothelial interactions compromise blood flow to the outer medulla to a greater extent than to the cortex.

Contribution of Tubular Cells to Inflammatory Injury

Both the S3 segment of the proximal tubule and the medullary thick ascending limb of the loop of Henle generate pro-inflammatory and chemotactic cytokines, such as TNF-α and macrophage chemotactic factors. In addition, inflamed tubular epithelial cells express receptors of the innate immune response after ischemia and reperfusion, produce complement and express complement receptors. Proximal tubular epithelia are also postulated to acquire the ability to regulate T-lymphocyte activity through expression of co-stimulatory molecules. Therefore, instead of being a passive victim of injury in AKI, the tubular epithelium is an active participant in the inflammatory response that occurs during the pathogenesis of AKI.

Tubular Factors

Whether the injury is related to oxygen deprivation, toxin exposure, or a combination of factors, there are many common features of the epithelial cell response. The processes of injury and repair to the kidney epithelium are depicted schematically in **Figure 32-2**. Injury results in rapid loss of cell polarity and cytoskeletal integrity. With severe injury, cells are desquamated, leaving regions where the basement membrane remains as the only barrier between the filtrate and the peritubular interstitium. This allows backleak of the filtrate, which can further contribute to decreased clearance of metabolic waste by the kidney. Backleak is especially prominent when the pressure in the tubule is increased by intratubular obstruction resulting from cellular debris in the lumen that interacts with matrix proteins such as fibronectin that enter the lumen.

Mechanisms of Tubular Injury

The breakdown in the structural integrity of the renal tubular epithelial cells is brought about by one or more specific pathogenic mechanisms of cellular injury that are triggered by relative oxygen deprivation or toxin exposure. A major consequence of acute ischemia and tissue hypoxia is depletion of intracellular adenosine triphosphate (ATP) levels due to ATP degradation and a switch in some epithelia to anaerobic metabolism. Hypoxia and exposure to certain toxins, such as endotoxin, can also result in mitochondrial dysfunction. The duration of ischemia is a critical determinant of cell survival after reperfusion because prolonged ischemia can lead to irreversible mitochondrial dysfunction. The major consequences of ATP depletion that lead to cellular injury include the loss of ion gradients, abnormalities of the tight and adherence

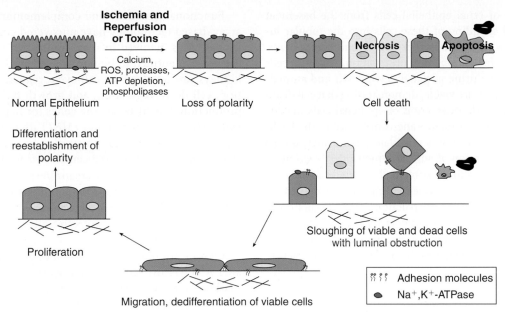

FIGURE 32-2 With ischemia or reperfusion injury to the kidney, an early response is loss of the brush border and polarity of the epithelial cell, with mislocation of adhesion molecules, Na^+,K^+-ATPase, and other proteins. With increasing injury, cell death occurs by means of necrosis or apoptosis. Some of the necrotic debris is released into the lumen, where it interacts with luminal proteins and can ultimately result in obstruction. Because of the mislocation of adhesion molecules, viable epithelial cells lift off the basement membrane and are found in the urine. The kidney can respond to the injury by initiating a repair process if provided sufficient nutrients and sufficient oxygen delivery and if the basement membrane integrity has not be altered irreparably. Viable epithelial cells migrate and cover denuded areas of the basement membrane. The source of these cells appears to be the kidney itself, not the bone marrow. Bone marrow cells may contribute to the interstitial cellular infiltrate and may produce factors that modulate inflammation and facilitate repair. Cells replacing the epithelium may be derived from dedifferentiated epithelial cells or from a subpopulation of progenitor cells in the tubule. The cells then undergo division and replace lost cells. Ultimately, the cells differentiate and re-establish the normal polarity of the epithelium. ATP, adenosine triphosphate; ROS, reactive oxygen species.

junctions between epithelial cells, cell swelling, increased intracellular calcium, and activation of intracellular proteases.

Reactive oxygen species (ROS) that are generated during reperfusion and as a result of the inflammatory response play a major role in cell injury in both ischemic and toxic AKI. ROS are generated by activated, infiltrating leukocytes and by epithelial cells, and they are directly toxic to tubular cells through the peroxidation of lipids, denaturation of proteins, and damage to DNA.

Activation of phospholipases is a well-documented mode of cellular injury after ischemia in various organs, including the kidney. Increased phospholipase activity leads to marked loss of phospholipid mass and intracellular accumulation of free fatty acids, lysophospholipids, diacylglycerol, and inositol phosphates. Lysophospholipids serve as substrates for eicosanoid production, which act as vasoactive and chemotactic mediators that contribute to functional and cytotoxic injury to the kidney during AKI.

Fate of Individual Renal Tubular Cells in Acute Kidney Injury

In most cases of AKI, many tubular cells remain viable or are sublethally injured and are able to recover functionally and structurally. The cells within the straight segment (i.e., S3 segment or pars recta) of the proximal tubule and the thick ascending limb in the outer medulla are more susceptible to injury than cells in the cortical region.

The renal tubule consists of highly polarized cells that line the tubular basement membrane. These cells have microvilli that constitute the brush border on their apical side, an array of focal adhesion molecules on the basolateral side that mediate crucial matrix–cell interactions, and tight junctions at cell–cell borders that mediate barrier function. The complex architecture and polarity of the renal tubular cells is supported by an intricate cytoskeletal network. Sublethal damage to tubular cells results in actin cytoskeletal derangements, leading to loss of cell polarity, loss of the brush border, and disruption of cell–cell and cell–substratum adhesion. The actin cytoskeleton is composed of bundles of microfilaments made of G-actin monomers woven into polymers of filamentous F-actin. ATP depletion induces disassembly of actin bundles and microfilaments. With loss of cell polarity, the expression of Na^+, K^+-ATPase, which normally is restricted to the basolateral surface, is rapidly redistributed to the apical membrane during anoxia. Data from ischemia and reperfusion animal models suggest that ischemia causes loss of the junctional complex; this, together with the loss of epithelial cells, explains the backleak of glomerular filtrate and contributes to the functional decline in GFR.

The loss of polarity and tethering of adhesion molecules to the actin network (i.e., loss of focal adhesion plaques) results in detachment of renal epithelial cells from the basement membrane and shedding of these cells into the tubular lumen together with brush border membrane components, leading to cast formation and obstruction. Tubular cells recovered from the urine of patients with AKI and animals with ischemic injury are viable, demonstrating that cell death is not required for desquamation of epithelial cells matrix. The denuded basement membrane contributes to the back-leak of filtrate. Moreover, it is postulated that detached cells with aberrant expression of adhesion molecules (e.g., integrins) become attached to the sublethally injured tubular cells that remain attached to the basement membrane, contributing further to intraluminal obstruction. Thus, disruption of the actin cytoskeleton and loss of polarity during ischemic or toxic injury may have profound consequences for the cell and plays a fundamental role in tubular backleak and obstruction observed in AKI.

CELL DEATH, REPAIR, AND REGENERATION

Cell Death by Necrosis and Apoptosis in Acute Kidney Injury

Although most cells remain viable after AKI because they escape injury or because they recover from sublethal injury, a significant amount of cell death does occur in severe AKI, as evidenced by histologic analysis of biopsy specimens and the presence of cellular debris in the casts that are in the urine. Death can occur by necrosis, which is a chaotic process that can elicit a profound inflammatory response in the organ. An alternative form of cell death, apoptosis, is a highly regulated program that leads to DNA fragmentation and cytoplasmic condensation, without triggering an inflammatory response. Inflammation is circumvented by efficient removal of apoptotic cells by phagocytes, which sequester the potentially immunogenic debris. Proteins upregulated during AKI, such as kidney injury molecule 1 (KIM-1), can confer on tubular epithelial cells the ability to phagocytose apoptotic tubular cells. There have been considerable efforts to elucidate the apoptotic mechanisms in AKI in the hope of identifying potential therapeutic strategies to ameliorate recovery.

Repair and Regeneration

Unlike the brain and the heart, the kidney possesses a remarkable capacity for regeneration and recovery after acute injury. Some patients who require dialysis and survive their episode of AKI can often recover function sufficiently to avoid long-term renal replacement therapy. The efficient reparative process is attributable to the unique capacity of surviving tubular epithelial cells to dedifferentiate, expand rapidly, and redifferentiate to restore the functional integrity of the kidney. Repair of the postnatal kidney parallels organogenesis in the high rate of proliferation and apoptosis and in patterns of gene expression.

Functional genomics and complementary DNA micro-array–based technology have uncovered complex molecular pathways involved in renal injury and repair. Many of the genes identified to be upregulated in the postischemic kidneys are involved in cell-cycle regulation, inflammation, cell death regulation, and growth factor or cytokine production. For instance, the genes for hepatocyte growth factor *(HGF)* and its receptor *(MET)* are rapidly upregulated after renal injury. Administration of recombinant HGF at the time of injury has been shown to accelerate renal recovery (based on serum creatinine level and severity of pathologic score) in animal models. It is not clear, however, with HGF and other growth factors, whether accelerated recovery results from a protective effect against injury or hastening of repair.

Identification of genes upregulated early and specifically after AKI has also led to the discovery of novel protein biomarkers, such as KIM-1, neutrophil gelatinase–associated lipocalin (NGAL), and interleukin 18, which may revolutionize early detection and possible intervention in AKI. Apart from their utility as biomarkers, these genes may also participate in the injury and/or repair of the kidney after AKI.

Stem Cells in Regeneration and Repair in Acute Kidney Injury

An exciting area of AKI research is identification of the origin of the cells that contribute to regeneration of the kidney after injury. Recent studies support the notion that intrinsic tubular epithelial cell proliferation accounts for replenishment of the tubular epithelium lost after ischemia, Bone Marrow derived stem cells migrate to the injured kidney and likely generate factors which are anti-inflammatory and which may influence the proliferative response of the repairing epithelium. Whether intrinsic renal stem cells participate in repair remains a subject of intense investigation.

THERAPEUTIC CONSIDERATIONS

Preconditioning

An important finding in animal models of ischemic renal injury is that previous ischemic or toxic injury protects from future injury. This preconditioning effect lasts for several weeks. These studies indicate that the kidney can activate endogenous protective mechanisms, which appear to protect vessels and tubules from injury. Exploiting these mechanisms will likely lead to new therapies.

Although the deliberate induction of sublethal renal ischemia has little practical clinical application, studies of preconditioning in the myocardium have shown that several pharmacologic agents can mediate the same protection as ischemic preconditioning. Cardiac studies have highlighted signaling pathways involving protein kinase A, protein kinase D, and mitogen-activated kinase in preconditioning. Nitric oxide, a pluripotential molecule derived from inducible nitric oxide synthase (iNOS), is a key mediator of protection associated with preconditioning in the kidney.

Bench to Bedside

Dialysis and conservative measures remain the foundation of therapy for severe AKI. The unraveling of the novel mechanisms of pathogenesis and repair in AKI has led to the development of novel therapeutic strategies to curb acute injury to the kidney (**Table 32-1**). Numerous experimental therapies have been explored, but few have been brought to fruition in humans for several reasons. First, the pathogenesis of AKI in animal models usually is less complex than it is in humans, because patients often have many causes of injury and multiorgan dysfunction. Second, AKI in humans often occurs in the setting of sepsis, and it has been difficult to establish good models of sepsis and AKI in animals. Third, many of the tested strategies in AKI might have been applied too late because the serum creatinine level was used as the biomarker for onset of AKI. Trials that take these barriers into consideration are now being conducted to test new compounds and to retest previously studied agents and maneuvers.

TABLE 32-1 Examples of Potential Therapies Based on Pathophysiologic Mechanisms

VASCULAR	TUBULAR
Vasodilation	**Cell Death/Inflammation**
CO-releasing compounds	Erythropoietin
Natriuretic peptides	Statins
Calcium channel blockers	PPAR agonists
Endothelin receptor antagonists	Caspase inhibitors
Adenosine antagonists	Iron chelators
Growth factors	Acetylcysteine
Nitric oxide	Fibrate
Fenoldopam	Sphingosine-1-phosphate analogues
Leukocyte-Endothelial Interactions	IL-10, IL-6 antagonists
Anti–ICAM-1, CD11a antibody	Minocycline
α-MSH	Edaravone
PAF antagonists	**Repair**
A_{2A} adenosine receptor agonists	Growth factors
C5a receptor antagonist	EGF
Iron Chelation	Heparin-binding EGF
NGAL	IGF-1
Apotransferrin	HGF
	Resolvins, protectins

CO, carbon monoxide; EGF, epidermal growth factor; HGF, hepatocyte growth factor; ICAM, intercellular adhesion molecule; IGF, insulin-like growth factor; IL, interleukin; MSH, melanocyte-stimulating hormone; NGAL, neutrophil gelatinase-associated lipocalin; PAF, platelet activating factor; PPAR, peroxisome proliferator-activated receptor.

BIBLIOGRAPHY

Ali ZA, Callaghan CJ, Lim E, et al: Remote ischemic preconditioning reduces myocardial and renal injury after elective abdominal aortic aneurysm repair: A randomized controlled trial. Circulation 116: 105–198, 2007.

Basile DP: The endothelial cell in ischemic acute kidney injury: Implications for acute and chronic function. Kidney Int 72: 151-156, 2007.

Bonventre JV: Dedifferentiation and proliferation of surviving epithelial cells in acute renal failure. J Am Soc Nephrol 14(Suppl 1):S55-S61, 2003.

Bonventre JV, Weinberg JM: Recent advances in the pathophysiology of ischemic acute renal failure. J Am Soc Nephrol 14: 2199-2210, 2003.

Bonventre JV, Zuk A: Ischemic acute renal failure: an inflammatory disease. Kidney Int. 66:480-485, 2004.

Chertow GM, Burdick E, Honour M, et al: Acute kidney injury, mortality, length of stay, and costs in hospitalized patients. J Am Soc Nephrol 16:3365-3370, 2005.

Conger JD, Schrier RW: Renal hemodynamics in acute renal failure. Annu Rev Physiol 42:603-614, 1980.

Devarajan P: Update on mechanisms of ischemic acute kidney injury. J Am Soc Nephrol 17:1503-1520, 2006.

Duffield JS, Bonventre JV: Kidney tubular epithelium is restored without replacement with bone marrow-derived cells during repair after ischemic injury. Kidney Int 68:1956-1961, 2005.

Duffield JS, Hong S, Vaidya VS, et al: Resolvin D series and protectin D1 mitigate acute kidney injury. J Immunol 177:5902-5911, 2006.

Huang Y, Rabb H, Womer KL: Ischemia-reperfusion and immediate T cell responses. Cell Immunol 248:4-11, 2007.

Humphreys BD, Bonventre JV: Mesenchymal stem cells in acute kidney injury. Annu Rev Med 59:311-325, 2008.

Humphreys BD, Valerius MT, Kosayashi A et al: Intrinsic epithelial cells repair the kidney after injury. Cell Stem Cell 2:284-291, 2008.

Jo SK, Rosner MH, Okusa MD: Pharmacologic treatment of acute kidney injury: Why drugs haven't worked and what is on the horizon. Clin J Am Soc Nephrol 2:356-365, 2007.

Johnson GB, Brunn GJ, Platt JL: Activation of mammalian Toll-like receptors by endogenous agonists. Crit Rev Immunol 23:15-44, 2003.

Kelly KJ, Williams WW Jr, Colvin RB, et al: Antibody to intercellular adhesion molecule 1 protects the kidney against ischemic injury. Proc Natl Acad Sci U S A 91:812-816, 1994.

Kelly KJ, Williams WW Jr, Colvin RB, et al: Intercellular adhesion molecule-1–deficient mice are protected against ischemic renal injury. J Clin Invest 97:1056-1063, 1996.

Leemans JC, Stokman G, Claessen N, et al: Renal-associated TLR2 mediates ischemia/reperfusion injury in the kidney. J Clin Invest 115:2894-2903, 2005.

Linas S, Whittenburg D, Repine JE: Nitric oxide prevents neutrophil-mediated acute renal failure. Am J Physiol 272:F48-F54, 1997.

Niemann-Masanek U, Mueller A, Yard BA, et al: B7-1 (CD80) and B7-2 (CD 86) expression in human tubular epithelial cells in vivo and in vitro. Nephron 92:542-556, 2002.

Nigam S, Lieberthal W: Acute renal failure. III. The role of growth factors in the process of renal regeneration and repair. Am J Physiol Renal Physiol 279:F3-F11, 2000.

Schrier RW, Wang W, Poole B, et al: Acute renal failure: Definitions, diagnosis, pathogenesis, and therapy. J Clin Invest 114:5-14, 2004.

Thurman JM: Triggers of inflammation after renal ischemia/reperfusion. Clin Immunol 123:7-13, 2007.

Togel F, Hu Z, Weiss K, et al: Administered mesenchymal stem cells protect against ischemic acute renal failure through differentiation-independent mechanisms. Am J Physiol Renal Physiol 289:F31-F42, 2005.

Zuk A, Bonventre JV, Brown D, et al: Polarity, integrin, and extracellular matrix dynamics in the postischemic rat kidney. Am J Physiol 275:C711-C731, 1998.

CHAPTER 33

Clinical Approach to the Diagnosis of Acute Renal Failure

Jean L. Holley

Acute renal failure (ARF) is a sudden reduction in the glomerular filtration rate (GFR) that is expressed clinically as the retention of nitrogenous waste products (e.g., urea, creatinine) in the blood. The accumulation of these nitrogenous waste products is sometimes called *azotemia*.

Specific criteria for defining the degree of ARF have been proposed and seem to correlate with prognosis. These standards, called the *RIFLE criteria*, include risk (R), injury (I), failure (F), loss (L), and end-stage renal disease (E). Risk is defined as a 1.5-fold increase in serum creatinine concentration, or a 25% reduction in GFR, or urine output less than 0.5 mL/kg/hr for 12 hours. Injury is defined as a twofold increase in serum creatinine concentration, or a 50% reduction in GFR, or urine output less than 0.5 mL/kg/hr for 12 hours. Failure is defined as a threefold increase in serum creatinine concentration, or a 75% reduction in the GFR, or urine output less than 0.5 mL/kg/hr for 24 hours or anuria for 12 hours. Loss is complete loss of kidney function for more than 4 weeks. End-stage renal disease is complete loss of kidney function for more than 3 months.

Some authorities have suggested that the term *acute kidney injury* (AKI) should be used instead of ARF, because kidney injury does not always result in renal failure. However, AKI has not been widely adopted, and the two terms can be used interchangeably. Using the RIFLE criteria, a patient may be described as having AKI or ARF, depending on the degree of impairment in kidney function. Although the RIFLE criteria may not yet be in widespread use, they are gaining acceptance, and use of a common definition can aid investigative efforts in the pathophysiology and treatment of ARF. In this chapter, the term ARF is used to encompass AKI and ARF as defined by the RIFLE criteria.

In most cases of ARF, the serum creatinine level increases 1 to 2 mg/dL/day. Depending on the clinical circumstances and the patient's symptoms, renal replacement therapy (i.e., dialysis) may be required. Despite the widespread availability of dialysis, the mortality rate for patients who develop ARF remains high, between 10% and 50%, depending on the patient's comorbidities and the medical setting in which the kidney dysfunction occurs (e.g., intensive care unit, obstetric case, surgical procedure). At least half of all episodes of ARF are iatrogenic and related to medications or procedures. The cause of ARF can be determined, in most cases, by following an algorithm that focuses on the patient's history, physical examination, urinalysis findings, basic laboratory results, and in some instances, radiologic imaging of the kidneys and determination of the urine sodium level and fractional excretion of sodium (FE_{Na}) and urea (FE_{UN}). The patient's history (especially medications, procedures, and changes in blood pressure), findings on physical examination (particularly assessment of volume status), ratio of blood urea nitrogen (BUN) to creatinine, and urinalysis results usually provide the information necessary to determine whether the ARF is a prerenal, intrinsic renal, or postrenal event. In some cases, a spot urine sodium concentration or ultrasonography of the kidneys may be needed in the initial evaluation. After the appropriate classification (i.e., prerenal, intrinsic renal, or postrenal) has been determined, the need for additional diagnostic tests and therapeutic interventions becomes clear.

ACUTE VERSUS CHRONIC KIDNEY DISEASE

Because ARF usually resolves and chronic kidney disease often progresses to end-stage renal disease and the need for chronic dialysis, it is useful to determine whether a patient's elevated creatinine concentration is the result of an acute insult or a progressive loss of functioning nephrons. If past serum creatinine values are not available, it may be difficult to differentiate acute from chronic kidney disease. In such cases, an ultrasound study to document the size of the kidneys may be helpful. The kidneys often are small (<10 cm longitudinally in a person of normal stature) and echogenic if the kidney disease is chronic and slowly progressive. The presence of normal-sized kidneys on ultrasound scans does not absolutely exclude chronic kidney disease, but small, echogenic kidneys are not consistent with ARF. An individual may have concomitant ARF and chronic kidney disease, and in such cases the kidney size is less helpful.

Laboratory features that suggest chronic kidney disease (but are not diagnostic) include a normocytic anemia, hyperphosphatemia, and hypocalcemia. The presence of nonspecific symptoms of uremia (e.g., nausea, vomiting, pruritus, fatigue) may also suggest chronic kidney disease rather than ARF, but there is no single variable other than kidney size or serial elevated creatinine values over time that conclusively establishes that kidney function impairment is chronic and not acute. Patients with chronic kidney disease may also develop episodes of ARF. In such cases, the kidneys usually are small, and the baseline creatinine value is elevated. An abrupt and unexpected rise in the baseline creatinine value in such patients should prompt an evaluation for superimposed, potentially reversible ARF.

CLASSIFICATION OF ACUTE RENAL FAILURE

All cases of ARF can be classified as prerenal, intrinsic (intrarenal), or postrenal (**Table 33-1**). Classification of each episode of ARF directs appropriate diagnostic and therapeutic strategies. ARF is also clinically described as oliguric (<400 mL of urine output in 24 hours), nonoliguric (>400 mL/24 hr), or anuric (<100 mL/24 hr). These categories help to establish cause and predict prognosis. Anuria is uncommon and suggests either complete obstruction or a major vascular event, such as bilateral renal infarction, renal vein thrombosis (RVT), cortical necrosis, or high-grade ischemic acute tubular necrosis (ATN). Prerenal, intrinsic renal, and postrenal ARF can each manifest with oliguria or nonoliguria. Nonoliguric ARF is common in intrarenal ARF (e.g., nephrotoxin-induced ATN, acute glomerulonephritis, acute interstitial nephritis). Oliguria more commonly characterizes obstruction and prerenal azotemia. Regardless of the cause of decreased kidney function, management is more difficult with oliguria, because volume overload occurs earlier in the course. Patients with nonoliguric ARF have a more favorable prognosis and reduced mortality rates.

PRERENAL ACUTE RENAL FAILURE

Prerenal abnormalities are physiologic responses that lead to decreased kidney function (i.e., decreased GFR). They manifest as elevated BUN and creatinine concentrations resulting from decreased perfusion of the kidney. The reduced renal perfusion that results in prerenal ARF may occur as a consequence of inadequate volume (e.g., blood loss, overly aggressive diuresis), inadequate cardiac output due to impaired myocardial function (e.g., cardiogenic shock after an acute myocardial infarction, progressive cardiomyopathy), or marked vasodilatation (e.g., sepsis). In each situation, the underlying kidney is normal, but ARF occurs because the primary disorder compromises renal blood flow enough to reduce the GFR. In cases of depleted intravascular fluid volume and congestive heart failure (the two most common causes of prerenal azotemia), the kidney initially compensates for the diminished perfusion to preserve filtration function.

Mechanisms of self-preservation include autoregulatory afferent arteriolar dilation and attenuation of afferent vasoconstriction by intrarenal prostaglandin-mediated vasodilatation. These and other physiologic maneuvers comprise renal compensation or autoregulation and are ultimately an attempt by the kidney to maintain the GFR in the face of hypoperfusion. When renal compensation is maximized and the conditions causing hypoperfusion remain uncorrected,

TABLE 33-1 **Classification of Acute Renal Failure**

Prerenal Acute Renal Failure (Reduced Renal Perfusion)

Volume depletion
  Renal loss: diuretics, osmotic diuresis (e.g., DKA), addisonian crisis
  Extrarenal loss: vomiting, diarrhea, skin losses (e.g., burns, sweating)

Hypotension (regardless of cause)

Cardiovascular causes
  Congestive heart failure, reduced myocardial function, arrhythmias

Hemodynamic causes (e.g., intense intrarenal vasoconstriction)

Radiographic contrast
Prostaglandin inhibition (e.g., NSAIDs)
Cyclosporine and tacrolimus
ACE inhibitors and ARBs
Amphotericin B

Hypercalcemia

Hepatorenal syndrome (i.e., bland urinary sediment, oliguria, low urine sodium, not reversed with volume repletion, reversible with successful liver transplantation)

Abdominal compartment syndrome

Intrinsic or Intrarenal Acute Renal Failure

Vascular causes
  Renal infarction, renal artery stenosis, renal vein thrombosis
  Malignant hypertension, scleroderma renal crisis, atheroemboli

Tubular
  Ischemic: prolonged prerenal state, sepsis syndrome, systemic hypotension
  Nephrotoxic: aminoglycosides, methotrexate, cisplatin, myoglobin (e.g., rhabdomyolysis), hemoglobin

Glomerular
  Acute glomerulonephritis
  Vasculitis (Wegener's granulomatosis, polyarteritis)
  Thrombotic microangiopathy (hemolytic uremic syndrome, TTP)

Interstitium
  Medications: penicillins, cephalosporins, ciprofloxacin, NSAIDs, phenytoin, PPIs
  Tumor infiltration (e.g., lymphoma, leukemia)

Postrenal Acute Renal Failure (Obstruction)

Prostate hypertrophy, neurogenic bladder

Intraureteral obstruction: crystals (e.g., uric acid, acyclovir, indinavir), stones, clots, tumor

Extraureteral obstruction: tumor (e.g., cervical, prostate), retroperitoneal fibrosis

ACE, angiotensin-converting enzyme; ARBs, angiotensin receptor blockers; DKA, diabetic ketoacidosis; NSAIDs, nonsteroidal anti-inflammatory drugs; PPIs, proton pump inhibitors; TTP, thrombotic thrombocytopenic purpura.

renal compensation becomes decompensation, and ARF occurs. The development of ARF after ingestion of a nonsteroidal anti-inflammatory drug (NSAID) by a patient who has congestive heart failure is a common clinical example of this type of hemodynamic insult. In this situation, the prostaglandin-mediated compensatory renal vasodilatation that occurs because the kidneys are hypoperfused from poor cardiac output is inhibited by the NSAID, and a consequent reduction in GFR occurs, manifested by rising BUN and creatinine values.

Intense intrarenal vasoconstriction may result in ARF, causing reduced renal blood flow and subsequent reduction

TABLE 33-2 Results of Urinalysis and Sodium, Urea, Blood Urea Nitrogen, and Creatinine Measurements in Acute Renal Failure

TYPE OF ACUTE RENAL FAILURE	URINALYSIS	U_{Na}* (mEq/L)	FE_{Na}* (%)	FE_{UN}* (%)	BUN-TO-CREATININE RATIO
Prerenal	High specific gravity Normal or hyaline casts	<20	<1	≤35	≥20:1
Intrarenal					
Acute tubular necrosis	Low specific gravity Muddy brown casts Renal tubular epithelial cells	>40	≥1	>50	≤20:1
Vascular disorders	Normal or hematuria	>20	Variable		
Glomerulonephritis	Proteinuria, hematuria RBC casts, dysmorphic RBCs	<20	<1		
Interstitial nephritis	Mild proteinuria, hematuria WBCs, WBC casts, eosinophils	>20	≥1		
Postrenal	Normal or hematuria WBCs, occasional granular casts	>20	Variable		≥20:1

*U_{Na}, FE_{Na}, and FE_{UN} vary with postrenal failure, interstitial nephritis, and glomerulonephritis.

BUN, blood urea nitrogen; FE_{Na}, fractional excretion of sodium; FE_{UN}, fractional excretion of urea; RBCs, red blood cells; U_{Na}, urinary sodium concentration; WBCs, white blood cells.

of glomerular perfusion. This hemodynamically mediated form of ARF resembles prerenal azotemia and is seen with exposure to radiographic contrast materials, cyclosporine, tacrolimus, amphotericin, and NSAIDs (see **Table 33-1**). Uncorrected, such episodes of prerenal azotemia may progress to ischemic ATN. Like other forms of prerenal azotemia, the urinalysis in cases of vasoconstrictor or hemodynamically mediated prerenal azotemia is bland, and the urinary sodium level often is low.

Evidence of preserved renal functional ability and the kidney's attempt to compensate for the reduced perfusion in prerenal states is the maximum tubular sodium resorption that occurs and is reflected in a low urine sodium level (<20 mEq/L) or low FE_{Na}(<1%) or FE_{UN} (<35%), or both (**Table 33-2**). The FE_{Na} is a quantitative measure of the fraction of filtered sodium that is excreted and is not influenced by changes in water resorption that can affect the simple urine sodium concentration. The filtered sodium is the product of the GFR (estimated by creatinine clearance) and the concentration of plasma sodium. Therefore, using U_x for the urinary concentration of any substance x, P_x for the plasma concentration of x, and V for urine volume, FE_{Na} is defined as follows:

$$FE_{Na} = \frac{\text{Na excreted}}{\text{Na filtered}} \times 100$$

$$= \frac{U_{Na} \times V}{P_{Na} \times GFR} \times 100$$

Because GFR is equal to $U_{creat}/P_{creat} \times V$,

$$FE_{Na} = \frac{U_{Na} \times V}{P_{Na} \times (U_{creat}/P_{creat}) \times V} \times 100$$

$$= \frac{U_{Na}/P_{Na}}{U_{creat}/P_{creat}} \times 100$$

Although the urine sodium level and the FE_{Na} are typically low in ARF as a result of prerenal causes, and typically high

(>40 mEq/L and ≥1%, respectively) in the setting of ATN, a FE_{Na} that is less than 1% occasionally may be seen with nonoliguric ATN, with ARF related to use of radiographic contrast agents, or with sepsis. Diuretics are often given as part of the treatment of prerenal conditions (e.g., congestive heart failure) to increase urine output. In such settings, the FE_{UN} may be a more sensitive and specific indicator of a prerenal state. The FE_{UN} is calculated by substituting urea nitrogen for sodium in the equation previously given. A result less than or equal to 35% is consistent with a prerenal state (see **Table 33-2**).

In patients with prerenal azotemia, the renal insult, which results from hypoperfusion, is indirect. The kidney's intrinsic ability to function is preserved. Glomeruli and the glomerular basement membrane are intact, and there is no tubular or interstitial damage. The urine usually is concentrated, with a high specific gravity and osmolality, but it is otherwise unremarkable. The dipstick shows no proteinuria or blood, and the microscopic examination result is bland, with no red blood cells (RBCs), white blood cells (WBCs), or cellular casts. Hyaline casts may be present. Mild qualitative proteinuria (e.g., trace or 1+ on the dipstick) may sometimes be seen in highly concentrated urines.

The history usually suggests volume loss or cardiac failure (**Table 33-3**; see **Table 33-1**). The most important aspect of the physical examination is to assess the patient's volume status. In terms of renal perfusion, intravascular volume overload with a decrease in effective arterial volume (e.g., congestive heart failure, cirrhosis) and intravascular volume depletion are identical; each leads to renal hypoperfusion. In these situations, which are clinically quite different, the renal response is the same: maximal sodium retention in an attempt to compensate for the reduced perfusion. The appropriate treatment for ARF in such cases is to increase the renal perfusion, and rapid reversal of the prerenal azotemia occurs if appropriate treatment is given (e.g., volume repletion). Unlike creatinine, urea diffuses across membranes,

TABLE 33-3 Using the History and Physical Examination as Tools to Categorize Acute Renal Failure

TYPE OF ACUTE RENAL FAILURE	HISTORY	PHYSICAL EXAMINATION
Prerenal	Volume loss (e.g., vomiting, diarrhea, diuretics, burns)	Weight, supine and standing blood pressure and pulse
	Past weights, daily intake and output values	
	Cardiac disease, liver disease	Mucous membranes, axillary moisture
	Thirst	Neck veins, S_3 heart sound, lung examination, edema
	Medications (e.g., NSAIDs, ACE inhibitors, ARBs, cyclosporine)	
	Radiographic contrast (e.g., CT, angiography)	
Intrarenal		
ATN	Medications (e.g., aminoglycosides)	Neck veins, S_3 heart sound, lung examination, edema, volume status
	Alcohol abuse, trauma, muscle necrosis (e.g., rhabdomyolysis)	Compartment syndrome, examination of extremities
	Hypotension episode	
Vascular	Trauma, known nephrotic syndrome, flank pain	Blood pressure, livedo reticularis
	Vessel catheterization, anticoagulation (e.g., atheroemboli)	Funduscopic examination (e.g., malignant hypertension)
	Progressive systemic sclerosis	Thickened skin, sclerodactyly, telangiectasia
Glomerular	Systemic disease (e.g., SLE, vasculitis), arthritis, rash	Oral ulcers, arthritis, skin lesions, footdrop
	Uveitis, weight loss, fatigue, intravenous drug use (e.g., hepatitis C)	Pleural and pericardial rubs
	Cough, hemoptysis (e.g., Goodpasture's syndrome), foamy urine	Periorbital, leg, and presacral edema
Interstitial	Medications (e.g., antibiotics, PPIs, allopurinol, phenytoin)	Fever, drug-related rash
	Arthralgias	
Postrenal	Urinary urgency, hesitancy, gross hematuria	Bladder distention, pelvic masses, prostate
	Intermittent polyuria, history of stones	
	Medications (e.g., indinavir, acyclovir, anticholinergics)	

ACE, angiotensin converting enzyme; ARBs, angiotensin receptor blockers; ATN, acute tubular necrosis; CT, computed tomography; NSAIDs, nonsteroidal anti-inflammatory drugs; SLE, systemic lupus erythematosus; PPIs, proton pump inhibitors.

and active urea resorption occurs when there is reduced urine flow. Therefore, prerenal ARF is characterized by an elevated BUN-to-creatinine ratio (>20:1). Other causes of a BUN/creatinine ratio greater than 20:1 include postrenal ARF, gastrointestinal blood loss (i.e., digested protein from an upper gastrointestinal bleed is absorbed and metabolized by the liver), high-dose corticosteroid therapy, and intense catabolism.

Another type of hemodynamically mediated ARF that can be seen in acutely ill patients is intra-abdominal hypertension or abdominal compartment syndrome. In the setting of trauma, abdominal surgery, or cases in which massive fluid or blood product resuscitation has occurred (e.g., septic shock, orthotopic liver transplantation complicated by severe bleeding), elevated intra-abdominal pressure may occur and ultimately lead to reduced renal perfusion and ARF, as well as multiorgan system failure. A high body mass index and high volumes of fluid resuscitation are the primary risk factors for susceptible patients. Measuring pressure in the bladder by means of a transducer can be a simple method for detecting an elevated intra-abdominal pressure. An intravesicular pressure of more than 20 to 25 mm Hg suggests abdominal compartment syndrome and may prompt consideration of laparoscopic evaluation or laparotomy for decompression. Because the elevation in intra-abdominal pressure leads to reduced renal perfusion, a low urine sodium level is common in this situation. The elevated intra-abdominal pressure also leads to elevated intrathoracic pressure, which may confound central venous pressure measurements. The confusing clinical picture of an oliguric patient with high central venous pressure, low urine sodium concentration, and normal left ventricular function may occur. In ICU patients who have abdominal trauma or have undergone surgery and have had more than 10 L of fluid or blood product resuscitation complicated by ARF, intra-abdominal hypertension and abdominal compartment syndrome should be considered and an intravesicular pressure measured.

POSTRENAL ACUTE RENAL FAILURE: OBSTRUCTIVE UROPATHY

The extent of pathology in postrenal ARF (i.e., obstructive uropathy) is determined by the level at which the obstruction occurs (see Chapter 46). However, the end point of all obstructive lesions is the potential destruction of functioning kidney parenchyma. The elevated pressures in obstructed conduits results in adaptive dilatation (e.g., hydroureter, hydronephrosis), which ultimately progresses to nephron destruction (i.e., atrophy of the tubular epithelium, interstitial fibrosis, and ultimately glomerular scarring) if unrelieved. Postrenal causes of ARF necessarily involve obstruction of both kidneys or both ureters, unless the patient has only a single functioning kidney. In patients with two functioning kidneys, unilateral obstruction (e.g., an obstructing kidney stone) rarely causes ARF because the glomerular filtration of the unobstructed kidney is not reduced.

In postrenal azotemia, the patient's history can identify predisposing factors and symptoms (see **Tables 33-1** and **33-3**). Reduced urine output (i.e., oliguria) and anuria are common in patients with postrenal ARF. The physical examination, like the history, should focus on the possibility of obstruction (e.g., pelvic masses, distended bladder, prostatic enlargement). Because there is reduced urine flow with obstruction, the BUN/creatinine ratio is usually elevated, as is the case in prerenal azotemia. Development of type IV renal tubular acidosis may sometimes be a diagnostic clue in obstructive uropathy. Values for urine sediment and concentration vary and usually are not helpful in the diagnosis of obstruction, except that hematuria may be seen with stones or tumor and gross hematuria due to urothelial tumors may obstruct the collecting system with clots. Renal ultrasonography usually shows hydronephrosis if obstruction is causing the ARF. Bladder catheterization with a marked urine volume or a postvoid residual amount of more than 100 mL confirms the presence of postrenal ARF. Rarely, despite the presence of obstruction, hydronephrosis may not be identified on ultrasound studies. Retroperitoneal fibrosis is often present in such cases, and it can be confirmed by computed tomography (CT) scan or magnetic resonance imaging (MRI). If the clinical suspicion of obstruction is high and hydronephrosis is not observed on ultrasound, additional kidney imaging, such as CT, MRI, or retrograde nephrography, should be done.

Like the external obstruction that occurs with tumor or prostate enlargement, intraureteral obstruction also may cause ARF (see **Table 33-1**). Kidney stones, endogenous crystals (i.e., uric acid such as in acute tumor lysis), exogenous crystals (i.e., medications such as indinavir or acyclovir), or other material (i.e., blood clots, renal papillae such as in papillary necrosis, or uroepithelial tumors of the ureter or renal pelvis) can cause postrenal ARF by intraureteral obstruction. ARF caused by obstruction usually resolves with relief of the obstruction by placement of a bladder catheter or nephrostomy tube. However, prolonged obstruction may cause irreversible nephron destruction and lead to chronic kidney disease.

INTRINSIC OR INTRARENAL ACUTE RENAL FAILURE

Intrinsic ARF can be categorized anatomically by the area of the kidney parenchyma involved: vascular, glomerular, tubular, or interstitial areas. Differences in the clinical setting and presentation, and particularly in the history, physical examination findings, and urinalysis results, can distinguish among these types of ARF. Determining whether a patient has ATN, acute interstitial nephritis, or acute glomerulonephritis as the cause of ARF is necessary, because the treatment and prognosis for each is different.

With all types of intrarenal ARF, the kidney is the site of the abnormality. Unlike prerenal and postrenal ARF, the decrement in the GFR is directly linked to kidney damage and is not the result of reduced renal perfusion or elevated pressures in the renal conduits. Because urea resorption is not preferentially increased, urea and creatinine concentrations rise in parallel, and the BUN-to-creatinine ratio is usually preserved (10:1 to 20:1). Similarly, because the impaired kidney function results from direct kidney injury, the urinalysis result is usually abnormal. Specific findings on dipstick and microscopic examination of the urine provide important clues to the location of the parenchymal injury responsible for the kidney dysfunction (see **Table 33-2**). In some cases, despite a careful history, physical examination, urinalysis, and additional specific tests (see **Table 33-3**), the type of the kidney disorder (tubular, vascular, glomerular, or interstitial) remains undefined, and a percutaneous kidney biopsy is needed to determine the cause.

ATN is the most common type of acute intrinsic ARF seen in hospitalized patients. The term ATN is sometimes used interchangeably with ARF, but, in fact, ATN is only one form of intrinsic ARF (see **Table 33-1**).

Acute Tubular Necrosis as a Cause of Intrinsic Acute Renal Failure

At least 45% of the cases of ARF are caused by ATN. Because the two major causes of ATN are ischemia and nephrotoxins, ATN can be characterized as ischemic or nephrotoxic. Important clues to these kidney insults are in the patient's history. Ischemia is the most common cause of ATN and often occurs after a prolonged prerenal state with associated renal hypoperfusion. The history may reveal systemic hypotension, marked volume depletion, or reduced effective circulating volume. Distinguishing between ongoing prerenal azotemia that is reversible and ATN may be difficult. However, the hallmark of prerenal ARF is its reversibility with restoration of renal perfusion (e.g., appropriate volume repletion); ATN does not improve with only volume repletion. The point at which a patient moves from prerenal azotemia to ischemic ATN depends on the patient and the clinical situation. Unless the patient is clearly volume overloaded, a fluid challenge to exclude a prerenal state usually is an integral part of the diagnosis of and therapy for suspected ischemic ATN.

Clinical features that may help to differentiate ischemic ATN from prerenal azotemia include the urinalysis results, urinary sodium concentration, FE_{Na} and FE_{UN} (see **Table 33-2**). Because the kidney is essentially normal in prerenal ARF, the urinalysis findings are unremarkable. In contrast, with ATN, evidence of the damaged tubules is usually seen in the urinary sediment: renal tubular epithelial cells and granular casts characterize ATN. The hallmark of ATN is the presence of dirty (or muddy) brown casts, a urinalysis finding that is pathognomonic of ATN. Because the tubules are the only site of renal injury in ATN, urinary findings that typify glomerular injury (e.g., proteinuria, RBCs [often dysmorphic], RBC casts) or interstitial injury (e.g., hematuria, WBCs, WBC casts) are not seen. Prerenal azotemia is characterized by intact tubular function, reduced renal blood flow, and maximal tubular resorption of sodium and urea (see **Table 33-2**). In patients with ATN, there is direct tubular damage and a loss of tubular function manifested by a high urine sodium level, FE_{Na} and FE_{UN}.

These characteristic findings on urinalysis and urinary sodium determinations occur with both ischemic and nephrotoxic forms of ATN. Aminoglycosides are among the most common causes of nephrotoxic ATN (see Chapter 34). With aminoglycoside-induced ATN, the creatinine level usually begins to rise 5 to 10 days after administration. Other nephrotoxins that may cause ATN include methotrexate, cisplatin, and endogenous pigments such as hemoglobin and myoglobin (as seen with rhabdomyolysis; see Chapter 36). The values for FE_{Na} and FE_{UN} are usually high in ATN. In most cases, both nephrotoxic and ischemic forms of ATN resolve. However, depending on the level of kidney dysfunction that occurs, temporary dialysis may be necessary.

Vascular Damage Resulting in Intrinsic Acute Renal Failure

Acute events involving the main renal arteries or veins can cause ARF. As with obstruction, bilateral involvement is required for ARF to develop, unless at baseline the patient has a solitary functioning kidney. Bilateral kidney infarction, RVT, or acute occlusion of the renal arteries may lead to acute intrinsic renal failure. Because the kidney parenchyma may not be initially directly injured, some authorities would classify these forms of ARF as prerenal azotemia rather than intrinsic ARF. Involvement of smaller blood vessels may also cause intrinsic ARF. Examples of this kind of ARF include malignant hypertension, scleroderma renal crisis, and cholesterol atheroembolic disease. In some systems of classification, ARF due to vasculitis also is included among the vascular types of intrinsic ARF. However, because glomerular involvement with its associated proteinuria and active urinary sediment is common with vasculitis, vasculitides are classified under glomerular causes of intrinsic ARF (see **Table 33-1**).

Historical data that suggest an acute vascular event as the cause of ARF include trauma, underlying nephrotic syndrome with significant proteinuria (a predisposition to RVT), and acute flank pain with hematuria. Microscopic hematuria, with or without proteinuria, is the most common finding on urinalysis in intrinsic ARF caused by vascular problems. Disease of the renal arteries or veins that results in ARF usually requires imaging to confirm the diagnosis. For example, MRI may reveal RVT or renal artery stenosis, CT may show renal infarction, and a radionuclide renal scan or Doppler ultrasound study may confirm the presence or absence of renal blood flow. Atheroemboli are the most common vascular problem causing intrinsic ARF. Important historical features of atheroembolic ARF include catheterization of the arterial system and anticoagulation. The physical examination in atheroembolic ARF may suggest widespread atheroemboli by demonstrating livedo reticularis in the skin of the toes and feet and Hollenhorst plaques in the retina (see Chapter 35).

RVT, although uncommon, is seen most often in patients with nephrotic syndrome. Nephrotic patients with severe hypoalbuminemia (serum albumin < 2 g/dL) and those with membranous glomerulonephritis are at highest risk for RVT. Hemoconcentration due to diuretic use in these patients may increase the risk of RVT. Non-nephrotic patients may develop RVT in the setting of trauma, use of oral contraceptives, hypovolemia (especially in infants), and coagulopathies (i.e., inherited procoagulant defects and antiphospholipid antibody syndrome). Acute RVT usually manifests with flank pain, microscopic or gross hematuria, a marked elevation in the serum lactate dehydrogenase (LDH) level (with normal transaminases), and enlargement of the kidneys on imaging. When there is bilateral RVT, ARF may occur. Chronic RVT is probably more common than acute RVT, is often asymptomatic, and occurs in association with pulmonary embolism. Acute RVT is diagnosed by imaging (i.e., spiral CT, MRI, or Doppler ultrasonography), and selective renal venography is the gold standard. The imaging study chosen depends on the institutional expertise, but CT is used most often. Treatment of acute RVT, like any other thrombotic process, is anticoagulation with or without local thrombolytic therapy and catheter thrombectomy, depending on the presentation and duration of the thrombosis.

Occlusion of the renal arteries may cause ARF due to vascular compromise. Renal infarction usually results from clot emboli and, although rare, most commonly occurs in patients with atrial fibrillation who experience clot embolization from the left atrium. Clot embolization from left ventricular thrombus in the setting of acute myocardial infarction, thromboemboli from complex plaque in the aorta, emboli from valvular vegetations, and rarely, tumor and fat emboli may lead to renal infarction. Other causes of renal infarction include cocaine use, dissection of the aorta or renal arteries, complication of endovascular intervention, and antiphospholipid antibody disease. Patients with acute renal infarction usually have acute onset of nausea, vomiting, flank or generalized abdominal pain, fever, and an acute rise in blood pressure (which is renin mediated). Patients may have signs of extrarenal embolization (e.g., focal neurologic defects). Abnormal laboratory results include an elevated WBC count and serum LDH level, which is often four times the normal value. Microscopic or gross hematuria occurs in one third to one half of patients, and mild proteinuria is possible. ARF can occur, especially with bilateral disease or a large embolus. Because of the nonspecific presenting symptoms and signs, the diagnosis is often delayed. Renal colic from nephrolithiasis and pyelonephritis are the primary diagnoses to exclude. Renal infarction is confirmed by spiral CT, which classically shows a wedge-shaped perfusion defect. If the CT study is not definitive, a radioisotope scan often can demonstrate segmental or generalized reduction in renal perfusion. Treatment most often involves anticoagulation after the cause of the thrombi has been determined.

Glomerular Type of Intrinsic Acute Renal Failure

Acute inflammation of vessels and glomeruli causing ARF may reflect renal involvement of a systemic illness (e.g., systemic lupus erythematosus, Wegener's granulomatosis, polyarteritis nodosa), which is suggested by the medical history and physical examination findings (see **Table 33-3**) (see Chapters 16, 23, and 24). Because proteinuria occurring with glomerular involvement is often in the nephrotic range (>3 g/24 hr), edema is common in patients with acute glomerulonephritis, who often also have hypertension and volume overload.

The urinalysis provides the most important clues to intrinsic ARF due to glomerulonephritis. Proteinuria and blood on the urine dipstick test, microscopic hematuria, RBC casts, and dysmorphic-appearing RBCs are characteristic (see **Table 33-2**). Probably because renin and, consequently, aldosterone are stimulated in the setting of glomerulonephritis, the urine sodium level may be low. However, the urinalysis and supporting history and physical examination findings are the keys to diagnosing acute glomerulonephritis. Because the abnormal urinalysis results in acute glomerulonephritis essentially excludes prerenal azotemia and ATN, the urine sodium level is rarely a diagnostic key to ARF caused by glomerulonephritis.

Interstitial Type of Intrinsic Acute Renal Failure

Involvement of the interstitium can cause ARF on an intrarenal basis (see Chapter 45). Acute interstitial nephritis is associated with a variety of medications, such as penicillin, other antibiotics, allopurinol, and proton pump inhibitors. The history of exposure to a new medication is the key to the diagnosis of this kind of intrinsic ARF. In about one third of patients with acute interstitial nephritis, a systemic illness may occur that is characterized by fever, a maculopapular erythematous rash, arthralgias, and eosinophilia. These clinical features have led some to refer to this entity as *allergic interstitial nephritis*. The urinalysis with acute interstitial nephritis usually shows mild proteinuria, microscopic hematuria, WBCs, and sometimes, WBC casts. Eosinophiluria may be identified by Hansel or Wright staining of urine. However, eosinophiluria is not pathognomonic of acute interstitial nephritis, because urine eosinophils also may be seen in cholesterol atheroembolic ARF, glomerulonephritis, and prostatitis. Percutaneous kidney biopsy may sometimes be needed to distinguish between interstitial nephritis and other forms of acute intrinsic renal failure, notably ATN.

BIBLIOGRAPHY

Bellomo R, Ronco C, Kellum JA, et al: Acute renal failure—Definitions, outcome measures, animal models, fluid therapy and information technology needs. The Second International Consensus Conference of the Acute Dialysis Quality Initiative (ADQI) Group. Crit Care 8:R204-R212, 2004.

Carvounis CP, Nisar S, Guro-Razuman S: Significance of the fractional excretion of urea in the differential diagnosis of acute renal failure. Kidney Int 62:2223-2229, 2002.

Esson ML, Schrier RW: Diagnosis and treatment of acute tubular necrosis. Ann Intern Med 137:744-752, 2002.

Hazanov N, Somin M, Attali M, et al: Acute renal embolism. Forty-four cases of renal infarction in patients with atrial fibrillation. Medicine (Baltimore) 83:292-299, 2004.

Himmelfarb J, Ikizler TA: Acute kidney injury: Changing lexicography, definitions, and epidemiology. Kidney Int 71:971-976, 2007.

Hou SH, Bushinsky DA, Wish JB, et al: Hospital-acquired renal insufficiency: A prospective study. Am J Med 74:243-248, 1983.

Liano F, Pascual J: Epidemiology of acute renal failure: A prospective, multicenter community-based study. Madrid Acute Renal Failure Study Group. Kidney Int 50:811-818, 1996.

Malbrain ML: Is it wise not to think about intraabdominal hypertension in the ICU? Curr Opin Crit Care 10:132-145, 2004.

Miller TR, Anderson RJ, Linas SL, et al: Urinary diagnostic indices in acute renal failure: A prospective study. Ann Intern Med 89:47-50, 1978.

Nolan CR, Anderson RJ: Hospital-acquired acute renal failure. J Am Soc Nephrol 9:701-718, 1998.

Singhal R, Brinble KS: Thromboembolic complications in the nephrotic syndrome: Pathophysiology and clinical management. Thromb Res 118:397-407, 2006.

Uchino S, Bellomo R, Goldsmith D, et al: An assessment of the RIFLE criteria for acute renal failure in hospitalized patients. Crit Care Med 34:1913-1917, 2006.

CHAPTER 34

Kidney Function Impairment Caused by Therapeutic Agents

Thomas M. Coffman

Compounds used for diagnostic and therapeutic purposes are major causes of acute and chronic renal failure. Because it is a major route of excretion for a variety of drugs, the kidney is a frequent target for toxic injury. The potential of many exogenous agents to cause nephrotoxicity is increased because they are greatly concentrated in the urinary space and within renal tubules. The rate of blood flow per gram of tissue weight in the kidney is relatively high, resulting in exaggerated exposure of renal endothelial cells and glomeruli to circulating substances. Because most renal functions depend on tightly regulated blood flow patterns, agents that impair these hemodynamic relationships may interfere with the ability of the kidney to maintain normal homeostasis.

Drug toxicity in the kidney is manifested through the prototypical clinical syndromes that are associated with kidney diseases of other causes, including acute renal failure (ARF), chronic kidney disease, and nephrotic syndrome (**Table 34-1**). Moreover, a single agent can cause more than one of these clinical syndromes. The particular clinical manifestation of nephrotoxicity is determined by the chemical properties of the agent and the dose and duration of exposure, along with individual patient factors such as age, volume status, and genetic background. This chapter describes a general approach to nephrotoxicity and reviews the renal effects of some common causative agents. Individual agents or syndromes associated with toxic renal injury are discussed elsewhere in this *Primer* (for example, Chapters 36, 38, and 45).

DIAGNOSIS

The possibility of drug-induced nephrotoxicity should be considered whenever the serum creatinine concentration rises during administration of a therapeutic agent and therefore should be included in the differential diagnosis for almost all hospitalized patients who develop ARF. Because of the nonlinear relationship between the serum creatinine level and the glomerular filtration rate (GFR), a substantial reduction in GFR is necessary before toxic injury can be appreciated clinically. This point is particularly important to consider in the context of agents that may cause chronic nephropathy. In this case, kidney injury may not be detected until 40% to 50% of kidney function has been irreversibly lost. A number of diagnostic markers, such as urinary excretion of tubular enzymes, have been evaluated as biomarkers of renal toxicity that might be more sensitive and specific than serum creatinine concentration. However, none of these has yet found widespread clinical application.

The clinical syndromes caused by drugs mimic those associated with kidney diseases of other causes. When the cause of reduced kidney function is being investigated, the possible role of therapeutic agents should always be considered, and a detailed medication history is an essential component of the clinical evaluation. Temporal associations between the appearance of a kidney abnormality and medication changes must be documented. For patients who are receiving compounds known to be nephrotoxic, the plan for clinical management should include avoidance of clinical risk factors, careful monitoring of kidney function, and when appropriate, monitoring of serum drug levels. In addition, the role of nephrotoxins in exacerbating kidney dysfunction induced by other causes should be appreciated. For example, in patients with acute tubular necrosis, the potential aggravating consequences of aminoglycosides or radiocontrast must be recognized. Renal clearance of certain drugs can be substantially reduced in these patients, and dosing must be adjusted appropriately (see Chapter 39).

TABLE 34-1 Representative Renal Syndromes Caused by Therapeutic Agents

CLINICAL SYNDROME	CAUSATIVE AGENTS
Acute renal failure Prerenal or hemodynamic	Cyclosporine, tacrolimus, radiocontrast, amphotericin B, ACE inhibitors, ARBs NSAIDs, interleukin 2
Intrarenal failure Acute tubular necrosis	Aminoglycosides, amphotericin B, cisplatin, certain cephalosporins
Acute intterstitial nephritis	Penicillins, cephalosporins, sulfonamides, rifampin, NSAIDs, interferon, interleukin 2
Postrenal or obstructive	Acyclovir, analgesic abuse, methysergide, methotrexate, indinavir, sulfadiazine
Chronic kidney disease	Lithium, analgesic abuse, cyclosporin, tacrolimus, cisplatin, nitrosourea
Nephrotic syndrome	Gold, NSAIDs, penicillamine, captopril, interferon

ACE, angiotensin-converting enzyme; ARBs, angiotensin receptor blockers; NSAIDs, nonsteroidal anti-inflammatory drugs.

DRUG-RELATED RENAL FAILURE

In epidemiologic studies, pharmacologic agents are implicated as a cause for acute kidney injury (AKI) in up to 20% of cases. As shown in **Table 34-1**, mechanisms of ARF related to drugs can be roughly categorized as prerenal or hemodynamic, intrarenal, and postrenal or obstructive syndromes. As described in Chapter 33, this separation can be extremely helpful in identifying the source and directing the management of ARF from any cause.

Prerenal Azotemia: Hemodynamically Mediated Renal Functional Impairment Associated with Drugs

As shown in **Table 34-1**, several classes of therapeutic agents, including cyclosporine, tacrolimus, radiocontrast, nonsteroidal anti-inflammatory drugs (NSAIDs), angiotensin-converting enzyme (ACE) inhibitors, and angiotensin receptor blockers (ARBs), can cause a syndrome of abnormal kidney function that resembles prerenal azotemia. Similar to prerenal azotemia from other causes, hemodynamic renal dysfunction caused by drugs can be associated with low levels of urine sodium excretion. Generally, renal dysfunction rapidly remits when the offending agent is discontinued, but persistent injury may result if exposure is prolonged or if aggravating factors are present.

Drugs cause hemodynamically mediated renal dysfunction through several mechanisms. Agents such as cyclosporine, tacrolimus, radiocontrast, and amphotericin B cause intense vasoconstriction in the kidney, reducing renal blood flow and glomerular perfusion. These compounds do not seem to affect vascular tone directly, but they may stimulate production of other vasoconstrictors such as endothelin or thromboxane A_2. Cyclosporine, tacrolimus, and amphotericin B can produce renal dysfunction in normal subjects with no underlying kidney abnormalities.

Hemodynamic kidney dysfunction associated with NSAIDs usually occurs in patients with preexisting impairment of renal perfusion. NSAIDs inhibit the cyclooxygenase isoenzymes, turning off the synthesis of prostaglandins. In normal subjects, renal prostaglandin production is low, and administration of NSAIDs has little effect on renal function. However, as an adaptive mechanism, production of vasodilator prostaglandins increases when renal perfusion is threatened. In these circumstances, inhibiting production of these vasodilator compounds by NSAIDs can cause precipitous declines in renal blood flow and GFR. This syndrome is most often seen in patients with volume depletion, heart failure, and preexisting kidney disease (see Chapter 38).

Similarly, ARF occurring after administration of ACE inhibitors or ARBs is seen almost exclusively in patients with underlying abnormalities of the renal vasculature and circulation. This syndrome is most commonly seen in patients who have congestive heart failure treated with diuretics; severe, bilateral renal artery stenosis; critical renal artery stenosis in a single functioning kidney; or vascular disease and nephrosclerosis. ACE inhibitors lower blood pressure by inhibiting the conversion of angiotensin I to angiotensin II. ARBs block the actions of angiotensin II at the type 1 (AT_1) angiotensin receptor. Activation of AT_1 receptors by angiotensin II causes potent vasoconstriction, increasing peripheral resistance. Within the glomerular circulation, angiotensin II preferentially constricts efferent arterioles to preserve glomerular pressure and maintain GFR when renal blood flow is compromised. In the clinical settings described earlier, ACE inhibitors cause ARF by reducing systemic blood pressure while simultaneously reducing glomerular pressure through the fall in postglomerular, efferent arteriolar resistance. As with other forms of drug-induced hemodynamic renal insufficiency, kidney function usually returns to baseline when the ACE inhibitor or ARB is discontinued.

Intrarenal Acute Renal Failure: Acute Tubular Necrosis and Acute Interstitial Nephritis Caused by Drugs

Drug-induced ARF from intrarenal mechanisms can be divided into two entities with distinct clinical and pathophysiologic characteristics: acute tubular necrosis (ATN) and acute interstitial nephritis (AIN). ATN associated with drug administration shares many of the clinical features of ATN from other causes. This form of ARF can be seen after administration of agents that are primarily excreted by the kidney, such as aminoglycoside antibiotics, amphotericin B, and chemotherapeutic agents such as cisplatin. Nephrotoxicity usually reflects the direct toxic effects of the compound on renal tubular cells, although hemodynamic mechanisms may play a role. In this setting, the onset of ARF is often nonoliguric and may be slow to develop. If nephrotoxicity is not detected and administration of the causative agent is continued, oliguric ARF may develop. The urinalysis is characteristically bland and may show modest proteinuria, tubular epithelial cells, and noncellular casts. Tubular toxicity usually abates after the offending agent is discontinued, although there may be a lag before complete recovery of renal function occurs. However, chronic, irreversible renal impairment may result from repetitive exposure to tubular toxins.

In AIN, drug exposure causes ARF through a syndrome of intrarenal inflammation. This disorder is described in Chapter 45 and is characterized by inflammatory cell infiltration of the renal interstitium with a reduced GFR and renal blood flow. Systemic signs of hypersensitivity, including rash, arthralgias, and fever, may occur. The urinalysis reflects active renal inflammation, and the urine usually contains red blood cells, white blood cells, and occasional cellular casts along with nonglomerular levels of proteinuria. Eosinophiluria can also be observed. Common causative agents include penicillins, cephalosporins, sulfonamide analogues, rifampin, and NSAIDs. AIN usually resolves after the offending agent is removed.

These drugs, which are significantly more expensive than conventional amphotericin, cause fewer constitutional symptoms, such as fever and chills, while retaining antifungal activity. Their renal toxicity, as indicated by increased serum creatinine levels, appears to be less than with other preparations.

Antiviral Drugs

Acyclovir

Acyclovir is an effective and relatively nontoxic antiviral agent that is widely used to treat herpesvirus infections. When given by the oral route, acyclovir is essentially devoid of significant renal toxicity. However, nephrotoxicity has been described in a small number of patients who have received intravenous courses of acyclovir, particularly at high doses (>500 mg/m^2). Acyclovir undergoes tubular secretion in the kidney, and renal tissue levels increase substantially during treatment. The mechanism of ARF is thought to be precipitation of the relatively insoluble drug within tubular lumens, causing obstruction. The urine sediment may contain red blood cells, white blood cells, and needle-shaped birefringent crystals.

Renal failure usually resolves when the acyclovir is discontinued. Risk factors for toxicity are volume depletion and bolus administration of the drug, but ARF has been observed even with adequate fluid repletion and the use of continuous infusion protocols.

Pentamidine

Approximately 25% of patients treated with pentamidine experience a reversible decrease in the GFR. Nephrotoxicity with pentamidine may be more common in patients with acquired immunodeficiency syndrome (AIDS), and it has been associated with significant hyperkalemia. Although the incidence of renal problems is reduced with inhaled preparations, reduced renal function has been reported as a complication of aerosolized pentamidine. Nonetheless, a specific role for pentamidine is often difficult to identify because of the presence of other drugs or comorbid conditions that also can affect kidney function.

Drugs for Treating Human Immunodeficiency Virus Infection

Patients infected with HIV have an increased risk for developing ARF. This is related in part to HIV infection and its secondary infectious complications. In addition, several of the drugs commonly used to control HIV infection can cause ARF directly or indirectly (see Table 29-2 in Chapter 29). Crystal nephropathy with obstruction caused by deposition of insoluble crystals in the kidney has been observed with indinavir. Moreover, adefovir and tenofovir have been associated with the development of proximal tubule injury with Fanconi's syndrome and ATN. The mechanism of toxicity seems to involve direct inhibition of mitochondrial function. Finally, the antiretroviral drug zidovudine has been associated with severe myopathy and rhabdomyolysis.

Radiocontrast Agents

The administration of radiocontrast agents is a frequent cause of nephrotoxic AKI, accounting for up to 10% of cases among hospitalized patients. Variations in the reported incidence of contrast nephropathy from published studies seem to be related to differences in the criteria for defining the syndrome, the period of observation after contrast administration, and the prevalence of risk factors in the population studied. The major risk factors are listed in **Table 34-3**. Preexisting reduced kidney function is the most important and best-documented risk factor, and significant contrast-induced nephropathy is rare in patients with normal kidney function.

The vasoactive effects of radiocontrast contribute to the pathogenesis of nephropathy. In animals, contrast injection initially causes vasodilatation of the renal circulation, followed by intense and persistent vasoconstriction. The cause of this vasoconstrictive phase is not clear, but it may include reduced production of vasodilator prostaglandins, enhanced endothelin release, or changes in intracellular calcium levels. Patients with contrast nephrotoxicity typically develop an increased serum creatinine level within 24 hours after radiocontrast administration that peaks within 3 to 4 days. Radiocontrast nephropathy is typically nonoliguric, but it can be associated with oliguria in severe cases. The urinary sediment is unremarkable, and, in contrast to many other forms of drug-induced ARF, the fractional excretion of sodium is typically very low ($<1\%$), reflecting the hemodynamic component of renal impairment.

The typical patient with radiocontrast nephropathy develops a mild, transient reduction in kidney function. Clinically significant kidney dysfunction is less common, but a few patients may require acute dialysis. Because radiographic studies usually are planned in advance, the clinician's efforts should be directed toward prevention of contrast nephropathy by avoiding unnecessary studies, particularly in patients with risk factors. In the high-risk patient, alternate approaches to imaging should be considered. However, because of reported associations between gadolinium administration and the development of nephrogenic systemic

TABLE 34-3 **Risk Factors for Development of Acute Renal Failure after Radiocontrast Administration**

Preexisting renal dysfunction
Diabetic nephropathy
Severe congestive heart failure
Volume depletion
Elderly age group
Multiple myeloma
Large volumes of radiocontrast
Concomitant treatment with ACE inhibitors, NSAIDs, or exposure to other nephrotoxins

ACE, angiotensin-converting enzyme; NSAIDs, nonsteroidal anti-inflammatory drugs.

fibrosis, magnetic resonance imaging with gadolinium should be avoided as an alternative approach in patients with preexisting impairment of kidney function (see Chapter 5).

If contrast administration is unavoidable, the amount of contrast used during the study should be kept to a minimum, and concomitant administration of other nephrotoxic agents should be avoided. Low-osmolality radiocontrast agents may provide some benefit in reducing risks for nephrotoxicity in patients with preexisting renal insufficiency. Hypovolemia should be corrected, and medications such as NSAIDs should be discontinued. In patients who are not hypervolemic, current data favor a trial of modest volume expansion. One common protocol is to infuse saline intravenously at a rate of 1 mL per kilogram of body weight per hour, beginning 12 hours before the procedure and continuing for an additional 12 hours afterward. In this circumstance, 0.9% saline appears to provide more benefit than 0.45% saline. Saline infusion regimens provide better protection against acute impairment of renal function than hydration plus mannitol or furosemide.

Other agents have been tested for potential benefits in preventing radiocontrast nephropathy. In two randomized clinical studies, *N*-acetylcysteine ameliorated the rise in serum creatinine concentration after radiocontrast administration, but it did not alter the development of severe ARF. Another study suggested that isotonic bicarbonate infused for 1 hour before contrast administration and 6 hours afterward might have added benefits compared with hydration with sodium chloride. However, some subsequent analyses failed to confirm the benefits of *N*-acetylcysteine and bicarbonate. Likewise, clinical trials of other agents, such as dopamine, fenoldopam, and atrial natriuretic peptide, failed to demonstrate clearcut benefits in preventing severe radiocontrast nephropathy. Prophylactic hemodialysis does not appear to be beneficial as a preventive measure. In the absence of definitive studies, most clinicians recommend prehydration with isotonic saline or bicarbonate solution, as described previously, and many also use *N*-acetylcysteine. Although the benefit of the latter has not been established conclusively, the drug is well tolerated and is relatively inexpensive.

Calcineurin Inhibitor Immunosuppressive Drugs

Cyclosporine and tacrolimus are immunosuppressive agents that inhibit the early events involved in T-cell activation, effectively suppressing transplant rejection. These agents have distinct chemical structures; cyclosporine is a cyclic peptide, and tacrolimus is a macrolide. Despite these marked structural differences, they have identical mechanisms of action. Both compounds produce potent inhibition of calcineurin, an intracellular phosphatase that plays a central role in coordinating T-cell activation by foreign antigens. Based on their efficacy as antirejection therapies, calcineurin inhibitors are the cornerstone of immunosuppressive regimens for patients with virtually every type of organ graft. However, the frequent occurrence of nephrotoxicity and the

concern about the potential for developing chronic, irreversible renal injury have complicated their clinical use.

The clinical manifestations of nephrotoxicity are similar for cyclosporine and tacrolimus, consisting of acute, reversible renal dysfunction and chronic interstitial nephropathy. Acute nephrotoxicity is the predominant renal abnormality seen within the first 6 to 12 months after initiating treatment, and it is characterized by an acute or subacute reduction in renal function that is often dose dependent. Generally, renal dysfunction is nonprogressive and remits when the dose is lowered or the drug is discontinued. Almost every patient who receives therapeutic doses of a calcineurin inhibitor experiences a component of persistent, reversible reduction in the GFR and renal blood flow. The mechanism of this acute nephrotoxicity is hemodynamic and results from the ability of these agents to induce intense renal vasoconstriction. Calcineurin inhibitors do not cause renal vasoconstriction directly, but they may act by stimulating production of other vasoconstrictor compounds, such as thromboxane A_2, endothelin, and leukotrienes.

In renal transplant recipients within the first year after transplantation, it is often difficult to differentiate acute nephrotoxicity from acute rejection. A stable or slowly progressive increase in serum creatinine concentration that reverses when the cyclosporine or tacrolimus dose is reduced suggests nephrotoxicity. Renal biopsy can be helpful in this setting. Aggressive inflammatory cell infiltrates are usually absent in acute nephrotoxicity, and their presence in a biopsy specimen suggests ongoing rejection. Conversely, findings characteristic of calcineurin inhibitor toxicity, such as isometric tubular vacuolization, favor a diagnosis of drug toxicity. Although serum drug levels frequently are used to monitor therapeutic efficacy and to prevent toxicity, there is only a rough correlation between conventional serum levels and clinical events.

Chronic nephrotoxicity is defined by the development of interstitial fibrosis with a reduced GFR in patients receiving long-term treatment with calcineurin inhibitors. The clinical features of chronic calcineurin inhibitor nephrotoxicity are well characterized. Usually, 6 to 12 months of treatment is required before signs of chronic nephropathy become apparent. Because of the irreversible nature of the morphologic abnormalities, this form of toxicity is more ominous than the acute form. Histologically, chronic nephrotoxicity is characterized by focal or striped medullary interstitial fibrosis. These alterations often are accompanied by tubular atrophy and obliterative arteriolar changes. In more advanced cases, diffuse interstitial fibrosis with focal and segmental glomerular sclerosis can be seen. In renal transplant recipients, these changes may be difficult to differentiate from the typical features of chronic allograft nephropathy. Although the mechanism of chronic nephrotoxicity is unknown, it is likely that cumulative dose, arterial hypertension, and immunologic injury contribute to the development of the lesion. Animal studies suggest that severe sodium depletion may potentiate the development of renal fibrosis associated with the administration of calcineurin inhibitors.

Cyclosporine and tacrolimus are metabolized primarily by the action of hepatic cytochrome P-450 (CYP) microsomal enzymes. Agents that influence the activity of this enzyme system can cause significant changes in their metabolism. In general, drugs or substances that reduce the rate of calcineurin inhibitor metabolism, such as erythromycin, clarithromycin, azole antifungal agents, non-dihydropyridine calcium channel blockers, and grapefruit juice, produce increased serum levels and can potentiate nephrotoxicity. However, agents that increase CYP activity, such as phenytoin, phenobarbital, rifampin, and St. John's wort, may reduce serum levels and thereby blunt therapeutic efficacy and precipitate rejection episodes.

Lithium

Because of its superior efficacy, lithium has been a cornerstone of therapy for bipolar disorders since the 1950s. However, it has a narrow therapeutic index and a number of problematic toxicities affecting a range of organ systems, including the kidney. The major route of excretion is the kidney, where lithium is handled much like sodium. The most common renal complication of lithium therapy is diabetes insipidus, which is manifested by polyuria, polydipsia, and an inability to concentrate urine normally in as many as 20% to 30% of patients. Lithium interferes with the actions of antidiuretic hormone to increase water permeability in the distal nephron. This effect occurs through inhibition of the generation or actions of cyclic adenosine monophosphate (cAMP), which decreases expression and attenuates apical targeting of aquaporin-2 water channels in renal epithelial cells. The polyuria caused by lithium typically is resistant to exogenous vasopressin agonists and represents a nephrogenic form of diabetes insipidus. Although this condition usually improves when lithium is discontinued, treatment with amiloride can mitigate the lithium effect by blocking lithium uptake in the collecting duct. This can effectively increase urinary osmolality and reduce urine volume in patients with diabetes insipidus who must continue on lithium therapy.

A more ominous form of renal toxicity associated with lithium is chronic interstitial nephritis, which clinically manifests as an insidious loss of renal function without significant proteinuria. Characteristic pathologic features include tubular atrophy and interstitial fibrosis that is out of proportion to the degree of glomerulosclerosis or vascular disease. Cortical and medullary tubular cysts are commonly seen, and these microcysts can be detected with noninvasive studies such as magnetic resonance imaging or ultrasound. The propensity for lithium to cause progressive chronic kidney disease has been a controversial issue. However, several studies have documented a slow reduction of GFR with time, and progression to end-stage renal disease has been reported in a small number of patients. Although renal function may improve in some patients after cessation of lithium, continued irreversible renal dysfunction with progression may be observed despite discontinuing therapy. Therefore, patients who require long-term lithium treatment should have frequent monitoring of their kidney function and careful attention to maintaining therapeutic serum lithium levels.

Acute lithium intoxication is a life-threatening emergency manifested by a range of systemic symptoms from nausea and tremor to seizures and coma; ATN also may occur. The severity of lithium intoxication correlates reasonably well with serum lithium concentrations for mild (1.5 to 2.5 mEq/L), moderate (2.5 to 3.5 mEq/L), and severe (>3.5 mEq/L) forms. However, patients may have significant symptoms when levels are within the therapeutic range. Along with gastric lavage and protection of the airway, saline should be administered to reverse extracellular fluid volume deficits and to induce diuresis, thereby facilitating lithium excretion. Lithium is efficiently removed by hemodialysis, which can reduce plasma lithium levels by about 1 mEq/L per 4-hour treatment. Hemodialysis is indicated in patients with severe neurologic symptoms or renal failure, and it should be considered for any patient with a serum level greater than 4.0 mEq/L.

Antineoplastic Agents and Cancer-Related Metabolic Derangements

Several compounds used in the treatment of cancer may be toxic to the kidney, and treatment of certain types of tumors with chemotherapy can cause kidney damage through tumor lysis syndrome and acute uric acid nephropathy. As with other nephrotoxic drugs, recognizing and anticipating the potential for renal injury is critical so that appropriate preventative measures may be implemented. A representative list of antineoplastic agents that affect the kidney is provided in **Table 34-4**. In the following sections, the renal effects of four commonly used antitumor drugs are discussed along with the syndrome of acute urate nephropathy.

Cisplatin

Cis-diamminedichloroplatinum II (cisplatin) is a very effective antineoplastic agent with a broad range of activity against a number of malignancies. Cisplatin also has a substantial capacity for nephrotoxicity. The drug is primarily excreted by the kidney, where it is concentrated in glomerular ultrafiltrate and accumulates in renal tubular epithelium. Tubular injury seems to be mediated by direct effects on epithelial cell metabolism and by the generation of free oxygen radicals. The development of cisplatin nephrotoxicity is dose related and cumulative. Although the drug can cause reversible ARF, irreversible decline of renal function associated with repeated cisplatin administration is the most problematic clinical manifestation of toxicity. The development of chronic cisplatin injury may be associated with dense interstitial fibrosis. Another common sequela of cisplatin-induced tubular injury is renal magnesium wasting that often produces clinically significant hypomagnesemia. Hypomagnesemia may be exacerbated by concomitant administration of aminoglycoside antibiotics, and it may persist for months after cisplatin has been discontinued.

TABLE 34-4 Nephrotoxicity of Selected Antineoplastic Agents

DRUG	CLINICAL SYNDROME
Alkylating Agents	
Cisplatin	Tubular injury, acute and chronic renal failure, renal Mg^{2+} wasting
Carboplatin	Less nephrotoxicity than cisplatin
Cyclophosphamide	Hemorrhagic cystitis, hyponatremia
Streptozotocin	Acute renal failure, tubular dysfunction
Antibiotics	
Mitomycin C	Hemolytic uremic syndrome
Mithramycin	Acute tubular necrosis
Antimetabolites	
Methotrexate	Acute renal failure with high-dose therapy
Cytosine arabinoside (ara-C)	Interstitial nephritis
5-Fluorouracil (5-FU)	Acute renal failure
Gemcitabine	Thrombotic microangiopathy
Biologic Response Modifiers	
Interleukin 2 (IL-2)	Hemodynamically mediated acute renal failure
Antiangiogenic Agents	
Bevacizumab	Proteinuria, thrombotic microangiopathy

Maneuvers that increase urine volume during cisplatin administration reduce the risk of nephrotoxicity. Vigorous intravenous fluid administration is indicated for prophylaxis. Increasing urine flow may prevent cisplatin toxicity by limiting the duration of contact between the drug and the renal epithelium. Because increasing the extracellular chloride concentration may inhibit the conversion of cisplatin to a more toxic metabolite, inclusion of isotonic sodium chloride in hydration protocols has been advocated. Infusions of mannitol also seem to be effective. Fluids should be administered to maintain urine flows of at least 100 mL/hr, and preferably greater than 200 ml/hr, for 12 hours before and 12 to 18 hours after cisplatin is administered. Second-generation platinum compounds such as carboplatin appear to have a reduced potential for nephrotoxicity, but renal failure and hypomagnesemia have been observed with carboplatin.

Cyclophosphamide

Cyclophosphamide is widely used for treating lymphomas and other hematologic malignancies. Its common adverse effects are bone marrow suppression, gastrointestinal toxicity, and hemorrhagic cystitis. Hyponatremia has been observed with high doses of cyclophosphamide ($\geq$50 mg/kg). High doses of cyclophosphamide inhibit renal water excretion, causing increased urine osmolality in the presence of reduced plasma osmolality. Because vasopressin levels are not elevated, the defective water handling appears to be a direct effect of the drug on the distal nephron. Although this defect generally resolves within 24 hours after drug administration, hypotonic fluids should not be included as a part of the intravenous fluid regimens administered to prevent bladder hemorrhage.

Methotrexate

Methotrexate is an antimetabolite that is used to treat a variety of solid tumors and leukemias. In the absence of preexisting renal dysfunction, nephrotoxicity is uncommon with standard doses of methotrexate. However, significant nephrotoxicity has been observed with high-dose methotrexate regimens. Intratubular precipitation of the drug causing obstruction may contribute to renal dysfunction. In addition, methotrexate has direct toxic effects on renal epithelial cells. Fluid administration to achieve urine volumes of more than 3 L/day reduces the potential for nephrotoxicity. Because the solubility of methotrexate and its metabolites is increased in alkaline solutions, alkalinization of urine during drug administration is recommended.

Bevacizumab

Bevacizumab is a monoclonal antibody against VEGF, a critical factor regulating blood vessel growth. Bevacizumab is a potent inhibitor of angiogenesis that is effective in the treatment of a wide range of cancers, including carcinoma of the colon, lung, breast, and kidney. Proteinuria and hypertension have been observed in a number of patients given bevacizumab. Nephrotic-range proteinuria has been reported in up to 1% to 2% of patients receiving the drug, and several case series have suggested that thrombotic microangiopathy may be a relatively common pathologic lesion in this setting. Hypertension with bevacizumab treatment occurs with a greater frequency than proteinuria, in up to 30% of patients in some series, and it may have a different pathogenesis. Because several inhibitors of the VEGF pathway are under development and bevacizumab use is expanding rapidly, the causes and long-term renal consequences of inhibiting VEGF actions require further scrutiny.

Acute Uric Acid Nephropathy

Acute urate nephropathy is most commonly seen in patients with tumor lysis syndrome. Tumor lysis syndrome is defined by the metabolic complications of rapid tumor cell turnover and dramatic lysis of tumor cells associated with antineoplastic treatment. It is characterized by hyperuricemia, hyperkalemia, hyperphosphatemia, and acidosis. Although tumor lysis syndrome may arise with a variety of tumor types, it occurs most commonly with poorly differentiated lymphomas such as Burkitt's lymphoma or with leukemias such as acute lymphoblastic leukemia. Rarely, this disorder may develop spontaneously, but most cases are associated with administration of chemotherapy.

Uric acid is the final end product of purine metabolism in humans. Serum uric acid levels increase dramatically in tumor lysis syndrome as a consequence of enhanced nucleoprotein turnover and the obligatory increase in purine nucleotide metabolism. Because uric acid is relatively insoluble in urine at acid pH, the subsequent marked increase in uric acid excretion results in precipitation of uric acid crystals within tubules, causing intranephron obstruction, oliguria, and ARF. Markedly elevated serum uric acid levels and uric acid crystalluria are typical clinical features of acute urate nephropathy. However, because uric acid excretion depends on glomerular filtration, an elevated serum uric acid concentration alone is not a useful predictor of acute urate nephropathy in the general population of patients with AKI. Alternatively, it has been suggested that a uric acid-to-creatinine ratio greater than 1 mg/mg in urine may be more indicative of this disorder.

Because acute urate nephropathy most commonly occurs after chemotherapy, major efforts should be directed toward prevention, beginning with the identification of high-risk patients. Because enhanced production of urate is a key feature in the pathogenesis of this disorder, the xanthine oxidase inhibitor allopurinol should be administered before starting chemotherapy. The risk for intrarenal precipitation of urate also can be reduced by increasing the urine flow rate and by alkalinizing the urine. Fluid deficits should be replaced and saline diuresis induced with intravenous fluids containing sodium bicarbonate. Uricosuric agents, including radiocontrast agents, should be avoided. In patients who develop ARF with indications for dialysis, hemodialysis and continuous venovenous hemodialysis can effectively remove urate, whereas clearance by peritoneal dialysis is much less efficient.

Unlike most other mammals, humans lack the enzyme uricase, which metabolizes uric acid to allantoin, a highly soluble and nontoxic compound. Accordingly, a recombinant uricase preparation, rasburicase, has been developed as an alternative approach for prevention and treatment of acute urate nephropathy. This preparation has been found to be safe and effective and is approved for prevention of tumor lysis syndrome in pediatric patients. Case reports have suggested that it may also be beneficial in patients who have established acute urate nephropathy and AKI.

Sodium Phosphate Cathartic Agents

Oral sodium phosphate solutions (OSPS) are widely prescribed for bowel preparation before colonoscopy because of their tolerability, low cost, and efficacy. However, it has become apparent that these agents can cause AKI in a subgroup of susceptible individuals. The mechanism of injury is related to transient elevation of serum phosphorous levels that, in extreme cases, results in deposition of calcium phosphate crystals in the kidney. In patients who develop AKI with OSPS, typical renal pathologic characteristics include signs of tubular injury with diffuse tubular deposits of calcium phosphate and interstitial inflammation. Based on the cause and pathologic appearance, this syndrome has been called *acute phosphate nephropathy*.

Although millions of individuals undergo screening colonoscopies in the United States each year, the precise incidence of acute phosphate nephropathy is not clear. Retrospective, observational studies suggest that age, female sex, excessive doses of OSPS, and concomitant use of ACE inhibitors and NSAIDs may be associated with increased risk. Renal functional impairment is often reversible, but persistent chronic kidney injury has been observed, with progression to end-stage renal disease in a few patients. Because most cases of OSPS-associated AKI occur in the setting of elective colonoscopy, prevention is critical. Preventive measures include an emphasis on adequate hydration, increased intervals between OSPS administration, appropriate dose reductions, and use of alternative agents such as polyethylene glycol in high-risk groups, including elderly patients and patients with chronic kidney disease.

BIBLIOGRAPHY

Bates DW, Su L, Yu DT, et al: Correlates of acute renal failure in patients receiving parenteral amphotericin B. Kidney Int 60:1452-1459, 2001.

Daugas E, Rougier JP, Hill G: HAART-related nephropathies in HIV-infected patients. Kidney Int 67:393-403, 2005.

Davidson MD, Thakkar S, Hix JK, et al: Pathophysiology, clinical consequences, and treatment of tumor lysis syndrome. Am J Med 116:546-554, 2004.

DeMattos AM, Olyei AJ, Bennett WM: Nephrotoxicity of immunosuppressive drugs: Long term consequences and challenges for the future. Am J Kidney Dis 35:333-346, 2000.

Deray G: Amphotericin B nephrotoxicity. J Antimicrob Chemother 49(Suppl S1):37-41, 2002.

Izzedine H, Isnard-Bagnis C, Launay-Vacher V, et al: Gemcitabine-induced thrombotic microangiopathy: A systematic review. Nephrol Dial Transplant 21:3038-3045, 2006.

Ermina V, Jefferson A, Kowalewska J, et al: VEGF inhibition and renal thrombotic microangiopathy. N Engl J Med 358:1129-1136, 2008.

Fishbane S: N-Acetylcysteine in the prevention of contrast-induced nephropathy. Clin J Am Soc Nephrol 3:281-287, 2008.

Humphreys BD, Soiffer RJ, Magee CC: Renal failure associated with cancer and its treatment: an update. J Am Soc Nephrol 16:151-161, 2005.

Hurst FP, Bohen EM, Osgard EM, et al: Association of oral sodium phosphate purgative use with acute kidney injury. J Am Soc Nephrol 18:3192-3198, 2007.

Kaloyanides GJ: Antibiotic-related nephrotoxicity. Nephrol Dial Transplant 9(Suppl 4):130-134, 1994.

Katzberg RW, Haller C: Contrast-induced nephrotoxicity: Clinical landscape. Kidney Int 69:S3-S7, 2006.

Markowitz GS, Stokes MB, Radhakrishnan J, D'Agati VD: Acute phosphate nephropathy following oral sodium phosphate bowel purgative: An underrecognized cause of chronic renal failure. J Am Soc Nephrol 16:3389-3396, 2005.

Merten GJ, Burgess WP, Gray LV, et al: Prevention of contrast-induced nephropathy with sodium bicarbonate: A randomized control trial. JAMA 291:2328-2334, 2004.

Meyer KB, Madias NE: Cisplatin nephrotoxicity. Miner Electrolyte Metab 20:201-213, 1994.

Murphy SW, Barrett BJ, Parfrey PS: Contrast nephropathy. J Am Soc Nephrol 11:177-182, 2000.

Perazella MA, Rodby RA: Gadolinium-induced nephrogenic systemic fibrosis in patients with kidney disease. Am J Med 120:561-562, 2007.

Presne C, Fakhouri F, Noel LH, et al: Lithium-induced nephropathy: Rate of progression and prognostic factors. Kidney Int 64:585-592, 2003.

Reis F, Klastersky J: Nephrotoxicity induced by cancer chemotherapy with special emphasis on cisplatin. Am J Kidney Dis 8:368-379, 1986.

Robinson RF, Nahata MC: A comparative review of conventional and lipid formulations of amphotericin B. J Clin Pharm Ther 24:249-257, 1999.

Solomon R, Werner C, Mann D, et al: Effects of saline, mannitol, and furosemide on acute decreases in renal function induced by radiocontrast agents. N Engl J Med 331:1416-1420, 1994.

Swan SK: Aminoglycoside nephrotoxicity. Semin Nephrol 17:27-33, 1997.

Tepel M, van der Giet M, Schwazfeld C, et al: Prevention of radiographic contrast agent-induced reductions in renal function by acetylcysteine. N Engl J Med 343:180-184, 2000.

Timmer RT, Sands JM: Lithium intoxication. J Am Soc Nephrol 10:666-674, 1999.

Tune BM, Hsu C-Y, Fravert D: Cephalosporin and carbacephem nephrotoxicity: Roles of tubular cell uptake and acylating potential. Biochem Pharmacol 51:557-561, 1996.

Weisbord SD, Palevsky PM: Prevention of contrast-induced nephropathy with volume expansion. Clin J Am Soc Nephrol 3:273-280, 2008.

CHAPTER 35

Cholesterol Atheroembolic Kidney Disease

Arthur Greenberg

Cholesterol atheroembolic kidney disease results when cholesterol crystals and other debris separate from atheromatous plaques, flow downstream, and lodge in small renal arteries, producing luminal occlusion, ischemia, and kidney dysfunction. Depending on the source and distribution of emboli, kidney disease may be the sole or predominant manifestation or only one feature of a systemic illness characterized by multiorgan ischemia or infarction. Early, autopsy-derived descriptions of renal atheroembolism overemphasized a catastrophic presentation with irreversible kidney failure, intestinal infarction, and death from intra-abdominal sepsis. Atheroembolism can also lead to occult or reversible declines in kidney function. Recovery of function may follow extended survival on renal replacement therapy.

PATHOLOGY

The initial lesion in cholesterol atheroembolism is obstruction of a medium-sized or small artery by atheromatous debris. Arterioles and capillaries are less commonly affected. Lesions may occur in any organ. Cholesterol dissolves during routine processing of tissue for histologic examination; crystals are not seen in tissue sections unless special fixatives are used. However, a characteristic cleft marks the space formerly occupied by the needle-like crystals (**Fig. 35-1**). The size of the artery affected is typically about 200 μm, but it can range from 55 to 900 μm. The earliest lesion consists of cholesterol crystals and thrombi. After dissolution of the thrombi, macrophages engulf the cholesterol, but the predominant reaction is endothelial. New endothelium covers the crystals. If the vessel wall is eroded by the crystals, an intense perivascular inflammatory response with giant cells is established (see **Fig. 35-1**). Concentric fibrosis, particularly involving the adventitia, occurs later. There is recanalization of small vascular channels. Crystal dissolution in vivo is slow; in experimental models, cholesterol clefts persist as long as 9 months after embolization. Although crystals may reach the glomerular capillary loops (**Fig. 35-2**), the principal glomerular finding is ischemia with glomerular collapse and basement membrane wrinkling. Focal segmental glomerulosclerosis with glomerular collapse and epithelial cell prominence may occur. These findings account for some of the atheroembolism cases associated with nephrotic range proteinuria. Antineutrophil cytoplasmic antibody (ANCA)-positive pauci-immune crescentic glomerulonephritis has been reported in a few patients who also had biopsy evidence of atheroembolism.

PATHOGENESIS

In his classic autopsy description, Flory observed cholesterol atheroembolism solely in patients with erosive plaques. The prevalence of atheroembolism paralleled the severity of aortic disease. Less severe atherosclerotic lesions or plaques covered by thrombus do not pose a risk of atheroembolism.

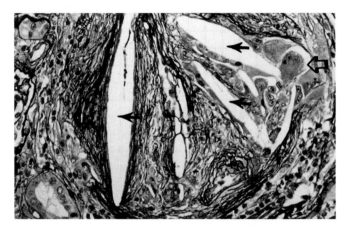

FIGURE 35-1 A cholesterol atheroembolus occludes the lumen of an interlobular renal artery. Needle-like clefts (*solid arrows*) can be seen, along with a macrophage–multinucleated giant cell reaction (*open arrow*) (methenamine silver–trichrome stain, original magnification ×450). (Courtesy of Dr. S. I. Bastacky. From Greenberg A, Bastacky SI, Iqbal A, et al: Focal segmental glomerulosclerosis associated with nephrotic syndrome in cholesterol atheroembolism: Clinicopathologic correlations. Am J Kidney Dis 29:334-344, 1997, with permission.)

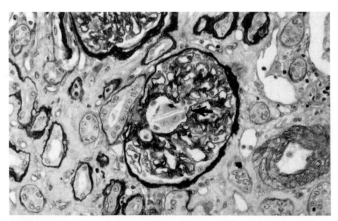

FIGURE 35-2 The glomerulus has cholesterol clefts at the hilum (*arrow*). The remainder of the glomerulus shows capillary loop thickening and wrinkling caused by ischemia. Adjacent tubules show acute ischemic injury (hematoxylin-eosin stain, original magnification ×250). (Courtesy of Dr. S. I. Bastacky.)

TABLE 35-1 Risk Factors for Cholesterol Atheroembolic Kidney Disease

Iatrogenic Embolization

Manipulation of the Aorta Proximal to the Renal Arteries

Angiography or angioplasty

Aortic aneurysm repair

Aortic aneurysm or other endovascular stenting

Coronary artery bypass grafting

Cardiac valve surgery

Intra-aortic balloon pump circulatory augmentation

Other causes

Anticoagulation or Thrombolytic Therapy

Heparin

Low-molecular-weight heparin

Warfarin

Tissue plasminogen activator

Streptokinase

Urokinase

Spontaneous Embolization

Severe ulcerating atherosclerosis

TABLE 35-2 Associated Findings in 354 Patients with Cholesterol Atheroembolism

ASSOCIATED FINDINGS	PERCENTAGE OF CASES
Hypertension	83
Male gender	83
Chronic kidney disease (stage ≥3)	82
Smoking history	70
Coronary artery disease	62
Peripheral vascular disease	58
Cerebrovascular disease	34
Congestive heart failure	30
Diabetes mellitus	18

Modified from Scolari F, Ravani P, Gaggi R, et al: The challenge of diagnosing atheroembolic renal disease: Clinical features and prognostic factors. Circulation 116;298-304, 2007.

TABLE 35-3 Histologic Involvement of Cholesterol Atheroembolic Kidney Disease Found at Autopsy

ORGAN	PERCENTAGE OF CASES
Kidney	75
Spleen	52
Pancreas	52
Gastrointestinal tract	31
Adrenal glands	20
Liver	17
Brain	14
Skin	6

Embolization may be spontaneous, particularly with severe aortic disease, but mechanical disruption of plaque during angiographic or surgical procedures, including conventional and endovascular aortic aneurysm repair, usually precedes it. **Table 35-1** lists predisposing factors. Irrespective of the area primarily targeted for imaging, passage of a catheter along the ascending or descending aorta proximal to the renal arteries confers a risk of embolization to the kidneys. Renal artery angioplasty or revascularization may pose a particular risk, and patients who develop atheroembolism in this setting have worsened outcomes. The site of any concurrent nonrenal embolization depends on the path of the catheter.

Thrombus overlying atheromatous plaque can bind and immobilize friable debris. Anticoagulation or thrombolysis removes this protective covering. Atheroembolism has been reported after heparin, warfarin, or thrombolytic therapy without angiography.

CLINICAL FEATURES

As expected of a process that complicates severe atherosclerosis, risk factors for atherosclerosis and evidence of disseminated atherosclerotic disease are commonly present. Most patients have a history of tobacco abuse, and the incidence is higher in tobacco users. Up to 83% of patients are male. The mean age of patients at diagnosis is in the mid-60s. Fewer than 5% of patients are younger than 50 years old. **Table 35-2** lists other accompanying or predisposing features. Notably, diabetes mellitus is a feature of only 2.5% to 31% of reported cases. In a large, prospective study of patients undergoing cardiac catheterization, among the 1.4% of patients who

developed cholesterol atheroembolism, multivariate analysis identified an increased C-reactive protein level, presence of an aortic aneurysm, smoking, hypertension, multivessel coronary artery disease, and acute coronary syndrome as predisposing factors.

The severity of cholesterol atheroembolism varies, and manifestations of the disorder depend on the extent of renal involvement and the extrarenal sites affected. The frequency of organ involvement is summarized in **Table 35-3**. Massive and widespread embolization in the multiple cholesterol emboli syndrome manifests catastrophically with fever, stroke, acute renal failure, abdominal pain, and gastrointestinal bleeding due to bowel infarction, intra-abdominal sepsis, and death. In contrast, spontaneous embolization can have an indolent course. Embolization during kidney transplantation may be isolated to the allograft.

Autopsy reports are skewed toward patients with severe involvement. In milder disease, kidney and cutaneous involvement predominate. Typically, the renal course is characterized by slowly deteriorating kidney function. The daily increase in serum creatinine concentration may be as little as 0.1 to 0.2 mg/dL, and progression to end-stage disease may occur over a period of 30 to 60 days or longer. Patients also may present with an insidious deterioration of kidney function occurring over many months. Some patients present with heavy proteinuria, with or without associated clinical features of atheroembolism.

The severity of skin involvement varies widely. In some patients, digital necrosis and gangrene with pain are prominent features. The classic "blue toes" lesion comprises livedo reticularis of the lower extremities caused by occlusion of small arteries and cyanosis of the toes. The distal pulses are typically preserved. In other patients, cutaneous involvement may be overlooked unless specifically sought. Livedo that is very subtle when the patient is supine can be made more conspicuous by asking the patient to dangle the feet below the bed or to stand. Features of gastrointestinal involvement include abdominal pain, anorexia, weight loss, and bleeding that can range from a positive stool test result for occult blood to brisk hemorrhage. Pancreatitis and acalculous cholecystitis may occur if emboli reach these organs. Bowel infarction and sepsis may also follow an episode of embolization. Central nervous system involvement includes stroke or diffuse cortical dysfunction due to widespread embolization and spinal cord lesions and the scotomata, field cuts, or blindness that accompany the classic, but rare, retinal Hollenhorst plaque.

DIAGNOSIS

The diagnosis of atheroembolism relies on a high index of suspicion about patients at risk. During the acute phase, patients may have leukocytosis and an elevated erythrocyte sedimentation rate. Eosinophilia is observed in 25% to 50% of affected individuals; hypocomplementemia is also reported, occurring in one study with a high prevalence. However, all of these findings are transient, and reports of their prevalence vary widely. Their absence cannot be taken as evidence to exclude the diagnosis. Hyperamylasemia suggests pancreatic involvement. Although nephrotic-range proteinuria may occur, proteinuria is typically modest and the urine sediment nonspecific.

Cholesterol atheroembolism is often confused with radiocontrast nephropathy (see Chapter 34). The course of the latter is much more rapid, a feature that permits the two to be readily distinguished. In radiocontrast nephropathy, renal failure occurs immediately, kidney function reaches a nadir within 3 to 4 days, and substantial recovery usually occurs over a similar period. In atheroembolism, the onset of renal failure may be delayed, and progression is slower. Recovery occurs after many weeks or months, if at all. A protracted episode of what appears to be radiocontrast nephropathy occurring after an arteriogram is instead probably cholesterol atheroembolism. Other disorders that can be mimicked by atheroembolic disease include ischemic acute tubular necrosis, systemic vasculitis, allergic interstitial nephritis, cryoglobulinemia, myeloma, hypertensive nephrosclerosis, and renal artery stenosis.

Most instances of cholesterol atheroembolism are diagnosed clinically, and it is not necessary to obtain biopsy confirmation when the presentation is typical. A positive biopsy is highly specific, because cholesterol clefts are never a normal finding. A kidney biopsy showing cholesterol atheroemboli is definitive, but alternative means of diagnosis or sites of biopsy should be considered first. Skin biopsy of an area of livedo reticularis has a high yield and is the least invasive approach. Muscle biopsy in a limb affected by cutaneous changes may be employed if a kidney biopsy is deemed too risky. Some cases of cholesterol atheroembolism with minimal or no extrarenal findings are diagnosed by a kidney biopsy done to evaluate unexplained acute kidney injury or chronic kidney disease.

PREVENTION

No controlled trials address prevention. Conventional measures to limit development of atherosclerosis, including smoking cessation and treatment of hypercholesterolemia with diet, statins, and other drugs, are of presumed benefit. If possible, manipulation of the vasculature and use of anticoagulants and thrombolytic drugs should be avoided. This is particularly important for secondary prevention in patients who have already sustained an episode of cholesterol atheroembolism. Embolization to the kidneys after renal arteriograms and angioplasty or stenting is well documented; this risk should be strongly considered whenever renal artery studies are contemplated. Some studies suggest a benefit from the use of downstream filter devices to protect organs at risk during aortic manipulation or catheterization.

THERAPY AND OUTCOME

Spontaneous atheroembolism occurs only in patients with more severe vascular involvement. Shedding of atheromatous debris often continues with a progressively downhill course. In patients with atheroembolism after vascular surgery or angiography, embolization may be limited to the initial episode. Stabilization and gradual improvement may follow as small-vessel inflammation subsides and recanalization with restoration of blood flow occurs. A typical patient who recovers will have gradually lessening anorexia and abdominal and digital pain with subsequent healing of digital ischemic lesions. Not surprisingly, patients with preexisting kidney function impairment have a worse prognosis for dialysis-free survival and mortality. Recent series report 1-year survival rates of 62% to 87%, in contrast to historical controls with 1-year survival rates of 19% to 36%. In an Italian series of 354 cases confirmed by biopsy or ophthalmoscopy, 23% of cases were spontaneous, and the remaining cases were iatrogenic. At 24 months of follow-up, 77% of patients were still alive, but 33% overall had required dialysis at some point, mostly within the first 4 months. Notably, 28% of initially dialysis-dependent patients recovered enough kidney function to stop dialysis at least transiently. To some extent, this striking improvement results from meticulous supportive care. Some of the improvement in survival compared with older trials reflects the availability of renal replacement therapy. Ascertainment bias and the changing cause of cholesterol atheroembolism are also responsible for some of the apparent improvement. Current cases are mainly provoked by angiography, whereas older series reported spontaneous cases with a fulminant course.

Management focuses on several issues. Patients require local care of digital ischemia, analgesia for pain, and digital amputation if tissue is not viable. Anticoagulation should be stopped and repeat angiographic procedures scrupulously avoided. Careful attention to supplemental nutrition is beneficial for patients with anorexia due to gastrointestinal tract involvement. Hemodialysis or peritoneal dialysis may be successfully employed, and up to one third of patients recover sufficient kidney function to permit discontinuation of dialysis. Several series document that the use of statins is associated with improved survival. Glucocorticoids and cytotoxic agents have been employed for patients with ANCA-positive glomerulonephritis. Low-dose glucocorticoids have been used in some patients with the rationale of diminishing vascular inflammation and improving tissue blood flow. Vasodilator prostaglandin infusions also have been used to increase blood flow. Controlled trials are lacking, and the benefit of such treatments has not been proved. Although abdominal or transesophageal ultrasonography may be used to localize diseased areas of the aorta, cholesterol atheroembolism occurs in an elderly population with extensive atherosclerotic disease and a high prevalence of hypertensive cardiovascular disease. These patients present a formidable surgical risk. The roles of endarterectomy, resection of diseased aortic segments, and use of endovascular stents to cover affected endothelial segments have not been established.

BIBLIOGRAPHY

Aviles B, Ubeda I, Blanco J, Barrientos A: Pauci-immune extracapillary glomerulonephritis and atheromatous embolization. Am J Kidney Dis 40:847-851, 2002.

Belenfant X, Meyrier A, Jacquot C: Supportive treatment improves survival in multi visceral cholesterol crystal embolism. Am J Kidney Dis 33:840-850, 1999.

Carroccio A, Olin JW, Ellosy SH, et al: The role of aortic stent grafting in the treatment of atheromatous embolization syndrome: Results after a mean of 15 months follow-up. J Vasc Surg 40:424-429, 2004.

Elinav E, Chajek-Shaul T, Stern M: Improvement in cholesterol emboli syndrome after iloprost therapy. BMJ 324:268-269, 2002.

Fine MJ, Kapoor W, Falanga V: Cholesterol crystal embolization: A review of 221 cases in the English literature. Angiology 38:769-784, 1987.

Flory CM: Arterial occlusions produced by emboli from eroded aortic atheromatous plaques. Am J Pathol 21:549-565, 1945.

Fukumoto Y, Tsutsui H, Tsuchihashi M, et al, for the Cholesterol Embolism Study (CHEST) Investigators: The incidence and risk factors of cholesterol embolization syndrome, a complication of cardiac catheterization: A prospective study. J Am Coll Cardiol 42:211-216, 2003.

Greenberg A, Bastacky SI, Iqbal A, et al: Focal segmental glomerulosclerosis associated with nephrotic syndrome in cholesterol atheroembolism: Clinicopathologic correlations. Am J Kidney Dis 29:334-344, 1997.

Kasinath BS, Corwin HL, Bidani AK, et al: Eosinophilia in the diagnosis of atheroembolic renal disease. Am J Nephrol 7:173-177, 1987.

Krishnamurthi V, Novick AC, Myles JL: Atheroembolic renal disease: Effect on morbidity and survival after revascularization for atherosclerotic renal artery stenosis. J Urol 161:1093-1096, 1999.

Lai CK, Randhawa PS: Cholesterol embolization in renal allografts. A clinicopathologic study of 12 cases. Am J Surg Pathol 31:536-545, 2007.

Meyrier A: Cholesterol crystal embolism: Diagnosis and treatment. Kidney Int 69:1308-1312, 2006.

McGowan JA, Greenberg A: Cholesterol atheroembolic renal disease. Report of 3 cases with emphasis on diagnosis by skin biopsy and extended survival. Am J Nephrol 6:135-139, 1986.

Modi KS, Rao VK: Atheroembolic renal disease. J Am Soc Nephrol 12:1781-1787, 2001.

Parodi JC, Mura RL, Ferreira LM: Safety maneuvers to prevent embolism complicating endovascular aortic repair. J Vasc Surg 36:1076-1078, 2002.

Scolari F, Ravani P, Gaggi R, et al: The challenge of diagnosing atheroembolic renal disease. Clinical features and prognostic factors. Circulation 116:298-304, 2007.

Scolari F, Ravani P, Pola A, et al: Predictors of renal and patient outcomes in atheroembolic renal disease: A prospective study. J Am Soc Nephrol 14:1584-1590, 2003.

Thadhani RI, Carmago CA, Xavier RJ, et al: Atheroembolic renal failure after invasive procedures: Natural history based on 52 histologically proven cases. Medicine (Baltimore) 74:350-358, 1995.

Tunick PA, Perez JL, Kronzon I: Protruding atheromas in the thoracic aorta and systemic embolization. Ann Intern Med 115:423-427, 1991.

CHAPTER 36

Myoglobinuric and Hemoglobinuric Acute Kidney Injury

Karl A. Nath and Narayana S. Murali

Acute kidney injury (AKI) may develop when the kidney is exposed to myoglobin, as occurs in myoglobinuria, or to hemoglobin, as occurs in hemoglobinuria. However, kidney function may be entirely unperturbed in myoglobinuria and hemoglobinuria, and not all forms of kidney dysfunction occurring in such states reflect heme pigment nephropathy.

RHABDOMYOLYSIS

Rhabdomyolysis is the syndrome arising from the loss of integrity of skeletal muscle and the release of contents of muscle into the extracellular fluid (ECF). The clinical manifestations of this disorder occupy a diverse spectrum, from asymptomatic elevation of the serum creatine kinase (CK) concentration to AKI requiring renal replacement therapy in the setting of multiorgan failure. Rhabdomyolysis accounts for 5% to 15% of all cases of AKI and is variably complicated by AKI, with the latter occurring in 5% to 50% of patients with this disease.

A fundamental contribution to the current understanding of this disorder was provided by Bywaters and Beall in their description of the crush syndrome in four patients who died during the blitz of London in 1940. These investigators noticed that the pathologic changes in the kidneys of these patients resembled those previously described in patients who died from mismatched blood transfusions, and in a series of clinical and experimental studies, they provided evidence for the pathogenetic role of myoglobin, especially in aciduric states, in damaging the kidney after muscle injury. Diverse traumatic and medical conditions are now recognized causes of rhabdomyolysis (**Table 36-1**).

Pathogenesis of Rhabdomyolysis

Most causes of rhabdomyolysis listed in Table 36-1 involve one or a combination of the following mechanisms occurring in the muscle cell: a demand for adenosine triphosphate (ATP) that outstrips the supply of ATP; increased permeability of the plasma membrane (i.e., sarcolemma); and sustained increments in calcium concentrations in the cytoplasm (i.e., sarcoplasm). In health, concentrations of sodium and calcium in the sarcoplasm are markedly lower than those in the ECF. Because the sarcoplasm is electronegative, an electrochemical gradient thus favors the intracellular influx of sodium and calcium. There is also an osmotic gradient that promotes the influx of water because of the hyperoncotic nature of the sarcoplasm. Finally, the sarcoplasm is continually exposed to intermittent elevations in calcium concentration during muscle contractions. Under these conditions, cellular homeostasis is maintained, at least in part, by the relative impermeability of the sarcolemma and by an adequate supply of ATP. ATP is required for the extracellular extrusion of sodium, the sequestration of calcium in the sarcoplasmic reticulum and mitochondria, and the extrusion of calcium from the cell.

When ATP is depleted, the attendant increase in cellular concentrations of calcium can activate assorted enzymes that damage cellular organelles and the sarcolemma. Accretion of sodium in the sarcoplasm due to depletion of ATP may lead to the intracellular movement of calcium and water, cell swelling, and cell injury. Such intracellular flux of calcium, sodium, and water can also occur when the impermeability of the sarcolemma is impaired by physical trauma or toxic substances (e.g., alcohol). Cell swelling may also be driven by the added osmotic effect of an increasing number of products from protein breakdown. Swelling of muscle is restricted by the surrounding fascia and other structures, leading to increased compartmental pressures and predisposing to muscle ischemia and necrosis (i.e., compartment syndrome). This pathogenetic sequence also accounts for the second wave of elevation of the CK concentration that follows the initial peak of CK after rhabdomyolysis.

Other mechanisms contributing to muscle injury after the original insult include the ischemia-reperfusion pathway and inflammatory processes. Both can generate oxidants, reactive nitrogen species, and diverse cytokines.

Causes of Rhabdomyolysis

Rhabdomyolysis is usually multifactorial and involves combinations of etiologic factors listed in Table 36-1. The more common causes are alcohol abuse, illicit and prescribed drugs, immobilization, trauma, seizures, and exertion. Rhabdomyolysis may recur, especially in patients with metabolic or myopathic diseases.

TABLE 36-1 Differential Diagnosis of Rhabdomyolysis

Physical Trauma to Muscle

Crush injury

Contact sports

Physical abuse

Compression (e.g., immobilization, restraint, confinement)

Inordinate or Aberrant Muscular Activity

Exercise and sports

Seizures, electroconvulsive therapy

Delirium tremens

March myoglobinuria

Movement disorders

Compromised Blood Flow to Muscle

Arterial thrombus, embolus, dissection, or clamping

Compartment syndrome

Shock

Disseminated intravascular coagulation

Capillary leak syndrome

Sickle cell disease

Multiple myeloma

Electrolyte and Metabolic Disturbances

Hypokalemia

Hypophosphatemia

Hyponatremia or hypernatremia

Hyperosmolar states

Hypothyroidism or thyroid storm

Diabetic ketoacidosis

Diabetic muscle infarction

Pheochromocytoma

Prescribed and Illicit Drugs

HMG-CoA reductase inhibitors (statins)

Fibrates

Isoniazid

Colchicine

Antihistamines

Antipsychotics

Selective serotonin reuptake inhibitors

Phenytoin

Propofol

Antimalarials

Zidovudine

Trimethoprim-sulfamethoxazole in HIV infection

Cocaine

Amphetamines

Heroin

Methadone

Phencyclidine

Dietary or Herbal Supplements

Creatine

Ephedra

Licorice

Wormwood oil

Toxins

Ethanol

Carbon monoxide

Hydrocarbons

Solvents

Toluene

Fish poisoning (e.g., Haff's disease, eating buffalo fish)

Venom (e.g., snakes, bees, spiders)

Quail poisoning

Mushroom poisoning

Deranged Temperature

Heat stroke

Hyperthermia

Burns

Electrical injury and lightning

Malignant hyperthermia

Neuroleptic malignant syndrome

Serotonergic syndrome

Saunas (e.g., after exercise, patients with sickle cell disease or trait)

Hypothermia

Frostbite

Deficiencies in Metabolic Enzymes

Glycogenolysis (e.g., myophosphorylase)

Glycolysis (e.g., phosphofructokinase)

Fat metabolism (e.g., carnitine palmitoyl transferase)

Mitochondrial metabolism (e.g., respiratory chain enzymes)

Inflammatory Conditions

Dermatomyositis and polymyositis

Vasculitis

Systemic inflammatory response syndrome

Infectious Causes

Bacterial infections (e.g., Legionnaires' disease, tularemia, toxic shock syndrome, streptococci, staphylococci, *Clostridium, Salmonella*)

Viral infections (e.g., influenza, parainfluenza, coxsackie, HIV, EBV, herpes, CMV)

Protozoal infections (e.g., *Plasmodium falciparum* malaria)

Septicemia

CMV, cytomegalovirus; EBV, Epstein-Barr virus; HIV, human immunodeficiency virus; HMG-CoA, 3-hydroxy-3-methylglutaryl-coenzyme A.

Trauma and Exertion

Muscle trauma may be obvious (e.g., after motor vehicle accidents) or less apparent (e.g., after immobilization). Muscle compression during surgical procedures can cause rhabdomyolysis and AKI, and it is recognized as a significant complication after bariatric surgery for morbid obesity.

Conditioning by regular exercise avoids the rise in the CK level that may occur after vigorous exercise in healthy individuals unused to such activity. A lack of adequate physical conditioning contributes to exertional "white collar rhabdomyolysis," which occurs in otherwise healthy individuals, usually men, who undergo intense, protracted, or recurrent bursts of exercise, especially exercise that involves eccentric (e.g., downhill running) rather than concentric (e.g., uphill running) activity. Inadequate hydration, fasting, concomitant or resolving viral infections, potassium deficiency, sickle cell disease or trait, certain muscle enzyme deficiencies, and hot and humid conditions are some of the additional risk factors for exertional rhabdomyolysis.

Potassium deficiency predisposes to exertional rhabdomyolysis for at least two reasons. First, during muscular contraction, cellular potassium is released into the ECF; by its vasorelaxant effects, the increased potassium concentration in the interstitium maintains blood flow to exercising muscle. Second, potassium stimulates glycogen synthesis, which provides a rapid supply of ATP. Enzyme deficiencies in ATP-generating pathways such as anaerobic glycolysis and oxidative phosphorylation also predispose to exertional rhabdomyolysis. Two of the more common deficiencies involve carnitine palmitoyl transferase, an enzyme that facilitates the import of fatty acids into mitochondria, and myophosphorylase, an enzyme that breaks down glycogen.

Drugs, Toxins, and Other Causes

The 3-hydroxy-3-methylglutaryl-coenzyme A (HMG-CoA) reductase inhibitors (i.e., statins) may induce asymptomatic elevations in the CK concentration, myalgia without an increase in the CK level, and frank rhabdomyolysis. Although the risk of rhabdomyolysis with cerivastatin (Baycol) led to its withdrawal, the risk of muscle injury and rhabdomyolysis with currently prescribed statins is quite low and is outweighed by the benefit of these agents. Statins may induce muscle injury through mechanisms such as impaired cell membrane integrity due to decreased cholesterol content, impaired lipid modification of proteins leading to perturbed cell signaling, and compromised mitochondrial function due to decreased mitochondrial content of ubiquinone (i.e., coenzyme Q_{10}). Supplementation with coenzyme Q_{10} may reduce myopathic symptoms associated with the use of statins. The risk for statin-induced muscle injury may be increased by the dose and type of statin employed, kidney disease, hepatic disease, hypothyroidism, the concomitant use of drugs (e.g., fibrates, cyclosporine, macrolide antibiotics), and increased intake of grapefruit juice. The potentiating effects of these compounds reflect, in part, their inhibition of metabolism

of statins by the cytochrome P-450 (CYP) system and glucuronidation. For example, cyclosporine may inhibit the CYP3A4 isozyme, whereas gemfibrozil inhibits the glucuronidation pathway.

Ethanol predisposes to rhabdomyolysis through several mechanisms, including intrinsic myotoxicity, associated malnutrition and poor caloric intake, potassium and phosphate depletion, hyperactivity and delirium tremens, trauma, and muscle compression due to unconsciousness. Illicit drugs, particularly cocaine and derivatives of amphetamines, commonly provoke rhabdomyolysis. Cocaine-induced muscle injury arises from intrinsic myotoxicity, vasoconstriction, hyperthermia, seizures, agitation and hyperactivity, and muscle compression in obtunded patients.

Rhabdomyolysis occurs in hyperthermic states, such as heat stroke, sepsis, neuroleptic malignant syndrome (inducible by butyrophenones and phenothiazines), and malignant hyperthermia. Malignant hyperthermia may be precipitated by anesthetics in patients with a genetic abnormality involving the calcium channel in the sarcoplasmic reticulum that incurs the leakage of calcium into the sarcoplasm; clinical features of this syndrome include hyperthermia, muscular rigidity, tachycardia, hypotension, and acidosis. Hyperthermia predisposes to myolysis because of direct myotoxicity and increased metabolic demand in conjunction with an inability to adequately supply ATP due to uncoupling of oxidative phosphorylation. Several mechanisms can contribute to myolysis after infectious processes, including direct muscle involvement, toxins produced by the infectious agent, cytokines elaborated in response to the infection, and employed drug therapy (e.g., zidovudine for human immunodeficiency virus [HIV] infection).

Consequences of Rhabdomyolysis

The pathophysiologic consequences of rhabdomyolysis largely reflect the release of cellular contents of muscle into the ECF and the uptake of ECF into muscle (**Fig. 36-1**). Hyperkalemia, which is often severe, commonly occurs because 70% of total body stores of potassium reside in muscle and at concentrations approximately 30-fold higher than plasma potassium. Hyperphosphatemia promotes the deposition of calcium phosphate in injured muscle, thereby contributing to hypocalcemia. Hyperuricemia reflects the generation of uric acid from purines derived from damaged muscle, whereas lactic acid and other organic acids contribute to a metabolic acidosis with an increased anion gap. The movement of large amounts of ECF into muscle induces ECF contraction and predisposes to a compartment syndrome. Hypoalbuminemia may occur, in part, from the leakage of plasma albumin across injured capillaries in muscle, and disseminated intravascular coagulation may be induced by thromboplastin from damaged muscle.

At least three mechanisms resulting from rhabdomyolysis converge on the kidney to induce pigment nephropathy: release of myoglobin, ECF depletion, and systemic acidosis or aciduria. The role of hyperuricemia in pigment nephropathy

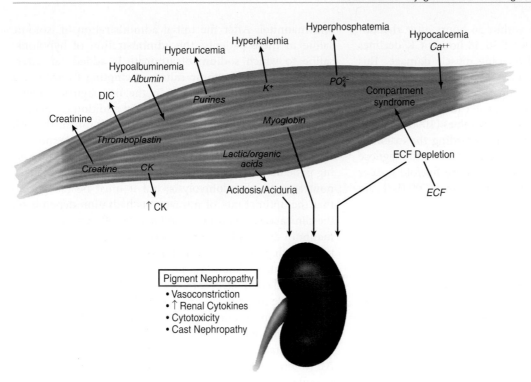

FIGURE 36-1 Complications of rhabdomyolysis occur as a consequence of either the release of muscle contents into the extracellular fluid (ECF) or the uptake of ECF into muscle. Ca^{++}, calcium; CK, creatine kinase; DIC, disseminated intravascular coagulation; K$^+$, potassium; PO$_4{}^{2-}$, phosphate. For detailed discussion, see text.

is uncertain. CK, an index of muscle damage, may not consistently predict AKI in patients with rhabdomyolysis, a finding that likely reflects the multifactorial nature of AKI in this setting.

Pathogenesis of Pigment Nephropathy

The kidney is particularly vulnerable to the toxicity of heme proteins (i.e., myoglobin and hemoglobin) for several reasons. First, renal blood flow depends on the availability of nitric oxide, and the latter is avidly scavenged by heme proteins. Second, heme proteins stimulate the production of potent renal vasoconstrictors (i.e., endothelin and isoprostanes). Third, the kidney concentrates and internalizes heme proteins. Fourth, hydrogen peroxide present in urine oxidizes heme proteins, thereby increasing their toxicity. Fifth, reduced urinary pH also denatures heme proteins and facilitates the interaction of heme proteins and Tamm-Horsfall protein to form urinary casts.

ECF depletion, acidosis, and sepsis increase the nephrotoxicity of heme proteins and thereby increase the likelihood of pigment nephropathy after rhabdomyolysis. Pigment nephropathy involves four major mechanisms: renal vasoconstriction, renal cytokine production (i.e., endothelin-1 and monocyte chemoattractant protein-1), cytotoxic effects of heme proteins, and cast formation. Renal vasoconstriction and attendant ischemia predispose toward cell injury and the sloughing of cellular debris into the nephron, thereby promoting cast formation. Not only do tubular casts occlude nephrons, but also, by inhibiting the urinary excretion of heme proteins, tubular casts prolong the exposure of renal epithelial cells to denatured heme proteins, thereby fostering cellular uptake of heme proteins and the risk of cytotoxicity.

When incorporated within renal epithelial cells, heme proteins are split into their heme and protein moieties, and heme, directly or through its released iron, can damage cells and their organelles. Heme proteins also can directly promote oxidant stress. In this manner, vasoconstriction, cell injury, and cast formation interact in the pathogenesis of pigment nephropathy.

Diagnosis

Patients with rhabdomyolysis may present with features of the underlying disease, the inciting cause, or a systemic process. Patients also may present with localizing symptoms and signs such as muscle pain, swelling, stiffness, weakness, bruising, features of a compartment syndrome, or a neurologic deficit. However, because these findings are absent in a significant number of affected patients, rhabdomyolysis should be considered even in largely asymptomatic patients presenting with dark urine, decreased urinary output, abnormalities in serum electrolytes, an acid-base disorder, or AKI.

Myoglobinuria may darken the color of urine, and in approximately 50% of patients, the urinalysis reveals the presence of heme proteins on dipstick testing in the absence of red blood cells (<5 RBCs/high-power field). The urinalysis may also show an acid pH, tubular epithelial cells, granular casts, or dark-pigmented casts. Proteinuria is present in 50% of cases and may attain nephrotic-range values. The fractional excretion of sodium may be low (<1%), especially in the early stages of the disease.

Myoglobinuria is transient, and the demonstration of myoglobin in urine by specific assays is rarely required to make the diagnosis. The diagnosis of rhabdomyolysis is readily confirmed by measuring the serum CK concentration, because the CK level peaks within 36 hours after rhabdomyolysis, and with a half-life of 36-48 hours, CK declines thereafter in the absence of ongoing muscle damage. This decline in the CK concentration assists in differentiating rhabdomyolysis from other myopathic conditions. Whereas values of CK of 100,000 IU/L or greater may be seen, rhabdomyolysis also occurs with lower CK values (1000 to 10,000 IU/L). There is a lack of consensus regarding the extent to which the CK concentration should be elevated to diagnose rhabdomyolysis. Serum CK values that are fivefold greater than the upper limit of normal, or greater than 500 IU/L, are employed in the literature, and national advisory committees on the administration of statins use a 10-fold increase in CK above the upper limit of normal in their definition of rhabdomyolysis. Mild elevations in the CK level may result from cardiac and neurologic disorders, and these diseases should be excluded by appropriate tests, including troponins for suspected cardiac disease. A second-wave CK profile should raise the suspicion of an evolving compartment syndrome. The extent and severity of rhabdomyolysis can be visualized by magnetic resonance imaging, avoiding the use of gadolinium when renal function is significantly impaired.

Other helpful diagnostic features in rhabdomyolysis include a pentad of alterations in the electrolyte and acid-base profile (i.e., hyperkalemia, hyperphosphatemia, hypocalcemia, hyperuricemia, and increased anion gap metabolic acidosis) and a low ratio of blood urea nitrogen (BUN) to creatinine (<10). After rhabdomyolysis, the rate of increase in the level of serum creatinine may outstrip that of BUN, a finding ascribed to enhanced conversion of creatine (from damaged muscle) to creatinine. However, it has been suggested that the low BUN-to-creatinine ratio observed in rhabdomyolysis indicates that patients with greater muscle mass (e.g., younger men) are more susceptible to rhabdomyolysis. Eventually, the BUN-to-creatinine ratio becomes greater as the rate of generation of urea increases as a result of the catabolism of protein from damaged muscle.

Management of Rhabdomyolysis and Pigment Nephropathy

Patients with rhabdomyolysis or suspected rhabdomyolysis require vigorous hydration with isotonic saline begun as soon as possible after muscle injury. Administration of isotonic saline expands the ECF, may increase urinary flow rate and the glomerular filtration rate, and may diminish the risk of cast formation. For example, intravenous hydration should be initiated in patients with the crush syndrome even before they are extricated from the debris, giving as much as 1 to 2 L of 0.9% saline within the first hour; within the first 24 hours, up to 12 L of total intravenous fluid may be given to monitored patients with the crush syndrome in whom there is adequate urinary output, with the intent of achieving urinary flow rates of 200 to 300 mL/hr or more.

Clinical experience in treating patients with the crush syndrome has suggested a beneficial effect of bicarbonate and mannitol. After the initial administration of isotonic saline in these patients, the administration of hypotonic saline to which sodium bicarbonate is added can alternate with that of isotonic saline, attempting to achieve a urinary pH greater than 6.5. In the nonoliguric patient, mannitol also may be administered; in addition to increasing the urinary flow rate, mannitol may diminish the risk of urinary cast formation and decrease the movement of ECF into injured muscle. This approach, employed in treating patients with the crush syndrome, is broadly applied to nontraumatic rhabdomyolysis, but it must be recognized that the optimal rate of intravenous hydration depends on the clinical case and context, and that the efficacy of alkaline-mannitol diuresis is an unresolved issue. In general, in patients with nontraumatic rhabdomyolysis, hydration with isotonic saline should be prompt and vigorous so as to rapidly and completely correct ECF depletion, to expand the ECF (while avoiding pulmonary edema), and to stimulate and maintain an ongoing diuresis. Alkalinization of urine may be achieved in several ways, including the use of 0.45% saline containing 75 mmol of sodium bicarbonate per liter. An isotonic solution that administers both bicarbonate and mannitol can be prepared by adding sodium bicarbonate (100 mL of 100 mEq $NaHCO_3$) and mannitol (100 mL of 25% mannitol) to 800 mL of 5% dextrose. One liter of this solution can be infused over 4 hours; if the urinary flow rate significantly improves, the rate of infusion can then be adjusted to match the urinary flow rate. If the urinary flow rate remains low (i.e., urine output <20 mL/hr), mannitol should not be administered. Initiation of renal replacement therapy may be required for persisting oligoanuria and increasing uremia, hyperkalemia not readily responsive to conservative treatment (e.g., insulin and glucose, β_2-agonists, sodium polystyrene sulfonate exchange resin), and systemic acidosis. The administration of alkali may worsen hypocalcemia, which usually is asymptomatic and does not require treatment. Intravenous calcium salts, however, may be required to treat symptomatic hypocalcemia, hypocalcemia-induced seizures, or hyperkalemia.

During the recovery from AKI, hypercalcemia may occur, reflecting mainly the mobilization of calcium deposited in muscle during the oliguric phase. Plasma levels of 1,25-dihydroxyvitamin D, which are elevated for unclear reasons during the recovery phase, may contribute to the hypercalcemia.

Manometric measurement of compartmental pressure in muscle may aid in the diagnosis of a compartment syndrome, which is likely to occur when pressures exceed 30 to 40 mm Hg (normal values: 0 to 10 mm Hg) or attain values 30 to 20 mm Hg less than the diastolic blood pressure. Tissue viability may be salvaged in a compartment syndrome by a timely fasciotomy. However, the indications for fasciotomy for a crush-induced compartment syndrome are more stringent because of the high risk for bleeding and sepsis. In this setting, and in nonoliguric patients, there is renewed interest in the use of mannitol in decreasing compartmental edema and pressure.

HEMOGLOBINURIC ACUTE KIDNEY INJURY

Hemoglobinuria describes the presence in urine of hemoglobin that is filtered by the kidney and has escaped uptake and degradation by the renal tubules. After intravascular hemolysis, hemoglobin avidly binds plasma haptoglobin and is retained in plasma as part of a large hemoglobin-haptoglobin complex, which is cleared by monocytes and macrophages. When the binding capacity of haptoglobin is exceeded, free hemoglobin appears in plasma, existing as a tetramer (two α and two β chains; molecular weight [MW], 68 kDa) and also as a dimer (one α and one β chain; MW, 32 kDa). Dimeric hemoglobin, unlike tetrameric hemoglobin, undergoes appreciable glomerular filtration, whereas the large size of the hemoglobin-haptoglobin complex precludes such filtration. Therefore, depending on the stage and severity of intravascular hemolysis, plasma may contain variable amounts of the hemoglobin-haptoglobin complex, tetrameric hemoglobin, and dimeric hemoglobin. The presence of free hemoglobin imparts a reddish color to plasma. In contrast, myoglobin (MW, 18 kDa) does not substantially accumulate in plasma after rhabdomyolysis, because myoglobin lacks a specific binding protein in plasma and is rapidly cleared by renal filtration. Red discoloration of plasma may occur in hemoglobinuria, but it is most unlikely in myoglobinuria.

Like myoglobin, filtered hemoglobin is taken up by megalin and cubulin receptors in renal proximal tubules and then split into the heme and globin moieties. The heme moiety is degraded by heme oxygenase, leading to the release of iron, which enters the cellular iron pool or is stored as ferritin or hemosiderin. In hemoglobinuria, hemosiderin may be detected in tubular epithelial cells shed into urine, and hemosiderinuria is used as a diagnostic aid. Hemoglobinuria does not occur after extravascular hemolysis, because the quantities of hemoglobin released are effectively and completely handled by the reticuloendothelial system. In contrast, intravascular hemolysis may release amounts of hemoglobin that overwhelm the binding capacity of haptoglobin and the renal tubular uptake of hemoglobin, giving rise to hemoglobinuria. The pathogenesis of hemoglobin-induced AKI is broadly similar to that of myoglobin-induced AKI and is described earlier in this chapter.

Differential Diagnosis of Hemoglobinuria

Hemoglobinuria may originate from stresses intrinsic or extrinsic to the RBC (**Table 36-2**). In paroxysmal nocturnal hemoglobinuria, the abnormal erythrocyte is unduly sensitive to complement-mediated lysis, which occurs spontaneously, after infections, or after blood transfusions. Deficiencies in erythrocyte enzymes, such as glucose-6-phosphate dehydrogenase, promote the oxidation of hemoglobin to methemoglobin and, ultimately, the release of the heme moiety; the buildup of oxidatively denatured hemoglobin and heme can induce hemolysis. Individuals who are deficient in glucose-6-phosphate dehydrogenase are prone to hemoglobinuria,

TABLE 36-2 Differential Diagnosis of Hemoglobinuria

Mechanisms Intrinsic to Red Blood Cells

Abnormalities in erythrocyte membrane or cytoskeleton (e.g., PNH)

Abnormalities in erythrocyte metabolism (e.g., G6PD deficiency)

Abnormalities in hemoglobin (e.g., sickle cell disease)

Mechanisms Extrinsic to Red Blood Cells

Immune-mediated mechanisms
   Transfusion reactions
   Autoimmune hemolytic anemia

Drugs or chemicals
   Oxidant stressors
   Immune injury
   Other agents

Osmotic stressors
   Hypotonic solutions
   Hypertonic solutions

Mechanical injury
   Heart valves, extracorporeal circulation or device, left ventricular assist device
   Transcatheter coil embolization, mechanical thrombectomy
   March hemoglobinuria, conga drumming, karate
   Physical abuse

Thermal injury
   Burns
   Radiofrequency ablation

Microangiopathies
   Disseminated intravascular coagulation
   TTP/HUS
   Vasculitides

Severe hypophosphatemia

Bone marrow transplantation

Infections
   Parasitic
   Bacterial

Venoms or toxins

Hemoglobin-based red blood cell substitute

G6PD, glucose-6-phosphate dehydrogenase; PNH, paroxysmal nocturnal hemoglobinuria; TTP/HUS, thrombotic thrombocytopenic purpura and hemolytic uremic syndrome.
Modified from Nath KA: Hemoglobinuria. In Molitoris B, Finn WF (eds): Acute Renal Failure: A Companion to Brenner and Rector's The Kidney. Philadelphia, WB Saunders, 2001, pp 214-219.

especially when exposed to oxidizing drugs (e.g., quinine) or unfavorable conditions (e.g., sepsis).

Immune-mediated processes include acute transfusion reactions caused by intravascular hemolysis of transfused cells by preformed antibodies in the recipient. Autoimmune hemolytic anemia may be caused by warm- or cold-associated antibodies; the former are induced by hematologic malignancies, connective tissue diseases, or medications. Viral or mycoplasmal infections may lead to a cold-reacting antibody and paroxysmal cold hemoglobinuria.

Drugs and chemicals used in clinical practice can induce hemoglobinuria, and these include antibiotics (e.g., penicillin, cefotetan, rifampicin, minocycline, dapsone), nonsteroidal anti-inflammatory agents, ribavirin, interferon-gamma, intravenous immunoglobulin, iron dextran, fluorescein, and ethanolamine oleate (used in sclerotherapy for varicose veins). Hemolysis may be induced by chemicals in industrial and other uses (e.g., benzene, phenol, naphthalene, copper, mercuric salts). Hypotonic solutions used to irrigate the genitourinary tract or inadvertently employed in plasmapheresis may cause hemolysis. Hypertonic stress and attendant hemolysis may arise from the use of contrast agents in dehydrated patients, hypertonic saline as an abortifacient, hypertonic glycerol to reduce intracranial pressure, or propylene glycol employed as a vehicle for medications.

Infectious causes of hemoglobinuria include *Plasmodium falciparum* malaria, in which extravascular hemolysis of parasitized and nonparasitized cells can occur in conjunction with intravascular hemolysis, especially in the setting of glucose-6-phosphate dehydrogenase deficiency and antimalarial agents that are pro-oxidant. Fulminant hemolysis in malaria leading to hemoglobinuria and dark urine is described as *blackwater fever*. Hemoglobinuria also may result from hemolysins produced by bacteria (e.g., *Clostridium perfringens*) and by venoms derived from certain species of snakes, spiders, scorpions, and jellyfish.

Diagnosis and Treatment

In hemoglobinuria and myoglobinuria, the urinalysis characteristically reveals a red supernatant that is heme positive by dipstick testing and a sediment that may contain pigmented casts but lacks RBCs. Hemoglobinuria (but not myoglobinuria) may be accompanied by red discoloration of plasma. Evidence of hemolysis is provided by elevated serum levels of lactate dehydrogenase and unconjugated bilirubin, reduced serum levels of haptoglobin, and elevated free hemoglobin concentrations. Reticulocytosis may be present, and the peripheral smear may demonstrate, depending on the underlying cause, fragmented RBCs, spherocytes, and other abnormalities in RBC morphology. Hyperkalemia may be prominent even in the absence of AKI.

The therapeutic approach in hemoglobinuria is similar to that employed in myoglobinuria: vigorous hydration and forced mannitol-alkaline diuresis. In certain instances, renal replacement therapy may be temporarily required if AKI of sufficient severity develops; recovery of kidney function usually occurs. Specific therapies should target, when possible, the underlying mechanism accounting for the destruction of RBCs, including cessation of exposure to the offending drug or agent, employing appropriate protocols for transfusion reactions, the use of eculizumab to inhibit hemolysis in paroxysmal nocturnal hemoglobinuria, and surgical correction for cardiac or vascular prostheses.

BIBLIOGRAPHY

Antons KA, Williams CD, Baker SK, et al: Clinical perspectives of statin-induced rhabdomyolysis. Am J Med 119:400, 2006.

Baer AN, Wortmann RL: Myotoxicity associated with lipid-lowering drugs. Curr Opin Rheumatol 19:67, 2007.

Better OS, Rubinstein I, Reis DN: Muscle crush compartment syndrome: Fulminant local edema with threatening systemic effects. Kidney Int 63:1155, 2003.

Brown CV, Rhee P, Chan L, et al: Preventing renal failure in patients with rhabdomyolysis: Do bicarbonate and mannitol make a difference? J Trauma 56:1191, 2004.

Bywaters EG, Beall D: Crush injuries with impairment of renal function. BMJ 1:427, 1941.

Fernandez WG, Hung O, Bruno GR, et al: Factors predictive of acute renal failure and need for hemodialysis among ED patients with rhabdomyolysis. Am J Emerg Med 23:1, 2005.

Fine DM, Gelber AC, Melamed ML, et al: Risk factors for renal failure among 72 consecutive patients with rhabdomyolysis related to illicit drug use. Am J Med 117:607, 2004.

Gabardi S, Munz K, Ulbricht C: A review of dietary supplement-induced renal dysfunction. Clin J Am Soc Nephrol 2:757, 2007.

Gabow PA, Kaehny WD, Kelleher SP: The spectrum of rhabdomyolysis 61:141, 1982.

Knochel JP: Mechanisms of rhabdomyolysis. Curr Opin Rheumatol 5:725, 1993.

Knochel JP: Catastrophic medical events with exhaustive exercise: "White collar rhabdomyolysis." Kidney Int 38:709, 1990.

Malinoski DJ, Slater MS, Mullins RJ: Crush injury and rhabdomyolysis. Crit Care Clin 20:171, 2004.

Melli G, Chaudhry V, Cornblath DR: Rhabdomyolysis: An evaluation of 475 hospitalized patients. Medicine (Baltimore) 84:377, 2005.

Nath KA: Hemoglobinuria. Acute Renal Failure: A Companion to Brenner and Rector's The Kidney. Philadelphia, WB Saunders, 2001, pp 214-219.

Nath KA, Balla G, Vercellotti GM, et al: Induction of heme oxygenase is a rapid, protective response in rhabdomyolysis in the rat. J Clin Invest 90:267, 1992.

Sever MS, Vanholder R, Lameire N: Management of crush-related injuries after disasters. N Engl J Med 354:1052, 2006.

Sharp LS, Rozycki GS, Feliciano DV: Rhabdomyolysis and secondary renal failure in critically ill surgical patients. Am J Surg 188:801, 2004.

Vanholder R, Sever MS, Erek E, et al: Rhabdomyolysis. J Am Soc Nephrol 11:1553, 2000.

Warren JD, Blumbergs PC, Thompson PD: Rhabdomyolysis: A review. Muscle Nerve 25:332, 2002.

Zager RA: Rhabdomyolysis and myohemoglobinuric acute renal failure. Kidney Int 49:314, 1996.

CHAPTER 37

Management of Acute Kidney Injury

Kerry C. Cho and Glenn M. Chertow

Despite many advances in nephrology, renal replacement therapy, and intensive care medicine, the mortality and morbidity rates for acute kidney injury (AKI) remain high. Mortality rates of 50% to 80% for AKI requiring dialytic support are commonly cited in observational studies. Although mortality rates have changed only modestly since the advent of hemodialysis, evidence suggests that comorbidities and illness severity have increased, masking real improvements in the care and outcomes for AKI. Successful management of AKI requires early recognition, management of uremic complications, timely renal replacement therapy, prevention of ongoing kidney injury, aggressive supportive care, and correction of the primary disorders. In this chapter, we focus primarily on acute tubular necrosis (ATN), one of the most common causes of AKI in hospitalized patients.

AKI is usually diagnosed by non-nephrologists such as internists, intensivists, and surgeons. Recognition of AKI and its severity is often missed or delayed. Increases in the serum creatinine level may not be noticed for 24 to 48 hours after the onset of AKI. The serum creatinine concentration is deceptive in patients with malnutrition, cachexia, or decreased muscle mass; small absolute changes in serum creatinine levels may reflect large changes in the glomerular filtration rate (GFR). Predictive formulas for creatinine clearance, such as the Cockcroft-Gault formula, may be used inappropriately in AKI, potentially delaying diagnosis and therapy. Changes in urine output, especially oliguria and anuria, may reflect kidney dysfunction before changes in serum creatinine concentration, but some physicians may mistake nonoliguria for preserved kidney function. A response to diuretics may be interpreted as recovering kidney function or the absence of kidney injury. The misperception that nephrologists have little to offer therapeutically except renal replacement therapy also may delay appropriate consultation, allowing uremic complications and further kidney injury to occur. One study showed that delayed nephrology consultation was associated with increased mortality and increased length of hospital and intensive care unit (ICU) stays. A low serum creatinine level and nonoliguria were the two conditions significantly associated with delayed consultation.

After AKI has been identified, management begins with prompt diagnosis and correction of the underlying cause (see Chapter 33). Correction of prerenal or postrenal causes often leads to rapid recovery. Prerenal AKI resolves with restoration of normal hemodynamics and kidney perfusion by fluid resuscitation, cardiovascular support, and withdrawal of offending medications. The lack of complete or even partial recovery after restoration of perfusion requires a re-examination of other potential diagnoses. Postrenal AKI results from urinary obstruction; relief of obstruction may lead to kidney recovery and profound diuresis (see Chapter 46). Early involvement of urologists and interventional radiologists for stone removal, ureteral stents, or nephrostomy tube placement may prevent the development of intrinsic kidney disease from long-standing obstruction. For patients with prerenal and postrenal AKI, nephrologists may cautiously withhold dialytic support in anticipation of imminent kidney recovery. However, the diagnosis of intrarenal (or intrinsic) AKI portends a less favorable prognosis, longer time to recovery, and a higher likelihood for dialysis or continuous renal replacement therapy (CRRT).

NONDIALYTIC KIDNEY SUPPORT

The goals of nondialytic management of AKI are prevention of further kidney injury and supportive care to allow potential functional recovery. Successful management requires meticulous attention to many details: volume status, hemodynamics, fluid and electrolyte management, acid-base status, nutrition, and medication dose adjustment or discontinuation (**Table 37-1**). Adjuvant therapy for concomitant sepsis, shock, and the systemic inflammatory response may also be required.

Kidneys of patients with AKI have impaired autoregulation; they are unable to maintain perfusion and the GFR over

TABLE 37-1 Nondialytic Management of Acute Kidney Injury

Treat or reverse underlying causes of acute kidney injury.

Achieve and maintain normal hemodynamics and euvolemia, avoiding hypovolemia and prerenal states.

Adjust medication dosages and frequency for level of kidney function.

Avoid nephrotoxic agents if possible, including aminoglycosides, radiocontrast, NSAIDs, ACE inhibitors, and angiotensin receptor blockers.

Provide adjuvant therapy, including antibiotics, mechanical ventilation, enteral or parenteral nutrition, intensive insulin therapy, and adrenal corticosteroid replacement as indicated.

Enlist the assistance of nephrologists and intensivists for supportive care and to determine the need for and timing of renal replacement therapy.

ACE, angiotensin-converting enzyme; NSAIDs, nonsteroidal anti-inflammatory drugs.

a range of mean arterial pressures. Maintaining adequate hemodynamics and kidney perfusion is essential for functional recovery. Successful volume management requires a careful physical examination, attention to daily weights and overall fluid balance, recognition of insensible losses, correct interpretation of hemodynamic parameters (including central pressure measurements), and selection of appropriate fluids. The goal is to achieve and maintain euvolemia while restoring effective circulating volume to allow adequate tissue and kidney perfusion. The physician may use crystalloids, colloids, blood products, vasopressors, or inotropes, incorporating information from the physical examination and central venous and pulmonary artery catheters as necessary toward this goal. Except possibly in the case of cirrhosis, colloids have not been found superior to crystalloids for volume expansion and AKI prevention. Identification and correction of hypovolemia may rapidly reverse prerenal AKI.

Optimal hemodynamic targets for resuscitation are not well defined. A trial of goal-oriented hemodynamic therapy (i.e., using specific hemodynamic and physiologic parameters as resuscitation end points) in critically ill patients (with and without AKI) to raise the cardiac index and oxygen delivery failed to improve survival, decrease ICU length of stay, or decrease the number of dysfunctional organs. However, another trial of early goal-directed therapy in patients with severe sepsis or septic shock used a protocol algorithm to maintain hemodynamic parameters (i.e., central venous pressure, mean arterial pressure, and central venous oxygen saturation) at specified targets using fluid resuscitation, inotropes, vasoactive agents, and red blood cell transfusions. Instituted before ICU admission, this protocol therapy reduced in-hospital mortality and organ dysfunction, although patients with AKI were not specifically highlighted. A prospective, cohort study of ICU patients showed increased mortality rates, length of stay, and costs in those who received pulmonary artery catheterization compared with those who did not.

Large, randomized clinical trials of fluid composition, hemodynamic targets, and invasive monitoring specifically in AKI have not been conducted, and there is no consensus on optimal strategies. However, adequate hydration to correct possible hypovolemia is recommended to diagnose and treat prerenal AKI. Monitoring with central venous pressures or pulmonary artery catheterization may help to guide volume management with fluid resuscitation, diuretics, or ultrafiltration. The management of shock may require vasopressors and inotropic agents.

Often preceded or exacerbated by the oliguria of AKI, volume overload may complicate patient mobility, mechanical ventilation, extubation, wound healing, central venous access, and abdominal compartment syndrome. Total parental nutrition and intravenous medications (in bolus or continuous forms) are often overlooked sources of fluid intake. Nutrition and blood products usually should not be restricted solely because of volume concerns. However, renal replacement therapy may be necessary even among patients with relatively preserved or recovering kidney function to optimize nutritional therapy or correct coagulopathy. One such example is the patient with hepatic failure requiring fresh-frozen plasma.

Diuretics may be useful to manage volume overload in AKI, but they have toxicities and potential pitfalls. Loop diuretics are ototoxic in high doses, and concomitantly administered aminoglycosides may increase the ototoxicity. Continuous infusions of loop diuretics may reduce drug toxicity by reducing cumulative dose requirements and peak serum concentrations. Although oliguria has been established as a poor prognostic sign in AKI, conversion of oliguria to nonoliguria (with diuretics or vasoactive substances) has not been shown to reduce mortality or facilitate kidney recovery. Conversion of oliguria to nonoliguria with diuretics may simply reflect less severe AKI or AKI with impending recovery. Ultimately, a trial of diuretics should not delay the initiation of dialysis when otherwise required in a nonoliguric patient.

Dopamine has been shown in animal and human trials to increase renal blood flow, GFR, and urine output. Some investigators have argued that low doses of dopamine (<3 μg/kg/min) provide selective renal vasodilation with few inotropic and vasoactive effects. Despite these theoretical physiologic benefits, randomized clinical trials and meta-analyses of dopamine in AKI have failed to demonstrate any benefit on outcomes, including prevention of or enhanced recovery from AKI. Some authorities may recommend a brief trial of diuretics and low-dose dopamine, but administration of dopamine commonly leads to arrhythmias, tachycardia, and myocardial ischemia. Furthermore, there is evidence that dopamine may cause intestinal ischemia, anterior pituitary dysfunction, and decreased T-cell function.

Because renal water and sodium handling may be abnormal in AKI, dysnatremias are common. Hyponatremia and hypernatremia in hospitalized patients with AKI are often iatrogenic; improper volume management and fluid composition unmasks the damaged kidney's inability to maintain sodium and water homeostasis. Hyponatremia usually results from excess free water relative to sodium and solute intake. Hypernatremia may result from hypotonic fluid losses through nasogastric suctioning, stool output, osmotic diuresis (including glucose, mannitol, and urea), and insensible losses. Overly aggressive normal saline resuscitation and inadequate free water intake are iatrogenic causes. Hypernatremia is usually associated with hypovolemia. Hypervolemic hypernatremia is rare and typically the result of hypertonic solute administration (e.g., sodium bicarbonate, hypertonic saline).

Metabolic acidosis is commonly seen in AKI because of reduced renal acid excretion. Dietary protein restriction to 0.6 to 0.8 g/kg/day may reduce acid production and ameliorate the metabolic acidosis, but this strategy may not be desirable in hypercatabolic patients. Alkaline intravenous fluids such as isotonic sodium bicarbonate can correct acidosis, especially if concomitant hypovolemia allows large-volume resuscitation. An alternative buffer is sodium acetate, which is found in parenteral nutrition. However, the exogenous sodium load with the potential for complications of hypervolemia, including pulmonary edema, often limits the capacity for aggressive alkali replacement. Hemodialysis or CRRT should be employed in cases of severe or refractory acidemia, especially in the setting of shock, multiorgan dysfunction, and other indications for renal support.

Hyperkalemia associated with electrocardiographic changes or clinical manifestations requires emergent therapy (see Chapter 12). Exogenous sources of potassium should be discontinued immediately, including nutrition (i.e., oral, enteral, or parenteral), potassium supplements, and intravenous fluids. The medical management of hyperkalemia includes immediate temporizing measures such as intravenous calcium gluconate (when electrocardiographic changes are present), insulin, sodium bicarbonate, and the inhaled β-agonist albuterol. Unless kidney function can be restored quickly (as in cases of acute obstruction), therapy to remove potassium should be initiated. Administered orally or rectally, sodium polystyrene sulfonate is an exchange resin that binds and removes potassium. However, its onset of action is measured in hours. It is relatively contraindicated in postoperative patients, including those recovering from kidney transplantation, because of the risk of bowel necrosis and perforation. Hemodialysis is the definitive treatment for hyperkalemia, and it rapidly corrects the serum potassium and electrocardiographic changes. Unfortunately, electrolyte testing, nephrology consultation, dialysis catheter placement, activation of a dialysis nurse and technician, and preparation of a dialysis machine can delay the initiation of hemodialysis by hours. Although some CRRT modalities (e.g., continuous venovenous hemodiafiltration) may be initiated soon after line placement, potassium removal by these therapies is less efficient per unit time and may not rapidly correct acute hyperkalemia.

Hyperphosphatemia and hypermagnesemia may occur in the course of AKI, particularly with direct tissue injury (e.g., rhabdomyolysis). Exogenous phosphorus in the diet, tube feedings, and parenteral nutrition should be reduced. Oral phosphorus binders, including calcium acetate and calcium carbonate, reduce phosphorus absorption from the intestinal tract. Aluminum hydroxide is an effective phosphorus binder, but its use should be limited to short courses (<2 to 3 weeks) to decrease the possibility of aluminum toxicity. Citrate salts increase aluminum absorption and should never be used with aluminum hydroxide. Sevelamer hydrochloride is a non-calcium, non-aluminum–containing phosphate binder; its physical structure as a hydrogel (i.e., expanding within a feeding tube) makes its use with forced enteral feeding problematic. Hypermagnesemia is often iatrogenic, caused by overzealous magnesium replacement or administration of magnesium-containing medications.

Bleeding diatheses may complicate AKI. Synthetic analogues of arginine vasopressin may be used acutely to correct uremic platelet dysfunction, but repeated doses result in tachyphylaxis. Estrogens and cryoprecipitate have been used for the treatment of uremic bleeding. Estrogens have an onset of action measured in hours, whereas cryoprecipitate

must be given repeatedly for a sustained effect. Hemodialysis is the definitive therapy for uremic bleeding. Patients with intracranial, gastrointestinal, retroperitoneal, or surgical bleeding should receive prompt dialytic support. Anticoagulation for hemodialysis or CRRT can be reduced or withheld for these patients. Heparin-induced thrombocytopenia is a real concern for patients requiring intermittent hemodialysis or continuous therapy. Other anticoagulants, such as citrate and prostacyclin, may be used. When this diagnosis is being considered, all heparin products, including flushes used to lock dialysis catheters between treatments, should be withheld.

Medications, especially antimicrobials, should be appropriately dosed for the level of kidney function or the modality of renal replacement (see Chapter 39). A rapidly changing serum creatinine concentration or oligoanuria suggests markedly diminished kidney function; dosing medications for an assumed GFR of less than 10 mL/min is prudent. Drug levels for vancomycin and aminoglycosides should be monitored to avoid toxicity and to ensure therapeutic levels. The doses of most penicillins (including extended-spectrum penicillins used against *Staphylococcus* and *Pseudomonas* spp.) and many cephalosporins and quinolones require adjustment. Imipenem should be avoided if other alternatives exist because imipenem metabolites can lead to seizures. If acute interstitial nephritis is a diagnostic possibility, the most likely offending agent and other potential culprits should be discontinued. Narcotic analgesics and their metabolites usually have prolonged half-lives in patients with AKI, potentially exacerbating uremic encephalopathy. Like imipenem, meperidine should be avoided in severe AKI because of its epileptogenic primary metabolite, normeperidine.

Potentially nephrotoxic agents should be avoided entirely if possible. Medications that adversely affect renal and systemic hemodynamics should be avoided. Nonsteroidal anti-inflammatory drugs reduce kidney perfusion and the GFR. Angiotensin-converting enzyme inhibitors and angiotensin receptor blockers tend to reduce the GFR, although kidney perfusion usually is maintained. The use of these drugs in AKI may confound the severity of injury or rate of potential recovery. To decrease the possibility of hypotension and prerenal AKI, antihypertensive agents should be carefully titrated. Intravenous radiocontrast may be required for diagnostic or therapeutic purposes. Other diagnostic modalities, such as ultrasonography, magnetic resonance imaging, and nuclear medicine, should be explored in consultation with radiologists. If there are no alternatives to intravascular radiocontrast, physicians should consider gentle volume expansion before radiocontrast administration, if tolerated. The use of agents to further reduce the rate of radiocontrast-associated nephropathy, including *N*-acetylcysteine, should be considered, recognizing that clinical trial results have been mixed. Maneuvers to prevent radiocontrast-induced nephropathy are discussed in Chapter 34. Any prophylactic strategy should not delay imaging studies in critically ill patients.

NUTRITION, ERYTHROPOIETIN, AND THERAPEUTIC AGENTS

AKI that occurs in the setting of multiorgan dysfunction is a hypercatabolic state with muscle and visceral protein wasting and negative nitrogen balance. Isolated AKI, however, has not been conclusively proved to be a catabolic state. Although total parenteral nutrition (TPN) is commonly used, clear evidence of its benefits in critically ill patients is lacking. One meta-analysis concluded that TPN might have a positive effect on nutritional end points and possibly on minor complications, but there was no evidence for decreased mortality or major complication rates (including organ failure). Randomized and nonrandomized trials of TPN specifically in the setting of AKI have been largely inconclusive. Nonetheless, it is axiomatic that nutrition is superior to no nutrition. General recommendations for TPN include a calorie intake of 30 to 35 kcal/kg/day and a maximum protein intake of 1.5 g/kg of body weight per day for hypercatabolic patients and 0.6 g/kg/day for noncatabolic patients. Potassium, phosphorus, and magnesium are typically withheld from parenteral nutrition solutions for patients with AKI. If electrolyte deficiencies develop, they can be quickly corrected with supplements. Energy and protein requirements should be estimated (often by an experienced registered dietitian), adjusting for dialysis-related losses of amino acids when appropriate. CRRT is associated with the largest dialytic losses of amino acids, often necessitating the administration of an additional 10 to 30 g of protein per day.

Experimental models of AKI have shown decreased synthesis and secretion of erythropoietin. Decreased circulating levels combined with bone marrow hyporesponsiveness to erythropoietin produce the anemia of AKI and critical illness. Recombinant human erythropoietin (rHuEpo) in rat models of AKI reverses anemia and leads to earlier recovery of kidney function. However, investigators have only begun to study rHuEpo in patients with AKI and critical illness. A trial of rHuEpo in critically ill patients found that weekly rHuEpo (40,000 units SC) increased hemoglobin and reduced red blood cell transfusions. Clinical outcomes such as mortality and organ failure were not studied, and a subgroup analysis of AKI patients was not performed. Therefore, the risk-benefit profile and cost-benefit ratio of rHuEpo in human AKI remain undefined.

The search for effective therapeutic agents for AKI has been frustrating. Despite encouraging results in experimental models, many agents with favorable phase II study results have shown no benefit in randomized clinical trials, including atrial natriuretic peptide, thyroxine, insulin-like growth factor 1, loop diuretics, and dopamine. Other biologic agents that have shown no benefit in experimental or human sepsis trials are antibodies to tumor necrosis factor-α, nitric oxide synthase inhibitors, tissue factor pathway inhibitor, endothelin antagonists, epidermal growth factor, inhibitors of arachidonic acid metabolism, and antithrombin. Other agents currently under study are fenoldopam (a selective dopamine$_1$-receptor agonist), platelet-activating factor inhibitors, and leukocyte adhesion inhibitors.

Some interventions have been shown to be effective in the treatment of critically ill patients, a population at risk for the development of AKI. These interventions include activated protein C, intensive insulin therapy, hemodynamic goal-directed therapy, the combination of hydrocortisone and fludrocortisone, and low-tidal-volume mechanical ventilation. Although these interventions have not been tested directly in an AKI population, they should be considered the standard of care and adjuvant therapy for AKI patients with critical illness. Recombinant activated protein C was the first drug approved by the U.S. Food and Drug Administration for the treatment of sepsis, and its use decreased the mortality rate in a large, randomized trial enrolling patients with known or suspected infection, organ failure, and signs of systemic inflammation. Intensive insulin therapy to maintain a glucose concentration between 80 and 110 mg/dL increased overall survival compared with conventional glucose control in a randomized trial of mechanically ventilated patients in a surgical ICU, although benefits appeared to be limited to populations that cannot be identified in advance. Intensive insulin also reduced the incidence of AKI and the need for renal replacement therapy. The combination of hydrocortisone and fludrocortisone reduced mortality rates for adult septic shock patients identified with relative adrenal insufficiency. Low-tidal-volume mechanical ventilation improved survival for patients with acute respiratory distress syndrome. Unless there are specific contraindications, patients with AKI and other complications should enjoy the potential benefits of these advances in critical care medicine.

RENAL REPLACEMENT THERAPY

Traditional indications for renal replacement therapy in AKI include acid-base disturbances, electrolyte abnormalities, volume overload refractory to diuretics, and uremic complications (**Tables 37-2** and **37-3**). Urgent hemodialysis should be considered in all cases of AKI with serum potassium concentrations of 6.0 mEq/L or higher, especially if nondialytic treatment is unsuccessful, kidney recovery is not imminent, the patient is oligoanuric, or the electrocardiogram shows evidence of hyperkalemia (e.g., peaked T waves, PR prolongation, QRS widening, ventricular arrhythmias). However, electrocardiographic manifestations correlate poorly with the severity of hyperkalemia. A patient with severe hyperkalemia and a normal electrocardiographic pattern still requires

---

TABLE 37-2 Uremic Complications

Platelet dysfunction and uremic bleeding

Pericarditis and pleuritis

Neuropathy, including asterixis, myoclonus, and wristdrop or footdrop

Encephalopathy

Seizures

TABLE 37-3 Renal Replacement Therapy in Acute Kidney Injury

Traditional Indications

Acid-base disturbances, most commonly metabolic acidosis

Electrolyte imbalances, especially hyperkalemia (serum potassium ≥6.0 mEq/L) with or without electrocardiographic abnormalities

Volume overload refractory to diuretics, especially in patients with pulmonary edema and respiratory compromise

Uremia, including cases of encephalopathy, pericarditis, or coagulopathy

Proactive Indications

Impending acid-base or electrolyte disturbances

Oligoanuria with large obligate fluid intake for medications and nutrition

Moderate to severe acute kidney injury with poor prognosis for immediate renal recovery

Acute kidney injury in the setting of sepsis or systemic inflammatory response syndrome

Goals of Renal Replacement Therapy

Acid-base, electrolyte, and volume homeostasis

Prevention of uremia and its complications

Maintenance of optimal cardiopulmonary performance and normal hemodynamics

Maximum nutritional support

---

cardiac monitoring, immediate conservative treatment for hyperkalemia, and possibly emergent hemodialysis.

The development of uremic complications correlates poorly with serum markers such as creatinine and blood urea nitrogen, and delay of renal replacement while attempting conservative management may be detrimental to the patient. Waiting for uremic complications to develop before initiating dialysis does not make intuitive sense. Some nephrologists believe that the initiation of kidney support should be anticipatory; that is, support should be started before uremic complications arise to allow optimal care, especially if prolonged or delayed kidney recovery is expected. However, few data are available on early or prophylactic initiation of renal replacement and its effects on outcomes (e.g., survival, kidney recovery). The optimal timing of initiation of kidney support is unknown and varies widely, often depending on local practice patterns. Observational data suggest that, among critically ill patients with AKI, initiation of kidney support at higher levels of serum urea is associated with an increased risk for death, even after adjustments for comorbidities and other confounders.

There are two major types of renal replacement therapy for AKI. CRRT includes hemodialysis, hemofiltration, and hemodiafiltration modalities. *Intermittent hemodialysis* includes standard hemodialysis and alternative forms such as sustained low-efficiency dialysis (SLED). Alternative forms usually are used when continuous therapies are not available or are undesirable (possibly because of patient immobility or the requirement for continuous anticoagulation). The extended treatment times allow more gradual ultrafiltration rates and improved solute clearance. Peritoneal dialysis is infrequently used for AKI in the United States, but it may be the only available modality in other areas or in certain emergency circumstances. External variables, such as modality availability and the training and expertise of the physician prescribing kidney support, often determine the selection of support modality.

Regardless of the hemodialysis modality, vascular access must be achieved, usually through a dual-lumen dialysis catheter placed in a central vein. The femoral vein is suitable for ventilated, immobilized, and sedated patients in the ICU, but the internal jugular vein may be preferred for ambulatory patients, especially if prolonged dialytic support is anticipated. The subclavian vein should be avoided because of the high incidence of venous stenosis that precludes using the ipsilateral extremity for future arteriovenous fistulas and grafts. Vein preservation from subclavian venous catheters, unnecessary phlebotomy, and intravenous access is important for patients with AKI who may require permanent vascular access for end-stage renal disease (ESRD). Patients requiring permanent or indefinite dialysis should have long-term vascular access before hospital discharge. Peritoneal catheter insertion and internal jugular tunneled catheter placement are relatively minor procedures. Vascular surgical consultation for creation of an arteriovenous fistula and graft should be considered for suitable candidates.

Continuous therapy has several real and theoretical advantages and disadvantages compared with intermittent hemodialysis. The advantages include hemodynamic stability, continuous correction of electrolyte and acid-base disorders, volume homeostasis, improved solute clearance, and the ability to provide maximal nutrition therapy. For example, TPN often requires large fluid volumes, which may be difficult or impossible to manage with intermittent hemodialysis. Other investigators have suggested that continuous therapies remove and adsorb cytokines and other important biologic agents in the inflammatory state of sepsis and AKI. It remains controversial whether removal and absorption of these agents by continuous therapies is significant relative to their production or whether CRRT has a therapeutic role in critical illness among patients without AKI.

The potential disadvantages of CRRT include limited availability, patient immobilization, need for continuous anticoagulation, and hypocalcemia with hemofiltration or citrate regional anticoagulation. CRRT is heavily resource dependent, requiring ICU monitoring and labor-intensive nursing care, which may be temporarily unavailable even in centers that offer CRRT therapy. Some investigators have argued that CRRT is more expensive than intermittent hemodialysis, although it is difficult to calculate infrastructure expenses and other embedded costs of hemodialysis. Others have suggested that CRRT may facilitate kidney recovery, resulting in fewer days of kidney support and potentially lower costs. Ultimately, patient outcomes, not cost considerations, should determine the selection of one modality over another.

Neither intermittent hemodialysis nor CRRT has been conclusively shown to be superior in terms of survival and

Drugs and the Kidney

CHAPTER 38

Analgesics and the Kidney

Fang-Ying Lin, Biff F. Palmer, and William L. Henrich

Nonsteroidal anti-inflammatory drugs (NSAIDs) are some of the most widely utilized therapeutic agents in clinical practice today. In fact, the Slone survey revealed that, of all prescription and over-the-counter medications, the three most commonly used in any given week were acetaminophen, aspirin, and ibuprofen. According to data from the National Health and Nutrition Examination Survey (NHANES), 76% of the U.S. population aged 17 years and older reported use of nonprescription analgesics during a 1-month period. This figure translates into about 143 million consumers, including 79 million women and 64 million men. These numbers and the number of adverse events are expected to increase as the population ages. Although the gastrointestinal toxicity of these medications is well known, it is also apparent that the kidney is an important target for many untoward clinical events.

The kidney toxicity associated with the use of NSAIDs can be classified into several distinct clinical syndromes (**Table 38-1**). These include a form of vasomotor acute renal failure, nephrotic syndrome associated with interstitial nephritis, chronic kidney disease (CKD), and abnormalities in sodium, water, and potassium homeostasis. The common link in these syndromes is a disruption in the metabolism of prostaglandins, the class of compounds whose synthesis is inhibited by these agents.

PROSTAGLANDIN BIOSYNTHESIS AND ACTIONS

NSAIDs act by inhibiting cyclooxygenase, which is the rate-limiting enzyme in the metabolic conversion of arachidonic acid into prostanoids. The cyclooxygenase enzyme exists as two isoforms, termed cyclooxygenase 1 (COX-1) and cyclooxygenase 2 (COX-2). The COX-1 enzyme is constitutively expressed in most tissues and is responsible for producing

TABLE 38-1	Renal Syndromes Associated with Use of Nonsteroidal Anti-inflammatory Drugs
Vasomotor acute renal failure	
Nephrotic syndrome with tubulointerstitial nephritis	
Chronic kidney disease	
NaCl retention	
Hyponatremia	
Hyperkalemia	

prostaglandins involved in maintaining normal tissue homeostasis. The COX-2 enzyme is principally an inducible enzyme that is rapidly upregulated in response to a variety of stimuli, such as growth factors and cytokines, typically found in the setting of inflammation. In the kidney, both COX-1 and COX-2 are constitutively expressed and are upregulated in response to various physiologic stimuli. As a result, the kidney toxicity of both nonselective and selective COX-2 inhibitors is similar. COX-2 plays an important role in maintaining kidney function in states of prostaglandin dependency. Therefore, a drug acting as a specific COX-2 inhibitor may not offer any distinct advantage over traditional NSAIDs with respect to kidney toxicity. As with other NSAIDs, such agents should be used with caution and require close monitoring of kidney function in patients at high risk for adverse renal outcomes. Because COX-2 inhibitors have been associated with an increased risk of cardiovascular events, these medications are less widely used today.

Prostacyclin (PGI_2) is the most abundant prostaglandin produced in the renal cortex and is primarily synthesized in cortical arterioles and glomeruli. This location corresponds to the known effects of PGI_2 in regulating renal vascular tone, glomerular filtration rate (GFR), and renin release. The most abundant prostaglandin synthesized in the tubules is prostaglandin E_2 (PGE_2), which is produced mainly in the collecting duct. This location provides the anatomic basis for PGE_2 to modulate sodium and chloride transport in the loop of Henle, arginine vasopressin (AVP)-mediated water transport, and vasa recta blood flow.

Prostaglandins play an important role in the maintenance of kidney function, primarily in the setting of a systemic or intrarenal circulatory disturbance. They have no role in renal hemodynamics under healthy, volume-repleted conditions. In the setting of volume depletion (**Fig. 38-1**), renal blood flow is decreased while sodium reabsorption, renin release, and urinary concentrating ability are increased. To a large extent, these changes are mediated by the effects of increased circulating levels of vasoconstrictive hormones such as angiotensin II, AVP, and catecholamines. At the same time, these hormones stimulate the synthesis of renal prostaglandins, which act locally to dilate the renal microvasculature and to inhibit salt and water reabsorption. Under these conditions, prostaglandin release serves to antagonize the physiologic effects of the hormones that elicit their production. As a result, renal blood flow and GFR are maintained at near-normal levels despite the clamping down of the

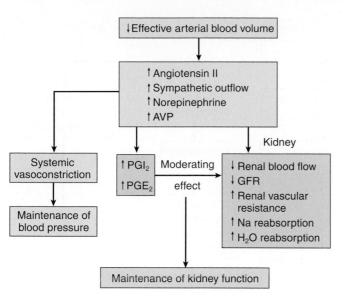

FIGURE 38-1 In the setting of absolute or effective volume depletion, a number of effectors are activated that serve to defend the circulation and at the same time, stimulate the synthesis of renal prostaglandins. In turn, renal prostaglandins function to moderate the effects of these hormonal systems so that kidney function is maintained in the setting of systemic vasoconstriction. AVP, arginine vasopressin; GFR, glomerular filtration rate; PGE_2, prostaglandin E_2; PGI_2, prostacyclin.

TABLE 38-2	Risk Factors for Acute Vasomotor Renal Failure Induced by Nonsteroidal Anti-inflammatory Drugs	
DECREASED EABV	**NORMAL OR INCREASED EABV**
Congestive heart failure	Chronic kidney disease
Cirrhosis	Glomerulonephritis
Nephrotic syndrome	Elderly patient
Sepsis	Contrast-induced nephropathy
Hemorrhage	Obstructive uropathy
Diuretic therapy	Cyclosporin, tacrolimus
Postoperative patients with "third space" fluid	
Volume depletion/hypotension	

EABV, effective arterial blood volume.

systemic circulation. Predictably, inhibition of prostaglandin synthesis leads to unopposed hormonal activity that results in exaggerated renal vasoconstriction and magnified antinatriuretic and antidiuretic effects. In fact, many of the renal syndromes that are associated with the use of NSAIDs can be explained by the predictions of this vasoconstrictive model.

VASOMOTOR ACUTE RENAL FAILURE INDUCED BY NONSTEROIDAL ANTI-INFLAMMATORY DRUGS

Acute renal failure induced by NSAIDs occurs under conditions in which maintenance of kidney function is critically dependent on vasodilatory prostaglandins (**Table 38-2**). For example, with decreased real or effective circulatory volume (e.g., diarrhea, congestive heart failure, cirrhosis), prostaglandins act to oppose the vasoconstrictive effects of sympathetic nervous activity and circulating effectors such as angiotensin II and catecholamines. A similar dependency can occur when effective circulatory volume is normal or expanded, but in such cases (e.g., urinary obstruction, radiocontrast administration, acute glomerulonephritis), there is an increased production of intrarenal vasoconstrictors. Under these circumstances, prostaglandins act to oppose the vasoconstrictive effect of substances such as endothelin, leukotrienes, thromboxane, and platelet-activating factor.

Acute renal failure induced by NSAIDs is most commonly an oliguric form that begins within several days after initiation of the drug. The urinalysis is unremarkable in most cases. In contradiction to other causes of acute oliguric renal failure, the fractional excretion of sodium is often less than 1%, reflecting the underlying hemodynamic nature of the kidney function impairment. Hyperkalemia out of proportion to the

decrement in kidney function is also a typical feature of this lesion (see later discussion). If the renal functional impairment is recognized early, it is reversible with discontinuation of the NSAID, and dialysis usually is not required.

IMPACT OF NONSTEROIDAL ANTI-INFLAMMATORY DRUGS ON SODIUM AND WATER BALANCE

Sodium retention is a characteristic feature of almost all NSAIDs and occurs in as many as 25% of patients who use them. The physiologic basis of this effect is directly related to the natriuretic properties of prostaglandins (**Fig. 38-2**). It would at first seem paradoxic that, under conditions of volume depletion, the kidney would elaborate a compound with further natriuretic properties. The role of prostaglandins in this setting, however, is to moderate the avid salt retention that would otherwise occur with unopposed activation of the renin-angiotensin-aldosterone (RAS) and adrenergic systems. By virtue of their natriuretic properties, prostaglandins ensure adequate delivery of filtrate to more distal nephron segments under conditions in which distal delivery is threatened (e.g. renal ischemia, hypovolemia). In addition, diminished NaCl reabsorption in the thick ascending limb of Henle reduces the energy requirements of this segment. This reduction in thick limb workload, in conjunction with a prostaglandin-mediated reallocation in renal blood flow, helps to maintain an adequate oxygen tension in the medulla under conditions that would otherwise have resulted in substantial hypoxic injury. Most individuals develop a transient positive sodium balance, but in some instances, the edematous state persists.

Likewise, prostaglandins have important modulatory effects on renal water metabolism. The primary effect of prostaglandins is to reduce maximal concentrating ability by interfering with two processes that are central in the elaboration of a concentrated urine: the generation of a hypertonic interstitium and maximal collecting-duct water permeability. AVP is known to stimulate PGE_2 synthesis in cells of the collecting ducts; by doing so, AVP induces its own antagonist. This interaction is another example in which prostaglandins

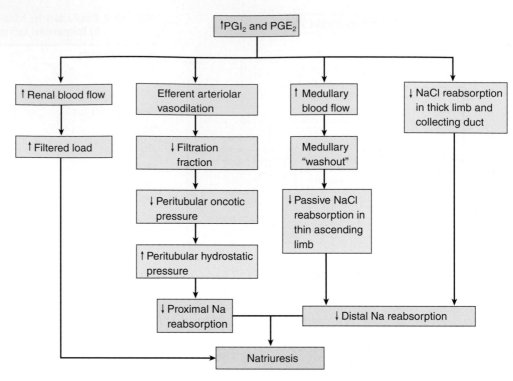

FIGURE 38-2 The direct and indirect mechanisms by which renal prostaglandins exert a natriuretic effect. PGE_2, prostaglandin E_2; PGI_2, prostacyclin.

exert a moderating effect on an effector mechanism that elicits their synthesis. Similar to their effect in salt-retentive states, prostaglandins play an important role in minimizing the water retention that would otherwise occur if the action of AVP were unopposed. In most circumstances, hyponatremia does not develop with use of NSAIDs, because a decrease in serum osmolality would result in inhibition of AVP release. This complication typically occurs in the setting of nonsuppressible AVP release. Removal of the counterbalancing effect of renal prostaglandins allows for any given level of AVP to exert a greater hydro-osmotic effect, thereby risking hyponatremia (**Fig. 38-3**). Patients at some increased risk for this complication include those with high circulating levels of AVP driven by a decreased effective arterial blood volume (e.g., congestive heart failure, cirrhosis). Patients with the syndrome of inappropriate antidiuretic hormone secretion (SIADH) and those taking medications capable of stimulating AVP secretion or impairing urinary dilution by other mechanisms are also at risk.

In considering the natriuretic and vasodilatory properties of prostaglandins, it is not surprising that the administration of NSAIDs has been shown to interfere with blood pressure control. In several studies, administration of NSAIDs was associated with an average increase in blood pressure of between 5 and 10 mm Hg. Of the various subgroups examined, this effect was most pronounced in patients who were already hypertensive, and much less so in those who were normotensive at baseline. Among the hypertensive patients, those receiving β-blockers seemed to be the most vulnerable to the hypertensive effect of NSAIDs. Less interaction occurred with diuretics and angiotensin-converting enzyme

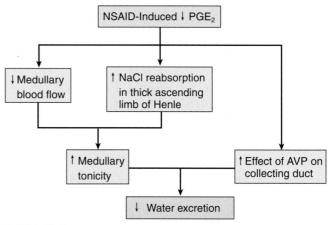

FIGURE 38-3 The mechanisms by which use of nonsteroidal anti-inflammatory drugs (NSAIDs) leads to decreased water excretion. AVP, arginine vasopressin; PGI_2, prostacyclin.

inhibitors, and no effect was seen with calcium channel blockers or angiotensin II receptor antagonists. Further subgroup analysis showed that patients with low-renin hypertension (e.g., elderly, African American) were also at higher risk for this hypertensive effect. The pathogenesis of NSAID-induced hypertension is not known with certainty. In one recent meta-analysis, NSAIDs were not found to alter body weight or urinary sodium excretion significantly, implying that mechanisms other than salt retention were responsible for the increased blood pressure. In this regard, elimination of the vasodilator PGI_2 from the resistance blood vessels is believed to play some role in the development of hypertension in individuals at risk.

GLOMERULAR AND INTERSTITIAL DISEASE INDUCED BY NONSTEROIDAL ANTI-INFLAMMATORY DRUGS

The use of NSAIDs can be associated with the development of a distinct syndrome characterized by interstitial nephritis and nephrotic-range proteinuria. Although virtually all NSAIDs have been reported to cause this syndrome, most cases have been reported in association with use of the propionic acid derivatives (fenoprofen, ibuprofen, and naproxen). Of these, fenoprofen has been implicated in more than 60% of reported cases. Interstitial nephritis with and without nephrotic syndrome has also been reported with the COX-2 inhibitors, rofecoxib and celecoxib.

In contrast to hemodynamically mediated acute renal failure, there are no obvious risk factors that identify those who are susceptible to developing this syndrome. The reported mean age of patients is 65 years. The presence of an underlying kidney disease before exposure to the NSAID has been notably absent. A number of features distinguish this form of interstitial kidney disease from that observed with other pharmacologic agents (**Table 38-3**). First, the average duration of exposure before the onset of disease is typically measured in months and can be as long as 1 year. By contrast, allergic interstitial nephritis caused by other drugs usually manifests within several days to weeks after exposure to the offending drug. Second, nephrotic-range proteinuria is found in more than 90% of cases of NSAID-induced interstitial disease, whereas this degree of proteinuria is distinctly uncommon in classic acute allergic interstitial nephritis. Third, symptoms of hypersensitivity commonly seen in acute allergic interstitial nephritis, such as rash, fever, arthralgias, or peripheral eosinophilia, are rare in NSAID-associated disease. Fourth, most cases associated with use of NSAIDs have been reported in older patients; in contrast, allergic interstitial nephritis is seen in all age groups.

Renal biopsy findings in NSAID-related interstitial disease typically show a diffuse or focal lymphocytic infiltrate consisting mainly of T lymphocytes. The number of eosinophils in the infiltrate is variable but usually is sharply increased. The glomerular changes are most commonly those seen in minimal change disease, although a few patients have been described with changes typical of membranous glomerulopathy. In particular, the glomeruli are normal by light microscopy, whereas podocyte effacement is seen with electron microscopy. In some cases, there is evidence of glomerulosclerosis. Because most patients who develop this syndrome are older, this latter finding may simply represent a normal age-related change. Immunofluorescence studies are typically nonspecific. There has been an occasional report of weak and variable staining for immunoglobulin G (IgG) and complement C3 along the tubular basement membrane. Mesangial electron-dense deposits have been observed in only three patients, suggesting that this is typically not an immune-mediated disease.

The usual clinical course is spontaneous remission after removal of the offending NSAID. The time until resolution is variable but ranges from a few days to several weeks. In some patients, the degree of kidney function impairment is severe enough to require dialytic support. Steroid therapy has been used in many of the reported cases; however, the efficacy and necessity of this therapy are unknown. Relapses have been reported after inadvertent exposure to the same NSAID or after exposure to a different NSAID.

RENIN RELEASE, HYPERKALEMIA, AND NONSTEROIDAL ANTI-INFLAMMATORY DRUGS

The use of NSAIDs has been associated with the development of hyperkalemia in the setting of CKD as well as normal kidney function. The physiologic basis for this effect is primarily inhibition of prostaglandin-mediated renin release with subsequent development of hyporeninemic hypoaldosteronism. The development of hyperkalemia in patients receiving NSAIDs is most likely to occur in the setting of impaired kidney function or baseline abnormalities in the RAS system. In particular, diabetic patients are at risk because of their increased incidence of hyporeninemic hypoaldosteronism. Compounding the propensity for hyperkalemia is insulin deficiency. Similarly, the elderly are at higher risk by virtue of the normal age-related decrease in circulating renin and aldosterone levels. Particular caution should be used when NSAIDs are combined with other pharmacologic agents known to interfere with the RAS cascade. Examples include β-blockers, calcineurin inhibitors, renin inhibitors, angiotensin-converting enzyme inhibitors, angiotensin receptor blockers, heparin, ketoconazole, high-dose trimethoprim, and potassium-sparing diuretics.

CLASSIC ANALGESIC NEPHROPATHY

Analgesic nephropathy is reported to be the most common form of drug-induced CKD and has been prominent in Australia, Europe, and the United States. This disease results from the habitual consumption over several years of analgesics, often preparations containing at least two antipyretic agents and usually codeine or caffeine. It is characterized by renal papillary necrosis (RPN) and chronic

TABLE 38-3 Comparison of Clinical Characteristics of NSAIDs-Induced and Typical Drug-Induced Forms of Tubulointerstitial Nephritis

CHARACTERISTIC	NSAID-INDUCED TIN	TYPICAL DRUG-INDUCED TIN
Duration of exposure	5 days to >1 yr	5-26 days
Hypersensitivity symptoms	7-8%	80%
Eosinophilia	17-18%	75-80%
Proteinuria >3.5 g/24 hr	>90%	<10%
Eosinophiluria	0-5%	80-85%
Peak serum creatinine	1.5 to >10 mg/dL	3.7 to >10 mg/dL

NSAIDs, nonsteroidal anti-inflammatory drugs; TIN, tubulointerstitial nephritis.

interstitial nephritis. This lesion has most commonly been associated with chronic ingestion of compound analgesics containing aspirin, phenacetin, and caffeine. The identification of phenacetin as the cause of the syndrome prompted many countries to remove the drug from the over-the-counter and prescription markets over the past 3 to 4 decades. However, removal of phenacetin was not uniformly followed by the expected reduction in the incidence of the syndrome in some countries, particularly Belgium. The isolated effects of phenacetin are unknown, because it was marketed only as a part of a combination analgesic. The lack of a uniform decline in analgesic nephropathy after substitution of other agents for phenacetin suggests that other combination mixtures could be responsible. In Belgium, a geographic correlation exists between the prevalence of analgesic nephropathy and sales of analgesic mixtures that do not contain phenacetin but do have a minimum of two analgesic components.

Numerous epidemiologic studies performed in the past demonstrated a wide variation in the worldwide incidence of analgesic nephropathy. Much of this variability could be explained by differences in the annual per capita consumption of phenacetin. In those countries with the highest consumption rates, such as Australia and Sweden, analgesic nephropathy was found to be responsible for up to 20% of cases of end-stage renal disease (ESRD) in the 1970s. In Canada, which had the lowest per capita consumption, analgesic nephropathy accounted for only 2% to 5% of ESRD patients during that era. It has been estimated that between 2% and 3% of all ESRD cases in the United States may be attributable to habitual analgesic consumption. Even within the United States, there are also regional differences in the reported incidence of analgesic nephropathy that most likely reflect differences in analgesic consumption. For example, the use of combination analgesics is more common in the southeastern United States, and analgesic nephropathy is thought to be more common as a cause of ESRD in North Carolina than in Philadelphia.

The development of analgesic nephropathy is associated with a number of well-defined clinical characteristics. The disease is usually more common in women by a factor of 2 to 6. The peak incidence is at age 53 years. Patients typically consume compound analgesics on a daily basis, often for chronic complaints such as headache or arthritis, or to improve work productivity. It has been estimated that nephropathy occurs after the cumulative ingestion of 2 to 3 kg of the index drug. Often patients exhibit a typical psychiatric profile characterized by addictive behavior. Gastrointestinal complications such as peptic ulcer disease are common. Anemia is frequently present as a result of gastrointestinal blood loss as well as CKD. Ischemic heart disease and renal artery stenosis have both been reported to occur with higher frequency in these patients. Finally, long-term use of analgesics is known to be a risk factor for the subsequent generation of uroepithelial tumors. Transitional cell carcinoma has been most closely associated with analgesic nephropathy, but renal cell carcinoma and sarcoma have also been reported.

Patients with analgesic nephropathy have predominantly tubulomedullary dysfunction characterized by impaired concentrating ability, acidification defects, and, rarely, a salt-losing state. Proteinuria tends to be low to moderate in quantity. The pattern of proteinuria is typically a mixture of glomerular and tubular origin. Pyuria is common and is often sterile. Occasionally, hematuria is noted, but if persistent, the possibility of a uroepithelial tumor should be raised.

There are many features of analgesic nephropathy that make it difficult to diagnose. The disease is slowly progressive, and the symptoms and signs are nonspecific. Patients are often reluctant to admit to heavy usage of analgesics and, therefore, are either misdiagnosed or not diagnosed at all until CKD is far advanced. In addition, the lack of a simple and noninvasive test that reliably implicates analgesics as the cause of the renal injury has been an important limiting factor. The noncontrasted abdominal computed tomogram was previously thought to be a helpful diagnostic tool in this setting, given its usefulness in the diagnosis of RPN. Characteristic findings include varying degrees of renal volume loss, cortical scarring, and papillary damage with calcification (**Fig. 38-4**). However, the recent National Analgesic Nephropathy Study examined the sensitivity of these findings in detecting analgesic-associated renal injury and found that this constellation did not occur frequently enough among heavy analgesic users to render the computed tomogram useful for diagnosis. In the United States, most heavy analgesic users had a negative "small indented calcified kidney" (SICK) scan.

RPN is a characteristic finding in individuals who abuse analgesics, particularly in Belgium. Although classic analgesic nephropathy has a greater association with RPN, several NSAIDs, either alone or in combination with aspirin, have also been associated with the development of this lesion through similar mechanisms. The parenchyma in this region of the kidney has a poor blood supply compared to the cortex and outer medulla. Furthermore, the vasculature here is highly dependent on prostanoids. In fact, the rate of prostaglandin synthetase activity of the papilla is 10 times higher than that of the medulla and 100 times higher than that of the cortex. Therefore, agents that inhibit cyclooxygenase activity, such as NSAIDs, can compromise blood flow and induce ischemia in this already underperfused region. Another reason why the papilla is vulnerable is the tubule's function of concentrating solutes to establish medullary hypertonicity. As a result, analgesics can accumulate in the medulla and lead to papillary injury. Usually, analgesic abuse alone does not cause RPN. Also required is a predisposing condition, such as diabetes, urinary tract obstruction, sickle hemoglobinopathy, or renal transplant rejection. Most lesions are asymptomatic, but patients can present with flank pain, ureteral colic, and hematuria, which can be confused for nephrolithiasis. Diagnosis can be obtained by visualizing necrotic tissue in the urine or, if the lesions are advanced, by imaging. Treatment is supportive and should include cessation of the offending analgesics.

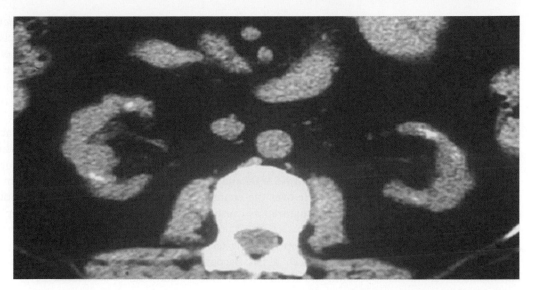

FIGURE 38-4 Computed tomographic findings in a patient with small indented calcified kidneys (SICK). Note the bilateral small kidneys, irregular contours, parenchymal scars, and coarse papillary calcifications. From Henrich WL, Clark RL, Kelly JP, et al: Non-contrast enhanced computerized tomography and analgesic-related kidney disease: Report of the National Analgesic Nephropathy Study. J Am Soc Nephrol 17:1472-1480, 2006.

CHRONIC KIDNEY DISEASE INDUCED BY NONSTEROIDAL ANTI-INFLAMMATORY DRUGS AND ACETAMINOPHEN

It is unresolved as to whether long-term and habitual use of NSAIDs alone can result in a progressive and/or irreversible form of CKD. The clinical characteristics of NSAID-induced CKD are sufficiently different from those of analgesic nephropathy to suggest that this is a distinct clinical entity (**Table 38-4**). Some observations have emerged to suggest that caution with regard to long-term use is warranted. In one multicenter case-control study, daily use of NSAIDs was associated with a twofold increase in the risk of newly diagnosed CKD, defined as a serum creatinine concentration of 1.5 mg/dL or greater. This increased risk was primarily limited to older men. An additional report linking chronic use of NSAIDs with development of CKD described 56 patients from Australia. These patients had taken only NSAIDs over a period of 10 to 20 years for treatment of a variety of rheumatic diseases. In 19 patients (34%), radiographic evidence of RPN was found. In 37 patients, kidney biopsy material was available and disclosed evidence of chronic interstitial nephritis. The clinical characteristics of these patients were quite different from those with analgesic nephropathy. In particular, patients with NSAID-associated kidney disease were older, had a 1:1 gender ratio, had a lower incidence of RPN, had less severe kidney functional impairment, and had a lower incidence of urinary tract infections.

More recently, however, multiple studies have challenged the belief that NSAIDs lead to CKD. The Physicians' Health Study was a large cohort study that examined self-reporting of analgesic use. Although the majority of the respondents were without renal dysfunction, the study found that moderate analgesic use conferred no increased risk of reduction in renal function. Even with a cumulative consumption of more than 2500 pills, mean creatinine concentrations were similar between users and nonusers. Likewise, the Nurses'

TABLE 38-4 Clinical Characteristics of Patients with Analgesic Nephropathy versus Chronic Kidney Disease Induced by NSAIDs

CHARACTERISTIC	ANALGESIC NEPHROPATHY	NSAID-INDUCED CHRONIC KID-NEY DISEASE
Age (yr)	40-50	>60
Gender ratio (female:male)	6:1	1:1
Psychiatric disorder	Common	Not a feature
Papillary necrosis (%)	90	30
Creatinine clearance (mL/min)	<20	40-60
Urinary tract infection	Common	Not a feature
Uroepithelial tumors	Increased risk	Not a feature
Ischemic heart disease	Common	Not a feature

NSAIDs, nonsteroidal anti-inflammatory drugs.

Health Study of healthy women showed that use of NSAIDs or aspirin was not associated with a reduction in GFR. Over a decade, no significant renal decline was noted. In examining the association between analgesic use and ESRD, a Spanish case-control study investigated an incident dialysis population. Patients were categorized as "users" if they had consumed any analgesics daily or every other day for 30 days or longer at any time before the diagnosis of kidney disease. Analysis was performed around this index date, and no association was found between ESRD and the use of nonaspirin products.

The inconsistent results from these studies assessing the effects of NSAIDs on CKD underscore their limitations. Many were retrospective and based on questionnaires or surveys of analgesic use and therefore were vulnerable to recall bias. Because of the time lag between drug exposure and the event of a diagnosis of renal insufficiency, lead time bias is generated. In most cases, the exact moment of toxic exposure cannot be identified. Furthermore, differing methodologies make comparisons of these studies difficult.

Each study established different criteria for defining abnormal creatinine concentration, creatinine clearance rate, and GFR. Dissimilar populations were examined, some healthy and some with preexisting renal disease to a varying degree. Future studies are needed to overcome these limitations. At this time, based on the studies that do show a positive association, it appears that some patients who use analgesics chronically may develop a change in kidney function over time. The number of people affected is likely to be relatively small, given the millions who take analgesics regularly. Nevertheless, given the abuse potential of NSAIDs and the fact that many preparations are available over-the-counter, chronic NSAID abuse may become recognized as cause of CKD in the future.

In considering the possible linkage between long-term NSAID use to the development of CKD, it has become common clinical practice to recommend acetaminophen for analgesia. Because acetaminophen is the major active metabolite of phenacetin, concern has been raised as to whether it, as a single ingredient, is nephrotoxic when consumed regularly. Two case-control studies examining the use of over-the-counter analgesics as a risk factor for ESRD found that acetaminophen was associated with CKD when used on a continual basis. In one study, heavy average use of acetaminophen (>1 pill/day) and medium to high cumulative intake (≥1000 pills in a lifetime) each doubled the odds of ESRD. The other study, a report from Sweden regarding analgesic use among patients with newly diagnosed renal dysfunction (creatinine clearance, 2.8 to 3.4 mg/dL), found that regular acetaminophen users were 2.5 times more likely to develop CKD. In contrast to these findings, the recent National Analgesic Nephropathy Study did not find a link between acetaminophen and ESRD. Discrepancies in the results may be attributed to several methodologic problems, such as confounding by indication, particularly in the earlier studies.

Because no data address the safety of chronic NSAID use in regard to renal function, the decision as to which analgesic to recommend is left to the realm of opinion. Taken as a whole, the current information favors acetaminophen as likely to be a safer alternative to NSAIDs if ingested in moderate quantities. If chronic use is required, then frequent monitoring of renal function is warranted.

Acute renal failure due to acetaminophen, though rare (<2% of all acetaminophen poisonings), has been better defined. It can occur either alone or in conjunction with hepatic necrosis. The primary renal manifestation is acute tubular necrosis, which is particularly notable in the proximal tubule. Risk factors are glutathione-depleted states (e.g., chronic alcohol abuse, fasting, starvation) and drugs that induce the cytochrome P-450 enzymes (e.g., anticonvulsants). The usual treatment regimen of gastric aspiration, activated charcoal, and oral N-acetylcysteine is recommended, although the latter may not expedite renal recovery if the nephrotoxicity is isolated. Most of these acute renal failure improve with supportive care within 7 to 10 days, with only a minority requiring dialysis. Because acetaminophen toxicity is the most commonly reported poisoning, nephrologists need to be aware of the drug's effects on the kidney.

Although the renal effects of NSAIDs and other analgesics are many, the chronic consequence of their use is an unsettled area of clinical medicine. The acute deleterious effects of NSAIDs in vulnerable populations is better defined. With regard to the risks engendered by chronic habitual use of any analgesic, common sense would dictate that the drugs should be consumed in the lowest effective dose and for the shortest period possible. For individuals who must consume analgesics, frequent (at least every 6 months) monitoring of renal function seems prudent. For patients with established CKD, acetaminophen is still the safest drug to consume, at least for short periods of time.

BIBLIOGRAPHY

Blakely P, McDonald BR: Acute renal failure due to acetaminophen ingestion. J Am Soc Nephrol 6:48-53, 1995.

Catella-Lawson F, McAdam B, Morrison B, et al: Effects of specific inhibition of cyclooxygenase-2 on sodium balance, hemodynamics, vasoactive eicosanoids. J Pharmacol Exp Ther 289:735-741, 1999.

Curhan GC, Knight EL, Rosner B, et al: Lifetime nonnarcotic analgesic use and decline in renal function in women. Arch Intern Med 164:1519-1524, 2004.

DeBroe ME, Elseviers M: Analgesic nephropathy. N Engl J Med 338:446-452, 1998.

Eknoyan G: Renal papillary necrosis. In Greenberg A (ed): Primer on Kidney Diseases. 4th ed., Philadelphia, Elsevier Saunders, 2005, pp 385-388.

Elseviers M, De Broe M: A long-term prospective controlled study of analgesic abuse in Belgium. Kidney Int 48:1912-1919, 1995.

Fored CM, Ejerblad E, Lindblad P, et al: Acetaminophen, aspirin, and chronic renal failure. N Engl J Med 345:1801-1801, 2001.

Henrich WL, Agodoa L, Barrett B, et al: Analgesics and the kidney: Summary and recommendations to the Scientific Advisory Board of the National Kidney Foundation from an Ad Hoc Committee of the National Kidney Foundation. Am J Kidney Dis 27:162-165, 1996.

Henrich WL, Anderson RJ, Berns AS, et al: The role of renal nerves and prostaglandins in control of renal hemodynamics and plasma renin activity during hypotensive hemorrhage in the dog. J Clin Invest 61:744-750, 1978.

Henrich WL, Clark RL, Kelly JP, et al: Non-contrast-enhanced computerized tomography and analgesic-related kidney disease: Report of the national analgesic nephropathy study. J Am Soc Nephrol 17:1472-1480, 2006.

Ibanez L, Morlans M, Vidal X, et al: Case-control study of regular analgesic and nonsteroidal anti-inflammatory use and end-stage renal disease. Kidney Int 67:2393-2398, 2005.

Kaufman DW, Kelly JP, Rosenberg L, et al: Recent patterns of medication use in the ambulatory adult population of the United States: the Slone survey. JAMA 387:337-344, 2002.

Palmer BF: Renal complications associated with use of non-steroidal antiinflammatory agents. J Invest Med 43:516-533, 1995.

Palmer BF, Henrich WL: Clinical acute renal failure secondary to non-steroidal antiinflammatory drugs. Semin Nephrol 15:214-227, 1995.

Paulose-Ram R, Hirsch R, Dillon C, et al: Prescription and non-prescription analgesic use among the US adult population: Results from the third National Health and Nutrition Examination Survey (NHANES III). Pharmacoepidemiol Drug Saf 12:315-326, 2003.

Perneger TV, Whelton PK, Klag MJ: Risk of kidney failure associated with the use of acetaminophen, aspirin, and nonsteroidal antiinflammatory drugs. N Engl J Med 331:1675-1679, 1994.

Rexrode , KM, Buring JE, Glynn RJ et al: Analgesic use and renal function in men. JAMA 286:315-321, 2001.

Rossat J, Maillard M, Nussberger J, et al: Renal effects of selective cyclooxygenase-2 inhibition in normotensive salt-depleted subjects. Clin Pharmacol Ther 66:76-84, 1999.

Sandler DP, Smith JC, Weinberg CR et al: Analgesic use and chronic renal disease. N Engl J Med 320:1238-1243, 1989.

Schlondorff D: Renal complications of nonsteroidal anti-inflammatory drugs. Kidney Int 44:643-653, 1993.

Segasothy M, Samad SA, Zulfigar A et al: Chronic renal disease and papillary necrosis associated with the long-term use of non-steroidal anti-inflammatory drugs as the sole or predominant analgesic. Am J Kidney Dis 24:17-24, 1994.

CHAPTER 39

Principles of Drug Therapy in Patients with Reduced Kidney Function

Gary R. Matzke

Reduced kidney function may occur in many situations, including chronic kidney disease (CKD) resulting from such disorders as diabetes mellitus, hypertension, and glomerulonephritis as well as age-related diminution of kidney function. In adults, these conditions have been associated with a high use of medications, making these patients particularly susceptible to the accumulation of a drug or its active or toxic metabolites. As clinicians strive to optimize the clinical outcomes of their patients they must have a thorough understanding of the impact of reduced kidney function on drug disposition and the appropriate methods by which to individualize drug therapy.

Individualization of therapy for those agents that are predominantly (>70%) eliminated unchanged by the kidney can be accomplished with a proportional dose reduction or dosage interval prolongation adjustment based on the fractional reduction in glomerular filtration rate (GFR) or its more commonly evaluated clinical counterpart, creatinine clearance (CL_{Cr}). However, because diminished kidney function has been associated with progressive alterations in the bioavailability, plasma protein binding, distribution volume, and metabolism of many drugs, a more complex adjustment scheme may be required for medications that are extensively metabolized by the liver or for which changes in protein binding and/or distribution volume have been noted. Patients with diminished kidney function may also respond to a given dose or serum concentration of a drug (e.g., phenytoin) differently from those with normal kidney function because of the physiologic and biochemical changes associated with progressive CKD.

Using a sound understanding of basic pharmacokinetic principles, the pharmacokinetic characteristics of a drug, and the pathophysiologic alterations associated with impaired kidney function, clinicians can design individualized therapeutic regimens. This chapter describes the influence of impaired kidney function resulting from CKD, and, when information is available, from acute kidney injury (AKI), on drug absorption, distribution, metabolism, and elimination. The chapter also provides a practical approach to drug dosage individualization for patients with reduced kidney function and those receiving continuous renal replacement therapy (CRRT), peritoneal dialysis, or hemodialysis.

EFFECT OF REDUCED KIDNEY FUNCTION ON DRUG ABSORPTION

There is little quantitative information about the influence of reductions in kidney function in CKD patients on drug absorption. Several variables, including changes in gastrointestinal transit time and gastric pH, edema of the gastrointestinal tract, vomiting and diarrhea (frequently seen in those with stage 5 CKD), and concomitant administration of phosphate binders, have been associated with alterations in the absorption of some drugs, such as digoxin and many of the fluoroquinolone antibiotics. Although the fraction of a drug that reaches the systemic circulation after oral versus intravenous administration (termed *absolute bioavailability*) is rarely altered in CKD patients, alterations in the peak concentration (C_{max}) and in the time at which the peak concentration was attained (t_{max}), have been noted for a few drugs. Although the bioavailability of some drugs, such as furosemide or pindolol, has been reported to be reduced, there are no consistent findings in patients with CKD to indicate that absorption is impaired. However, an increase in bioavailability as the result of a decrease in metabolism during the drug's first pass through the gastrointestinal tract and liver has been noted for some β-blockers and for dextropropoxyphene and dihydrocodeine.

EFFECT OF REDUCED KIDNEY FUNCTION ON DRUG DISTRIBUTION

The volume of distribution of many drugs is significantly altered in patients with stage 4 or stage 5 CKD (**Table 39-1**), and changes in patients with oliguric AKI have also been reported. These changes are predominantly the result of altered plasma protein or tissue binding, or of volume expansion secondary to reduced renal sodium and water excretion. The plasma protein binding of acidic drugs such as warfarin and phenytoin is decreased in patients with CKD. This decrease in binding of acidic drugs has been attributed to changes in the conformation of the binding sites, accumulation of endogenous inhibitors of binding, and decreased concentrations of albumin. In addition, the high concentrations of metabolites of some drugs that accumulate in CKD patients may interfere with the protein binding of the parent compound.

TABLE 39-1 Volume of Distribution of Selected Drugs in Patients with Stage 5 CKD

DRUG	NORMAL (L/kg)	STAGE 5 CKD (L/kg)	CHANGE FROM NORMAL (%)
Amikacin	0.20	0.29	45
Azlocillin	0.21	0.28	33
Cefazolin	0.13	0.17	31
Cefoxitin	0.16	0.26	63
Cefuroxime	0.20	0.26	30
Clofibrate	0.14	0.24	71
Dicloxacillin	0.08	0.18	125
Digoxin	7.3	4.0	-45
Erythromycin	0.57	1.09	91
Gentamicin	0.20	0.32	60
Isoniazid	0.6	0.8	33
Minoxidil	2.6	4.9	88
Phenytoin	0.64	1.4	119
Trimethoprim	1.36	1.83	35
Vancomycin	0.64	0.85	33

CKD, chronic kidney disease.

The plasma concentration of the principal binding protein for several basic drug compounds, α_1-acid glycoprotein, is increased in kidney transplantation patients and in hemodialysis patients. For this reason, the unbound fraction of some basic drugs (e.g., quinidine) may be increased, and, as a result, the volume of distribution in these patients is reduced. The net effect of changes in protein binding is usually an alteration in the relationship between unbound and total drug concentrations, an effect frequently encountered with phenytoin. The increase in unbound fraction, to values as high as 20% to 25% from the normal of 10%, results in increased hepatic clearance and decreased total concentrations. Although the unbound concentration therapeutic range is unchanged, the therapeutic range for total phenytoin concentration is reduced to 4 to 10 µg/mL (normal, 10 to 20 µg/mL) as the degree of kidney impairment increases. Therefore, the maintenance of therapeutic unbound concentrations of 1 to 2 µg/mL provides the best target for individualizing phenytoin therapy in patients with reduced kidney function. The optimal approach to management in these patients relies on the measurement of unbound phenytoin serum concentrations.

Altered tissue binding may also affect the apparent volume of distribution of a drug. For example, the distribution volume of digoxin has been reported to be reduced by 30% to 50% in patients with severe CKD. This may be the result of competitive inhibition by endogenous or exogenous digoxin-like immunoreactive substances that bind to and inhibit membrane adenosine triphosphatase (ATPase). The absolute amount of digoxin bound to the tissue digoxin receptor is reduced, and the resultant serum digoxin concentration observed after the administration of any dose is greater than expected.

Therefore, in patients with CKD, a normal total drug concentration may be associated with either serious adverse reactions secondary to elevated unbound drug concentrations or subtherapeutic responses because of an increased plasma-to-tissue drug concentration ratio. Monitoring of unbound drug concentrations is suggested for those drugs that have a narrow therapeutic range, those that are highly protein bound (>80%), and those for which marked variability in the bound fraction has been reported (e.g., phenytoin, disopyramide).

EFFECT OF REDUCED KIDNEY FUNCTION ON METABOLISM

The relationship of CKD to cytochrome P-450 (CYP)-mediated metabolism in the liver and other organs has been reviewed. In rat models of CKD, protein expression in the liver of several CYP enzymes, including CYP3A1 and CYP3A2 (equivalent to human CYP3A4), is reduced by as much as 75%; in addition, CYP2C11 and CYP3A2 activity is significantly reduced, whereas CYP1A2 activity is unchanged. In humans, CYP2C19 and CYP3A4 activity is reduced, but CYP2D6 and CYP2E1 activity appears to be unaffected by the presence of CKD. The reduction of nonrenal clearance (CL_{NR}) of several drugs in patients with stage 4 or stage 5 CKD supports this premise. These studies must be interpreted with caution, however, because concurrent drug intake, age, smoking status, and alcohol intake were often not taken into consideration. Furthermore, pharmacogenetic variations in drug-metabolizing enzyme activity that may have been present in the individual before the onset and progression of CKD must be considered, if known. For these reasons, prediction of the effect of reduced kidney function on the metabolism of a particular drug is difficult, and a general quantitative strategy to adjust drug dosage regimens for extensively metabolized agents is not yet available. However, some insight may be gained if one knows which enzymes are involved in the metabolism of the drug of interest and how those enzymes are affected by the reduction in kidney function.

The effect of CKD on the metabolism of a particular drug is difficult to predict even for drugs within the same pharmacologic class. The reductions in CL_{NR} for those with CKD have frequently been noted to be proportional to the reductions in GFR. In the small number of studies that have evaluated CL_{NR} in critically ill patients with AKI, residual CL_{NR} was higher than in CKD patients with similar levels of CL_{Cr}, whether measured or estimated from the Cockcroft-Gault equation. Because a patient with AKI may have a higher CL_{NR} than a CKD patient, the resultant plasma concentrations will be lower than expected, and possibly subtherapeutic, if classic CKD-derived dosage guidelines are followed.

EFFECT OF REDUCED KIDNEY FUNCTION ON RENAL EXCRETION

Renal clearance (CL_R) is the net result of glomerular filtration of unbound drug plus tubular secretion minus tubular reabsorption. An acute or chronic reduction in GFR results in a decrease in CL_R. The degree of change in total body clearance of a drug is dependent on the fraction of the dose that is eliminated unchanged in individuals with normal kidney function, the intrarenal drug transport pathways, and the degree of functional impairment of each of these pathways. The primary renal transport systems of clinical significance include the organic anionic (OAT), organic cationic (OCT), and P-glycoprotein transporters. Diuretics, β-lactam antibiotics, nonsteroidal anti-inflammatory drugs, and glucuronide metabolites of many different drugs are eliminated by the family of OAT transporters. The OCT transporters contribute to the secretion and excretion of cimetidine, famotidine, and quinidine, and the P-glycoprotein transport system in the kidney is involved in the secretion of cationic and hydrophobic drugs (e.g., digoxin, *Vinca* alkaloids). The clearance of drugs that are extensively secreted by the kidney (CL_R >300 mL/min) may be significantly reduced as the result of impairment in one or more of these renal transporters.

Despite the different mechanisms involved in the elimination of drugs by the kidney, the clinical estimation of CL_{Cr} remains the guiding index for drug dosage regimen design, because there is no clinical means to estimate the activity of the key secretory pathways. The importance of an alteration in kidney function on drug elimination therefore usually depends primarily on two variables: (1) the fraction of drug normally eliminated by the kidney unchanged and (2) the degree of kidney functional impairment as assessed by CL_{Cr}. There are a few drugs for which a metabolite is the primary active entity; in that situation, a key variable is the degree of renal clearance of the metabolite. The calculation of CL_{Cr} from a timed urine collection with creatinine measurement in serum and urine has been the standard clinical measure of kidney function for decades. However, urine is difficult to collect accurately in most clinical settings, and the interference of many commonly used medications with creatinine measurement limits the utility of this approach. The administration of radioactive markers ($[^{125}I]$iothalamate, ^{51}Cr-EDTA, or ^{99m}Tc-DTPA) or nonradioactive markers (aminoglycosides, iohexol, iothalamate, and inulin) of GFR, although scientifically sound, is clinically impractical, because intravenous or subcutaneous administration of the marker and the multiple timed blood and urine collections make the procedures expensive and cumbersome.

Estimation of CL_{Cr} or GFR, in contrast, requires only routinely collected laboratory and demographic data. The Cockcroft-Gault equation for CL_{Cr} and the two Modification of Diet in Renal Disease (MDRD) equations for GFR estimation correlate well with CL_{Cr} and GFR measurements in individuals with stable kidney function and average body composition (see Chapter 2). The traditional approach of estimating CL_{Cr} and using it as a continuous variable of renal function is now being supplemented and, in some institutions, replaced by estimation of GFR using the four-variable MDRD equation with categorical CKD staging. The four-variable version of the MDRD (MDRD4) equation was introduced in 2000 and has demonstrated precision and accuracy similar to its six-variable predecessor. This version of the MDRD equation, referred to here as the *estimated GFR (eGFR)* does not include albumin or blood urea nitrogen, resulting in wider application in most outpatient clinical settings. This measurement is endorsed by the National Kidney Foundation's Kidney Disease Outcomes Quality Initiative (K/DOQI) and the Kidney Disease Evaluation Program (KDEP) of the National Institutes of Health for use in identification and stratification of individuals with CKD (see Chapter 53.)

The validity of the eGFR equation for clinical use in all patient settings and as a guide for drug dosage adjustment is controversial at best. This equation has not been validated in children, pregnant women, the elderly (age >70 years), racial or ethnic subgroups other than Caucasian and African Americans, patients with diabetes, and those with "normal" kidney function. Therefore, the CL_{Cr} is still the standard for drug dosing, because, in addition to the shortcomings of the eGFR approach for the estimation of true GFR, almost all of the primary literature has used CL_{Cr} to derive the relationship between kidney function and renal and total body clearance of a drug. However, all of these methods (including the Cockcroft-Gault equation) are extremely poor predictors of kidney function in individuals with liver disease, and their use is not recommended for such patients. Finally, although several methods for CL_{Cr} estimation in patients with unstable kidney function (e.g., AKI) have been proposed, the accuracy of these methods has not been rigorously assessed, and at the present time their use cannot be recommended.

STRATEGIES FOR DRUG THERAPY INDIVIDUALIZATION

The design of the optimal dosage regimen for a patient with reduced kidney function depends on the availability of an accurate characterization of the relationship between the pharmacokinetic parameters of the drug and kidney function, as well as the patient's CL_{Cr}. Before 1998, there was no consensus regarding the criteria for characterization of the pharmacokinetics of a drug in patients with CKD. An industry guidance report issued by the U.S. Food and Drug Administration in May of 1998 provided guidelines regarding when a study should be considered and provided recommendations for study design, data analysis, and assessment of the impact of the study results on drug dosing. As a result, the quantity and quality of data available to clinicians has improved in the last 10 years. The key unresolved question is whether this improvement in information has made its way into clinical practice.

Most dosage adjustment reference sources for clinical use have proposed the use of a fixed dose or interval for patients with a broad range of renal function. Indeed, "normal" renal function has often been ascribed to anyone who has a CL_{Cr} greater than 50 mL/min, even though many individuals (e.g., early hyperfiltering diabetics) have values in the range of 120 to 180 mL/min. The "moderate renal function impairment" category in many guides encompasses a fivefold range of CL_{Cr}, from 10 to 49 mL/min, whereas severe renal function impairment or end-stage renal disease is defined as a CL_{Cr} of less than 10 to 15 mL/min. Each of these categories encompasses a broad range of renal function, and the calculated drug regimen may not be optimal for all patients within that range. The American Hospital Formulary Service's Drug Information Service, the *British National Formulary,* Aronoff's *Drug Prescribing in Renal Failure,* and Martindale's *Complete Drug Reference* are considered by many to be excellent resources for drug dosage recommendations for patients with impaired renal function. However, a recent systematic comparison of these four sources revealed remarkable variation in recommendations, along with a paucity of details of the methods used to generate the dosing advice and a lack of reference to primary literature. Therefore, these sources of drug information are not consistent and do not provide an optimal approach for drug dosage selection for individual patients.

If specific literature recommendations or data on the relationship of the pharmacokinetic parameters of a drug to CL_{Cr} are not available, then these parameters can be estimated for a particular patient using the method of Rowland and Tozer, provided that the fraction of the drug that is eliminated unchanged by the kidney (f_e) in subjects with normal kidney function is known. This approach assumes that the change in drug clearance is proportional to the change in CL_{Cr}, that kidney disease does not alter the drug's metabolism that any metabolites produced are inactive and nontoxic, that the drug obeys first-order (linear) kinetic principles, and that it is adequately described by a one-compartment model. If these assumptions are true, the kinetic parameter or dosage adjustment factor (Q) can be calculated as follows:

$$Q = 1 \simeq [f_e(1 \simeq KF)]$$

where KF is the ratio of the patient's CL_{Cr} to the assumed normal value of 120 mL/min. As an example, the Q factor for a patient who has a CL_{Cr} of 10 mL/min and a drug that is 85% eliminated unchanged by the kidney would be

$$Q = 1 - [0.85(1 - 10/120)]$$
$$= 1 - [0.85(0.92)]$$
$$= 1 - 0.78$$
$$= 0.22$$

The estimated clearance rate of the drug in this patient (CL_{PT}) would then be calculated as

$$CL_{PT} = CL_{norm} \times Q$$

where CL_{norm} is the respective value in patients with normal kidney function derived from the literature.

For antihypertensive agents, cephalosporins, and many other drugs for which there are no target values for peak or trough concentrations, attainment of an average steady-state concentration similar to that in normal subjects is appropriate. The principal means to achieve this goal is to decrease the dose or prolong the dosing interval. If the dose is reduced and the dosing interval is unchanged, the desired average steady-state concentration will be near-normal; however, the peak will be lower and the trough higher. Alternatively, if the

dosing interval is increased and the dose remains unchanged, the peak, trough, and average concentrations will be similar to those in the patients with normal kidney function. This interval adjustment method is often preferred, because it is likely to yield significant cost savings as the result of less frequent drug administration. If a loading dose is not administered, it will take 4 to 5 half-lives for the desired steady-state plasma concentrations to be achieved in any patient; this may require days rather than hours because of the prolonged half-life of many drugs in patients with reduced kidney function. Therefore, to achieve the desired concentration rapidly, a loading dose (D_L) should be administered for most patients with reduced kidney function. D_L can be calculated as follows:

$$D_L = (C_{peak}) \times (V_D) \times (\text{Body weight in kilograms})$$

The loading dose is usually the same for patients with reduced kidney function as it is for those with normal kidney function. However, if the V_D in patients with reduced kidney function is significantly different from that V_D in patients with normal kidney function (see **Table 39-1**), then the modified value should be used to calculate the D_L.

The adjusted dosing interval (τ_{RKF}) and maintenance dose (D_{RKF}) for the patient can then be calculated from the normal dosing interval (τ_n) and normal dose (D_n), respectively:

$$\tau_{RKF} = \tau_n/Q$$

$$D_{RKF} = D_n \times Q$$

If these approaches yield a time interval or a dose that is impractical, a new dose can be calculated using a fixed, prespecified dose interval (τ_{RKF}) such as 24 or 48 hours, as follows:

$$D_{RKF} = [D_n \times Q \times \tau_{RKF}]/\tau_f$$

Patients Receiving Continuous Renal Replacement Therapy

CRRT is used primarily in patients with AKI. Drug therapy individualization for the patient receiving CRRT must take into account the fact that patients with AKI may have a higher residual CL_{NR} of a drug than do CKD patients with a similar CL_{Cr}. In addition to patient-specific differences, there are marked differences in the efficiency of drug removal (see Chapter 54) among the three primary types of CRRT: continuous venovenous hemofiltration (CVVH), continuous venovenous hemodialysis (CVVHD), and continuous venovenous hemodiafiltration (CVVHDF). The primary variables that influence drug clearance during CRRT are the ultrafiltration rate (UFR), the blood flow rate (BFR), and the dialysate flow rate (DFR), as well as the type of hemofilter used. For example, clearance during CVVH is directly proportional to the UFR as a result of convective transport of drug molecules. The clearance of a drug in this situation is a function of the membrane permeability of the drug, which is called the sieving coefficient (SC), and the UFR. The SC can be approximated by the fraction of drug that is unbound to plasma proteins (f_u), so the clearance can be calculated as follows:

$$CL_{CVVH} = UFR \times SC$$

or

$$CL_{CVVH} = UFR \times f_u$$

Clearance during CVVHD also depends on the DFR and the SC of the drug. If UFR is negligible, CL_{CVVHD} can be estimated to be maximally equal to the product of DFR and f_u or SC.

Clearance of a drug by CVVHDF is generally greater than by CVVHD, because drug is removed by diffusion as well as by convection/ultrafiltration. The CL_{CVVHDF} in many clinical settings can be mathematically approximated as

$$CL_{CVVHDF} = (UFR + DFR) \times SC$$

provided that the DFR is less than 33 mL/min and BFR is at least 75 mL/min. Changes in BFR typically have only a minor effect on drug clearance by any mode of CRRT, because BFR is usually much larger than the DFR and is therefore not the limiting factor for drug removal.

Individualization of therapy for a patient receiving CRRT is based on the patient's residual kidney function and the clearance of the drug by the mode of CRRT employed. The patient's residual drug clearance can be predicted as described earlier in this chapter. The CRRT clearance can also be approximated from published literature reports, although many of these reports did not specify all the operating conditions, and it may thus be hard to directly apply the findings to a given patient situation. The clearances of several frequently used drugs by CVVH and CVVHDF are summarized in **Tables 39-2** and **39-3**, respectively. Whenever feasible, plasma drug concentration monitoring for certain drugs such as aminoglycosides and vancomycin is highly recommended.

Patients Receiving Chronic Hemodialysis

Drug therapy in hemodialysis patients should be guided by careful evaluation of the patient's residual renal function in addition to the added clearance associated with the patient's dialysis prescription. Literature-derived dosing recommendations are useful for many agents, especially those with a wide therapeutic index. However, for those drugs with a narrow therapeutic index, individualization of the drug therapy regimen is highly recommended based on prospective serum concentration monitoring. Although many new hemodialyzers have been introduced in the past 10 years and the average delivered dose of hemodialysis has increased, the effect of hemodialysis on the disposition of a drug is rarely re-evaluated after its initial introduction to the market, and

TABLE 39-2 Drug Clearance and Dosing Recommendations for Patients Receiving Continuous Venovenous Hemofiltration (CVVH)

DRUG	HEMOFILTER	CL_T (mL/min, mean or range)	CL_{CVVH} (mL/min, mean or range)	DOSAGE RECOMMENDATION
Acyclovir	PS	0.39	NR	5 mg/kg q12h
Amikacin	PS	10.5	10-16	IND*
Amrinone	PS	40.8	2.4-14.4	None provided
Atracurium	PA	502.5	8.25	None provided
Ceftazidime	AN69, PMMA, PS	NR	7.5-15.6	500 mg q12h
Ceftriaxone	AN69, PMMA, PS	NR	NR	300 mg q12h
	PA	39.3	17	1000 mg q24h
Cefuroxime	PS	32	11	0.75-1.0 g q24h
Ciprofloxacin	AN69	84.4	12.4	400 mg q24h
Fluconazole	AN69	25.3	17.5	400-800 mg q24h
Gentamicin	PS	11.6	3.47	IND*
Imipenem	PS	108.3	13.3	500 mg q6-8h
Levofloxacin	AN69	42.3	11.5	250 mg q24h
Meropenem	PA	76	16-50	0.5-1.0 g q12h
Phenytoin	PS	NR	1.02	IND*
Piperacillin	NR	42	NR	4 g q12h
Ticarcillin	PS	29.7	12.3	2 g q8-12h
Tobramycin	PS	11.7	3.5	IND*
Vancomycin	PA, PMMA, PS	14-29	12-24	750-1250 mg q24h

*Serum concentrations may vary markedly depending on the patient's condition, therefore dose individualization is recommended.
AN69, acrylonitrile; CL_{CVVH}, CVVH clearance; CL_T, total body clearance; IND, individualize; NR, not reported; PA, polyamide filter; PMMA, polymethylmethacrylate filter; PS, polysulfone filter.
Adapted from Matzke GR, Clermont G: Clinical pharmacology and therapeutics. In Murray P, Brady HR, Hall JB [eds]: Intensive Care Nephrology. London, Taylor and Francis, 2006.

TABLE 39-3 Drug Clearance and Dosing Recommendations for Patients Receiving Continuous Venovenous Hemodiafiltration (CVVHDF)

DRUG	HEMOFILTER	CL_T (mL/min, mean or range)	CL_{CVVHDF} (mL/min, mean or range)	DOSAGE RECOMMENDATION
Acyclovir	AN69	1.2	NR	5 mg/kg q12h
Ceftazidime	AN69, PMMA, PS	25-31	13-28	0.5-1 g q24h
Ceftriaxone	AN69	—	11.7-13.2	250 mg q12h
	PMMA, PS	—	19.8-30.5	300 mg q12h
Cefuroxime	AN69	22	14-16.2	750 mg q12h
Ciprofloxacin	AN69	264	16-37	300 mg q12h
Fluconazole	AN69	21-38	25-30	400-800 mg q12h
Ganciclovir	AN69	32	13	2.5 mg/kg q24h
Gentamicin	AN69	20	5.2	IND*
Imipenem	AN69, PS	134	16-30	500 mg q6-8h
Levofloxacin	AN69	51	22	250 mg q24h
Meropenem	PAN	55-140	20-39	1000 mg q8-12h
Mezlocillin	AN69, PS	31-253	11-45	2-4 g q24h
Sulbactam	AN69, PS	32-54	10-23	0.5 g q24h
Piperacillin	AN69	47	22	PIP: 4 g q12h
				PIP/TAZO: 3.375 g q8-12h
Teicoplanin	AN69	9.2	3.6	LD: 800 mg
				MD: 400 mg q24h × 2, then q48-72h
Vancomycin	AN69	17-39	10-17	7.5 mg/kg q12h
	PMMA	—	15-27.0	1.0-1.5 gm q24h
	PS	36	11-22	0.85-1.35 gm q24h

*Serum concentrations may vary markedly depending on the patient's condition, therefore dose individualization is recommended.
AN69, acrylonitrile; CL_{CVVHD}, CVVHD clearance; CL_T, total body clearance; IND, individualize; LD, Loading dose; MD, Maintenance dose; NR, not reported; PA, polyamide filter; PAN, polyacrylonitrile filter; PMMA, polymethylmethacrylate filter; PS, polysulfone filter; TAZO, Tazobactam.
Adapted from Matzke GR, Clermont G: Clinical pharmacology and therapeutics. In Murray P, Brady HR, Hall JB [eds]: Intensive Care Nephrology. London, Taylor and Francis, 2006.

most of the published dosing guidelines probably present an underestimation of the impact of hemodialysis on drug disposition. Therefore, clinicians should cautiously consider the prescription of doses that are larger than those conventionally recommended for their critically ill patients. The effect of hemodialysis on a patient's drug therapy depends on the molecular weight, protein binding, and distribution volume of the drug; the composition of the dialyzer membrane; its surface area; BFR and DFR; and whether the dialyzer is reused. Drugs that are small molecules but are highly protein bound usually are not well dialyzed, because both of the principal binding proteins (α_1-acid glycoprotein and albumin) are high-molecular-weight entities. Finally, those drugs that have a large volume of distribution are poorly removed by hemodialysis.

Conventional or low-flux dialyzers are relatively impermeable to drugs with a molecular weight greater than 1000 Da. High-flux hemodialyzers allow the passage of most drugs that have a molecular weight of 10,000 Da or less. The effect of reuse of dialyzers on clearance has been reported for only a few "model" drugs (cefazolin, ceftazidime, tobramycin, and vancomycin). Minimal to no change in clearance was reported with several low-flux dialyzers. Modest clearance decrements of up to 13% were noted after 5 to 10 reuses of high-flux polysulfone dialyzers. In contrast, significant clearance decreases of 25% to 45% were evident after 5 to 10 reuses of high-flux cellulose triacetate dialyzers.

The determination of drug concentrations at the start and end of dialysis, with subsequent calculation of the half-life during dialysis, has historically been used as an index of drug removal by dialysis. A more accurate means of assessing the effect of hemodialysis is to calculate the dialyzer clearance rate (CL_D) of the drug. Because drug concentrations are generally determined in plasma, the plasma clearance of the drug by hemodialysis (CL_{pD}) can be calculated as follows:

$$CL_{pD} = Q_p([A_p - V_p]/A_p)$$

where p represents plasma, A_p is arterial plasma concentration, V_p is venous plasma concentration, and Q_p is the plasma flow rate calculated as PFR = BFR × (1 − Hematocrit). This clearance calculation accurately reflects dialysis drug clearance only if the drug does not penetrate or bind to formed blood elements.

For patients receiving hemodialysis, the usual objective is to restore the amount of drug in the body at the end of dialysis to the value that would have been present if the patient had not been dialyzed. The supplementary dose (D_{postHD}) is calculated as follows:

$$D_{postHD} = [V_D \times C](e^{-k \cdot t} - e^{-k_{HD} \cdot t})$$

where ($V_D \times C$) is the amount of drug in the body at the start of dialysis, $e^{-k \cdot t}$ is the fraction of drug remaining as a result of the patient's residual total body clearance during the dialysis procedure, and $e^{-k_{HD} \cdot t}$ is the fraction of drug remaining as a result of elimination by the dialyzer: $k_{HD} = CL_{pD}/V_D$. Recently, some clinicians have evaluated alternative dosing strategies for some drugs, such as gentamicin and vancomycin, that include administration of the drug before or during the dialysis procedure. These approaches may save time in the ambulatory dialysis setting, but they increase drug cost, because more drug will have to be given to compensate for the increased removal by dialysis. Values for CL_{pD} of some commonly used drugs are listed in **Table 39-4**, and data for others can be obtained for specific dialysis procedures from literature cited in the bibliography. This information only serves as the initial dosing guidance for the patient's course of therapy. Measurement of predialysis serum concentrations is highly recommended to guide subsequent drug dosing considerations.

The impact of hemodialysis on drug therapy must not be viewed as a "generic procedure" that will result in removal of a fixed percentage of the drug from the body with each dialysis session; neither should simple "yes/no" answers on the dialyzability of drug compounds be considered sufficient information for therapeutic decisions. Compounds considered nondialyzable with low-flux dialyzers may in fact be significantly removed by high-flux hemodialyzers.

Patients Receiving Chronic Peritoneal Dialysis

Peritoneal dialysis, like other dialysis modalities, has the potential to affect drug disposition; however, drug therapy individualization is often less complicated in these patients because of the relative inefficiency of the procedure per unit time. Variables that influence drug removal in peritoneal dialysis include drug-specific characteristics such as molecular weight, solubility, degree of ionization, protein binding, and volume of distribution, as well as peritoneal membrane characteristics such as splanchnic blood flow, surface area, and permeability. The contribution of peritoneal dialysis to total body clearance is often low and, for most drugs, markedly less than the contribution of hemodialysis per unit time. Anti-infective agents are the most commonly studied drugs because of their primary role in the treatment of peritonitis and the dosing recommendations for the management of peritonitis and exit site infection, which are regularly updated, should be consulted as necessary. Most other drugs can generally be dosed according to the residual kidney function of the patient, because clearance by peritoneal dialysis is small.

If there is a significant relationship between the desired peak (C_{peak}) or trough (C_{trough}) concentration of a drug for a given patient with reduced kidney function (RKF) and the potential clinical response (e.g., aminoglycosides) or toxicity (e.g., quinidine, phenobarbital, phenytoin), then attainment of the target plasma concentration value is critical. In these situations, the adjusted dosage interval (τ_{RKF}) and maintenance dose (D_{RKF}) for the patient can be calculated as follows:

$$\tau_{RKF} = ([1/k_{PT}] \times \ln[C_{peak}/C_{trough}]) + t_{inf}$$

$$D_{RKF} = [k_{PT} \times V_D \times C_{peak}] \times [1 - e^{-(k_{PT})(\tau_{RKF})}/1 - e^{-(k_{PT})(t_{inf})}]$$

where t_{inf} is the infusion duration, k_{PT} is the elimination rate constant of the drug for that patient, which can be estimated as $K_{PT} = K_{norm} \times Q$, and V_D is the volume of distribution of the drug which can be obtained from literature values such as those in Table 39-1. This estimation method assumes that the drug is administered by intermittent intravenous infusion and that its disposition is adequately characterized by a one-compartment linear model.

TABLE 39-4	Drug Disposition during Dialysis Depends on Dialyzer Characteristics			
	Hemodialysis Clearance (mL/min)		**Half-Life during Dialysis (hr)**	
DRUG	**CONVENTIONAL**	**HIGH-FLUX**	**CONVENTIONAL**	**HIGH-FLUX**
Ceftazidime	55-60	155 (PA)	3.3	1.2 (PA)
Cefuroxime	NR	103 (PS)	3.8	1.6 (PS)
Foscarnet	183	253 (PS)	NR	NR
Gentamicin	58.2	116 (PS)	3.0	4.3 (PS)
Tobramycin	45	119 (PS)	4.0	NR
Ranitidine	43.1	67.2 (PS)	5.1	2.9 (PS)
Vancomycin	9-21	31-60 (PAN)	35-38	12.0 (PAN)
		40-150 (PS)		4.5-11.8 (PS)
		72-116 (PMMA)		NR

NR, not reported; PA, polyamide filter; PAN, polyacrylonitrile filter; PMMA, polymethylmethacrylate; PS, polysulfone filter.

TABLE 39-5	Key Recommendations for Clinicians

1. Over-the-counter and herbal products as well as prescription medications should be assessed to ensure that they are indicated.

2. The least nephrotoxic agent should be used whenever possible.

3. If a drug interaction is suspected and the clinical implication is significant, alternative medications should be used.

4. Although the MDRD eGFR equation may be used for staging CKD, the Cockcroft-Gault equation remains the standard renal function index for drug dosage adjustment.

5. The dosage of drugs that are more than 30% renally eliminated unchanged should be verified to ensure that appropriate initial dosage adjustments are implemented in CKD.

6. Maintenance dosage regimens should be adjusted based on patient response and serum drug concentration determinations when indicated and available.

CKD, chronic kidney disease; eGFR, estimated glomerular filtration rate; MDRD, Modification of Diet in Renal Disease.

CONCLUSIONS

The adverse outcomes associated with inappropriate drug use and dosing are largely preventable if the principles illustrated in this chapter are used by the clinician in concert with reliable population pharmacokinetic estimates to design rational initial drug dosage regimens for patients with reduced kidney function and those needing dialysis. Subsequent individualization of therapy should be undertaken whenever clinical therapeutic monitoring tools, such as plasma drug concentrations, are available. These key recommendations for practice are highlighted in **Table 39-5**.

BIBLIOGRAPHY

Aronoff GR, Bennetl WM, Berns JS, et al: Drug Prescribing in Renal Failure: Dosing Guidelines for Adults and Children, 5th ed. Philadelphia, American College of Physicians-American Society of Internal Medicine, 2007.

Joy MS, Matzke GR, Armstrong DK, et al: A primer on continuous renal replacement therapy for critically ill patients. Ann Pharmacother 32:362-375, 1998.

Lee W, Kim RB: Transporters and renal drug elimination. Annu Rev Pharmacol Toxicol 44:137-166, 2004.

Matzke GR: Status of hemodialysis of drugs in 2002. J Pharm Practice 15:405-418, 2002.

Matzke GR, Clermont G: Clinical pharmacology and therapeutics. In Murray PT, Brady HR, Hall JB (eds): Intensive Care in Nephrology. Boca Raton, FL, Taylor and Francis, 2006, pp 245-265.

Matzke GR, Comstock TJ. Influence of renal disease and dialysis on pharmacokinetics. In Evans WE, Schentag JJ, Burton ME (eds.): Applied Pharmacokinetics: Principles of Therapeutic Drug Monitoring, 4th ed. Baltimore, Lippincott Williams and Wilkins, 2005.

Matzke GR, Dowling TD: Dosing concepts in renal dysfunction. In Murphy JE (ed): Clinical Pharmacokinetics Pocket Reference, 4th ed. Bethesda, MD, American Society of Health-System Pharmacists, 2008, pp 475-501.

McEvoy GK, Litvak K, Welsh OH, et al: American Hospital Formulary Service, Drug Information. Bethesda, MD, American Society of Hospital Pharmacists, 2004.

Mueller BA, Pasko DA, Sowinski KM: Higher renal replacement therapy dose delivery influences on drug therapy. Artif Organs 27:808-814, 2003.

Munar MY, Singh H: Drug dosing adjustments in patients with chronic kidney disease. Am Fam Physician 75:1487-1496, 2007.

Nolin TD, Frye RF, Matzke GR: Hepatic drug metabolism and transport in patients with kidney disease. Am J Kidney Dis 42:906-925, 2003.

Piraino B, Bailie GR, Bernardini J, et al: Peritoneal dialysis related infections: 2005 Update. Perit Dial Int 25:107-131, 2005.

Rowland M, Tozer TN: Clinical Pharmokinetics: Concepts and Applications, 3rd ed. Philadelphia, Lea and Febiger, 1995.

Spruill WJ, Wade WE, Cobb HH: Estimating glomerular filtration rate with a Modification of Diet in Renal disease equation: Implications for pharmacy. Am J Health-Syst Pharm 64:652-660, 2007.

Taylor CA, Abdel-Rahman E, Zimmerman SW, Johnson CA: Clinical pharmacokinetics during continuous ambulatory peritoneal dialysis. Clin Pharmacokinet 31:293-308, 1996.

Thummel KE, Shen DD Isoherranen N, Smith HE: Design and optimization of dosage regimens: Pharmacokinetic data. In Burton LL, Laszo JS, Parker KL (eds): Goodman & Gilman's The Pharmacological Basis of Therapeutics, 11th ed. New York, McGraw-Hill, 2006.

van dijik EA, Drabbe NRG, Kruijtbosch M, De Smet PAGM: Drug dosage adjustments according to renal function at hospital discharge. Ann Pharmacother 40:1254-1260, 2006.

Veltri MA, Neu AM, Fivush BA, et al: Drug dosing during intermittent hemodialysis and continuous renal replacement therapy: Special considerations in pediatric patients. Pediatr Drugs 6:45-65, 2004.

Vidal L, Shavit M, Fraser A, et al: Systematic comparison of four sources of drug information regarding adjustment of dose for renal function. BMJ 331:263-266, 2005.

Wargo KA, Eiland EH, Hamm W, English TM, Phillippe HM. Comparison of the Modification of Diet in Renal Disease and Cockroft-Gault equations for antimicrobial dosage adjustments. Ann Pharmacother 40:1248-1253, 2006.

Hereditary Kidney Disorders

CHAPTER 40

Genetically Based Renal Transport Disorders

Steven J. Scheinman

The coming of age of clinical chemistry in the latter half of the 20th century, bringing with it the routine measurement of electrolytes and minerals in patient samples, produced descriptions of distinct inherited syndromes of abnormal renal tubular transport. Clinical investigation led to speculation, often ingenious and sometimes controversial, regarding the underlying causes of these syndromes. In the past decade, the tools of molecular biology made possible the cloning of mutated genes found in patients with these monogenic disorders of renal tubular transport. These diseases represent experiments of nature, and the discoveries they have revealed are exciting. Some have provided gratifying confirmation of our existing knowledge of transport mechanisms along the nephron. Examples include mutations in diuretic-sensitive transporters in the Bartter and Gitelman syndromes. In other cases, positional cloning led to the discovery of previously unknown proteins, often surprising ones, that appear to play important roles in epithelial transport. For example, the chloride channel transporter CLC-5 (also called CLCN5), the tight junction claudin 16 (i.e., paracellin 1), and the phosphaturic hormone fibroblast growth factor 23 (FGF-23) were discovered through positional cloning in the study of Dent's disease, inherited hypomagnesemic hypercalciuria, and autosomal dominant hypophosphatemic rickets, respectively.

Table 40-1 summarizes genetic diseases of renal tubular transport for which the molecular basis is known. The diseases listed are explained by abnormalities in the corresponding proteins. Such monogenic conditions tend to be uncommon or rare. Common conditions often can have important genetic components, but they usually are polygenic. In those settings, inheritance is often complex and involves polymorphisms in several genes, each of which contributes to the disease phenotype. Some genes responsible for the rare monogenic diseases may also contribute in subtle ways to the common polygenic conditions, but determining the contributions of these genes, and presumably others that remain unidentified, for complex conditions such as hypertension will be the next major challenge for genetics.

DISORDERS OF PROXIMAL TUBULAR TRANSPORT FUNCTION

Selective Proximal Transport Defects

Sodium resorption in the proximal tubule occurs through secondary active transport processes in which the entry of sodium is coupled to that of glucose, amino acids, or phosphate or to the exit of protons. Autosomal recessive conditions of impaired transepithelial transport of glucose and dibasic amino acids have been shown to be caused by mutations in sodium-dependent transporters that are expressed in both kidney and intestine, resulting in urinary losses and intestinal malabsorption of these solutes. Other disorders with renal-selective transport defects are thought to result from mutations in transporters expressed specifically in kidney.

Impaired Proximal Phosphate Reabsorption

X-linked (dominant) hypophosphatemic rickets (XLHR) is characterized by impaired sodium-dependent phosphate reabsorption, in which the maximal transport capacity for phosphate is reduced. This is reflected in a reduced number of units of the sodium-dependent phosphate transporter type 2 (NaPi2) in the apical membrane of proximal tubular cells. XLHR is the most common form of hereditary rickets. Mutations in XLHR involve not the gene encoding NaPi2 but rather a phosphate-regulating gene with homologies to a neutral endopeptidase on the X chromosome (PHEX) that is expressed in bone and is thought to be involved in the processing of a circulating phosphate transport-regulating hormone designated *phosphatonin*.

The rare autosomal dominant form of hypophosphatemic rickets (ADHR) is associated with mutations in the gene encoding a member of the fibroblast growth factor family, FGF-23, that protect FGF-23 from proteolytic cleavage. It is not clear whether FGF-23 is a substrate for the PHEX enzyme or why mutations in *PHEX* are associated with high FGF-23 levels, but the physiologic effects of FGF-23 are consistent with its being a phosphatonin, because it inhibits renal phosphate reabsorption by inhibiting expression of two sodium-dependent phosphate transporters in proximal tubule, SLC34A1 (formerly Npt2a) and SLC34A3 (formerly Npt2c). Serum levels of uncleaved FGF-23 are excessive in XLHR, ADHR, and tumor-induced hypophosphatemic osteomalacia, all of which are characterized by impaired renal phosphate reabsorption. FGF-23 inhibits the 1-hydroxylation of 25-hydroxyvitamin D, and this probably explains why the hypophosphatemia in these three conditions is not associated with elevated levels of 1,25-dihydroxyvitamin D or hypercalciuria.

Recently, autosomal recessive inheritance of hypophosphatemic rickets has been reported. Patients with this condition resemble those with autosomal dominant (i.e., *FGF23* mutations) and X-linked forms (*PHEX* mutations), with

TABLE 40-1 Molecular Bases of Genetic Disorders of Renal Transport

INHERITED DISORDER	DEFECTIVE PROTEIN
Proximal Tubule	
X-linked hypophosphatemic rickets (XLHR)	Phosphate-regulating gene with homologies to endopeptidases on the X chromosome (PHEX)
Autosomal dominant hypophosphatemic rickets (ADHR)	Fibroblast growth factor 23 (FGF-23) (excess)
Autosomal recessive hypophosphatemic rickets	Dentin matrix protein 1
Hereditary hypophosphatemic rickets with hypercalciuria (HHRH)	Sodium-phosphate cotransporter Npt2c (SLC34A3)
Familial hyperostosis-hyperphosphatemia	Fibroblast growth factor 23 (FGF-23) (deficiency)
	N-acetylglucosaminyl (GalNac) transferase 3
Autosomal recessive proximal RTA	Basolateral sodium bicarbonate cotransporter NBC1
Fanconi's syndrome	Aldolase B (hereditary fructose intolerance)
Oculocerebrorenal syndrome of Lowe	OCRL1, an inositol polyphosphate-5-phosphatase
Dent's disease (X-linked nephrolithiasis)	Chloride channel transporter ClC-5 (CLCN5)
	Phosphatidylinositol-4,5-bisphosphate-5-phosphatase (OCRL1)
Cystinuria	Apical cystine dibasic amino acid transporter rBAT (SLC3A1)
	Light subunit of rBAT/SLC3A1
Dibasic aminoaciduria	Basolateral dibasic amino acid transporter (lysinuric protein intolerance)
Fanconi-Bickel syndrome	Facilitated glucose transporter GLUT2
Glucose-galactose malabsorption syndrome	Sodium-glucose cotransporter 1 (SGLT1)
Thick Ascending Limb of Henle's Loop	
Bartter syndrome	
Type I	Bumetanide-sensitive Na$^+$-K$^+$-2Cl$^-$ cotransporter (NKCC2 [SLC12A1])
Type II	Apical potassium channel ROMK (KCNJ1)
Type III	Basolateral chloride channel ClC-Kb (CLCNKb)
Type IV, with sensorineural deafness	Barttin (CLCNKb–associated protein)
Familial hypocalcemia with Bartter features	Calcium-sensing receptor (activation)
Familial hypomagnesemia with hypercalciuria	
Without ocular abnormalities	Claudin 16 (also called paracellin 1)
With ocular abnormalities	Claudin 19
Familial hypocalciuric hypercalcemia	Calcium-sensing receptor (heterozygous inactivation)
Neonatal severe hyperparathyroidism	Calcium-sensing receptor (homozygous inactivation)
Familial hypercalciuric hypocalcemia	Calcium-sensing receptor (activation)
Familial juvenile hyperuricemic nephropathy	Uromodulin (Tamm-Horsfall protein)
Distal Convoluted Tubule	
Gitelman's syndrome	Thiazide-sensitive Na-Cl cotransporter (NCCT [SCL12A3])
Familial hypomagnesemia with secondary hypocalcemia	TRPM6 cation channel[†]
Isolated recessive renal hypomagnesemia	Epidermal growth factor (EGF)
Isolated renal magnesium loss	γ subunit of Na$^+$, K$^+$-ATPase
Pseudohypoparathyroidism type Ia*	Guanine nucleotide-binding protein (Gs)
Collecting Duct	
Liddle's syndrome	β and γ subunits of epithelial sodium channel (ENaC)
Pseudohypoaldosteronism	
Type 1	
Autosomal recessive	α, β, and γ subunits of ENaC
Autosomal dominant	Mineralocorticoid (type 1) receptor
Type 2 (Gordon's syndrome)	WNK1 and WNK4 kinases
Syndrome of apparent mineralocorticoid excess	11β-hydroxysteroid dehydrogenase type II
Glucocorticoid-remediable aldosteronism	11β-hydroxylase and aldosterone synthase (encoded by a chimeric gene)[‡]

(Continued)

TABLE 40-1 Molecular Bases of Genetic Disorders of Renal Transport — cont'd

INHERITED DISORDER	DEFECTIVE PROTEIN
Distal RTA	
Autosomal dominant	Basolateral anion exchanger (AE1, now called SLC4A1), band 3 protein
Autosomal recessive with hemolytic anemia	Basolateral anion exchanger (AE1, now called SLC4A1), band 3 protein
Autosomal recessive with hearing deficit	β_1 subunit of H$^+$-ATPase
Autosomal recessive with variable hearing deficit	α_4 isoform of the α subunit of H$^+$-ATPase
Carbonic anhydrase II deficiency§	Carbonic anhydrase type II
Nephrogenic diabetes insipidus	
X-linked	Arginine vasopressin type 2 (V$_2$) receptor
Autosomal	Aquaporin 2 water channel

RTA, renal tubular acidosis.

*Gene also is expressed in the proximal tubule, where functional abnormalities are clinically apparent.

†Gene also is expressed in the intestine.

‡Gene is expressed in the adrenal gland.

§Clinical phenotype can be proximal RTA, distal RTA, or a combined form.

renal phosphate wasting, inappropriately normal levels of 1,25-dihydroxyvitamin D, absence of hypercalciuria, and elevated serum levels of FGF-23. In this autosomal recessive form, the mutated gene *(DMP1)* encodes the dentin matrix protein 1 (DMP-1), a bone matrix protein.

Hereditary hypophosphatemic rickets with hypercalciuria (HHRH), an autosomal recessive disorder, is different from XLHR and ADHR, which are associated with reduced urinary calcium excretion. Unlike XLHR and ADHR, the hypophosphatemia in HHRH is associated with appropriate elevations of 1,25-dihydroxyvitamin D levels, and FGF-23 levels are normal or reduced. This profile in HHRH is consistent with a primary defect in phosphate transport. The most abundant phosphate transporter in the proximal tubule, SLC34A1, is not mutated in any of the families with HHRH studied, but several pedigrees have been reported with mutations in SLC34A3. Expression of both SLC34A1 and SLC34A3 responds to physiologic stimuli such as parathyroid hormone (PTH) and dietary phosphate. Knockout of the mouse homologue of SLC34A1 reproduces the features of human HHRH except for rickets; a mouse knockout of SLC34A3 has not been described.

Excessive Proximal Phosphate Reabsorption

Inherited hyperphosphatemia in the familial hyperostosis-hyperphosphatemia syndrome represents a mirror image of ADHR and XLHR, with excessive renal phosphate reabsorption, persistent hyperphosphatemia, inappropriately normal levels of 1,25-dihydroxyvitamin D, and low levels of FGF-23. Recent reports document that this can result from mutations in FGF-23 itself or in a Golgi-associated biosynthetic enzyme, *N*-acetylglucosaminyl (GalNac) transferase 3, that is involved in glycosylation of FGF-23, which is necessary for its secretion. Together, these discoveries are fleshing out our understanding of the role of bone in the complex regulation of mineral metabolism.

Impaired Proximal Bicarbonate Transport

Proximal renal tubular acidosis (RTA) is inherited in an autosomal recessive manner and is associated with mutations that inactivate the basolateral sodium bicarbonate cotransporter SLC4A4 (also called NBC1). These patients often suffer blindness from ocular abnormalities, including band keratopathy, cataracts, and glaucoma, probably as a consequence of impaired bicarbonate transport in the eye. Mutations in the *SLC4A4* gene result in impaired transporter function or aberrant trafficking of the protein to the basolateral surface. This gene belongs to the same group as the gene encoding the anion exchanger AE1 (now designated SLC4A1), which is mutated in distal RTA.

Inherited Fanconi's Syndrome

The Fanconi syndrome results from the generalized impairment in reabsorptive function of the proximal tubule and comprises proximal RTA with aminoaciduria, renal glycosuria, hypouricemia, and hypophosphatemia. Some or all of these abnormalities are present in individual patients with Fanconi's syndrome. Inherited causes of the Fanconi syndrome include hereditary fructose intolerance, Lowe's syndrome, and Dent's disease.

Hereditary fructose intolerance is caused by mutations that result in deficiency of the aldolase B enzyme, which cleaves fructose-1-phosphate. Symptoms are precipitated by intake of sweets. Massive accumulation of fructose-1-phosphate occurs, leading to sequestration of inorganic phosphate and deficiency of adenosine triphosphate (ATP). Acute consequences can include hypoglycemic shock, severe abdominal symptoms, and impaired function of the Krebs cycle that produces metabolic acidosis, and this is exacerbated by impaired renal bicarbonate reabsorption. ATP deficiency leads to impaired proximal tubular function in general, including the full expression of the Fanconi syndrome with consequent rickets and stunted growth. ATP breakdown can be so dramatic as to produce hyperuricemia, as well as hypermagnesemia from the dissolution of the magnesium-ATP complex. Acute symptoms and chronic consequences such as liver disease can be minimized by avoiding dietary sources of fructose.

Characteristic features of the oculocerebrorenal syndrome of Lowe include congenital cataracts, mental retardation, muscular hypotonia, and the renal Fanconi syndrome. In contrast, Dent's disease is confined to the kidney. In both syndromes, low-molecular-weight (LMW) proteinuria is a prominent feature, together with other evidence of proximal tubulopathy such as glycosuria, aminoaciduria, and phosphaturia. One important difference is that proximal RTA with growth retardation can be severe in patients with Lowe's syndrome, but it is not a part of Dent's disease. Some patients with Lowe's syndrome or Dent's disease may have rickets, which is thought to be a consequence of hypophosphatemia and, in Lowe syndrome, of acidosis. Hypercalciuria is a characteristic feature of Dent's disease. It is associated with nephrocalcinosis in most or kidney stones in many patients, but these are less evident in Lowe's syndrome. Renal failure is common in both, progressing to end-stage disease in young adulthood in Dent's disease and even earlier in patients with Lowe's syndrome.

Dent's disease is caused by mutations that inactivate the chloride transporter CLC-5. This transport protein is expressed in the proximal tubule, the medullary thick ascending limb (MTAL) of Henle's loop, and the alpha-intercalated cells of the collecting tubule. In the cells of the proximal tubule, CLC-5 colocalizes with the proton-ATPase in subapical endosomes. These endosomes are important in the processing of proteins that are filtered at the glomerulus and taken up by the proximal tubule through adsorptive endocytosis. The activity of the proton-ATPase acidifies the endosomal space, releasing the proteins from membrane binding sites and making them available for proteolytic degradation. CLC-5 mediates electrogenic exchange of chloride for protons in these endosomes, dissipates the positive charge generated by proton entry, and may provide a brake or set point for endosomal acidification. Mutations that inactivate CLC-5 in patients with Dent's disease interfere with the mechanism for reabsorption of LMW proteins and explain the consistent finding of LMW proteinuria. Glycosuria, aminoaciduria, and phosphaturia are less consistently seen and may be consequences of CLC-5 inactivation, possibly through alterations in membrane trafficking. Lowe's syndrome is associated with mutations in *OCRL1,* which encodes a phosphatidylinositol-4, 5-bisphosphate-5-phosphatase. In renal epithelial cells, this phosphatase is localized to the *trans*-Golgi network, which plays an important role in directing proteins to the appropriate membrane. The CLC-5 protein and the OCRL1 phosphatase interact with the actin cytoskeleton and are involved in assembly of the endosomal apparatus. Similarities in the renal features of these two syndromes may be the result of defective membrane trafficking. Still to be explained is why some patients with mutations in *OCRL1* have no cataracts or cerebral dysfunction, and no RTA.

DISORDERS OF TRANSPORT IN THE MEDULLARY THICK ASCENDING LIMB OF HENLE

Bartter's Syndrome

Solute transport in the MTAL involves the coordinated functions of a set of transport proteins depicted in **Figure 40-1.** These proteins are the bumetanide-sensitive Na^+-K^+-$2Cl^-$ cotransporter (NKCC2) and the renal outer medullary potassium channel (ROMK) on the apical surface of cells of the MTAL, and the chloride channel ClC-Kb on the basolateral surface. Optimal function of the ClC-Kb chloride channel requires interaction with a subunit called *barttin*. Mutations in any of the genes encoding these four proteins lead to the phenotype of Bartter's syndrome. In addition, activation of the epithelial calcium-sensing receptor (CaSR) inhibits activity of the ROMK potassium channel. Mutations producing constitutive activation of the CaSR cause familial hypocalcemic hypercalciuria. Some patients with hypocalcemic hypercalciuria have the phenotype of Bartter's syndrome, and mutations in the CaSR may be considered a fifth molecular cause of this syndrome. Together, these five genes still do not account for all patients with Bartter's syndrome.

The ClC-Kb basolateral chloride channel provides the route for chloride exit to the interstitium. Flow of potassium through the ROMK channel ensures that potassium concentrations in the tubular lumen do not limit the activity of the Na^+-K^+-$2Cl^-$ cotransporter, and it maintains a positive electrical potential in the lumen of this nephron segment. This positive charge is the driving force for paracellular reabsorption of calcium and magnesium.

Bartter's syndrome manifests in infancy or childhood with polyuria and failure to thrive, often occurring after a pregnancy with polyhydramnios. It is characterized by hypokalemic metabolic alkalosis, typically with hypercalciuria, and these patients resemble patients chronically taking loop diuretics that inhibit activity of NKCC2 pharmacologically. Defective function of NKCC2, ROMK, ClC-Kb, or barttin leads to impaired salt reabsorption in the MTAL, resulting in volume contraction and activation of the renin-angiotensin-aldosterone axis, which stimulates distal tubular secretion of potassium and protons and produces hypokalemic metabolic alkalosis. Despite impaired reabsorption of magnesium, serum magnesium levels are usually normal in patients with Bartter's syndrome, but levels occasionally are mildly depressed. Severity, age of onset of symptoms, and particular clinical features vary with the gene abnormality. For example, nephrocalcinosis as a consequence of hypercalciuria is seen especially in patients with mutations in genes encoding NKCC2 and ROMK. Barttin is expressed in the inner ear, and patients with mutations in its gene have sensorineural deafness. Bartter's syndrome is discussed further in Chapter 9.

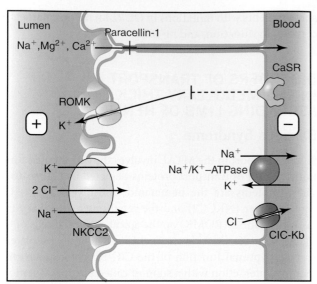

FIGURE 40-1 Transport mechanisms in the thick ascending limb (TAL) of Henle's loop transport proteins affected by mutations in genetic diseases. Reabsorption of sodium chloride occurs through the electroneutral activity of the bumetanide-sensitive $Na^+-K^+-2Cl^-$ cotransporter, NKCC2. Activity of the basolateral sodium-potassium adenosine triphosphatase (Na^+,K^+-ATPase) provides the driving force for this transport and also generates a high intracellular concentration of potassium, which exits through the ATP-regulated apical potassium channel. ROMK. This ensures an adequate supply of potassium for the activity of the NKCC2 and also produces a lumen-positive electrical potential, which itself is the driving force for paracellular reabsorption of calcium, magnesium, and sodium ions through the tight junctions, involving the protein paracellin 1. Chloride transported into the cell by NKCC2 exits the basolateral side of the cell through the voltage-gated chloride channel, ClC-Kb. Activation of the extracellular calcium-sensing receptor, CaSR, inhibits solute transport in the TAL by inhibiting activity of the ROMK and possibly by other mechanisms. Mutations that inactivate the CaSR are associated with enhanced calcium transport and hypocalciuria in familial benign hypercalcemia, and mutations that activate the CaSR occur in patients with familial hypercalciuria with hypocalcemia. (Adapted from Scheinman SJ, Guay-Woodford LM, Thakker RV, Warnock DG: Genetic disorders of renal electrolyte transport. N Engl J Med 340:1177-1187, 1999, with permission. Copyright © 1999, Massachusetts Medical Society.)

Inherited Hypomagnesemic Hypercalciuria

Reabsorption of calcium and magnesium in the MTAL occurs through the paracellular route, driven by the positive electrical potential in the tubular lumen. Selective movement of cations (i.e., calcium, magnesium, and sodium) is determined by the tight junctions between the epithelial cells. Disturbance of this selective paracellular barrier would be expected to produce parallel disorders in the reabsorption of calcium and magnesium.

Familial hypomagnesemia with substantial renal magnesium losses, hypercalciuria, and nephrocalcinosis (FHHNC) is inherited in an autosomal recessive fashion. These patients develop renal failure and kidney stones. Investigation of families led to identification by positional cloning of the gene encoding a tight junction protein designated claudin 16 (also called paracellin 1). It is expressed at the tight junction between cells of the MTAL (see Fig. 40-1) and in the distal convoluted tubule. This was the first instance of

a disease shown to result from mutations that alter a tight junction protein. Another member of this family, claudin 19, is mutated in other pedigrees in whom FHHNC is associated with ocular abnormalities (e.g., macular colobomas, myopia, horizontal nystagmus) with severe visual impairment. Both claudin 16 and claudin 19 are expressed in the thick ascending limb (TAL), but claudin 19 also is expressed in the retina. These two proteins interact in the tight junction to regulate cation permeability. It is not clear, however, why a defect in tight junctions is associated with hyperuricemia, a consistent finding in this disease.

Familial Hypocalciuric Hypercalcemia

The extracellular CaSR is expressed in many tissues in which ambient calcium concentrations trigger cellular responses. In the parathyroid gland, activation of the CaSR suppresses synthesis and release of parathyroid hormone. In the kidney, the CaSR is expressed on the basolateral surface of cells of the TAL (cortical more than medullary), on the luminal surface of the cells of the papillary collecting duct, and in other portions of the nephron. Activation of the CaSR in the TAL probably mediates the known effects of hypercalcemia to inhibit the transport of calcium, magnesium, and sodium in this nephron segment. For example, CaSR activation inhibits activity of the ROMK potassium channel (see Fig. 40-1). This can be expected to reduce the positive electrical potential in the lumen and thereby suppress the driving force for reabsorption of calcium and magnesium. In the papillary collecting duct, activation of the apical CaSR may explain the effects of hypercalciuria to impair the hydro-osmotic response to vasopressin. The more dilute urine produced in this situation is potentially protective against development of nephrocalcinosis or nephrolithiasis in the setting of hypercalciuria due to hypercalcemia and an increased filtered load.

In familial hypocalciuric hypercalcemia (FHH), loss-of-function mutations of the *CASR* gene increase the set point for calcium sensing, resulting in hypercalcemia with relative elevation of parathyroid hormone levels. Urinary calcium excretion is low because of enhanced calcium reabsorption in the TAL and PTH-stimulated calcium transport in the distal convoluted tubule. FHH occurs in patients heterozygous for such mutations, and it is benign, because tissues are resistant to the high serum calcium levels. A family history helps to differentiate FHH from primary hyperparathyroidism, and parathyroidectomy should not be performed. Infants of consanguineous parents with FHH can be homozygous for these mutations, resulting in a syndrome of severe hypercalcemia with marked hyperparathyroidism, fractures, and failure to thrive, known as *neonatal severe hyperparathyroidism*.

Other mutations result in constitutive activation of the CaSR, and this produces hypocalcemia with hypercalciuria without elevated PTH concentrations. As discussed earlier, these circumstances also can produce the phenotype of Bartter's syndrome. One polymorphism (R990G) in the *CASR* gene that produces a mild gain-of-function expression of the CaSR without frank hypocalcemia has been associated with idiopathic hypercalciuria.

Familial Juvenile Hyperuricemic Nephropathy

Mutations in the *UMOD* gene encoding uromodulin (i.e., Tamm-Horsfall protein) occur in families in which children present with hyperuricemia and gout. This syndrome overlaps with medullary cystic kidney disease type 2, which also is associated with *UMOD* mutations. Cytosolic inclusions seen on electron microscopy in the epithelial cells of the MTAL appear to be crystallized uromodulin. A physiologic explanation for the hyperuricemia has not been offered. The occurrence of hyperuricemia in this disease and in the syndrome associated with mutations in paracellin indicates that our understanding of the role of the MTAL in uric acid transport is not fully understood. Families with an indistinguishable phenotype have been identified in whom linkage to the *UMOD* locus is excluded, indicating that genetic heterogeneity is likely.

DISORDERS OF TRANSPORT IN THE DISTAL CONVOLUTED TUBULE

Gitelman's Syndrome

Reabsorption of sodium chloride in the distal convoluted tubule occurs through electroneutral transport mediated by the thiazide-sensitive sodium chloride cotransporter (NCCT). Mutations in the NCCT gene *(SLC12A3)* are associated with Gitelman's syndrome, another condition of hypokalemic metabolic alkalosis. Gitelman's syndrome was viewed as a variant of Bartter's syndrome. An essential distinction between these two conditions is the hypocalciuria in Gitelman's syndrome, in contrast to the hypercalciuria that occurs in Bartter's syndrome or in patients taking loop diuretics. Hypocalciuria in Gitelman's syndrome resembles the reduction in calcium excretion that occurs in patients taking thiazide diuretics. These findings are satisfying in that they connect the clinical physiology with molecular physiology. However, our understanding of renal transport does not allow us to explain the fact that significant hypomagnesemia with renal magnesium wasting is typical of Gitelman's syndrome, whereas in Bartter's syndrome it is much less common and, when it does occur, milder.

Familial Hypomagnesemia with Secondary Hypocalcemia

Patients with familial hypomagnesemia with secondary hypocalcemia have severe hypomagnesemia, often with neonatal seizures and tetany. If not recognized and treated early, the hypomagnesemia can be fatal. Serum magnesium levels fall to levels low enough to impair PTH release or responsiveness, and this is presumed to be the mechanism of the hypocalcemia that commonly accompanies the

hypomagnesemia in these patients. The primary defect appears to be in intestinal magnesium absorption, although renal magnesium conservation also is deficient. These patients have mutations in a gene *(TRPM6)* encoding the TRPM6 protein. TRPM6 is a member of the long transient receptor potential channel family and is expressed in both the intestine and the distal convoluted tubule. Under experimental conditions, TRPM6 forms functional heteromers with its close homologue TRPM7 (which has not been associated with renal disease) and may function as both a cation channel and a kinase, although its role in normal physiology remains to be defined.

Isolated Recessive Renal Hypomagnesemia

Isolated recessive renal hypomagnesemia has been described in a single consanguineous Dutch pedigree, in which two sisters presented with hypomagnesemia with renal magnesium wasting, otherwise normal serum and urinary electrolyte metabolism, and associated mental retardation. This disease is linked to the locus encompassing the gene encoding the epidermal growth factor (EGF), and both patients had homozygous mutation in this gene. The mutation leads to abnormal basolateral sorting of pro-EGF. EGF receptors are expressed on distal convoluted tubule cells and elsewhere in the renal epithelium and vasculature. Activation of EGF receptors stimulates activity of TRPM6 magnesium channels, and blockade of EGF receptors with the monoclonal antibody cetuximab prevents this stimulation. This observation is consistent with the clinical experience with cetuximab used as therapy for colon cancer, because it is associated with hypomagnesemia.

DISORDERS OF TRANSPORT IN THE COLLECTING TUBULE

Liddle's Syndrome

Sodium reabsorption by the principal cells of the cortical collecting duct is physiologically regulated by aldosterone. As in other cells, low intracellular sodium concentrations are maintained by the basolateral Na^+,K^+-ATPase, and this drives sodium entry through amiloride-sensitive epithelial sodium channels (ENaC) on the apical surface. Mutations that render the ENaC persistently open produce a syndrome of excessive sodium reabsorption and low-renin hypertension (i.e., Liddle's syndrome). This autosomal dominant condition often manifests in children with severe hypertension and hypokalemic alkalosis. It resembles primary hyperaldosteronism, but serum aldosterone levels are quite low, and for this reason, the disease also has been called *pseudohyperaldosteronism*. In their original description of the syndrome, Liddle and colleagues demonstrated that aldosterone excess was not responsible for this disease and that, although spironolactone had no effect on the hypertension, patients did respond well to triamterene or dietary sodium restriction. They proposed that the primary abnormality was excessive renal salt conservation and potassium secretion independent of mineralocorticoid. This hypothesis proved to be correct, and it is explained by excessive sodium channel activity. Renal transplantation in Liddle's original proband led to resolution of the hypertension, consistent with correction of the defect intrinsic to the kidneys.

In Liddle's syndrome, gain-of-function mutations in the ENaC produce channels that are resistant to downregulation by physiologic stimuli such as volume expansion. The ENaC is formed by three homologous subunits, designated αENaC, βENaC, and γENaC. Missense or truncating mutations in patients with Liddle's syndrome alter the carboxyl-terminal cytoplasmic tail of the β or γ subunit in a domain that is important for interactions with the cytoskeletal protein that regulates activity of the ENaC. In addition to the severe phenotype of Liddle's syndrome resulting from these mutations, it has been speculated that polymorphisms in the ENaC sequence that have less dramatic effects on sodium channel function may contribute to the much more common low-renin variant of essential hypertension.

Pseudohypoaldosteronism Types 1 and 2

Pseudohypoaldosteronism types 1 and 2 are referred to as *pseudohypoaldosteronism,* because they feature hyperkalemia and metabolic acidosis without aldosterone deficiency. Type 1 disease is associated with salt wasting and results from mutations that inactivate either the mineralocorticoid receptor (autosomal recessive) or the ENaC (autosomal dominant). The autosomal recessive form is milder and resolves with time, but the autosomal dominant form is more severe and persistent. Type 2 disease is a hypertensive condition, which provides an important difference between these patients and those with hypoaldosteronism. Type 2 pseudohypoaldosteronism (i.e., Gordon's syndrome) is a mirror image of Gitelman's syndrome, with hyperkalemia, metabolic acidosis, and hypercalciuria, although serum magnesium levels are normal.

Gordon's syndrome is caused by mutations in two kinases known as WNK1 and WNK4 (with no lysine [K]). Both are expressed in the distal convoluted tubule and collecting duct. WNK4 downregulates the activity of the NCCT sodium chloride cotransporter and of the ENaC. Inactivating mutations in *WNK4* result in increased activity of both pathways for sodium reabsorption. WNK4 also regulates the ROMK potassium channel, but mutations that relieve WNK4's inhibition of sodium transport enhance its inhibition of ROMK, contributing to the hyperkalemia in Gordon's syndrome. WNK1 is a negative regulator of WNK4, and gain-of-function *WNK1* mutations indirectly increase NCCT activity. Coordinated regulation of distal ion transport by these WNK kinases may explain how the kidney balances the two effects of aldosterone on sodium reabsorption and potassium secretion, and polymorphisms in this pathway may be relevant to the mechanisms of essential hypertension.

Other Disorders Resembling Primary Hyperaldosteronism

Two other hereditary conditions produce hypertension in children with clinical features resembling primary hyperaldosteronism. The syndrome of apparent mineralocorticoid excess (AME) is an autosomal recessive disease in which the renal isoform of the 11β-hydroxysteroid dehydrogenase enzyme is inactivated by mutation. In a sense, this is a genetic analogue of ingestion of black licorice, which contains glycyrrhizic acid that inhibits this enzyme. Inactivation of the enzyme results in failure to convert cortisol to cortisone locally in the collecting duct, allowing cortisol to activate mineralocorticoid receptors and produce a syndrome resembling primary hyperaldosteronism but, like Liddle's syndrome, with low circulating levels of aldosterone. As in Liddle's syndrome, renal transplantation has resulted in resolution of hypertension in patients with AME syndrome.

The autosomal dominant condition known as glucocorticoid-remediable aldosteronism (GRA) is caused by a chromosomal rearrangement that produces a chimeric gene in which the regulatory region of the gene encoding the steroid 11β-hydroxylase (which is part of the cortisol biosynthetic pathway and normally is regulated by adrenocorticotropic hormone [ACTH]) is fused to distal sequences of the aldosterone synthase gene. This results in production of aldosterone that responds to ACTH rather than normal regulatory stimuli. Patients with GRA may have variable elevations in plasma aldosterone levels and are often normokalemic. Aldosterone levels are suppressed by glucocorticoid therapy. Elevated urinary levels of 18-oxacortisol and 18-hydroxycortisol are characteristic of GRA.

Hereditary Renal Tubular Acidosis

Secretion of acid by the alpha-intercalated cells of the collecting duct is accomplished by the apical proton-ATPase. Cytosolic carbonic anhydrase catalyzes the formation of bicarbonate from hydroxyl ions, and the bicarbonate then exits the cell in exchange for chloride through the basolateral anion exchanger, AE1 (now called SLC4A1). Mutations affecting each of these proteins have been documented in patients with hereditary forms of RTA. Autosomal recessive distal RTA is associated with mutations in the β_1 subunit of the proton-ATPase. This form of RTA is often severe, manifesting in young children and often with hearing loss, consistent with the fact that this ATPase is expressed in the cochlea, endolymphatic sac of the inner ear, and kidney. Other patients with autosomal recessive distal RTA have mutations in the gene encoding a noncatalytic α_4 isoform of the α accessory subunit of the ATPase, and these patients have less severe or no hearing deficit. Autosomal dominant RTA, a milder disease that often is undetected until adulthood, is associated with mutations in the AE1, which is also the band 3 erythrocyte membrane protein. In Asian patients, mutations in the AE1 occur with recessive inheritance of distal RTA and hemolytic anemia.

Other genetic loci appear to be responsible for additional familial cases of distal RTA. Familial deficiency of carbonic anhydrase II is also characterized by cerebral calcification and osteopetrosis, and the latter condition reflects the important role of carbonic anhydrase in osteoclast function. The acidification defect in carbonic anhydrase II deficiency affects bicarbonate reabsorption in the proximal tubule and the collecting duct.

Nephrogenic Diabetes Insipidus

Reabsorption of water across the cells of the collecting duct occurs only when arginine vasopressin (AVP) is present. AVP activates V_2 receptors on the principal cells and cells of the inner medullary collecting duct, initiating a cascade that results in fusion of vesicles containing aquaporin 2 (AQP-2) water channel pores into the apical membranes of these cells. The V_2 receptor is encoded by a gene on the X chromosome, and the most common form of nephrogenic diabetes insipidus is caused by inactivating mutations in the V_2 receptor gene. This results in vasopressin-resistant polyuria that typically is more severe in male patients and is associated with impaired responses to the effects of AVP that are mediated by extrarenal V_2 receptors, specifically vasodilatation and endothelial release of von Willebrand's factor. Less commonly, families have been described with autosomal recessive inheritance of nephrogenic diabetes insipidus, and these patients have mutations in the gene encoding AQP-2 that result in either impaired trafficking of water channels to the plasma membrane or defective pore function. Rare autosomal dominant occurrence of nephrogenic diabetes insipidus with a mutation in AQP-2 has also been reported.

BIBLIOGRAPHY

Bichet DG: Hereditary polyuric disorders: New concepts and differential diagnosis. Semin Nephrol 26:224-233, 2006.

Fry AC, Karet FE: Inherited renal acidoses. Physiology (Bethesda) 22:202-211, 2007.

Groenestege WM, Thebault S, van der Wijst J, et al: Impaired basolateral sorting of pro-EGF causes isolated recessive renal hypomagnesemia. J Clin Invest 117:2260-2267, 2007.

Hou J, Renigunta A, Konrad M, et al: Claudin-16 and claudin-19 interact and form a cation-selective tight junction complex. J Clin Invest 118:619-628.,

Jonsson KB, Zahradnik R, Larsson T, et al: Fibroblast growth factor 23 in oncogenic osteomalacia and X-linked hypophosphatemia. N Engl J Med 348:1656-1663, 2003.

Kahle KT, Ring AM, Lifton RP: Molecular physiology of the WNK kinases. Annu Rev Physiol 70:329-355, 2007.

Karet FE: Inherited distal renal tubular acidosis. J Am Soc Nephrol 13:2178-2184, 2002.

Kleta R, Bockenhauer D: Bartter syndromes and other salt-losing tubulopathies. Nephron Physiol 104:73-80, 2006.

Konrad M, Weber S: Recent advances in molecular genetics of hereditary magnesium-losing disorders. J Am Soc Nephrol 14:249-260, 2003.

Scheinman SJ: Dent's disease. In Lifton R, Somlo S, Giebisch G, Seldin D (eds): Genetic Diseases of the Kidney. San Diego, Elsevier, 2008.

Scheinman SJ, Guay-Woodford LM, Thakker RV, Warnock DG: Genetic disorders of renal electrolyte transport. N Engl J Med 340:1177-1187, 1999.

Simon DB, Lu Y, Choate KA, et al: Paracellin-1, a renal tight junction protein required for paracellular Mg resorption. Science 285:103-106, 1999.

Tenenhouse HS: Phosphate transport: Molecular basis, regulation and pathophysiology. J Steroid Biochem Mol Biol 103:572-577, 2007.

Thakker RV: Diseases associated with the extracellular calcium-sensing receptor. Cell Calcium 35:275-282, 2004.

Torres VE, Scheinman SJ: Genetic diseases of the kidney. NephSAP 3:54-70, 2004.

Vezzoli G, Terranegra A, Arcidiacono T, et al: R990G polymorphism of calcium-sensing receptor does produce a gain-of-function and predispose to primary hypercalciuria. Kidney Int 71:1155-1162, 2007.

Walder RY, Landau D, Meyer P, et al: Mutation of TRPM6 causes familial hypomagnesemia with secondary hypocalcemia. Nat Genet 31:171-174, 2002.

Warnock DG: Liddle syndrome: Genetics and mechanisms of Na^+ channel defects. Am J Med Sci 322:302-307, 2001.

Wilson FH, Kahle KT, Sabath E, et al: Molecular pathogenesis of inherited hypertension with hyperkalemia: The Na-Cl cotransporter is inhibited by wild-type but not mutant WNK4. Proc Natl Acad Sci U S A 100:680-684, 2003.

CHAPTER 41

Sickle Cell Nephropathy

Antonio Guasch

The sickle hemoglobinopathies are caused by the homozygous (Hb SS disease) or heterozygous (Hb AS or sickle cell trait) inheritance of the sickle β-globin gene. The substitution of valine for glutamic acid at position 6 of the β chain of hemoglobin leads to production of an unstable isoform that, when slowly deoxygenated, can polymerize, leading to the production of sickle cells. These cells lack the fluidity of normal erythrocytes and can impede or block capillary flow, resulting in tissue ischemia. Other hemoglobin variants (e.g., Hb C, Hb D, Hb E or β-thalassemia) may coexist with sickle cell anemia (SCA), producing double heterozygosity. In the United States, the sickle cell trait occurs in about 8% of individuals of African American origin, and Hb SS disease affects about 1 in 500 African American newborns.

Because the kidney is a highly vascular organ with a low oxygen tension (Po_2) in the renal medullary interstitium, the kidney is one of the sites vulnerable to vaso-occlusive events. Renal involvement in SCA is common and is summarized in **Table 41-1**.

RENAL HEMODYNAMICS IN SICKLE CELL ANEMIA

The glomerular filtration rate (GFR) is increased in children with SCA (i.e., glomerular hyperfiltration), as are renal plasma and blood flows (i.e., renal hyperperfusion), all consequences of renal vasodilation. A marked glomerular hypertrophy, which is present histologically in individuals with no clinical disease, contributes to the glomerular hyperfiltration. The hypertrophy can be observed in individuals as young as 2 years of age. Analogous to what is observed in individuals with chronic hypoventilation due to obesity, the elevated GFR is presumed to be a compensation for hypoxia. The supernormal GFR returns to normal values after the second or third decade, but renal blood flow rates continue to be higher than in healthy individuals. The mechanisms mediating the renal vasodilation are not known, but some evidence supports a role for vasodilatory prostaglandins or enhanced activity of the nitric oxide system. Treatment of SCA patients with a dose of indomethacin that does not affect the GFR or renal plasma flow in normal individuals normalizes the GFR and decreases renal plasma flow, which approaches a normal value.

TABLE 41-1 Kidney Involvement in Sickle Cell Anemia

Glomerular Conditions

Glomerular hyperfiltration and hyperperfusion

Sickle cell glomerulopathy (focal segmental glomerulosclerosis)
  Microalbuminuria and macroalbuminuria
  Progressive reduction in glomerular filtration rate
  End-stage renal disease

Membranoproliferative glomerulonephritis

Medullary Conditions

Concentrating defects with preserved diluting capacity

Renal papillary necrosis

Hematuria

Tubular Dysfunction

Incomplete distal renal tubular acidosis

Hyperkalemic hyperchloremic acidosis
  Type IV renal tubular acidosis
  Distal renal tubular acidosis with hyperkalemia
  Selective aldosterone deficiency

Decreased potassium excretion without aldosterone deficiency

Increased sodium and phosphate reabsorption

Increased urate secretion

Malignancy

Renal medullary carcinoma

BLOOD PRESSURE IN SICKLE CELL ANEMIA

Despite a higher prevalence of hypertension in the African American population, hypertension is uncommon in SCA. Average blood pressure values are 5 to 15 mm Hg lower in Hb SS patients than in healthy African Americans matched for age and gender, probably as a consequence of a low systemic vascular resistance. A higher mortality rate attributed to vascular events occurs in SCA individuals with blood pressure values higher than the 90th percentile of the blood pressure distribution for the SCA population. In patients with Hb SS disease, this increase in mortality occurs when blood pressure values are higher than 130/84 mm Hg. Blood pressure values higher than 130/84 mm Hg should be considered abnormal in adult patients with SCA and should be treated. Age-appropriate values should be used in assessing children (see Chapter 49.)

SICKLE CELL GLOMERULOPATHY

Glomerular involvement, manifested by proteinuria or progressive loss of kidney function, occurs commonly in SCA patients. Dipstick-positive proteinuria occurs in 25% to 30% of adult SCA patients, and 14% have proteinuria values of 2+ or more. The proteinuria results from enhanced glomerular passage of albumin and larger proteins (of glomerular origin), and it is not the result of tubular failure to reabsorb low-molecular-weight proteins. Proteinuria occurs more frequently in patients with Hb SS disease than in other sickle hemoglobinopathies (i.e., Hb SC or Sβ-thalassemia) and is uncommon in sickle cell trait.

Albuminuria in Sickle Cell Anemia

Abnormal albumin excretion rates may occur in children with SCA. In one series, microalbuminuria was diagnosed in 19% of children, and dipstick proteinuria was identified in 6%. In older teenagers, the prevalence of dipstick-confirmed clinical proteinuria was 12%. The development of albuminuria is age dependent, and microalbuminuria was identified in 24% of children between the ages of 7 and 14 years and in 29% of children older than 15 years. In children, the development of abnormal albuminuria is inversely correlated with hemoglobin levels and is associated with other complications, such as stroke, episodes of acute chest syndrome, and hospitalizations.

Cross-sectional studies indicate that the prevalence of abnormal albuminuria in adults is higher than in the pediatric population, and the severity of albuminuria increases with age. Systematic examination showed that 27% of adults with Hb SS disease had macroalbuminuria and 41% had microalbuminuria, for a combined prevalence of abnormal albuminuria of 68%. The clinical significance of microalbuminuria in SCA patients is unknown, but they may be at risk for progression to macroalbuminuria or even loss of kidney function. However, macroalbuminuria in SCA patients indicates the presence of a glomerulopathy. In other sickle hemoglobinopathies (e.g., Hb SC, Sβ-thalassemia), abnormal albuminuria is much less common than in Hb SS disease, with prevalences of macroalbuminuria and microalbuminuria of 10% and 32% of adult patients, respectively. A lower prevalence of glomerular involvement occurs in patients with Hb SS disease with combined inheritance of α-thalassemia.

Pathophysiology

Some SCA patients may develop chronic kidney disease with progressive loss of kidney function associated with worsening proteinuria. Detailed studies of glomerular filtration using neutral dextrans of graded size as filtration markers show an increase in glomerular pore size in SCA patients with proteinuria, indicative of impaired membrane permselectivity. Initially, the glomerular capillary ultrafiltration coefficient (K_f) is increased, in keeping with the increase in membrane surface area associated with the glomerular hypertrophy observed. With progression of disease, the GFR and renal plasma flow fall to normal and then subnormal values. Proteinuria increases, and the K_f decreases. At this stage, the histologic findings consist of focal glomerulosclerosis (see "Pathology"). As sclerosis progresses, glomerular membrane surface area decreases, accounting for the decrease in K_f.

Clinical Presentation

Sickle cell glomerulopathy occurs more frequently in Hb SS disease than in other sickle hemoglobinopathies, and it is usually detected by the finding of proteinuria at the time of a routine urinalysis. In the initial stages, the only clinically evident abnormality is proteinuria; the serum creatinine level and creatinine clearance rate are in the normal range. As disease progresses, kidney function begins to decline. The rate of proteinuria is usually between 0.5 and 2.5 g/day, but it can be in the nephrotic range. Urinalysis usually reveals no hematuria or pyuria. The presence of hematuria or red blood cell casts should alert the physician to the possibility of other causes for the glomerular disease. Because of the long-term exposure of these patients to blood products and higher incidence of infections, other glomerulopathies (e.g., hepatitis-associated glomerulonephritis, human immunodeficiency virus [HIV] nephropathy) should be excluded. Acute glomerulonephritis has been reported in association with parvovirus infection.

The reported prevalence of impaired kidney function in adult patients with SCA is between 4% and 7%, based on abnormal serum creatinine values. Reduced GFR is more common in Hb SS patients than in patients with Hb SC disease. Caution should be exercised, however, when the assessment of kidney function in SCA patients is based on the serum creatinine norms for healthy individuals. SCA patients have a lower muscle mass than healthy individuals, and serum creatinine values are lower in SCA patients than in healthy controls. As a result, serum creatinine values greater than 1.0 to 1.1 mg/dL can be abnormal in this population. Determination of the creatinine clearance from a 24-hour urine collection or the estimation of kidney function using the Cockcroft-Gault formula or Modification of Diet in Renal Disease (MDRD) equation (see Chapter 2) may be valuable in this population, although neither formula has been specifically validated in this setting.

Pathology

Early descriptions of the pathologic features of SCA individuals with heavy proteinuria emphasized the occurrence of a membranoproliferative glomerulonephritis, possibly a reflection of an unrecognized infection-related glomerulonephritis. Current reports indicate that focal segmental glomerulosclerosis (FSGS) rather than membranoproliferative glomerulonephritis predominates in proteinuric SCA individuals. Quantitative morphometric analysis of biopsy specimens obtained in this population show a significant increase in glomerular diameter and cross-sectional area compared with age-matched autopsy controls. These observations are in accord with the conventional histologic findings of FSGS in SCA, which include hypertrophy of unaffected glomeruli, segmental sclerotic lesions that are more prominent in juxtamedullary nephrons and in the perihilar region, global nephrosclerosis, and tubular atrophy with interstitial fibrosis in regions downstream from the affected glomeruli. As with other cases of FSGS, minor deposits of immunoglobulin M (IgM), Clq, and C3 may be found in sclerotic areas by immunofluorescence assay, but immune complex deposits are absent on electron microscopy. Electron-lucent subendothelial expansion with mesangial interposition is observed in some cases.

Treatment

Because of the findings of proteinuria and focal glomerulosclerosis, angiotensin-converting enzyme (ACE) inhibitors are a logical choice in patients with sickle cell glomerulopathy. In proteinuric patients with mild to moderate impairment of kidney function, low-dose enalapril (5 to 10 mg/day) given over a 2-week period produced a 50% reduction in proteinuria without lowering the GFR or reducing systemic blood pressure. In patients with microalbuminuria, ACE inhibitors reduced albumin excretion when given short term. Data specifically on the long-term effects of ACE inhibition in SCA are not available, but it is reasonable to continue long-term therapy, titrating to maximal tolerated doses as in other microalbuminuric or proteinuric disorders.

Hypertension, even in relative terms, should be treated to achieve blood pressure levels lower than 130/80 mm Hg. Diuretics should be avoided as initial antihypertensive agents, because they may cause volume depletion and precipitate sickle cell crises. Patients may also benefit from moderate protein restriction (0.7 to 0.8 g/kg/day), although the benefit of protein restriction has not been proved (see Chapters 52 and 57). In patients with more advanced chronic kidney disease, potassium levels should be monitored closely. Many SCA patients have selective tubular excretion defects for potassium, which can be worsened by ACE inhibitor therapy. Other potentially nephrotoxic drugs, such as nonsteroidal anti-inflammatory drugs (NSAIDs), should be avoided. Metabolic acidosis can be treated with alkali supplementation. Erythropoietin has been used with moderate success to correct worsening anemia and reduce the need for transfusions.

Patients who develop kidney failure and end-stage renal disease can be successfully treated with dialysis or organ transplantation. The reported survival of SCA patients on dialysis is poor, with a median survival time of only 2 years, although there is a clinical impression that survival has improved lately. In transplanted patients, data from the United States Renal Data System (USRDS) database (see Chapter 56) indicate that the 1-year kidney allograft survival rate in individuals with SCA is similar to that in African American recipients without SCA (78% versus 77%), but their 3-year allograft survival rate is lower (48% versus 60%). SCA recipients tolerate immunosuppressive treatment relatively well, but the frequency of sickle pain crises is higher after successful transplantation. Caution should be used with anti-lymphocyte preparations to prevent or treat acute rejections, because they can precipitate acute vaso-occlusive episodes or the acute chest syndrome. Despite these potential drawbacks, the USRDS data indicate a trend toward better survival in transplanted patients than in patients who remained on the transplant waiting list.

Apart from survival data, quality of life is better with transplantation. Patients with SCA-related kidney failure should be fully informed of the risks but encouraged to undergo transplant evaluation. Although a high level of panel-reactive antibodies resulting from repeated prior blood transfusions may significantly prolong the wait time for transplantation, the high prevalence of stroke, iron overload, and other disorders makes careful screening essential.

RENAL CONCENTRATING DEFECTS

One of the most common renal abnormalities in SCA is an inability to maximally concentrate the urine. The hypertonic and relatively hypoxic environment in the renal medulla is conducive to sickling in the vasa recta. Obstruction of flow and the associated concentration defect can be reversed by early transfusion, which reduces the number of sickled cells. By age 15, however, the concentration defect is fixed and is associated with fibrosis and obliteration of the medullary vasa recta with papillary shortening, as shown by microangiographic studies. Impairment of vasa recta flow interferes with the formation of the medullary urea and sodium gradient necessary for water reabsorption along those segments of the nephron. Patients with SCA cannot achieve urinary osmolalities greater than 400 mOsm/kg and have obligatory water losses of 1.5 to 2.0 L/day. A less severe defect occurs in patients with sickle cell trait. Maximal urinary concentration in older children and young adults with Hb AS is 800 mOsm/kg and reaches 450 to 500 mOsm/kg in older individuals. SCA patients should drink 2 to 3 L of water daily to prevent dehydration, which can precipitate sickle cell pain crises. The free water clearance and urinary diluting ability are preserved in SCA.

HEMATURIA

Hematuria is a relatively common manifestation of SCA and may occur in both sickle cell trait and Hb SS disease. Hematuria usually is painless and originates from the left kidney in about 70% to 80% of cases, but it is bilateral in about 10% of cases. It results from sickling in the vasa recta, causing microinfarctions or severe stasis in peritubular capillaries with extravasation into the renal parenchyma and collecting system. The differential diagnosis includes glomerulonephritis, nephrolithiasis, renal papillary necrosis, urinary tract infections, and urologic malignancies. Initial episodes should be evaluated thoroughly to rule out malignancies. After the initial workup is negative, subsequent episodes may be treated without performing imaging studies, but periodic re-evaluation may be necessary because of the longer life expectancy of SCA patients and the possibility of a higher frequency of renal medullary carcinoma in this population.

The treatment is bed rest and forced diuresis with hypotonic intravenous fluid administration to decrease the tendency to clot formation in the urinary system. Alkalinization of the urine or diuretics can be used to reduce medullary sickling. The benign nature and the possible relapsing nature of the condition should be explained to patients to avoid unnecessary procedures. In persistent cases, ε-aminocaproic acid (EACA) at a dose of 4 to 12g/day in four divided doses can be administered. When EACA is used, a high urinary flow rate should be maintained to avoid clot formation in the renal collecting system. Chronic relapsing hematuria can be treated with exchange transfusion, EACA administration, iron supplementation, and the avoidance of strenuous physical activity. Severe cases may require selective embolization, but nephrectomy is warranted only in case of life-threatening hemorrhage because of the tendency for recurrence in the contralateral kidney.

RENAL PAPILLARY NECROSIS

Renal papillary necrosis is a common manifestation of SCA, and intravenous pyelography demonstrates unilateral or bilateral papillary necrosis in as many as 67% of unselected patients without a prior history of urinary symptoms. Papillary necrosis usually is asymptomatic, but it may manifest with microscopic hematuria or renal colic. It is caused by localized medullary ischemia and necrosis of the medullary tip as a result of obliteration of the medullary vessels from sickling. The diagnosis is made with intravenous pyelography or ultrasound studies. There are radiographic irregularities in the renal calyces, with formation of a sinus tract that with time progresses to complete sequestration of the affected area, producing the radiographic "ring sign." In late stages, there is clubbing due to the sloughing or reabsorption of the papillae. On ultrasound, there is increased echogenicity of the inner medulla. In more advanced cases, a filling defect can be seen in the area of the medullary tip. In symptomatic patients with renal papillary necrosis, an associated urinary tract infection should be ruled out. In contrast to other forms of renal papillary necrosis, the prognosis for long-term renal function is good. NSAIDs should be avoided.

ACIDIFICATION AND POTASSIUM EXCRETION DEFECTS

Under normal conditions, most SCA patients have a normal acid-base balance or a mild respiratory alkalosis. Metabolic acidosis can occur when SCA patients are given an acute acid load or when they are stressed by intercurrent illness such as diarrhea that results in gastrointestinal bicarbonate loss. This incomplete form of distal renal tubular acidosis (RTA) results from an inability to lower the urinary pH normally, i.e. below 5.3, with a resultant decrease in titratable acid and ammonium excretion. Proximal tubular bicarbonate reabsorption is normal.

Other variants have been described. Some patients with SCA, including those with sickle cell trait, may develop a hyperkalemic hyperchloremic metabolic acidosis. In some patients, selective aldosterone deficiency or hyporeninemic hypoaldosteronism leads to hyperkalemia, impaired ammoniagenesis, and proton retention despite a normal ability to lower urine pH. Other patients have hyperkalemic distal RTA, an inability to generate the tubular transepithelial electrical gradient that permits normal potassium or proton secretion. Treatment consists of sodium bicarbonate, a low-potassium diet, mineralocorticoids, and loop diuretics.

OTHER TUBULAR ABNORMALITIES

Proximal tubular transport processes are typically increased in patients with SCA, but the change usually has little clinical significance. In some patients, hyperphosphatemia may occur as a result of increased proximal tubular phosphate reabsorption. Uric acid excretion is increased as a result of an increased red blood cell turnover rate and an increase in uric acid production. Even so, gout is uncommon in SCA.

RENAL MEDULLARY CARCINOMA

Reports suggest an increased incidence of renal medullary carcinoma among SCA patients. This rare, highly aggressive tumor occurs in young people; the reported age at diagnosis ranges from the second to the fifth decade. The tumor arises in the medulla, but in the reported series, it had already extended beyond the capsule, and metastases were present at diagnosis. Patients may present with hematuria, abdominal pain, a flank mass, or weight loss. Diagnosis requires demonstration by renal imaging studies, such as a computed tomography (CT) followed by excision.

Chromosomal abnormalities in the tumor tissue have been localized to chromosome 11 and, less often, to chromosome 3. The former is the locus of the gene encoding the hemoglobin β chain. The latter is the site of the mutation for von Hippel-Lindau syndrome, which is also associated with renal cell carcinoma.

Renal medullary carcinoma has a poor prognosis. In one study, mean survival after excision was only 15 weeks (range, 2 to 52 weeks). Neither radiotherapy nor chemotherapy has proved useful. The available studies are retrospective, and clinical details were not available for all patients. These findings require confirmation in more carefully conducted studies. Nevertheless, a urologic evaluation should be performed in patients with SCA presenting with hematuria or abdominal pain, but screening asymptomatic SCA patients with CT or ultrasound to uncover urologic malignancies is not indicated.

BIBLIOGRAPHY

Allon M, Lawson L, Eckman JR, et al: Effects of nonsteroidal antiinflammatory drugs on renal function in sickle cell anemia. Kidney Int 34:500-506, 1988.

Batlle D, Itsarayoungyuen K, Arruda JA, Kurtzman NA: Hyperkalemic hyperchloremic metabolic acidosis in sickle cell hemoglobinopathies. Am J Med 72:188-192, 1982.

Falk RJ, Scheinman J, Phillips G, et al: Prevalence and pathologic features of sickle cell nephropathy and response to inhibition of angiotensin-converting enzyme. N Engl J Med 326:910-915, 1992.

Figenshau RS, Easier JW, Ritter JH, et al: Renal medullary carcinoma. J Urol 159:711-713, 1998.

Guasch A, Cua M, Mitch WE: Extent and the course of glomerular injury in patients with sickle cell anemia. Kidney Int 49:786-791, 1996.

Guasch A, Cua M, You W, Mitch WE: Sickle cell anemia causes a distinct pattern of glomerular dysfunction. Kidney Int 51:826-833, 1997.

Guasch A, Navarrete J, Nass K, et al: Glomerular involvement in adults with sickle cell hemoglobinopathies: Prevalence and clinical correlates of progressive renal failure. J Am Soc Nephrol 17:2228-2235, 2006.

Guasch A, Zayas CF, Eckman JR, Elsas L: Evidence that microdeletions in the α globin gene protect against the development of sickle cell glomerulopathy. J Am Soc Nephrol 10:1014-1019, 1999.

McBurney PG, Hanevold CD, Hernadez CM, et al: Risk factors for microalbuminuria in children with sickle cell anemia. J Pediatr Hematol Oncol 24:473-477, 2002.

McKie KT, Hanevold CD, Hernandez C, et al: Prevalence, prevention, and treatment of microalbuminuria and proteinuria in children with sickle cell disease. J Pediatr Hematol Oncol 29:140-144, 2007.

Ojo AO, Govaerts TC, Schmouder RL, et al: Renal transplantation in end-stage sickle cell nephropathy. Transplantation 67:291-295, 1999.

Pandya KK, Koshy M, Brown N, Presman D: Renal papillary necrosis in sickle cell hemoglobinopathies. J Urol 115:497-501, 1976.

Pegelow CH, Colangelo L, Steinberg M, et al: Natural history of blood pressure in sickle cell disease: Risks for stroke and death associated with relative hypertension in sickle cell anemia. Am J Med 102:171-177, 1997.

Pham PT, Pham PC, Wilkinson AH, Lew SQ: Renal abnormalities in sickle cell disease. Kidney Int 57:1-8, 2000.

Powars DR, Elliot-Mills DD, Chan L, et al: Chronic renal failure in sickle cell disease: Risk factors, clinical course, and mortality. Ann Intern Med 115:614-620, 1991.

Saborio P, Scheinman JI: Sickle cell nephropathy. J Am Soc Nephrol 10:187-192, 1999.

Statius van Eps LW, Pinedo-Veels C, Vries GH: de Koning J: Nature of concentrating defect in sickle-cell nephropathy: Micro-radioangiographic studies. Lancet 1:450-452, 1970.

Wigfall DR, Ware RE, Burchinal MR, et al: Prevalence and clinical correlates of glomerulopathy in children with sickle cell disease. J Pediatr 136:749-753, 2000.

Zayas CF, Platt J, Eckman JR, et al: Prevalence and predictors of glomerular involvement in sickle cell anemia [abstract]. J Am Soc Nephrol 7:1401, 1996.

CHAPTER 42

Polycystic and Other Cystic Kidney Diseases

Arlene B. Chapman

Significant advances have been made in understanding the genetics and molecular pathogenesis of inherited cystic disorders of the kidney. Many of the genes and their respective proteins have been identified (**Table 42-1**). Final common pathways regarding the formation and development of cysts are being elucidated. Most cystic diseases develop because of abnormal function of the primary cilium that resides in all epithelial cells. Newer, molecularly targeted therapies being tested offer hope for improved outcome or cure of these disorders.

AUTOSOMAL DOMINANT POLYCYSTIC KIDNEY DISEASE

Autosomal dominant polycystic kidney disease (ADPKD) is the most common inherited kidney disease, affecting 1 in 400 to 1000 people. It has similar prevalence rates in all ethnic groups. ADPKD is a systemic disease resulting in kidney, liver, pancreas, thyroid, and subarachnoid cysts and in intracranial aneurysms (ICAs). It accounts for 5% of the end-stage renal disease (ESRD) population in the United States and Europe. The clinical hallmark of ADPKD is gradual and massive cystic enlargement of the kidneys, ultimately resulting in kidney failure.

Pathogenesis

At least two genes (*PKD1* and *PKD2*) are responsible for ADPKD. Mutations in either gene have prognostic implications, with patients with *PKD2* mutations developing renal cysts, hypertension, and ESRD at a later age than those with *PKD1* mutations (mean age of onset of ESRD, 53 years for *PKD1* patients and 69 years for *PKD2* patients). Families with ADPKD not linked to *PKD1* or *PKD2* have been reported, but a third locus has not been identified.

In 85% of families affected with ADPKD, the disorder is linked to a mutation in the *PKD1* gene located on the short arm of chromosome 16 (16p13.3). *PKD1* codes for an integral membrane protein (i.e., polycystin 1) made up of 4304 amino acids with as an incompletely defined function. Polycystin 1 is localized in the membrane, specifically in the base and tip of the primary cilia of epithelial cells. The known properties of polycystin 1 are those of a ligand with extracellular interactions and cell cycle regulation. Mutations in the *PKD2* gene located on the long arm of chromosome 4 (4q21.2) account for 15% of affected families. *PKD2* codes for a 968–amino acid protein (i.e., polycystin 2), which is structurally similar to polycystin 1. It colocalizes with polycystin 1 in primary cilia and independently in the membrane of the endoplasmic reticulum. Polycystin 2 belongs to the family of voltage-activated calcium channels (e.g., transient receptor potential polycystin 2 [TRPP-2]) and is involved in intracellular calcium regulation through several pathways. Polycystin 1 and 2 in the primary cilium of renal epithelial cells function as mechanical sensors, and the physical interaction between polycystin 1 and 2 is required for the membrane calcium channel to operate properly. Primary cilia create a transmembrane calcium current in the presence of stretch or luminal flow. This interaction increases intracellular calcium, which

TABLE 42-1 Genes and Proteins of Inherited Cystic Disorders of the Kidney

DISEASE	FREQUENCY	CHROMOSOME	GENE LOCUS	PROTEIN	FUNCTION
ADPKD	1:1,000	16p13.3	PKD1	Polycystin 1, which colocalizes with polycystin 2 in the primary cilium	Regulates intracellular cAMP, mTOR, planar polarity
	1:15,000	4q21.2	PKD2	Polycystin 2, which colocalizes with polycystin 1 in the primary cilium and ER	Regulates intracellular Ca levels through ER Ca release, activates Ca channels
ARPKD	1:20,000	6q24.2	PKHD	Fibrocystin or polyductin, located throughout the primary cilium	Serves as receptor to maintain intracellular cAMP levels
VHL	1:25,000	3p25	VHL	VHL, located at the base of the primary cilium	Inhibits HIF-1α and cell turnover, maintains planar polarity, allows ciliogenesis
TSC	1:20,000	9q34.3	TSC1	Hamartin	Interacts with tuberin to suppress mTOR activity
		16p13.3	TSC2	Tuberin	Interacts with hamartin to suppress mTOR activity

ADPKD, autosomal dominant polycystic kidney disease; ARPKD, autosomal recessive polycystic kidney disease; Ca, calcium; ER, endoplasmic reticulum; HIF, hypoxia-inducible factor, mTOR, mammalian target of rapamycin; TSC, tuberous sclerosis complex; VHL, von Hippel-Lindau disease.

function becomes impaired, progression is universal, with an average decline in the GFR of 4.0 to 5.0 mL/min/yr (similar to the rate of decline found in those with large kidney volumes in the CRISP study). Predictors of progression to ESRD include male gender, *PKD1*, hypertension, increased kidney size, and increased level of proteinuria. However, increased proteinuria is not a major feature, with an average level of 260 mg of protein excretion per day in adults with ADPKD. Consistent with other tubulointerstitial diseases, only 18% of adults have urinary protein excretion rates greater than 300 mg/day. In individuals whose urine protein excretion exceeds 2 g/24 hr, evaluation for a second kidney disease is warranted.

Hypertension is a common and early manifestation of ADPKD, occurring in 60% of patients with normal kidney function. The mean age at onset of hypertension is 31 years. It is associated with larger kidney size in children and adults. Unlike the difference between *PKD1* and *PKD2* patients, hypertension is associated with a greater rate of kidney enlargement (6.2%/year versus 4.5%/year), suggesting a relationship between elevated blood pressure and cyst expansion.

Given that polycystins are also expressed in vascular smooth muscle cells, *PKD* mutations involving this protein may contribute directly to a vasculopathy or hypertensive state, independent of their effects on the kidney. The renin-angiotensin system is activated early in the course of ADPKD as a result of cyst expansion, causing bilateral intrarenal ischemia. Hypertension contributes to an accelerated loss of kidney function and should be treated aggressively. There is no evidence that angiotensin-converting enzyme (ACE) inhibitors or angiotensin receptor blockers (ARBs) are more effective than other antihypertensive agents in retarding progression to ESRD in ADPKD; however, the Halt Progression of Polycystic Kidney Disease clinical trial is determining whether rigorous control of blood pressure or maximal inhibition of the renin-angiotensin system is effective in slowing progression of ADPKD.

Kidney transplant recipients with ESRD due to ADPKD survive longer than patients transplanted for other causes. Potential transplant recipients are screened for the possible presence of an ICA. Native polycystic kidneys do not have to be removed before transplantation unless chronic infections are present or their large size interferes with nutritional intake or quality of life.

Extrarenal Manifestations

Polycystic Liver Disease

Hepatic cysts are the most common extrarenal manifestation in ADPKD. MRI shows universal presence of hepatic cysts in individuals with ADPKD by the age of 30 years, with equal gender representation. Hepatic function is preserved even in the presence of massive cystic disease, and biochemical test results are normal except for a mild elevation in the serum concentration of alkaline phosphatase. Hepatic enlargement is the predominant complication of polycystic liver disease, resulting in symptoms of shortness of breath, pain, early

satiety, decreased mobility, ankle swelling, and rarely, inferior vena cava compression. This severe form of polycystic liver disease is unusual and occurs in less than 10% of patients. It predominantly affects women and may require surgical cyst deroofing, fenestration and resection, or liver transplantation. Isolated autosomal dominant polycystic liver disease independent of ADPKD has been linked to two genetic defects for the gene *PRKCSH* (19p13.2-13.1) encoding β-glucosidase II and SEC-63. Both proteins are part of the molecular machinery involved in the translocation, folding, and quality control of newly synthesized glycoproteins in the endoplasmic reticulum.

Cardiovascular Manifestations

ICAs occur in 4% to 8% of asymptomatic ADPKD patients. Other vascular abnormalities, including intracoronary aneurysms, may occur in this group. ICAs cluster in ADPKD families and occur in 10% of individuals with a family history of a nonruptured ICA and 20% of individuals with a family history of a ruptured ICA. The aneurysms occur most often in the anterior circulation, similar to the general population; however, multiple ICAs are common in ADPKD patients, similar to the manifestation of non-ADPKD familial ICAs. Individuals who underwent screening with magnetic resonance angiography (MRA) and were found to be aneurysm free did not demonstrate a new ICA when screened 7 years later.

Rupture of an ICA is associated with an immediate mortality rate of more than 50% and permanent morbidity rate of more than 80%. Screening is indicated in asymptomatic patients with a positive family history for ICA, previous history of intracranial hemorrhage, those with high-risk occupations, or before major elective surgery that would affect intracranial hemodynamics. Persons without a family history and without these additional concerns do not warrant routine screening and should be so advised. The imaging modality of choice for screening is time-of-flight, three-dimensional MRA. Although gadolinium has been used for arteriographic imaging, the occurrence of nephrogenic systemic fibrosis makes routine use of gadolinium complicated, particularly in those with impaired renal function.

Although rupture of an ICA is associated with significant morbidity and mortality, only 50% of individuals with ICA have a rupture during their lifetimes. Postoperative complications related to surgical clipping are common, and recovery from elective surgery can be prolonged. For larger aneurysms (>10 mm), the risk of rupture is significant, and elective surgical intervention is recommended. For those with an ICA smaller than 5 mm, longitudinal studies have not demonstrated significant growth of the ICA, and the risk of rupture is relatively small. The current indications for repair of these smaller ICAs are unclear. With the development of less invasive and safer therapies (i.e., coiling or stenting), successful treatment of small, asymptomatic ICAs may become available.

Mitral valve prolapse and regurgitation is common in ADPKD, occurring in 26% of individuals compared with

3% of the general population. Aortic insufficiency also occurs more frequently (11%) in people with ADPKD.

Effects on Fertility and Pregnancy

Overall, fertility rates in ADPKD men and women not yet on dialysis are similar to those in the general population despite a higher incidence of ectopic pregnancies, congenital absence of the seminiferous tubules, and amotile spermatozoa. Affected women with a normal GFR and normal blood pressure have pregnancy outcomes similar to those of the general population. Hypertensive ADPKD women have a higher incidence of worsening hypertension and preeclampsia during pregnancy and higher rate of premature delivery. Those with a decreased GFR before pregnancy are at high risk for mid-trimester fetal loss.

Autosomal Dominant Polycystic Kidney Disease in Children

Renal manifestations of ADPKD in children are similar to those in adults. The percentage of at-risk individuals diagnosed as part of a family screening program while still asymptomatic has increased from 40% in the 1980s to almost 59% since the year 2000. This corresponds in part to the development of more advanced ultrasound imaging devices. Children present more often with diffuse abdominal pain instead of flank or back pain.

Hypertension is the most common feature leading to a diagnosis of ADPKD, occurring in 5% to 44% of newly diagnosed patients. The presence of hypertension correlates with disease severity; hypertensive children have larger kidneys that grow at a faster rate than their normotensive counterparts. Other vascular abnormalities in ADPKD children include abnormal circadian blood pressure patterns with a loss of the normal nocturnal decline in blood pressure (33%). In addition to mitral valve prolapse, increased left ventricular mass and hypercholesterolemia occur with increased frequency in ADPKD children. Cerebral aneurysms have been described, albeit rarely, in this age group. At-risk offspring should have regular blood pressure measurements and urinalyses. However, there are no guidelines for systematic screening of asymptomatic ADPKD children.

Therapy

Randomized, controlled clinical trials evaluating ACE inhibitors, rigorous blood pressure control, and dietary protein restriction have failed to demonstrate statistically significant renal protection in ADPKD. Other dietary modifications, including abstinence from caffeine intake and increased water intake, have been suggested but not formally tested in a prospective, randomized clinical trial. However, the trials performed have been inadequately designed or powered to definitely determine whether the therapies tested are effective. A meta-analysis of randomized, controlled trials involving at least 142 hypertensive patients with ADPKD showed that ACE inhibitors were associated with significant

slowing in the rate of decline in renal function and urinary protein reduction in those with greater degrees of proteinuria. A prospective, randomized, 3-year study involving 36 ADPKD individuals treated with amlodipine or candesartan therapy demonstrated a significantly greater decline in creatinine clearance and increase in proteinuria in the amlodipine group compared with the candesartan group.

Current recommendations for target blood pressure level and the initial drug of choice for ADPKD are based on the Seventh Joint National Committee (JNC7) recommendations for all patients with chronic kidney disease, targeting blood pressure below 130/80 mm Hg using ACE inhibitors or ARBs. A promising therapy aimed at reducing intracellular cAMP accumulation by blocking the vasopressin V_2 receptor has successfully retarded renal cyst progression in four distinct genetic forms of cystic disease: the PKD2 WS25 mouse, the Han:SPRD rat, the pcy mouse (a mouse model for familial juvenile nephronophthisis), and the polycystic kidney (pck) rat (a murine model for autosomal recessive polycystic kidney disease [ARPKD]). Phase II studies of vasopressin V_2 receptor antagonists in ADPKD subjects demonstrate effective inhibition of the V_2 receptor, resulting in decreased water reabsorption and urinary osmolality over 24 hours. This medication is well tolerated, with patients maintaining serum sodium concentrations and tolerating mild increases in the frequency of nocturia. Large, prospective, randomized, phase III studies are being conducted to determine whether long-term therapy with V_2 receptor antagonists effectively reduces the rate of increase in kidney size over time in ADPKD patients.

Other small, prospective studies evaluating somatostatin, another inhibitor of intracellular cAMP accumulation through inhibition of the G protein and adenylate cyclase pathway, in a randomized, placebo-controlled fashion have demonstrated reduction in the rate of increase in kidney volume in 12 ADPKD patients treated for 6 months compared with controls ($2.2 \pm 3.7\%$ versus $5.9 \pm 5.4\%$; $P < .05$). Recent evidence indicates that normal polycystin 1 interacts with the tuberous sclerosis complex (TSC1/TSC2), and the interaction between polycystin 1 and the TSC complex plays a role in the inhibition of mammalian target of rapamycin (mTOR) activity. In support of these findings, the inhibitor of mTOR, sirolimus, has been shown to decrease kidney cyst burden in the Han:SPRD rat. ADPKD patients who received sirolimus for kidney transplantation demonstrate a significant decline in the size of their native kidneys over time.

AUTOSOMAL RECESSIVE POLYCYSTIC KIDNEY DISEASE

ARPKD affects approximately 1 in 20,000 individuals (see **Table 42-1**). At-risk offspring have a 25% chance of being affected. ARPKD has been linked to a mutation in the *PKHD1* gene on the short arm of chromosome 6 (6p21.1). The protein product is a 4074–amino acid protein called polyductin or fibrocystin, which is characterized by a single transmembrane segment and a short cytoplasmic C-terminal segment. This protein is thought to act as a membrane receptor involved in transducing intracellular signals. Similar to the *PKD1* and *PKD2* gene products, polyductin colocalizes to primary epithelial cilia, usually at their base.

ARPKD is characterized by ectatic dilatation of the distal collecting ducts, leading to renal cysts. Mutations have been identified in the *PKHD1* gene in approximately 60% of affected individuals. Most mutations are heterogeneic, with the most severe disease associated with homozygous mutations that predict immediate stop codons or a truncated protein. Congenital hepatic fibrosis is a universal feature of ARPKD and often predominates in children who survive the perinatal period.

Clinical Features

Prenatally, the disease is diagnosed by the presence of echogenic, enlarged kidneys. The level of kidney enlargement for ARPKD in utero is significantly greater than for ADPKD. Renal cysts are more likely to appear in utero in ARPKD than in ADPKD. Oligohydramnios, with resultant lung hypoplasia and compressed (Potter) facies, is a poor prognostic indicator for patient survival. Perinatal death usually is attributed to respiratory failure resulting from delayed pulmonary development and difficulties with ventilation due to large kidneys. In a contemporary series from 34 centers of 166 ARPKD infants born after 1990, 50% of whom were diagnosed prenatally, 74.7% survived the neonatal period. Among the children who died, respiratory failure and sepsis were the most common causes of death. Predictors of outcome included the degree of oligohydramnios and amniotic cystatin C levels.

In infancy, affected children present with pneumomediastinum, pneumothorax due to poor fetal lung development related to oligohydramnios, hypertension, cardiac hypertrophy, congestive heart failure from endomyocardial fibrosis, and impaired kidney function. In a recent series, 40% required mechanical ventilation at birth, and 12% developed chronic lung disease. Beyond infancy, several clinical features are observed. Growth retardation occurs in approximately 25% of patients. Hypertension is common, occurring in more than 60% of ARPKD patients. Reduced kidney function is present in 42%, with an additional 21% requiring dialysis or transplantation. Hepatic fibrosis and portal hypertension and its complications (i.e., ascending cholangitis and variceal bleeding), predominate as ARPKD patients age.

Treatment

Hypertension should be treated with salt restriction and ACE inhibitors, targeting blood pressure below the 75th percentile for age and gender. Anemia and growth management should be provided for all ARPKD children with decreased kidney function with an erythropoiesis-stimulating agent, correction of acidosis, and growth hormone therapy. Dialysis should be offered when needed. Liver involvement rarely leads to hepatocellular damage or

synthetic dysfunction, but portal hypertension usually develops between the ages of 5 and 10 years. Therapy includes portosystemic shunts for severe varices, and children with advanced disease are candidates for liver or combined liver and kidney transplantation.

TUBEROUS SCLEROSIS COMPLEX

TSC is an autosomal dominant disorder affecting 40,000 Americans and about 2 million people worldwide. Its prevalence is about 1 case per 6000 individuals. TSC is caused by mutations in the *TSC1* or *TSC2* gene. The spontaneous mutation rate is high (65% to 75%) in individuals with the mutated *TSC1* gene. The spontaneous mutation rate is lower and the phenotype is less severe in individuals with the mutated *TSC2* gene.

Two genes can lead to the tuberous sclerosis clinical phenotype. *TSC1* is located on the long arm of chromosome 9 (9q34). It is composed of 23 exons spanning 55 kb of genomic DNA that encode for a ubiquitously expressed 8.6-kb mRNA. The gene's product is hamartin, a 1164–amino acid protein of 130 kDa. *TSC2* is on the short arm of chromosome 16 (16p13.3). It consists of a 5.4-kb coding region with 41 exons spanning 40 kb of genomic DNA. Its protein product is a 200-kDa protein, tuberin, which contains 1807 amino acids. *TSC2* is only 48 base pairs distant from the *PKD1* gene, and a contiguous deletion of both *TSC2* and *PKD1* genes leads to the severe phenotype of very-early-onset polycystic kidney disease.

The *TSC* genes are tumor suppressor genes that coassemble and interact with each other. No phenotypic features distinguish TSC type 1 patients from TSC type 2 patients. Many of the renal cell carcinomas in TSC show a loss of heterozygosity, suggesting a "two-hit" process. Genetic mosaicism has been documented and includes somatic mutations (not found in all cell lines) or germline mutations (found only in gonadal cells and transmitted to all offspring while parents are spared from any disease manifestation). The mechanisms through which the *TSC1* and *TSC2* gene products control cellular growth and proliferation have been partially elucidated. The two proteins, hamartin and tuberin, are responsible for regulation of cell growth and tumorigenesis. These proteins demonstrate a tight binding interaction, forming a tumor suppressor heterodimer. In its active GTP-bound state, RHEB, a RAS-related small GTPase that is enriched in the brain, stimulates mTOR, promoting protein synthesis and cell growth. RHEB is the direct target of the TSC1/TSC2 complex, and through a critical GTPase-activating protein domain, the TSC1/TSC2 heterodimer switches RHEB from an active GTP-bound state to an inactive GDP-bound state, leading to cell growth arrest. Mutations in the *TSC1* or *TSC2* genes result in activation of the mTOR metabolic pathway and are associated with the growth of tuberous sclerosis lesions, suggesting that sirolimus or analogues may be useful in the treatment of this disease.

In July 1998, the National Institutes of Health sponsored a consensus conference of international experts to review the literature on TSC and to determine diagnostic criteria (**Table 42-2**). A definite diagnosis of TSC entails the presence of any two of the major features.

Renal angiomyolipomas occur in 70% to 80% of affected individuals and are detected based on their fat content by CT or MRI. They are histologically similar to the lymphangiomyolipomas found in the lung. Hemorrhage from these lesions is the most common cause of death and kidney failure in adults with TSC. Complications commonly occur after the angiomyolipomas reach 4 cm in diameter. Longitudinal imaging using ultrasound indicates that more than one half of TSC children have detectable growth in kidney angiomyolipomas over 1 year. As the angiomyolipomas increase in size, the vascular supply becomes more tortuous and ultimately aneurysmal. Aneurysmal dilation is a cause of hemorrhage of kidney angiomyolipomas and is more predictive than kidney size, although increased size and aneurysmal vascular change tend to occur together.

Management of kidney angiomyolipomas is evolving rapidly. Given that disinhibition of the mTOR pathway is central to the pathogenesis of TSC, clinical studies have been initiated to determine the potential benefit of sirolimus in reducing the size of angiomyolipomas. Case reports have demonstrated significant reductions in angiomyolipomas over a short period.

Arterial embolization frequently is used as a kidney-sparing approach to reduce the size of angiomyolipomas. Regrowth of angiomyolipomas does not occur after successful embolization. However, postembolectomy syndrome occurs in most cases during the first 48 hours after the procedure, and these patients have nausea, pain fever, and hemodynamic instability. Postembolization enucleation to remove residual debris and percutaneous drainage of liquefied material are commonly needed.

VON HIPPEL-LINDAU DISEASE

Von Hippel-Lindau (VHL) disease is a rare, autosomal dominant disorder affecting 1 in 35,000 individuals. VHL disease is caused by inactivation of the *VHL* (tumor suppressor) gene located on chromosome 3 (3p25). Affected individuals do not develop the disease without a somatic mutation or second hit. Genetic screening of at-risk family members is considered the standard of care. There appears to be a genotype-phenotype relationship in VHL, and the development of renal cell carcinoma correlates with a specific missense mutation.

The wild-type *VHL* gene encodes for the VHL protein (VHL), which under normoxic conditions is involved in the degradation of hypoxia-inducible factors such as vascular endothelial growth factor and erythropoietin. In the absence of a functional VHL protein, these factors accumulate, despite the presence of oxygen, which may explain the vascular nature of the tumors in VHL and the presence of polycythemia as a paraneoplastic syndrome in some cases. The VHL protein plays an essential role in primary ciliary function. Microtubules involved in establishing planar polarity that contribute to the formation of the internal skeleton of primary cilia require VHL for proper orientation and organization. Lack of VHL results in nonciliated epithelial cells and cyst development, potentially through a lack of centromere attachment to the cell membrane and proper microtubule alignment.

VHL disease is clinically characterized by the development of benign and malignant tumors in many organs. Benign cysts of the kidneys, pancreas, and epididymis are common and rarely lead to kidney or pancreatic dysfunction or to infertility. The lifetime risk of renal cell carcinoma is greater than 70%. These are clear cell tumors that are widely metastatic by the time patients have symptoms. Management strategies include annual screening of VHL patients with CT or ultrasonography, or both. The treatment of choice remains parenchymal-sparing renal surgery.

Other common manifestations are hemangioblastomas, which are highly vascular, nonmetastatic, noninvading tumors that occur almost exclusively in the cerebellum, the spinal cord, or the brainstem. They affect 21% to 72% of VHL patients and are often multiple. Compression of adjacent neurologic structures determines the presenting symptoms.

TABLE 42-2 Diagnostic Criteria for Tuberous Sclerosis Complex*

Major Features

Facial angiofibromas or forehead plaque

Nontraumatic ungulas or periungual fibromas

Hypomelanotic macules (≥3)

Shagreen patches (connective tissue nevus)

Multiple retinal nodular hamartomas

Cortical tuber[†]

Subependymal nodule

Subependymal giant cell astrocytoma

Cardiac rhabdomyoma (single or multiple)

Lymphangiomyomatosis[‡]

Renal angiomyolipoma[‡]

Minor Features

Multiple, randomly distributed pits in dental enamel

Hamartomatous rectal polyps[§]

Bone cysts [¶]

Cerebral white matter radial migration lines[‡]

Gingival fibromas

Nonrenal hamartomas[§]

Retinal achromic patch

Confetti skin lesions

Multiple renal cysts[§]

*Definite tuberous sclerosis complex (TSC) is defined by two major features or one major feature plus two minor features. Probable TSC is defined by one major feature plus one minor feature. Possible TSC is defined by one major feature or two or more minor features.

[†]If cerebral cortical dysplasia and cerebral white matter migration tracts occur together, they should be counted as one rather than two features of TSC.

[‡]If both lymphangiomyomatosis and renal angiomyolipomas occur, other features of TSC should be identified before a definite diagnosis is assigned.

[§]Histologic confirmation is suggested.

[¶]Radiographic confirmation is suggested.

Surgical intervention is the treatment of choice, with or without radiation therapy. Patients should be screened annually for these tumors using gadolinium-enhanced MRI.

Other tumors include retinal angiomas (50%), which can lead to retinal detachment and blindness. Tumors are treated by laser photocoagulation. Endolymphatic sac tumors (10%), which arise from the membranous labyrinth of the inner ear, are usually bilateral, leading to vertigo, tinnitus, and hearing loss. Current therapeutic recommendations are surgical. Pheochromocytomas are seen in 7% to 20% of patients, tend to occur at a young age, and are often bilateral, multiple, and extra-adrenal. Patients with suggestive symptoms should be screened biochemically and radiologically for pheochromocytomas. Asymptomatic patients scheduled for any elective surgery should be screened to prevent fatal hemodynamic and cardiac complications associated with anesthesia and surgery.

ACQUIRED CYSTIC KIDNEY DISEASE

Acquired cystic kidney disease (ACKD) refers to the development of cysts during a period of chronic kidney disease or ESRD. A finding of more than three to five cysts in each kidney in the setting of chronic kidney disease and small kidneys with no family history of cystic disease is required to make the diagnosis. Cysts are usually bilateral and small (<3 cm in diameter). Between 8% and 13% of patients initiating renal replacement therapy have ACKD, and the prevalence increases with increased duration of replacement therapy. Significant associations with ACKD include gender and race, with African American men more frequently affected.

Cyst microdissection and analysis suggest that the cysts in ACKD arise from the proximal tubule and demonstrate epithelial hyperplasia and hypertrophy. Two murine models of proximal cyst formation similar to that in ACKD are the Han: SPRD rat and the congenital polycystic kidney (cpk) mouse.

Most patients with ACKD are asymptomatic; however, cyst rupture can lead to hematuria or perinephric hematomas with flank pain. The most feared complication of ACKD is the development of renal cell carcinoma, estimated to affect 2% to 7% of patients. The risk of renal cell carcinoma in association with ACKD is possibly a result of mutations and dysregulation of proto-oncogenes. Whereas most sporadic cases of renal cell carcinoma are clear cell or granular carcinomas, papillary tumors are found with increased frequency in the setting of ACKD.

Screening of ESRD patients for ACKD is controversial. A decision-analysis model revealed that screening provided significant benefits only for patients with a life expectancy of at least 25 years. However, it may be beneficial to screen high-risk individuals (i.e., male, African American patients who have been on dialysis for more than 3 years). Anyone with signs or symptoms of ACKD should also be investigated.

Ultrasonography is a good screening tool for detecting ACKD; however, CT and MRI should be performed in patients who develop symptoms suggesting carcinoma (e.g., hematuria, unexplained anemia, back pain), because these modalities are more sensitive for detecting small tumors. Irregular appearance and enhancement with iodinated contrast or gadolinium usually suggest the presence of a neoplasm. When detected, tumors larger than 3 cm should be treated surgically with total nephrectomy.

An evaluation of 194 transplant recipients found that ACKD is common, occurring more frequently in those with previous dialysis exposure or longer duration of ESRD. Renal cell carcinoma occurred in 4.8% of this group, most often in those with ACKD. The risk factors for renal cell carcinoma included male gender, significant cardiovascular disease, and calcification in the allograft. These findings suggest that transplant recipients, similar to ESRD patients, should be screened for the presence of ACKD, and if diagnosed, they should be followed regularly with imaging studies.

BIBLIOGRAPHY

Choyke PL: Acquired cystic kidney disease. Eur Radiol 10:1716-1721, 2000.

Couch V, Lindor NM, Karnes PS, et al: Von Hippel-Lindau disease. N Engl J Med 75:265-272, 2000.

Dabora SL, Jozwiak S, Franz DN, et al: Mutational analysis in a cohort of 224 tuberous sclerosis patients indicates increased severity of TSC2 compared to TSC1 disease in multiple organs. Am J Hum Genet 68:64-80, 2001.

El-Hashemite N, Zhang H, Henske EP, Kwiatkoski DJ: Mutation in TSC2 and activation of mammalian target of rapamycin signaling pathway in renal angiomyolipoma. Lancet 361:1348-1349, 2003.

Gattone VH II, Wang X, Harris PC, et al: Inhibition of renal cystic disease development and progression by a vasopressin V_2 receptor antagonist. Nat Med 9:1323-1326, 2003.

Grantham JJ, Torres VE, Chapman AB, et al: Volume progression in polycystic kidney disease. N Engl J Med 354:2122-2130, 2006.

Guay-Woodford LM, Desmand RA: Autosomal recessive polycystic kidney disease: The clinical experience in North America. Pediatrics 111:1072-1080, 2003.

Hyman MH, Whittemore VH: National Institutes of Health consensus conference: Tuberous sclerosis complex. Arch Neurol 57:662-665, 2000.

Kaelin WG Jr: Molecular basis of VHL hereditary cancer syndrome. Nat Rev Cancer 2:673-682, 2002.

Nutahara K, Higashihara E, Horie S, et al: Calcium channel blocker versus angiotensin II receptor blocker in autosomal dominant polycystic kidney disease. Nephron Clin Pract 99:c18-c23, 2005.

Pirson Y, Chauveau D, Torres V: Management of cerebral aneurysms in autosomal dominant polycystic kidney disease. J Am Soc Nephrol 13:269-276, 2002.

Ravine D, Gibson RN, Walker RG, et al: Evaluation of ultrasonographic diagnostic criteria for autosomal dominant polycystic kidney disease 1. Lancet 343:824-827, 1994.

Rossetti S, Turca R, Coto E, et al: A complete mutation screen of PKDH1 in autosomal recessive polycystic kidney disease (ARPKD) pedigrees. Kidney Int 64:391-403, 2003.

Ruggenenti P, Remuzzi A, Ondei P, et al: Safety and efficacy of long-acting somatostatin treatment in autosomal dominant polycystic kidney disease. Kidney Int 68:206-216, 2005.

Schwarz A, Vatandaslar S, Merkel S, Haller H: Renal cell carcinoma in transplant recipients with acquired cystic kidney disease. Clin J Am Soc Nephrol 2:750-756, 2007.

Serra AL, Kistler AD, Poster D, et al: Clinical proof-of-concept trial to assess the therapeutic effect of sirolimus in patients with autosomal dominant polycystic kidney disease: SUISSE ADPKD study. BMC Nephrol 8:13-18, 2007.

Shillingford JM, Murcia NS, Larson CH, et al: The mTOR pathway is regulated by polycystin-1, and its inhibition reverses renal cystogenesis in polycystic kidney disease. Proc Natl Acad Sci U S A 103:5466-5471, 2006.

Tantravahi J, Steinman TI: Acquired cystic kidney disease. Semin Dial 13:330-334, 2000.

Tao Y, Kim J, Schrier RW, Edelstein CL: Rapamycin markedly slows disease progression in a rat model of polycystic kidney disease. J Am Soc Nephrol 16:46-51, 2005.

Torres VE, Harris PC, Pirson Y: Autosomal dominant polycystic kidney disease. Lancet 369:1287-1301, 2007.

Wiesener MS, Eckardt KU: Erythropoietin, tumors and the von Hippel-Lindau gene: Towards identification of mechanisms and dysfunction of oxygen sensing. Nephrol Dial Transplant 17:356-359, 2002.

Wilson PD: Polycystic kidney disease. N Engl J Med 350:151-162, 2004.

Zhang MJ, Mai W, Li C, et al: PKHD1 protein encoded by the gene for autosomal recessive polycystic kidney disease associates with basal bodies and primary cilia in renal epithelial cells. Proc Natl Acad Sci U S A 101:2311-2316, 2004.

Nephronophthisis and Medullary Cystic Kidney Disease

John F. O'Toole and Friedhelm Hildebrandt

Nephronophthisis and medullary cystic kidney disease (MCKD) represent a set of rare genetic kidney diseases with a similar renal histopathology, which includes interstitial fibrosis with tubular atrophy, tubular basement membrane disruption, and cyst formation. Nephronophthisis and MCKD can be distinguished clinically by their inheritance pattern and usually by age of onset. Nephronophthisis has an autosomal recessive inheritance pattern and results in end-stage renal disease (ESRD) within the first three decades of life. MCKD has an autosomal dominant inheritance pattern and usually results in ESRD between the fourth to seventh decades of life (**Table 43-1**).

EPIDEMIOLOGY

Nephronophthisis has long been recognized as a rare cause of ESRD worldwide and is one of the most common genetic causes of ESRD in the pediatric population. Historically, the incidence of nephronophthisis alone has been quoted as between 1 in 50,000 to 1 in 1 million live births. The 2007 Annual Data Report of the United States Renal Data System indicated

that the incidence and prevalence of ESRD related to NPHP or MCKD were both about 0.1% in the United States.

The incidence and prevalence of these diseases may be an underestimate, because patients often come to clinical attention only after reaching ESRD, and a definitive diagnosis may not be established. In addition, urinalysis for patients with these disorders is typically bland, without significant proteinuria or hematuria, making aggressive diagnostic procedures such as biopsy less likely to be pursued. Although a presumptive diagnosis of nephronophthisis or MCKD can be made on the basis of clinical features and the renal histopathology seen on biopsy, the only way to definitively diagnose these disorders and ascertain the type of nephronophthisis or MCKD (see **Table 43-1**) is through genetic testing, which until recently has been unavailable.

PATHOLOGY

The similar appearance of the renal histology in cases of nephronophthisis and MCKD led to the historical association of these two disorders. The classic triad of renal

TABLE 43-1 Genetic Causes and Extrarenal Manifestations of Nephronophthisis and Medullary Cystic Kidney Disease

DISEASE	GENE	PROTEIN	INHERITANCE PATTERN	CHROMOSOMAL LOCATION	EXTRARENAL MANIFESTATIONS
NPHP1	NPHP1	Nephrocystin 1	AR	2q13	Retinitis pigmentosa Oculomotor apraxia
NPHP2	INVS	Inversin	AR	9q31	Retinitis pigmentosa Situs inversus
NPHP3	NPHP3	Nephrocystin 3	AR	3q22.1	Retinitis pigmentosa Liver fibrosis
NPHP4	NPHP4	Nephrocystin 4	AR	1p36.22	Retinitis pigmentosa Oculomotor apraxia
NPHP5	NPHP5/IQCB1	Nephrocystin 5	AR	3q13.33	Retinitis pigmentosa
NPHP6	NPHP6/CEP290	Nephrocystin 6	AR	12q21.32	Retinitis pigmentosa Vermis cerebellar aplasia Meckel-Gruber syndrome
NPNP7	NPHP7/GLIS2	GLIS2	AR	16p13.3	None
NPHP8	NPHP8/RPGRIP1L	RPGRIP1L	AR	16q12.2	Vermis cerebellar aplasia Meckel-Gruber syndrome
MCKD1	Unknown	Unknown	AD	1q21	Hyperuricemia, gout
MCKD2	UMOD	Uromodulin	AD	16p13.11	Hyperuricemia, gout

AD, autosomal dominant; AR, autosomal recessive; NPHP, nephronophthisis; MCKD, medullary cystic kidney disease.

pathology, which is shared by all of the genetic types of nephronophthisis except nephronophthisis type 2 (NPHP2), includes interstitial fibrosis with tubular atrophy, tubular basement membrane (TBM) disruption, and corticomedullary cysts. Periglomerular fibrosis and sclerosis also have been identified. Cysts range in size from 1 to 15 mm and usually arise from the distal convoluted tubule or medullary collecting duct. The kidney size is normal or reduced in these types of nephronophthisis, and the cysts may not be apparent by imaging early in the course of the disease. In contrast to autosomal dominant polycystic kidney disease (ADPKD), cysts have not been observed in other organs.

NPHP2, or infantile nephronophthisis, is caused by mutations in the inversin gene *(INVS),* and its renal pathology and clinical course are distinct from those of other types of nephronophthisis. NPHP2 results in ESRD in the first decade of life, often within the first 2 years, and it is characterized by the cystic enlargement of the kidneys bilaterally. Renal pathology is characterized by more remarkable cyst formation, which appears more prominent in the cortex but can also be present in the medulla. Cysts seem to arise from the proximal and distal tubules, and cystic enlargement of the glomerulus has been observed. Tubulointerstitial nephritis is another prominent finding in NPHP2, which it shares with the other forms of nephronophthisis. TBM disruption is a less consistent finding in the setting of NPHP2.

The gross appearance of the kidney in MCKD is normal to slightly reduced in size, as in nephronophthisis. Histologically, the renal pathology of MCKD is virtually indistinguishable from that of nephronophthisis, which has led to the historical nomenclature of these diseases as the *nephronophthisis–medullary cystic kidney disease complex.*

PATHOGENESIS

Eight genes that cause nephronophthisis have been identified (see **Table 43-1**). All of them have a broad tissue expression pattern. The presence of two recessive mutations in any one of these genes results in the corresponding nephronophthisis type, which is completely penetrant, consistent with an autosomal recessive inheritance pattern. The most common form of nephronophthisis is type 1 (NPHP1), which accounts for roughly 25% of all cases. Approximately 85% of mutations in *NPHP1* consist of large deletions, which typically include the whole gene. The remaining genetic causes of nephronophthisis each account for between 1% and 4% of diagnosed cases of nephronophthisis.

The use of positional cloning has resulted in identification of eight genetic causes of nephronophthisis. The study of their gene products, the nephrocystins, has provided important insights into the pathogenetic mechanism underlying nephronophthisis. Many of the nephrocystin proteins have been found to participate in multiple protein–protein interactions. Several of the nephrocystin proteins are present in a precipitable complex with other nephrocystin proteins. The many interactions among the nephrocystin proteins suggest that they may be a part of a common functional network.

Another striking finding has been the common subcellular localization of the nephrocystin proteins to the primary cilia–basal body–centrosome complex. The primary cilia are nonmotile, microtubule-based cilia that arise from the basal body in most polarized cell types. Localization to the primary cilia–basal body–centrosome complex is a feature the nephrocystins have in common with other renal cystoproteins, including the products of genes mutated in Bardet-Biedl syndrome and in autosomal dominant and autosomal recessive polycystic kidney disease. The common localization of many renal cystoproteins to the primary cilia–basal body–centrosome complex has led to the development of several hypotheses regarding the role of this complex in the pathogenesis of cystic kidney disease.

The primary cilia extend from the apical surface of the renal tubular epithelial cells into the tubular lumen. Flexion of the primary cilia results in Ca^{2+} entry into the cell mediated by polycystin 1 and polycystin 2, the products of the genes mutated in ADPKD. Increased intracellular Ca^{2+} functions as a second messenger, transmitting information about urine flow in the tubular lumen back to the cell body, where it may have a role in cell cycle regulation. Another study has linked increased urine flow detected by the primary cilia to increased expression of inversin, the gene product of *INVS* (formerly designated *NPHP2*). Inversin participates in intracellular signaling pathways, which may be important for appropriate cell division. These signaling pathways may be disrupted, as in the case of *INVS* mutations in NPHP2, resulting in cyst formation and ESRD.

Localization of the nephrocystin proteins to the primary cilia–basal body–centrosome complex has implicated them in the pathogenesis of cystic kidney disease. However, interstitial fibrosis and tubular atrophy are more prominent than cyst formation in the histopathology of nephronophthisis. The examination of an NPHP7 mouse model showed that, when the transcription factor GLIS2 (formerly designated NPHP7) is knocked out, there are increased rates of apoptosis in renal tubular epithelial cells, and genes promoting fibrosis and epithelial-to-mesenchymal transition are upregulated. Dysregulation of the renal cystoproteins and the primary cilia may perturb the cell cycle regulation in renal tubular epithelial cells, leading to hyperproliferation in ADPKD or senescence in nephronophthisis.

The precise pathogenetic mechanisms by which mutations in the nephrocystin proteins result in kidney disease are not known. However, as noted earlier, recent research has implicated the nephrocystins in the regulation of signaling pathways important for the regulation of cell division and transcriptional pathways important for the regulation of mediators of kidney fibrosis. The nephrocystin proteins appear to be important for the control of fibrosis in the kidney and the maintenance of the tubulointerstitial space. They probably function in several different pathways, which, when dysregulated, result in a common renal histopathology of renal fibrosis and tubular atrophy.

Two genetic loci have been identified for MCKD: *MCKD1* on 1q21 and *MCKD2* on 16p12. The causative gene for

MCKD type 1 (MCKD1) has not been identified. Mutations in uromodulin, the Tamm-Horsfall protein, have been shown to cause MCKD type 2 (MCKD2), familial juvenile hyperuricemic nephropathy (FJHN), and glomerulocystic kidney disease (GCKD). Uromodulin is expressed in the thick ascending limb of the nephron; it is the matrix protein for casts and is the most abundant protein found in the urine. The excretion of uromodulin is reduced in these patients as a result of abnormal intracellular trafficking. Pathologic intracellular accumulation of uromodulin occurs in the tubular epithelial cells of the thick ascending limb.

CLINICAL FEATURES AND DIAGNOSIS

The age at onset of renal impairment and the pattern of inheritance in familial cases are different in nephronophthisis and MCKD (see **Table 43-1**). Renal impairment in nephronophthisis occurs early, resulting in a slow decline in renal function toward ESRD within the first 3 decades of life. The earliest clinical manifestation of nephronophthisis is a urinary concentrating defect that results in the clinical symptoms of polyuria, secondary enuresis, and consistently drinking throughout the night. These findings may precede the onset of reduced kidney function. A family history of affected siblings with an autosomal recessive inheritance pattern strongly suggests the diagnosis, but, given the rarity of the disease, sporadic cases are more common.

Historically, the age at onset has been considered an important clinical distinction among the various types of nephronophthisis, leading to categorization of the disease as infantile (NPHP2), juvenile (NPHP1 and NPHP4), or adolescent (NPHP3). However, with the exception of NPHP2, which leads to ESRD in the first decade of life, it is not clear that there is truly a predictable difference in the age of onset for nephronophthisis.

The extrarenal manifestations of nephronophthisis (see **Table 43-1**) include retinitis pigmentosa, which has been present in all cases of NPHP5 and NPHP6 thus far identified but can be present in any NPHP type. Many cases of NPHP6 and NPHP8 are identified as a component of Joubert's syndrome. Cogan-type congenital oculomotor apraxia is associated with mutations in *NPHP1* and *NPHP4* genes. Situs inversus can occur with NPHP2 disease. Liver fibrosis can occur with NPHP3. Several additional clinical syndromes have been described that can include a renal phenotype similar to nephronophthisis, including the Jeune, COACH, Arima, Sensenbrenner, and Bardet-Biedl syndromes.

Physical findings of nephronophthisis include growth retardation related to reduced kidney function and high blood pressure, although the latter is less prevalent than expected from the degree of kidney functional impairment.

The laboratory evaluation of nephronophthisis patients includes a urinalysis of the first morning void, which usually is normal except for a low specific gravity reflecting a urinary concentrating defect. The absence of proteinuria or of hematuria may differentiate nephronophthisis from other heritable kidney diseases, such as focal segmental glomerulosclerosis and Alport's syndrome, respectively. Anemia is commonly observed at the time of presentation, and it is often related to the severely reduced kidney function at that time. However, in diagnosed patients with relatively preserved kidney function, the anemia may be related to the significant interstitial infiltration often seen on biopsy, with nephronophthisis resulting in reduced erythropoietin secretion. Other laboratory abnormalities are commensurate with the degree of renal insufficiency.

The most relevant diagnostic test is ultrasound examination of the kidneys, which demonstrates normal to slightly reduced kidney size, increased echotexture, and loss of the corticomedullary border. Cysts, when present, may be observed at the corticomedullary junction, but cysts visible on imaging are not required for the diagnosis of nephronophthisis. The imaging findings for patients with NPHP2 are substantially different from those for patients with other types of nephronophthisis: kidney size is often increased, and cysts are a prominent finding.

In summary, the diagnosis of nephronophthisis should be entertained when an individual presents in the first 3 decades of life with reduced kidney function, a bland urine sediment result, and normal to small kidneys on ultrasound with increased echotexture and loss of the corticomedullary junction. Cysts may be observed on ultrasound examination of the kidneys, but that finding is not required for the diagnosis. The most common extrarenal manifestation associated with nephronophthisis is retinitis pigmentosa, which often leads to blindness in the first decade of life and occurs in about 10% of patients. The occurrence of similarly affected siblings in the family strongly suggests the diagnosis of nephronophthisis. The parents of affected individuals are not affected, because nephronophthisis is inherited as an autosomal recessive disease. The recessive inheritance pattern differentiates nephronophthisis from MCKD, which is transmitted as an autosomal dominant disease (i.e., one parent of the affected individual should also be affected).

MCKD usually manifests in the fourth to seventh decades of life. Two exceptions to this pattern are FJHN and GCKD, which are allelic (i.e., caused by mutations in the same gene) to MCKD2 but manifest within the first 3 decades of life. MCKD, FJHN, and GCKD are inherited in an autosomal dominant pattern. The only extrarenal manifestation associated with these diseases, aside from those attributable to declining kidney function, is hyperuricemia with gouty arthritis.

No other distinctive findings on physical examination are associated with MCKD. Laboratory evaluation findings are notable for a urinary concentrating defect, with a reduced fractional excretion of uric acid, but the urinalysis is otherwise unremarkable. Ultrasound examination demonstrates normal to slightly reduced kidney size, increased echogenicity, loss of corticomedullary differentiation, and medullary cysts, but these abnormalities may be too subtle for detection with ultrasound or computed tomographic studies. Ultrasound examination of GCKD patients may reveal normal to small kidney size and cortical cysts.

Although biopsy findings in conjunction with the appropriate clinical and historical presentation can suggest a diagnosis of nephronophthisis or MCKD, the only definitive diagnostic modality is genetic testing. Most genetic testing is done on a research basis, but recently commercial testing has also become available. A list of research and clinical laboratories offering genetic testing is available online at http://www.genetests.org (accessed July 25, 2008).

TREATMENT

No systematic trials have been undertaken to examine treatment regimens for nephronophthisis or MCKD in humans. Some studies have been done on the effect of treatment in a mouse model of nephronophthisis. The *Pcy* mouse is a model of NPHP3. A missense mutation has been identified in the murine homologue of *NPHP3* that, when present homozygously, results in renal cystic disease and ESRD at about 40 weeks of age. In various studies, these mice have been treated with soy proteins, glucocorticoids, probucol, and an antagonist of the vasopressin 2 (V_2) receptor. All of these treatments produced a reduction in cyst formation and slower progression of renal failure in the mouse model. The antagonist of the V_2 receptor was tested in the same trial on a rat model of autosomal recessive polycystic kidney disease and demonstrated efficacy there also. The mechanism by which antagonism of the V_2 receptor inhibits cystic changes in the renal parenchyma remains incompletely understood, but decreased levels of cyclic adenosine monophosphate (cAMP) were observed in the renal tubules of both animal models, suggesting that cAMP is functioning as a second messenger in the abnormal proliferation of renal epithelial cells in cystic kidney diseases.

It is not known whether blockade of the rennin-angiotensin-aldosterone axis slows the progression of nephronophthisis, as has been observed in several other kidney diseases. Knockout mice in which the angiotensin-converting enzyme gene *(Ace)* has been deleted develop a kidney phenotype resembling that of nephronophthisis.

Until human trials become available for the treatments that appear promising in rodent models of cystic kidney diseases, no disease-specific therapies can be recommended. Conservative therapies known to slow the progression of kidney disease and those appropriate to treat the attendant manifestations of reduced kidney function (including anemia, acidosis, and hyperparathyroidism) remain the standard of care. Patients with nephronophthisis and MCKD have successfully undergone kidney transplantation without evidence of recurrent disease.

BIBLIOGRAPHY

Arts HH, Doherty D, van Beersum SEC, et al: Mutations in the gene encoding the basal body protein RPGRIP1L, a nephrocystin-4 interactor, cause Joubert syndrome. Nat Genet 39:882-888, 2007.

Attanasio M, Uhlenhaut NH, Sousa VH, et al: Loss of GLIS2 causes nephronophthisis in humans and mice by increased apoptosis and fibrosis. Nat Genet 39:1018-1024, 2007.

Bernascone I, Vavassori S, Di Pentima A, et al: Defective intracellular trafficking of uromodulin mutant isoforms. Traffic 7:1567-1579, 2006.

Dahan K, Devuyst O, Smaers M, et al: A cluster of mutations in UMOD gene causes familial hyperuricemic nephropathy with abnormal expression of uromodulin. J Am Soc Nephrol 14:2883-2893, 2003.

Delous M, Baala L, Salomon R, et al: The ciliary gene *RPGRIP1L* is mutated in cerebello-oculo-renal syndrome (Joubert syndrome type B) and Meckel syndrome. Nat Genet 39:875-881, 2007.

Gattone VH, Wang X, Harris PC, Torres VE: Inhibition of renal cystic disease development and progression by a vasopressin V_2 receptor antagonist. Nat Med 9:1323-1326, 2003.

Hart TC, Gorry MC, Hart PS, et al: Mutations of the *UMOD* gene are responsible for medullary cystic disease 2 and familial hyperuricemic nephropathy. J Med Genet 39:882-892, 2002.

Hildebrandt F: Nephronophthisis-medullary cystic kidney disease. In Avner ED, Harmon WE, Niaudet P (eds): Pediatric Nephrology, 5th ed. Philadelphia, Lippincott, Williams & Wilkins, 2004, pp 665-673.

Hildebrandt F, Otto E: Cilia and centrosomes: A unifying pathogenetic concept for cystic kidney disease? Nat Rev Genet 6:928-940, 2005.

Hildebrandt F, Zhou W: Nephronophthisis associated ciliopathies. J Am Soc Nephrol 18:1855-1871, 2007.

Nauli SM, Alenghat FJ, Luo Y, et al: Polycystins 1 and 2 mediate mechanosensation in the primary cilium of kidney cells. Nat Genet 33:129-137, 2003.

Otto EA, Loeys B, Khanna H, et al: A novel ciliary IQ domain protein, NPHP5, is mutated in Senior-Loken syndrome (nephronophthisis with retinitis pigmentosa) and interacts with RPGR and calmodulin. Nat Genet 37:282-288, 2005.

Rampoldi L, Caridi G, Santon D, et al: Allelism of MCKD, FJHN and GCKD caused by impairment of uromodulin export dynamics. Hum Mol Genet 12:3369-3384, 2003.

Sayer JA, Otto EA, O'Toole JF, et al: A novel centrosomal protein, nephrocystin-6, is mutated in Joubert syndrome and activates transcription factor ATF4/CREB2. Nat Genet 38:674-681, 2006.

Simons M, Gloy J, Ganner A, et al: Inversin, the gene product mutated in nephronophthisis type II, functions as a molecular switch between Wnt signaling pathways. Nat Genet 37:537-543, 2005.

CHAPTER 44

Alport's Syndrome and Related Disorders

Martin C. Gregory

Alport's syndrome is a disease of collagen that affects the kidneys always, the ears usually, and the eyes often. Cecil Alport described the association of hereditary hematuric nephritis with hearing loss in a family whose affected male members died in adolescence. Genetic advances have broadened the scope of the condition to include optical defects, platelet abnormalities, late-onset kidney failure, and normal hearing in some families. At least 85% of kindreds have X-linked disease, and most or all of those cases result from a mutation of COL4A5, the gene located at Xq22 that codes for the α5 chain of type IV collagen, α5(IV). Autosomal recessive inheritance occurs in perhaps 15% of cases, and autosomal dominant inheritance has been shown in a handful of cases.

JUVENILE AND ADULT FORMS

The distinction between juvenile and adult forms is fundamental to the understanding of Alport's syndrome. Kidney failure tends to occur at a similar age in all male members in a kindred, but this age varies widely among kindreds. Uremia in male patients occurs in childhood or adolescence in some families and in adulthood in others. Forms with early onset of kidney failure in affected males are called *juvenile*, and those with kidney failure in middle age are called *adult*-type nephritis. Extrarenal manifestations tend to be more prominent in the juvenile kindreds. Because boys in juvenile kindreds do not commonly survive to reproduce, these kindreds tend to be small and frequently arise from new mutations. Adult-type kindreds are typically much larger, and new mutations occur infrequently.

BIOCHEMISTRY

The open mesh of interlocking molecules of type IV collagen that forms the framework of the glomerular basement membrane (GBM) is composed of heterotrimers of α chains. In fetal life, these heterotrimers consist of two α1(IV) chains and one α2(IV) chain, but early in postnatal development, production switches toward α3(IV), α4(IV), and α5(IV) chains. The primary chemical defect in Alport's syndrome most commonly involves the α5(IV) chain, but faulty assembly of the α3,4,5-heterotrimer produces similar pathology in glomerular, aural, and ocular basement membranes, regardless of which α chain is defective. As an illustration of failure of normal heterotrimer formation, most patients whose genetic defect is in the gene coding for the α5(IV) chain lack demonstrable α3(IV) chains in GBMs.

CLASSIC GENETICS

In most kindreds, inheritance of Alport's syndrome is X-linked. This was suggested by classic pedigree analysis, strengthened by tight linkage to restriction-fragment-length polymorphisms (RFLPs), and proved by identification of mutations.

MOLECULAR GENETICS

Causative mutations of COL4A5, the gene coding for α5(IV), appear consistently in many kindreds. These mutations include deletions, point mutations, and splicing errors. There is poor correlation between the mutation type and the clinical phenotype, but deletions and some splicing errors cause severe kidney disease and early hearing loss. Missense mutations may cause juvenile disease with hearing loss or adult disease with or without hearing loss. Deletions involving the 5′ end of the COL4A5 gene and the 5′ end of the adjacent COL4A6 gene occur consistently in families with esophageal and genital leiomyomatosis.

Homozygotes or mixed heterozygotes for mutations of the COL4A3 or COL4A4 genes (chromosome 2) develop autosomal recessive Alport's syndrome. Heterozygotes for these mutations account for many cases of benign familial hematuria (i.e., familial thin basement membrane disease [TBMD]). Patients with autosomal dominant Alport's syndrome, usually with thrombocytopenia and giant platelets, have mutations of the nonmuscle myosin heavy chain 9 gene (MYH9) on chromosome 22.

Patients with autosomal dominant hematuria and kidney failure with thrombocytopenia, giant platelets (Epstein's syndrome), and leukocyte inclusions (Fechtner's syndrome) have mutations of the MYH9 gene on chromosome 22. These patients should no longer be considered to have Alport's syndrome but should instead be classified with MYH9-related disorders.

IMMUNOCHEMISTRY

Male patients with X-linked Alport's syndrome and patients with autosomal recessive Alport's syndrome frequently lack the α3, α4, and α5 chains of type IV collagen in the GBM, and hemizygous males with X-linked Alport's syndrome often lack α5(IV) chains in the epidermal basement membrane (EBM). Monoclonal antibodies specific to the α2 and α5 chains of type IV collagen are commercially available and can be used to assist in the diagnosis of Alport's syndrome. The GBM and EBM of normal individuals, as well as those of all Alport's patients, react with the α2 antibody, but most male and female patients with autosomal recessive Alport's syndrome and most male patients hemizygous for a *COL4A5* mutation show no staining of the GBM with the α5 antibody. Males with X-linked disease commonly show no staining of EBM with antibody to α5; females heterozygous for a *COL4A5* mutation show interrupted staining of the GBM and EBM, consistent with mosaicism.

After kidney transplantation, about 10% of male patients with Alport's syndrome develop anti-GBM nephritis, presumably because they are exposed for the first time to normal collagen chains, including a normal 26-kDa monomer of the α3(IV) chain to which tolerance has never been acquired. Recurrences of anti-GBM nephritis are usual but not inevitable after repeat transplantation. The serum antibodies to GBM developing after transplantation are heterogeneous; all stain normal GBM, and some stain EBM.

PATHOLOGY

In young children, results of light microscopy of the kidneys may be normal or near-normal. Glomeruli with persisting fetal morphology may be seen. As disease progresses, interstitial and tubular foam cells, which arise for reasons that are unclear, may become quite prominent (**Fig. 44-1**), although they can also be found in many other conditions. Eventually, progressive glomerulosclerosis and interstitial scarring develop. The results of routine immunofluorescence examination for immunoglobulins and complement components are negative, but staining for the α5(IV) chain may be informative (see "Immunochemistry"). The GBM is up to two or

three times its normal thickness, split into several irregular layers, and frequently interspersed with numerous electron-dense granules about 40 nm in diameter (**Fig. 44-2**). In florid cases of juvenile types of the disease, the basement membrane lamellae may branch and rejoin in a complex basket-weave pattern. Early in the development of the lesion, thinning of the GBM may predominate or may be the only abnormality visible. The abnormalities in children or adolescents with adult-type Alport's syndrome may be unimpressive or indistinguishable from those of TBMD disease (discussed later).

CLINICAL FEATURES

Renal Features

Uninterrupted microscopic hematuria occurs from birth in affected males. Hematuria may become visible after exercise or during fever; this is more common in juvenile kindreds. Microscopic hematuria has a penetrance of approximately 90% in heterozygous females in adult-type kindreds. In juvenile kindreds, the penetrance of hematuria in females has been studied less extensively, but it appears to be common. Urinary erythrocytes are dysmorphic, and red cell casts usually can be found in affected males. The degree of proteinuria varies, but it occasionally reaches nephrotic levels.

Hemizygous males inevitably progress to end-stage renal disease (ESRD). This occurs at widely different ages in the

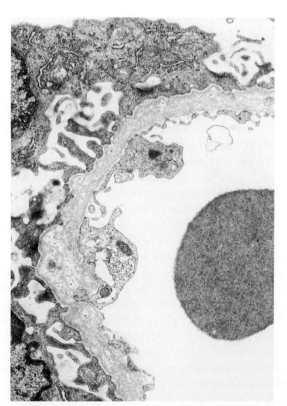

FIGURE 44-2 High-resolution electron micrograph shows a glomerular basement membrane (GBM) from a patient with Alport's syndrome that varies in thickness. It is split into several layers, which in some areas are separated by lucent areas containing small, dense granules. (Courtesy of Dr. Theodore J. Pysher.)

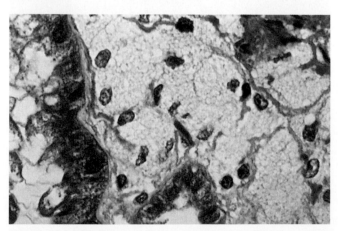

FIGURE 44-1 High-power photomicrograph shows foam-filled tubular and interstitial cells in a kidney biopsy specimen from a patient with Alport's syndrome. Relatively normal proximal tubular cytoplasm stains red in the tubules on the left and at the bottom. The remaining cells appear "foamy" because of the spaces left where lipids have been eluted during processing.

broader population, but the age is fairly constant within each family. Heterozygous females usually are much less severely affected. About one fourth of them develop ESRD, usually after the age of 50 years, but ESRD does occur in girls in their teens or even younger.

In families with autosomal inheritance, females are affected as severely and as early as males. Kidney failure often occurs before the age of 20 years in those who are homozygous for autosomal recessive Alport's syndrome.

Extrarenal Features

Hearing Loss

Bilateral, high-frequency cochlear hearing loss occurs in many kindreds, but X-linked nephritis progressing to ESRD can occur in families without overt hearing loss. Expectation of hearing loss causes many missed diagnoses of Alport's syndrome. In families with juvenile-type disease, hearing loss is almost universal in male hemizygotes and common in severely affected female heterozygotes.

Patterns of hearing loss vary. Often, the most severe loss is at 2 to 6 kHz, but it may occur at a higher frequency if there has been superimposed noise damage. The loss is also severe at 8 to 20 kHz, but these frequencies are not covered by conventional audiometry. In adult-type Alport's syndrome with hearing loss, there is typically no perceptible deficit until age 20 years, but loss progresses to 60 to 70 dB at 6 to 8 kHz after 40 years of age. Hearing loss occurs earlier in juvenile kindreds. The rate at which hearing is lost is not well established in juvenile kindreds, but many children of grade-school age and adolescents require hearing aids.

Ocular Defects

Ocular defects appear to be confined to juvenile kindreds. Myopia, arcus juvenilis, and cataracts occur but lack diagnostic specificity. Three changes that are present in a minority of kindreds but that are almost diagnostic are anterior lenticonus, posterior polymorphous corneal dystrophy, and retinal flecks. Anterior lenticonus is a forward protrusion of the anterior surface of the ocular lens. It results from a weakness of the type IV collagen forming the anterior lens capsule. The resulting irregularity of the surface of the lens causes an uncorrectable refractive error. The retina cannot be clearly seen by ophthalmoscopy, and with a strong positive lens in the ophthalmoscope, the lenticonus often can be seen through a dilated pupil as an "oil drop" or circular smudge on the center of the lens **Fig. 44-3**. Retinal flecks are small, yellow or white dots scattered around the macula or in the periphery of the retina **Fig. 44-4**. If sparse, they may be difficult to distinguish from small, hard exudates. Macular holes occur rarely but can severely affect sight. Ocular manifestations are often subtle, and consultation with an ophthalmologist familiar with Alport's syndrome is invaluable.

Leiomyomatosis

Members of several families with X-linked Alport's syndrome develop striking leiomyomas of the esophagus and female genitalia at early ages. Patients frequently have large

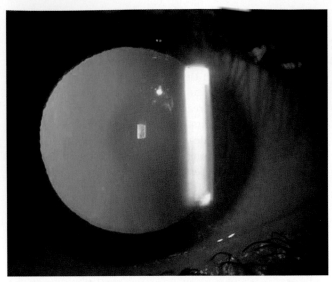

FIGURE 44-3 Retroilluminated lens photography shows the "oil-drop" appearance of anterior lenticonus, a pathognomonic feature of Alport's syndrome. The bulging area of the lens is the darker circular area just to the left of the vertical reflected light artifact from the slit-lamp examination. This is similar to the view obtained through a direct ophthalmoscope using a strong positive lens.

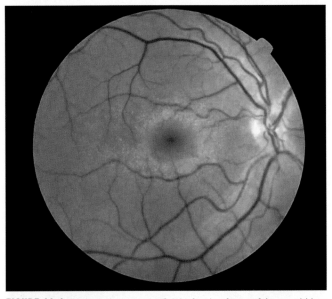

FIGURE 44-4 Retinal photograph of right fundus from a 14-year-old boy with Alport's syndrome shows perimacular dots and flecks that spare the foveola and are more discrete at the outer margin of the ring. Alport's retinopathy varies from occasional dots and flecks in the temporal macula to this appearance. (Courtesy of Dr. Judith Savige and Dr. Deb Colville.)

and multiple tumors. They may bleed or obstruct, and their resection can be difficult. All families described have had a deletion at the 5' ends of the contiguous *COL4A5* and *COL4A6* genes.

DIAGNOSIS

No single clinical feature is pathognomonic. The diagnosis is based on finding hematuria in many family members, a history of kidney failure in related males, and biopsy results showing characteristic ultrastructural changes in the proband or a relative. Immunofluorescence examination of the biopsy specimen should include staining with antibodies specific to GBM or to α5(IV); the lack of staining in most male patients with Alport's syndrome helps to differentiate Alport's syndrome from familial TBMD, in which staining is normal. In large families without a known mutation, segregation analysis can show whether a particular individual carries a defective gene. If the skin of affected family members is known to lack immunofluorescent staining with antibodies to α5(IV), an α5(IV) immunofluorescence examination of a biopsy specimen of skin from a suspected case in the family may be diagnostic.

Molecular diagnosis is almost 100% sensitive and specific but only after a mutation has been found in the family. Sequencing the *COL4A5* gene is at least 80% sensitive for mutations, but it is not widely available, and it cannot find mutations in the other causative genes. In some families with a previously defined *COL4A5* mutation, molecular diagnosis of affected males and gene-carrying females is possible. Specific genetic tests are available for mutations (i.e., C1564S, L1649R, and R1677Q) that commonly cause kidney failure in middle age. These tests are useful in the investigation of potentially affected individuals when a family member is known to carry one of these mutations. It is not clear whether these tests can be useful in the investigation of otherwise unexplained hematuria or chronic kidney disease.

The key to diagnosis is to suspect the possibility of Alport's syndrome in any patient with otherwise unexplained hematuria, glomerulopathy, or kidney failure. In many cases, the familial nature of the condition is not immediately apparent. Inquiry into the family history must be detailed and insistent. The patient is usually a boy or young man. Chances are that he knows little about his distant relatives, but his mother probably knows more about the family details. Male relatives linked to the patient through one or more female relatives may have kidney failure. Urine samples from both of the patient's parents, particularly his mother, should be checked for microscopic hematuria. Hearing loss is a helpful clue, but it is crucial to remember that hearing loss is neither a sensitive nor a specific marker of Alport's syndrome; it is neither necessary nor sufficient for the diagnosis. Many patients with hearing loss and kidney disease do not have Alport's syndrome but instead have a variety of other kidney disorders, most often glomerulonephritis, and have a more common cause for hearing loss, such as noise exposure, aminoglycoside therapy, or inherited hearing loss unrelated to Alport's syndrome.

TREATMENT

There is no specific treatment for Alport's syndrome. General measures to retard the progression of kidney failure, such as effective treatment of hypertension, appear warranted, but are unproven. As for other forms of progressive kidney disease, angiotensin-converting enzyme inhibitors and angiotensin receptor blockers may offer a specific advantage, but this has

yet to be demonstrated in patients with Alport's syndrome. Unconfirmed reports claim benefit from cyclosporine in reducing proteinuria and retarding progression of kidney disease; however, other investigators have found little benefit but evidence of cyclosporine nephrotoxicity.

Male patients should wear hearing protection in noisy surroundings. Hearing aids improve but do not completely correct the hearing loss. Tinnitus usually is resistant to all forms of therapy; hearing aids may make it less disruptive by amplifying ambient sounds. Retinal lesions do not commonly affect vision and require no therapy. The serious impairment of vision caused by lenticonus or cataract cannot be corrected with spectacles or contact lenses. Lens removal with reimplantation of an intraocular lens is standard and satisfactory treatment.

RELATED DISORDERS

Autosomal Recessive Alport's Syndrome

A few children have homozygous or mixed heterozygous mutations of the genes for the α3(IV) or α4(IV) chains of type IV collagen. Boys and girls are equally affected. They may develop severe kidney disease before the age of 10 years. The heterozygous parents commonly have TBMD (discussed later), but not all have persistent hematuria.

Autosomal Dominant Alport's Syndrome

Rare families have autosomal dominant Alport's syndrome as a consequence of heterozygous mutations of the genes for the α3(IV) or α4(IV) chains of type IV collagen.

Alport's Syndrome with Thrombocytopathy: Epstein's Syndrome and Fechtner's Syndrome

The Epstein and Fechtner syndromes are uncommon, autosomal dominant syndromes of hematuria and progressive kidney failure associated with moderate thrombocytopenia, severe hearing loss, and kidney failure in males and females. The platelets (about 7 μm in diameter) are much larger than normal (1 to 1.5 μm), and there is a mild or moderate bleeding tendency. In families with Fechtner's syndrome, an additional feature is inclusion bodies (i.e., Fechtner's bodies) in leukocytes. These syndromes are caused by a mutation in the nonmuscle myosin heavy chain 9 gene *(MYH9)* on chromosome 22q12.3-13.1.

Familial Thin Basement Membrane Disease

TBMD or benign familial hematuria is an autosomal dominant basement membrane glomerulopathy. Many cases result from heterozygous mutations of the *COL4A3* or *COL4A4* gene at chromosome 2q35-2q37; those who carry homozygous or compound heterozygous mutations in these same genes develop autosomal recessive Alport's syndrome. Ultrastructurally, the GBM is uniformly thinned to about one half of its normal thickness. There is no disruption or lamellation of the GBM, nor are any other abnormalities of the glomeruli, tubules, vessels, or interstitium visible by light, immunofluorescence, or electron microscopy. Kidney failure does not occur. Longevity is unaffected by this condition, and survivors into the ninth decade are recorded. Minor degrees of lamellation of the GBM and hearing loss have been described in some families, but these families might have had unrecognized Alport's syndrome.

After the precise diagnosis is established, the patient and family can be spared further invasive tests, and an appropriate prognosis can be given to them and to health insurers. However, the distinction between Alport's syndrome and benign familial hematuria is not always easy to make. Being certain of the pattern of inheritance requires a large pedigree with accurate diagnoses for all family members. A single mistaken diagnosis from incidental kidney disease, inaccurate urinalysis, or incomplete penetrance may vitiate conclusions about the pattern of inheritance in the entire pedigree. Even biopsy evidence is fallible. Early cases of Alport's syndrome may show ultrastructural changes indistinguishable from those of benign familial hematuria. This is particularly likely if a child from an adult-type Alport's kindred is diagnosed based on a biopsy result. Stability of serum creatinine for several years in a child does not exclude adult-type Alport's syndrome. Testing for mutations for the common adult types of X-linked Alport's syndrome (discussed earlier) may avoid some diagnostic errors. The situation is further complicated because some cases of autosomal recessive Alport's syndrome appear in families with TBMD. In these families, autosomal dominant TBMD and autosomal recessive Alport's syndrome are caused by the same mutations (see "Autosomal Recessive Alport's Syndrome").

APPROACH TO THE PATIENT WITH HEREDITARY NEPHRITIS

Although Alport's syndrome is less common than polycystic kidney disease, it is probably more common than is generally appreciated. Important differential diagnoses of hematuria in young persons are IgA nephropathy or other glomerulonephritis, renal calculi, and medullary sponge kidney. The differential diagnosis of familial kidney disease with hematuria includes TBMD, familial IgA nephropathy, and polycystic disease. Familial kidney diseases without hematuria that may be confused with Alport's syndrome include polycystic kidney disease, medullary cystic disease, and rare forms of inherited glomerular and tubulointerstitial kidney disease.

If a patient with unexplained hematuria or kidney failure has a family history of hematuria or kidney failure, the family history should be extended, concentrating particularly on the mother's male relatives. Finding hearing loss strengthens and finding a specific ocular lesion greatly strengthens suspicion for Alport's syndrome. Kidney biopsy usually is indicated for one family member, but after the diagnosis of a basement membrane nephropathy is established in a family, it is difficult to justify further biopsies in other members unless there are features that suggest another diagnosis. The extent of investigation is guided by clinical judgment and relates inversely to the strength of the family history. For example, a young man on the line of descent of a known Alport's family whose urine contains dysmorphic erythrocytes needs minimal investigation. He may need no further workup other than an assessment of the glomerular filtration rate and urine protein measurement, unless there are additional clinical features suggesting a systemic disease. A patient with hematuria and an uncertain family history may merit the standard nephrologic workup for hematuria. If available and if suspicion of Alport's syndrome is moderate or strong, a skin biopsy with staining for the $\alpha 5(IV)$ chain may be considered.

Genetic testing is of limited applicability in sporadic cases and small kindreds because most families have unique mutations. For three large kindreds in the United States, specific mutation tests are available (i.e., C1564S, L1649R, and R1677Q). In these families, direct mutation analysis can quickly establish whether an individual is a gene carrier and spare the need for a kidney biopsy.

Patients with any hereditary nephropathy should be informed about the nature of the disease and perhaps given a copy of the genetic analysis or kidney biopsy report to avoid unnecessary further investigation. Similar recommendations apply to family members who are potential gene carriers. Those with Alport's syndrome should be followed regularly for elevation of blood pressure and serum creatinine levels. The frequency of follow-up depends on the anticipated age of onset of kidney functional deterioration in the family, and periods between examinations become shorter as this age is approached. Those with familial TBMD should be checked about every 2 years, because some may ultimately turn out to have Alport's syndrome.

BIBLIOGRAPHY

Barker DF, Hostikka SL, Zhou J, et al: Identification of mutations in the *COL4A5* collagen gene in Alport's syndrome. Science 248:1224-1227, 1990.

Gleeson MJ: Alport's syndrome: Audiological manifestations and implications. J Laryngol Otol 98:449-465, 1984.

Govan JA: Ocular manifestations of Alport's syndrome: A hereditary disorder of basement membranes? Br J Ophthalmol 67:493-503, 1983.

Gregory MC: Alport's syndrome and thin basement membrane nephropathy: Unraveling the tangled strands of type IV collagen. Kidney Int 65:1109-1110, 2004.

Gregory MC, Shamshirsam A, Kamgar M, Bekhernia MR: Alport's syndrome, Fabry's disease, and nail-patella syndrome. In Schrier RW (ed): Diseases of the Kidney, 8th ed. Boston, Little Brown, 2007, pp 540-569.

Heath KE, Campos-Barros A, Toren A, et al: Nonmuscle myosin heavy chain IIA mutations define a spectrum of autosomal dominant macrothrombocytopenias: May-Hegglin anomaly and Fechtner, Sebastian, Epstein, and Alport-like syndromes. Am J Hum Genet 69:1033-1045, 2001.

Jais JP, Knebelmann B, Giatras I, et al: X-Linked Alport syndrome: Natural history in 195 families and genotype-phenotype correlations in males. J Am Soc Nephrol 11:649-657, 2000.

Jais JP, Knebelmann B, Giatras I, et al: X-Linked Alport syndrome: Natural history and genotype-phenotype correlations in girls and women belonging to 195 families. A "European Community Alport Syndrome Concerted Action" study. J Am Soc Nephrol 14:2603-2610, 2003.

Kashtan CE, Kleppel, MM, Gubler M-C: Immunohistologic findings in Alport's syndrome. In Tryggvason K (ed): Molecular Pathology and Genetics of Alport's syndrome. Basel, Karger, 1996, pp 142-153.

Lemmink HH, Nielsson WN, Mochizuki T, et al: Benign familial hematuria due to mutation of the type 4 collagen gene. J Clin Invest 98:1114-1118, 1996.

Tiebosch TA, Frederik PM, van Breda Vriesman PJ, et al: Thin basement membrane nephropathy in adults with persistent hematuria. N Engl J Med 320:14-18, 1989.

Tubulointerstitial Nephropathies and Disorders of the Urinary Tract

CHAPTER 45

Acute and Chronic Tubulointerstitial Disease

Catherine M. Meyers

Primary interstitial nephropathies make up a diverse group of diseases that elicit interstitial inflammation associated with renal tubular cell damage. Traditionally, interstitial nephritis has been classified morphologically and clinically into acute and chronic forms. Acute interstitial nephritis (AIN) generally induces rapid deterioration in kidney function and elicits marked interstitial inflammatory responses characterized by interstitial edema with varying degrees of tubular cell damage, as well as mononuclear cell infiltrates consisting primarily of lymphocytes (**Fig. 45-1**). This process typically spares both glomerular and vascular structures. Eosinophils, macrophages, plasma cells, and neutrophils may also be apparent within these infiltrates. In some cases of AIN, interstitial granuloma formation is also observed. Most commonly, this form of granulomatous interstitial nephritis is associated with either drug- or infection-induced renal inflammation. AIN is not an uncommon cause of kidney dysfunction and should always be considered in the differential diagnosis of acute kidney injury (AKI). Moreover, estimates from large hospital series suggest that AIN accounts for at least 10% to 15% of reported cases of AKI.

By contrast, chronic interstitial nephritis (CIN) follows a more indolent course and is characterized by tubulointerstitial fibrosis and atrophy associated with interstitial mononuclear cell infiltration. Over time, glomerular and vascular structures are involved, with progressive fibrosis and sclerosis

within the kidney. The United States Renal Data System (USRDS) 2007 Annual Report indicates that approximately 4000 (0.8%) incident and 6000 (1.2%) prevalent cases of end-stage renal disease (ESRD) in the United States in 2005 were induced by primary CIN. The mean age of incident cases was 65 years, whereas that for prevalent cases was 56 years. Patients who develop ESRD as a result of CIN are predominantly Caucasian (80%).

ACUTE TUBULOINTERSTITIAL NEPHRITIS
Histopathology

Despite the varied inciting factors of acute tubulointerstitial nephritis in humans (**Table 45-1**), the striking similarity of induced interstitial infiltrates, which consist primarily of T-cell lymphocytes, suggests that immune-mediated mechanisms are important either in initiating the interstitial damage or in amplifying primary interstitial injury from nonimmune causes. Studies in experimental models of interstitial disease suggest that both humoral and cell-mediated immune mechanisms are relevant effector pathways for inducing interstitial injury. Cell-mediated events probably

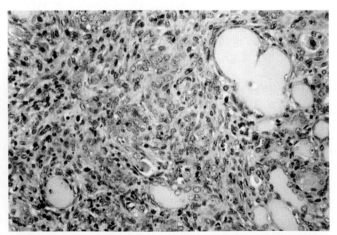

FIGURE 45-1 Acute interstitial nephritis. Light microscopy demonstrates the loss of normal tubulointerstitial architecture with a dense mononuclear cell infiltrate and some evidence of tubular dilation and atrophy. Note that the renal tubules are displaced by infiltrating mononuclear cells, edema, and mild interstitial fibrosis (original magnification × 100).

TABLE 45-1 Acute Interstitial Nephritis

Drugs

Antibiotics (most commonly penicillin analogues, cephalosporins, sulfonamides, and rifampin)

Nonsteroidal anti-inflammatory drugs

Proton pump inhibitors (most commonly omeprazole)

Diuretics (most commonly thiazides and furosemide)

Infections

Direct infection of renal parenchyma

Associated with a systemic infection

Immunologic disorders

Systemic lupus erythematosus

Sjögren's syndrome

Sarcoidosis

Tubulointerstitial nephritis and uveitis (TINU) syndrome

Mixed essential cryoglobulinemia

Acute allograft rejection

Idiopathic

play a prominent role in most forms of human disease, in view of the preponderance of T-cell lymphocytes (CD4$^+$ and CD8$^+$) present within interstitial infiltrates, generally in the absence of antibody deposition. Circulating or deposited antibodies against tubular basement membrane (TBM) have also been reported in some settings (e.g., rifampin-induced lesions, systemic immune disorders). Significant in vitro T-cell proliferation responses to suspected drug pathogens have been noted in peripheral blood samples isolated from patients with drug-induced AIN, further suggesting a drug specificity of cell-mediated responses in this disorder.

Immunohistochemical studies conducted on biopsy specimens obtained in drug-induced AIN also indicate the importance of cell–cell interactions in intrarenal inflammation, because there is a significant increase in interstitial expression of cellular adhesion molecules. In AIN, increased expression of leukocyte function-associated antigen 1 and very late antigen 4 cell surface receptors, as well as their respective ligands, intercellular adhesion molecule 1 and vascular cell adhesion molecule 1, is generally observed in areas of mononuclear cell infiltration. Published studies have extended these observations by examining the role of chemokines, a family of proinflammatory chemotactic mediators, in a number of kidney disease models associated with marked tubulointerstitial infiltration. The chemoattractants for inflammatory cells known as RANTES (*regulated on activation normal T-cell expressed and secreted*), osteopontin, and monocyte chemotactic peptide 1 have been best characterized, and studies demonstrate that their expression is markedly upregulated in AIN, correlating directly with the level of monocyte infiltration and interstitial damage.

Clinical Features

AIN occurs in four distinct clinical settings (see **Table 45-1**). It may occur as a consequence of drug or toxin exposure, systemic or local infection, or immunologic disease or as an idiopathic lesion without an apparent precipitating cause. Large retrospective studies of kidney biopsy findings revealed that drug-induced AIN has accounted for 70% to 90% of all cases of AIN, whereas infections induced 0% to 15% and immune disorders induced 0% to 6% of cases. It is noteworthy that between 0% and 8% of biopsy-proven AIN cases were idiopathic. AIN is observed in all age groups; however, older patients appear more predisposed to development of AKI. Systemic manifestations of a hypersensitivity reaction, such as fever, rash, and arthralgias, are nonspecific findings that may accompany AIN. In such cases, an erythematous maculopapular rash involves the trunk and proximal extremities. Hypertension and edema are not characteristic of AIN but have been reported in specific drug-induced lesions. Other nonspecific constitutional symptoms, as well as flank pain with gross hematuria, have been variably reported.

The spectrum of urinary laboratory abnormalities (**Table 45-2**) consists primarily of microscopic hematuria that at times may be macroscopic, sterile pyuria, and white blood cell casts. Red blood cell casts have also been reported, albeit rarely, in AIN. Eosinophiluria, with greater than 1% of urinary leukocytes positive by Hansel's stain, is suggestive of AIN but can be seen in other forms of renal injury and inflammation, such as rapidly progressive glomerulonephritis, urinary tract infection, and renal atheroemboli. A review of four retrospective patient series suggested that the sensitivity of eosinophiluria for AIN overall was 67%, and the specificity was 82%. Because considerable variability was apparent between series and not all diagnoses were biopsy-confirmed, the presence of eosinophiluria is best considered as being consistent with, but not diagnostic of, AIN.

Mild proteinuria, usually less than 1 g/day, is frequently observed in AIN. Nephrotic-range proteinuria with acute disease has been reported, however, with nephropathies induced by nonsteroidal anti-inflammatory drugs (NSAIDs) (see Chapter 38) or, rarely, by ampicillin, rifampin, or interferon-alfa therapy. Serologic studies in AIN, such as anti-DNA antibodies, antinuclear antibodies (ANA), and complement levels, are typically normal, except when AIN occurs in the setting of a systemic autoimmune disorder. Case reports also have described antineutrophil cytoplasmic antibody (ANCA) positivity, a serologic marker for systemic vasculitis, in some patients during the acute phase of interstitial nephritis. Elevated perinuclear ANCA (P-ANCA) titers have been observed in AIN induced by some drugs (omeprazole, ciprofloxacin, and cimetidine), and cytoplasmic ANCA (C-ANCA) in the tubulointerstitial nephritis and uveitis (TINU) syndrome, although the clinical relevance of ANCA titers in AIN is unclear.

Urinary fractional excretion of sodium is greater than 1% in many patients with AIN, but this is not a reliable diagnostic indicator. Biochemical abnormalities reflective of the tubular damage induced by the inflammatory process are also observed in these patients (see **Table 45-2**). The pattern of tubular dysfunction varies depending on the principal site of injury. Lesions affecting the proximal tubule result in renal glucosuria, aminoaciduria, phosphaturia, uricosuria, and proximal renal tubular acidosis (type II RTA). Distal tubular lesions result in an inability to acidify urine (type I RTA) and appropriately regulate potassium and sodium

TABLE 45-2 Laboratory Findings in Acute Interstitial Nephritis

PARAMETER	FINDING
Urinary sediment	Erythrocytes, leukocytes (eosinophils), leukocyte casts
Urinary protein excretion	<1 g/day; rarely, >1 g/day (NSAIDs)
Fractional excretion of sodium	Usually >1%
Proximal tubular defects	Glucosuria, bicarbonaturia, phosphaturia, aminoaciduria, proximal RTA
Distal tubular defects	Hyperkalemia, sodium wasting, distal RTA
Medullary defects	Sodium wasting, urine-concentrating defects

NSAIDs, nonsteroidal anti-inflammatory drugs; RTA, renal tubular acidosis.

balance. Medullary lesions interfere with maximal urinary concentration and promote polyuria. A considerable degree of overlap in these proximal and distal abnormalities may be apparent clinically. Kidney ultrasonography in affected patients typically reveals normal or enlarged kidneys, depending on the degree of interstitial edema. Renal gallium scanning has been advocated in some centers to distinguish AIN from other causes of AKI, primarily acute tubular necrosis, but this test lacks both sensitivity and specificity. In view of the nonspecific nature of many of these clinical features of AIN, a definitive diagnosis can be made only by kidney biopsy.

Clinical Course and Therapy

The spectrum of kidney dysfunction in AIN ranges from mild, self-limited disease to oliguric renal failure requiring dialysis therapy. Because this kidney lesion is usually reversible, even despite initial severe renal functional impairment, the overall prognosis is quite favorable. Recovery of kidney function may occur over weeks to several months. Some patients have persistent tubular defects and/or residual renal functional impairment, and progression to ESRD has been reported with all forms of AIN. The USRDS 2007 Annual Report relates that almost 1000 (0.2%) incident cases and 550 (0.1%) prevalent cases of ESRD in the United States in 2005 were caused by AIN. The mean ages for incident and prevalent ESRD cases were 67 years and 64 years, respectively. Similar to the observations for ESRD in the setting of CIN, reported cases are noted predominantly in Caucasians (80%).

Clinical studies suggest that a less favorable prognosis in AIN correlates with extensive interstitial infiltrates, interstitial fibrosis, tubular atrophy, and interstitial granuloma formation on kidney biopsy. Other variables that correlate with chronic kidney disease are advanced patient age, preexisting kidney disease, and a protracted course of oliguric AKI (>3 weeks). In general, chronic kidney disease after a bout of AIN is most commonly induced by NSAIDs or proton pump inhibitors (PPIs).

The treatment of AIN consists primarily of supportive measures, after elimination of possible inciting influences such as drugs or infections. Patients with mild renal functional impairment and evidence of recovery of kidney function a few days after discontinuation of the inciting drug do not require further therapy. The role of corticosteroids in treating more severe cases of AIN has not been clearly elucidated. Rapid improvement and complete recovery of kidney function after steroid therapy in several cases of drug-induced lesions has suggested their therapeutic usefulness in AIN. Two empirically derived steroid regimens have been implemented in drug-induced (primarily antibiotic-induced) AIN, typically after biopsy findings have confirmed the diagnosis. One protocol, for patients with severely impaired kidney function, consists of administration of parenteral methylprednisolone (0.5 to 1.0 g) for 1 to 3 days, followed by daily high-dose oral prednisone (1 mg/kg of body weight per day). The other, more commonly used regimen consists only of high-dose daily oral

prednisone therapy or alternate-day oral prednisone (2 mg/kg every other day), administered for approximately 2 to 3 weeks, with gradual tapering initiated after plasma creatinine levels return to near-baseline levels. A few published reports have suggested that steroid-unresponsive (after 2 to 3 weeks of therapy), steroid-intolerant, or steroid-dependent patients may respond to cyclophosphamide (2 mg/kg/day) or to mycophenolate mofetil (up to 1000 mg twice daily). Recognizing that interstitial fibrosis, a lesion unresponsive to current therapies, can begin occurring in AIN as soon as 10 to 14 days after disease induction, many clinicians are reluctant to expose patients to potentially more toxic drugs after steroid treatment failure.

Some clinical reports have not corroborated the steroid responsiveness of this kidney lesion, particularly for NSAID-induced cases. It should also be noted that prospective, randomized studies have not been conducted. Steroids are not used in infection-related AIN but may be helpful in the treatment of nephritogenic responses in systemic immunologic disorders. Although experimental models have suggested a disease-protective role for cyclophosphamide and cyclosporine in interstitial nephritis, similar studies have not been conducted in human subjects. Anecdotal reports have also suggested efficacy of adjunctive plasmapheresis therapy, with immunosuppressant therapy, for the rare occurrence of AIN associated with circulating or deposited antibodies against TBM.

DISTINCT CAUSES OF ACUTE INTERSTITIAL NEPHRITIS

Drugs Associated with Acute Interstitial Nephritis

The list of drugs that reportedly induce AIN is extensive (**Table 45-3**). Many of these have been reported from only a single case, however, and have developed in patients exposed to a number of different medications. Drug-induced AIN is a rare idiosyncratic reaction that occurs in a small subset of patients exposed to a particular medication. It is not dose-dependent, and it typically recurs on repeat exposure to the same or a closely related drug. As seen in **Table 45-3**, implicated drugs have diverse chemical structures, although, within a class of related drugs, structural similarity can lead to cross-reactive sensitivities. This has been observed particularly with β-lactam drugs, in that penicillin-induced nephropathies have been exacerbated with cephalosporin therapy. A few drugs, most notably penicillins (cephalosporins), NSAIDs, PPIs, sulfonamide derivatives, and rifampin, account for the majority of reported cases of AIN. NSAID-induced AIN is discussed in detail in Chapter 38. Characteristic features of AIN associated with other drugs are discussed later in this chapter.

Penicillins

β-Lactam antibiotics, predominantly penicillins, are the most common cause of drug-induced AIN. The largest number of cases has occurred with methicillin, which is no longer used in clinical practice. AIN has been reported with most of the routinely prescribed penicillin analogues (see **Table 45-3**), although at much lower incidence than with methicillin. Marked impairments in kidney function in this setting have been observed most commonly in older children and young adults. A recent case series from a single center reported four cases in 1 year of nafcillin-associated AIN in adults treated for methicillin-sensitive *Staphylococcus aureus* infections. This report is of interest, because nafcillin has not previously been considered a common inducer of this disorder. The classic hypersensitivity triad of fever, rash, and eosinophilia in the setting of AKI occurs in up to 30% of patients with β-lactam–induced AIN. Oliguric renal failure has been reported in approximately 30% of the cases. Clinical studies have suggested a beneficial role for steroids in this patient population; however, as already stated, randomized, controlled studies have not been performed. AIN has developed during treatment of a variety of infections, although an underlying infection is clearly not requisite for inducing this reaction, because several patients given prophylactic antibiotics have subsequently developed AIN.

Proton Pump Inhibitors

Since the introduction of omeprazole in 1989 for treatment of acid-related gastrointestinal disorders, PPIs have become widely prescribed in the United States. The first case report of omeprazole-induced AIN appeared in 1992, and there have been almost 90 published cases in the literature to date. Currently, five different PPIs are marketed in the United States: omeprazole, pantoprazole, esomeprazole, lansoprazole, and rabeprazole. All marketed PPIs have been associated with AIN, although most reports are related to omeprazole use, perhaps because it has been available most widely for clinical practice. Case reports suggest that AIN is induced after one to several weeks of PPI exposure, and that patients present with nonspecific constitutional symptoms in the setting of AKI. Although recovery of kidney function is common after discontinuation of the PPI, many reports indicate that recovery is incomplete, particularly in older patients (>60 years). The utility of corticosteroids in PPI-induced AIN is not established; early detection of AKI and cessation of the offending drug is critical to limiting the extent of kidney damage.

Rifampin

Numerous cases of rifampin-induced AIN have occurred during treatment of tuberculosis. Most of these cases have developed with intermittent therapy or on restarting of rifampin after a lapse in uneventful daily therapy. Patients typically complain of flulike symptoms such as fever, chills, malaise, and headache. In contrast to other drug-induced lesions, flank pain and hypertension are common in this form of AIN. Moreover, oliguric AKI occurs frequently, and dialysis is required in approximately two thirds of affected patients. In many cases, this reaction has occurred within hours after a single dose of rifampin. Some patients have developed thrombocytopenia, hemolysis, or abnormalities in liver function in addition to AIN. Histologically, evidence of acute tubular necrosis may be apparent in addition to AIN. In a few cases, an associated proliferative glomerulonephritis has also been observed. Circulating rifampin-specific antibodies, as well as immunoglobulin G (IgG) deposition along the TBM, have been reported in some affected patients. Because AIN has developed in patients receiving concurrent rifampin and prednisone therapy, there is no evidence to suggest that steroids can play a therapeutic role in this disease.

Sulfonamide Derivatives

Drug-induced AIN was first described in the setting of sulfonamide administration. Most cases of AIN induced by sulfonamide derivatives have been reported with combination sulfamethoxazole and trimethoprim therapy. Thiazides and furosemide have also been associated with a few cases of AIN, some of which have developed in patients with preexisting kidney disease. The associated hypersensitivity triad of fever, rash, and eosinophilia with kidney dysfunction is variably present in affected patients. In addition to the characteristic histologic features of AIN, some biopsy specimens have revealed a predominance of eosinophils within interstitial infiltrates, as well as interstitial granuloma formation. Isolated case reports have suggested beneficial effects of steroid therapy in treating this drug-induced AIN.

TABLE 45-3 Drug-Induced Acute Interstitial Nephritis*

Antibiotics

Penicillin analogues: *methicillin, ampicillin, penicillin, nafcillin,* carbenicillin, oxacillin, amoxicillin, mezlocillin, flucloxacillin

Cephalosporins: cephalothin, cefotetan, cephradine, cephalexin, cefoxitin, cefazolin, cefaclor, cefotaxime

Sulfonamide derivatives: *sulfamethoxazole,* cotrimoxazole

Other antibiotics: *rifampin, ciprofloxacin,* gentamicin, kanamycin, vancomycin, acyclovir, indinavir, aztreonam, erythromycin, azithromycin, ethambutol, tetracyclines, nitrofurantoin

Analgesics

Fenoprofen, ibuprofen, indomethacin, piroxicam, tolmetin, naproxen, rofecoxib, celecoxib, zomepirac, diflunisal, sulindac, *phenylbutazone,* aspirin, phenacetin, mefenamic acid, 5-amino-salicylates

Proton Pump Inhibitors

Omeprazole, pantoprazole, esomeprazole, lansoprazole, rabeprazole

Diuretics

Thiazides, furosemide, triamterene, chlorthalidone

Miscellaneous medications

Phenytoin, allopurinol, cimetidine, ranitidine, famotidine, phenobarbital, azathioprine, cyclosporine, α-methyldopa, carbamazepine, diazepam, phenylpropanolamine, captopril, clofibrate, interferon-alfa, interleukin-2, α-CD4 monoclonal antibodies, ticlopidine, quinine, propylthiouracil, streptokinase, Chinese herbs (aristolochic acid), clozapine, phentermine/phendimetrazine, pranlukast

*Drugs reported with greatest frequency are shown in *italics.*

Infections Associated with Acute Interstitial Nephritis

AIN was first described in the preantibiotic era in the setting of diphtherial and streptococcal infections. It is now apparent that AIN complicates the clinical course of a number of bacterial, viral, fungal, and parasitic infections, as listed in **Table 45-4**. This inflammatory response within the kidney may occur as a result of direct renal infection (i.e., pyelonephritis) or as a reaction to a systemic infection. Pyelonephritis, the most common cause of infection-related AIN, typically manifests with fever, costovertebral tenderness, dysuria, pyuria, bacteriuria, and leukocytosis. Kidney function is unimpaired unless there is urinary tract obstruction. Characteristic renal parenchymal lesions consist of focal areas of neutrophils throughout the interstitium. Pyelonephritis responds well to antibiotic therapy and is discussed more extensively in Chapter 48.

Transplant centers have reported interstitial nephritis associated with human polyomaviruses (BK and JC) occurring in kidney allografts, typically within 1 year after transplantation and with a 1% to 10% prevalence in published series. Human polyomaviruses, predominantly BK virus, induce interstitial nephritis in immunosuppressed patients after reactivation of latent virus in renal epithelium. Diagnosis is established by allograft biopsy. Histologic features of this lesion are interstitial inflammatory cell infiltration with extensive tubulitis, basophilic or amphophilic intranuclear inclusions, and in situ evidence of virally infected cells on kidney biopsy. Distinguishing polyomavirus–related interstitial nephritis from acute rejection is critical in this setting, because therapeutic interventions in these disorders are vastly different. Viral infection–associated graft dysfunction dictates a prudent decrease in immunosuppression, whereas acute rejection requires more intensive immunosuppression. Specific BK virus therapy is not currently available, although some centers have reported anecdotal experience with antiviral agents such as cidofovir, leflunomide, intravenous immunoglobulin, and quinolones. Further discussion of kidney allograft therapeutics is provided in Chapter 63.

TABLE 45-4   Infections Associated with Acute Interstitial Nephritis*

Bacterial infections

Streptococcus, diphtheria, brucella, legionella, pneumococcus, *tuberculosis*

Viral infections

Epstein-Barr virus, *cytomegalovirus*, *polyomavirus*, *Hantaan virus*, measles (rubeola), human immunodeficiency virus, herpes simplex virus type 1

Fungal Infections

Candidiasis, histoplasmosis

Other infections

Toxoplasmosis, leishmaniasis, schistosomiasis, *Rocky Mountain spotted fever*, ehrlichiosis, malaria, mycoplasma, *leptospirosis*, syphilis, ascaris lumbricoides

*Infections associated with direct renal infection are shown in *italics*.

In contrast to pyelonephritis, other infection-associated interstitial processes occur in the absence of urinary tract infection. Interstitial infiltrates are frequently perivascular and composed of mononuclear cells, predominantly T-cell lymphocytes. As already discussed, the pathogenesis of such immune targeting in these infections is not well understood, although cross-reactive determinants may play a role in immune recognition of interstitial structures.

Infection-associated interstitial nephritis is usually transient, and kidney function improves with appropriate treatment of the systemic illness; however, chronic kidney disease has been reported.

Immune Disorders Associated with Acute Interstitial Nephritis

Although glomerulonephritis is the most common renal manifestation of systemic immunologic disorders, predominant interstitial pathology can be seen in systemic lupus erythematosus, sarcoidosis, Sjögren's syndrome, TINU, and mixed essential cryoglobulinemia. Most affected patients present with nonoliguric renal failure and biochemical evidence of tubular dysfunction. In addition to the typical pathologic features of AIN, biopsy samples from many of these patients also reveal immune-complex and complement deposition along the TBM and, occasionally, within interstitial vessels. Concurrent glomerular pathology may also be apparent. Interstitial inflammation and granuloma formation associated with uveitis are observed in Sjögren's syndrome, sarcoidosis, and the TINU syndrome, and such patients require further evaluation to distinguish these disorders. Standard therapeutic modalities in these immunologic disorders consist of corticosteroids and/or cytotoxic agents. Such therapy is beneficial unless irreversible tubulointerstitial damage has occurred.

The TINU syndrome, which has been reported in approximately 140 patients, has occurred with a median age of 15 years at presentation, although cases have also been reported in adults and in the elderly. A 3:1 female-to-male predominance has been observed. TINU is associated with a variety of systemic complaints, such as fever, malaise, rash, arthralgias, and weight loss. Anterior uveitis can precede, accompany, or follow AIN. Although the cause of TINU syndrome is not known, an autoimmune nature is suggested by occasional positive serologic findings, such as C-ANCA, rheumatoid factor, hypocomplementemia, and ANA, in affected patients. Diminished cellular immune responses have also been observed, as well as anergy and an increased CD4/CD8 ratio, perhaps associated with concurrent viral infection. An association with specific major histocompatibility complex class II genes was described in one patient series. Kidney disease in the TINU syndrome is frequently reversible and typically responds to a brief course of corticosteroid therapy, although a few patients have developed chronic kidney disease. Relapse of ocular problems has been commonly reported.

Acute kidney allograft rejection, a distinct subset of immunologic disorders, also induces acute interstitial inflammation and is discussed further in Chapter 63.

Idiopathic Acute Interstitial Nephritis

In up to 8% of biopsy-proven cases of AIN from retrospective renal biopsy studies, no precipitating cause was detected. Systemic manifestations of a hypersensitivity reaction are typically absent in these idiopathic cases, which often manifest with nonoliguric renal failure. As with other causes of AIN, the role of corticosteroids in treating the idiopathic lesion is not yet established.

CHRONIC TUBULOINTERSTITIAL NEPHRITIS

Histopathology

The histopathology of CIN is remarkably consistent despite the varied apparent causes (**Table 45-5**). In addition to tubular cell damage and predominantly mononuclear cell inflammation, CIN is characterized by the development of tubulointerstitial fibrosis and scarring. Interstitial granulomatous disease has also been observed in certain forms of CIN (sarcoidosis). Glomerular and vascular structures may be relatively preserved early in the course of disease, but ultimately they become involved in progressive fibrosis and sclerosis. Observations from the experimental literature suggest that renal tubular epithelial-myofibroblast transition (TEMT) may play a pivotal role in initiation and progression of tubulointerstitial fibrosis. Although the processes relevant for primary CIN in humans have not been elucidated, experimental models of injury have implicated a large role for transforming growth factor-β and other fibrogenic mediators such as fibroblast growth factor 2, advanced glycation end-products, and angiotensin II, in regulating renal TEMT and thereby propagating chronic interstitial damage and fibrosis.

As in AIN, mononuclear cell infiltrates typically accompany CIN, further suggesting a pathogenic immune-mediated mechanism for disease progression. One hypothesis concerning immune recognition of the interstitium suggests that portions of infectious particles or drug molecules may cross-react with or alter endogenous renal antigens. An immune response directed against these inciting agents would theoretically target the interstitium as well. Intriguing results of a study examining a series of kidney biopsy samples obtained over 8 years at a single center suggested a prominent role of Epstein-Barr virus (EBV) in cases of CIN previously deemed idiopathic. Investigators detected EBV DNA and its receptor, CD21, primarily in proximal tubular cells of specimens from all 17 patients with primary idiopathic interstitial nephritis but not in 10 control kidney biopsy specimens. Such observations imply a more prominent role than previously appreciated for EBV infection in eliciting chronic deleterious immune responses that target the interstitium.

Clinical Features

As shown in **Table 45-5**, CIN occurs in a variety of clinical settings, most commonly after exposure to drugs or toxins or in the setting of hereditary disorders, metabolic disorders,

immune-mediated diseases, hematologic disturbances, infections, or obstruction. Because CIN tends to occur as a slowly progressive disease, most patients diagnosed

TABLE 45-5 Causes of Chronic Interstitial Nephritis

Drugs/Toxins

Analgesics

Heavy metals (lead, cadmium)

Lithium

Chinese herbs (aristolochic acid)

Calcineurin inhibitors (cyclosporine, tacrolimus)

Cisplatin

Nitrosoureas

Hereditary Disorders

Polycystic kidney disease

Medullary cystic disease–juvenile nephronophthisis

Hereditary nephritis

Metabolic Disturbances

Hypercalcemia/Nephrocalcinosis

Hypokalemia

Hyperuricemia

Hyperoxaluria

Cystinosis

Immune-Mediated Disorders

Renal allograft rejection

Systemic lupus erythematosus

Sarcoidosis

Wegener's granulomatosis

Vasculitis

Sjögren's syndrome

Hematologic Disturbances

Multiple myeloma

Light chain disease

Dysproteinemias

Lymphoproliferative disease

Sickle cell disease

Infections

Renal

Systemic

Obstruction/Mechanical Disorders

Tumors

Stones

Vesicoureteral reflux

Miscellaneous Disorders

Endemic nephropathy

Radiation nephritis

Aging

Hypertension

Renal ischemia

with CIN present with systemic complaints of the primary underlying disease, if present, or with signs of chronic kidney disease. Laboratory findings in these patients include non–nephrotic-range proteinuria, microscopic hematuria, and pyuria. As listed in **Table 45-2**, other urinary abnormalities such as glucosuria, phosphaturia, and sodium wasting are frequently reported and are reflective of tubular defects. Affected patients also may have elevated urinary excretion of low-molecular-weight proteins that are commonly associated with tubular injury and damage, such as lysozyme, β_2-microglobulin, and retinol-binding protein, as well as increased enzymuria with N-acetyl-β-D-glucosaminidase, alanine aminopeptidase, and intestinal alkaline phosphatase. Routine assessment of urinary low-molecular-weight proteins and enzymes is not typically conducted, however, because it is of little diagnostic or prognostic use. Hypertension is another common clinical feature, although in many forms of CIN it is not apparent until the patient approaches ESRD. With progressive CIN, kidney ultrasonography in patients without significant structural abnormalities (e.g., cystic kidney disease) typically reveals shrunken kidneys. Irregular renal contours and renal calcifications are seen in some forms of CIN.

Clinical Course and Therapy

In view of the slowly progressive loss of kidney function observed in most cases of CIN, general therapeutic considerations include treating an underlying systemic disorder (e.g., sarcoidosis), avoiding the drug or toxin exposure (e.g., analgesics, lead), or eliminating the condition that has induced the chronic interstitial lesion (e.g., obstruction). The interstitial fibrosis and scarring in CIN, and resultant impairment in kidney function, are not currently amenable to therapeutic intervention. Although definitive diagnosis of CIN requires kidney biopsy, it is probably of limited usefulness in patients with kidney failure. Therapy for CIN is therefore largely supportive, with renal replacement therapy initiated for patients who develop ESRD. More specific treatments for interstitial lesions associated with lead exposure or sarcoidosis are discussed in the next section.

DISTINCT CAUSES OF CHRONIC TUBULOINTERSTITIAL NEPHRITIS

Many causes of CIN listed in **Table 45-5** are more fully described in other chapters 24, 38, 42, and 63 of this *Primer*. This section focuses on a few common causes of CIN.

Lead

Chronic exposure to high levels of lead, over several years to decades, is associated with a progressive CIN. Most such chronic exposures are occupational and include the manufacturing and use of lead-containing paints, ammunitions, radiators, batteries, wires, ceramic glazes, solder, and metal cans. In addition, environmental lead exposure can occur in several settings, such as drinking water from lines containing lead pipes and solder joints, consuming crops grown in lead-contaminated soil, or ingesting lead-based paint scraps or moonshine generated in lead-lined car radiators. Recent population-based studies have also noted a trend of increased blood lead levels in the general population and a related inverse trend in creatinine clearance. It is unclear whether these population-based observations reflect an increase in chronic lead nephropathy or an increase in kidney disease that induces lead retention.

An early histologic lesion observed with chronic lead exposure is proximal tubular intranuclear inclusion bodies composed of a lead-protein complex, so the early stage of lead-induced kidney damage probably results from proximal resorption with subsequent intracellular lead accumulation. Early clinical manifestations reflect proximal tubular dysfunction with hyperuricemia, aminoaciduria, and glucosuria. Because the kidney disease is slowly progressive, affected patients typically present with signs of chronic kidney disease and with hypertension, hyperuricemia, and gout. This symptom complex might suggest a diagnosis of either chronic urate nephropathy or hypertensive nephrosclerosis. Chronic urate nephropathy with tophaceous gout is currently an uncommon condition, and some studies suggest that previously reported cases were actually associated with chronic lead exposure. By contrast, hypertensive nephrosclerosis is not typically associated with hyperuricemia and gout. Patients presenting with hypertension, hyperuricemia, and chronic kidney disease should therefore be questioned about lead exposure.

The diagnosis of chronic lead intoxication is usually established by means of a lead mobilization test, which is performed by measuring urinary lead excretion after administration of ethylenediamine tetra-acetic acid (EDTA). X-ray fluorescence may also be used to determine bone lead levels. However, the diagnosis of lead nephropathy is frequently made on the basis of a history of lead exposure in the setting of hyperuricemia, hypertension, and slowly progressive kidney disease consistent with CIN. Treatment of lead intoxication consists of chelation therapy with EDTA or oral succimer. Although chronic lead nephropathy has been considered an irreversible process, recent studies from Taiwan suggested that chelation therapy may slow progression of kidney disease in patients with excessive total body lead levels.

Chinese Herb Nephropathy

Rapidly progressive fibrosing interstitial nephritis has been described in clusters of patients in weight loss programs who ingested Chinese herbal preparations tainted with a plant nephrotoxin derived from *Aristolochia fangchi* (aristolochic acid). More than 150 cases have been reported in the literature, although some involved patients who ingested herb preparations that did not contain aristolochic acid. Other reports from Asia suggest that herbal therapy–induced kidney damage is not uncommon. Kidney disease in affected individuals is typically progressive and irreversible despite withdrawal of toxin exposure; many patients require dialysis therapy or transplantation within 1 year after presentation. The mechanism of herb-induced nephrotoxicity has not been delineated. The observation that some patients who are exposed to toxic herbs do not develop kidney disease suggests variability in patient susceptibility to kidney injury. Studies in animal models indicate that both toxin exposure and concurrent renal vasoconstriction may be required to precipitate the characteristic progressive kidney disease. A frequent association of cellular atypia and urothelial cell malignancies of the genitourinary tract has also been reported in patient series.

Endemic Nephropathy

Endemic or Balkan nephropathy is a form of CIN endemic to the areas of Bulgaria, Romania, Serbia, Croatia, Bosnia, and Herzegovina. It occurs most commonly along the confluence of the Danube River and has been reported almost exclusively among farmers. Although the cause of the disease has not been elucidated, several environmental toxins (i.e., plant nephrotoxins, mycotoxins, trace metals, and aromatic hydrocarbons) have been explored. The tendency for clustering of cases in families also suggests that genetic variables play a role in disease susceptibility. Like many forms of CIN, endemic nephropathy is a slowly progressive kidney disease, and patients present with blood and urinary evidence of tubular dysfunction. It is typically observed in the fourth decade of life or later and rarely affects patients younger than 20 years of age. Patients usually present with normal blood pressure and either normal-sized or slightly reduced kidneys on ultrasonography. A specific diagnostic test has not yet been developed, and there is no specific treatment or preventive regimen for the disorder. Like Chinese herb nephropathy,

endemic nephropathy is associated with urothelial tumors. Studies have reported a wide range of tumor incidence, ranging from 2% to 47% of patients with endemic nephropathy. A recent study of renal and urothelial cancer tissue isolated from patients with endemic nephropathy identified DNA adducts from aristolochic acid as well as *TP53* gene mutations—two features that characterize aristolochic acid–induced tumors in rodents. After it is activated, aristolochic acid reacts directly with DNA, forming covalently bound aristolactam-DNA adducts. Such compounds persist in tissues for long periods and are considered potential mutagens. These observations further implicate aristolochic acid in the pathogenesis of endemic nephropathy.

Sarcoidosis

The most common renal manifestation of sarcoidosis is mediated through disordered calcium metabolism resulting in hypercalcemia and hypercalciuria. Patients occasionally present with nephrolithiasis. Although interstitial disease, at times with formation of noncaseating granulomas, is relatively common in sarcoidosis (15% to 30% of cases), autopsy series indicate that it is unusual for the interstitial abnormalities to result in clinically significant kidney dysfunction. It is also unusual to observe interstitial disease in the absence of extrarenal involvement in sarcoidosis. Although most patients with impaired kidney function respond well to corticosteroid therapy (1 mg/kg/day), recovery of kidney function is frequently incomplete because of chronic interstitial inflammation and fibrosis. Relapse of renal functional impairment during steroid taper has been reported, but progression to ESRD is rare.

BIBLIOGRAPHY

Baker RJ, Pusey CD: The changing profile of acute tubulointerstitial nephritis. Nephrol Dial Transplant 19:8-11, 2004.

Becker JL, Miller F, Nuovo GJ, et al: Epstein-Barr virus infection of renal proximal tubule cells: Possible role in chronic interstitial nephritis. J Clin Invest 104:1673-1681, 1999.

Brause M, Magnusson K, Degenhardt S, et al: Renal involvement in sarcoidosis: A report of 6 cases. Clin Nephrol 57:142-148, 2002.

Brewster UC, Perazella MA: Acute kidney injury following proton pump inhibitor therapy. Kidney Int 71:589-593, 2007.

Clarkson MR, Giblin L, O'Connell FP, et al: Acute interstitial nephritis: Clinical features and response to corticosteroid therapy. Nephrol Dial Transplant 19:2778-2783, 2004.

Crew RJ, Markowitz G, Radhakrishnan J: Therapeutic options in BK virus-associated interstitial nephritis. Kidney Int 70:399-402, 2006.

De Vriese AS, Robbrecht DL, Vanholder RC, et al: Rifampicin-associated acute renal failure: Pathophysiologic, immunologic, and clinical features. Am J Kidney Dis 31:108-115, 1998.

Grollman AP, Shibutani S, Moriya M, et al: Aristolochic acid and the etiology of endemic (Balkan) nephropathy. Proc Natl Acad Sci U S A 104:12129-12134, 2007.

Hoppes T, Prikis M, Segal A: Four cases of nafcillin-associated acute interstitial nephritis in one institution. Nat Clin Prac Nephrol 3:456-461, 2007.

Kannerstein M: Histologic kidney changes in the common acute infectious diseases. Am J Med Sci 203:65-73, 1942.

Kim R, Rotnitsky A, Sparrow D, et al: A longitudinal study of low-level lead exposure and impairment of renal function. The Normative Aging Study. JAMA 275:1177-1181, 1996.

Lin JL, Lin-Tan DT, Hsu KU, et al: Environmental lead exposure and progression of chronic renal diseases in patients without diabetes. N Engl J Med 348:277-286, 2003.

Liu Y: Epithelial to mesenchymal transition in renal fibrogenesis: Pathologic significance, molecular mechanism, and therapeutic intervention. J Am Soc Nephrol 15:1-12, 2004.

Meyers CM: New insights into the pathogenesis of interstitial nephritis. Curr Opin Nephrol Hypertens 8:287-292, 1999.

Muntner P, He J, Vupputuri S, et al: Blood lead and chronic kidney disease in the general United States population: Results from NHANES III. Kidney Int 63:1044-50, 2003.

Nortier JL, Martinex M-C, Schmeiser HH, et al: Urothelial carcinoma associated with the use of a Chinese herb (*Aristolochia fangchi*). N Engl J Med 342:1686-1692, 2000.

Preddie DC, Markowitz GS, Radhakrishnan J, et al: Mycopheno-late mofetil for the treatment of interstitial nephritis. Clin J Am Soc Nephrol 1:718-722, 2006.

Rossert J: Drug-induced interstitial nephritis. Kidney Int 60: 804-817, 2001.

Spanou Z, Keller M, Britschgi M et al: Involvement of drug-specific T cells in acute drug-induced interstitial nephritis. J Am Soc Nephrol 17:2919-27, 2006.

Takemura T, Okada M, Hino S, et al: Course and outcome of tubu-lointerstitial nephritis and uveitis syndrome. Am J Kidney Dis 34:1016-1021, 1999.

US Renal Data System, USRDS 2007 Annual Data Report: Atlas of Chronic Kidney Disease and End-stage Renal Disease in the United States. National Institutes of Health, National Institute of Diabetes and Digestive and Kidney Diseases, Bethesda, MD, 2007.

CHAPTER 46

Obstructive Uropathy

Michelle Krause

The term *obstructive uropathy* refers to structural changes that prevent urinary flow anywhere along the genitourinary tract, including the renal pelvis, ureters, bladder, or urethra. Often "obstructive uropathy" and "obstructive nephropathy" are used interchangeably. However, the term *obstructive nephropathy* should be reserved for those individuals who have chronic kidney disease (CKD) as a result of blockage or impairment of urinary flow. The incidence of obstructive uropathy varies with age and follows a bimodal distribution pattern. The highest incidence is in the first decade of life, predominately as a result of congenital anomalies of the urinary tract, and there is a second peak after the sixth decade, most commonly resulting from obstructive disorders of the prostate. Obstructive uropathy or nephropathy has been described in 3% to 4% of individuals in autopsy studies, and these disorders account for an estimated 4% of adult patients and approximately one third of children with end-stage renal disease (ESRD) requiring renal replacement therapy.

Obstructive uropathy may be classified based on several criteria, such as degree, duration, and site of the obstruction. The degree of obstruction refers to whether the blockage of urinary flow is complete (high grade) or partial (low grade). The duration of obstruction is either acute or chronic. Acute obstruction is that occurring over a short period of time, most commonly from nephrolithiasis; chronic obstruction occurs insidiously over weeks to months. Chronic obstruction, as seen in congenital anomalies of the genitourinary tract and prostatic disease, is more likely to contribute to the development of obstructive nephropathy and CKD, whereas acute obstruction is more likely to be promptly recognized. The site of obstruction is also an important factor in the classification. Obstruction that occurs above the level of the ureterovesical junction is termed upper tract obstruction and typically is unilateral in nature; obstruction that occurs below the level of the ureterovesical junction is called lower tract obstruction and is more often bilateral in nature.

PATHOGENESIS

The pathogenesis of obstructive uropathy is complex and involves changes in intratubular pressure, glomerular filtration, and renal vascular resistance. In acute complete obstruction, there is a rise in the intratubular pressure from approximately 10 to 25 mm Hg, and as high as 50 to 70 mm Hg with hydration or diuresis. This rise in intratubular pressure is sustained for only a few hours, and in unilateral obstruction it falls to preobstructive values within a day or so. The mechanism by which the intratubular pressure declines is thought to involve a decrease in the amount of tubular fluid within the nephron, which results from loss of glomerular filtration, increased sodium reabsorption in the tubules, and an increase in tubular fluid removal via lymphatic drainage.

The glomerular filtration rate (GFR) is determined from the change in transcapillary hydrostatic pressure (ΔP) and the change in transcapillary osmotic pressure ($\Delta \Pi$) by the following formula:

$$GFR = LpA(\Delta P - \Delta \Pi)$$

where LpA is the ultrafiltration coefficient. The rise in intratubular pressure is transmitted to Bowman's space. As a result, ΔP falls, leading to a reduction in GFR. Alterations in renal blood flow further reduce the GFR. In early acute obstruction, there is an increase in renal blood flow which is thought to be secondary to an increase in prostaglandins and prostacyclin caused by compression of the intramedullary vasculature from increased intratubular pressure. The increase in renal blood flow is transient; within 1 to 2 hours, there is a progressive fall in renal blood flow by as much as 50%. This reduction in renal blood flow is caused by increased renal vascular resistance, synthesis of vasoconstrictors such as thromboxane A_2 and angiotensin II from lymphocytic infiltration, and a reduction in tubular delivery of solute to the macula densa. As renal blood flow falls, the net filtration pressure within the glomerulus decreases, and there is a further decline in the GFR. Administration of inhibitors of thromboxane A_2 and angiotensin-converting enzyme have been shown to reverse the effects of renal blood flow in obstructive uropathy in animal models.

Individuals with obstructive uropathy also have changes in distal tubular function characterized by defects in urinary acidification and concentration. During acute obstruction, there is an initial increase in sodium reabsorption by the tubules, with a spot urine sodium concentration of less than 10 mEq/L and a fractional excretion of sodium of less than 1%, mimicking prerenal acute renal failure. As the obstruction persists, marked sodium wasting occurs, predominately because of tubular injury and decreased activity of the sodium-potassium adenosine triphosphatase (Na^+,K^+-ATPase) enzyme. The inability to reabsorb sodium in the distal nephron limits generation of the electronegative tubular lumen potential that ordinarily favors excretion of hydrogen and potassium ions. The net retention of hydrogen and potassium results in the "voltage-dependent" renal tubular acidosis commonly seen in patients with obstructive uropathy. The inability to reabsorb sodium along the loop of Henle also affects the ability of the distal nephron to effectively concentrate the urine. The loss of sodium reabsorption at the Na^+-K^+-$2Cl^-$ (NKCC2) transporter in the thick ascending limb results in inability to maintain a concentrated medullary interstitium, which produces a "washed out" medulla. In conjunction with downregulation of aquaporins along the entire nephron and tubular resistance to the effects of antidiuretic hormone (ADH), defects in water reabsorption also contribute to the decline in urinary concentration. The fall in urinary concentration contributes to the postobstructive diuresis that is seen after relief of the acute obstructive process and continues until solute balance is re-established in the recovering nephron.

The histologic changes that are seen in obstructive uropathy and nephropathy are identical for all causes of obstruction. The hallmark of the renal pathologic changes is tubulointerstitial disease with interstitial fibrosis and atrophy. As intratubular pressure rises and is maintained, focal areas of ischemia occur in the interstitium, resulting in the generation of oxidant free radicals that result in tubular injury. As tubular injury occurs, there is activation of the renin-angiotensin system. Increased levels of angiotensin II recruit inflammatory lymphocytes and macrophages into the interstitium; they, in turn, promote the release of transforming growth factor-β (TGFB1), which results in cellular apoptosis and interstitial fibrosis. There is evidence from animal studies that the use of angiotensin-converting enzyme inhibitors, angiotensin receptor blockers, and neutralizing anti-TGFB1 antibodies may slow the progression of CKD in obstructive nephropathy.

ETIOLOGY AND RISK FACTORS
Intrinsic Causes of Obstructive Uropathy

The causes of obstructive uropathy are classified according to the site of obstruction to urine flow, which may be *intrinsic* to the genitourinary tract or *extrinsic,* resulting from abnormalities in the gastrointestinal tract, reproductive tract, abdominal vasculature, or retroperitoneum. The intrinsic causes of obstruction may be further subdivided by the blockage of urine flow either intraluminally or intramurally. *Intraluminal* obstruction occurs when the blockage is within the urinary space, in the tubular lumen, ureters, or urethra; *intramural* obstruction is defined by conditions such as ureteropelvic junction (UPJ) or ureterovesicular junction (UVJ) obstruction or bladder outlet obstruction that result in obstruction to urine flow outside the urinary space. Multiple myeloma with cast nephropathy is the most common cause of intraluminal obstruction within the kidney (see Chapter 27).

Another cause of intraluminal intraparenchymal obstruction occurs with acute urate nephropathy. Acute urate nephropathy is characterized by uric acid crystallization within the tubular lumen resulting in cast formation and obstruction of urine flow. Approximately 10% of individuals with hematologic malignancies (e.g., leukemias, lymphomas) will have acute urate nephropathy, most commonly when the serum uric acid level is greater than 15 mg/dL. Treatment of these hematologic malignancies with chemotherapy results in rapid tissue breakdown and release of uric acid into the bloodstream. Glomerular filtration and proximal tubule secretion of uric acid into an acidic urine favors precipitation and intraluminal cast formation that results in kidney failure. Dehydration may further increase the risk of acute urate nephropathy. Pretreatment with hydration, lowering the serum uric acid level with administration of allopurinol or rasburicase, and alkalinization of the urine have been shown to reduce the likelihood of acute urate nephropathy. Another, less common cause of intraluminal obstruction is crystal deposition from medications, including sulfonamides, ciprofloxacin, and antiviral agents such as acyclovir and indinavir.

Extrarenal causes of intraluminal obstruction include nephrolithiasis, papillary necrosis, and, occasionally, blood clots that form from cyst rupture in individuals with polycystic kidney disease or from gross hematuria during a flare of immunoglobulin A nephropathy. Nephrolithiasis is a common condition that is estimated to occur in 10% of adults, with typical age at onset in the third or fourth decade of life (see Chapter 47). Most kidney stones are composed of calcium oxalate; like urate stones, they typically cause acute obstruction. Infected stones and struvite staghorn calculi are more likely to cause chronic obstructive nephropathy because of their large size and difficulty eradicating the nidus of infection with antibiotic therapy. Most stones pass spontaneously or with supportive care including hydration and analgesic therapy. Stones larger than 7 mm often require urologic intervention to relieve obstruction. Unilaterally obstructing stones usually are not associated with a rise in the serum creatinine concentration, as long as the unaffected kidney is normally functioning and compensates for the fall in GFR in the obstructed kidney. If acute renal failure occurs, then one should consider bilateral obstruction, unilateral obstruction in a solitary kidney, another cause of kidney disease in the unobstructed kidney, or other disorders such as primary hyperoxaluria or cystinuria with extensive stone formation.

Papillary necrosis is a less common cause of intraluminal extraparenchymal obstruction. Conditions that result in medullary ischemia, such as analgesic use, diabetes mellitus, acute pyelonephritis, and sickle cell disease, may be associated with papillary necrosis. Papillary necrosis may be limited to the papillae, or it may more diffusely involve ischemic damage to the medulla. Papillary necrosis tends to be bilateral. It is estimated that 50% to 75% of the cases occur in diabetics, and one third to one half of these are associated with severe obstruction and acute renal failure. The incidence of papillary necrosis is not well known, unrecognized as a cause of acute renal failure, given that of papillary necrosis is not well known as its presenting signs and symptoms such as fever, Flank pain, and hematuria may be attributed to infection and/or renal ischemia. Papillary necrosis is typically self-limited and improves with hydration and antibiotic therapy if a coexistent infection is present. Chronic forms do exist and contribute to obstructive nephropathy and CKD. With severe bilateral obstruction, invasive measures such as ureteral stents or percutaneous nephrostomy tubes may be required to manage the acute renal failure in papillary necrosis.

Other causes of obstructive uropathy intrinsic to the genitourinary tract include intramural functional and anatomic abnormalities of the ureter and bladder. Disorders that cause bladder dysfunction with urinary retention and reflux occur in children with spina bifida and in adults with diabetes mellitus, multiple sclerosis, Parkinson's disease, and other disorders associated with autonomic neuropathy. These conditions may result in obstructive nephropathy and CKD. Rarely, diverticula or cancers of the bladder can cause an anatomic obstruction by preventing urinary flow out of the urethra or creating increased pressure in the bladder, leading to reflux. More commonly, functional disorders of the ureter are caused by abnormalities occurring at the level of the UPJ or the UVJ. UPJ obstruction is the most common cause of fetal hydronephrosis during pregnancy. UPJ obstruction is more likely to occur in male infants, and it unilaterally involves the left kidney more often than the right kidney. UPJ obstruction is thought to result from abnormal smooth muscle and connective tissue development at the level of the UPJ, possibly from a reduction in nerve growth factors, malrotation of the kidney, aberrant insertion of the ureter into the renal pelvis, or, more likely in adults, extrinsic compression on the UPJ from vasculature or tumors. Individuals with UPJ obstruction may be completely asymptomatic, or they may present with recurrent urinary tract infections, flank pain, failure to thrive, and progressive kidney failure. The classic description of UPJ obstruction is Dietl's crisis with nausea, vomiting, and flank pain during intermittent bouts of obstruction, often occurring during times of large urine volumes (e.g., use of diuretic agents or caffeinated beverages). The diagnosis of UPJ obstruction relies on imaging studies, particularly after hydronephrosis is discovered in utero.

The Society of Fetal Urology developed a grading system that classifies hydronephrosis into five categories of severity (**Table 46-1**). In general, the lower the grade of dilatation, the better the outcome; grades 3 and 4 may require more aggressive interventions to relive the obstruction. If hydronephrosis is discovered in utero, it is recommended that the kidney ultrasound study be repeated within 1 week after birth to determine the severity of obstruction.

Management of UPJ obstruction relies heavily on the severity of the patient's clinical symptoms; those who are asymptomatic may improve spontaneously over time. In asymptomatic patients, observation with serial ultrasound studies (quarterly in the first year of life, biannually in the second year, and annually thereafter) is recommended to evaluate for progression. Symptomatic UPJ obstruction, such as failure to thrive, recurrent urinary tract infections, abdominal or flank pain, hematuria, or a reduction in GFR, warrants more aggressive intervention. Patients whose GFR is reduced to less than 40% in the obstructed kidney and those with declining renal function in the affected kidney based on serial diuretic renal scans should have surgical repair of the obstructing lesion. Diuretic renal scans are helpful in the evaluation of UPJ obstruction because they provide both a qualitative and quantitative assessment for the severity of obstruction. The gold standard surgical treatment of UPJ obstruction is either a laparoscopic or an open pyeloplasty. Surgical repair is curative in more than 90% of the cases and is confirmed by resolution of the hydronephrosis on ultrasonography performed 1 month after the procedure.

Vesicoureteral reflux (VUR) is another common cause of hydronephrosis and obstruction. It occurs predominately in children and young adults and is defined by the backward flow of urine from the bladder into the ureters and kidneys. VUR is estimated to affect 1% of newborns, but the incidence increases to 30% to 50% of children who develop urinary tract infections. VUR is more common in Caucasians, in younger children, and in girls. There appears to be a familial inheritance pattern in VUR, because two thirds of infants with VUR have a parent with VUR, and up to one third have affected siblings. The term *reflux nephropathy* refers to the chronic scarring and damage to the renal parenchyma with loss of GFR associated with VUR.

The pathogenesis of VUR is classified into primary and secondary causes. Primary VUR is more common than secondary types, is present at birth, and is associated with a normal genitourinary tract. Reflux is thought to occur because of a short intramural ureter, abnormalities of the ureteral orifice, or bladder detrusor dysfunction. Secondary causes of VUR are associated with abnormalities of the genitourinary tract, including posterior urethral valves, neurogenic bladder, bladder diverticula, and bladder outlet obstruction. Posterior urethral valves are the most prevalent cause of secondary VUR. They occur exclusively in males and result from abnormal development of the posterior urethra; tissue folds at the junction with the bladder prevent the normal passage of urine. In addition to hydronephrosis, infants with

TABLE 46-1	Society of Fetal Urology Grading System for Hydronephrosis
GRADE	DESCRIPTION
0	No dilation of the genitourinary system
I	Mild splitting of the renal pelvis
II	Dilatation of the renal pelvis without calyceal involvement
III	Dilatation of both the renal pelvis and calyces
IV	Dilatation of the renal pelvis and calyces with renal parenchymal thinning

Adapted from the Society of Fetal Urology www.fetalurology.org (accessed July 21, 2008).

Noncontrast abdominal computed tomographic (CT) scanning is now being used more commonly for the diagnosis of obstructive uropathy, particularly in nephrolithiasis and cases in which the clinical suspicion is high and the renal ultrasound is negative for obstruction. Because they are invasive or require the administration of potentially nephrotoxic radiographic contrast agents, intravenous and retrograde pyelography are less frequently used today. Nonetheless, intravenous pyelography may be helpful if abdominal CT scanning is unable to confirm the diagnosis or location of the obstruction, especially with small kidney stones or papillary necrosis. Magnetic resonance imaging (MRI) typically is not used in the diagnosis of obstruction unless detailed anatomy is required in conditions that preclude the use of radiation (e.g., pregnancy). MRI may be useful in detecting retroperitoneal fibrosis if iodinated contrast studies (e.g., retrograde pyelography, CT) are contraindicated due to the risk of contrast-induced nephropathy in patients with CKD.

More functional radiographic imaging techniques include VCUG and diuretic renography. As discussed earlier, VCUG can establish both the presence and the severity of VUR (**Fig. 46-2**). VCUG may be used to monitor individuals serially to determine severity and progression of obstruction, but the technique is invasive, requiring catheterization and significant radiation exposure. Renal ultrasonography may be used in the place of VCUG to determine changes in kidney size and severity of hydronephrosis. Because ultrasound lacks the ability to reliably detect renal scars, radionuclide scans are now favored as the imaging procedure of choice to serially monitor patients with VUR, particularly children. Diuretic renography involves the administration of intravenous furosemide before a radionuclide scan. A prolonged washout period (>20 minutes) confirms the diagnosis of obstruction. Symptomatic pain during the administration of furosemide is also considered a positive test result in obstructive uropathy. Diuretic renograms are less sensitive and less specific in individuals with bilateral obstruction or reduced GFR. They can be helpful to differentiate between obstruction and a patulous, nonobstructed collecting system, particularly in asymptomatic individuals in whom hydronephrosis was discovered as an incidental finding .

TREATMENT

The treatment of obstructive uropathy relies on relief of the obstruction, either medically or with more invasive techniques such as ureteral stenting, percutaneous nephrostomy tubes, or surgery. Medical therapy includes the administration of antibiotics for obstruction associated with infections such as pyelonephritis in VUR, papillary necrosis, intraabdominal abscesses, and prostatitis. Pharmaceutical therapy directed at reducing prostate hypertrophy or treatment of prostate cancer in men with obstructive uropathy may prevent the need for more invasive measures. Analgesic therapy and the administration of intravenous fluids are indicated for acute nephrolithiasis when the stone is likely to pass spontaneously. Invasive techniques to relieve obstruction include the placement of ureteral stents via cystoscopy or the placement of percutaneous nephrostomy tubes to allow for the temporary passage of urine until the cause of the obstruction is corrected. Surgical procedures such as transurethral resection of the prostate (TURP), open reimplantation of the ureters in primary VUR, valve ablation in posterior urethral valves, and radiation or chemotherapy of malignant disease in extrinsic causes of obstructive uropathy are the treatments of choice for long-term management of obstruction.

Relief of obstruction may be complicated by hematuria, hypotension from systemic vasodilatation (especially in the elderly and those with concomitant volume depletion), and postobstructive diuresis. The incidence of postobstructive diuresis is variable because of lack of consensus in the definition based on volume of urine output. Most authorities agree that polyuria in excess of 250 mL/hr after relief of obstruction is indicative of diuresis. Postobstructive diuresis is thought to occur as a result of the physiologic excretion of retained solute including sodium and urea, decreased resorption of sodium in the proximal tubule, and secretion of systemic diuretic factors such as atrial natriuretic peptide during the obstructive process. Typically, once the accumulated solute is excreted and tubular function is restored, the diuresis resolves and metabolic balance is restored. Rarely, there may be a more sustained salt-wasting nephropathy and impairment of urinary concentration capacity lasting for months after relief of the obstruction. Gradual rather than complete decompression of the bladder was once thought to decrease the risk of bladder hemorrhage and postobstructive diuresis.

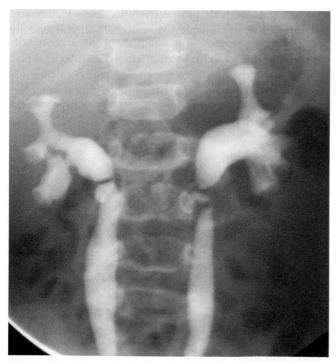

FIGURE 46-2 Grade III vesicoureteral reflux on voiding cystoureterogram. (Courtesy of Dr. Muhammad Yousaf.)

However, the literature has failed to support this notion, and complete decompression of the bladder is now recommended. The necessity of fluid resuscitation to treat postobstructive diuresis depends on the development of clinical symptoms from volume loss, such as hypotension, orthostasis, or a decline in renal function consistent with prerenal acute renal failure. In those instances, replacement of urinary salt and water losses is required until the diuresis has resolved.

PROGNOSIS

The duration of obstruction is one of the most important determinants in the development of obstructive nephropathy and loss of GFR. Most investigators agree that more than 6 weeks of obstruction results in irreversible CKD. Failure to recover renal function within 1 week after relief of the obstruction also increases the risk for obstructive nephropathy and CKD. Once obstructive nephropathy develops, there is progressive loss of kidney function leading to ESRD. Individuals with a higher risk for development of ESRD include those with hypertension, proteinuria, and an elevated serum creatinine concentration at diagnosis. There is evidence that angiotensin-converting enzyme inhibitors may protect against the development of obstruction-related renal fibrosis. Once obstructive nephropathy develops, the mainstay of treatment is aggressive blood pressure lowering to less than 130/80 mm Hg, attempts to reduce proteinuria to less than 500 mg/day, and avoidance of nephrotoxic agents such as iodinated contrast agents and nonsteroidal anti-inflammatory medications. Care appropriate to the stage of CKD and the patient's underlying disease is also in order.

BIBLIOGRAPHY

The American Urological Association Pediatric Vesicoureteral Reflux Guidelines Panel: Caring for Children with Primary Vesicoureteral Reflux. American Urological Association. Available at http://www.auanet.org/content/guidelines/patient_guides/PedRefluxptguide.pdf (accessed July 21, 2008).

Bander SJ, Buerkert JE, Martin D, Klahr S: Long term effects of 24-hr unilateral obstruction on renal function in the rat. Kidney Int 28:614-620, 1985.

Batlle DC, Arruda JA, Kurtzman NA: Hyperkalemic distal renal tubular acidosis associated with obstructive uropathy. N Engl J Med 304:373-380, 1981.

Chevalier RL: Specific molecular targeting of renal injury in obstructive nephropathy. Kidney Int 70:1200-1201, 2006.

Garin EH, Campos A, Homsy A: Primary vesicoureteral refux: Review of current concepts. Pediatr Nephrol 12:249-256, 2004.

Klahr S: Pathophysiology of obstructive nephropathy. Kidney Int 23:414-426, 1983.

Klahr S, Morrissey J: Obstructive nephropathy and renal fibrosis. Am J Physiol Renal Physiol 238:F861-F875, 2002.

Nyman MA, Shcwenk NM, Silverstein MD: Management of urinary retention: Rapid versus gradual decompression and risk of complications. Mayo Clin Proc 72:951-956, 1997.

Sabatini S, Kurtzman NA: Enzyme activity in obstructive uropathy: Basis for salt wastage and the acidification defect. Kidney Int 37:79-84, 1990.

Wilson DR: Pathophysiology of obstructive nephropathy. Kidney Int 18:281-292, 1980.

CHAPTER 47

Nephrolithiasis

Gary Curhan

SCOPE OF THE PROBLEM

Nephrolithiasis is a major cause of morbidity involving the urinary tract. The prevalence of nephrolithiasis in the U.S. population increased from 3.8% in the late 1970s to 5.2% in the early 1990s. The increase in prevalence was observed in both men and women, and both whites and blacks. There were almost 2 million physician office visits for stone disease in 2000. Surprisingly, the estimated annual costs have remained at approximately $2 billion, probably as a result of the shift from inpatient to outpatient procedures.

The lifetime risk of nephrolithiasis is about 12% in men and 6% in women. In men, the first episode of renal colic is most likely to occur after age 30, but can occur earlier. The incidence for men who have never had a stone is about 0.3% per year between the ages of 30 and 60 years and diseases thereafter with age. For women, the rate is about 0.2% per year between the ages of 20 and 30 years and then declines to 0.1% for the next 4 decades.

The risk of the first recurrent stone after the incident stone in untreated patients remains controversial. Reported frequencies of stone recurrence in uncontrolled studies have ranged from 30% to 50% at 5 years. However, data from the control groups of recent randomized, controlled trials suggest much lower rates of first recurrence after an incident calcium oxalate stone, ranging from 2% to 5% per year. Sex-specific rates are not available from the randomized trials.

ACUTE RENAL COLIC

With the passage of a stone from the renal pelvis into the ureter resulting in partial or complete obstruction, there is sudden onset of unilateral flank pain of sufficient severity that the individual usually seeks medical attention. Despite the use of the misnomer "colic," the pain does not completely remit but rather waxes and wanes. Nausea and vomiting may accompany the pain. The pattern of pain depends on the location of the stone: if it is in the upper ureter, pain may radiate anteriorly to the abdomen; if it is in the lower ureter, pain may radiate to the ipsilateral testicle in men or labium in women; if it is lodged at the ureterovesical junction (UVJ), the primary symptoms may be urinary frequency and urgency. A less common acute presentation is gross hematuria without pain.

The symptoms from a ureteral stone may mimic those of several other acute conditions. A stone lodged in the right ureteropelvic junction can mimic acute cholecystitis. A stone lodged in the lower right ureter as it crosses the pelvic brim can mimic acute appendicitis. A stone lodged at the UVJ can mimic acute cystitis. A stone lodged in the lower left ureter as it crosses the pelvic brim can mimic diverticulitis. An obstructing stone with proximal infection can mimic acute pyelonephritis. Note that infection in the setting of obstruction is a medical emergency ("pus under pressure") that requires emergent drainage, by placement of a ureteral stent or a percutaneous nephrostomy tube. However, because nephrolithiasis is common, the simple presence of a kidney stone does not confirm the diagnosis of renal colic in a patient presenting with acute abdominal pain.

Other conditions to consider in the differential diagnosis of suspected renal colic include muscular or skeletal pain, herpes zoster, duodenal ulcer, abdominal aortic aneurysm, gynecologic causes, ureteral obstruction due to other intraluminal factors (e.g., blood clot, sloughed papilla), and ureteral stricture. Extraluminal factors causing compression tend not to result in a presentation with symptoms of renal colic.

The physical examination alone rarely makes the diagnosis, but clues guide the evaluation. The patient typically is in obvious pain and unable to achieve a comfortable position. There may be ipsilateral costovertebral angle tenderness, or, in cases of obstruction with infection, signs and symptoms of sepsis may be present.

Although blood tests are typically normal, there may be a leukocytosis resulting from stress or infection. The serum creatinine concentration is typically normal but may be elevated in the setting of volume depletion, bilateral ureteral obstruction, or unilateral obstruction in a patient with a solitary kidney. The urinalysis classically reveals red blood cells and white blood cells and may occasionally show crystals. If ureteral obstruction by the stone is complete, there may be no red blood cells, because no urine will be flowing through that ureter into the bladder.

Because of the often nonspecific physical examination and laboratory findings, imaging studies play a crucial role in making the diagnosis. The imaging modality of choice is helical (spiral) computed tomography (CT), because it does not require a radiocontrast agent and can detect stones as small as 1 mm, even pure uric acid stones (traditionally considered "radiolucent"). Typically, the study shows a ureteral stone or evidence of recent passage, such as perinephric stranding or hydronephrosis. A plain abdominal radiograph of the kidney, ureter, and bladder (KUB) can miss a stone in the ureter or kidney, even one that is radiopaque, and it provides no information on obstruction. Although KUB is often used to monitor the progress of a ureteral stone or the growth of asymptomatic kidney stones, its sensitivity is limited. An intravenous pyelogram (IVP) requires contrast and can miss small stones; it should be ordered only rarely for the evaluation and treatment of nephrolithiasis. Although there is a general belief that the osmotic diuresis induced by the radiocontrast agent can facilitate stone passage, there is insufficient confirmatory evidence. Ultrasonography, while avoiding radiation, can image only the kidney and proximal ureter.

Renal colic is one of the most excruciating types of pain; therefore, pain control is essential. Narcotics and parenteral nonsteroidal anti-inflammatory drugs are effective, and the latter are preferable because they cause fewer side effects. Other treatments that may be effective include α-adrenergic blockers and calcium channel blockers. Urinary alkalinization may be effective for a uric acid stone, but this type is relatively rare and there must be adequate urine flow past the stone.

TYPES OF STONES

Almost 90% of stones in men and 70% of stones in women contain calcium, most commonly as calcium oxalate (**Fig. 47-1**). Other types of stones, such as cystine, pure uric acid, and struvite, are much less common. However,

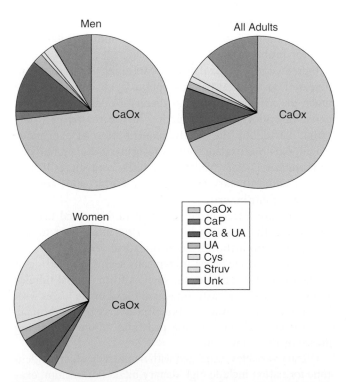

FIGURE 47-1 Types of stones and their frequency in adults. Ca & UA, calcium and uric acid; CaOx, calcium oxalate; CaP, calcium phosphate; Cys, cystine; Struv, struvite; UA, uric acid; Unk, unknown. (From Coe F, Parks J [eds]: Nephrolithiasis: Pathogenesis and Treatment. Chicago, Year Book Medical, 1988, with permission.)

these types of stone also deserve careful attention, because recurrences are common. No information is available on the frequencies from first-time stone formers, in part because the first stone typically is not retrieved or sent for analysis.

PATHOGENESIS

The urinary concentrations of calcium, oxalate, and other solutes that influence stone formation are high enough that they should result in crystal formation in the urine of most individuals, but this is clearly not the case. This condition is termed *supersaturation*. Substances in the urine, called *inhibitors*, prevent crystal formation. The most common inhibitor is citrate, which works by chelating calcium cations in the urine, thereby decreasing the free calcium available to bind with oxalate or phosphate anions. If the supersaturation is sufficiently high or there are insufficient inhibitors, precipitation occurs with resulting crystalluria.

The causes of stone formation differ for different stone types. Cystine stones form only in individuals with the autosomal recessive disorder of cystinuria. Uric acid stones form only in those who have persistently acid urine, with or without hyperuricosuria. Struvite stones form only in the setting of an upper urinary tract infection with a urease-producing bacterium. These stones are seen in individuals with recurrent urinary tract infections, particularly those with abnormal urinary tract anatomy, such as patients who have urinary diversions or who require frequent catheterization. Stones may occasionally result from precipitation of medications such as acyclovir and indinavir in the urinary tract.

Calcium-based stones have a multifactorial etiology. Traditionally, stone formation was believed to occur from (1) crystal formation in the renal tubule, followed by (2) attachment of the crystal to the tubular epithelium, usually at the tip of the papilla, and (3) growth of the attached crystal by deposition of additional crystalline material. However, it now appears that the initial crystal forms in the medullary interstitium and is composed of calcium phosphate. This may then erode through the papilla, and calcium oxalate is subsequently deposited. Several medical conditions increase the likelihood of calcium oxalate stone formation. With primary hyperparathyroidism, urinary calcium is increased. Crohn's disease and other malabsorptive states in which the colon is intact are associated with increased urinary oxalate excretion. With fat malabsorption, calcium is bound in the small bowel to free fatty acids, leaving a smaller amount of free calcium to bind to oxalate. An increased amount of unbound oxalate is then available for absorption in the colon. The accompanying low urine volume presents an additional risk factor. Citrate resorption is increased by metabolic acidosis, leaving less urinary citrate to serve as a calcium chelator. For this reason, distal renal tubular acidosis predisposes to stone formation as well.

Calcium phosphate stones are more likely to form in the presence of high urine calcium, low urine citrate, and alkaline urine. Systemic conditions that are present more frequently in patients with calcium phosphate stones include renal tubular acidosis and primary hyperparathyroidism. The remainder of this chapter focuses on calcium oxalate stones except where noted.

Urinary variables that increase the risk of calcium oxalate stone formation are higher levels of calcium and oxalate; higher levels of citrate and higher total volume decrease the risk (**Table 47-1**). Although higher urine uric acid concentration has been thought to increase the risk of calcium oxalate stone formation, results from a recent large study did not support this belief and raised the possibility that a higher urine uric acid level may actually reduce the risk. The traditional approach to urinary abnormalities is based on 24-hour urinary excretion. There are generally accepted definitions of "abnormal" values for hypercalciuria (≥250 mg/day for women, ≥300 mg/day for men), hyperoxaluria (≥45 mg/day for both women and men), hyperuricosuria (≥750 mg/day for women, ≥800 mg/day for men), and hypocitraturia (≥320 mg/day for both women and men). After being evaluated, patients have typically been classified into categories according to their urinary abnormalities, and treatment and advice have been directed at correcting the abnormalities.

Although this approach has been used for decades, it has several limitations. Stone formation is a disease of concentration. Therefore, it is not just the absolute amount of substances that determines the likelihood of stone formation. The traditional definitions of "abnormal" excretion must be applied cautiously for several reasons. First, there are insufficient data supporting the cutoff points used regarding the risk of actual stone formation. For example, the traditional definition of hypercalciuria is 50 mg/day greater in men than in women, but there is no justification with respect to stone formation for having a higher upper limit of normal in men, particularly because the mean 24-hour urine volume is lower

in men than in women. Similarly, another common definition of hypercalciuria is urinary calcium excretion in excess of 4 mg/kg of body weight per day. However, by this definition, an individual who is heavier or gains weight can excrete more calcium than someone who is thinner but still be below the cutoff point. Second, an individual could have "normal" absolute excretion of calcium but still have a high urinary calcium concentration due to low urine volume. This situation has therapeutic implications, because the goal is to modify the concentration of the lithogenic factors. Finally, the risk of stone formation is a continuum, so the use of a specific cutoff point may give the false impression that a patient with "high-normal" urinary calcium excretion is not at risk for stone recurrence. Just as cardiovascular risk increases with increasing blood pressure (even in the "normal" range), the risk of stone formation increases with increasing urine calcium levels.

Pak and colleagues advocated subdividing cases of elevated urinary calcium into three categories: (1) absorptive (caused by increased gastrointestinal absorption of ingested calcium), (2) resorptive (caused by increased bone resorption), and (3) renal (caused by increased urinary excretion of filtered calcium). However, there is not general agreement on the clinical importance of this approach. A substantial proportion of cases cannot be classified, and there is evidence that individuals may change categories when studied years later. Therefore, most clinicians do measure 24-hour urine chemistries as part of the metabolic evaluation but do not subclassify patients. The underlying mechanisms for idiopathic hypercalciuria remain unknown, although hormones and their receptors involved in calcium metabolism, such as 1,25-dihydroxyvitamin D and the vitamin D receptor, probably play important roles.

Increased urinary oxalate concentrations may result from increased gastrointestinal absorption (high dietary oxalate intake or increased fractional dietary oxalate absorption), increased endogenous production, or decreased gastrointestinal secretion. The relative contribution of exogenous and endogenous oxalate sources to urinary oxalate remains controversial. Dietary oxalate most likely contributes 10% to 30%, but other dietary factors (e.g., ascorbic acid) are also important contributors.

Purines are metabolized to uric acid. Increased urinary uric acid is the result of higher purine intake and higher endogenous production from purine turnover.

Low urine citrate levels are typically seen in the setting of a systemic metabolic acidosis, such as from a renal tubular acidosis or excessive gastrointestinal bicarbonate losses with diarrhea. Because citrate is a potential source of bicarbonate, it is actively reclaimed in the proximal tubule after being filtered by the glomerulus.

Dietary variables associated with decreased risk of incident stone formation include high dietary intakes of calcium, oxalate, potassium, and fluid; those associated with increased risk include high intakes of supplemental calcium, animal protein, sodium, and sucrose (see **Table 47-1**). Although dietary oxalate intake has been generally believed to be important for stone

TABLE 47-1 **Risk Factors for Calcium Oxalate Stone Formation**

HIGH LEVELS	LOW LEVELS
Urinary Risk Factors	
Calcium	Citrate
Oxalate	Total volume
Dietary Risk Factors	
Oxalate	Calcium, dietary
Animal protein	Potassium
Sodium	Phytate
Sucrose	Fluid
Fructose	
Calcium, supplemental	
Vitamin C	
Other Risk Factors	
Obesity	
Gout	
Diabetes	
Anatomic abnormalities	

formation, the magnitude of the risk is not very high. Many foods contain small amounts of oxalate, but foods that are high in oxalate are less common. Only recently have measurements of the oxalate content of foods become more reliable.

Data from observational and randomized, controlled studies support the concept that dietary calcium intake is inversely associated with risk of stone formation. The mechanism by which dietary calcium may reduce the risk of stone formation is unknown but may involve calcium binding to oxalate in the intestine, blocking oxalate absorption. It is also possible that there is some other protective substance in dairy products, the major source of dietary calcium.

Differences in timing of ingestion may explain the apparent contradiction between the protective effect of dietary calcium and the detrimental effect of supplemental calcium. A protective effect would not be expected unless the calcium supplement were taken with meals containing oxalate; in this case the observed increase in risk might rather be a result of increased urinary calcium excretion without any change in urinary oxalate excretion.

Nondietary factors that increase the risk for kidney stone formation include genitourinary anatomic abnormalities; medical conditions such as medullary sponge kidney, primary hyperparathyroidism, gout, and diabetes mellitus; and larger body size.

CLINICAL EVALUATION

Evaluation after the first kidney stone appears to be cost-effective, although there is some lack of agreement on how much should be done. The decision to proceed depends on several variables. First, what is the stone burden? Even though the episode that brought the patient to medical attention may have been the first symptomatic event, an appreciable proportion of patients have remaining kidney stones and could be considered "recurrent" stone formers. If such a patient had only a KUB or even an IVP during the acute evaluation, either of which could miss small stones, it would seem prudent to obtain a CT scan (preferably a helical CT) or kidney ultrasonogram to determine whether there are any residual kidney stones. Second, if the initial stone was large (e.g., >10 mm) or required an invasive intervention to remove, an evaluation would be indicated. Finally, and most important, are the patient's preferences.

A detailed history provides information crucial for treatment recommendations. The following points should be covered: total number of stones, evidence of residual stones, number and types of procedures, types and success of previous preventive treatments, family history of stone disease, and dietary intake and medication use before the stone event. After having experienced acute renal colic, a patient may attribute a variety of types of chronic back or flank pain to the kidney or to a residual stone. Further questioning often reveals other causes, particularly musculoskeletal. The physical examination may reveal findings of systemic conditions associated with stone formation, but these signs are uncommon.

LABORATORY (METABOLIC) EVALUATION

Retrieval of the stone for chemical analysis is an often overlooked but essential part of the evaluation, because treatment recommendations vary by stone type. The stone composition cannot be predicted with certainty from imaging or other laboratory studies. The decision to proceed with a metabolic evaluation should be guided by the patient's willingness to make lifestyle changes to prevent recurrent stone formation. Some experts advocate proceeding with an evaluation only after the second stone. However, safe and inexpensive interventions (e.g., modifying fluid intake) can be prescribed based on results of the relatively inexpensive 24-hour urine collection. If a metabolic evaluation is pursued, it is identical for first-time and recurrent stone formers. Serum chemistry values that should be measured include electrolytes, kidney function markers, and calcium and phosphorus concentrations. The decision to measure parathyroid hormone or vitamin D concentrations is based on results of the serum and urine chemistries. If the patient has high serum calcium, low serum phosphorus, or high urine calcium, then a parathyroid hormone level should be measured. The cornerstone of the evaluation is the 24-hour urine collection. Two 24-hour urine collections should be done while the patient is consuming his or her usual diet. Because individuals often change their dietary habits soon after an episode of renal colic, a patient should wait at least 6 weeks before carrying out the collections. Two collections are needed because there is substantial day-to-day variability in the values.

The variables that should be measured in the 24-hour urine collections are total volume, calcium, oxalate, citrate, uric acid, sodium, potassium, phosphorus, pH, and creatinine. Some laboratories calculate the relative supersaturation from measurements of the urine factors, which can be used to gauge the impact of therapy.

MEDICAL TREATMENTS

Because stones can remain asymptomatic for years, the actual time of formation of the stone that brought the patient to medical attention is usually unknown. The current metabolic evaluation may, in fact, be completely normal, and no changes in lifestyle would be needed. Whether the patient is an active stone former influences the decision to treat. The likelihood of recurrence cannot be definitely predicted from the urine chemistry results; a repeat imaging study 1 year later helps determine whether the patient is an active stone former. For patients who are at risk for stone recurrence, lifestyle modification should be attempted first, tailoring the recommendation according to stone type and urine chemistry findings. Lifelong changes are needed to prevent recurrence of this chronic condition. Because the supersaturation required for an existing stone to grow is lower than that needed for a new stone to form , recommendations to prevent stone growth may be more aggressive than those to prevent new stone formation.

Dietary Recommendations

Dietary recommendations that are useful in preventing nephrolithiasis are listed in **Table 47-2**. There is no evidence that dietary calcium restriction is helpful in preventing stone formation, and there is substantial evidence that it is harmful. Decreasing intake of animal protein (meat, chicken, and seafood) may be helpful. Patients who have low urine citrate concentrations should increase their intake of potential alkali (fruits and vegetables) and decrease intake of acid-producing foods such as animal protein. The role of calcium supplements deserves comment, because their use is common. In someone who has never had a kidney stone, the risk attributable to the supplement is low. For a patient who has had a calcium-containing stone and wishes to continue taking the supplement, 24-hour urine chemistry values should be measured while the patient is taking and not taking the supplement. Increased fluid intake decreases the risk of stone formation and recurrence. On the basis of the urine volume, the patient should be instructed how many additional 8-ounce glasses of fluid to drink each day, with the goal of producing approximately 2 L of urine daily.

For patients with high urine oxalate levels, the benefit of a low-oxalate diet is less clear because of the previously addressed issues regarding the oxalate content of food; however, spinach should be avoided. There is no accepted definition of a low-oxalate diet. An increase in dietary calcium with meals may reduce oxalate absorption and thereby reduce urine oxalate excretion. In addition, vitamin C supplementation should be avoided, because higher vitamin C intake may increase urine oxalate excretion.

Pharmacologic Options

The use of medication is indicated if dietary recommendations are unsuccessful in adequately modifying the urine composition. The three most commonly used classes of medications for stone prevention are (1) thiazides, which are used to reduce urine calcium excretion (e.g., chlorthalidone, hydrochlorothiazide); (2) alkali, which is used to increase urine citrate excretion (e.g., potassium citrate); and (3) allopurinol, which is used to reduce urine uric acid excretion.

For patients who have elevated urinary calcium levels but do not have an excessive calcium intake (i.e., not more than 1500 mg/day), a thiazide diuretic has been demonstrated to reduce the likelihood of stone recurrence and also to help maintain bone density. The dosages required to reduce urinary calcium adequately are substantially higher than those typically used for treatment of hypertension (at least 25 mg/day, and often 50 to 100 mg/day). Randomized trials of at least 3 years' duration have consistently shown a 50% reduction in the risk of recurrence. Adequate sodium restriction (to <3 g/day) is necessary to achieve maximum benefit from the thiazides; a higher sodium intake leads to greater distal sodium delivery, which minimizes or negates the beneficial effect of the thiazides. For patients who are unable to increase their fluid intake, a thiazide may be helpful even if the total urine calcium excretion is not high, because it will reduce the urinary calcium concentration. In addition, a thiazide may be more readily prescribed if there is evidence of low bone density.

For patients with low urine citrate levels, any form of alkali will increase the urine citrate. However, citrate is the base of choice, because it is better tolerated than bicarbonate. Potassium salts are preferred over sodium because of the potential effect on urinary calcium excretion. The alkali preparations must be taken at least twice daily to maintain adequate citrate levels. Randomized trials suggest a greater than 50% reduction in risk of recurrence with alkali supplementation.

In one randomized trial, allopurinol reduced the recurrence rate by 50% among individuals with a history of recurrent calcium oxalate stones and isolated hyperuricosuria. Given the epidemiologic observation that higher urine uric acid levels do not increase a person's likelihood of being a stone former, it is unclear whether the benefit was caused by the reduction in urine uric acid concentration or by some other mechanism.

NONCALCIUM STONES

For the less common types of stones (uric acid, struvite, and cystine), there is little or no information on the influence of dietary factors on actual stone formation (rather than simply changes in urine composition). The following recommendations are based our current understanding of

---

TABLE 47-2 Dietary and Pharmacologic Treatments to Prevent Nephrolithiasis, According to Urinary Abnormality

URINARY ABNORMALITY	DIETARY CHANGES	MEDICATION
High calcium concentration	Avoid excessive intake of calcium supplements	Thiazide
	Maintain adequate dietary calcium intake	
	Reduce intake of animal protein	
	Reduce sodium intake to <3 g/day	
	Reduce sucrose intake	
High oxalate concentration	Avoid high-oxalate foods	
	Maintain adequate dietary calcium intake	High-dose pyridoxine?
	Avoid vitamin C supplements	
High uric acid concentration	Reduce purine intake (i.e., meat, chicken, fish)	Allopurinol
Low citrate concentration	Increase intake of fruits and vegetables	Alkali (e.g., K citrate)
	Reduce intake of animal protein	
Low volume	Increase total fluid intake	Not applicable

the pathophysiology of these stone types, but caution is warranted because they are based on studies of urine composition rather than actual stone formation.

Uric Acid Stones

A higher intake of animal protein may increase the risk of uric acid stone formation. Consumption of meat, chicken, and seafood increases uric acid production because of the purine content of animal flesh. Animal protein has a greater content of sulfur-containing amino acids than vegetable protein, and their metabolism leads to increased acid production with a subsequent lowering of the urinary pH. Both increased uric acid excretion and the lower urine pH increase the risk of uric acid crystal formation. Higher intake of fruits and vegetables, which are high in potential base such as citrate, may raise the urine pH, thereby reducing the risk of uric acid crystal formation.

Alkali supplementation is the most effective treatment of existing uric acid stones. If the urine pH is maintained at 6.5 or higher (which often requires 90 to 120 mEq of supplemental alkali per day), pure uric acid stones will actually dissolve. Slightly lower doses may be used to prevent new uric acid stone formation. Allopurinol is the second-line choice if the patient has marked hyperuricosuria or is unable to maintain a urine pH of 6.5 or higher.

Cystine Stones

Higher sodium intake may increase urine cystine excretion. Because the solubility of cystine increases as pH rises, a higher consumption of fruits and vegetables may have a beneficial effect by increasing urine pH. Although the restriction of proteins high in cystine (e.g., animal protein) seems advisable, there is little evidence to support this recommendation as a means of directly lowering urinary cystine levels; however, reducing animal protein intake may be beneficial because it raises the urine pH.

Medications such as tiopronin and penicillamine increase the solubility of the filtered cystine. The effectiveness of these drugs is limited by the amount of cystine excreted daily and the high side-effect profile. If adequate amounts of the medication enter the urine, cystine stones can be dissolved. Supplemental potassium alkali salts may also provide some additional benefit by increasing the urine pH.

Struvite Stones

Because struvite stones form only in the setting of an infection in the upper urinary tract with urease-producing bacteria, it is very unlikely that dietary factors can directly influence struvite stone formation. Struvite stones are almost always large and may fill the renal pelvis (referred to as "staghorn calculi"); these stones should be removed by an experienced urologist. In addition to complete removal of all residual fragments, prevention of urinary tract infections is the cornerstone for preventing recurrence. Acetohydroxamic acid is the only drug available that inhibits urease; however,

it should be used with extreme caution because of its very common and serious side effects.

Calcium Phosphate Stones

Information on dietary issues related to actual calcium phosphate stone formation is limited. However, on the basis of the known physicochemical aspects, nutrients that might stimulate calcium phosphate crystal formation include excessive calcium intake (resulting in higher urinary calcium excretion), higher phosphate intake (resulting in higher urinary phosphate excretion), and higher intake of fruits and vegetables (resulting in a higher urinary pH). Nonetheless, caution is advised, because the "theoretical" benefits of limiting these nutrients may not be realized and there are, of course, other reasons to maintain an adequate intake of calcium, fruits, and vegetables.

Reduction in urine calcium can be achieved with thiazides, using a similar approach to that recommended for calcium oxalate stones. Because patients who form calcium phosphate stones may also have low urine citrate concentrations, alkali supplementation may be used with caution. Alkali supplementation often increases urine pH and therefore could increase the risk of calcium phosphate crystal formation.

SURGICAL MANAGEMENT OF STONES

In the acute setting, the urologist will assist in the management. If the stone does not pass rapidly, the patient can be sent home with appropriate oral analgesics, an α-blocker or calcium channel blocker to increase the likelihood of stone passage, and instructions to return in case of fever or uncontrollable pain. Most urologists wait several days before intervening for a ureteral stone unless one of the following conditions exists: urinary tract infection, stone greater than 6 mm in size, presence of an anatomic abnormality that would prevent passage, or intractable pain. A cystoscopically placed ureteral stent is typically used but requires anesthesia. The stent can be quite uncomfortable and not infrequently causes gross hematuria. Although it is debatable whether a stent helps with stone passage, the cystoscopy or stent placement may push the stone back up into the renal pelvis, thus relieving the obstruction and permitting its management on a nonemergent basis.

Stone size, location, and composition; the urinary tract anatomy; availability of technology; and the experience of the urologist determine the method of stone removal. Extracorporeal shock wave lithotripsy (ESWL) is the least invasive method. Cystoscopic stone removal, by either basket extraction or fragmentation, is invasive but more effective than ESWL, and newer instruments allow removal of stones even in the kidney. Percutaneous nephrostolithotomy, an approach requiring the placement of a nephrostomy tube, is more invasive but is necessary for large stone burdens and for kidney stones that cannot be removed cystoscopically; this is the gold standard for freeing a patient of stones. Open procedures such as ureterolithotomy or nephrolithotomy are rarely needed.

The surgical treatment of asymptomatic stones is controversial. The availability of ESWL has lowered the threshold for treating asymptomatic stones; most urologists consider treating only asymptomatic stones that are at least 1 cm in size.

With the increasing prevalence of obesity in the United States, the treatment of existing stones in morbidly obese individuals deserves mention. The ability to image the urinary tract may be limited if the patient's size prohibits access to scanning by CT. ESWL may not be an option, because morbid obesity can impede stone localization and the ability of the shock waves to reach the calculus; therefore, more invasive approaches, such as ureteroscopy, are used.

LONG-TERM FOLLOW-UP

The nephrologist or primary care provider should assume responsibility for the long-term prevention program and should consult with the urologist as needed for further surgical interventions. The plan should include recommendations for prevention based on the evaluation; interventions should be followed by repetition of the metabolic measurements to assess their success, adjustment of recommendations, and follow-up imaging.

Adherence to recommendations frequently declines over time. In addition, the long-term sequelae of the treatments and the underlying abnormalities may have other implications for the health of the patient. For example, individuals with higher urine calcium excretion typically have lower bone density and are at increased risk for osteoporosis. With appropriate attention and evaluation, the morbidity and cost of recurrent stone disease can be dramatically reduced.

BIBLIOGRAPHY

Borghi L, Schianchi T, Meschi T, et al: Comparison of two diets for the prevention of recurrent stones in idiopathic hypercalciuria. N Engl J Med 346:77-84, 2002.

Coe FL, Evan A, Worcester E: Kidney stone disease. J Clin Invest 115:2598-2608, 2005.

Coe FL, Favus MJ, Pak CY, et al (eds): Kidney Stones: Medical and Surgical Management. Philadelphia, Lippincott Williams & Wilkins, 1996.

Curhan GC, Willett WC, Rimm EB, Stampfer MJ: A prospective study of dietary calcium and other nutrients and the risk of symptomatic kidney stones. N Engl J Med 328:833-838, 1993.

Curhan GC, Willett WC, Speizer FE, Stampfer MJ: Beverage use and the risk for kidney stones in women. Ann Intern Med 128:534-540, 1998.

Evan AP, Lingeman JE, Coe FL, et al: Randall's plaque of patients with nephrolithiasis begins in basement membranes of thin loops of Henle. J Clin Invest 111:607-616, 2003.

Pearle MS, Calhoun EA, Curhan GC: Urolithiasis. In Litwin MS, Saigal CS (eds): Urologic Diseases in America. U.S. Department of Health and Human Services, Public Health Service, National Institutes of Health, National Institute of Diabetes and Digestive and Kidney Diseases. Washington, DC: U.S. Government Publishing Office, 2004, pp 3-39.

Taylor EN, Curhan GC: Differences in 24-hour urine composition between black and white women. J Am Soc Nephrol 18:654-659, 2007.

Taylor EN, Curhan GC: Oxalate intake and the risk for nephrolithiasis. J Am Soc Nephrol 18:2198-2204, 2007.

Taylor EN, Stampfer MJ, Curhan GC: Dietary factors and the risk of incident kidney stones in men: New insights after 14 years of follow-up. J Am Soc Nephrol 15:3225-3232, 2004.

Taylor EN, Stampfer MJ, Curhan GC: Obesity, weight gain, and the risk of kidney stones. JAMA 293:455-462, 2005.

Teichman JMH: Acute renal colic from ureteral calculus. N Engl J Med 350:684-693, 2004.

CHAPTER 48

Urinary Tract Infection

Lindsay E. Nicolle

Urinary tract infection (UTI) is the presence of microbial pathogens within the normally sterile urinary tract. Infections are overwhelmingly bacterial, although fungi, viruses, and parasites may occasionally be pathogens (**Table 48-1**). UTI is the most common bacterial infection in humans and can be either symptomatic or asymptomatic. Symptomatic infection is associated with a wide spectrum of morbidity, from mild irritative voiding symptoms to bacteremia, sepsis, and, occasionally, death.

Asymptomatic UTI is isolation of bacteria from urine in quantitative counts consistent with infection but without localizing genitourinary or systemic signs or symptoms attributable to the infection. It is often used interchangeably with the term *bacteriuria*, which simply means bacteria present in the urine but is generally used to imply isolation of a significant quantitative count of organisms. Recurrent UTI is common in individuals who experience an initial infection. It may be either a relapse (i.e., recurrence after therapy with the pretherapy isolate) or a reinfection (i.e., recurrence with a different organism). An important consideration in the management of UTI is whether the patient has a functionally or structurally normal genitourinary tract (uncomplicated UTI or acute nonobstructive pyelonephritis) or an abnormal tract (complicated UTI).

The microbiologic diagnosis of UTI requires isolation of a pathogenic organism in sufficient quantitative amounts from a urine specimen collected to minimize contamination with vaginal or periurethral organisms. A quantitative bacterial count of 10^5 colony-forming units per milliliter (CFU/mL) or higher is the usual standard to distinguish infection from organisms present as contaminants. Use of the quantitative urine culture is important in diagnosis of a UTI and description of the natural history, but the single quantitative standard of 10^5 CFU/mL is not currently considered valid for all potential clinical presentations.

ACUTE UNCOMPLICATED URINARY TRACT INFECTION

Acute uncomplicated UTI, or acute cystitis, is infection occurring in individuals with a normal genitourinary tract and no recent instrumentation. It is a common syndrome that occurs almost exclusively in women; 60% of all women experience at least one infection in their lifetime. The highest incidence is in young, sexually active women. Between 1% to 2% of women have frequent recurrent infections. Risk factors for infection in these women are both genetic and behavioral. Women with recurrent acute uncomplicated UTI are more likely to have first-degree female relatives with UTI and to be nonsecretors of blood group substances. Sexual activity is strongly associated with infection. The frequency of infection correlates with frequency of intercourse. The use of spermicides or a diaphragm for birth control also increases the risk of infection, but use of the birth control pill or condoms without spermicide does not. For young women, behavioral practices such as postvoid personal hygiene, type of underwear, postcoital voiding, and bathing rather than showering are not associated with infection. For postmenopausal women, frequency of sexual intercourse is not a risk factor for infection. The most important predictor of infection in older women is a history of prior UTI at a younger age.

Escherichia coli is isolated in 80% to 85% of episodes. *Staphylococcus saprophyticus,* a coagulase-negative staphylococcus, occurs in 5% to 10% of episodes. This organism is rarely isolated in any other clinical syndromes, and it has a unique seasonal variation, with increased occurrence in the late summer and early fall. *Klebsiella pneumoniae* and *Proteus mirabilis* are each isolated in 2% to 3% of cases. Organisms that cause infection originate from the normal gut flora, colonize the vagina and periurethral area, and ascend to the bladder. Women who experience this syndrome frequently have alterations in vaginal flora characterized by decreased or absent H_2O_2-producing lactobacilli, consequent increased

TABLE 48-1 Nonbacterial Pathogens That Cause Urinary Tract Infection

FUNGI	VIRUSES	PARASITES
Candida albicans	JC virus, BK virus	Schistosoma hematobium
Candida parapsilosis	Adenovirus types 11, 21	
Candida glabrata	Mumps	
Candida tropicalis	Hantavirus[†]	
Blastomyces dermatitidis*		
Aspergillus fumigatus*		
Cryptococcus neoformans*		
Histoplasma capsulatum*		

*With disseminated infection.
[†]Hemorrhagic fever and renal syndrome.

TABLE 48-3 Prophylactic Antimicrobial Therapy for Women with Frequent Recurrence of Acute Uncomplicated Urinary Tract Infection

	Regimen	
AGENT	**LONG-TERM**	**POSTCOITAL (ONE DOSE)**
TMP-SMX*	40/200 mg daily or 3 times/wk	40/200 mg
TMP*	100 mg daily	100 mg
Nitrofurantoin*	50-100 mg daily	50-100 mg
Cephalexin	125 mg daily	250 mg
Norfloxacin	200 mg every other day	200-400 mg
Ciprofloxacin	—	250 mg

TMP-SMX, trimethoprim-sulfamethoxazole.
*Recommended first-line agents.

TABLE 48-4 Abnormalities of the Genitourinary Tract Associated with Complicated Urinary Tract Infection

ABNORMALITY	EXAMPLES
Metabolic or structural	Medullary sponge kidney
	Nephrocalcinosis
	Malakoplakia
	Xanthogranulomatous pyelonephritis
Congenital	Cystic disease
	Duplicated drainage system with obstruction
	Urethral valves
Obstruction	Vesicoureteral reflux
	Pelvicalyceal obstruction
	Papillary necrosis
	Ureteral fibrosis or stricture
	Bladder diverticulum
	Neurogenic bladder
	Prostatic hypertrophy
	Tumors
	Urolithiasis
Instrumentation	Indwelling catheter
	Intermittent catheterization
	Cystoscopy
	Ureteric stent
Other	Nephrostomy tube
	Immunocompromised host
	Renal transplant recipient
	Neutropenia

of illness and concern about compliance with outpatient therapy. The parenteral antimicrobial treatment can usually be replaced by oral therapy once clinical improvement has occurred, usually by 48 to 72 hours. The urine culture results are also available by this time and will direct optimal selection of a specific oral antimicrobial agent for continuing therapy.

By 48 to 72 hours after initiation of effective antimicrobial therapy, there should be evidence of clinical improvement, including decreased costovertebral angle discomfort and a decrease in or resolution of fever. If there has been no improvement, an abnormality within the genitourinary tract causing urinary obstruction or abscess formation should be excluded. Women with early symptomatic recurrence after therapy should also be evaluated for a potential complicating abnormality of the genitourinary tract. An initial ultrasonographic examination is helpful to exclude obstruction, although it may not identify small stones. Computed tomography scanning is superior to ultrasonography for identifying small stones or an intrarenal abscess. The selection of an imaging approach should be individualized depending on presentation, clinical course, and access to diagnostic testing.

COMPLICATED URINARY TRACT INFECTION

The most important host defense preventing UTI is intermittent, unobstructed voiding of urine. Any abnormality of the genitourinary tract that impairs voiding may increase the frequency of UTI. UTI in individuals with structural or functional abnormalities of the urinary tract, including those who have undergone instrumentation, is considered to be "complicated" UTI (**Table 48-4**). The frequency of infection is determined by the underlying abnormality and is independent of gender or age. For some abnormalities, infection is infrequent but difficult to manage (e.g., an infected cyst in a patient with polycystic kidney disease). For others, infection is very frequent (e.g., 5% per day in patients with an indwelling catheter).

The clinical presentation of symptomatic complicated UTI varies along a spectrum from mild lower-tract irritative symptoms to systemic manifestations such as fever and even septic shock. Individuals who have complete obstruction of urine flow or mucosal bleeding are at greatest risk for the most severe clinical presentations. A quantitative count of organisms in the urine of 10^5 CFU/mL or greater remains the standard for microbiologic diagnosis of complicated UTI. The microbiology findings are characterized by a greater diversity of organisms and increased prevalence of antimicrobial resistance when compared with uncomplicated infection. Organisms isolated are less likely to express virulence factors, because the host abnormality of impaired voiding is itself sufficient for infection. Increased antimicrobial resistance is common in infecting organisms because of nosocomial acquisition or repeated prior courses of antimicrobial therapy for recurrent infection. If broad-spectrum antimicrobial therapy has been given for prolonged periods, reinfection may occur with yeast species or with highly resistant bacteria, such as some *Pseudomonas aeruginosa* strains.

Antimicrobial treatment is based on the clinical presentation, patient tolerance, and known or suspected susceptibilities of the infecting organism. If possible, antimicrobial therapy should be delayed until urine culture results are available. However, patients with moderate to severe symptoms usually require empiric therapy before culture results are available. The recent history of antimicrobial use and prior urine culture results in the individual patient are helpful in directing the choice of empiric therapy. Parenteral therapy may initially be required for ill patients with severe systemic manifestations, for those who cannot tolerate oral therapy, or if the infecting organism is suspected or known to be resistant to any available oral therapy. For patients with a clinical presentation of lower-tract symptoms, 7 days of therapy is usually adequate. If fever or other systemic symptoms are present, 10 to 14 days of therapy is recommended.

Complicated UTI can be prevented if the underlying genitourinary abnormality is corrected, and there is a high likelihood of recurrent infection if it cannot be corrected. For instance, 50% of patients with a neurogenic bladder and voiding managed by intermittent catheterization experience recurrent infection within 4 to 6 weeks after antimicrobial therapy. Prophylactic antimicrobials are not recommended, because long-term antimicrobial therapy has not been shown to decrease infections, and reinfection will be with organisms resistant to the antimicrobial agent given. In selected patients with frequent, severe symptomatic recurrences and an abnormality that cannot be corrected, long-term suppressive therapy may be considered. This therapy is individualized in every case. Full therapeutic antimicrobial doses are initiated and may subsequently be decreased to one-half the regular dose if the urine culture remains negative and the clinical course is satisfactory.

ASYMPTOMATIC URINARY TRACT INFECTION

The term *asymptomatic bacteriuria* refers to isolation of uropathogens in quantitative counts consistent with UTI ($\geq 10^5$ CFU/mL) in a patient who has no localizing genitourinary signs or symptoms. Pyuria is present in 50% to 90% of patients. Asymptomatic bacteriuria occurs with increased frequency in persons who also experience symptomatic UTI, suggesting that the biologic defect promoting UTI is similar. Asymptomatic infection, with or without pyuria, does not usually require treatment. Long-term cohort studies have not documented adverse effects attributable to bacteriuria, and prospective randomized trials have not reported clinical benefits of treatment. In fact, adverse antibiotic effects and reinfection with organisms of increased resistance are observed with treatment. The important exception to the recommendation for nontreatment is bacteriuria in pregnant women. Identification and treatment of asymptomatic bacteriuria in early pregnancy prevents pyelonephritis and negative fetal outcomes of premature delivery and low birth weight. Antimicrobial therapy is also indicated before an invasive genitourinary procedure; in this situation, however, prophylaxis is given to prevent perioperative sepsis rather than as treatment of asymptomatic bacteriuria.

SPECIAL POPULATIONS

Urinary Tract Infection in Children

UTI occurs more frequently in boys than in girls during the first year of life. Infection in boys often occurs before 3 months of age and may be associated with congenital anomalies of the urinary tract. The clinical presentation is usually of neonatal sepsis without localizing signs to the genitourinary tract, and these episodes are treated as neonatal sepsis. After the first year of life, UTI occurs more frequently in girls than in boys, and the clinical presentation is with genitourinary symptoms. Most episodes in girls are acute uncomplicated UTI, and these girls will also experience UTI more frequently as adults. Vesicoureteral reflux, which may lead to impaired kidney function, must be excluded for girls with recurrent UTI. Imaging studies, including voiding cystourethrography, ultrasonography, and technetium 99m–labeled dimercaptosuccinic acid (^{99m}Tc-DMSA) scanning are indicated for any child who presents with pyelonephritis, for a first UTI in a boy of any age or a girl younger than 3 years of age, for a second UTI in a girl older than 3 years, and for a first UTI at any age in a patient with a family history of urinary tract abnormalities, abnormal voiding, hypertension, or poor growth.

Treatment of acute lower-tract infection in young girls consists of 3 to 7 days of therapy. Pyelonephritis should be treated for 10 to 14 days. The antimicrobials used are similar to those used in adults, with appropriate dose adjustments for weight. The quinolones are not recommended for children younger than 16 years of age because of potential adverse effects on cartilage. Long-term low-dose prophylactic therapy is indicated for young girls who have frequent symptomatic recurrences or severe vesicoureteral reflux (grade IV or V) and recurrent UTIs. Asymptomatic UTI is common in schoolgirls. Treatment of asymptomatic UTI does not alter the natural history of kidney disease in young girls nor prevent renal scarring. In fact, treatment of asymptomatic bacteriuria with antimicrobial drugs appears to increase the frequency of symptomatic infection. Therefore, it is not recommended to screen for or treat asymptomatic bacteriuria in girls.

Urinary Tract Infection in Pregnancy

Hormonal changes in pregnancy produce hypotonicity of the autonomic musculature, leading to urine stasis. In addition, obstruction at the pelvic brim, more marked on the right than on the left side, occurs as the fetus enlarges. These changes are maximal at the beginning of the third trimester and probably explain the increased risk of pyelonephritis at this stage of gestation. Acute pyelonephritis may precipitate premature labor and delivery, as may any febrile illness in later pregnancy. Women who have asymptomatic bacteriuria in early pregnancy have as much as a 30% risk of developing acute pyelonephritis later in the pregnancy. Between 75% and 90% of episodes of acute pyelonephritis in pregnancy can be prevented by identification and treatment of asymptomatic bacteriuria early in pregnancy. Premature delivery and low birth rate are also prevented with treatment.

Because of these benefits of treatment of asymptomatic bacteriuria in pregnancy, all pregnant women should be screened for bacteriuria by urine culture at 12 to 16 weeks' gestation. If significant bacteriuria is identified, it should be confirmed with a second urine culture and, if confirmed, treated. The antimicrobial agent is selected with consideration for the susceptibilities of the infecting organism and safety of the drug for use in pregnancy. A 3-day course of amoxicillin, nitrofurantoin, or cephalexin is usually sufficient. TMP-SMX has been widely used and is effective, but it may be associated with increased fetal abnormalities when used in the first trimester and should be avoided early in pregnancy. Fluoroquinolones are contraindicated. Women with either symptomatic or asymptomatic infection treated in early pregnancy should be monitored with monthly urine cultures throughout the remainder of the pregnancy to identify recurrent infection. If a second episode occurs, it should be treated and low-dose prophylactic therapy, usually with nitrofurantoin or cephalexin, should be continued until delivery.

Urinary Tract Infection in Men

Men rarely present with acute uncomplicated UTI or acute nonobstructive pyelonephritis. Lack of circumcision, acquisition of infection from a sexual partner, and having sex with men are potential risk factors in the few cases that do occur. *E. coli* is the usual infecting organism. However, uncomplicated infection is so uncommon in men that any man presenting with UTI should be investigated for the possibility of an underlying abnormality. Pelvic and kidney ultrasonography is the most useful initial test.

Elderly men have an increased frequency of UTI due to prostatic hypertrophy leading to obstruction and turbulent urine flow. These men also develop chronic bacterial prostatitis. Once bacteria are established in the prostate, they are often impossible to eradicate, due to poor diffusion of antibiotics into the prostate and formation of prostate stones. The prostate then serves as a nidus for recurrent symptomatic or asymptomatic bladder infections. If recurrent symptomatic infections occur, suggesting chronic bacterial prostatitis, a more prolonged antimicrobial course of therapy (6 to 12 weeks) may increase the likelihood of long-term cure. TMP-SMX or fluoroquinolones are recommended first-line agents.

Urinary Tract Infection in the Elderly

UTI is the most common infection occurring in both ambulatory and institutionalized elderly populations. The prevalence of bacteriuria is 5% to 10% for women and 5% for men older than 65 years of age who are living in the community, and the prevalence increases with advancing age. In long-term care facilities, 25% to 50% of all elderly residents have asymptomatic bacteriuria at any given time. The prevalence increases with increasing functional impairment, including dementia and bladder and bowel incontinence.

Asymptomatic bacteriuria in elderly patients should not be treated with antimicrobials. Antimicrobial treatment does not decrease morbidity or mortality but is associated with increased adverse drug effects, increased cost, and increasing antimicrobial resistance. It follows that asymptomatic elderly populations should not be screened for bacteriuria.

The clinical presentation of symptomatic infection may be similar in the elderly to that in younger populations. However, the diagnosis may not be straightforward, particularly in the institutionalized or functionally impaired population. Difficulties in communication, comorbid illnesses with chronic symptoms, and the high frequency of asymptomatic bacteriuria all impair diagnostic acumen. A decreased fever response and lower frequency of leukocytosis characterize infection in the elderly, and acute confusion may be a prominent presenting symptom.

Antimicrobial selection for treatment of symptomatic UTI in elderly patients is similar to that in younger populations. The dosage should be adjusted for kidney function but not for age per se. The duration of treatment is also similar to that recommended for younger populations. Cure rates with any duration of therapy for older women are lower. Post-treatment urine cultures to document microbiologic cure are not recommended unless symptoms persist or recur. Some women with frequent, recurrent, symptomatic infections may have a decreased number of infections with the use of topical intravaginal estradiol, although this treatment is less effective for prevention than prophylactic antimicrobials. Systemic estrogen therapy does not prevent infections and, in several studies, has been associated with an increased risk of infection.

Urinary Tract Infection in Patients with Impaired Kidney Function

Treatment of UTI requires adequate concentrations of effective antimicrobial agents in the kidneys or urine. When kidney function is decreased, there is decreased excretion of antimicrobials into the urine, and anticipated urinary drug levels may not be achieved. With severe bilateral impairment, it is difficult to cure UTI. Antimicrobial agents such as nitrofurantoin and tetracyclines (other than doxycycline) are toxic in the presence of impaired kidney function and should be avoided. Aminoglycosides may not penetrate nonfunctioning kidneys sufficiently to provide effective therapy. The penicillins and cephalosporins, as well as fluoroquinolones, constitute effective treatment for most individuals with impaired kidney function. Dosage adjustments appropriate for the level of kidney function are necessary. In some situations, such as infected native kidneys in transplant recipients, infection cannot be eradicated and long-term suppressive therapy may be necessary to prevent frequent symptomatic recurrences.

If renal functional impairment is unilateral, the better-functioning kidney will preferentially excrete the antimicrobial. If the nonfunctioning kidney is infected, effective antimicrobial levels may not be achieved at the site of infection despite adequate levels in the excreted urine. This may explain relapsing infection in some individuals.

Fungal Urinary Tract Infection

Fungal UTI has been increasing in frequency. It is primarily a nosocomial infection and occurs in the setting of diabetes, indwelling urethral catheters, and intense broad-spectrum antimicrobial therapy. *Candida albicans* is the species most frequently isolated, but other *Candida* species, such as *glabrata, krusei, parapsilosis,* and *tropicalis,* also are observed. The clinical importance of fungal UTI is often difficult to assess, in part because the affected patients have multiple complex medical problems. If there are no symptoms, treatment is not necessary. If there is an indwelling urethral catheter, it should be discontinued if possible. Fungus balls may lead to obstruction and should be excluded in individuals with obstructive uropathy and candiduria or candidemia.

If repeated cultures have grown yeast organisms at concentrations of 10^4 CFU/mL or greater and there are symptoms referable to the genitourinary tract, funguria should be treated.

Fluconazole 100 to 400 mg/day for 7 days is recommended, because it is excreted in the urine and may be given as oral therapy. Itraconazole (100 to 400 mg/day), 5-fluorocytosine (50 to 150 mg/kg/day for 7 days), and amphotericin B have also been effective. There is limited experience with newer antifungal drugs such as caspofungin and voriconazole, but none of these agents are excreted in the urine. *Candida* species other than *C. albicans* are more likely to be resistant to fluconazole, and amphotericin B may be necessary for treatment. Amphotericin B bladder irrigation (50 mg/L continuously for 5 days) is no longer considered first-line therapy because it requires urethral catheterization and is no more effective than other therapeutic options. However, in selected situations, particularly in subjects with chronic renal failure and bladder infection, the washout method may still be useful. The cure rate with any treatment is only 70% to 75%, but assessment of outcome is often limited by serious accompanying illnesses.

BIBLIOGRAPHY

Bent S, Nallamothu BK, Simel DL, et al: Does this woman have an acute uncomplicated urinary tract infection? JAMA 287:2701-2710, 2002.

Cardenas DD, Hooton TM: Urinary tract infection in persons with spinal cord injury. Arch Phys Med Rehab 76:272, 1995.

Collins TR, Devries CR: Recurrent urinary tract infections in children: A logical approach to diagnosis, treatment, and long-term management. Compr Ther 23:44-48, 1997.

Fihn SD: Acute uncomplicated urinary tract infection in women. N Engl J Med: 349:259-266, 2003.

Hooton TM: The current management strategies for community-acquired urinary tract infection. Infect Dis Clin North Am 17:303-332, 2003.

Johnson JR: Microbial virulence determinants and the pathogenesis of urinary tract infection. Infect Dis Clin North Am 17:261-178, viii,2003.

Johnssen TE: The role of imaging in urinary tract infections. World J Urol 22:392-398, 2004.

Lipsky BA: Urinary tract infection in men: Epidemiology, pathophysiology, diagnosis, and treatment. Ann Intern Med 110:138-150, 1989.

Naber KG, Bishop MC, Bjerklund-Johansen TE, et al: Guidelines on the management of urinary and male genital tract infections. In Grabe M, Bishop MC, Bjerklund-Johansen, et al (eds): European Association of Urology: Guidelines, 2007 edition. ISBN-13:978-90-70244-59-D. Arnhem, The Netherlands, European Association of Urology, 2008, pp 1-126.

Nicolle LE: A practical guide to the management of complicated urinary tract infection. Drugs 53:583-592, 1997.

Nicolle LE: SHEA Long Term Care Committee. Urinary tract infections in long term care facilities. Infect Control Hosp Epidemiol 22:167-175, 2001.

Nicolle LE, Bradley S, Colgan R, et al: Infectious Diseases Society of America guidelines for the diagnosis and treatment of asymptomatic bacteriuria in adults. Clin Infect Dis 40:643-654, 2005.

Schaeffer AJ: Chronic prostatitis and the chronic pelvic pain syndrome. N Engl J Med 355:1690-1698, 2006.

Sobel JD, Kauffman CA, McKinsey D, et al: Candiduria: A randomized, double-blind study of treatment with fluconazole or placebo. The National Institute of Allergy and Infectious Diseases Mycoses Study Group. Clin Infect Dis 30:19-24, 2000.

Stapleton A: Novel approaches to prevention of urinary tract infections. Infect Dis Clin North Am 17:457-471, 2003.

Warren JW: Catheter-associated urinary tract infections. Infect Dis Clin North Am 11:609-622, 1997.

Warren JW, Abrutyn E, Hebel JR, et al: Guidelines for antimicrobial therapy of uncomplicated acute bacterial cystitis and acute pyelonephritis in women. Clin Infect Dis 29:745-758, 1999.

The Kidney in Special Circumstances

CHAPTER 49

The Kidney in Infants and Children

Sharon Phillips Andreoli

KIDNEY DEVELOPMENT AND MATURATION

The development of the kidney in utero begins at approximately 5 to 6 weeks of gestation, with the first metanephric glomeruli appearing at 9 weeks' gestation. Nephron formation proceeds until 34 to 36 weeks of gestation, when nephrogenesis is complete. Full-term neonates are born with their full complement of nephrons, whereas premature infants are born with less than the full complement, depending on their gestational age at the time of birth. As described later, prenatal and postnatal insults in premature neonates may interfere with nephron development and lead to interrupted nephrogenesis, setting the stage for kidney complications in later life. Although the full-term newborn has the same number of nephrons as an adult, the kidney of the newborn is anatomically and physiologically quite immature compared to the adult kidney. The deeper glomeruli are the most mature, because they are formed first; the cortical glomeruli are formed last. Fetal urine is produced at 10 weeks' gestation, and aminotic fluid is largely composed of fetal urine. Decreased in utero urine production resulting from severe renal dysplasia, cystic kidney disease, obstructive uropathy, or other renal diseases can cause oligohydramnios and Potter's syndrome, which consists of pulmonary hypoplasia, flattened nasal bridge, low-set ears, and joint contractures due to fetal constraint. Severe pulmonary hypoplasia from oligohydramnios can be lethal.

The full-term newborn kidney measures 4 to 5 cm in length and continues to grow, reaching 10 to 12 cm by adolescence. The glomerular filtration rate (GFR) is low in the full-term newborn and rises to approximately 50 mL/min/1.73 m^2 by the end of the first week of life. The GFR continues to increase in the infant and reaches approximately 100 to 130 mL/min/1.73 m^2 at 2 years of age. The most common method of calculating GFR in the child is with the Schwartz formula:

$$GFR = k \times L/SCr$$

where k is a constant (0.33 in the preterm neonate, 0.45 in the term neonate, 0.55 in children in the first decade of life and adolescent girls, and 0.70 in adolescent boys); L is the length of the infant or height of the child or adolescent in centimeters; and SCr is the serum creatinine concentration measured in milligrams per deciliter. The normal creatinine value in children is lower than in the adult and is age and gender dependent. The creatinine concentration increases throughout childhood as the child's muscle mass increases with growth; normal values for serum creatinine for girls and boys are shown in **Figure 49-1**.

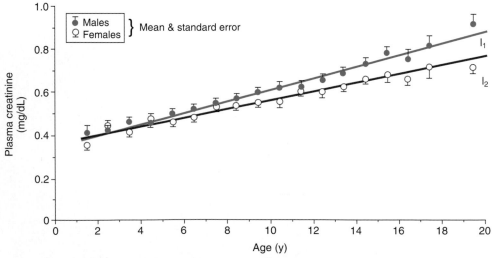

FIGURE 49-1 Normal plasma creatinine values for males and females according to age. Normal plasma creatinine values gradually increase with age. (From Schwartz GJ, Brion LP, Spitzer A: The use of plasma creatinine concentration for estimating glomerular filtration rate in infants, children, and adolescents. Pediatr Clin North Am 34:571-590, 1987.)

FLUID AND ELECTROLYTE BALANCE

The physiologic development of the kidney is also not complete at the time of birth in the full-term neonate. The ability of the kidney to concentrate urine is decreased for several reasons, including immature tubules with a lower response to antidiuretic stimuli. The ability to concentrate urine increases throughout the first year of life. The maximum urine osmolality is 400 to 500 mOsm/L in premature neonates and 500 to 600 mOsm/L in full-term neonates; it reaches approximately 1100 mOsm/L by 12 months of age. Similarly, premature neonates are unable to conserve sodium normally. The fractional excretion of sodium (FE_{Na}) is a percentage calculated by the formula

$$FE_{Na} = (U_{Na}/S_{Na}) \times (S_{Cr}/U_{Cr}) \times 100$$

where U is the urinary concentration of a substance, S is its serum concentration, Na is sodium, and Cr is creatinine. The FE_{Na} is higher in premature infants compared to full term neonates at any given level of sodium intake. The mechanism for sodium wasting in premature infants is thought to be related to the inability of the tubules to respond to aldosterone. Sodium requirements for growth are 2 to 3 mEq/kg/day in normal neonates and higher in the premature infant.

The normal range for serum potassium levels is slightly higher in neonates than in adults, and children require approximately 2 mEq/kg/day of potassium for normal growth. The normal serum calcium level is slightly lower in neonates (7 to 10 mEq/L) than in children (8.5 to 10.5 mEq/L). In contrast, the normal range for serum phosphorus is 4 to 9 mg/dL in neonates, 4 to 6.5 mg/dL in infants, 3.5 to 6.8 mg/dL in children in the first decade of life, and 3.0 to 4.5 mg/dL in older children and adolescents. Newborns are also unable to maximally reabsorb sodium bicarbonate due to immature tubular function, and newborns have a physiologic renal tubular acidosis which is further accentuated with prematurity.

The threshold for reabsorption of bicarbonate is approximately 18 mEq/L for premature neonates and 21 mEq/L for full-term neonates. The normal threshold of 22 to 26 mEq/L is reached by 1 year of age.

ACUTE KIDNEY INJURY

The causes of acute kidney injury (AKI) in the infant and child are substantially different than in the adult patient. The more common causes are listed in **Table 49-1** by age. Some causes of AKI, such as cortical necrosis and renal vein thrombosis, occur much more commonly in neonates, whereas hemolytic uremic syndrome (HUS) is more frequent in young children, and rapidly progressive glomerulonephritis (RPGN) typically occurs in older children and adolescents. An important cause of AKI in neonates is exposure to drugs in utero that interfere with nephrogenesis, such as angiotensin-converting enzyme inhibitors, angiotensin receptor blockers, and nonsteroidal anti-inflammatory drugs (NSAIDs). Hypoxic/ischemic AKI is relatively common at any age; it is listed under vascular and tubulointerstitial diseases because the pathophysiology is characterized by an initial vascular component and a later tubular cell necrosis.

With some diseases, such as the tumor lysis syndrome, drug-induced interstitial nephritis, aminoglycoside nephrotoxicity, and other toxic nephropathies, recovery from AKI is usual; other diseases, such as RPGN, may manifest as AKI but persist as chronic kidney disease (CKD). Several renal diseases, such as HUS, Henoch-Schönlein purpura, and obstructive uropathy with associated renal dysplasia, may manifest as AKI and show improvement of renal function to normal or near-normal levels with therapy, but after the initial recovery the child's renal function may slowly deteriorate, leading to CKD in later life. As described later, children with a history of AKI from any cause (with the exception of acute postinfectious glomerulonephritis) need long-term

---

TABLE 49-1	Common Causes of Acute Kidney Injury According to Age Group		
AGE (YR)	**GLOMERULAR DISEASES**	**VASCULAR DISEASES**	**DEVELOPMENTAL/TUBULOINTERSTITIAL DISEASES**
≤2	—	Cortical necrosis Renal artery thrombosis Renal vein thrombosis Hypoxic/ischemic AKI	In utero exposure to ACE inhibitors, ARBs, NSAIDs Obstructive uropathy Dysplastic kidneys Hypoxic/ischemic AKI Nephrotoxic AKI
2-6	Postinfectious GN HSP	HUS Hypoxic/ischemic AKI	Obstructive uropathy Hypoxic/ischemic AKI Nephrotoxic AKI Tumor lysis syndrome
6-12	Postinfectious GN HSP RPGN	HUS Hypoxic/ischemic AKI	Obstructive uropathy Hypoxic/ischemic AKI Nephrotoxic AKI Tumor lysis syndrome Interstitial nephritis
12-18	RPGN SLE HSP	—	Obstructive uropathy Hypoxic/ischemic AKI Nephrotoxic AKI Interstitial nephritis

ACE, angiotensin-converting enzyme; AKI, acute kidney injury; ARBs, angiotensin receptor blockers; HSP, Henoch-Schönlein purpura; HUS, hemolytic uremic syndrome; GN, glomerulonephritis; NSAIDs, nonsteroidal anti-inflammatory drugs; RPGN, rapidly progressive glomerulonephritis; SLE, systemic lupus erythematosus.

follow up and are at risk for CKD in later childhood or as adults.

The incidence of AKI in pediatric patients appears to be increasing. Over the past several decades, the etiology of AKI in children has shifted from primary renal disease to multifactorial causes including hypoxic, ischemic, nephrotoxic, and other insults, particularly in hospitalized children. Very low birth weight (<1500 g), a low Apgar score, a patent ductus arteriosus, and maternal administration of antibiotics and NSAIDs have each been associated with the development of AKI. Although environmental factors are important, some children may also be genetically predisposed to develop AKI. For example, in newborns, the frequency of a combination of genetic polymorphisms involved in the inflammatory response was greater in newborns with AKI. A similar result was found with a genetic polymorphism of heat shock proteins.

Oliguria is defined as urine output less than 1 mL/kg/hr in infants and young children and less than 0.5 to 1 mL/kg/hr in older children. As described earlier, several urinary parameters, including the ability to concentrate the urine or to conserve sodium, are decreased in the full-term infant and are further depressed in the premature newborn. This must be taken into account when using urinary indices to differentiate prerenal causes of AKI from intrinsic renal disease in newborns. In older children whose renal tubules are working appropriately, prerenal azotemia is suggested if the urine osmolality is greater than 400 to 500 mOsm/L, the urine sodium is less than 10 to 20 mEq/L, and the FE_{Na} is less than 1%. The corresponding values suggestive of renal hypoperfusion in the newborn are urine osmolality greater than 350 mOsm/L, urine sodium less than 20 to 30 mEq/L, and FE_{Na} less than 2.5%. If the renal tubules have sustained injury, as occurs in acute tubular necrosis, they cannot conserve sodium and water appropriately, so that the urine osmolality is less than 350 mOsm/L, the urine sodium concentration is greater than 30 to 40 mEq/L, and the FE_{Na} is greater than 2.0% to 3.0%. These values are further accentuated in premature newborns with AKI.

In the past, it was thought that AKI from hypoxic/ischemic and nephrotoxic insults was typically reversible, with full return of kidney function to normal the rule. However, it is now known that hypoxic/ischemic insults can lead to CKD. Importantly, AKI is likely to be particularly deleterious if the kidney is not yet grown to adult size or before the full complement of nephrons have been developed. As described earlier, nephrogenesis is not complete until 34 to 36 weeks' gestation, and AKI during this interval might lead to a decreased nephron number. AKI can interfere with the completion of nephrogenesis. Some premature infants develop nephromegaly and decreased nephron number after AKI. Similarly, AKI in the full-term neonate is associated with impaired kidney function later in life, and studies in older children have shown that AKI leads to CKD in a higher percentage of children than previously appreciated. Therefore, children with a history of AKI need long-term follow-up and are at risk for CKD as adults.

A relatively common cause of AKI in children that is rare in adults is diarrhea-positive HUS, which occurs in association with hemorrhagic colitis from infection with *Escherichia coli* O157:H7 (see Chapter 28). HUS is a systemic disease in which the kidney and gastrointestinal tract are the organs most commonly affected; however, evidence of central nervous system, pancreatic, skeletal, and myocardial involvement may also be present. Gastrointestinal involvement may lead to rectal prolapse, ischemic colitis, and transmural colonic necrosis. Pancreatic involvement, manifested as elevated pancreatic enzymes, occurs in 10% to 20% of affected children, and glucose intolerance due to pancreatic islet cell involvement occurs in fewer than 10% of children. Central nervous system disease may manifest as seizures, coma, lethargy, and irritability. Laboratory studies demonstrate the characteristic triad of HUS: microangiopathic hemolytic anemia, thrombocytopenia, and renal disease. The renal disorder is manifested as hematuria or proteinuria with elevated blood urea nitrogen (BUN) and creatinine in most cases. The role of the administration of antibiotics to children with hemorrhagic colitis associated with Shiga toxin–producing *E. coli* is controversial. Some studies have suggested that antibiotic therapy precipitates HUS, but a meta-analysis failed to demonstrate an adverse effect. Antimotility agents are clearly not indicated, because they may increase the systemic absorption of toxin due to the slower gastrointestinal transit time. Currently, therapy for HUS is only supportive. Oliguria and anuria occur in about 30% to 50% of affected children, and 40% to 75% of children with HUS will need dialysis therapy. In some children, HUS leads to substantial long-term complications, including CKD due to irreversible damage to glomeruli that may not become apparent until adulthood.

Any form of severe glomerulonephritis may manifest as AKI and RPGN. The clinical features include hypertension, edema, hematuria that is typically gross, and rapidly rising BUN and creatinine concentrations. For example, acute postinfectious glomerulonephritis can cause AKI, typically occurring in late childhood and early adolescence, but it has an excellent long-term prognosis and does not typically lead to CKD. In contrast, RPGN secondary to antineutrophil cytoplasmic antibody (ANCA)-positive glomerulonephritis, systemic lupus erythematosus, Goodpasture's syndrome, or idiopathic RPGN typically manifests with AKI and may persist as CKD. Serologic tests including complement studies and titers for ANCA, antineutrophil antibodies, and anti-glomerular basement membrane antibodies may be required to evaluate the cause of AKI with glomerulonephritis. Because specific therapy depends on the pathologic findings, a biopsy should be performed promptly if a child presents with AKI and RPGN.

CHRONIC KIDNEY DISEASE

The causes of CKD in the infant, child, and adolescent are markedly different from those in adult patients. Diabetes and hypertensive nephrosclerosis are distinctly unusual causes, accounting for fewer than 0.1% of the cases of stage 5 CKD in children. **Table 49-2** lists the common causes of CKD in

TABLE 49-2 Common Causes of Chronic Kidney Disease According to Age Group

AGE (YR)	GLOMERULAR DISEASES	VASCULAR DISEASES	TUBULOINTERSTITIAL DISEASES	CYSTIC DISEASES
≤2	Congenital nephrotic syndrome	Cortical necrosis Renal artery thrombosis Renal vein thrombosis	Obstructive uropathy Dysplastic kidneys Prune-belly syndrome Reflux nephropathy	ARPKD
2-6	—	HUS	Obstructive uropathy Dysplastic kidneys Prune-belly syndrome Reflux nephropathy	ARPKD
6-12	FSGS Primary GN MPGN types I, II, III	HUS	Obstructive uropathy Dysplastic kidneys Prune-belly syndrome Reflux nephropathy Cystinosis	ARPKD Juvenile nephronophthisis
12-18	FSGS Primary GN SLE MPGN types I, II, III	—	Obstructive uropathy Dysplastic kidneys Prune-belly syndrome Reflux nephropathy Cystinosis	Juvenile nephronophthisis

ARPKD, autosomal recessive polycystic kidney disease; FSGS, focal segmental glomerulosclerosis; GN, glomerulonephritis; HUS, hemolytic uremic syndrome; MPGN, membranoproliferative glomerulonephritis; SLE, systemic lupus erythematosus.

children according to age. Younger children are more likely to have a renal dysplasia (with or without obstructive uropathy) or cystic kidney disease, whereas in older children primary renal disease (including focal segmental glomerulosclerosis) and primary and secondary glomerulonephritides are more common causes of CKD.

Compared with adults, children are more commonly treated with peritoneal dialysis or kidney transplantation as the initial therapy for end-stage renal disease (ESRD). However, the use of hemodialysis is increasing, and, according to the most recent North American Pediatric Renal Trial Cooperative Study, almost 60% of children with ESRD were receiving hemodialysis as renal replacement therapy. Like adults, children with CKD have comorbidities affecting their quality of life, morbidity, and mortality. The pediatric patient with CKD has a cumulative higher exposure to the abnormal milieu of CKD, compared with an adult patient. Therefore, pediatric patients with CKD have a substantial risk for complications of CKD.

Although cardiovascular disease as a comorbid condition is less prevalent in children than in adults with CKD, cardiovascular events are still an important cause of morbidity and mortality, and the death rate among children with CKD is 1000 times the rate in the general population. Anemia is treated with recombinant human erythropoietin and oral or intravenous iron therapy. Because children have growing skeletons, renal bone disease is an important complication of CKD that contributes substantially to morbidity. In many children, symptoms are minor to absent. Others develop bone pain, skeletal deformities, and slipped epiphyses. High-turnover bone lesions are associated with secondary and tertiary hyperparathyroidism, whereas low-turnover bone disease is associated with suppressed parathyroid activity. The pathogenesis of hyperparathyroid bone disease is multifactorial and is related to phosphate retention, decreased synthesis

of 1,25-dihydroxyvitamin D, decreased intestinal absorption of calcium, increased parathyroid gland activity, and alterations in the calcium sensing receptor (see Chapter 58).

Growth failure is a common complication of CKD in children. The pathogenesis is complex and multifactorial and includes poorly controlled bone disease, inadequate nutrition, chronic acidosis, and abnormalities of the growth hormone axis. Despite adequate nutrition and good control of bone disease and acid-base balance, many children remain substantially growth retarded. Treatment with human recombinant growth hormone accelerates growth, induces persistent catch-up growth, and can lead to normal adult height in children with CKD. Indications for growth hormone therapy include a height below the 3rd percentile or a declining growth velocity. Complications of growth hormone therapy are rare but include glucose intolerance, hyperinsulinemia, pseudotumor cerebri, and exacerbation of poorly controlled renal bone disease. Growth hormone is also beneficial in the child with growth failure after renal transplantation.

NORMAL BLOOD PRESSURE AND HYPERTENSION

When measuring the blood pressure of an infant or child, it is important to use age- and size-appropriate measurement devices. The cuff should cover at least two thirds of the upper arm and the bladder should encircle 80% to 100% of the circumference of the arm (**Table 49-3**). Automated devices based on oscillometric methods are commonly used in newborns and young infants.

The normal range for blood pressure is lower in children than in adults. Because blood pressure increases with age and with body size, it is essential to interpret the measurements according to normal values for age, gender, and height, as recommended by the Fourth Report on the Diagnosis,

CHAPTER 50

The Kidney in Pregnancy

Phyllis August and Tiina Podymow

Pregnancy, in the setting of significant maternal kidney disease, is hazardous and frequently unsuccessful. Pregnancy imposes a hemodynamic strain on the maternal kidney; in some cases, kidney function deteriorates irreversibly in women with preexisting kidney disease during or after pregnancy. Alterations in immune function and increased inflammation associated with pregnancy may also contribute to worsening of kidney disease during gestation. In general, the closer to normal the glomerular filtration rate (GFR) and blood pressure, the greater the likelihood of successful pregnancy. Management of gravidas with kidney disease may be complicated and requires an understanding of the physiologic changes associated with pregnancy as well as close cooperation between obstetrician and nephrologist.

KIDNEY ANATOMY AND PHYSIOLOGY IN PREGNANCY

Anatomic and Functional Changes in the Urinary Tract

Kidney length increases by approximately 1 cm during normal gestation, and overall kidney volume increases by up to 30%. The major anatomic alterations of the urinary tract during pregnancy occur in the collecting system, where calyces, renal pelves, and ureters dilate, often giving the erroneous impression of obstructive uropathy. The cause of the ureteral dilation is disputed and has been attributed to hormonal mechanisms or to mechanical obstruction by the enlarging uterus. These morphologic changes result in stasis in the urinary tract and a propensity of pregnant women with asymptomatic bacteriuria to develop pyelonephritis, especially if they have a history of prior urinary tract infection.

Renal Hemodynamics

Pregnancy is characterized by marked generalized vasodilatation, which is detectable early in the first trimester (by 6 weeks' gestation). This early vasodilation is accompanied by a decrease in blood pressure, am increase in cardiac output, and increases in renal plasma flow and GFR, all of which persist until late gestation. Because renal plasma flow increases slightly more than GFR, the filtration fraction remains constant or is slightly reduced in pregnancy. Increases in blood flow and GFR reach a maximum during the first trimester and are approximately 50% greater than nonpregnant levels. Increased progesterone, estrogen, nitric oxide, prostacyclin, vascular endothelial growth factor (VEGF), placental hormones, and relaxin have all been implicated as mediators of the systemic and renal vasodilation of pregnancy. Although GFR is significantly increased throughout the duration of normal pregnancy, there is little evidence for increased intraglomerular pressure.

Creatinine production is unchanged during pregnancy, so the increase in clearance results in decreased serum creatinine levels. There is also increased excretion of glucose, amino acids, calcium, and urinary protein, resulting in an increase in the upper limit of normal for urinary protein excretion (from 150 to 300 mg/day).

Acid-Base Regulation in Pregnancy

In the resting state, pregnant women have increased respiratory rate, tidal volume, and alveolar ventilation, resulting in a reduced arterial carbon dioxide tension (P_{CO_2}). Augmented respiratory sensitivity in pregnancy has been attributed to the increased circulating level of progesterone, which directly stimulates the medullary respiratory center. There is a partially compensated respiratory alkalosis, with reductions in hydrogen ion concentration, P_{CO_2}, and serum bicarbonate, which are apparent in the first trimester. Finally, it should be appreciated that a "normal" P_{CO_2} of 40 mm Hg would signify considerable carbon dioxide retention in a pregnant woman.

Water Metabolism

Pregnancy is associated with a decrease in serum sodium and plasma osmolality, to values 5 to 10 mOsm/kg below those of nongravid women. This decrease in plasma osmolality is associated with appropriate responses to water loading and dehydration and suggests resetting of the osmoreceptor system and thirst to a lower serum osmolality. Clinical studies demonstrating decreased osmotic thresholds for thirst and for release of arginine vasopressin (AVP) in pregnant women support this hypothesis. In addition, pregnant women metabolize AVP more rapidly as a consequence of vasopressinases produced by the placenta. Some pregnant women develop diabetes insipidus because of the increased metabolism of AVP. This disorder may be treated with desmopressin acetate (dDAVP), a synthetic analogue of AVP that is resistant to the circulating vasopressinases because of its altered N-terminus.

Volume Regulation

Total body water increases by 6 to 8 L during pregnancy, and 4 to 6 L of the increase is extracellular. Plasma volume increases by 50% during gestation, with the largest rate of increment occurring in midpregnancy. There is a gradual cumulative retention of about 900 mEq of sodium, which is distributed between the products of conception and the maternal extracellular space. Despite the increase in plasma volume, there is no evidence for a hypervolemic (i.e., overfilled) circulation state during pregnancy. Indeed, the marked vasodilation that is observed as early as the first trimester may be the stimulus for increased sodium retention and increased plasma volume. The observations that blood pressure is significantly lower and that the renin-angiotensin system (RAS) is stimulated during normal pregnancy are consistent with a primary vasodilation that precedes and causes the increase in plasma volume.

Blood Pressure Regulation

Normal pregnancy is characterized by generalized vasodilation so marked that, despite increases in cardiac output and plasma volume in the range of 40%, mean arterial pressure decreases by approximately 10 mm. Reduced blood pressure is apparent in the first trimester, reaches a nadir at midpregnancy, and then increases gradually to approach prepregnancy values at term. The RAS is markedly stimulated in pregnancy. Increases in plasma renin activity are apparent early in pregnancy and reach a maxim by midpregnancy of about four times the nonpregnant values. The increase in plasma renin activity is accompanied by increases in aldosterone secretion. Despite the increased renin and aldosterone levels, blood pressure and electrolytes are normal during pregnancy. Indeed, normotensive gravidas demonstrate exaggerated responses to acute angiotensin-converting enzyme (ACE) inhibition, suggesting that the stimulated RAS is an important defense against hypotension during pregnancy.

Assessment of Kidney Function in Pregnancy

GFR and creatinine clearance increase by 40% to 65% in pregnancy. Creatinine production is unchanged, so increments in clearance result in decreased serum creatinine levels. Calculation of GFR by serum creatinine–based formulas are confounded by increasing maternal weight which is not muscle weight, and neither the Modification of Diet in Renal Disease (MDRD) nor the Cockcroft-Gault GFR estimates have been validated in pregnancy.

The gold standard for evaluation of abnormal proteinuria in pregnancy is the 24-hour urine protein measurement. A 24-hour protein excretion of greater than 300 mg is abnormal in pregnancy and correlates with a urine dipstick 1+ protein measurement. Although urine dipstick testing is commonly used to detect proteinuria, it is susceptible to error because of variations in urine concentration; therefore, if the level of suspicion is high, 24-hour urine testing should be performed. The ratio of total protein to creatinine ratio has been shown to accurately estimate 24-hour urine protein excretion in nonpregnant patients, but in pregnancy it does not adequately exclude the equivalent of 0.3 g/24 hr proteinuria and underestimates severe proteinuria.

HYPERTENSIVE DISORDERS OF PREGNANCY

Hypertension in pregnancy is defined as a blood pressure of 140/90 mm Hg or greater (Korotkoff V). In the United States, approximately 8% to 10% of all pregnancies are complicated by hypertension, with half of these cases attributable to the pregnancy-specific disorder known as preeclampsia. The four types of hypertensive disorders in pregnancy are preeclampsia, chronic hypertension, chronic hypertension with superimposed preeclampsia, and gestational hypertension.

Preeclampsia

Preeclampsia is a maternal syndrome characterized by hypertension, proteinuria, and edema, at times accompanied by coagulation and liver function abnormalities, and a fetal syndrome characterized by poor placentation, growth restriction, and, in rare cases, death. The characteristic renal histologic lesion seen in preeclampsia is called *glomerular capillary endotheliosis*. The glomerular capillary endothelial cells are swollen, and the appearance is that of a "bloodless glomerulus." Several alterations in kidney function occur in women with preeclampsia, although preeclampsia is rarely associated with significant impairment in kidney function. Both GFR and renal plasma flow are reduced in preeclampsia, by an average of about 25% in most instances. Nonetheless, GFR remains above pregravid values in most cases. Serum creatinine is therefore usually in the range of 0.8 to 1.2 mg/dL in women with preeclampsia; although these values are within normal range for nonpregnant women, they are above normal in pregnancy. Increased proteinuria is an important feature of preeclampsia, and if proteinuria is absent, the diagnosis should be strongly questioned.

Changes occur in the renal handling of other solutes in preeclampsia. There is decreased uric acid clearance accompanied by an increase in blood levels, which may precede other clinical signs of the disease. In pregnancy, serum urate levels greater than 4.5 mg/dL should raise the index of suspicion for preeclampsia. The level of hyperuricemia may correlate with the severity of the preeclamptic renal lesion. Calcium handling is also altered. Marked hypocalciuria is often observed, possibly as a result of increased proximal and distal tubular reabsorption, which may be mediated by excess parathyroid hormone.

Current research suggests that the pathogenesis of preeclampsia involves release of excessive amounts of a splice variant of a receptor for VEGF, called soluble fms-like tyrosine kinase 1 (sFlt-1), from the placenta into the maternal circulation. This leads to decreased bioavailability of VEGF, maternal vascular endothelial cell dysfunction, and the characteristic clinical features such as hypertension and proteinuria. Administration of sFlt-1 to pregnant rats recapitulates the classic renal histologic findings of glomerular endotheliosis.

Eclampsia is the convulsive form of preeclampsia. The pathogenesis of the eclamptic seizure is not well understood. It may be a variant of hypertensive encephalopathy, although seizures may occur in women with only moderately elevated blood pressure. Seizures may develop antepartum or in the immediate postpartum period. Rarely, eclamptic seizures occur as remotely as 2 weeks after deliver ("late postpartum eclampsia"). Preeclampsia usually develops in the third trimester, less frequently in the second trimester, and extremely rarely as early as 20 weeks' gestation. The syndrome is more common in nulliparous women. Preexisting kidney disease, hypertension, diabetes, and obesity also increase risk. Additional risk factors include multiple gestations, positive family history, extremes of reproductive age, and hydatidiform mole. Thrombophilic disorders, particularly the factor V Leiden mutation, and anti-phospholipid antibody (APA) syndrome are also associated with an increased risk of preeclampsia. Preeclampsia that develops close to term in a previously healthy nulliparous woman is not likely to recur. However, women with early, severe preeclampsia, particularly those who are multiparous, may have a recurrence rate as high as 50%.

Management of Preeclampsia

Management of preeclampsia includes accurate early diagnosis, bed rest, judicious use of antihypertensive therapy, close monitoring of maternal and fetal condition, prevention of convulsions with magnesium sulfate, and appropriately timed delivery. Once the diagnosis of preeclampsia is suspected, hospitalization is advisable in all but the mildest cases. Rest is an important aspect of therapy, because it improves uteroplacental perfusion. Delivery should be considered in all cases at term and in cases remote from term if there are signs of impending eclampsia (hyperreflexia, headaches, epigastric pain) or uncontrollable blood pressure elevation. Most obstetricians also consider the development of significant thrombocytopenia (platelet count <100,000/μL) or elevated liver enzymes (features of the HELLP syndrome, discussed later) to be an indication for delivery. The rationale for lowering blood pressure is to prevent the adverse consequences of accelerated hypertension in the mother. Lowering blood pressure does not "cure" preeclampsia, and there is even some concern that aggressive lowering of blood pressure may compromise uteroplacental perfusion, which could be hazardous to fetal well-being. Although there is no consensus as

TABLE 50-1 **Antihypertensive Therapy in Preeclampsia**

DELIVERY IMMINENT	DELIVERY POSTPONED
Hydralazine (IV, IM)	Methyldopa
Labetalol (IV)	Labetalol, other β-blockers
Calcium channel blockers	Calcium channel blockers
Diazoxide (IV; rarely used)	Hydralazine
	α-blockers
	Clonidine

to what level of blood pressure should be treated in women with preeclampsia, levels that exceed 150/100 mm Hg may be hazardous in women who previously had low-normal blood pressures. Parenteral therapy is recommended if delivery is likely to take place within the next 24 hours (**Table 50-1**). If it appears that delivery can be safely postponed, an oral agent is advisable.

There is strong evidence from randomized trials to support the use of magnesium sulfate for prevention and treatment of eclampsia. This agent reduces the incidence of eclampsia in women with preeclampsia and lowers the risk of maternal death in women with eclampsia. It is superior to other agents such as phenytoin and diazepam. Although it is not considered to be an antihypertensive agent, it does lower blood pressure to a mild degree in some women. It is usually prescribed immediately after delivery, because convulsions are most likely to occur in the immediate postpartum period. Magnesium is rarely administered before delivery. It can not only slow the progress of labor but also complicate anesthesia and intraoperative monitoring during cesarean section.

Prevention of Preeclampsia

Many strategies have been investigated in well-conducted clinical trials (involving thousands of women) of antiplatelet therapy, nutritional supplementation, and antioxidant vitamins for the prevention of preeclampsia. These trials and subsequent meta-analyses demonstrated a small benefit (10% to 15% reduction in relative risk) for low-dose aspirin in the prevention of preeclampsia and meaningful adverse maternal and fetal outcomes. With respect to nutritional strategies, calcium supplementation appeared to have a small benefit in women who had a low-calcium diet at baseline but not much benefit in those consuming normal amounts of calcium. In two large, randomized, controlled trials, antioxidant supplementation with vitamins C and E did not demonstrate benefit.

Chronic Hypertension

Most women with stage 1 or 2 essential hypertension do well during pregnancy, although they are at increased risk (as high as 25%) for the development of superimposed preeclampsia. Preexisting maternal hypertension is also associated with increased risks of placental abruption, intrauterine growth restriction, and mid-trimester fetal death. Women with chronic hypertension often have reductions in blood pressure into the normal range by the end of the first trimester. A failure of this reduction to occur or an increase in blood pressure during the early or mid-trimester indicates a guarded prognosis for the pregnancy. Fetal outcome is certainly worse in hypertensive women with superimposed preeclampsia, compared with previously normotensive women who develop preeclampsia. Chronic hypertension with superimposed preeclampsia also seems to be responsible for most cases of cerebral hemorrhage in pregnancy.

The treatment of chronic hypertension during pregnancy differs from the approach in the nonpregnant individual. During pregnancy, the concern is preservation of maternal health during the period of gestation and maintenance of a favorable intrauterine environment to allow fetal maturity while minimizing fetal exposure to potentially harmful drugs. Few data support a specific target level of blood pressure that should be attained during pregnancy. There are also no data to suggest that maintaining blood pressure levels close to normal prevents the development of superimposed preeclampsia. Therefore, a reasonable strategy is to treat maternal hypertension when the blood pressure exceeds 145 to 150 mm Hg systolic, or 95 to 100 mm Hg diastolic. The antihypertensive agents that are currently recommended during pregnancy and those that are contraindicated are listed in **Table 50-2**).

Although secondary hypertension is considerably less common than essential hypertension, failure to recognize the presence of the primary cause can result in adverse pregnancy outcomes. Therefore, it is preferable to diagnose secondary hypertension before conception. Kidney disease is the most common cause of secondary hypertension. Both pheochromocytoma and renovascular hypertension are associated with poor maternal and fetal prognosis. Accelerated hypertension, superimposed preeclampsia, and fetal demise are more common with these disorders. Women with primary aldosteronism may have relatively uncomplicated pregnancies, particularly if hypertension is only stage 1. However, if more severe hypertension is present, then pregnancy may be complicated and dangerous. If a hypertensive woman is first seen after conception, then blood and urine tests can be performed to rule out pheochromocytoma and to screen for primary aldosteronism. However, in view of the normal stimulation of the RAS in pregnancy, plasma renin and aldosterone levels may be difficult to interpret, making diagnosis of hyperaldosteronism extremely difficult. Renovascular hypertension is also difficult to diagnose during pregnancy. Improved technical results with magnetic resonance angiography can aid in anatomic diagnosis of renal artery lesions. Angioplasty has been performed successfully in the early second trimester, and it should be considered in women with severe, poorly controlled hypertension, particularly if previous pregnancies have been complicated by severe preeclampsia in

TABLE 50-2 Antihypertensive Drugs and Pregnancy

DRUG GROUP	COMMENTS
α_2-Adrenergic receptor agonists	Methyldopa is the most extensively used drug in this group. Its safety and efficacy are supported by evidence from randomized trials and a 7.5-year follow-up study of children born to mothers treated with this agent.
β-Adrenergic receptor antagonists	These drugs appear to be safe and efficacious in late pregnancy, but fetal growth restriction has been reported when treatment was started in early or mid-gestation. Fetal bradycardia can occur, and animal studies suggest that the fetus' ability to tolerate hypoxic stress may be compromised.
α-Adrenergic receptor and β-adrenergic receptor antagonists	Labetalol is as effective as methyldopa, but there is limited information regarding follow-up of children born to mothers given labetalol. Rare cases of hepatotoxicity have been reported.
Arterial vasodilators	Hydralazine is frequently used as adjunctive therapy with methyldopa and β-adrenergic antagonists. Rarely, neonatal thrombocytopenia has been reported. The experience with minoxidil is limited, and this drug is not recommended.
Calcium channel blockers	Small, uncontrolled studies and a meta-analysis suggested that these agents are safe and effective in pregnancy. There is limited information regarding follow-up of children exposed to calcium channel blockers in utero.
Angiotensin-converting enzyme inhibitors	Captopril causes fetal death in diverse animal species, and several converting enzyme inhibitors have been associated with oligohydramnios and neonatal renal failure when administered to humans. Do not use in pregnancy.
Angiotensin II receptor blockers	These drugs have not been used in pregnancy. In view of the deleterious effects of blocking angiotensin II generation, angiotensin II receptor antagonists are also considered to be contraindicated in pregnancy.
Diuretics	Many authorities discourage the use of diuretics, but others continue these medications if they were prescribed before conception or there is evidence of salt sensitivity.

association with fetal complications (e.g., early delivery, growth restriction, fetal demise).

Gestational Hypertension

The term *gestational hypertension* refers to high blood pressure that appears first after mid pregnancy; it is distinguished from preeclampsia by the absence of proteinuria. This category is broad and includes women who later develop preeclampsia as well as women with chronic hypertension who experienced a decrease in blood pressure in early pregnancy, masking the true diagnosis. Women with gestational hypertension that resolves after delivery and was not caused by preeclampsia are more likely to develop essential hypertension later in life.

Hypertension in Pregnancy and Long-Term Risk

Several recent analyses of large databases demonstrated that women with hypertension during pregnancy, particularly preterm preeclampsia, are at increased risk of developing cardiovascular disease later in life, including stroke, coronary heart disease, and hypertension. Studies have not clarified whether the reason for the increased risk is that preeclampsia and cardiovascular disease have common risk factors (e.g. obesity, diabetes) or that preeclampsia itself induces changes that increase the risk of cardiovascular disease.

KIDNEY DISEASE IN PREGNANCY

Kidney disease during pregnancy may be (1) preexisting kidney disease that was diagnosed before conception, (2) CKD that was unappreciated before pregnancy and diagnosed for the first time during pregnancy, or (3) kidney disease that develops for the first time during pregnancy. There is some overlap with respect to the diseases that are typical of the three categories. For example, lupus nephritis may be a chronic condition, or it may develop for the first time during pregnancy.

Chronic Kidney Disease in Pregnancy

General Principles

Fertility and the ability to sustain an uncomplicated pregnancy are related to the degree of kidney function impairment, rather than to the specific underlying disorder. The greater the functional impairment, and the higher the blood pressure, the less likely it is that the pregnancy will be successful. Moderate impairments in kidney function (serum creatinine concentration, 1.2 to 2.5 mg/dL) confer increased risk for preeclampsia (20% to 30%) and preterm delivery. Women with moderate to severe kidney dysfunction should be discouraged from conceiving, because up to 40% of these pregnancies are complicated by hypertension or deterioration in kidney function that may be irreversible.

In patients with CKD, the level of blood pressure at the time of conception is an important variable in pregnancy outcome. In the absence of hypertension at conception, there is significantly less chance of irreversible deterioration in kidney function during pregnancy. If hypertension is present, and especially if it is severe, pregnancy outcome is rarely uncomplicated. Preterm delivery and deterioration in kidney function are expected. Urine protein excretion may increase markedly in pregnant women with underlying kidney disease. A recent prospective cohort study of women with CKD found that women with proteinuria at conception (>1 g/day) were also at increased risk for adverse maternal and fetal outcomes, including worsening kidney function after delivery.

Diabetic Nephropathy

Diabetes is one of the most common medical disorders encountered during pregnancy, and most cases are gestational diabetes. Preexisting diabetes poses significant risks to pregnancy. Many younger women with pregestational diabetes have type 1 diabetes; if their disease has been present for 10 to 15 years, they may show early signs of diabetic nephropathy. Women with microalbuminuria rather than macroalbuminuria, well preserved kidney function, and normal blood pressure have a good prognosis for pregnancy, although they are at increased risk for transient, pregnancy-associated increases in proteinuria, preeclampsia, and urinary tract infection. Therefore, women with type 1 diabetes who have microalbuminuria, normal kidney function, and normotension should be encouraged *not* to postpone pregnancy, because the prognosis is worse once overt nephropathy develops. Published studies of pregnancy and nephropathy associated with type 2 diabetes are lacking. However, given the increasing prevalence of this condition, it is an important area for future study.

Systemic Lupus Erythematosus

Women with systemic lupus erythematosus are advised not to conceive unless their disease has been "inactive" for the preceding 6 months, because there is a higher incidence of maternal and fetal complications with active disease. An additional complication associated with lupus and pregnancy is placental transfer of maternal autoantibodies, which can cause a neonatal lupus syndrome characterized by heart block, transient cutaneous lesions, or both. Women with lupus are also more likely to have clinically significant titers of APAs and the lupus anticoagulant, which are associated with spontaneous fetal loss, hypertensive syndromes indistinguishable from preeclampsia, and thrombotic events including deep vein thrombosis, pulmonary embolus, myocardial infarction, and strokes. All women with systemic lupus erythematosus should be screened for APAs early in gestation. If titers are elevated, daily aspirin (80 mg) is recommended. If there is a history of thrombotic events, then heparin in combination with aspirin is recommended.

Increased activity of lupus in the latter part of pregnancy may be difficult to distinguish from preeclampsia. Both are characterized by an increase in proteinuria, a decrease in GFR, and hypertension. Thrombocytopenia may also be observed in both conditions. Hypocomplementemia is not a feature of preeclampsia, whereas increases in liver function tests may be observed in preeclampsia but are not characteristic of lupus activity. If disease activity is present before 20 weeks of gestation, then the diagnosis is more likely to be a lupus flare. In the latter half of pregnancy, it may be impossible to distinguish between a renal lupus flare and preeclampsia. In fact, frequently both are present simultaneously, and what starts as increased lupus activity appears to trigger preeclampsia. The presence of red blood cell casts in the urine can also signify lupus nephritis activity. Delivery may be necessary if immunosuppressive therapy and supportive care fail to stabilize the condition.

The approach to treatment of lupus nephritis during pregnancy is based largely on anecdotal experience and knowledge regarding treatment of lupus in nonpregnant patients, as well as information on fetal toxicity of immunosuppressants gained from treatment of other conditions such as organ transplantation. Corticosteroids and azathioprine are the mainstays of treatment. Hydroxychloroquine has also been associated with improved pregnancy outcomes and absence of fetal toxicity. Cyclophosphamide and mycophenolate mofetil are not recommended during pregnancy because of potential fetal toxicity.

Chronic Glomerulonephritis

Glomerulonephritides in women of childbearing age include immunoglobulin A nephropathy, focal segmental glomerulosclerosis (FSGS), membranoproliferative glomerulonephritis, minimal change nephritis, and membranous nephropathy. There are no data to support the notion that histologic subtype confers a specific prognosis for pregnancy. Rather, the previously mentioned principles are applicable to women with chronic glomerulonephritis. When kidney function is normal and hypertension is absent, the prognosis is good.

Polycystic Kidney Disease

Young women with autosomal dominant polycystic kidney disease (ADPKD) are frequently asymptomatic, with normal kidney function and normal blood pressure, and indeed may be unaware of their diagnosis. An increased incidence of maternal complications has been reported in patients with ADPKD compared with unaffected family members who also became pregnant. Preexisting hypertension was the most common risk factor for maternal complications during pregnancy. Pregnant women with polycystic kidney disease are also at increased risk of urinary tract infection. Estrogen is reported to cause liver cysts to enlarge, and repeated pregnancies may result in symptomatic enlargement of liver cysts. Given the association between cerebral aneurysms and ADPKD in some families, screening for such aneurysms should be considered before natural labor in a woman with a family history of cerebral aneurysm. All patients should undergo genetic counseling before pregnancy to ensure they are aware that their offspring have a 50% chance of being affected.

Vesicoureteral Reflux

Reflux nephropathy caused by vesicoureteral reflux may result in CKD in young women. A prospective study of 54 pregnancies in 46 women with reflux nephropathy found that preeclampsia occurred in 24% and was more common in women with hypertension. Nine women (18%) experienced deterioration in kidney function during pregnancy, and those with preexisting reduced kidney function were at greater risk. One third of the infants were delivered preterm, and 43% had vesicoureteral reflux. High-risk women should be screened with urine cultures and should be treated promptly if infection is present, with consideration to suppressive antibiotic therapy for the duration of pregnancy in some cases.

Chronic Kidney Diseases First Diagnosed during Pregnancy

The presence of CKD may first be appreciated during pregnancy, in part because pregnant women are scrutinized more closely and also because the renal hemodynamic alterations during pregnancy may cause proteinuria to increase into the clinically detectable range. Furthermore, the presence of even mild preexisting kidney disease is associated with an increased risk of preeclampsia, so underlying kidney disease may first become apparent after preeclampsia has developed. Kidney diseases that may be relatively silent before conception and then "manifest" during pregnancy include immunoglobulin A nephropathy, FSGS, polycystic kidney disease, and reflux nephropathy. Renal diagnostic testing during pregnancy can include blood and urine testing and ultrasonography. Kidney biopsy is usually deferred until after delivery unless acute deterioration in kidney function or morbid nephrotic syndrome occurs. Although experienced operators have reported few complications of kidney biopsy during pregnancy, increased renal blood flow, hypertension, and difficulty positioning the patient are concerns.

Kidney Diseases Developing for the First Time during Pregnancy

Pregnant women are at risk for any of the kidney diseases that occur in women of childbearing age, including pyelonephritis, glomerulonephritis, interstitial nephritis, and acute renal failure. Pyelonephritis in pregnant women is more likely to be associated with significant azotemia compared with nonpregnant women, and it should be treated aggressively. Glomerulonephritis and interstitial nephritis are not more likely to develop during pregnancy, although they do occur. Acute kidney injury (AKI) in association with pregnancy, a rare complication in developed countries, is also decreasing in incidence in the developing world. Recent estimates suggest that the incidence of AKI from obstetric causes is less than 1 in 20,000 pregnancies.

If acute renal failure occurs early in pregnancy (12 to 18 weeks), it is usually in association with septic abortion or prerenal azotemia caused by hyperemesis gravidarum. Most cases of AKI in pregnancy occur between gestational week 35 and the puerperium and are primarily caused by preeclampsia and bleeding complications. Preeclampsia, particularly the HELLP variant (*h*emolysis, *e*levated *l*iver enzymes, *l*ow *p*latelet count) is an important cause of AKI in pregnancy. Although most cases of preeclampsia are not associated with renal failure, significant kidney dysfunction may be seen in the HELLP syndrome, especially if it is not treated promptly. Most women without preexisting kidney or hypertensive disease who develop AKI in the setting of preeclampsia/HELLP do not require long-term renal replacement therapy. Additional important clinical entities causing renal failure during pregnancy are the thrombotic microangiopathies, acute tubular necrosis (ATN), acute fatty liver of pregnancy, and urinary tract obstruction.

Thrombotic Microangiopathy

Although they are rare, the thrombotic microangiopathies (thrombotic thrombocytopenic purpura [TTP] and hemolytic uremic syndrome [HUS]) are important causes of pregnancy-related AKI because they are associated with considerable morbidity. They also share several clinical and laboratory features of pregnancy-specific disorders such as the HELLP variant of preeclampsia and acute fatty liver of pregnancy, and distinction of these syndromes is important for therapeutic and prognostic reasons. Features that may be helpful in making the correct diagnosis include timing of onset and the pattern of laboratory abnormalities. Preeclampsia typically develops in the third trimester, with only a few cases developing in the postpartum period, usually within a few days after delivery. TTP usually occurs before delivery, with many cases developing in the second trimester. HUS is usually a postpartum disease. Symptoms may begin before delivery, but most cases are diagnosed afterward. Women who develop postpartum HUS often have had features of preeclampsia before delivery.

Preeclampsia is much more common than TTP/HUS, and it is characterized by hypertension and proteinuria. Renal failure is unusual, even with severe cases, unless significant bleeding, hemodynamic instability, or marked disseminated intravascular coagulation (DIC) occurs. In some cases, preeclampsia develops in the immediate postpartum period, and, if thrombocytopenia is severe, it may be indistinguishable from HUS. However, preeclampsia spontaneously remits, whereas TTP/HUS is often associated with CKD and hypertension, with many patients requiring dialysis or transplantation in the long term.

Laboratory features that are more consistent with preeclampsia or HELLP syndrome and not with TTP/HUS include evidence of mild DIC, prolongation of prothrombin and partial thromboplastin times, and, occasionally, marked elevations in liver enzymes. The presence of fever is more consistent with a diagnosis of TTP than preeclampsia or HUS. The main distinctive features of HUS are its tendency to occur in the postpartum period and the severity of the associated renal failure. Treatment of preeclampsia/HELLP syndrome consists of delivery and supportive care; more aggressive treatment is rarely indicated. Some centers have used corticosteroids in cases of severe HELLP syndrome, although this therapy has not been rigorously evaluated in placebo-controlled clinical trials. Treatment of TTP/HUS includes plasma infusion or exchange and other modalities used in nonpregnant patients with these disorders.

Acute Tubular Necrosis

ATN may occur during pregnancy, although the incidence is low. In the first trimester, ATN is usually associated with hyperemesis gravidarum; later in pregnancy and in the peripartum period, it is usually associated with abruptio placentae or other causes of obstetric hemorrhage. Occasionally, nonsteroidal anti-inflammatory agents, used for postpartum analgesia, may precipitate AKI in patients who are volume depleted. In cases of severe obstetric hemorrhage, acute cortical necrosis with associated DIC may be present, and ultrasonography or computed tomography may demonstrate hyperechoic or hypodense areas in the renal cortex. Most patients ultimately require dialysis, but 20% to 40% have partial recovery of kidney function.

Acute Fatty Liver of Pregnancy

Acute fatty liver of pregnancy is a rare complication of late pregnancy that is characterized by rapidly progressive liver failure. Women usually present with nausea, vomiting, and anorexia, and many have coincident diagnoses of preeclampsia or HELLP syndrome. Other laboratory abnormalities that are frequently observed (in addition to marked elevations in aspartate and alanine aminotransferase) include elevated bilirubin, hypofibrinogenemia, prolonged partial thromboplastin time, hypoglycemia, anemia, and low platelet count. Many cases are associated with significant azotemia. One series compared acute fatty liver of pregnancy with HELLP syndrome and observed that AKI was significantly more common with the former condition.

Urinary Tract Obstruction

Pregnancy is associated with dilation of the collecting system, which is not usually accompanied by kidney dysfunction. Ultrasonography often demonstrates mild to moderate hydronephrosis in later pregnancy. Rarely, complications such as bulky uterine fibroids that enlarge in the setting of pregnancy can lead to obstructive uropathy. Occasionally, acute urinary tract obstruction in pregnancy is caused by a kidney stone.

Management of Acute Kidney Disease in Pregnancy

Management of AKI occurring in pregnancy or immediately after delivery is generally similar to that in nongravid subjects, although there are several important considerations unique to pregnancy. Uterine hemorrhage near term may be concealed, and blood loss underestimated, so any overt blood loss should be replaced early. Both peritoneal dialysis and hemodialysis have been used successfully in patients with obstetric AKI. Neither pelvic peritonitis nor the enlarged uterus is a contraindication to the former method. In fact, this form of treatment is more gradual than hemodialysis and therefore is less likely to precipitate labor. Because urea, creatinine, and other metabolites that accumulate in uremia traverse the placenta, dialysis should be undertaken early, with the aim of maintaining the blood urea nitrogen concentration at approximately 50 mg/dL. In essence, the advantages of early dialysis in nongravid patients are even more important for the pregnant patient. Excessive fluid removal should be avoided, because it may contribute to hemodynamic compromise, reduction of uteroplacental perfusion, and premature labor. On the other hand, polyhydramnios is also thought to contribute to premature labor. In some cases, it may be advisable to perform continuous fetal monitoring during dialysis, particularly after midpregnancy.

TREATMENT OF END-STAGE RENAL DISEASE DURING PREGNANCY

Dialysis

Fertility is reduced in dialysis patients, because abnormalities of pituitary release of luteinizing hormone leads to anovulation. Pregnancy that does occur in patients undergoing maintenance dialysis is extremely high risk, and conception should be strongly discouraged because of the very high fetal mortality rate; in large surveys, only 42% to 60% of such pregnancies resulted in a live-born infant. Prematurity, very low birth weight, and intrauterine growth restriction are common, and approximately 85% of infants born to women who conceive after starting dialysis are born before 36 weeks' gestation.

The single most important factor influencing fetal outcome in these patients is the maternal plasma urea level. In patients undergoing hemodialysis, both the number of sessions per week and the time per session must be increased to provide a minimum of 20 hr/wk, aiming for a predialysis urea concentration of 30 to 50 mg/dL (5 to 8 mmol/L). Heparinization should be minimized to prevent obstetric bleeding. Dialysate bicarbonate should be decreased to 25 mEq/L, in keeping with the expected low tCO_2 in pregnancy. If peritoneal dialysis is being used, it is recommended to decrease the exchange volumes by increasing exchange frequency or cycler use.

Adequate calorie and protein intake is required; 1 g/kg/day protein intake plus an additional 20 g/day has been suggested. After the first trimester, the maternal "dry" weight should be increased by approximately 1 pound (400 g) per week to adjust for the expected progressive weight increase in pregnancy. Antihypertensive therapy should be adjusted for pregnancy by discontinuing ACE inhibitors and angiotensin receptor blockers; methyldopa, labetalol, and sustained-release nifedipine in standard doses should be used to achieve a target maintenance maternal diastolic pressure of 80 to 90 mm Hg. Anemia should be treated with supplemental iron, folic acid, and erythropoietin. Erythropoietin is safe to use in pregnancy, and pregnancy-related erythropoietin resistance requires a dose increase of approximately 50% to maintain hemoglobin target levels of 10 to 11 g/dL. Because of placental conversion of 25-hydroxyvitamin D_3, decreased supplemental vitamin D may be required; this decision should be guided by the levels of vitamin D, parathyroid hormone, calcium, and phosphorus. Magnesium supplementation may be needed to maintain the serum magnesium level at 5 to 7 mg/dL (2 to 3 mmol/L). Low-dose aspirin to prevent preeclampsia has been suggested.

Babies born to mothers on dialysis may require monitoring for osmotic diuresis in the immediate postpartum period if maternal urea was high at the time of delivery.

Kidney Transplantation

Menstruation and fertility resume in most women between 1 and 12 months after kidney transplantation. Pregnancy is not uncommon after kidney transplantation, and the risk to mother and baby is much lower in this population than in pregnant patients on dialysis. Although pregnancy has become common after transplantation, there is little other than case reports, series, and voluntary databases to guide practice. A Consensus Conference produced a report in 2005 that summarized the literature, generated practice guidelines, and identified gaps in knowledge. Most pregnancies (>90%) that proceed beyond the first trimester succeed. However, there are maternal and fetal complications due to immunosuppressant effects, preexisting hypertension, and kidney dysfunction. These include maternal complications of glucocorticosteroid therapy, such as impaired glucose tolerance, hypertension (47% to 73% of cases), preeclampsia (30%), and increased infection. Fetal complications include a higher incidence of preterm delivery and intrauterine growth restriction with lower birth weight.

Best practice guidelines have outlined criteria for considering pregnancy in kidney transplant recipients, and it is suggested that those contemplating pregnancy should meet the following conditions:

1. Good health and stable kidney function for 1 to 2 years after transplantation with no recent acute or ongoing rejection or infections
2. Absent or minimal proteinuria (<0.5 g/day)
3. Normal blood pressure or easily managed hypertension
4. No evidence of pelvicaliceal distention on ultrasonography before conception
5. Serum creatinine concentration less than 1.5 mg/dL
6. Drug therapy: prednisone, 15 mg/day or less; azathioprine, 2 mg/kg or less; cyclosporine, less than 5 mg/kg/day.

Although cyclosporine levels tend to decrease during pregnancy, there is no information regarding whether drug dosage should be increased. Tacrolimus has not been used as widely in pregnancy as cyclosporine, although growing experience suggests that is safe, with a similar side effect profile to cyclosporine. Considerations regarding hypertension and growth restriction are important; there is no established blood pressure target, though 140/90 mm Hg is suggested, and antihypertensives should be switched to those that are safe in pregnancy. Mycophenolate mofetil has been reported to be embryotoxic in animals and is associated with ear and other deformities in humans; this drug should be discontinued before conception, and azathioprine should be substituted, if indicated. Sirolimus causes delayed ossification in animal studies, and, although successful live births have been reported in humans, its use is contraindicated until more data are available.

Finally, data from the National Transplantation Pregnancy Registry and the European Dialysis and Transplant Association suggest that, in women with stable, near-normal kidney function, pregnancy rarely negatively affects the graft, although there may be minor increases in serum creatinine concentration after delivery, compared with the prepregnancy level. On the other hand, women with significantly reduced transplant function before delivery are at risk for irreversible deterioration afterward, as observed with CKD in native kidneys. Rejection is difficult to diagnose in pregnancy, and kidney biopsy may be required; the consensus opinion is that corticosteroids and intravenous immunoglobulin are safe treatments for acute rejection, but the safety of antilymphocyte globulins or rituximab in pregnancy is unknown.

BIBLIOGRAPHY

Andrade RM, McGwin G Jr, Alarcon M, et al: Predictors of postpartum damage accrual in systemic lupus erythematosus: Data from LUMINA, a multiethnic US cohort (XXXVIII). Rheumatology (Oxford) 45:1380-1384, 2006.

August P, Mueller FB, Sealey JE, et al: Role of renin-angiotensin system in blood pressure regulation in pregnancy. Lancet 345:896-897, 1995.

Dashe JS, Ramin SM, Cunningham FG: The long-term consequences of thrombotic microangiopathy (thrombotic thrombocytopenic purpura and hemolytic uremic syndrome) in pregnancy. Obstet Gynecol 91:662-668, 1998.

Derksen RH, Bruinse HW, de Groot, PG, Kater K: Pregnancy in systemic lupus erythematosus: A prospective study. Lupus 3:149-155, 1994.

Duley L: Evidence and practice: The magnesium sulphate story. Best Pract Res Clin Obstet Gynaecol 19:57-74, 2005.

Duley L, Henderson-Smart DJ, Meher S, King JF: Antiplatelet agents for preventing pre-eclampsia and its complications. Cochrane Database Syst Rev (1):CD004659, 2004.

Ekbom P, Damm P, Felt-Rasmussen B, Feldt-Rasmussen U: Pregnancy outcome in type 1 diabetic women with microalbuminuria. Diabetes Care 24:1739-1744, 2001.

Erkan D: The relation between antiphospholipid syndrome-related pregnancy morbidity and non-gravid vascular thrombosis: A review of the literature and management strategies. Curr Rheumatol Rep 4:379-386, 2002.

Fesenmeier MF, Coppage KH, Lambers DS, et al: Acute fatty liver of pregnancy in 3 tertiary care centers. Am J Obstet Gynecol 192:1416-1419, 2005.

Gammill HS, Jeyabalan A: Acute renal failure in pregnancy. Crit Care Med 33(10 Suppl):S372-S384, 2005.

Girling JC: Re-evaluation of plasma creatinine concentration in normal pregnancy. J Obstet Gynaecol 20:128-131, 2000.

Hofmeyr GJ, Atallah AN, Duley L: Calcium supplementation during pregnancy for preventing hypertensive disorders and related problems. Cochrane Database Syst Rev (3):CD001059, 2006.

Holley JL, Reddy SS: Pregnancy in dialysis patients: A review of outcomes, complications, and management. Semin Dial 16:384-388, 2003.

Jensen DM, Damm P, Moelsted-Pedersen L, et al: Outcomes in type 1 diabetic pregnancies: A nationwide, population-based study. Diabetes Care 27:2819-2823, 2004.

Jones DC, Hayslett JP: Outcome of pregnancy in women with moderate or severe renal insufficiency. N Engl J Med 335:226-232, 1996.

Lindheimer MD, Davison JM: Osmoregulation: The secretion of arginine vasopressin and its metabolism during pregnancy. Eur J Endocrinol 132:133-143, 1995.

Maynard S, Min JY, Merchan J, et al: Excess placental soluble fms-like tyrosine kinase 1 (sFlt1) may contribute to endothelial dysfunction, hypertension, and proteinuria in preeclampsia. J Clin Invest 111:649-658, 2003.

McKay DB, Josephson MA: Pregnancy in recipients of solid organs: Effects on mother and child. N Engl J Med 354:1281-1293, 2006.

Petri M, Howard D, Repke J: Frequency of lupus flare in pregnancy: The Hopkins Lupus Pregnancy Center experience. Arthritis Rheum 34:1538-1545, 1991.

Poston L, Briley AL, Seed PT, et al: Vitamin C and vitamin E in pregnant women at risk for pre-eclampsia (VIP trial): Randomised placebo-controlled trial. Lancet 367:1145-1154, 2006.

Rossing K, Jacobsen P, Hommel E, et al: Pregnancy and progression of diabetic nephropathy. Diabetologia 45:36-41, 2002.

Ruiz-Irastorza G, Lima F, Alves J, et al: Increased rate of lupus flare during pregnancy and the puerperium: A prospective study of 78 pregnancies. Br J Rheumatol 35:133-138, 1996.

Rumbold AR, Crowther CA, Haslam RR, et al: Vitamins C and E and the risks of preeclampsia and perinatal complications. N Engl J Med 354:1796-1806, 2006.

Smith WT, Darbari S, Kwan M, et al: Pregnancy in peritoneal dialysis: A case report and review of adequacy and outcomes. Int Urol Nephrol 37:145-151, 2005.

van Runnard Heimel PJ, Franx A, Schobben AFAM, et al: Corticosteroids, pregnancy, and HELLP syndrome: A review. Obstet Gynecol Surv 60:57-70, 2005.

Vigil-De Gracia P: Acute fatty liver and HELLP syndrome: Two distinct pregnancy disorders. Int J Gynaecol Obstet 73:215-220, 2001.

Weissenbacher ER, Reisenberger K: Uncomplicated urinary tract infections in pregnant and non-pregnant women. Curr Opin Obstet Gynecol 5:513-516, 1993.

CHAPTER 51

The Kidney in Aging

Maya K. Rao and Sharon Anderson

The changes in kidney function during normal aging are among the most dramatic of any organ system. This chapter considers the progressive structural and functional deterioration of the kidney that occur with normal aging.

AGE-RELATED CHANGES IN KIDNEY FUNCTION AND STRUCTURE

By 2 years of age, the glomerular filtration rate (GFR) of a child nears adult levels, and it remains at 140 mL/min/1.73 m² until the fourth decade. Thereafter, GFR declines by about 8 mL/min/1.73 m² per decade, although the rate of decline is highly variable. Acceleration of age-related loss of kidney function has been noted in the setting of systemic hypertension, diabetes, lead exposure, smoking, and atherosclerotic vascular disease; male gender may be another factor. Research ranging from the classic inulin clearance studies of Davies and Shock (1950) to recent determinations based on the Third National Health and Nutrition Examination Survey (NHANES) confirm wide variability in the spectrum of loss of kidney function in aging (**Fig. 51-1**).

The age-related reduction in creatinine clearance rate (CrCl) is accompanied by a reduction in daily urinary creatinine excretion due to reduced muscle mass. Accordingly, the relationship between the serum creatinine concentration (SCr) and the CrCl changes. The net effect is near-constancy of SCr while true GFR (and CrCl) declines; consequently, substantial reductions of GFR occur despite a relatively normal SCr. The CrCl in adult men may be estimated from the SCr with the Cockcroft-Gault formula:

$$CrCl = \frac{(140 - Age) \times Weight}{SCr \times 72}$$

where age is given in years and weight in kilograms; in women, the resulting value is multiplied by 0.85. Alternatively, the Modification of Diet in Renal Disease (MDRD) formula is in common clinical usage and has been validated in subjects ranging from 18 to 70 years of age. However, there remains considerable controversy as to the most accurate method of estimating GFR in the elderly, and a number of alternative formulas have been proposed.

Population studies indicate that the incidence of both microalbuminuria and overt proteinuria increase with advancing age, even in the absence of diabetes, hypertension, or elevated SCr. In the NHANES study, the risk of age-associated microalbuminuria was highest in those of non-Hispanic black and Mexican American ethnicity.

In addition to an age-related decline in GFR, renal blood flow declines by about 10% per decade after the fourth decade. The decrease in renal blood flow is most profound in the renal cortex; redistribution of flow from cortex to medulla may explain the slight increase in filtration fraction seen in the elderly. Renal mass increases from about 50 g at birth to more than 400 g during the fourth decade, after which it declines to less than 300 g by the ninth decade, correlating with the reduction in body surface area. Loss of renal mass is primarily cortical, with relative sparing of the medulla.

Glomerular number also decreases, though studies differ on the size of the remaining glomeruli. Glomerular shape changes, with decreased lobulation and reduction in length of the glomerular tuft perimeter relative to total area. The glomerular basement membrane undergoes progressive folding and thickening and eventually condenses into hyaline material with glomerular tuft collapse. Degeneration of cortical glomeruli results in atrophy of both afferent and efferent arterioles, leading to global sclerosis. In the juxtamedullary

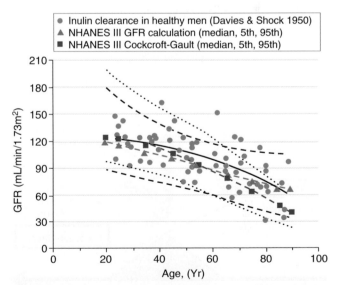

FIGURE 51-1 Percentiles of glomerular filtration rate (GFR, estimated by the MDRD equation) and creatinine clearance (calculated by the Cockcroft-Gault equation), by age, plotted on the same graph as data by Davies and Shock (J Clin Invest 29:496-507, 1950) representing measured inulin clearances in healthy men. Dashed lines without symbols show the 5th and 95th percentiles for GFR estimates. MDRD, Modification of Diet in Renal Disease; NHANES III, Third National Health and Nutrition Examination Survey. (Reproduced from Coresh J, Astor BC, Greene T, et al: Prevalence of chronic kidney disease and decreased kidney function in the adult U.S. population. Am J Kidney Dis 41:1-12, 2003, with permission.)

glomeruli, glomerular tuft sclerosis is accompanied by the formation of direct channels between the afferent and efferent arterioles, resulting in aglomerular arterioles.

The incidence of glomerular sclerosis increases with advancing age but, again, with wide variability. Sclerotic glomeruli make up less than 5% of the total before the age of 40 years, but as much as 30% of the glomerular population by the eighth decade. Therefore, both diminished glomerular lobulation and sclerosis of glomeruli reduce the surface area available for filtration and contribute to the observed age-related decline in GFR. Progressive increases in tubulointerstitial fibrosis contribute as well. In addition, age-related changes in cardiovascular hemodynamics, such as reduced cardiac output and systemic hypertension, are likely to play a role in reducing renal perfusion and filtration. Finally, it is hypothesized that increases in cellular oxidative stress that accompany aging result in endothelial cell dysfunction and changes in vasoactive mediators, resulting in increased atherosclerosis, hypertension, and glomerulosclerosis (**Fig. 51-2**).

AGE-RELATED ALTERATIONS IN FLUID AND ELECTROLYTE HOMEOSTASIS

There are no specific age-related changes in serum electrolyte or acid-base parameters in healthy subjects. However, hospitalized or ill elderly subjects frequently exhibit elevated values for blood urea nitrogen and creatinine, and alterations in serum electrolyte levels are more prominent (see later discussion). These observations indicate the ability of the aging kidney to maintain normal electrolyte homeostasis under steady-state conditions but impaired ability to respond to perturbations of fluid and electrolyte balance.

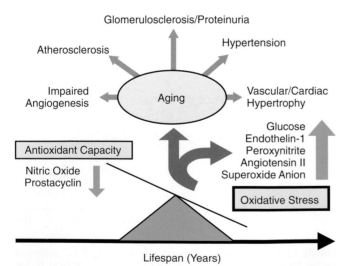

FIGURE 51-2 Proposed mechanisms of the vascular and renal aging process. A continuous increase in cellular oxidative stress with aging results in a shift that promotes activity and production of vasoactive mediators. Enhanced formation of growth-promoting factors such as superoxide anion, angiotensin II, and endothelin-1 counteracts the loss of anti-inflammatory and growth-inhibitory mediators such as nitric oxide and prostacyclin with increasing age. (Reproduced from Barton M: Ageing as a determinant of renal and vascular disease: role of endothelial factors. Nephrol Dial Transplant 20:485-490, 2005, with permission.)

Disorders of Sodium Balance

In the absence of acquired kidney disease, the aging kidney is able to adjust sodium handling appropriately in the face of extracellular sodium deficiency or excess; however, the response time is impaired, and management of these disorders is complicated accordingly. The renal response to dietary sodium deprivation in the elderly is blunted. When challenged with an acute reduction in sodium intake (from 100 to 10 mEq/day), elderly subjects can conserve sodium and achieve sodium balance, but at a slower rate than younger subjects. For example, study of acute dietary sodium restriction found that, compared with subjects younger than 25 years of age, those older than 60 years took longer to reduce their urinary sodium excretion rates and ultimately could not reduce levels down to those achieved by the younger group. Studies in the elderly suggest that sodium handling is fairly normal in the proximal tubule, but the capacity to reabsorb sodium in the ascending limb of the loop of Henle is markedly impaired. The reduced loop capacity to reabsorb sodium has two important consequences: (1) the amount of sodium delivered to the more distal segments increases, and (2) the capacity to concentrate the medullary interstitium is reduced, which further contributes to the inability to concentrate the urine.

Age-related abnormalities in several hormonal systems controlling sodium excretion play a role in this impaired ability to conserve sodium. Levels of plasma renin and of blood and urinary aldosterone fall significantly, and responses to appropriate stimuli such as sodium restriction are blunted. The tubular response to aldosterone is also reduced. Mechanisms for suppression of the renin-angiotensin system (RAS) are not well defined. It has been postulated that these age-related changes result from the loss of nephrons; compensatory hyperfiltration in the remaining nephrons leads to increased sodium chloride delivery to the macula densa, with suppression of renin synthesis and release, and, consequently, reduced formation of angiotensin II and aldosterone. Studies in aging animals indicate that both renal synthesis of renin and its release in response to volume stimuli are reduced, and that both aspects contribute to the observed fall in plasma renin concentration with aging. Other mechanisms may include the decrease in insulin secretion with aging. Whatever the mechanisms, the impaired response to sodium deprivation (relative salt-wasting) makes the elderly patient more susceptible to development of a cumulative sodium deficit and its attendant systemic complications.

Similarly, the renal response to a sodium load is sluggish in older patients. Natriuresis is impaired both by the reduced GFR, which leads to diminished delivery of sodium to the nephron, and by abnormalities in tubular handling of sodium. Studies in aging animals indicate a greater fall in renal perfusion and filtration with angiotensin II administration, as well as impaired natriuresis and augmented kaliuresis. Similarly, animal studies indicate impaired natriuretic responses to increased perfusion pressure, mediated in part by the renal nerves. Other vasoactive mediators are also involved, including altered levels of, or responsiveness to, various natriuretic stimuli including norepinephrine, atrial natriuretic peptide, kallikrein, and dopamine.

Disorders of Water Balance

Renal concentrating and diluting abilities are impaired in the aging kidney. In response to water deprivation, both the maximal decrease in urine volume and the increase in urine osmolality in healthy elderly subjects are significantly diminished, compared with responses in younger subjects. For example, one study found that the maximal urine osmolality after dehydration was 1109 mOsm/kg in subjects aged 20 to 39 years, 1051 mOsm/kg in those aged 40 to 59 years, and 882 mOsm/kg in those aged 60 to 79 years. Several conditions may contribute to this deficiency. The reduced number of functioning nephrons may contribute to an obligatory solute diuresis in the remaining intact nephrons. There is altered responsiveness to exogenous antidiuretic hormone (arginine vasopressin, or AVP), and the release of endogenous AVP in response to appropriate stimuli is abnormal. In some cases, there is decreased thirst perception after rising serum osmolality, so volume depletion or hyperosmolality stimuli are less effective. The increase in plasma AVP levels after infusion of hypertonic saline is greater in older than in younger subjects, indicating enhanced osmoreceptor sensitivity. In contrast to the response to an osmolar stimulus, the AVP response to volume-pressure stimuli (assumption of upright posture after overnight dehydration) is markedly impaired in some elderly subjects, as is the fall in plasma AVP after drinking water.

Similarly, the aging kidney demonstrates a modest inability to dilute urine appropriately, as determined by the maximal excretion of free water after water loading. This is most likely caused by the reduced GFR and renal perfusion, as well as by functional impairment in the diluting segment of the nephron. Studies in aging animals indicate that age-related polyuria is associated with downregulation of the aquaporin-2 and -3 water channels in the medullary collecting duct.

Hyponatremia

Serum sodium levels remain within the normal range in healthy elderly individuals, but defective sodium and water homeostatic mechanisms render this population markedly susceptible to perturbations. Hyponatremia is the most common electrolyte disorder in the elderly, occurring in as many as one quarter of all hospitalized elderly patients. Numerous mechanisms contribute to the susceptibility of elderly individuals to hyponatremia and may generally be deduced after clinical evaluation. The most common underlying mechanisms of geriatric hyponatremia are (1) decreased ability to excrete water, (2) water intoxication in the setting of diuretic therapy, and (3) oversecretion of AVP.

Elderly patients carry a disproportionate burden of illness associated with extracellular fluid volume deficit and excess. Extracellular volume depletion is common, particularly after administration of diuretics; in one series of 77 elderly patients, diuretic therapy accounted for two thirds of all cases of hyponatremia. In a survey of 631 hospitalized elderly patients, 12% of subjects taking thiazides were hyponatremic, with the percentage being higher in elderly women. Several age-related abnormalities probably contribute to this increased susceptibility: volume depletion, potassium depletion, and inhibition of urinary dilution. Compared with younger subjects, older patients challenged with a thiazide diuretic exhibited greater impairment of minimum urine osmolality and clearance of free water, possibly associated with lower prostaglandin production. It should also be noted that thiazide diuretics and nonsteroidal anti-inflammatory drugs (NSAIDs) may have an additive effect in causing hyponatremia in the elderly.

Hypervolemic hyponatremia is also common in elderly patients, with congestive heart failure being the most common cause of this disorder. Relatively isovolemic hyponatremia is also prominent in the elderly, who may exhibit increased plasma AVP levels in the absence of recognizable stimuli for AVP secretion. The presence of excessive levels of AVP, together with their AVP-independent impaired ability to excrete free water, render the elderly particularly susceptible to hyponatremia in numerous clinical settings, and particularly in the postoperative setting in the presence of narcotic administration and large amounts of intravenous hypotonic fluids. The incidence of hyponatremia due to antidepressant medication has been increasingly recognized.

Hypernatremia

Hypernatremia is also prominent in the elderly. At particularly high risk are institutionalized older patients with cognitive impairment, who often manifest failure to recognize thirst and/or physical inability to obtain fluids. In a study of hospital-acquired hypernatremia, 86% of the patients lacked free access to water. Additional evidence, albeit somewhat equivocal, suggests that hypodipsia, or failure to recognize thirst despite substantial elevations in serum osmolality, may be more common in elderly patients. Cerebrovascular disease may also inhibit thirst, as well as limiting the physical ability to gain access to fluids.

Alterations in Potassium Balance

Significant abnormalities in cellular and total body potassium occur with advancing age. The erythrocyte potassium concentration (a reflection of general intracellular potassium content) is decreased, and both total body potassium and total exchangeable body potassium are reduced by about 20% compared with younger subjects. Mechanisms include decreased muscle mass, alterations of cell membrane characteristics, nutritional deficiencies, and inability of the kidney to conserve potassium.

Hypokalemia is the most prominent potassium abnormality in the elderly population; one series found hypokalemia in 11% of elderly patients visiting an emergency department.

The most prominent cause of hypokalemia in the elderly is probably diuretic therapy; elderly patients appear to be more susceptible to the hypokalemic effects of these drugs.

In the absence of kidney disease or drugs that raise the potassium concentration, hyperkalemia is not usually a problem. The reduction in total body potassium stores may serve to offset the reduced GFR, thus protecting against significant hyperkalemia. However, studies in aging rodent models indicated impaired ability to excrete a potassium load, and studies in aging humans confirmed that the aldosterone response to hyperkalemia is impaired. These mechanisms, together with reduced activity of the RAS in the elderly, may serve to enhance the risk of hyperkalemia in the presence of excessive potassium intake or drugs that raise the potassium concentration. Indeed, hyperkalemia is more prominent in elderly than in younger subjects with administration of potassium supplements or drugs such as NSAIDs and trimethoprim-sulfamethoxazole. Furthermore, the increasing use of angiotensin-converting enzyme (ACE) inhibitors and aldosterone receptor antagonists for treatment of congestive heart failure is likely to induce further hyperkalemia in the setting of age-related reductions in GFR.

DISORDERS OF ACID-BASE BALANCE IN AGING

Abnormalities in both pulmonary and renal acid-base mechanisms may contribute to disorders in the elderly. The healthy elderly are generally able to maintain normal values for serum pH, carbon dioxide tension (P_{CO_2}), and bicarbonate concentration. There is a modest but significant decrease in serum bicarbonate levels (within the normal range) with aging. Although these systems adequately dispose of the normal daily acid load, studies of ammonium loading in elderly patients indicate a reduced ability to excrete an acute exogenous acid load. However, when corrected for the reduced GFR values, the response of elderly subjects is similar to that in younger subjects, indicating that nephron loss probably accounts for this difference. More chronic acid loading may be associated with delayed normalization, and the response to alkali loading may also be delayed in elderly subjects.

CALCIUM, PHOSPHORUS, AND MAGNESIUM DISORDERS IN AGING

Serum levels of total calcium, ionized calcium, phosphorus, magnesium, and parathyroid hormone usually remain within the normal range in the elderly, although there may be a tendency toward increased serum parathyroid hormone levels with advancing age. However, calcium metabolism is substantially impaired, as a result of age-related decreases in intestinal calcium absorption, reduced renal 1α-hydroxylase activity, diminished 1,25(OH)$_2$ vitamin D$_3$ (calcitriol) activity, and decreased intestinal adaptation to dietary calcium restriction. A decrease in vitamin D levels is frequently seen in elderly patients who are in poor health; contributing influences include lack of exposure to sunlight, dietary deficiency, and impaired conversion to calcitriol. Age-related changes in growth hormone and insulin-like growth factor 1 are among other influences that have been suggested to affect vitamin D levels in the elderly. However, renal tubular absorption of calcium does not seem to be affected in aging, which probably contributes to the observed constancy of serum calcium levels. The elderly exhibit decreased renal tubular reabsorption of phosphate, and experimental animals have shown decreased intestinal phosphate absorption and impaired renal tubular adaptation to dietary phosphate restriction. However, as with calcium, these defects do not appear to influence serum levels substantially. Serum magnesium levels do not change with age.

KIDNEY DISEASE IN THE ELDERLY

By itself, age-related kidney disease poses little threat to well-being, because even half of the normal GFR is ample for sustaining good renal health. However, the gradual loss of kidney function that accompanies normal aging may be greatly accelerated when acquired kidney disease is superimposed. The incidence of primary kidney disease in the elderly is not significantly different from that in young adults, although the preponderance of specific forms of glomerular injury varies in different age groups.

Several large series of biopsy results in elderly patients indicated the relative incidence of the major forms of glomerular injury. In published series of elderly patients with nephrotic syndrome, membranous glomerulonephritis was the most frequent cause, followed in varying degrees by proliferative or rapidly progressive glomerulonephritis and focal glomerular sclerosis. Most studies also found a substantial proportion of minimal change disease. Therefore, membranous glomerulonephritis remains the most common cause of nephrotic syndrome in the elderly, whereas rapidly progressive glomerulonephritis is the most common cause of an acute nephritic syndrome in the elderly population. The incidence of kidney disease secondary to systemic illness such as atherosclerosis, hypertension, cardiac failure, diabetes, and malignancy clearly increases with advancing age. Also to be considered are vasculitis and amyloidosis, which are relatively infrequent in younger patients. Particularly prominent in the elderly are deposition diseases, including amyloidosis, light chain deposition disease, and fibrillary glomerulonephritis.

Acute Kidney Injury in the Elderly

Elderly patients are at risk for all of the causes of acute kidney injury (AKI) seen in the general population, and susceptibility may be enhanced. In a study contrasting causes of AKI in 67 young and 298 elderly patients, the older patients had an increased incidence of AKI due to septic shock, volume depletion, nephrotoxins, and obstructive causes. This prevalence of hemodynamic renal failure was echoed in a retrospective study spanning the years 1975-1990 in an intensive care unit, where hemorrhagic, septic, or cardiogenic shock was the predominant cause of AKI in the elderly.

In the case of treatment-related AKI a prospective study found that the most prominent causes were nephrotoxic drugs (66% of cases, with aminoglycosides, NSAIDs, and ACE inhibitors as the top offenders), sepsis (45.7%), and hypoperfusion (45.7%). Presumably, the elderly are at higher risk for prerenal causes due to a tendency toward reduced sodium intake, diuretic administration, and inability to conserve sodium, predisposing to volume depletion. One representative study found volume depletion to be primarily responsible in 23.4% of cases of AKI in elderly patients, and preexisting volume depletion would also enhance the risk for AKI after administration of contrast agents or nephrotoxic drugs. Other causes are listed in **Table 51-1**.

Older age also increases the risks of AKI associated with surgical complications, aminoglycoside nephrotoxicity, NSAIDs, ACE inhibitor therapy, radiocontrast agents, and postrenal (obstructive) causes. Indeed, more than 80% of reported cases of NSAID-induced AKI are in patients older than 60 years of age. Certain other causes of AKI are also more frequent in the elderly, including multiple myeloma, carcinoma leading to obstruction, nephrotoxicity from chemotherapeutic interventions, polypharmacy with or without inappropriate drug dosing, obstructive uropathy due to prostatic disease, and atheroembolic renal disease.

Chronic Kidney Disease in the Elderly

The prevalence of chronic kidney disease (CKD) in the elderly is high compared with the younger population. Serial analyses of the NHANES survey data indicated that the prevalence of CKD in the United States was highest in the older age groups and was rising over time (**Fig. 51-3**). In addition, older age was a strong predictor of new-onset kidney disease. Whether age-related loss of kidney function represents a disease process distinct from other forms of CKD is a controversial question and is under active investigation. The number and relative frequency of entry of elderly patients into end-stage renal disease (ESRD) programs is increasing each year in the United States, as is the average age of dialysis patients, reflecting the aging of the population in general. In recent years, the highest annual increase in incidence of ESRD has been in patients older than 75 years of age (**Fig. 51-4**). In 2005, the median age of incident white ESRD patients was 67.4 years. In addition to the direct burden of kidney disease, ESRD at age 75 confers a threefold increased risk of death, compared with the population without kidney disease. All projections indicate that these trends will continue, posing a major challenge for the health care system in the coming years.

With regard to renal transplantation, 5% of dialysis patients aged 65 years or older were on the waitlist in 2005, and 35% of transplants in this age group were living donor transplants, compared with just 8% in 2003. There does not appear to be a consistent difference in outcomes for older versus younger patients if the data are adjusted for death with a functioning graft. However, it is clear that kidneys from older donors have shorter survival than those from younger donors.

TABLE 51-1 Pathologic Diagnoses in Elderly Patients with Acute Kidney Injury

DIAGNOSIS	PROPORTION OF BIOPSY SPECIMENS (%)
Pauci-immune crescentic GN	31.2
Acute interstitial nephritis	18.6
ATN with nephrotic syndrome	7.5
Atheroemboli	7.1
ATN necrosis alone	6.7
Light chain cast nephropathy	5.9
Postinfectious GN	5.5
Anti-GBM antibody GN	4.0
Immunoglobulin A nephropathy or Henoch-Schönlein nephritis	3.6
Nondiagnostic for acute renal failure	9.9

ATN, acute tubular necrosis; GBM, glomerular basement membrane; GN, glomerulonephritis.

Adapted from Kohli HS, Bhaskaran MC, Muftukumar T, et al: Treatment-related acute renal failure in the elderly: A hospital-based prospective study. Nephrol Dial Transplant 15:212-217, 2000.

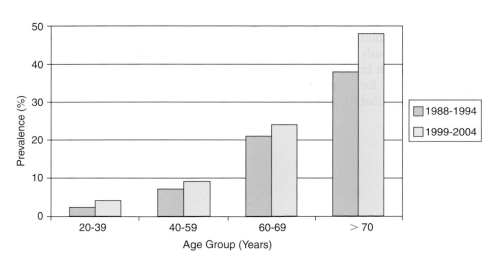

FIGURE 51-3 Prevalence of chronic kidney disease by age group in the National Health and Nutrition Examination Surveys (NHANES) for 1998-1994 and 1999-2004. (Adapted from Coresh J, Selvin E, Stevens LA, et al: Prevalence of chronic kidney disease in the United States. JAMA 298:2038-2047, 2007, with permission.)

Chronic Kidney Disease and its Therapy

CHAPTER 52

Pathophysiology of Chronic Kidney Disease

Arrigo Schieppati, Roberto Pisoni, and Giuseppe Remuzzi

STAGES OF PROGRESSION OF CHRONIC KIDNEY DISEASE

Most chronic nephropathies are characterized by a progressive course that leads, at a variable rate, to loss of kidney function and the need for renal replacement therapy. This final stage of chronic nephropathies is termed end-stage renal disease (ESRD). The progression of chronic kidney diseases (CKD) typically moves through phases from initial diminution of renal reserve to mild, moderate, and severe reductions in glomerular filtration rate (GFR), to ESRD.

In 2002, the National Kidney Foundation Kidney Disease Outcome Quality Initiative (NKF-K/DOQI) proposed a classification of CKD that is still widely used by both practicing physicians and clinical investigators. The K/DOQI classification establishes five stages, which are based on the estimation of GFR without regard to the cause of the CKD (see Table 53-2 in Chapter 53). This staging system for CKD was conceived to provide estimates of disease prevalence, to allow development of intervention plans for evaluation and management of each stage of CKD, and to define the characteristics of individuals who are at increased risk for developing CKD.

The staging of CKD and the assessment of progression are based on GFR measurements or estimates (see Chapters 2 and 53). The most reliable assessment of GFR is based on the measurement of kidney clearance of a filtration marker such as inulin. This method is not suitable for routine clinical practice and is cumbersome even for clinical research. Radionuclides that are handled by the kidney in a fashion similar to inulin and procedures using nonradioactive contrast agents (e.g., iothalamate, iohexol) can provide accurate GFR measurements and are used in clinical research, but their use is not practical for repeated measurements.

The K/DOQI classification is based on the estimation of GFR with an equation developed using data from the Modification of Diet in Renal Disease (MDRD) study. The equation requires the input of four simple variables: serum creatinine concentration (SCr), age in years, gender, and ethnicity. An earlier equation, the Cockcroft-Gault formula, estimates creatinine clearance rather than GFR. Creatinine clearance exceeds the GFR by the fraction of creatinine that is secreted by the tubules. The Cockcroft-Gault formula estimates creatinine clearance in milliliters per minute, and the MDRD equation estimates GFR in milliliters per minute per 1.73 m², and this difference should be kept in mind when comparing their outputs.

The estimates of GFR provided by these equations have limitations, including the calibration of the method of SCr assay and the population of patients from which these equations were originally derived. In a recent study, both the Cockcroft-Gault and MDRD equations significantly underestimated the GFR in newly diagnosed type 2 diabetic patients, particularly those with a GFR of 90 mL/min/1.73 m² or greater. This highlights a limitation in the use of estimated GFR in the majority of diabetic subjects outside the setting of CKD.

Another study evaluated the performance of nine equations, compared with the iothalamate clearance method, in 798 renal transplant recipients at 1 year after transplantation. Predictive performance was modest for all equations, although the MDRD equation came closest in predicting the GFR. Because the bias was significantly related to body mass index, age, and gender in most equations, the authors concluded that, at least in transplant patients, better equation models should be developed taking in account patient factors.

CKD is a worldwide threat to public health, but the precise dimension of this problem is not fully known. Approximately 1.8 million people are currently being treated with renal replacement therapy, which comprises primarily kidney transplantation, hemodialysis, and peritoneal dialysis. More than 90% of these individuals live in industrialized countries, because the availability of this therapy is scarce in developing countries and practically absent in underdeveloped areas, except for very wealthy individuals. A relevant question for health care planning is how many patients at an early stage of CKD will progress to ESRD?

The K/DOQI staging system has been used to estimate the prevalence of CKD in the United States. A survey was conducted as part of the Third National Health and Nutrition Examination Survey (NHANES III). A sample of 15,625 adults aged 20 years and older was analyzed. Kidney function, kidney damage, and stages of CKD were estimated from SCr levels, random urine albumin levels, age, gender, and race. The prevalence of CKD in the U.S. adult population was estimated to be 10.8% (approximately 19.2 million people).

In Europe, a similar screening program was conducted in the Prevention of Renal and Vascular End-Stage Disease (PREVEND) study. Eighty thousand people in Groningen, The Netherlands, were evaluated for kidney function and urinary abnormalities. Up to 12% of the adult population had some degree of kidney damage. If these data were to be extrapolated to the world population, the number of people with CKD could be estimated to be in the hundreds of millions.

During the past 2 decades there has been a major effort to understand the underlying mechanisms of CKD progression, and significant achievements have been made in the development of effective therapeutic strategies.

MECHANISMS OF RENAL DISEASE PROGRESSION

Glomerular Hypertension, Hyperfiltration, and the Role of Angiotensin II

In 1982, Brenner and coworkers put forward their hypothesis that progressive deterioration of kidney function was the result of compensatory glomerular hemodynamic changes in response to nephron loss. In their experimental model of renal mass reduction, the remaining nephrons underwent hypertrophy, with reduced arteriolar resistance and increased glomerular blood flow. It has also been shown that, with progression of kidney disease, afferent arteriolar tone decreases more than efferent tone. As a consequence, intraglomerular pressure and the amount of filtrate formed by each single nephron rise—in other words, glomerular hyperfiltration occurs (**Fig. 52-1**). Hyperfiltration has also been documented in rodent models of diabetic nephropathy. Angiotensin II appears to mediate this process through several mechanisms. In vivo, angiotensin II enhances the vascular tone of both afferent and efferent glomerular arterioles, modulating intraglomerular capillary pressure and GFR. Angiotensin II exerts its vasoconstrictor effect predominantly on the postglomerular arterioles, thereby increasing the glomerular hydraulic pressure and the filtration fraction. High glomerular capillary pressure increases the radius of the pores in the glomerular membrane, thus impairing the size-selective function of the membrane for macromolecules.

In addition to glomerular hemodynamic effects, studies have revealed several nonhemodynamic effects of angiotensin II that may also be important for CKD progression. In an experimental model of the isolated perfused kidney, infusion of angiotensin II resulted in a loss of glomerular size permselectivity and in proteinuria, an effect that has been attributed to both hemodynamic activity of angiotensin II and its direct effect on the glomerular membrane. Podocytes have a complex cytoskeleton with contractile properties, and there are angiotensin II receptors on their surface. Angiotensin II may alter permselective properties of the glomerular barrier by mediating contraction of the foot processes of the podocytes, ultimately changing the slit-diaphragm architecture (see Chapter 1) and allowing proteins to escape readily into the urinary space.

The observation that angiotensin II depolarizes podocytes by opening a chloride conductance channel related to cytoskeleton function via an angiotensin II type 1 (AT$_1$) receptor) is in line with such a possibility. The concentration of angiotensin II in Bowman's space is up to 1000-fold higher than in the vascular space, suggesting that angiotensin II is produced by a local renin-angiotensin system.

Angiotensin II also modulates renal cell growth, which, in turn, may contribute to tubulointerstitial injury. Proliferation of glomerular cells and fibroblasts induced by angiotensin II enhances structural renal damage and fibrosis. Increased expression of *FOS* and *EGR1*, the immediate early genes whose activation precedes cell proliferation, has been shown in proximal tubular cells exposed to angiotensin II. The peptide, acting through AT$_1$ receptors, also induces hypertrophy in tubular cells by upregulating the gene for transforming growth factor-β1 (TGFB1), which results in increased synthesis of collagen type IV. Remodeling of the

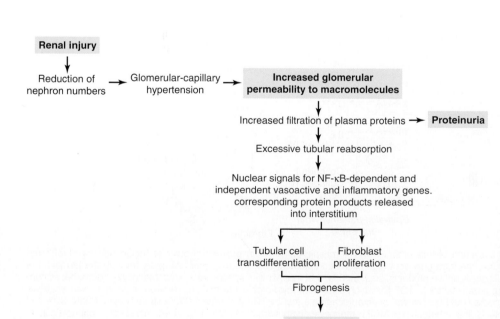

FIGURE 52-1 Schematic representation of the events leading to progressive kidney damage. Excessive resorption of proteins as a consequence of increased glomerular permeability results in the accumulation of proteins in proximal tubular cells, which may trigger activation of nuclear factor-κB (NF-κB)-dependent and NF-κB-independent genes encoding chemokines, cytokines, and endothelin. Excessive synthesis of inflammatory and vasoactive substances contributes to fibroblast proliferation and interstitial inflammation.

interstitial architecture may also occur as a result of transformation of tubular cells, an additional event promoted by the enhanced synthesis of TGFB1.

Angiotensin II also stimulates the production of plasminogen activator inhibitor 1 and may therefore further increase the accumulation of he extracellular matrix through inhibition of its breakdown by matrix metalloproteinases, which require conversion to an active form by plasmin. Angiotensin II upregulates genes and stimulates secretion of peptides with chemotactic and vasoactive properties. By stimulating macrophage activation and phagocytosis, angiotensin II may enhance the inflammatory component associated with chronic kidney injury.

The Role of Proteinuria

Proteinuria is not merely a consequence of glomerular hyperfiltration or a marker of altered glomerular barrier integrity. Abundant experimental evidence supports the notion that proteinuria itself contributes to progressive nephron damage (**Fig. 52-2**). Filtered proteins are reabsorbed by proximal tubular cells. Moreover, focal breaks in tubular basement membranes and leakage of the tubular contents into the renal interstitium can lead to protein overload in the interstitium, followed by macrophage infiltration and increased production by macrophages of inflammatory mediators such as endothelin 1, monocyte chemoattractant protein 1 (MCP-1), osteopontin, and RANTES (regulated on activation normal T-cell expressed and secreted), which is a chemotactic cytokine for monocytes and memory T cells.

Complement components may also play a major role in proteinuria-induced interstitial damage. Complement proteins are filtered through the glomerulus, and deposits of C3 and C5b-9 are found in proximal tubular cells. Activation of the complement system in tubular cells is associated with

alterations of the cytoskeleton, production of reactive oxygen species, and synthesis of pro-inflammatory mediators.

The activation of a variety of molecules, such as cytokines, growth factors, and vasoactive substances derived from tubular cells, may result in the abnormal accumulation of extracellular matrix collagen, fibronectin, and other components that are responsible for interstitial fibrosis. All forms of CKD are associated with tubulointerstitial injury, manifested by tubular dilatation and interstitial fibrosis, even if the primary process is a glomerulopathy. Furthermore, in almost all chronic progressive glomerular diseases, the degree of tubulointerstitial disease is a better predictor of GFR decline and long-term prognosis than is the severity of glomerular injury. It is possible in these settings that tubulointerstitial disease causes tubular atrophy or obstruction, eventually leading to nephron loss.

CLINICAL EVIDENCE OF THE ROLES OF HYPERTENSION AND PROTEINURIA IN PROGRESSION OF CHRONIC KIDNEY DISEASE

Systemic hypertension is both a cause and a consequence of CKD. The incidence of hypertension increases as CKD advances. The prevalence of hypertension requiring therapy in patients with stage 4 CKD is greater than 80%. There is strong evidence that high blood pressure is a risk factor for progression of CKD in humans. As an example, the Multiple Risk Factor Intervention Trial (MRFIT) documented that elevated blood pressure was a strong and independent risk factor for the development of ESRD in men. However, in this and several subsequent studies that showed a strong association between hypertension and CKD progression, information on baseline GFR was often lacking, so it was not always possible to exclude kidney disease present at the start of the study.

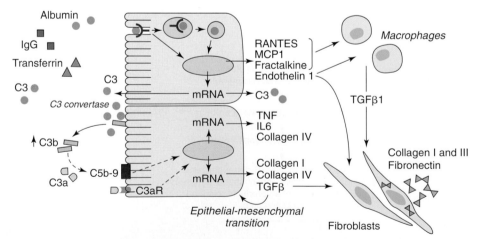

FIGURE 52-2 Mechanisms underlying the activation of inflammatory and fibrogenic pathways in proximal tubular epithelial cells by ultrafiltered protein load. As a consequence of proteinuria, the intrarenal activation of the complement cascade may promote injury through the formation of membrane attack complex (C5b-9) and biologically active products, such as C3a, that interact with specific receptors. Monocyte-macrophages contribute to fibrosis by release of transforming growth factor-β (TGF-β), which stimulates myofibroblast formation, collagen deposition, and epithelial mesenchymal transformation. The latter process could be induced in an autocrine manner by TGF-β of proximal tubular cell origin. C3aR, activated complement 3 receptor; IgG, immunoglobulin G; IL6, interleukin 6; MCP1, monocyte chemoattractant protein 1; mRNA, messenger ribonucleic acid; RANTES, regulated on activation normal T cell expressed and secreted; TNF, tumor necrosis factor. (From Abbate M, Zoja C, Remuzzi G: How does proteinuria cause progressive renal damage? J Am Soc Nephrol 17:2974-2984, 2006.

In a recent study, a cohort of more than 300,000 people enrolled in a health care delivery system was evaluated. These subjects had a GFR of 60 mL/min/1.73 m² or greater and no evidence of urinary abnormalities at baseline. During the follow-up, 1149 people developed ESRD. Compared with subjects whose blood pressure readings were less than 120/80 mm Hg, individuals with readings of 120-129/80-84 mm Hg had a 1.6-fold higher relative risk of developing ESRD, and those with readings greater than 210/120 mm Hg had a 4.2-fold increased risk. This study showed clearly that even a relatively modest increase in blood pressure is an independent risk factor for developing ESRD.

The role of proteinuria as a risk factor for progression of CKD is suggested by the strong correlation between the amount of urinary protein and kidney outcome. In 840 patients with nondiabetic kidney disease enrolled in the MDRD study, proteinuria was the strongest predictor of kidney disease progression. The Ramipril Efficacy in Nephropathy (REIN) study of 352 patients with chronic nondiabetic proteinuric nephropathies showed that the baseline urinary protein excretion rate was the best single predictor of GFR decline and ESRD, independent of the nature of the underlying disease. Patients with a baseline urinary protein excretion of less than 1.9 g/24 hr had the lowest rate of GFR decline and kidney failure during 3 years of follow-up. In contrast, patients with proteinuria greater than 3.9 g/24 hr lost more than 10 mL/min/l.73 m² GFR per year, and 30% developed ESRD within 3 years.

Besides predicting the rate of progression of the decline in kidney function, urinary protein excretion can be used to identify which patients would benefit most from renoprotective treatments. In the MDRD trial, the patients with higher baseline proteinuria were those whose rate of GFR decline was reduced the most by strict blood pressure control. Among patients with urinary protein excretion greater than 3 g/24 hr in the REIN study, the beneficial effect of ramipril, an angiotensin-converting enzyme (ACE) inhibitor, in slowing the GFR decline and in reducing the risk of ESRD increased as the baseline level of proteinuria increased.

TABLE 52-1 Risk Factors for Kidney Disease Progression

Proteinuria >1.5 g/24 hr or urinary protein-to-creatinine ratio >1 g/g

Hypertension

Type of underlying kidney disease (e.g., polycystic kidney, diabetic nephropathy)

African American race

Male gender

Obesity

Hyperlipidemia

Smoking

High-protein diet

Phosphate retention

Metabolic acidosis

There is also evidence that, in patients with nondiabetic proteinuric chronic nephropathies, the protein-to-creatinine (P/C) ratio in a single spot morning urine sample closely correlates with 24-hour protein excretion and predicts GFR decline and risk progression to ESRD even better than 24-hour protein excretion. In one study, the P/C ratio was measured in 177 nondiabetic patients with CKD. In the one third of subjects with the lowest P/C ratio (<1.7), there was 3% progression to renal failure, compared with 21.2% in the highest third (>2.7). This easy and inexpensive procedure can establish the severity and prognosis of kidney disease and is less time-consuming and less error prone than 24-hour collection.

Several other factors are also associated with an increased rate of progression of CKD. The type of kidney disease appears to be a risk factor. Glomerulonephritis, diabetic and hypertensive nephropathies, and polycystic kidney disease tend to progress faster than tubulointerstitial diseases. African American race, male gender, obesity, high serum low-density lipoprotein (LDL) cholesterol, cigarette smoking, metabolic acidosis, and phosphate retention may hasten CKD progression (**Table 52-1**).

PREVENTION OF PROGRESSION OF CHRONIC KIDNEY DISEASE

Early experiments in several animal models of kidney disease showed that inhibition of angiotensin II with an ACE inhibitor could slow the progressive loss of kidney function. The strategy to prevent progression of CKD has developed as a consequence of these studies and clinical observations. Central to the strategy is renoprotection via blockade of the renin-angiotensin system, with blood pressure control and reduction of proteinuria as the two targets.

The first robust demonstration of the validity of such an approach was provided by a U.S. collaborative study in patients with type 1 diabetes mellitus who had proteinuria greater than 500 mg/day and SCr of 2.5 mg/dL or less. Randomization to captopril treatment was associated with a 50% reduction in the risk of the combined end points of death, dialysis, and transplantation, compared with placebo. The role of proteinuria in promoting progression and its impact on kidney outcome was explored by the REIN study. This study was designed to assess the hypothesis that ACE inhibitors could be superior to other antihypertensive drugs in reducing proteinuria, limiting the decline in GFR, and preventing ESRD in patients with chronic nondiabetic nephropathies. Patients were randomly assigned to receive ramipril or conventional antihypertensive therapy to maintain diastolic blood pressure at 90 mm Hg or less. The REIN study showed that, although blood pressure control was similar in the two treatment groups, ACE inhibitor therapy decreased the progression to ESRD by 50% during 3 years of follow-up. Among patients with proteinuria of 3 g/24 hr or more, those who received the ACE inhibitor had a significantly slower rate of decline in GFR than did patients receiving conventional antihypertensive therapy.

In the REIN study, 186 patients (stratum 1) had baseline proteinuria between 1 and 3 g/24 hr, and the remainder (stratum 2) had proteinuria greater than 3 g/24 hr. In stratum 1 patients, progression to ESRD was significantly less common in those who were randomized to receive ramipril compared with conventional therapy (9/99 versus 18/87; relative risk, 2.72). Proteinuria decreased by 13% in the ramipril group and increased by 15% in the controls. As expected, the rate of decline in GFR and the frequency of ESRD were much lower in stratum 1 than in stratum 2. However, ACE inhibition conferred renoprotection in both strata. The study was continued for 2 years (the REIN follow-up study), during which time all patients previously receiving conventional antihypertensive medications were switched to ramipril. Among those patients who were randomized to ramipril and continued to receive ramipril during the 2-year extension, the rate of GFR decline decreased further, from approximately 5 mL/min/yr to 1 mL/min/yr during follow-up, a figure similar to that associated with normal aging. Patients who switched from conventional therapy to ramipril also benefited from the treatment. This analysis provides evidence that the tendency of GFR to decline with time can be halted and that remission is achievable in some patients with CKD.

Three large randomized studies later examined the role of drugs in the angiotensin receptor blocker (ARB) class in type 2 diabetic nephropathy. In one study (Irbesartan Diabetic Nephropathy Trial, or IDNT), 1715 patients with nephropathy from type 2 diabetes mellitus were randomized to receive the ARB irbesartan, the calcium channel blocker amlodipine, or placebo. With irbesartan, the risk of reaching the composite end point of doubling of SCr, ESRD, or death was 20% lower than with placebo and 23% lower than with amlodipine. In the second trial (Reduction of Endpoints in NIDDM with the Angiotensin II Antagonist Losartan, or RENAAL), the renoprotective effect of losartan versus placebo (in addition to conventional antihypertensive therapy) was evaluated in 1513 patients with overt type 2 diabetic nephropathy. The primary composite end point was doubling of SCr, ESRD, or death. Despite the attainment of equivalent blood pressure levels, losartan reduced the incidence of SCr doubling by 25% and the risk of ESRD by 28%. Proteinuria declined by 35% in the losartan group. However, the death rate was similar in the two groups. The third study evaluated the renoprotective effect of the ARB irbesartan in 1715 hypertensive patients with incipient diabetic nephropathy. The end point of the study was the time of onset of overt albuminuria. In 2 years of follow-up, only 5.2% of patients receiving 300 mg irbesartan reached the end point, compared with 14.9% of patients receiving placebo. The groups had similar blood pressure control, a finding that suggests that ARBs are renoprotective independent of their antihypertensive effect.

Although these studies showed that ARBs have a renoprotective effect, only relatively small-scale randomized studies have evaluated the role of ACE inhibitors specifically in type 2 diabetic nephropathy. With one exception, these studies demonstrated no significant difference between ACE inhibitors and other classes of antihypertensive agents in terms of prevention of GFR decline over time. On the other hand, a study by Canadian investigators showed that the use of ACE inhibitors was associated with a significant reduction in all-cause and cardiovascular-related mortality in a broad spectrum of patients with type 2 diabetes and no underlying cardiovascular disease (CVD).

Dual Blockade of the Renin-Angiotensin System

The combination of an ACE inhibitor and an ARB may afford greater renoprotection than each drug used alone. The rationale for the combined therapy rests on the evidence that long-term ACE inhibitor treatment results in the accumulation of angiotensin I, which may escape ACE inhibition and generate angiotensin II by means of alternative enzymes not sensitive to ACE inhibitors (e.g., chymase, serine proteases). Experimental studies of ACE inhibition have demonstrated compensatory angiotensin II formation at the kidney tissue level through such a nonsensitive pathway. ARBs antagonize angiotensin II by blocking its receptor, AT_1, so the non–ACE-dependent effects of angiotensin are also blocked by these drugs. On the other hand, inhibition of AT_1 results in increased angiotensin II levels, which may overcome in part the effect of the ARB.

In a study examining tissue angiotensin II levels, animals were treated with captopril, losartan, or a combination of the two. Both captopril alone and the combination treatment reduced plasma angiotensin II significantly, compared with control or with losartan alone. In contrast, in kidney tissue, angiotensin II values were reduced in the combination drug group more than with control or with either drug given singly. Small clinical studies support the concept that combination therapy is more potent in reducing proteinuria than single therapy in diabetic and nondiabetic CKD. A large trial, the COOPERATE study, was designed to compare combined treatment with an ACE inhibitor plus an ARB with monotherapy with each drug at its maximum dose in patients with nondiabetic kidney disease. Among patients receiving the dual treatment, 11% reached the combined primary end point of doubling of SCr or ESRD, compared with 23% of patients receiving trandolapril alone and 23% of those receiving on losartan alone, at 3 years of follow-up. Although these results are encouraging, they show that other strategies are needed to achieve complete prevention of progressive nondiabetic kidney disease, because some patients reached the primary end point even with combined treatment.

ACE inhibition results in an acute decrease in aldosterone concentration, but with continued use the suppression is not sustained, a phenomenon known as "aldosterone escape." Selective blockade of aldosterone, independent of renin-angiotensin blockade, reduces proteinuria and nephrosclerosis in experimental animals. Moreover, there is increasing evidence that aldosterone has a stimulatory effect on vascular remodeling and collagen formation by endothelial cells. Recently, there have been reports of an additive antiproteinuric effect of anti-aldosterone drugs combined with ACE inhibitor/ARB therapy. One study showed that spironolactone treatment, added to maximal doses of ACE inhibitors and other recommended renoprotective measures, may offer further renoprotection in patients with diabetic nephropathy who have nephrotic-range albuminuria. Another study demonstrated that spironolactone significantly increased the antiproteinuric effect of combined therapy with irbesartan and ramipril in patients with nondiabetic chronic nephropathies.

A number of side effects, such as gynecomastia and impotence, can limit the use of spironolactone. The novel aldosterone blocker, eplerenone, has been studied in experimental models of CKDs. In doxorubicin-induced nephrotic syndrome, early treatment with eplerenone or enalapril was effective in reducing daily and cumulative protein excretion and afforded preservation of the podocyte-related proteins, nephrin and podocin. More profound antiproteinuric effects were observed when enalapril and eplerenone were combined.

The combination of eplerenone with an ACE inhibitor was tested in patients with type 2 diabetes and albuminuria. Two-hundred sixty eight patients were randomized to three groups that received either placebo or eplerenone in two graded doses; in addition, all patients received enalapril at submaximal dose. After 12 weeks, albuminuria had significantly decreased in both groups given eplerenone but not in the placebo group, whereas blood pressure was reduced to the same extent in all three groups. The incidence of hyperkalemia, either sustained ($[K^+]$ >5.5 mmol/L) or severe ($[K^+]$ >6.0 mmol/L), was not significantly different among the three groups, even in the quartile with the lowest estimated GFR, and the rates of hyperkalemia were low.

Nonetheless, hyperkalemia is a significant concern with ACE inhibitor or ARB therapy, and several studies bear on this question. One study compared the effects of an ACE inhibitor versus an ARB on the changes in serum potassium concentration in patients with impaired kidney function. For the total group, these changes were not significantly different with lisinopril or valsartan treatment. However, patients with GFR values of 60 mL/min/1.73 m^2 or lower who received lisinopril showed a significant increase in serum potassium of 0.28 mEq/L above the mean baseline of 4.6 mEq/L. With valsartan, a smaller rise in serum potassium was observed, 0.12 mEq/L above baseline. In summary, in patients with renal insufficiency, the ARB valsartan seems to be less likely to increase serum potassium than ACE inhibitor therapy. In another study in patients undergoing chronic hemodialysis, the use of ACE inhibitors or ARBs was independently associated with an increased risk of developing hyperkalemia. However, the small size of the population involved in this study suggests that caution should be used in interpreting the data.

Aliskiren is the first member in a new class of antihypertensive drugs that are characterized by an exceptional affinity for the human renin enzymatic site. It is a potent, direct renin inhibitor with sufficient bioavailability to produce sustained suppression of plasma renin activity. When aliskiren is used alone, blood pressure reductions are similar to those provided by other drugs as monotherapies. When it is combined with

diuretics, additional blood pressure reduction is seen. When it is given with an ARB, aliskiren produces significant additional blood pressure reduction.

In one recent study, aliskiren was renoprotective in a model of advanced diabetic nephropathy in the rat. Recently, the results of the AVOID study were published, which evaluated the renoprotective effects of dual blockade of the renin-angiotensin-aldosterone system by adding treatment with aliskiren, to treatment with the maximal recommended dose of losartan and optimal antihypertensive therapy in patients who had hypertension and type 2 diabetes with nephropathy.

Treatment with 300 mg of aliskiren daily, as compared with placebo, reduced the mean urinary albumin-to-creatinine ratio by 20% , with a reduction of 50% or more in 24.7% of the patients who received aliskiren as compared with 12.5% of those who received placebo.

Other Measures to Prevent Progression of Chronic Kidney Disease

For patients with advanced CKD, the evidence from both experimental studies and clinical trials suggests that current practice can at best retard development of ESRD for a few years; it cannot altogether eliminate the need for dialysis for most patients during their lifetime. However, that goal may be attainable in some patients if a more complex strategy than intervention with a single pharmacologic agent is employed.

Lifestyle Changes

In seeking more effective treatments, the role of lifestyle changes should not be overlooked. Physical activity is instrumental to the loss of weight, but activity may also have an intrinsic favorable effect, as was documented by a small study in 20 patients with CKD who were assigned to 12-week regular aquatic exercise or a sedentary lifestyle. During this short period of time, body mass index did not change in either group. However, proteinuria decreased by 50% in those who performed aquatic exercise, while there was no change in the sedentary group.

The association between smoking and impaired kidney function was recently explored in a population-based study in Sweden. A cohort of 926 patients with CKD (defined as SCr >3.4 mg/dL in males or >2.8 mg/dL in females) were compared with 998 control subjects. Despite a modest, nonsignificant overall association between smoking and kidney disease, heavy smoking (>20 cigarettes per day), long duration (>40 years) and high cumulative dose (>30 pack-years) all were significantly associated with increased risk of progression. The association was strongest in the subgroup with an underlying diagnosis of nephrosclerosis.

The role of smoking on kidney function in apparently healthy subjects was investigated in Australia. In a randomized, population-based, cross-sectional study of more than 11,000 people, smoking was significantly associated with impaired kidney function after adjustment for confounding factors in men, but not in women. The risks of smoking in terms of CKD progression and the potential renoprotective benefit of smoking cessation are not well appreciated by many patients, or even by physicians.

Management of Hyperlipidemia

Hyperlipidemia is common in patients with CKD, especially in those with nephrotic syndrome. Experimental studies suggest that hyperlipidemia may not only be a risk factor in the development of systemic atherosclerosis, but it may also enhance the rate of progressive glomerular injury. The mechanisms of kidney injury by lipids are incompletely understood, but LDL stimulates mesangial cell proliferation and the synthesis of proinflammatory molecules by these cells, which could contribute to glomerular injury.

Robust clinical evidence that control of dyslipidemia is effective in preventing the progression of CKD is still lacking. A meta-analysis of 13 studies concluded that lipid-lowering interventions slowed the progressive loss of kidney function, but overall, only 362 patients with kidney disease were included in the analysis. A post hoc analysis of three randomized, controlled trials that compared pravastatin with placebo in subjects at high risk for coronary artery disease was performed to evaluate the effect of lipid-lowering treatment on CKD progression. These three studies enrolled more than 18,000 people, 18.3% of whom had CKD at baseline, as defined by a calculated GFR between 30 and 60 mL/min/1.73 m². In this pooled analysis, pravastatin had a positive, albeit small, effect on the rate of kidney function loss, compared with placebo.

The same group of authors examined data from the Veterans Affairs High-Density Lipoprotein Intervention Trial, a randomized trial that compared gemfibrozil with placebo in men with coronary disease and hypertriglyceridemia. Among the study subjects for whom baseline kidney function was available, 20% had moderately reduced GFR. During a median follow-up of 61 months, the rate of change in GFR did not differ between the two treatment groups, and therefore gemfibrozil did not seem to offer a significant renoprotective effect.

In summary, large clinical trials designed specifically to assess the role of lipid-lowering interventions on CKD progression are still needed. A well-powered study capable of definitively assessing the effect of lipid lowering would have to be very large-scale, very long-term, and therefore very expensive. Because patent protection for statins is expiring, pharmaceutical industry support for a trial of this sort seems unlikely.

In the meantime, the main goal of treatment of dyslipidemia in CKD is actually the prevention of atherosclerotic disease. In the non-uremic population, an LDL cholesterol target of less than 130 mg/dL has been recommended for patients without CVD, whereas plasma values of less than 100 mg/dL have been the target for those with CVDs. Diet and body weight reduction may help to improve the lipid profile, but often the use of statins, which are generally well tolerated, is necessary. The risk of liver and muscle toxicity, ranging from myalgias to myositis, possibly associated with myoglobinuric acute kidney injury, should be taken into account in CKD patients, but the side effect profile of statins

in patients with CKD seems to be comparable to that in the general population. The United Kingdom Heart and Renal Protection study (UK-HARP-I) involved 448 patients with CKD at various stages (including patients undergoing dialysis and transplant recipients) who were treated with simvastatin. There was no difference between those receiving active drug and the placebo group in term of elevation of liver enzyme or creatine kinase levels.

ACE inhibitors and ARBs often reduce serum LDL cholesterol levels, and the magnitude of these changes appears to be related to the degree of decrease in proteinuria.

Glycemic Control

The role of diabetic control in the development and progression of CKD has been extensively examined (see Chapters 25 and 26). Both interventional and population-based studies have linked hyperglycemia with the risk of development of albuminuria or diabetic nephropathy. Less strong evidence links hyperglycemia with progression of established diabetic nephropathy to ESRD. The effect of blood pressure control appears to be much greater than the effect of blood sugar control on CKD prevention. Hyperglycemia may play a more decisive role in the initiation of nephropathy, whereas other variables may be responsible for progression. Because randomized trials show that intensive therapy in patients with type 2 diabetes results in a decreased risk of microvascular complications, glycemic control should be as tight as feasible in patients with diabetic nephropathy, although the risk of hypoglycemic complications must be taken into account in individual patients.

Protein Restriction

In animal models of CKD, dietary restriction of protein intake protects against renal disease progression. The putative mechanism of the renoprotective effect of protein restriction is a reduction of glomerular hypertension, but other, nonhemodynamic mechanisms, such as reduction of cytokine release at the glomerular level, may participate.

The effect of dietary protein restriction on the progression of CKD has been assessed in clinical trials. Although early, small studies supported restriction of protein intake, at least in some diseases such as diabetic nephropathy and chronic glomerular diseases, a large controlled trial in Italy that included 456 patients with a variety of renal diseases showed that a low-protein diet produced only a small, statistically insignificant benefit at 2 years. This study had several shortcomings, including imprecise measurement of GFR, noncompliance with the diet, and the modest reduction in protein intake achieved. The MDRD study randomized 585 patients with nondiabetic CKD to a daily protein intake regimen of 1.1 or 0.7 g/kg. Compliance was good, but no significant benefit was observed in the low-protein diet group compared with controls. Even in a subgroup of patients with advanced renal function impairment who were randomized to receive a diet with a very low protein content (0.3 g/kg/day plus essential amino acids), there was only a small and statistically insignificant effect on progression.

In summary, the role of protein restriction in slowing progression remains unclear. Most of the studies on low-protein diets were conceived and conducted at a time when the effect of aggressive blood pressure reduction with ACE inhibitors on progression was not yet fully established. Some investigators maintain that protein restriction would be worthwhile if it produced a reduction in the rate of GFR decline that was sufficient to delay dialysis initiation by even a few months. Moreover, dietary protein restriction is helpful in controlling hyperphosphatemia and metabolic acidosis. The concern that a low-protein diet causes loss of protein stores and induces malnutrition is not supported by the clinical experience in properly monitored patients. Finally, because dietary protein restriction can reduce proteinuria, it can act synergistically with antiproteinuric agents.

We recommend dietary protein restriction to less than 0.8 g/kg/day for patients with CKD, and probably less in patients with uncomplicated progressive CKD as well. With proper monitoring by a physician and the help of a skilled dietitian, protein restriction is safe and can be made acceptable to most patients.

Multiple Drug Approach

The prevention of CKD progression requires a multidrug strategy to attain several goals, as summarized in **Table 52-2**. This multidrug approach has been formalized as an interventional protocol at our outpatient "remission clinic." Patients with CKD and proteinuria greater than 1 g/24 hr are initially treated with a low dose of an ACE inhibitor, which is then gradually increased to the maximum dose. If the goals of blood pressure less than 130/80 mm Hg and proteinuria less than 0.3 g/24 hr are not achieved, an ARB is added at half-maximum dose and increased stepwise. Throughout this process, the addition of a diuretic is usually needed to facilitate blood pressure control or prevent hyperkalemia. To exploit their specific antiproteinuric effect, even if the blood pressure target has been achieved, ACE inhibitors or ARBs may be used at greater doses than those usually recommended for antihypertensive effects. Their use should not be limited by the initial level of GFR, although SCr and potassium should be closely monitored. An increase over baseline of SCr of less than 30% that stabilizes within the first 2 months of treatment

is associated with long-term preservation of kidney function and should be considered acceptable. Withdrawal of an ACE inhibitor or ARB should be considered only for patients with a rise in SCr that exceeds 30% of baseline or for development of hyperkalemia greater than 5.5 mmol/L that is not controllable by other means. With such a reduction in GFR, the presence of renal artery stenosis should be suspected and investigated. The concomitant use of drugs that interfere with kidney function or promote potassium retention, such as nonsteroidal anti-inflammatory drugs (NSAIDs), should also be excluded.

COMPLICATIONS OF CHRONIC KIDNEY DISEASE

The stages of CKD reflect gradual adaptation to nephron loss. In the early phase, stages 1 and 2, the patient is asymptomatic, blood urea nitrogen (BUN) and SCr are normal or near-normal, and acid-base, fluid, and electrolyte balances are maintained through an adaptive increase of function in the remaining nephrons. A reduction of GFR to 30 to 59 mL/min/1.73 m^2 defines stage 3, moderate impairment of GFR. The patient usually has no symptoms, although SCr and BUN are increased, and the serum levels of hormones such as erythropoietin, calcitriol, and parathyroid hormone (PTH) are usually abnormal. Stage 4, severe impairment of GFR, involves a further loss of kidney function. Findings, if present, are mild; patients may have anemia, acidosis, hypocalcemia, hyperphosphatemia, and hyperkalemia. The final stage of kidney disease, stage 5 is defined by a GFR of less than 15 mL/min/1.73 m^2, is usually characterized by worsening of all the aforementioned findings, and symptoms including fatigue, dysgeusia, anorexia, nausea, and pruritus may develop.

At present, there is no clear consensus on when dialysis should start. The 2006 U.S. NKF-K/DOQI guidelines recommended starting dialysis when GFR falls to 14 mL/min/1.73 m^2, and a similar cutoff GFR was suggested by the European Best Practice Guidelines of 2002. This is especially reinforced if malnutrition, fluid overload, acidosis, or hypertension is present despite treatment. These guidelines have not been universally adopted. In any case, dialysis should be started before the GFR drops below 6 mL/min/1.73 m^2, even if there are no symptoms or signs.

As kidney function declines, the kidney progressively loses its regulatory capacity, so that both excretion and conservation of water and electrolytes are impaired. When sudden loads or losses of fluid or electrolytes occur, decompensation may result. These complications of CKD can be classified into water, electrolyte, acid-base, metabolic, and organ system disorders.

TABLE 52-2 Treatment Goals for Slowing Progression of Chronic Kidney Disease

Tight blood pressure control (<130/80) using stepwise treatment
  Low-sodium diet
  ACE inhibitors
  Angiotensin receptor antagonists
  Diuretics
  Nondihydropyridine calcium channel blockers

Dietary protein restriction to 0.8 g/kg/day

Glycemic control in diabetic patients (HbA1c <7.5%)

Treatment of dyslipidemia (goal LDL cholesterol <100 mg/dL)

ACE, angiotensin-converting enzyme; HbA1c, glycated hemoglobin; LDL, low-density lipoprotein.

Water

Free water clearance is maintained until the GFR is severely reduced. In advanced stages of CKD, the reduced capacity of the kidney to concentrate or dilute urine may lead to hypernatremia or hyponatremia. The reduced capacity for concentrating the urine is particularly common in patients with diseases affecting the renal medulla, such as interstitial nephritis and pyelonephritis. Patients with a normal thirst mechanism and access to fluid will usually ingest an appropriate amount of fluid to match obligate losses. Dehydration can occur readily, however, in patients with inadequate fluid intake because of persisting diuresis. Attention to the fluid prescription is necessary when access to water is impaired by intercurrent illnesses.

Sodium

Maintaining sodium balance is very important in patients with CKD. Both sodium retention, with signs of volume overload, and sodium depletion, with signs of volume depletion, are common. In most patients with stable CKD, the total body sodium content is increased but only slightly; more substantial sodium retention is common in patients with a GFR of less than 10 mL/min/1.73 m^2 and in those with concomitant nephrotic syndrome or cardiac failure. Sodium retention contributes to, or aggravates, hypertension, edema, and congestive heart failure. A sodium-restricted diet (<2 g/day) and loop diuretics are often required. On the other hand, sodium conservation may be impaired early in CKD. In some instances, particularly tubulointerstitial diseases, sodium wasting may be present. For the most part, this failure of conservation can be viewed as an adaptation to the need to maintain balance and excrete the daily load of ingested sodium despite the reduced GFR. The diseased kidney may be unable to abruptly reverse this compensatory increase in fractional sodium excretion. Therefore, in the setting of CKD, the fractional sodium excretion may be higher than 1% even in the presence of volume depletion.

Extrarenal causes of sodium loss (vomiting, diarrhea, fever) may lead to extracellular fluid volume depletion with thirst, dry mucous membranes, tachycardia, orthostatic hypotension, vascular collapse, dizziness, syncope, and a fall in GFR that is usually reversible. Apart from treating the underlying cause of sodium depletion, it may be necessary to give intravenous isotonic saline; diuretics, if used, must be temporarily withdrawn.

Potassium

Because of an adaptive increase in potassium excretion by the remnant nephrons, patients with CKD usually have a normal serum potassium concentration until oliguria occurs. However, in patients with metabolic acidosis, which is characterized by a shift in potassium from intracellular to extracellular fluids, and in those with hyporeninemic hypoaldosteronism (seen in tubulointerstitial disease and diabetes mellitus), hyperkalemia may develop early. Hyperkalemia can also arise from an acute potassium load or with drugs that alter potassium secretion, such as ACE inhibitors, ARBs, potassium-sparing diuretics, β-blockers, aldosterone antagonists, NSAIDs, cyclosporine, and tacrolimus. Short-term management of hyperkalemia is discussed in Chapter 12. Dietary restriction is the mainstay of long-term management of hyperkalemia. Loop diuretics and potassium-binding resins can be useful for long-term control, but they are seldom necessary and often carry side effects. Spontaneous hypokalemia is uncommon in CKD, but it can be seen in salt-wasting nephropathy, Fanconi's syndrome, hereditary or acquired tubulointerstitial diseases, and renal tubular acidosis. In patients with CKD, hypokalemia is usually caused by low dietary potassium intake combined with high doses of diuretics or by gastrointestinal loss.

Acid-Base Disorders

Acid-base balance is normally maintained by kidney excretion of the daily acid load, both as titratable acid (primarily phosphate) and as ammonium. With advanced CKD (stage 3 and beyond), ammoniagenesis is impaired, and hydrogen ion excretion by the kidney is often not sufficient to match endogenous acid production and exogenous acid loads. Chronic metabolic acidosis results. As the patient approaches ESRD, the plasma bicarbonate concentration tends to stabilize between 12 and 20 mEq/L and rarely falls below 10 mEq/L. In the early stages of CKD, hyperchloremic renal tubular acidosis with normal anion gap is common; with more advanced stages, a high anion gap may develop. The anion gap is elevated in this setting as a result of the retention of unmeasured anions such as phosphate, sulfate, urate, and hippurate.

The treatment of acidosis (serum bicarbonate concentration <22 mEq/L) is desirable to prevent osteopenia and muscle catabolism. In fact, bone buffering of some of the excess hydrogen ions leads to the release of calcium and phosphate from bone, which may worsen bone disease. Uremic acidosis increases muscle breakdown, which may be exacerbated by a low-protein diet and decreased albumin synthesis, leading to loss of lean body mass and muscle weakness. These abnormalities in muscle function and albumin metabolism can be reversed by alkali therapy. Although there are no definitive studies proving that alkali therapy is beneficial in preventing or delaying osteopenia and hyperparathyroid bone disease, its use is recommended in patients with CKD with the aim of maintaining a plasma bicarbonate concentration higher than 22 mEq/L. Concern about the safety of sodium bicarbonate administration is probably overstated. It is usually well tolerated and not associated with signs of sodium retention. Oral sodium bicarbonate (in a daily dose of 0.5 to 1 mEq/kg) is the agent of choice; it usually produces little or no sodium retention or increase in blood pressure. Sodium citrate (citrate is rapidly metabolized to bicarbonate) can be used in patients with CKD but should be avoided in those who are also receiving phosphate binders containing aluminum, because citrate increases intestinal aluminum absorption and the risk of aluminum intoxication.

Phosphate, Calcium, and Bone

Even during the early stages of CKD, phosphate retention contributes to the development of the secondary hyperparathyroidism that plays an important role in the pathogenesis of bone disease and in other uremic complications. Moreover, the excess phosphate may contribute to CKD progression. This topic is covered in detail in Chapter 58.

THE UREMIC SYNDROME

The uremic syndrome is the clinical manifestation of severe kidney failure. It is partly the result of a reduction in kidney excretory function with the retention of toxic substances that impair cell regulatory mechanisms involving the cardiovascular, gastrointestinal, hematopoietic, immune, nervous, and endocrine systems. It is also the consequence of derangements in endocrine and metabolic functions of the kidney. The uremic syndrome is characterized not only by solute accumulation but also by hormonal alterations such as decreased production of erythropoietin and calcitriol, decreased clearance of insulin, end-organ resistance to insulin and PTH, and excess production of PTH. The signs and symptoms vary from one patient to another, depending partly on the rate and severity of the loss of kidney function (**Table 52-3**).

Cardiovascular System

Cardiovascular disorders (see also Chapter 59) are the leading cause of death in patients with ESRD, accounting for more than half of the deaths among patients on dialysis. Hypertension and congestive heart failure are common; retention of salt and water is important in the pathogenesis of both. Hypertension is present in more than 80% of patients undergoing chronic dialysis, and it is presumably a major risk factor for CVD, congestive heart failure, and cerebrovascular disease, although definitive evidence for this concept is lacking. In addition to salt and water retention, in uremia there are several conditions that may contribute to the development of hypertension, including enhanced activity of the renin-angiotensin system, excess aldosterone secretion, increased sympathetic tone, and reduced production of vasodilatory hormones such as prostaglandins and kinins.

Risk factors for CVD in CKD have been divided into two broad categories: traditional and nontraditional risk factors. The former group includes a number of risk factors for atherosclerosis that were originally identified in the

TABLE 52-3 Major Clinical Abnormalities in Uremia	
Fluid and Electrolyte Abnormalities	**Neurologic Abnormalities**
Volume expansion and depletion	Malaise
Hypernatremia and hyponatremia	Headache
Hyperkalemia and hypokalemia	Irritability and sleep disorders
Metabolic acidosis	Muscle cramps
Hyperphosphatemia and hypocalcemia	Tremor
Hypermagnesemia	Asterixis
Cardiovascular Abnormalities	Seizures
Hypertension	Stupor and coma
Congestive heart failure	Peripheral neuropathy
Cardiomyopathy	Restless legs
Pericarditis	Motor weakness
Vascular medial calcification	**Endocrine and Metabolic Abnormalities**
Accelerated atherosclerosis	Carbohydrate intolerance
Arrhythmias	Hypertriglyceridemia
Sudden cardiac death	Protein malnutrition
Gastrointestinal Abnormalities	Impaired growth
Anorexia, nausea, and vomiting	Infertility, sexual dysfunction, and amenorrhea
Uremic fetor	Renal osteodystrophy
Stomatitis, gastritis, and enteritis	Secondary hyperparathyroidism
Peptic ulcer	Hyperuricemia
Gastrointestinal bleeding	**Dermatologic Abnormalities**
Hematologic and Immunologic Abnormalities	Pallor
Anemia	Hyperpigmentation
Bleeding	Pruritus
Phagocyte inhibition	Ecchymoses
Lymphocytopenia and lymphocyte dysfunction	Uremic frost
Increased susceptibility to infection and neoplasia	

Framingham study and are commonly associated with increased risk of CVD in the general population, such as hypertension, diabetes, elevated LDL cholesterol, smoking, and a family history of CVD. There are limited data exploring the role of these traditional CVD risk factors exclusively in a population of patients with CKD, so we must rely on information extrapolated from studies in the general population. However, there is no reason to believe that these risks factors should behave differently in patients with CKD.

Most of the nontraditional risk factors (see Table 59-2 in Chapter 59) are present in CKD, and they have biologic plausibility. However, convincing evidence is still lacking that they are independent predictors of increased CVD or that interventions aimed at modifying these risk factors indeed are protective in a representative population of patients with CKD. One study compared traditional and novel risk factors as predictors of cardiovascular mortality in a cohort of 5808 subjects, aged 65 years or older, who were enrolled in the Cardiovascular Health Study. The proportion of participants who had CKD at baseline (defined as an estimated GFR of <60 mL/min/1.73 m^2) was 22%. In this study, a mortality rate of 32 deaths per 1000 person-years among subjects with CKD was observed, twice the rate among those without CKD. In multivariate analyses, diabetes, systolic hypertension, smoking, low physical activity, non-use of alcohol, and left ventricular hypertrophy (traditional risk factors for CVD) were all predictors of cardiovascular mortality in persons with CKD. Among the novel risk factors examined—C-reactive protein, fibrinogen, interleukin-6, factor VIIIc, lipoprotein(a), and hemoglobin—only log C-reactive protein ($P = .05$) and log interleukin 6 ($P < .001$) were independently associated with the outcome.

In patients on hemodialysis, rapid extracellular fluid volume changes may be associated with episodes of hypotension and electrolyte imbalance. Increased intake of calcium to treat hyperphosphatemia may enhance coronary arterial calcification. In dialysis patients, nitric oxide synthesis is often inhibited, with subsequent vasoconstriction and hypertension.

As a consequence of electrolyte imbalance, left ventricular dysfunction, or coronary artery disease, serious arrhythmias occur frequently with uremia. Symptomatic myocardial ischemia usually results from coronary artery disease, but it is nonatherosclerotic in origin in about 25% of patients. Widespread arterial medial calcification is a common complication of CKD (see Chapter 59). Uremic cardiomyopathy, possibly caused by PTH-induced myocardial calcification and fibrosis, has been described. Uremic pericarditis has become rare because of earlier initiation of dialytic therapy.

Gastrointestinal System

Gastrointestinal complications are common in advanced CKD and in some cases may be the first or only complaint on presentation. Anorexia, nausea, vomiting, and uremic fetor, with its typical ammoniacal odor on the breath, are common manifestations of uremia. Vomiting may occur without nausea and is often prominent in the early morning. Stomatitis, gastritis, and enteritis can develop with ESRD in patients not treated with dialysis or transplantation. Mucosal ulcerations can occur at any level of the gastrointestinal tract and, given the bleeding tendency of uremia, they largely account for the gastrointestinal bleeding seen in untreated uremia. An altered gastric mucosal barrier may contribute to the development of ulcerative lesions. Peptic ulcer occurs in about one fourth of uremic patients. The parotitis that develops in some patients may be related to the high salivary urea content in the presence of the low salivary flow rates that characterizes kidney failure. Rarely, pancreatitis is a significant clinical problem. Drugs such as metoclopramide can control nausea and enhance gastric emptying. Ulcerogenic medications, especially NSAIDs, should be avoided.

Red Blood Cells and Hemostasis

Anemia develops early during kidney failure and is one of the major causes of malaise and fatigue as kidney function worsens. In CKD, the management of anemia has radically changed since the advent of recombinant human erythropoietin. Correction of anemia improves cardiac function, central nervous system symptoms, appetite, and sexual function (see Chapter 60).

Immune Response

Phenotypic and functional alterations in both humoral and cellular immunity have been identified at early stages of CKD. They worsen with the progression of uremia, and some features are exacerbated by the hemodialysis procedure. The enhanced susceptibility to infection is greater with unmodified cellulosic hemodialysis membranes than with synthetic membranes. The antibody response to antigens is impaired, and the serum level of complement may be depressed.

The peripheral leukocyte count is normal and increases appropriately in response to infection in uremia, but metabolic and functional abnormalities of polymorphonuclear leukocytes (PMNLs) contribute to an increased susceptibility to infection. These abnormalities include impairments in carbohydrate metabolism, adenosine triphosphate (ATP) generation, adherence to endothelial cells, generation of reactive oxygen species, release of lysosomal enzymes, and chemotactic functions. Intensive intravenous iron therapy may aggravate the reduction in PMNL activity. Hemodialysis patients with elevated ferritin levels in the setting of functional iron deficiency (see Chapter 60) show significant impairment of fundamental PMNL functions, just as patients with refractory anemia who become iron-overloaded after multiple transfusions and patients with hereditary hemochromatosis do.

Increased intracellular calcium is associated with alterations of PMNL function and metabolism, which improve with normalization of calcium content with administration of calcium channel blockers or correction of hyperparathyroidism. Several compounds isolated from uremic serum inhibit the biologic activity of PMNLs. Granulocyte inhibitory proteins I (GIP I) and II (GIP II) inhibit the uptake of deoxyglucose, chemotaxis, oxidative metabolism, and intracellular killing by PMNLs.

GIP I displays homology with immunoglobulin light chain protein and GIP II with β_2-microglobulin. Degranulation inhibitory proteins I and II inhibit spontaneous and stimulated PMNL degranulation and are identical in molecular structure to angiogenin and complement factor D respectively.

Moderate lymphocytopenia with reduced circulating T cells, increased suppressor cell activity, and reduced helper cell activity may be present in uremic patients. The ratio of CD4-positive to CD8-positive T cells may be reduced. The response of lymphocytes to mitogens is reduced. Interferon production is also decreased.

Typical of uremia are an increased incidence of infections, including tuberculosis and bacteremia; immunologically modulated disorders such as cancer; and inadequate antibody production in response to hepatitis B vaccination. Although impaired humoral and cell-mediated immunity contribute to suboptimal and short-lived antibody responses to vaccines, vaccination still has an important role in attenuating infection risk. Adequate response has been documented with standard or augmented regimens for vaccinations against influenza, hepatitis B, pneumococcus, and varicella. For example, various strategies have been attempted to improve seroconversion after hepatitis B vaccination, such as extra doses of vaccine, doubling the dose, or repeating the vaccine when the antibody titer falls to less than 10 IU/L. Also, treatment with drug such as interferon, timopentin, erythropoietin, and granulocyte-macrophage colony-stimulating factor (GM-CSF) has been attempted with the aim of improving seroconversion. GM-CSF as adjuvant therapy via intradermal injection appears promising. Monitoring of antibody titers helps to determine the need for booster vaccination. Immunization against hepatitis B virus has significantly decreased the prevalence and incidence of this infection in hemodialysis units. The use of influenza vaccine and of polyvalent pneumococcal vaccine has reduced the morbidity and mortality attributable to these infections in uremic patients.

Neurologic Manifestations

Central nervous system disorders are seen in advanced stages of CKD (see Chapter 61). The early symptoms are those of disturbances of mentation and cognition resulting from reduced general cerebral activity, such as apathy, fatigue, confusion, impaired memory, and decreased capacity for prolonged intellectual effort. As the disorder progresses, disorientation and irritability may manifest, followed by hallucinations, anxiety, depression, and mania. Finally, lethargy, stupor, and coma occur. Peripheral neuropathy is common in advanced CKD. It is usually symmetrical and slowly progressive, beginning distally and spreading proximally. Dialysis can control the progression of peripheral neuropathy.

Metabolic and Endocrine Disorders

Glucose intolerance develops in most patients with CKD, mainly as a result of resistance to the peripheral action of insulin, but release of insulin in response to hyperglycemia may also be impaired. In patients with GFR less than 10 to 15 mL/min/1.73 m², insulin clearance is reduced, so insulin requirements are often paradoxically lower. Alterations in lipid metabolism may be present early in the course of CKD. Hypertriglyceridemia is the hallmark of dyslipidemia in CKD, and there is a concomitant increase in serum total cholesterol in the presence of nephrotic syndrome (see Chapter 61). Protein synthesis gradually decreases with CKD. In addition, most uremic patients are catabolic and have a negative nitrogen balance (see Chapter 58). Malnutrition, insulin resistance, metabolic acidosis, and hyporesponsiveness to growth hormone may all contribute to the negative nitrogen balance.

Free thyroxine (T_4) and serum thyroid-stimulating hormone (TSH, or thyrotropin) are usually normal, whereas the serum triiodothyronine (T_3) concentration is low because of decreased peripheral conversion of T_4 to T_3. Most of these patients are clinically euthyroid and need no thyroid treatment. In uremic women, estrogen production is low and prolactin levels are high, leading to disturbances in menstruation and fertility. Men may be impotent, infertile, or oligospermic secondary to low plasma testosterone levels (see Chapter 61).

Skin Effects

The cutaneous manifestations of uremia include pallor (anemia), ecchymoses (impaired hemostasis), pruritus, pigmentation, and dehydration. Uremic patients have a characteristic sallow pallor caused by anemia, retention of urochrome pigments and urea, and increased melatonin. The skin is usually dry and atrophic. With severe azotemia, the precipitation of urea crystals secreted in sweat leads to uremic frost. Several factors have been proposed to have a pathogenic role in uremic pruritus, including secondary hyperparathyroidism, dry skin, increased calcium and phosphate deposition in the skin, anemia, peripheral neuropathy, high aluminum levels, and hypervitaminosis A. Pruritus sometimes improves with dialysis, but it is usually resistant to most systemic and topical therapies. The administration of recombinant erythropoietin has been inconsistently reported to improve pruritus, for reasons that are not understood. At present, the best therapy for severe pruritus is a combination of erythropoietin, ultraviolet phototherapy, topical ointments, and, if necessary, an antihistamine.

Uremic Toxins and Hormonal Deficiencies

The uremic syndrome is attributed to the retention of a number of organic and inorganic substances that are normally excreted in the urine. These compounds are commonly called *uremic toxins,* although the attribution of clinical manifestations of uremia to specific substances has been difficult. Uremic retention substances are classified according to their molecular masses: (1) low-molecular-mass solutes (10 to 3000 Da) such as urea, creatinine, and guanidine compounds; (2) middle-mass molecules (3000 to 15,000 Da) including PTH and β_2-microglobulin; and (3) larger solutes (>15,000 Da) such as complement factor D, leptin, and cytokines.

CHAPTER 53

Staging and Management of Chronic Kidney Disease

Lesley A. Stevens, Nicholas Stoycheff, and Andrew S. Levey

Chronic kidney disease (CKD) is a serious public health problem. The number of persons with kidney failure who are treated with dialysis and transplantation in the United States is expected to rise dramatically, with a projected increase from 470,000 in 2004 to more than 2.2 million in 2030. The poor outcomes of CKD are not restricted to kidney failure but also include the complications of decreased kidney function, such as hypertension, anemia, malnutrition, bone and mineral disorders, and neuropathy, as well as increased risk of cardiovascular disease (CVD).

In 2002, the Kidney Disease Outcomes Quality Initiative (K/DOQI) of the National Kidney Foundation (NKF) sponsored guidelines for the definition, classification, evaluation, and stratification of risk of CKD. The purpose of these guidelines was to create uniform terminology to improve communications among all involved in the care and management of CKD, including patients, physicians, researchers, and policymakers. Previous terms (e.g., renal insufficiency, predialysis, progressive renal disease) were often imprecisely defined, and it was recognized that consistent language was necessary for the public and medical community to address this problem at all levels. New features of the classification system were that the definition and stages do not depend on identification of the cause of kidney disease, that kidney function is expressed as the level of estimated glomerular filtration rate (GFR), and that higher stages are associated with an increasing prevalence of complications resulting from decreased kidney function and CVD.

The goals of this chapter are to describe the conceptual model for the progression of CKD; the NKF-K/DOQI definition, stages of CKD, and estimated prevalence; an associated clinical action plan; and the role of nephrologists in the care of these patients.

DEFINITION AND STAGING OF CHRONIC KIDNEY DISEASE

Course of Chronic Kidney Disease

A conceptual model for the course of CKD is shown in **Figure 53-1**. This model describes the natural history of CKD, beginning with antecedent conditions, followed by the stages of CKD (kidney damage, decreased GFR, and kidney failure), and other associated outcomes. The model stresses that kidney disease tends to worsen over time by transitions through a defined sequence of stages, regardless

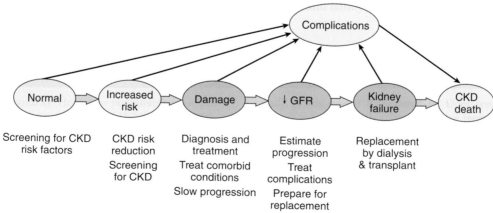

FIGURE 53-1 Conceptual model for stages in the initiation and progression of chronic kidney disease (CKD) and therapeutic interventions. Orange ellipses represent stages of CKD; yellow ellipses represent potential antecedents or consequences of CKD. Thick arrows between ellipses represent risk factors associated with initiation and progression of disease that can be affected or detected by interventions: susceptibility factors *(dark blue)*, initiation factors *(medium blue)*, progression factors *(pale blue)*, and end-stage factors *(white)* (see Table 53-1). Interventions for each stage are given beneath the stage. Complications refer to all complications of CKD and its treatment. (From the National Kidney Foundation, K/DOQI clinical practice guideline for chronic kidney disease; Evaluation, classification and stratification. Am J Kid Dis 39(supp2) 246; 2002, with permission.)

of the underlying susceptibility to disease, the specific cause of kidney damage, or the rate of progression through each stage. The earlier stages and the risk factors for progression to higher stages can be identified, permitting improvement in outcome by prevention, earlier detection, and initiation of therapies that can slow progression.

Susceptibility factors are characteristics that put an individual at risk for kidney damage (**Table 53-1**). These factors can be genetic, such as angiotensin-converting enzyme (ACE) polymorphisms, or developmental, such as low birth weight resulting in a reduced nephron mass. Demographic characteristics such as older age, minority race or ethnicity, and low financial income also describe individuals who are at increased risk for the development of kidney damage. The mechanisms underlying all of these associations have not been completely described or proven. For example, minority race or ethnicity may imply an underlying genetic tendency, or it may be a marker for lack of access to health care. Susceptibility factors may explain why a family history of kidney disease, regardless of the cause, places an individual at increased risk for development of kidney disease.

Initiation factors are conditions that can directly cause kidney damage, including diabetes, hypertension, autoimmune diseases, and kidney stones (see **Table 53-1**). Exposure to these conditions, together with the presence of susceptibility factors, determines whether an individual develops kidney damage. Individuals with susceptibility or initiation factors for CKD are at increased risk for development of CKD and should be tested for it on a regular basis.

In patients with kidney damage, *progression factors* influence the risk for and rate of decline in kidney function. Kidney disease may progress because the disorder responsible for inciting damage is continuous or as a result of pathways independent of the initial damage. Progression factors include elevated blood pressure, higher level of proteinuria, poor glycemic control in diabetes, and smoking. Current understanding of the mechanisms of progression; the risks conferred by specific progression factors; the interactions among susceptibility, initiation, and progression factors; and the variability of response in individual patients remains limited.

End-stage factors influence the risk for the development of adverse outcomes in patients with kidney failure. These factors relate to adequacy of dialysis, type of vascular access, compliance with dialysis prescription, nutritional status, and the presence of CVD.

Outcomes of CKD include loss of kidney function and CVD. Although kidney failure is the most visible outcome of CKD, decreased kidney function is more common and can lead to a myriad of systemic complications that may result in mortality, morbidity, or decreased quality of life. Also more common than kidney failure is CVD, which deserves special emphasis because CKD by itself is a risk factor for CVD. Conversely, CVD is a risk factor for CKD that is treatable and potentially preventable.

Definition of Chronic Kidney Disease

CKD is defined as either kidney damage or a GFR of less than 60 mL/min/1.73 m^2 of body surface area lasting for longer than 3 months. CKD can be diagnosed without knowledge of its cause.

Even with normal GFR, kidney damage is defined as CKD, because kidney damage may portend a poor prognosis for the major outcomes related to CKD. Kidney damage is usually ascertained by markers of damage without kidney biopsy. Because most kidney disease in North America is caused by diabetes or hypertension, persistent proteinuria or albuminuria is the principal marker. Numerous studies have shown that proteinuria is associated with a faster decline in GFR, increased risk of kidney failure, and CVD. Other markers of damage include abnormalities in urine sediment (e.g., tubular cells or casts), abnormal findings on imaging studies (e.g., hydronephrosis, asymmetry in kidney size, polycystic kidney disease, small echogenic kidneys), and abnormalities in blood and urine chemistry measurements (those related to altered tubular function, such as renal tubular acidosis). A history of kidney transplantation is also defined as a marker of kidney damage, and patients with a functioning transplant are considered to have CKD, irrespective of the presence of other markers of kidney damage or the level of GFR.

Reduced kidney function, specifically a GFR lower than 60 mL/min/1.73 m^2, is also defined as CKD. The level of GFR is usually accepted as the best overall index of kidney function in health and disease. A GFR level of less than 60 mL/min/

TABLE 53-1 Types of Risk Factors for Chronic Kidney Disease and Its Outcomes

RISK FACTORS	DEFINITION	EXAMPLES
Susceptibility factors	Increase susceptibility to kidney damage or education	Older age, family history of chronic kidney disease; reduction in kidney mass, low birth weight, racial or ethnic minority status, low income
Initiation factors	Directly initiate kidney damage	Diabetes, high blood pressure, autoimmune diseases, systemic infections, urinary tract infections, urinary stones, lower urinary tract obstruction, drug toxicity
Progression factors	Cause worsening of kidney damage and faster decline in kidney function	Higher levels of proteinuria, higher blood pressure, poor glycemic control in diabetes, smoking
End-stage factors	Increase morbidity and mortality in kidney failure	Lower dialysis dose (Kt/V), temporary vascular access, anemia, low serum albumin, late nephrology referral

Kt/V, dialysis dose as measured by urea clearance (K) multiplied by unit time (t) and divided byper volume of distribution of urea (V).

From the National Kidney Foundation, K/DOQI clinical practice guideline for chronic kidney disease; Evaluation, classification and stratification, Am J Kid Dis 39(supp2) 246; 2002, with permission.

$1.73 m^2$ represents the loss of half or more of the adult level of normal kidney function and is associated with an increased prevalence of systemic complications. The normal level of GFR varies according to age, gender, and body size. Normal GFR is approximately 120 to 130 mL/min/$1.73 m^2$ in a young adult and declines with age by approximately 1 mL/min/$1.73 m^2$ per year after the third decade. More than 25% of individuals aged 70 years and older have a GFR of less than 60 mL/min/$1.73 m^2$; this may be due to normal aging or to the high prevalence of systemic diseases that cause kidney disease. The definition of CKD does not vary with age. Whatever its cause, a GFR of less than 60 mL/min/$1.73 m^2$ in the elderly is an independent predictor of adverse outcomes such as death and CVD. As in younger patients, adjustment of drug doses is required in elderly patients with this level of GFR.

Kidney failure is defined as either a GFR of less than 15 mL/min/$1.73 m^2$ (which in most cases is accompanied by signs and symptoms of uremia) or a need to start kidney replacement therapy (dialysis or transplantation). Kidney failure is not synonymous with end-stage renal disease (ESRD), which is the administrative term used in the United States that indicates treatment by dialysis or transplantation and confers Medicare eligibility. ESRD does not include patients with kidney failure who are not treated with dialysis or transplantation.

Stages of Chronic Kidney Disease

The NKF-K/DOQI classification system for stages of CKD is based on the severity of the disease as indicated by the level of GFR, with higher stages representing lower GFR levels, regardless of the specific cause or the rate of progression (**Table 53-2**). The increased risk of complications with decreased GFR is demonstrated through analyses of the Third National Health and Nutrition Examination Survey (NHANES III), which showed an increasing prevalence of complications such as hypertension, anemia, malnutrition, bone and mineral

disorders, neuropathy, and decreased quality of life at higher stages of CKD (**Fig. 53-2**).

The risk of developing kidney failure is related to the stage of CKD as well as the rate of decline in GFR. The rate of decline of GFR varies among individuals and may even vary within an individual over time. For example, if the rate of decline is 4 mL/min/$1.73 m^2$ per year, then the interval from a GFR of 60 mL/min/$1.73 m^2$ to onset of kidney failure (<15 mL/min/$1.73 m^2$) will be 11 to 12 years. This rate of decline is considered fast. By contrast, if the rate of decline in GFR is 1 mL/min/$1.73 m^2$ per year, an elderly patient with a GFR of 60 mL/min/$1.73 m^2$ may not reach kidney failure in his or her lifetime. It is important to note that stage of CKD is only one metric for severity. CKD is a heterogenous disease, and patients may experience a wide range in severity of associated symptoms and conditions. Depending, in part, on the type of CKD and the comorbidities present, an individual patient may experience a wide variability in rate of progression or associated complications.

Prevalence

Table 53-2 shows the prevalence estimates of CKD derived from the most recent NHANES (1999-2004). The prevalence of CKD stages 1 through 4 appears to have increased to approximately 13% of the U.S. adult population, or 26 million people. This prevalence is more than 50 times greater than the prevalence of kidney failure (stage 5), which 0.2%. Because kidney disease usually begins late in life and progresses slowly, most people in the earlier stages of CKD die before they develop kidney failure. The burden of earlier stages of CKD in terms of mortality, morbidity, and reduced quality of life is now understood to be considerable for CVD and mortality; however, the impacts on other adverse outcomes (e.g., infectious diseases, malignancies) and complications of care (e.g., adverse drug reactions, perioperative complications) are also probably considerable. The systemic

---

TABLE 53-2 National Kidney Foundation K/DOQI: Classification, Prevalence, and Action Plan for Stages of Chronic Kidney Disease

STAGE	DESCRIPTION	GFR (mL/min/1.73 m²)	PREVALENCE,* n (%)	CLINICAL ACTION PLAN†
0	Individuals at increased risk	>60		Testing for the presence of CKD; CKD risk reduction
1	Kidney damage with normal or ↑ GFR	>90	3,600,000 (1.8)	Diagnosis and treatment; slowing progression; CVD risk reduction
2	Kidney damage with mild ↓ GFR	60-89	6,500,000 (3.2)	Estimation of progression
3	Moderate ↓ GFR	30-59	15,500,000 (7.7)	Evaluation and treatment of complications
4	Severe ↓ GFR	15-29	700,000 (0.4)	Preparation for kidney replacement therapy
5	Kidney failure	<15 (or dialysis)	400,000 (0.2)	Kidney replacement therapy (if uremia is present and patient wishes therapy)

CKD, chronic kidney disease; CVD, cardiovascular disease; GFR, glomerular filtration rate; K/DOQI, Kidney Disease Outcome Quality Initiative.

*Prevalence for stages 1 through 4 are projected from the 1999-2004 National Health and Nutrition Examination Survey for the population of 200 million adults aged 20 years or older in 2000. Prevalence for stage 5 is from United States Renal Data System for people treated with dialysis or transplantation, together with an estimate of 0.36 patients with untreated kidney failure for every treated patient.

†Action plan is cumulative in that each stage incorporates recommendations from the previous stage.

Updated and reprinted from the National Kidney Foundation, K/DOQI clinical practice guideline for chronic kidney disease; Evaluation, classification and stratification, Am J Kid Dis 39(supp2) 246; 2002, with permission.

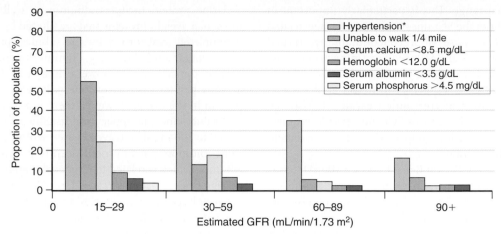

FIGURE 53-2 Estimated prevalence of selected complications, by category of estimated glomerular filtration rate (GFR), among participants aged 20 years and older in the Third National Health and Nutrition Examination Survey (NHANES III), 1988-1994. These estimates are not adjusted for age. A total of 10,162 participants with a mean age of 39 years had a GFR greater than 90 mL/min/1.73 m^2; 4404 participants with a mean age of 54 years had a GFR of 60 to 89 mL/min/1.73 m^2; 961 with a mean age of 72 years had a GFR of 30 to 59 mL/min/1.73 m^2; and 52 with a mean age of 75 years had a GFR of 15 to 29 mL/min/1.73 m^2. *Hypertension was defined as blood pressure of 140/90 mm Hg or higher or use of antihypertensive medication. The probably trend for was $P < .001$ for each abnormality. (From the National Kidney Foundation, K/DOQI clinical practice guideline for chronic kidney disease; Evaluation, classification and stratification, Am J Kid Dis 39(supp2) 246; 2002, with permission.)

complications of decreased GFR begin at levels well above those associated with kidney failure (see **Fig. 53-2**). In addition, increasing evidence shows that both albuminuria and decreased GFR are independent risk factors for CVD.

Clinical Action Plan

Associated with each stage of CKD is a clinical action plan (see **Table 53-2**). The action plan includes recommended care for each stage, as well as attention to the progression factors for the transition to a more advanced stage. Three key points must be emphasized. First, the action plan is cumulative, in that recommended care at each stage of disease includes care for less severe stages. Second, care for patients with CKD requires multiple interventions, and providing such care requires the coordinated, multidisciplinary effort of primary care physicians, allied health care workers, and other specialists in addition to nephrologists. Third, the management of each stage of disease must take into consideration CKD and CVD, as well as other comorbid conditions. The stage-specific clinical action plan is a guide, but not a replacement, for the physician's assessment of the needs of a specific patient.

EVALUATION AND MANAGEMENT

Diagnosis

Screening Procedures

As part of routine checkups, all patients should be evaluated to determine whether they are at increased risk for developing CKD because of the presence of susceptibility or initiation factors (see **Table 53-1**). Those deemed at high risk should at minimum have a measurement of serum creatinine concentration (SCr) to estimate GFR and assessment of proteinuria.

The recommended method for assessment of proteinuria in most individuals at increased risk is measurement of the albumin-to-creatinine ratio in an untimed ("spot") urine sample (see later discussion). Clinical judgment should determine the necessity of additional methods of detecting kidney damage, including imaging studies, other urine or serum markers, or biopsy of the kidney. The Joint National Committee on Prevention, Detection, Evaluation and Treatment of High Blood Pressure, the American Diabetes Association, and the Infectious Disease Society of America recommend yearly testing for CKD in patients with diabetes, hypertension, and human immunodeficiency virus (HIV) infection, respectively. The Kidney Disease Improving Global Outcomes (KDIGO) recommended annual testing for CKD in patients with hepatitis C as well as testing at the initiation of any cancer diagnosis and with each change in therapy. At resent, there are few data regarding the optimal frequency of testing for CKD in individuals who have risk factors other than diabetes and hypertension. Until evidence is available, it is reasonable to suggest that those at increased risk be tested at least every 3 years.

Assessment of Kidney Function

The National Institute of Diabetes, Digestive and Kidney Diseases, the NKF, and the American Society of Nephrology recommend the use of GFR, determined from the SCr with an estimating equation, as the primary assessment of kidney function in standard clinical practice. CKD is diagnosed when the estimated GFR is found to be less than 60 mL/min/1.73 m^2 on two occasions more than 3 months apart.

Current guidelines focus on estimated GFR rather than SCr alone, for a variety of reasons. SCr is affected by influences other than GFR (see Chapter 2). Consequently, there is a wide range of "normal" SCr, and in many patients GFR must decline by approximately 50% before SCr rises above the normal range. This is particularly important in the elderly, in whom the SCr does not reflect the age-related decline in GFR because of a concomitant age-related decline in muscle mass and reduced creatinine production. For these reasons, it is difficult to use the SCr alone to estimate the level of GFR, especially to detect earlier stages of CKD. Measurement of creatinine clearance (CrCl) can avoid some of the limitations of SCr; however, it requires collection of a timed urine sample, which is inconvenient and frequently inaccurate.

The Modification of Diet in Renal Disease (MDRD) Study equation and the Cockcroft-Gault equation provide useful estimates of GFR in adults. The MDRD study equation is more accurate and more precise than the Cockcroft-Gault equation or CrCl for persons with a GFR less than approximately 60 mL/min/1.73 m^2. However, as indicated in Chapter 2, these and other estimating equations do not perform as well in populations and settings other than those in which they were developed. GFR estimates may be inaccurate in populations without CKD; in other racial, ethnic, or geographic groups; or in individuals in whom creatinine production would be expected to differ from the general population (e.g., extremes of body size, high levels of dietary meat intake, malnutrition, spinal cord injury, amputation, or conditions associated with muscle wasting). GFR estimating equations should be used in conjunction with the clinical context. For example, given the imprecision in the GFR estimating equations, some people with estimated GFR of slightly less than 60 mL/min/1.73 m^2 would have a measured GFR that is actually greater than 60 mL/min/1.73 m^2. In these instances, a clinician must turn to alternative information, such as the presence of kidney damage or CKD risk factors, to guide clinical decisions about the presence of CKD. If an accurate estimate of GFR is required, a clearance measurement should be obtained, either a 24-hour urine collection for CrCl or clearance of an exogenous filtration marker, such as iothalamate or iohexol.

Cystatin C has been suggested as an alternative filtration marker to SCr. It has been reported to correlate better with GFR than the SCr alone; however, there is little or no improvement over GFR estimating equations. In addition, many studies now suggest that cystatin C generation, kidney handling, or assay may differ among populations, which would limit its widespread application as a filtration marker. Many studies have shown that cystatin C is a better predictor of adverse events than SCr or GFR estimated from SCr, particularly in elderly patients or those with CVD. Overall, more work is required to understand how to best use cystatin C as a filtration marker in clinical practice.

Kidney Damage

Markers of kidney damage include proteinuria, hematuria, other abnormalities of the urinary sediment, and radiologic evidence of damage. The most common causes of CKD in adults are diabetes (see Chapters 25 and 26) and hypertension (see Chapters 64 through 66), and therefore the most common marker for kidney damage is increased excretion of protein, and specifically of albumin.

Urine protein includes albumin as well as other low-molecular-weight proteins that are filtered by the kidney and incompletely reabsorbed by the tubules; proteins derived from tubular epithelium (e.g., Tamm-Horsfall protein); and proteins derived from the lower urinary tract (see Chapter 4). Healthy persons usually excrete only 50 to 100 mg/day of protein in the urine. However, there is a wide range of normal values, and the upper limit usually is extended as high as 200 to 300 mg/day to avoid false-positive evaluations. The most common type of protein seen in patients with CKD is albumin, which is related to glomerular injury. It is the earliest sign of kidney disease caused by diabetes, glomerular diseases, or hypertension. An elevated albumin excretion rate is a specific sign of kidney damage.

The ratio of concentrations of albumin or total protein to creatinine in a spot urine specimen has replaced 24-hour excretion rates as the preferred method for measuring albuminuria and proteinuria (**Table 53-3**). Use of such a ratio corrects for variations in urinary protein concentration due to hydration and is far more convenient than timed urine collections. A "positive" result for a spot urine albumin-to-creatinine (A/C) ratio is greater than 17 mg/g in men or 25 mg/g in women. Values between 17 and 250 mg/g are considered to be in the microalbuminuria range (i.e., not detectable by spot or timed urine collection for the detection of total protein) in men; in women, the corresponding range is 25 to 355 mg/g. Values greater than these upper limits are considered to represent macroalbuminuria. A positive result for the urine total protein to creatinine (P/C) ratio is 200 mg/g or higher. P/C ratios greater than 500 to 1000 mg/g usually indicate a glomerular disease (although such values may also be present in interstitial and vascular diseases). At this level of proteinuria, measurement of total protein, instead of albumin, on a spot urine sample is acceptable. Clinical features of the nephrotic syndrome typically arise when the spot urine P/C ratio is greater than 3000 mg/g.

Proteinuria can be seen intermittently in people without kidney disease secondary to vigorous exercise, fever, or infection. The algorithm for testing for proteinuria shown in **Figure 53-3** distinguishes persons with and without risk factors for CKD. A sample of urine from the first voiding after awakening is preferred, but a random specimen is acceptable. Ideally, patients should refrain from vigorous exercise for 24 hours before sample collection. The algorithm for adults who are at increased risk begins with testing of a random spot urine sample with an albumin-specific dipstick. Patients with a positive result on a dipstick test for albuminuria (≥20 mg/L or 1+) should undergo confirmation by measurement of the A/C ratio on a spot urine sample within 3 months. Alternatively, testing could begin with the A/C ratio. Patients with two or more positive results on quantitative tests temporally spaced over 3 months have persistent proteinuria and are considered to have CKD irrespective of the level of kidney function.

Urine dipstick or sediment examination (see Chapter 3) should also be performed in all patients who are at high risk for CKD. Imaging studies (see Chapter 5) should be performed in selected individuals, such as those with a

TABLE 53-3 Definitions of Proteinuria and Albuminuria

URINE COLLECTION METHOD	NORMAL VALUE	MICROALBUMINURIA	MACROALBUMINURIA OR PROTEINURIA
Total Protein			
24-Hour excretion (varies with method)	<300 mg/day	NA	>300 mg/day
Spot urine dipstick	<30 mg/dL	NA	>30 mg/dL
Spot urine P/C ratio (varies with method)	<200 mg/g	NA	>200 mg/g
Albumin			
24-Hour excretion	<30 mg/day	30-300 mg/day	>300 mg/day
Spot urine albumin-specific dipstick	<3 mg/dL	>3 mg/dL	NA
Spot urine A/C ratio (varies by gender*)	<17 mg/g (men)<25 mg/g (women)	17-250 mg/g (men)25-355 mg/g (women)	>250 mg/g (men)>355 mg/g (women)

A/C, albumin-to-creatinine; NA, not applicable; P/C, total protein-to-creatinine.

*Gender-specific cutoff values are derived from a single study. Use of the same cutoff value for men and women leads to higher values of prevalence for women. Current recommendations from the American Diabetics Association define cutoff values for spot urine A/C ratio as 30 mg/g for microalbuminuria and 300 mg/g for albuminuria, without regard to gender.

From National Kidney Foundation: K/DOQI Clinical Practice Guidelines for CKD: Evaluation, Classification, and Stratification. Part 4. Definition and Classification of Stages of Chronic Kidney Disease. Guideline 1. Definition and Stages of Chronic Kidney Diseases. Table 15. Definitions of Proteinuria and Albuminuria. Available at http://www.kidney.org/professionals/KDOQI/guidelines_ckd/Gif_File/kck_t15.gif (assessed July 25, 2008).

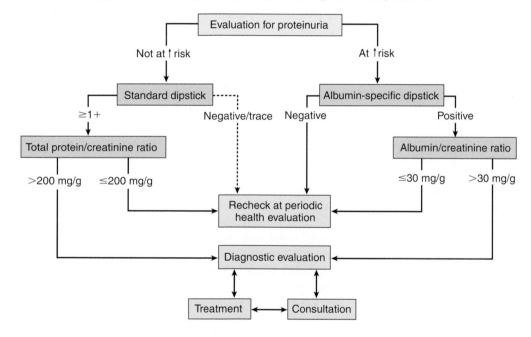

FIGURE 53-3 Evaluation of proteinuria in patients not known to have kidney disease. (From the National Kidney Foundation, with permission.)

family history of polycystic kidney disease or a history of vesicoureteral reflux in childhood, because they may have chronic scarring from the remote injury that increases their risk for ongoing progressive kidney disease.

Evaluation

Starting treatment early in CKD is essential to prevent adverse outcomes. The goals of evaluation are
1. To identify the stage of CKD
2. To diagnose the type of kidney disease
3. To detect reversible causes
4. To identify risk factors for progression of kidney disease
5. To identify risk factors for CVD
6. To detect complications of decreased GFR

Diagnosis of CKD is traditionally based on pathology and etiology. A simplified classification emphasizes diseases in native kidneys (diabetic or nondiabetic in origin) and diseases in transplanted kidneys. Diabetic nephropathy is the largest single cause of kidney failure in the United States, accounting for approximately one third of new cases. Its earliest manifestation is microalbuminuria with a normal or elevated GFR (CKD stage 1). Nondiabetic kidney disease includes glomerular, vascular, tubulointerstitial, and cystic kidney disorders.

Evaluation of CKD starts with a thorough history and physical examination to detect any signs and symptoms that may be clues to the cause of kidney disease and, in particular, any reversible elements or treatable risk factors for progression of CKD or for CVD (e.g., uncontrolled hypertension, use of nonsteroidal anti-inflammatory drugs). The physical examination should pay particular attention to details such as funduscopy, blood pressure, and vascular examination. Laboratory tests should be performed to detect disruptions of other kidney functions besides GFR, including maintenance of the filtration barrier for plasma proteins; resorption or excretion of water or specific solutes (e.g., sodium, potassium, bicarbonate); and endocrine functions. In individuals known to have CKD, urine protein should be quantified with spot urine examination for the P/C or A/C ratio, urine sediment examination, urine specific gravity, urine pH, and measurement of serum electrolytes. Imaging studies should be performed if indicated based on clinical clues. Ultrasonography should be performed in all cases to detect anatomic abnormalities and to exclude obstruction of the urinary tract. Further testing may be indicated if there is concern about anatomic abnormalities. Individuals with CKD stages 3 through 5 (GFR <60 mL/min/1.73 m^2) should have measurements of hemoglobin as well as serum calcium, phosphate, albumin, and parathyroid hormone. Laboratory evaluation should also include a search for traditional CVD risk factors, such as a lipid profile, and possibly tests for nontraditional risk factors such as insulin resistance and inflammation. Additional studies may be necessary to evaluate symptoms of CVD more fully or to detect asymptomatic CVD in patients with multiple risk factors.

Because of the age-related decline in GFR, many elderly individuals have an estimate GFR of less than 60 ml/min/1.73 m^2 and fulfill the criteria for a diagnosis of CKD stage 3. These individuals are at low risk for progression to kidney failure but are at increased risk for CKD complications and for CVD. In the absence of risk factors for CKD, markers of kidney damage, or complications of CKD, clinicians may elect to defer some parts of the evaluation for CKD. However, a search for reversible causes of decreased GFR, adjustment of medication dosages for decreased GFR, appropriate attention to CVD risk factor management, and subsequent monitoring of estimated GFR are appropriate measures.

Management

The essential features of management are as follows:
1. Treat specific causes of kidney disease.
2. Treat other reversible conditions causing kidney damage or decreased GFR.
3. Treat progression factors.
4. Treat uremic complications, and prepare for kidney replacement therapy if appropriate.
5. Treat CVD and its risk factors.
6. Avoid exposing the patient to medications that are toxic to the kidneys.

Treatment of progression factors is the cornerstone of care for patients with CKD. The details of their management are described elsewhere in this *Primer* (see Chapters 52, 57, 58, and 61). Close attention to returning the extracellular fluid volume to normal, achievement of the target blood pressure (see Chapter 65), and blockade of the renin-angiotensin system are key components of therapy. The usual target blood pressure for patients with CKD is below 130/80 mm Hg (**Table 53-4**). Use of ACE inhibitors or angiotensin receptor blockers (ARBs) is recommended for all patients with diabetic kidney disease and for those with nondiabetic kidney disease who have spot urine P/C ratios greater than 200 mg/g. Strong evidence documents the efficacy of these therapies to slow progression of CKD. Most patients require more than two antihypertensive agents to achieve this blood pressure target. For most diseases, diuretics are preferred as the second agent. Additional therapies may be considered for patients with spot urine P/C ratios greater than 500 to 1000 mg/g, including a lower blood pressure goal or initiation or increased dosage of agents that reduce proteinuria, including ACE inhibitors, ARBs, and nondihydropyridine calcium channel blockers. Other potential targets of intervention to slow kidney disease progression are dietary protein restriction, lipid-lowering therapy, strict glycemic control in diabetes, and smoking cessation.

Individuals with CKD are considered to be at high risk for development of CVD. As in patients without CKD, treatment of CVD risk factors is critical for the prevention of initial and

---

TABLE 53-4　National Kidney Foundation K/DOQI: Clinical Practice Guidelines on Hypertension and Antihypertensive Agents in Chronic Kidney Disease

TYPE OF KIDNEY DISEASE	BLOOD PRESSURE TARGET (mm Hg)	PREFERRED AGENTS FOR CKD, WITH OR WITHOUT HYPERTENSION	OTHER AGENTS TO REDUCE CVD RISK AND REACH BLOOD PRESSURE TARGET
Diabetic kidney disease	<130/80	ACE inhibitor or ARB	Diuretic preferred, then BB or CCBs
Nondiabetic kidney disease with spot urine P/C ratio ≥200 mg/g	<130/80	ACE inhibitor or ARB	Diuretic preferred, then BB or CCBs
Nondiabetic kidney disease with spot urine P/C ratio <200 mg/g	<130/80	None preferred	Diuretic preferred, then ACE inhibitor, ARB, BB, or CCB
Kidney disease in the kidney transplant recipient	<130/80	None preferred	CCB, diuretic, BB, ACE inhibitor, ARB

ACE, angiotensin-converting enzyme; ARB, angiotensin receptor blocker; BB, β-blocker; CCB, calcium channel blocker; CKD, chronic kidney disease; CVD, cardiovascular disease; K/DOQI, Kidney Disease Outcome Quality Initiative; P/C, total protein-to-creatinine.

From National Kidney Foundation: K/DOQI clinical practice guidelines for hypertension and antihypertensive agents in chronic kidney disease. Am J Kidney Dis. 43(5 suppl 1): S1-S290, 2004. Table 21 in these guidelines.

subsequent events. However, in patients with CKD there are several differences in management of these risk factor conditions. Hypertensive patients with CKD are recommended to have a blood pressure goal of less than 130/80 mm Hg, which is lower than the recommended goal of 140/90 mm Hg in other populations; also, as discussed earlier, an ACE inhibitor or ARB is the preferred first-line agent in the setting of proteinuria. The use of oral diabetes agents must often be altered when the GFR is low. Glipizide is preferred to other sulfonylureas because, unlike many of its counterparts, it is not degraded to a metabolite that is dependent on the kidneys for elimination. Dosages of incretin enhancers may need to be lowered, and metformin should be avoided. In the treatment of dyslipidemia, a plasma LDL cholesterol value of less than 100 mg/dL is recommended in patients with CKD, and care must be taken in the use of fibrates because of the increased risk of myopathy in combination therapy with statins. Investigations for the diagnosis of CVD must also be altered; careful consideration must be given in the use of iodinated contrast agents or gadolinium for angiography or magnetic resonance imaging (see chapters 5 and 34).

Uremic complications should be monitored and treated. These include electrolyte abnormalities (hyperkalemia, metabolic acidosis), anemia, hyperparathyroidism, hyperphosphatemia, bone disease, malnutrition, and nervous system disorders (neuropathy, cognitive changes). The details of their management are discussed elsewhere in this *Primer* (see Chapters 52 and 63 through 67).

Patient education is a central aspect of the management strategy, particularly in that CKD is a chronic and often asymptomatic disease and patients may not understand the importance of multidrug regimens and laboratory testing without explicit education. Complete management of chronic disease requires behavioral change by the patient, which may include lifestyle alterations, adherence to medication regimens, self-monitoring of blood pressure, and adherence to plans for medical follow-up. Patient education is also important with respect to avoidance of exposure to medications that are toxic to the kidneys. Patients must be aware that any drugs or herbal remedies may be directly nephrotoxic or may require a dosage adjustment for the level of kidney function.

Health Care Structure for Treatment of Chronic Kidney Disease

Nephrology Referral

CKD can be a life-threatening condition. Nephrologists have several functions in the diagnosis and care of patients at all stages of CKD, including determining the cause of CKD, recommending specific therapy, suggesting treatments to slow progression in patients who have not responded to conventional therapies, identifying and treating kidney disease–related complications, and preparing for dialysis.

Recommendations for referral to a kidney disease specialist are summarized in **Table 53-5**. Only a subset of patients with CKD in stages 1 to 3 are likely to require referral to a specialist. The strongest evidence for the importance of

TABLE 53-5 Indications for Referral to Kidney Disease Specialists for Consultation and Comanagement

Evaluation and management of CKD, as described in the National Kidney Foundation K/DOQI Clinical Action Plan (see Table 53-2)
GFR <30 mL/min/1.73 m^2
Spot urine total protein-to-creatinine ratio >500-1000 mg/g
Increased risk for progression of kidney disease
GFR decline >30% within 4 mo without explanation
Hyperkalemia (serum potassium concentration >5.5 mEq/L) despite treatment
Resistant hypertension
Difficult-to-manage drug complications

CKD, chronic kidney disease; GFR, glomerular filtration rate; K/DOQI, Kidney Disease Outcome Quality Initiative.
From Vassalotti, JA, Stevens LA, Levey AS, Testing for chronic kidney disease: a position statement from the National Kidney Foundation. Am J kidney Dis. 50: pp. 169-180, 2007. Table 10 in this article.

referral to a nephrologist is for management of CKD stages 4 and 5 (GFR <30 mL/min/1.73 m^2). Late referral to a nephrologist (i.e., <3 months before the start of dialysis therapy) has been associated with higher mortality after the initiation of dialysis. It is recommended that all patients with CKD stage 4 be referred to a nephrologist for comanagement. During stage 4, it is important to prepare the patient for the possible onset of kidney failure (CKD stage 5). Preparation involves estimating the risk of progression to kidney failure, holding discussions regarding kidney replacement therapy (dialysis and transplantation), and instituting conservative therapy for those who are not willing or are unable to undergo kidney replacement therapy. In patients who elect replacement therapy, timely creation of vascular access for hemodialysis, home dialysis training, and donor evaluation for preemptive transplantation should occur during stage 4.

Primary Care and Specialist and Comanagement

Optimal management of chronic disease requires coordination among all physicians, allied health care workers, and the patient. Primary care physicians and specialists each bring unique skills to patient management, and, for many patients, it is important to incorporate both into the care plan. A care delivery model in which primary care physicians and specialists share responsibility for the care of persons with CKD is recommended. In this model, most patients with CKD stages 1 through 3 would mainly under the care of primary care physicians, generalists, or specialists other than nephrologists, with referral to a nephrologist for assistance in the evaluation and in the development and implementation of the clinical action plan for the CKD. As kidney disease worsens, the need for consultation and comanagement with nephrologists increases (**Fig. 53-4**). The specific configuration of the comanagement depends not only on the structure of the health care system and the geographic location of the practice, but also on the needs of the individual patient and physician. In rural settings or where there is a shortage of nephrologists or other specialists, comanagement can be done

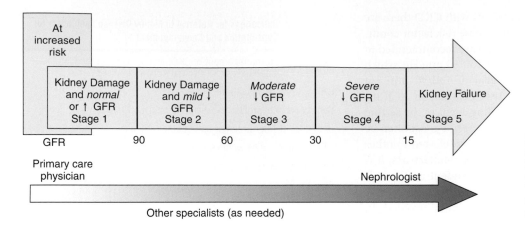

FIGURE 53-4 Primary care physicians and nephrologists are both important in the care of patients with chronic kidney disease (CKD). The relative contribution each makes to the care of a patient shifts as patients reach CKD stage 4.

via telephone, e-mail, or other forms of electronic information transfer in addition to visits in person.

Multidisciplinary Clinics

Complex, multifaceted disease processes require systematic approaches to care delivery. Optimal management of CKD requires coordination of antihypertensive and antiproteinuric strategies, smoking cessation, lipid-lowering therapies, management of diabetes, and other dietary and lifestyle modifications. This agenda is best accomplished by coordinated effort among practitioners. Allied health care workers such as nurse practitioners, nurses, dietitians, pharmacists, and social workers are integral to providing excellent care. Other aspects of chronic care management that can be facilitated in this framework are self-management by patients, decision support by physicians, case management, planned appointments with the multidisciplinary team and nephrologists, and routine laboratory tests.

A small but growing literature demonstrates the benefit of having CKD patients seen by nephrologists in a multidisciplinary clinic. Benefits include delay in need for initiation of kidney replacement therapy, increased rate of seroconversion after hepatitis B vaccination, improved biochemical parameters at the start of hemodialysis, and decreased left ventricular hypertrophy. In multidisciplinary clinics, patient education can be organized and appropriately delivered. The benefit of patient education was recently shown in a randomized trial of a short, patient-directed educational program that led to a prolongation by 17 months of the interval before the need for kidney replacement therapy.

Clinics need not be geographically based. Use of templates or pathways that involve different kinds of caregivers may allow for similar delivery of care. The use of information technology is important in the coordination of care among multiple caregivers, and it is particularly important for nongeographically based clinics and geographically isolated settings.

BIBLIOGRAPHY

Coresh J, Selvin E, Stevens LA, et al: Prevalence of chronic kidney disease in the U.S. during 1988-1994 and 1999-2004. JAMA 298:2038-2047, 2007.

Eknoyan G, Hostetter T, Bakris G, et al: Proteinuria and other markers of chronic kidney disease: A position statement of the National Kidney Foundation (NKF) and the National Institute of Diabetes and Digestive and Kidney Diseases (NIDDK). Am J Kidney Dis 42:617-622, 2003.

Go A, Chertow GM, Fan D, et al: Chronic kidney disease and the risks of death, cardiovascular events, and hospitalization. N Engl J Med 351:1296-1305, 2004.

Jafar T, Stark P, Schmid C, et al: Progression of chronic kidney disease: The role of blood pressure control, proteinuria, and angiotensin-converting enzyme inhibition—A patient-level meta-analysis. Ann Intern Med 139:244-252, 2003.

Klahr S, Levey AS, Beck GJ, et al: The effects of dietary protein restriction and blood-pressure control on the progression of chronic renal disease. N Engl J Med 330:877-884, 1994.

Levey A, Coresh J, Balk E, et al: National Kidney Foundation practice guidelines for chronic kidney disease: Evaluation, classification, and stratification. Ann Intern Med 139:137-147, 2003.

Levey AS, Coresh J, Greene T, et al: Using standardized serum creatinine values in the Modification of Diet in Renal Disease study equation for estimating glomerular filtration rate. Ann Intern Med 145:247-254, 2006.

Levin A, Lewis M, Mortiboy P, et al: Multidisciplinary predialysis programs: Quantification and limitations of their impact on patient outcomes in two Canadian settings. Am J Kidney Dis 29:533-540, 1997.

National Kidney Foundation: K/DOQI clinical practice guidelines for chronic kidney disease: Evaluation, classification, and stratification. Am J Kidney Dis 39(2 Suppl 1):S1-S266, 2002.

National Kidney Foundation: K/DOQI clinical practice guidelines for hypertension and antihypertensive agents in chronic kidney disease. Am J Kidney Dis 43(5 Suppl 1):S1-S290, 2004.

O'Hare A, Bertenthal D, Covinsky KE, et al: Mortality risk stratification in chronic kidney disease: One size for all ages? J Am Soc Nephrol 17:846-853, 2006.

Sarnak MJ, Greene T, Wang X, et al: The effect of a lower target blood pressure on the progression of kidney disease: Long-term follow-up of the modification of diet in renal disease study. Ann Intern Med 142:342-351, 2005.

Sarnak M, Levey A, Schoolwerth A, et al: Kidney disease as a risk factor for development of cardiovascular disease: A statement from the American Heart Association Councils on Kidney in Cardiovascular Disease, High Blood Pressure Research, Clinical Cardiology, and Epidemiology and Prevention. Circulation 42:1050-1065, 2003.

Standards of medical care in diabetes—2007. Diabetes Care 30 (Suppl 1):S4-S41, 2007.

Stevens LA, Coresh J, Feldman HI, et al: Evaluation of the modification of diet in renal disease study equation in a large diverse population. J Am Soc Nephrol 18:2749-2757, 2007.

Stevens LA, Coresh J, Greene T, et al: Assessing kidney function: Measured and estimated glomerular filtration rate. N Engl J Med 354:2473-2483, 2006.

Stevens LA, Manzi J, Levery AS, et al: Impact of creatinine calibration on performance of GFR estimating equations in a pooled individual patient database. Am J Kidney Dis 50:21-35, 2007.

United Kingdom Prospective Diabetes Study (UKPDS) Group: Intensive blood-glucose control with sulphonylureas or insulin compared with conventional treatment and risk of complications in patients with type 2 diabetes (UKPDS 33). Lancet 352:837-853, 1998.

United States Renal Data System: USRDS 2007 Annual Data Report: Atlas of End-Stage Renal Disease in the United States. Bethesda, MD, National Institutes of Health, National Institute of Diabetes and Digestive and Kidney Diseases, 2007.

Vassalotti, JA, Stevens LA, Levey AS: Testing for chronic kidney disease: A position statement from the National Kidney Foundation. Am J Kidney Dis 50:169-180, 2007.

Bioincompatibility of dialysis membranes refers to the interactions that occur as a result of contact of blood with the membrane. Examples include activation of proteins of the coagulation and complement systems as well as various peripheral blood leukocytes and platelets. Biocompatibility is relative, because all dialysis membranes induce reactions to a certain extent, which can manifest, for example, as thrombosis in the dialyzer and, rarely, as acute anaphylactoid reactions. When in vitro assays of blood collected during hemodialysis are used to determine biocompatibility, unmodified cellulosic membranes appear to be the least biocompatible type. Epidemiologic studies also suggest that unmodified low-flux membranes are associated with higher patient mortality compared to synthetic membranes—an adverse outcome that is not shared by modified cellulosic membranes. These studies, however, do not distinguish between the effect of biocompatibility and the effect of flux. The use of unmodified cellulosic dialysis membrane also appears to be associated with worse recovery in kidney function and greater patient mortality in cases of AKI. Although they are not definitive, these clinical studies and the plausible biologic basis of membrane incompatibility suggest that membrane materials could indeed affect clinical outcomes. Unmodified cellulosic membranes are rarely used in the United States at present. Hemofiltration membranes are always high flux and are usually made of synthetic materials. Although synthetic membranes are in general considered to be more biocompatible, they may still cause bioincompatibility reactions.

TABLE 54-1 Glossary of Extracorporeal Therapy for Kidney Failure

A. Hemodialysis (HD)

1. **Conventional hemodialysis**—hemodialysis using a conventional low-efficiency/low-flux membrane. Solute removal is primarily by diffusion.

2. **High-efficiency hemodialysis**—hemodialysis using a membrane with high efficiency in removal of small-size solutes (e.g., urea), which is typically achieved by a larger surface area

3. **High-flux hemodialysis**—hemodialysis using a membrane with large pore sizes. It is more efficient in removing middle molecules (e.g., β_2-microglobulin).

4. **Slow or sustained low-efficiency dialysis (SLED)**—continuous low-efficiency hemodialysis using a low blood flow rate and a low dialysate flow rate. The term **continuous venovenous hemodialysis (CVVHD)** is practically synonymous with SLED.

B. Hemofiltration (HF)

1. **Continuous arteriovenous or venovenous hemofiltration (CAVHF/CVVHF)**—removal of small-sized solutes and middle molecules using a high-flux membrane and convection rather than diffusion. Blood is accessed either from an artery using the driving force derived from the systemic arterial pressure or from a vein using an external blood pump. The blood is returned to a vein in either case. Because it is performed continuously (usually in the intensive care setting), it is also very effective in removing large amounts of fluid.

2. **Intermittent hemofiltration**—hemofiltration performed on an intermittent basis for end-stage renal disease

C. Hemodiafiltration (HDF)

1. **Continuous arteriovenous or venovenous hemodiafiltration (CAVHDF/CVVHDF)**—similar to CAVHF/CVVHF in that solutes are removed by convection using a high-flux membrane, usually in the intensive care setting. In addition, dialysate flows continuously through the dialysate compartment in order to enhance solute removal by diffusion (i.e., it is a combination of hemodialysis and hemofiltration).

2. **Intermittent hemodiafiltration**—hemodiafiltration performed on an intermittent basis for end-stage renal disease, often employing a hemodiafiltration machine that also generates sterile pyrogen-free replacement fluid on-line continuously.

D. Hemoperfusion (HP)—removal of solutes by adsorption to charcoal or resin, primarily for treatment of acute poisoning.

TABLE 54-2 Performance of Different Types of Dialyzers and Hemofilters

	UREA K_0A* (mL/min)	UREA CLEARANCE† (mL/min)	ULTRAFILTRATION COEFFICIENT‡ (mL/hr/mm Hg)	β_2M CLEARANCE† (mL/min)
Dialyzers				
Conventional	<450	<150	<12	<10
High-efficiency	>600	>200	Variable	Variable
High-flux	Variable	Variable	>12	>20
Hemofilters	Variable	Variable	>12	>20

β_2M, β_2-macroglobulin.
*The mass transfer coefficient-area product (K_0A) is the product of the mass transfer coefficient (K_0) times the surface area of the dialysis membrane (A). K_0 describes the capacity of the dialysis membrane to clear a specific solute of interest, such as urea, and can be viewed conceptually as the inverse of the resistance of the dialysis membrane to diffusive transport of the solute.
†Values observed under usual clinical operating conditions.
‡The ultrafiltration coefficient describes the capacity of the dialysis membrane to remove water and is usually calculated as the plasma water removal rate normalized by the transmembrane hydrostatic pressure.

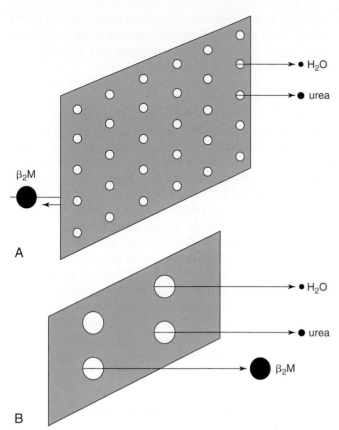

A

B

FIGURE 54-2 Diagrams of low-flux and high-flux dialysis membranes. **A,** Low-flux membranes have small pores that are highly permeable to small solutes such as water and urea (60 Da) but restrict the transport of middle molecules such as β_2-microglobulin (β_2M). Because of their small pores, they also tend to have low ultrafiltration coefficients, although the ultrafiltration coefficient can be increased by increasing the surface area of the membrane. A low-flux membrane can be either high efficiency or low efficiency for urea transport, depending on its surface area and, to a lesser extent, its thickness. **B,** High-flux membranes have large pores that facilitate the transport of middle molecules such as β_2M in addition to small molecules. Their ultrafiltration coefficients are high. A high-flux membrane can be either high efficiency or low efficiency, depending on its surface area and, to a lesser extent, its thickness.

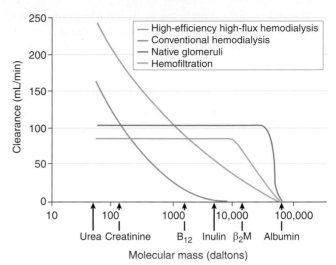

FIGURE 54-3 Solute clearance profile of various modalities. The curves are constructed based partially on data and partially on theoretical projection. The actual values may vary depending on the surface area of the membrane and operating conditions (e.g., blood flow rate). The curve for native glomeruli represents the summation of all the glomeruli in two normal kidneys. "Glomeruli" instead of "kidneys" are used because tubular reabsorption substantially lowers the kidney clearance of certain solutes, such as urea and glucose. Clearance of solutes by diffusion (via either conventional or high-efficiency/high-flux dialysis) deteriorates rapidly with increase in molecular mass of the solute. In contrast, clearance by convection (hemofiltration or glomeruli) remains constant over a wide range of molecular mass. B_{12}, vitamin B_{12}; β_2M, β_2-microglobulin.

WATER TRANSPORT AND SOLUTE CLEARANCE PROFILES

The ability of dialysis membranes to transport small-sized solutes, such as urea (60 Da) and potassium (31 Da), are usually expressed as the mass transfer coefficient-area product (K_oA), which is the product of the mass transfer coefficient (K_o) and membrane surface area (A). High-efficiency dialyzers are those with high K_oA values for urea (>600 mL/min) (see **Table 54-2**) which are usually achieved by having a large surface area, whereas low-efficiency dialyzers are those with low K_oA values (<450 mL/min). The clearance profile of solutes by hemodialysis membranes presented in **Figure 54-3** reflects primarily the K_oA of the membranes and provides only a rough estimation of what might be achieved clinically. The actual solute clearance depends also on the rate of blood flow that presents the solute to the dialyzer, the rate of dialysate flow that provides the diffusion gradient, and the rate of fluid removal that supplements the diffusion by convective

loss of the solute. Diffusive clearance of solutes by hemodialysis decreases rapidly with increasing molecular size. For small solutes such as urea, however, the removal per unit time by high-efficiency hemodialysis (180 to 240 mL/min) is approximately twice that achieved by the glomeruli in two native kidneys (90 to 120 mL/min for adults), which, in turn, is significantly higher than the urinary excretory rate of urea after kidney tubular resorption. However, patients spend only 9–15 hours per week on hemodialysis, whereas native kidneys function continuously for a total of 168 hours per week. As a result, the total weekly clearance of urea by hemodialysis is far lower than that achieved in a patient with normal functioning kidneys.

The effectiveness of water transport across a dialysis or hemofiltration membrane is measured as the ultrafiltration coefficient (defined as the volume of water transported per unit time) normalized by the transmembrane hydrostatic pressure gradient. Ultrafiltration coefficients for low-flux hemodialysis membranes are usually 2 to 5 mL/hr/mm Hg. With a transmembrane pressure of 200 mm Hg, a dialyzer with a coefficient of 2.5 mL/hr/mm Hg will remove 0.5 L of fluid per hour, or 2 L in 4 hours. Ultrafiltration coefficients for high-flux dialysis or hemofiltration membranes are much higher, 12 to 60 mL/hr/mm Hg. It should be noted that extracorporeal fluid removal from a patient is usually limited by the rate at which extravascular fluid can be transferred into the intravascular compartment, and almost never by the ultrafiltration coefficient of the dialysis membrane.

The ability of the membrane to clear middle molecules is governed by the size of the membrane pores and is closely related to the ultrafiltration coefficient (see **Fig. 54-2**). Middle molecules are solutes that are significantly larger than urea but smaller than albumin (60,000 Da); they are often represented by the protein β_2M (11,800 Da). Low-flux dialyzers are those with β_2M clearances that have been arbitrarily defined as less than 10 mL/min and are often close to nil, whereas high-flux dialyzers have β_2M clearances greater than 20 mL/min under normal operating conditions of blood and dialysate flow rates. Ideally, the capacity of dialysis membranes to remove β_2M should be expressed in terms of its K_oA, similar to the K_oA for urea, but this notion has not been adopted by the general dialysis community. Diffusive clearance of solutes decreases rapidly with increases in molecular size and is usually only 20 to 60 mL/min for β_2M even by high-flux hemodialysis, compared to more than 150 mL/min for urea. In contrast to diffusion, solute transport by convection through high-flux membranes is unrestricted and independent of solute size, up to a certain point. Therefore, the clearance of β_2M can be as high as the ultrafiltration rate during intermittent hemofiltration, which is often greater than 100 mL/min.

Efficiency (the ability to clear small solutes) and flux (the ability to clear middle molecules) are not related to each other. High-efficiency membranes can be either high flux (large surface area and large pores) or low flux (large surface area but small pores); likewise, low-efficiency membranes can be either low flux or high flux. Similarly, high-flux membranes can be either high efficiency (large pores and large surface area) or low efficiency (large pores but small surface area). Conventional membranes, those that were used most commonly in the 1970s and 1980s, are low flux and low efficiency. Although their popularity has significantly declined in the United States, they are still used in some parts of the world.

DIALYSATE

The dialysate creates solute concentration gradients to drive diffusion across the dialysis membrane. The typical composition of dialysate for hemodialysis is shown in **Table 54-3**. To avoid substantial changes in plasma sodium concentration, dialysate sodium is usually maintained at concentrations similar to those in plasma. Therefore, sodium is removed primarily by convection during hemodialysis. The ultrafiltration of 4 L of isotonic fluid results in removal of approximately 560 mEq (13 g) of sodium without a change in plasma sodium *concentration*. In contrast, the dialysate potassium concentration is often kept low (<4 mEq/L) in order to decrease the plasma potassium concentration. The use of potassium-free dialysate is associated with higher incidence of arrhythmias and should generally be avoided.

Because dialysis patients are usually acidemic, base in the form of either bicarbonate or acetate is offered. Proportioning systems in modern machines have made the delivery of bicarbonate dialysate a relatively easy task. Dialysates containing primarily acetate are rarely used in the United States because of associated intradialytic hypoxemia, hypotension, arrhythmia, and other complications, although they are still prevalent in some other countries.

Calcium concentration in the dialysate varies depending on the specific need of the patient to gain or lose calcium (see Chapter 58). In order to avoid hypercalcemia or a high plasma calcium-phosphate product that may predispose to vascular calcification, dialysate calcium concentrations are usually limited to 3.0 mEq/L (1.5 mmol/L of ionized calcium) or less, especially for patients who are taking oral calcium regularly as a phosphate binder. A low dialysate calcium concentration has the disadvantage of impairing cardiac contractility, which predisposes to intradialytic hypotension. If citrate is used as the anticoagulant in the extracorporeal circuit (see later discussion), the dialysate must be devoid of calcium to prevent thrombosis. The dialysate magnesium concentration is sometimes, although infrequently, lowered so that the patient can tolerate oral magnesium-containing phosphate binders. Glucose is usually provided at 200 mg/dL to maintain the plasma glucose level stable for both diabetic and nondiabetic patients and thereby avoid hypoglycemia and caloric loss into the dialysate.

HEMODIALYSIS AND HEMOFILTRATION MACHINES

The dialysis machine incorporates many important features, such as a pump to deliver blood to the dialyzer at a constant rate up to approximately 500 mL/min, monitors to ensure that the pressures inside the extracorporeal circuit are not excessive, a detector for leakage of red blood cells from the blood compartment into the dialysate compartment, an air detector and shut-off device to prevent air embolism, a pump to deliver dialysate, a proportioning system to properly dilute the dialysate concentrate, a heater to warm the dialysate to body temperature, an ultrafiltration controller to precisely regulate fluid removal, and conductivity monitors to check the ionic strength of the dialysate.

TABLE 54-3 **Composition of Dialysate Commonly Used in Clinical Hemodialysis**

ION	CONCENTRATION (mEq/L)
Na^+	132-145*
K^+	0-4.0
Cl^-	103-110
HCO_3^-†	0-40
Acetate†	2-37
Ca^{2+}	0-3.5‡
Mg^{2+}	0.5-1.0
Glucose	0-200 mg/dL

*Higher dialysate sodium concentration is sometimes used in sodium modeling.
†Either HCO_3^- or acetate is used as the primary buffer.
‡3.5 mEq/L of Ca^{2+} is equivalent to 1.75 mmol/L or 7.0 mg/dL of ionized calcium in the protein-free dialysate.

These devices ensure the proper, safe, and reliable delivery of blood and dialysate to the filter where exchange of water and solutes takes place. Some modern machines also incorporate more sophisticated features, such as devices that detect changes in the patient's intravascular volume (based on changes in the hematocrit due to hemoconcentration). Other features include computer software programs that can be preset to alter the ultrafiltration rate or the dialysate sodium concentration during the course of the dialysis treatment to maintain intravascular volume and prevent symptomatic hypotension; these techniques are known as ultrafiltration modeling and sodium modeling, respectively.

Machines employed for chronic intermittent (e.g., three times a week) hemofiltration and hemodiafiltration are similar to those used for hemodialysis, with the additional requirements for precise fluid replacement control and, in some machines, on-line generation of sterile replacement fluids. In contrast, continuous arteriovenous hemofiltration (CAVHF) used for the treatment of AKI does not require any machinery. Blood is delivered to the hemofilter from an artery, such as the femoral artery, via a large-bore (14- or 15-gauge) catheter and returned to a large vein, with the driving force derived from the systemic arterial blood pressure rather than a mechanical pump. Replacement fluid is provided by prepackaged sterile solutions. However, because blood flow, and therefore the hemofilter transmembrane pressure and ultrafiltration rate, are sometimes erratic in CAVHF, it is more customary nowadays to employ specially designed machines that pump blood from a vein through the hemofilter and back to a vein, a technique known as continuous venovenous hemofiltration (CVVHF). The machines for CVVHF are usually simpler in design than conventional hemodialysis machines, because dialysate production and some other features are absent. One disadvantage of CAVHF and CVVHF is that they are less efficient than hemodialysis in removing urea, potassium, and other small solutes, because there is no dialysate to permit diffusion. To improve solute clearance, continuous dialysate flow is sometimes added to these systems, techniques known, respectively, as continuous arteriovenous hemodiafiltration (CAVHDF) and continuous venovenous hemodiafiltration (CVVHDF). The addition of dialysate adds complexity to these systems, and as a result, CVVHDF machines are in fact quite similar to regular hemodialysis machines.

Home hemodialysis may employ standard machines that are used for in-center dialysis. However, these machines tend to be complicated and require longer training time for patients and family members to master them. They also require the installation of a water purification system at the home. Some newer home hemodialysis machines are smaller and simpler. Instead of a water purification system, these machines employ pre-prepared sterile dialysate in plastic bags. The disadvantage is the limitation in the dialysate volume that can be used, because of the financial costs and the necessary storage of dialysate bags at the home.

VASCULAR ACCESS

Maintenance of vascular access is a major challenge in chronic hemodialysis. An adequate vascular access should permit blood flow to the dialyzer of 200 to 500 mL/min in adults, depending on the size of the patient. In the United States, there is a tendency to use blood pump speeds of 350 to 500 mL/min, whereas speeds of 200 to 250 mL/min are common in Asia. This discrepancy is partly due to the smaller body size in the Asian population, longer dialysis sessions in some countries, and uncertainty regarding the clinical benefits of very high clearances of small solutes in chronic hemodialysis. A large-diameter venous catheter is necessary to perform acute hemodialysis in the absence of a functional permanent vascular access. Under these circumstances, a double-lumen catheter is placed, usually in the internal jugular vein or the femoral vein. One lumen is used to extract the blood from the patient (the so-called "arterial" side, even though it comes from the patient's vein), and the other lumen is used to return blood to the patient ("venous" side). Femoral catheters are seldom left in place for more than one dialysis session unless the patient is confined to bed, because catheters in this location are prone to kinking, dislodgement, and infection.

For usage of several weeks or longer, an indwelling double-lumen catheter or twin single-lumen catheters with a cuff for anchoring are tunneled under the skin and placed in an internal jugular or subclavian vein by a surgeon, an interventional radiologist, or an interventional nephrologist. These catheters sometimes allow blood flow rates in excess of 400 mL/min and are most suitable in the setting of AKI or as an intermediate measure while waiting for the maturation of a permanent arteriovenous access for chronic dialysis (discussed later). Although it is not desirable, they are often used as a form of permanent vascular access because of convenience, poor alternatives, or preference of patients who refuse repeated needle puncture of the fistula (see later discussion). Infection leading to systemic sepsis is a common complication of use of these catheters. They are also frequently occluded by thrombi and sometimes become kinked or dislodged. The instillation of fibrinolytic agents into the lumen of the catheter is sometimes effective in dissolving the thrombus. In addition, indwelling catheters predispose the vessels to stenosis, which precludes insertion of another catheter at those sites in the future. Stenosis of these vessels also causes obstruction to venous return, which is especially problematic if a permanent arteriovenous fistula, with arterialized venous pressure and augmented blood flow, is present in the ipsilateral arm. Severe swelling, pain, and dysfunction of the arteriovenous access in the ipsilateral arm may result. Stenosis of the superior vena cava sometimes occurs. Subclavian veins appear to be more likely to develop stenosis than internal jugular veins and therefore should be avoided if possible. Femoral veins and, very rarely, the hepatic vein and the inferior vena cava are also used if no other options are available.

Between dialysis sessions, the lumens of these catheters are filled with an anticoagulant, most often heparin. The anticoagulant is removed by aspiration immediately before use of the catheter at the next dialysis session. Failure to remove the heparin before infusion of fluids into the catheter, which sometimes occurs if medical personnel are unfamiliar with hemodialysis, can result in inadvertent systemic anticoagulation. If thrombosis inside the catheter lumen occurs despite the use of indwelling heparin between dialysis sessions, it can sometimes be resolved by local instillation of thrombolytic agents. Under no circumstances should high pressure with a syringe be applied, because dislodgement of the clot can result in pulmonary embolism.

Long-term vascular access for hemodialysis is usually established by the creation of an arteriovenous fistula in an upper extremity, although a lower extremity or even an axillary vessel may sometimes be employed. A fistula is established by connecting an artery to an adjacent vein, either by direct surgical anastomosis of the native vessels or with a synthetic graft, such as a graft made of polytetrafluoroethylene (PTFE). Rarely, a bovine arterial segment is used as the fistula. Native fistulas are preferred over PTFE grafts because of their relative longevity (approximately 80% in 3 years, versus <50% for PTFE grafts) and their lower susceptibility to infection. The disadvantages of native fistulas are the requirement for sufficiently large native veins and a 4- to 16-week maturation period, during which the wall of the fistula thickens and the lumen enlarges, before the fistula can be cannulated with large-bore needles for dialysis. Frequently, the native arteriovenous fistula fails to mature and cannot be used. In a recent U.S. multicenter trial, approximately 60% of fistulas had not matured adequately for clinical use even 5 months after placement. The chronic use of a potent antiplatelet agent, clopidogrel, for 6 weeks after creation of an arteriovenous fistula increased their patency rate but was not effective in increasing their usability at 5 months. The factors that predispose to the failure of native arteriovenous fistula maturation are unclear and are under investigation.

PTFE grafts can be used earlier, occasionally at 1 week or less. However, they tend to elicit acute transient local inflammatory reactions, manifested by pain, swelling, and redness, that resemble infectious cellulitis. These reactions usually subside spontaneously within a few weeks. PTFE grafts are also more prone to thrombosis and infection, but the convenience that they offer has continued to make them a popular choice among many dialysis personnel in the United States. Declotting of arteriovenous access can be accomplished surgically, with local infusion of thrombolytic agents or mechanical devices inserted percutaneously to break up the clot. In general, re-establishment of blood flow is more successful in a graft than in a native arteriovenous fistula.

Stenosis at the outflow tract of arteriovenous fistulas, especially PTFE grafts, occurs frequently and represents the major cause of failure of these accesses. The stenosis is almost exclusively caused by neointimal hyperplasia, which is composed of proliferating myofibroblasts and deposition of extracellular matrix, similar to that seen in coronary artery restenosis. Partial obstruction of the dialysis access impedes the flow of cleansed blood from the dialyzer back to the central veins; as a result, the blood recirculates back to the "arterial" (afferent) limb of the fistula and decreases the amount of fresh systemic blood delivered to the dialyzer, diminishing the overall efficiency of the dialysis process.

Several methods can be used to detect stenosis of arteriovenous fistulas and grafts. Obstruction of the vascular access outflow tract leads to an increase in pressure inside the "venous" (efferent) tubing during hemodialysis, which has been used as a clue to the presence of fistula outflow stenosis. Techniques involving noninvasive devices and the dilution principle have been developed to assess the total blood flow through arteriovenous fistulas. These monitoring techniques are performed during hemodialysis, and the monitoring equipment is sometimes built in as a component of the dialysis machine. Gradual decrease in blood flow rate through the fistula or graft over time provides a clue and allows earlier detection of stenosis. Duplex ultrasonography is also useful for the diagnosis of vascular access stenosis. The predominance of the evidence, however, suggests that regular monitoring of blood flow rates and prophylactic angioplasty intervention do not prolong the useful life of hemodialysis grafts. An angiogram (also called a "fistulogram" for arteriovenous fistulas) with injection of contrast dye remains the gold standard for confirmation and anatomic definition of vascular access stenosis. The fistulogram is also helpful in searching for collateral veins, which are impediments for the growth and maturation of the native fistula. Improvement in duplex ultrasound techniques has diminished the use of contrast fistulograms, unless an angioplasty procedure is being planned in conjunction with the fistulogram.

Fistula or graft stenosis can be treated surgically by replacing or bypassing the stenotic segment. Alternatively, the stenosis may be relieved by percutaneous balloon angioplasty with or without the placement of a stent to keep the lumen patent. A major problem with angioplasty, although it temporarily restores the flow and usefulness of the vascular access, is that the trauma induced by the balloon actually predisposes the vessel wall to further stenosis, setting up a vicious cycle. If left untreated, most stenotic vascular accesses eventually become totally occluded by thrombi. The value of systemic antiplatelet agents or anticoagulants to prolong the useful life of an arteriovenous fistula or graft is unproven. In a recent study, the combination of aspirin and clopidogrel did not result in longer survival of arteriovenous grafts but did increase the incidence of systemic bleeding. A large multicenter trial using the combination of aspirin and dipyridamole for grafts showed promising results. Various pharmacologic and radiation strategies are being investigated to prevent dialysis graft stenosis and make synthetic grafts a better option. Until those strategies materialize, the native arteriovenous fistula remains the preferred vascular access.

Vascular access infection is common and is particularly prevalent with catheters, which have an infection rate 15 times higher than in native fistulas. Further, bacteremia is frequently observed with catheter infections. The clinical manifestations of catheter infection, and even the bacteremia, can be indolent. Endocarditis and disseminated abscesses are detrimental complications of catheter infection and bacteremia when treatment is delayed; therefore, a high index of suspicion is required in these patients. Catheter infection without signs at the exit site is usually diagnosed by blood cultures obtained directly from the catheter. Graft infections are sometimes manifested by gross signs on the overlying skin, such as erythema, fluctuance, or purulent drainage. Deep infections can sometimes be detected using nuclear scans with radiolabeled leukocytes. The infecting organisms for catheter infections are most commonly *Staphylococcus aureus, Staphylococcus epidermidis,* or gram-negative bacilli. Graft infections are typically with *S. aureus.* Mild infection may be treated with antibiotics alone. Although they are more difficult to treat conservatively, infected catheters and PTFE grafts do not invariably require surgical removal. An adjunct measure for the treatment of catheter infection, in addition to systemic antibiotics, is instillation of antibiotics into the lumens of the catheters for dwell during the interdialytic period. This so-called antibiotic lock technique appears promising but has not been proven to have benefit in a large randomized trial.

The spontaneous blood flow through an arteriovenous fistula or graft often exceeds 1 L/min and occasionally 2.5 L/min, accounting for 20% to 40% of cardiac output, although the blood flow through the dialysis needle to the dialyzer is considerably lower. This diversion of cardiac output from the systemic capillary beds by the fistula can cause distal ischemia (i.e., steal syndrome). Rarely, it can precipitate or exacerbate congestive heart failure. Surgical ligation or banding to decrease the luminal cross-sectional diameter of the fistula is sometimes, albeit very infrequently, necessary.

Early planning and placement of a permanent native arteriovenous fistula should take place before the patient requires chronic dialysis, usually when the patient reaches stage 4 or 5 chronic kidney disease, to avoid emergency placement of catheters after the patient becomes frankly uremic. The actual timing for fistula placement depends partially on the rate of decline in kidney function. Mapping of the arm veins using ultrasound is useful to identify suitable vessels for the creation of native fistulas. In patients with poor veins or inadequate planning to allow time for the maturation of a native fistula, the synthetic graft is a reasonable alternative. Central venous catheters should be considered as a temporary measure, until the arteriovenous access is ready for use. For patients with a short life expectancy or if sites for arteriovenous access are no longer available, these catheters can be used for extended periods, sometimes exceeding 2 years, although infection and obstruction typically mandate that they be replaced periodically. The current trend in the United States to increase the placement of native arteriovenous fistulas and the inability of many of these fistulas to mature may have accounted for the substantial increase in the rate of dialysis catheter use in recent years, especially at the initiation of chronic dialysis. Therefore, placement of a native arteriovenous fistula may not be the first choice for all patients and its suitability must be evaluated individually. Percutaneous catheters that are not tunneled under the skin must be used only as a temporary access. It is preferable to use the internal jugular vein on the contralateral side of the planned arteriovenous fistula, to avoid the complications of central vein stenosis. Repeat catheterization of femoral veins for a few individual dialysis sessions is a reasonable alternative, although this is an uncommon practice currently, because of inconvenience.

ANTICOAGULATION

Exposure of blood to the extracorporeal circuit activates the clotting pathways in the blood. Unfractionated heparin is the anticoagulant ordinarily used for acute and chronic hemodialysis and hemofiltration. It is often given as an intravenous bolus of 1000 to 5000 units at the beginning of the session, followed by continuous infusion at 500 to 2000 units/hr. The monitoring of activated clotting time or partial thromboplastin time is mandatory for continuous renal replacement therapy in the intensive care unit (ICU) if full-dose heparin is used, but this is seldom done in the chronic dialysis setting because of the short duration of treatment. A single bolus of low-molecular-weight heparin at the beginning of the dialysis session has been used. The prolonged half-life of this type of heparin in end-stage renal disease (ESRD) should be taken into consideration.

For patients in whom systemic anticoagulation is risky, lower-dose heparin (termed by some "tight" or "minimum" heparin) can be used with careful observation of the extracorporeal circuit for clotting. Hemodialysis can sometimes be performed without the use of any anticoagulants. Underlying coagulation defects, high blood flow rates through the dialyzer, and periodic flushing of the blood tubing and dialyzer with saline are helpful to prevent clotting under these circumstances. The two latter maneuvers are most often used in patients who are actively bleeding or who have recently had dangerous systemic bleeding episodes.

Regional heparinization is another technique that may be used to minimize systemic anticoagulation. Heparin is infused into the "arterial" blood entering the dialyzer and then neutralized by infusion of protamine sulfate into the "venous" line. The beneficial effect of regional heparinization in preventing systemic bleeding has not been convincingly demonstrated. Regional citrate is a similar technique in which calcium-free dialysate is used. Citrate solution infused into the arterial tubing chelates serum calcium, inhibiting activation of the coagulation cascade. Calcium infused into the venous tubing restores the serum calcium concentration before the blood is returned to the patient. Besides patients who are at risk for systemic bleeding, regional citrate anticoagulation is also useful for patients with heparin-induced thrombocytopenia, in whom heparin cannot be used for extracorporeal anticoagulation. The disadvantages of regional citrate are that the serum concentration of ionized calcium needs to be carefully monitored, the dosages of citrate and calcium are sometimes difficult to titrate, and the additional volume and alkali associated with the citrate administration need to be accounted for. Lepirudin and argatroban (direct thrombin inhibitors) and danaparoid (a low-molecular-weight heparinoid) are alternative anticoagulants that can be used for hemodialysis in patients with heparin-induced thrombocytopenia, but their costs are substantial and often prohibitive for long-term chronic use.

INDICATIONS AND SCHEDULES FOR HEMODIALYSIS AND HEMOFILTRATION

Acute hemodialysis is performed primarily for AKI or drug overdose. Indications for emergency dialysis in the AKI setting include fluid overload (including pulmonary edema), hyperkalemia, and uremic signs and symptoms (see Chapter 37). Depending on the circumstances, the initiation of dialysis before onset of these problems is preferable. If reversal of the AKI does not appear to be imminent, dialysis is often instituted when the blood urea nitrogen concentration (BUN) is approximately 70 to 80 mg/dL or the estimated glomerular filtration rate is 5 to 10 mL/min, before overt clinical symptoms occur. On the other hand, if some return of kidney function is immediately expected (e.g., on relief of urinary tract obstruction), fluid overload and hyperkalemia are not necessarily absolute indications for acute dialysis. Intermittent hemodialysis is usually performed thrice weekly for AKI, although extra sessions may be added as needed. Some have advocated hemodialysis on a daily basis. Beyond the need in individual patients based on clinical judgment, the benefits of routine daily hemodialysis for AKI are unclear (see later discussion).

Continuous extracorporeal therapy, such as CVVHF, is particularly useful for patients in the ICU whose cardiovascular status is too unstable for rapid fluid removal, as may occur during intermittent hemodialysis. It is also used in patients from whom removal of substantial amounts of fluid on a continuous basis is desired, such as patients with multiorgan trauma who are receiving parenteral nutrition, blood products, and various intravenous medications. Clearances of urea and potassium by CVVHF are sometimes inadequate to maintain plasma concentrations of these solutes in the desirable range. Under such circumstances, continuous dialysate flow is added to the system (i.e., CVVHDF is employed). The limited available data have not demonstrated a clearly superior clinical outcome associated with continuous therapy compared with intermittent hemodialysis. Peritoneal dialysis is another form of continuous therapy that can be used in patients with AKI and unstable hemodynamics, but, for technical reasons and inconvenience, it has been largely replaced by extracorporeal modalities in this setting. Rarely, peritoneal dialysis is performed in the United States for AKI accompanying severe pancreatitis or when hemodialysis is not available. In most cases, AKI is still treated with hemodialysis, although there has been a gradual increase in the use of continuous extracorporeal modalities.

Maintenance dialysis for ESRD in the United States is usually started at a GFR of 7 to 8 mL/min, unless the clinical conditions dictate earlier intervention. Some have advocated earlier initiation of chronic dialysis; the optimal timing has not been established and is the objective of an ongoing Australian trial. Hemodialysis is used in approximately 90% of ESRD patients in the United States, with the remaining 10% using peritoneal dialysis. Hemodialysis is usually conducted in-center in a dialysis unit, with a thrice-weekly schedule and 3 to 5 hours of dialysis in each session. If fluid overload becomes a significant problem, a fourth session is sometimes added. Restrictions on reimbursement limit more frequent chronic dialysis in the United States. Infrequently, hemodialysis is performed for 2 to 4 hours per session, six times a week in the daytime (short daily hemodialysis) or for 6 to 10 hours per session, three to six times a week at night (nocturnal hemodialysis). A limited literature suggests that these more intense hemodialysis schedules are associated with better control of blood chemistry, lower blood pressure, fewer hospitalizations, and improved nutrition and quality of life. A recently completed, small, randomized trial from Canada reported an improvement in left ventricular hypertrophy, lower blood pressure, and decreased requirement for phosphate binders associated with nocturnal hemodialysis (at least 6 hours per session, four to five times per week). Two parallel U.S. multicenter, randomized trials, examining the intermediate outcomes of nocturnal and daily hemodialysis are ongoing.

Hemofiltration and hemodiafiltration are almost never used for ESRD in the United States, partly because of the reimbursement structure and partly because there is no equipment approved by the Food and Drug Administration for the on-line generation of replacement fluids. The advantage of hemofiltration or hemodiafiltration over hemodialysis is the greater clearance of middle molecules. Because the clinical benefits of greater removal of middle molecules have not been definitively established (see later discussion), there are no recommendations as to which modality should be employed for the ESRD patient. In Europe and Japan, intermittent hemofiltration or hemodiafiltration is used for ESRD more often than in the United States, but still far less than hemodialysis. In Hong Kong and Mexico, peritoneal dialysis is more prevalent than hemodialysis as ESRD therapy.

OUTCOMES OF HEMODIALYSIS

Fluid removal is a major goal of hemodialysis. Removal of fluid to maintain the patient in a euvolemic or slightly hypovolemic state after dialysis is often desirable, but this so-called "dry weight" for individuals is often defined arbitrarily as the weight below which the patient develops symptomatic hypotension or muscle cramps. There is much imprecision associated with this approach. For example, the likelihood of developing hypotension depends not only on the amount of fluid removed but also on the rate of fluid removal. Practice standards for fluid assessments and targets have not been established and are sorely needed.

Normalization of plasma concentrations of electrolytes, such as potassium and bicarbonate, is important. Because of the role of phosphorus in the pathogenesis of hyperparathyroidism and vascular calcification (see Chapter 58), extracorporeal removal of phosphorus is usually desirable, although removal of this ion is seldom used as a guide for dialytic therapies. Urea has been widely used as a marker to guide hemodialysis, because it is an index of the production and accumulation of nitrogenous waste products derived from protein metabolism. In addition, epidemiologic studies have suggested that the clearance of urea by hemodialysis correlates with clinical outcome to some extent. In urea kinetic modeling, the index Kt/V is often used for quantitation of the dose of dialysis therapy. K is the hemodialyzer urea clearance (in milliliters per minute), t is the duration of the dialysis session (in minutes), and V is the volume of distribution of urea in the body (in milliliters). A Kt/V value of 1.20 for each hemodialysis session is currently considered to be the minimum delivered dose. The value V as a fraction of total body weight varies significantly among patients. Therefore, Kt/V is therefore usually calculated with the help of a computer and is routinely presented in the chronic dialysis laboratory reports. The decrease in BUN during dialysis is often used as a simpler and alternative guide. A postdialysis-to-predialysis BUN ratio of 0.35, or a "urea reduction ratio" (calculated by subtracting the postdialysis BUN from the predialysis BUN and then dividing by the predialysis BUN) of 65% to 67%, is roughly equivalent to a Kt/V of 1.20 to 1.25. However, the relationship between urea reduction ratio and Kt/V varies depending on the ultrafiltration volume. Because the delivered Kt/V is sometimes lower than that intended, it is recommended that the prescribed Kt/V be empirically raised to allow for the inadequacy in delivery.

The results of a U.S. multicenter trial (the Hemodialysis or HEMO study) on the clinical effects of higher urea Kt/V and high-flux membrane were published in 2003. In that study, comparisons were made between a urea Kt/V of 1.25, which is the level recommended by practice guidelines in the United States, and a higher Kt/V of 1.65. Comparisons were also made between low-flux membranes (defined as dialyzer β_2M clearance of <10 mL/min) and high-flux membranes (β_2M clearance >20 mL/min). There were no statistically significant differences in all-cause mortality between the two levels of Kt/V or between the two flux arms. However, secondary analysis showed that high-flux dialysis was associated with a decrease in cardiac death. Further, higher urea Kt/V was associated with a decrease in all-cause mortality in women, but not in men. High-flux dialysis was associated with a decrease in all-cause mortality in patients who had been undergoing dialysis for a long period (>3.7 years). This study did not specifically address different hemodialysis schedules, such as daily or nocturnal dialysis, nor did it address urea Kt/V levels of less than 1.25. Nevertheless, there is no doubt that very low Kt/V levels (e.g., <0.50) would be associated with poor clinical outcome in anuric patients. Based on these results and other epidemiologic studies, it is recommended that urea Kt/V should be maintained at 1.25 or higher for all patients. Consideration should be given to a higher Kt/V for women and to the use of high-flux membranes in general. Preliminary results of a more recent multicenter trial in Europe also suggest the clinical benefits of high-flux membranes. These findings lend support to the concepts of the toxic effects of uremic middle molecules and the beneficial effects of removal of these molecules using plasma β_2M level as a marker. Further extrapolation of these data would suggest that intermittent hemodiafiltration is the preferred extracorporeal modality for ESRD, although this notion requires further confirmatory studies.

Longer-duration hemodialysis sessions offer the advantage of allowing more fluid removal at rates that are more tolerable by the patient. Observational studies suggest that longer dialysis sessions are associated with a lower mortality rate in ESRD patients, independent of the urea Kt/V values. Whether this apparent survival benefit is a result of greater fluid removal or clearance of uremic middle molecules (which is enhanced by longer treatment time) is unclear. The small nocturnal hemodialysis trial mentioned earlier provided corroboration for the notion that longer dialysis times may be beneficial, but outcome data involving clinical events are not available.

The best methods for quantifying hemodialysis and determining the optimal amount of hemodialysis that should be delivered are even less certain in AKI than in ESRD. Frequently, the dialysis prescription is empiric and depends largely on the experience and intuition of the nephrologists and the limitations of the clinical circumstances. For example, a temporary central venous catheter is usually the only available vascular access, so the extracorporeal blood flow rate and solute removal are restricted. Diagnostic tests, surgical procedures, unstable clinical conditions, and other activities in the ICU unit often limit the hemodialysis schedule. Net removal of body fluid is often the predominant goal and is guided on clinical grounds. The dosage of dialysis for the treatment of exogenous toxins (e.g., overdose of salicylates or lithium) is often guided by the plasma levels of the toxin and the clinical status. In addition to body fluid volume, the dosage of hemodialysis for AKI is guided by the plasma chemistry findings, including BUN, potassium, and bicarbonate concentrations, and other clinical signs and symptoms, with the objective of maintaining the BUN at less than 80 mg/dL most of the time. For example, a patient with transient oliguric AKI and significant hyperkalemia resulting from contrast-induced nephropathy should have correction of serum potassium as the primary goal.

Despite the apparent advantages of CRRT for AKI in the ICU setting, no data have convincingly demonstrated the superiority of CRRT over intermittent hemodialysis in clinical outcome. Whether hemodialysis or CRRT for AKI should be quantified using urea Kt/V is unclear. An observational study suggested that, when patients treated by either intermittent hemodialysis or CRRT were considered together, higher urea Kt/V was associated with improved patient survival only among those with moderate illness severity, and not among those who were very ill or only mildly ill. An earlier randomized study showed that the clinical outcome in AKI was also influenced by the total ultrafiltration volume in hemofiltration. Patients who were randomized to a volume of 35 mL/kg of body weight per hour had a lower mortality rate than those randomized to 20 mL/kg/hr. Because a higher ultrafiltration rate in hemofiltration increases removal of both small-size solutes and middle molecules, these results do not help elucidate the relative toxicity of these solutes. The frequency of hemodialysis may also affect the clinical outcome in AKI. In an earlier randomized trial conducted in Germany, daily hemodialysis was associated with lower short-term mortality than every-other-day hemodialysis. In contrast, a recent U.S. larger multi-center trial comparing a lower dose (ultrafiltration volume of 20 mL/kg/hr) of CRRT or thrice-weekly acute hemodialysis with a higher dose (ultrafiltration volume of 35 mL/kg/hr) of CRRT or six times per week hemodialysis failed to show differences in patient survival or recovery in kidney function.

Collectively, new data in the last few years have buttressed the notion that greater removal of small solutes (as indicated by urea Kt/V) and middle molecules (as indicated by $\beta_2 M$ clearance), longer hemodialysis durations, and more frequent hemodialysis sessions may improve clinical outcomes in ESRD, but not necessarily in AKI. This notion will be further examined in on-going and future clinical studies.

COMPLICATIONS OF HEMODIALYSIS

Although hemodialysis is a relatively safe procedure, a number of complications may arise. Some are inherent side effects of rapid fluid and solute removal and exposure to the normal extracorporeal circuit; some result from technical errors; and yet others are due to abnormal reactions of patients to the procedure. Intradialytic hypotension is common and has been attributed variably to body volume depletion, shifting of fluid from extracellular to intracellular spaces as a result of the decrease in serum osmolality induced by dialysis, impaired sympathetic activity, vasodilatation in response to warm dialysate, sequestration of blood in the muscles, and splanchnic pooling of blood while eating during dialysis. Avoidance of large interdialytic fluid gain; administration of normal saline, hypertonic saline, hypertonic glucose, mannitol, or colloids; decreasing the dialysate temperature to produce vasoconstriction, and avoidance of eating during dialysis are sometimes useful to reduce the frequency of hypotensive events. Other strategies that are used to minimize intravascular volume depletion include ultrafiltration modeling and sodium modeling, which tailors dialysate sodium concentrations (between 135 and 160 mEq/L) during the dialysis session. Another strategy is performing isolated ultrafiltration, which removes fluid in the absence of dialysate and therefore does not decrease plasma osmolality and cause intercompartmental fluid shifts; in addition, the loss of body heat that is dissipated along with the ultrafiltered fluid promotes vasoconstriction and, consequently, maintenance of blood pressure. None of these strategies is as reliable as minimizing interdialytic fluid gain and the need for dialytic fluid removal.

Cardiac arrhythmias may occur as a result of rapid electrolyte changes, especially in patients taking digitalis who are dialyzed against very low potassium dialysate (0 to 1 mEq/L). The use of acetate dialysate also appears to induce arrhythmias. Arrhythmias can induce or aggravate hypotension and overt or silent myocardial ischemia. Avoiding rapid changes in electrolytes and fluid volumes by increasing the dialysis duration is perhaps the best strategy to prevent intradialytic arrhythmias.

Muscle cramps, nausea, and vomiting occur commonly during hemodialysis and are often a consequence of rapid fluid removal. Too rapid removal of urea and other small solutes may lead to the disequilibrium syndrome (see Chapter 61), manifested by headache with nausea and vomiting, altered mental status, seizures, coma, and even death. The pathophysiology of this syndrome is complex and may be related to a rapid decrease in plasma urea concentration and osmolality that causes fluid shifts into the brain and cerebral edema. Severe disequilibrium syndrome is now rare, because hemodialysis is usually initiated at an early stage, when the BUN is not yet very high. Nonetheless, the practitioner should still be mindful of this possibility, and the efficiency of solute removal should be deliberately limited during the first hemodialysis session, as appropriate.

Dialyzers or dialysates that are contaminated with microorganisms or their toxins can cause fever or infection. Hepatitis B was prevalent in the 1970s, whereas hepatitis C infection is more common in hemodialysis units at present. The mode of transmission of hepatitis C in dialysis units has not been well established.

Anaphylactoid reactions during hemodialysis are rare. They are manifested by various combinations of hypertension or hypotension, pulmonary symptoms, chest and abdominal pain, vomiting, fever, chills, flushing, urticaria, and pruritus. Cardiopulmonary arrest and death rarely ensue. The causes are probably multifactorial and may involve activation of plasma proteins by dialysis membranes, allergy to disinfectants, or the release of noxious substances that have contaminated the dialyzers during the manufacturing or sterilization process. Another cause is the accumulation of vasoactive kinins as a result of enhanced activation of kininogen by dialysis membranes made of copolymers of acrylonitrile and methallyl sulfonate and decreased kinin degradation as a result of the simultaneous administration of angiotensin-converting enzyme inhibitors, which are also kininase inhibitors. Measures to prevent anaphylactoid reactions include thorough rinsing of the dialyzer before use to remove residual ethylene oxide and avoidance of the types of dialyzer, disinfectant, or medications to which a particular patient is hypersensitive. Ethylene oxide gas was popular in the past but has been largely replaced by steam and gamma irradiation for sterilization during the manufacturing of dialyzers.

Hypoxemia occurs commonly during hemodialysis when acetate is used, instead of bicarbonate, as the dialysate buffer. The primary mechanism appears to be the initial loss of bicarbonate and carbon dioxide by diffusion into the dialysate, which leads to hypoventilation. Dialysis membrane bioincompatibility may play a role by releasing mediators that impair gas exchange in some instances. A decrease in systemic partial oxygen pressure of 10 to 12 mm Hg sometimes occurs and could be deleterious for patients with underlying cardiopulmonary disease.

An array of technical errors associated with hemodialysis has been described, but they occur very rarely. Inadequate purification of municipal water before use may result in high levels of contaminants in the dialysate and cause intoxication with metals such as aluminum or calcium. Contamination of dialysate with disinfectant chloramines, improper proportioning or overheating of dialysate by the dialysis machine, and defective dialysis tubing can cause hemolysis. Rupture of the dialysis membrane by high transmembrane pressure causes blood loss into the dialysate and entry of microorganisms from the dialysate into the blood. Defective blood circuit and monitoring devices may result in air embolism. Difficult or improper puncture with the dialysis needle may cause a local hematoma around the vascular access or external bleeding, which can be aggravated by the intradialytic administration of heparin.

The most common posthemodialysis symptom is probably asthenia or a generalized "washed-out" sensation, which has been attributed to the relatively rapid changes in fluids or serum chemistry. Some patients appear to suffer from this symptom consistently, whereas others appear to be immune. It usually lasts for a few hours and disappears spontaneously.

DIALYZER REUSE

Hemodialyzers can be reused repeatedly on the same patient after thorough cleansing and disinfection. A variety of disinfectants have been used, including formaldehyde, glutaraldehyde, sodium hypochlorite (bleach), and the combination solution of hydrogen peroxide and peroxyacetic acid. The blood compartment must be thoroughly rinsed to remove all the sterilants before the next use, because infusion of residual disinfectants into the body can be harmful. Inadequate disinfection, on the other hand, has been associated with infection by common or rare microorganisms. In general, reused dialyzers can clear small-sized solutes, such as urea, almost as effectively as new dialyzers, unless a substantial number of the hollow fibers have been occluded by clotted blood. In contrast, middle molecule clearance is sometimes significantly impaired with reuse, even when the clearance of small-sized solutes is maintained. The total volume of patent hollow fiber lumens is checked with an automated machine after each processing, and the dialyzer is discarded if the residual volume is less than 80% of that of a new dialyzer. Other contraindications to reuse include a disrupted dialyzer casing and hepatitis B infection. Reports on the effect of dialyzer reuse on long-term clinical outcome are conflicting. Because of the economic benefits and lack of definite harmful effects when it is practiced properly, dialyzer reuse is common in the United States, although its popularity has declined in the last few years.

CHOICE OF HEMODIALYZERS

There are several considerations when choosing a hemodialyzer for clinical use. One of the most important is the capacity of the membrane to clear urea, as indicated by the index K_oA, because urea removal (Kt/V) correlates with clinical outcome to a certain extent, as discussed previously. Data presented earlier in this chapter suggested that the removal of middle molecules is also beneficial; however, middle molecule clearances are currently not quantified in clinical practice. Biocompatibility characteristics of dialysis membrane are taken into account by some but not all nephrologists. Instead, many dialysis units and nephrologists simply employ synthetic high-flux dialysis membranes. Purchase cost and reusability of the dialyzer are additional concerns.

DRUG USAGE IN HEMODIALYSIS

The removal of a drug by hemodialysis depends on the properties of the drug and dialysis membrane as well as the conditions of the dialysis procedure (see Chapter 39). Guidelines for dosing medications in kidney failure with or without dialysis have been published. It is imperative to refer to these publications if the physician is unfamiliar with the use of a particular drug in these settings. For example, different types of penicillins behave differently, and the clearance of a drug by low-flux hemodialysis can be substantially different from that by hemofiltration or peritoneal dialysis. It is also important to note that these publications provide only rough guidelines. Data derived from conventional, low-efficiency/low-flux hemodialysis might not be applicable to high-efficiency/high-flux dialysis, and vice versa. Finally, the efficacy of the particular dialysis session must be taken into account. A short and difficult dialysis session plagued by vascular access problems would remove only a small amount of aminoglycoside, and the postdialysis supplemental dose should be adjusted accordingly. Frequently, monitoring of drug levels is required.

CARE OF PATIENTS UNDERGOING CHRONIC HEMODIALYSIS

Dialysis care of ESRD patients in the United States is usually managed by the nephrologist, although, in rare instances, dialysis treatments are supervised instead by other physicians. The nephrologist sees the patient during dialysis rounds, the frequency of which varies from thrice weekly to once monthly, depending on the stability of the patient, the proximity of the dialysis unit, and the standard of practice in the community. The rounding nephrologist should evaluate a number of clinical and laboratory parameters that are particularly pertinent to the dialysis procedure or inherent to ESRD. These include uremic symptoms; dialysis dose (represented by urea Kt/V); intradialytic and postdialytic complications; vascular access; blood pressure; fluid status and estimated dry weight; anemia; iron stores and iron and erythropoietin dosage; serum levels of electrolytes, calcium, phosphorus, and parathyroid hormone; dosages of phosphate binders, vitamin D analogues, and cinacalcet; and nutritional status. Whenever possible, these routine evaluations should be conducted in the outpatient dialysis unit and not during acute hospitalization, because conditions in these two settings are often very

toward concentration equilibrium, and the ratio of dialysate to serum urea levels approaches 1.0. Because the peritoneal membrane has a net negative charge, negatively charged solutes, such as phosphate, move across it more slowly than positively charged solutes of similar size, such as potassium. Macromolecules such as albumin cross the peritoneum by mechanisms that are not completely understood but probably via lymphatics and through large pores in the capillary membranes. During a dwell, the osmotic gradient created by the dialysate within the abdominal cavity declines as the glucose is absorbed, In time this can result in fluid reabsorption into the systemic circulation because of the added effects of intraperitoneal hydrostatic pressure and intravascular oncotic pressure. Continuous lymphatic absorption also diminishes net fluid removal.

The rate of movement of small solutes between dialysate and blood differs from one patient to another. Peritoneal function characteristics are monitored by the peritoneal equilibration test (PET) (**Fig. 55-1**). In this standardized test, 2 L of dialysate containing 2.5 g/dL glucose is infused, and the ratio of dialysate to plasma creatinine (D/P$_{Cr}$ ratio) at the end of a 4-hour dwell is calculated. With this test, each patient's peritoneal membrane can be categorized as having high (D/P$_{Cr}$ >0.81), high-average (0.65 to 0.81), low-average

(0.50 to 0.65), or low (<0.5) peritoneal transport capability. Use of 2 L of dialysate containing 4.25 g/dL glucose during the same dwell period as in the PET permits assessment of ultrafiltration failure; an effluent volume of less than 2400 mL is diagnostic.

Removal of fluid and solutes is highly dependent on the type of transporter status as described by the PET (**Fig. 55-2**). Patients with a high D/P$_{Cr}$ ratio (high transporters) have rapid clearance of small molecules but poor ultrafiltration because of rapid glucose absorption and dissipation of the osmotic gradient between dialysate and blood. These patients require short-dwell peritoneal dialysis regimens to achieve adequate fluid removal. In addition, because the volume of fluid removed also contributes to the solute clearance of equilibrated dialysate via convection, high transporters also have reduced solute clearance over long dwells because of low drain volumes. Patients with a low D/P$_{Cr}$ ratio (low transporters) have low clearance rates for solutes and usually require more dialysis exchanges or increased volume per exchange, or both, to avoid uremic symptoms once residual kidney function is lost. Ultrafiltration in this category of patient is usually excellent. By virtue of the definition, most patients have high-average to low-average peritoneal transport and do well on either CAPD or APD.

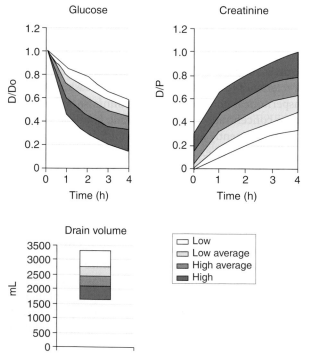

FIGURE 55-1 The peritoneal equilibration test (PET) measures the peritoneal transport characteristics of glucose from the peritoneal fluid to plasma and of creatinine from plasma to the peritoneal fluid. The instilled peritoneal fluid volume for the PET is 2 L. D/D$_0$ represents the ratio of dialysate glucose concentration (D) at a given time point to the dialysate glucose concentration at time 0 (D$_0$). D/P represents the ratio of dialysate (D) to plasma (P) concentrations. The rate of transport of these molecules depends on the permeability of the membrane: the higher the permeability (high transporter), the more rapid the transport of glucose, with dissipation of the osmotic gradient and therefore less drain volume.

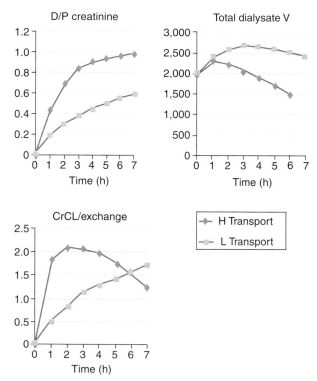

FIGURE 55-2 The profiles of intraperitoneal dialysate volume (V) and solute transport (CrCl/exchange), in relation to dwell time in hours, vary in high transporters (H) and low transporters (L). These profiles are used in prescription setting of dwell times and fluid volumes. For long-dwell continuous ambulatory peritoneal dialysis (CAPD), high transporters show both low fluid removal and low CrCl, compared with low transporters, CrCl, creatinine clearance; D/P creatinine, dialysate-to-plasma creatinine ratio.

TECHNIQUES OF PERITONEAL DIALYSIS

Continuous Ambulatory Peritoneal Dialysis

Compared with other forms of peritoneal dialysis, CAPD uses the smallest volume of dialysate to prevent uremia; this usually means a daily volume of 8 to 10 L of dialysate. The CAPD technique entails three to five daily exchanges of 0.5 to 3.0 L each, with dialysis occurring continuously and occupying the entire 24-hour period. The prescription (volume, dwell time, and number of exchanges) varies according to patient size, peritoneal permeability, and residual kidney function.

Peritoneal dialysis fluid is instilled by gravity into the peritoneal cavity and drained out after a dwell period of several hours. The basic CAPD system, which has remained largely unchanged for almost 3 decades, consists of a plastic bag containing 0.5 to 3.0 L of dialysis fluid, a transfer set (tubing between the catheter and the plastic bag), and a permanent, indwelling Silastic catheter, which is implanted so that the tip of the intraperitoneal portion lies in the pelvis. Because the connection between the bag and the transfer set is broken three to five times a day (approximately 1500 exchanges per year), the procedure must be performed using a strict, aseptic, non-touch technique, which the patient or helper performs at home. The most common connection device used today is based on a "Y"-disconnect system. This entails drainage of the effluent after the connection has been made with the new bag, which permits "flushing out" of any accidental touch contamination in the tubing before infusion of new fluid into the peritoneal cavity (**Fig. 55-3**). This system reduces the incidence of infection and also relieves the patient from carrying the empty bag and transfer set, thus improving the psychological aspects and quality of life of CAPD patients.

Automated Peritoneal Dialysis

APD is a broad term that is used to refer to all forms of peritoneal dialysis that utilize a mechanical device (called a *cycler*) to assist in delivery and drainage of the dialysis fluid. The simplest form of APD is IPD, which is performed in patients with acute or chronic kidney failure three times a week in sessions lasting 24 hours, with a total exchange of 20 to 60 L of dialysis fluid. More complicated APD regimens include

- Continuous cycling peritoneal dialysis (CCPD), which provides three exchanges during the night and one during the day (a reversal of the CAPD regimen)
- Nightly intermittent peritoneal dialysis (NIPD), which provides rapid exchanges during the night, with the abdomen kept dry during the "dry day"
- Nightly peritoneal dialysis plus two exchanges during the day to allow for increased small-solute and fluid clearance (NIPD with "wet day")
- Tidal peritoneal dialysis (TPD), in which only 40% to 60% of the intraperitoneal fluid volume is replaced with each exchange, so that continuous fluid-membrane contact improves the efficiency (but requires 20 to 30 L of fluid per 24 hours)

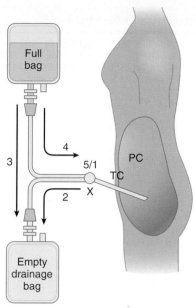

FIGURE 55-3 Diagrammatic representation of a continuous ambulatory peritoneal dialysis (CAPD) exchange using a Y-set disconnect system. The Y-set consists of tubing with a full bag of dialysate at one end and an empty drainage bag at the other, placed on the floor. Fluid flow is by gravity, and the direction of flow is controlled by clamps on the tubing. Between exchanges, the peritoneal cavity (PC) contains dialysate and only a short, capped extension tubing attached to the peritoneal Tenckhoff catheter (TC). The exchange procedure comprises five steps:
1. To begin the exchange, the patient connects the Y tubing to the short extension tubing at X.

2. Keeping the clamp on the full bag closed, the patient or caregiver opens the clamp on the peritoneal catheter extension to allow the fluid in the PC to drain into the drainage bag by gravity. Time required: 10-15 minutes

3. The patient then closes the clamp on the peritoneal catheter extension tubing and opens the clamp on the full bag, allowing fresh fluid to "flush" the tubing of air and any contamination into the drainage bag. Time required: a few seconds (count of 5).

4. Next, the patient closes the clamp on the drainage bag and opens the clamp on the peritoneal catheter extension tubing, allowing fresh dialysis fluid into the PC via the TC. Time required: 10 minutes.

5. The final step is to close the clamp on the peritoneal catheter extension tubing, disconnect the Y tubing, and cap the short extension tubing.

These regimens are illustrated in **Table 55-1**.

APD regimens usually entail an increased number of short-dwell exchanges to enhance solute and fluid removal. The cycler delivers a set number of exchanges over 8 to 10 hours, with the last fill constituting the long day dwell, which may be necessary to provide additional dialysis to achieve solute and fluid removal targets. The most obvious advantage of APD is that it eliminates the need for intensive manual involvement, because most of the dialysis occur at night during sleep. In essence, APD entails only two procedures daily: an initial connection of the catheter to the machine and a disconnection at the end of dialysis. APD is increasingly being used in the United States and Europe in lieu of CAPD. This trend may be related to the convenience of performing the dialysis connections and to the new cycler models, which are smaller, lighter, less expensive than previously, and more attractive to patients. In the past, APD tended to be offered only to patients who had been identified

TABLE 55-1 Regimens Used in Peritoneal Dialysis

TYPE OF DIALYSIS*	NUMBER OF DAYTIME EXCHANGES	NUMBER OF NIGHTTIME EXCHANGES	VOLUME OF EXCHANGES (L)
CAPD	2-3	1-2†	1.0-3.0
CCPD	1	3-4	1.0-3.0
NIPD	0	3-5	2.0-3.0
NIPD with "wet day"	1-2	3-5	2.0-3.0
TPD	0	20	1.0-1.5
IPD	5-10	5-10	1.0-2.0

CAPD, continuous ambulatory peritoneal dialysis; CCPD, continuous cycling peritoneal dialysis; IPD, intermittent peritoneal dialysis; NIPD, nocturnal intermittent peritoneal dialysis; TPD, tidal peritoneal dialysis.

*All regimens except CAPD utilize a cycler machine and are therefore variants of automated peritoneal dialysis.

†If an additional exchange is needed during CAPD to achieve adequate dialysis, a mechanical exchange device can be used to perform the exchange during the night while the patient is asleep.

TABLE 55-2 Composition of Standard Peritoneal Dialysis Fluids Including the Osmotic Agents Used

AGENT	AMOUNT
Sodium	132 mEq/L
Chloride	96-102 mEq/L
Calcium	1.25, 2.5, or 3.5 mEq/L
Magnesium	0.5 or 1.25 mEq/L
Lactate	35 or 40 mEq/L
Glucose	1.5, 2.5, or 4.25 g/dL*
Amino acids	1.1 g/dL†
Icodextrin	7.5 g/dL

*Newer glucose-based solutions with low levels of glucose degradation products (GDPs) are now available and are being used increasingly.

†Amino acid solutions are rarely used in practice, because definite nutritional benefits have never been proven and these solutions are expensive to produce.

by PET as high transporters and who therefore required shorter dwell times. However, lifestyle issues and freedom from daytime exchanges are now major factors in modality choice for both patient and physician.

Peritoneal Dialysis Solutions

Standard peritoneal dialysis solutions (**Table 55-2**) contain varying concentrations of glucose as the osmotic agent and of lactate, sodium, magnesium, and calcium. Lactate was initially used as the buffer, in preference to the more physiologic bicarbonate, because the low pH of the former prevented caramelization of the glucose from autoclaving for sterilization during the manufacturing process. The biocompatibility of standard solutions has been intensively studied. There is no doubt that their unphysiologically low pH, high osmolality, and presence of glucose degradation products (GDPs) generated during manufacture and autoclaving are harmful to peritoneal cells in vitro and are implicated in peritoneal neovascularization, collagen production, and peritoneal thickening, all of which may contribute to loss of function. Newer, more physiologic solutions have been developed that are low in GDPs, use bicarbonate as a buffer, or contain alternative osmotic agents.

Glucose is still the most common osmotic agent because of its low cost and ease of manufacture; however, larger molecules have interesting and attractive properties. Icodextrin is an isosmotic glucose polymer that produces ultrafiltration by colloid osmosis even with dwell periods of as long as 12 hours; it has been shown to improve fluid balance, particularly in patients with high peritoneal transport status. Amino acid–based solutions provide nutritional supplementation in peritoneal dialysis, although there is minimal evidence that they improve long-term outcome, except perhaps in severely malnourished patients. Used in combination with icodextrin, they have the potential to preserve peritoneal membrane integrity and to reduce the metabolic side effects of glucose absorption. This combination is currently

under investigation by the Nutrineal, Extraneal, Physioneal, Physioneal (NEPP) Study, but results so far have been reported only in abstract form.

Lactate in peritoneal dialysis fluid is gradually being replaced by bicarbonate, a more physiologic buffer, which is separated from the other constituents of the fluid during the manufacturing process by means of a multichamber bag. The bags have separate chambers for glucose and bicarbonate. This allows autoclaving without the risks of caramelization and generation of GDPs during the manufacturing process. The patient mixes the contents of the chambers immediately before infusion, producing a solution with relatively neutral pH and low GDPs. These newer solutions are being used increasingly, with a view to improving biocompatibility and prolonging peritoneal dialysis technique survival.

Peritoneal Catheters

The access for peritoneal dialysis is a catheter inserted into the abdominal cavity, typically by either a surgeon or a nephrologist using local anesthetic with sedation. General anesthesia is usually reserved for patients with previous abdominal surgery and complicated insertions. The catheter can be inserted surgically, under direct vision through a minilaparotomy, or percutaneously, using the Seldinger technique or with peritoneoscopic guidance. Although there are numerous catheter designs, such as the Swan-neck catheter (said to undergo less catheter tip migration and fewer exit-site infections) and curled catheters, none offers a significant proven advantage over the original double-cuffed Silastic Tenckhoff catheter. This original and simple design is still the most commonly used catheter. The intra-abdominal portion of the catheter has multiple perforations through which dialysate flows. With the deep cuff placed in a paramedian position in the rectus muscle, the extra-abdominal portion of the catheter is tunneled through the subcutaneous tissue to exit the skin, pointing laterally and caudally. The subcutaneous superficial cuff is located 2 to 3 cm from the exit site of the catheter. Peritoneal dialysis can be initiated immediately after catheter placement if exchange volumes are small and the patient is kept recumbent. Ideally, dialysis should be deferred for at least 4 weeks after insertion, until the exit site is well healed, at which time the patient may be trained to perform CAPD or APD. Hemodialysis can be used, if necessary, as a temporary measure until peritoneal dialysis is initiated.

MANAGEMENT OF PERITONEAL DIALYSIS

Peritoneal Dialysis Prescription

In arriving at a particular prescription for an individual patient, one needs to take into account the fixed components at the time, including residual kidney function, peritoneal membrane permeability, and size of the patient, as well as the variable components of dialysate volume, dwell times, concentration of glucose, and number of exchanges. A prescription entails modifications of the variable components to arrive at a regimen that provides for adequate solute and fluid removal to meet clinical needs and maintain reasonable quality of life. The setting of a peritoneal dialysis prescription is outlined in **Figure 55-4**. Dialysis adequacy regarding solute removal, fluid status, nutritional status and clinical well-being are monitored regularly (see later discussion), and the prescription is modified accordingly.

The overall clearance capacity of the peritoneum for small solutes is limited by the volume of dialysis fluid that can be provided daily. Many CAPD patients are prescribed four exchanges of 2 L of dialysate per day. Four 2-L CAPD exchanges

per day with 2 L daily net ultrafiltration represents a drain volume of 70 L/wk, which is inadequate in the absence of significant residual kidney function fo1421r most patients, especially those who weigh more than 80 kg. Initially, most patients have residual kidney function that contributes to the total solute clearance. As kidney function is gradually lost, the patients require larger exchange volumes (2.5 or 3.0 L) and may also need five daily exchanges to avoid uremic symptoms and reach the target values of urea Kt/V and creatinine clearance (see "Peritoneal Dialysis Adequacy"). In a CAPD regimen, the fifth exchange may be provided by use of an automated device that performs during the night. However, this technique is in decline, because it effectively introduces a mini-APD machine, and most patients and physicians would opt to switch completely at this point from CAPD to APD. Larger patients should be started on exchange volumes of 2.5 to 3.0 L. APD can achieve higher clearance of small solutes, but it may necessitate one or two day dwells ("wet day") in addition to three or four nocturnal exchange volumes of 2.5 to 3.0 L each.

Peritoneal Dialysis Adequacy

Adequacy of peritoneal dialysis is determined by clinical assessment, solute clearance measurements, nutritional status, and fluid removal. The well-dialyzed patient has a good appetite, no nausea, and minimal fatigue; is well nourished; and feels well. In contrast, the uremic patient is anorectic with dysgeusia, nausea, and complaints of fatigue. In addition to

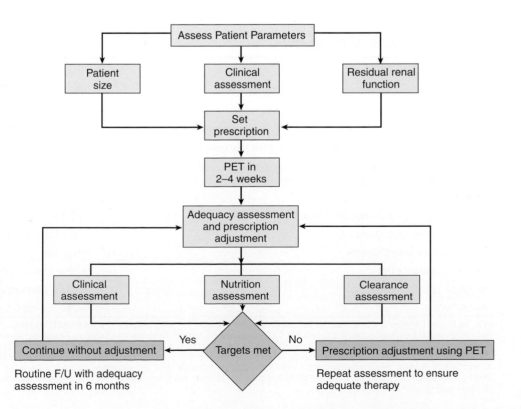

FIGURE 55-4 Algorithm for prescription setting. After the initial peritoneal equilibration test (PET) at 2 to 4 weeks, the prescription is altered according to the membrane permeability results. For high transporters, short-dwell automated peritoneal dialysis (APD) is appropriate; for high-average and low-average transporters, continuous ambulatory peritoneal dialysis (CAPD) would suffice. F/U, follow-up.

these clinical parameters, two primarily measures are used to assess adequacy of solute removal:

1. An index of peritoneal urea removal, expressed as Kt/V, which is urea clearance (K) multiplied by time (t) and related to total body water volume, which is assumed to be the urea distribution volume (V). Kt is obtained by multiplying the ratio of effluent dialysate to plasma urea nitrogen concentration (D/P$_{urea}$) by the 24-hour effluent drain volume. Kidney urea clearance is added to this value to yield the total daily body clearance. The daily value is multiplied by 7 to provide a weekly value. V can be estimated as 60% of weight in males or 55% of weight in females. A typical calculation is given in **Table 55-3**.

2. Creatinine clearance (CrCl), which is provided by both peritoneal clearance and that contributed by residual kidney function. Peritoneal CrCl is again obtained from the 24-hour collection of dialysate, but to this is added an estimate of the glomerular filtration rate (GFR) achieved by the residual kidney function. By tradition, residual kidney clearance is determined by averaging CrCl and urea nitrogen clearance as an estimate of the GFR. This is performed to correct for tubular secretion of creatinine, which substantially overestimates GFR at low levels of kidney function. An adjustment for body surface area is also usually applied.

Although the validity of these measurements and calculations continues to cause some controversy, they have become the accepted methods of estimating dialysis adequacy, and various national and international organizations have set minimum targets for both CrCl and urea clearance based on them. However, it is sometimes difficult for patients to achieve one or both targets, and doubt remains about the precise level at which the targets should be set. The National Kidney Foundation Kidney Disease Outcomes Quality Initiative (K/DOQI) Practice Guidelines for Peritoneal Dialysis were published in 1997 and updated in 2006. On the basis of recent studies, the target minimum Kt/V for urea was reduced from 2.0 to 1.7, and the target total weekly CrCl from 60 L to 50 L, largely as a result of one large, well-conducted and randomized prospective study (ADEMEX), which showed no survival advantage with the higher dialysis dose. It is thought that failure to achieve these guidelines is likely to lead to uremic symptoms, decreased protein intake, and an increase in mortality, but conclusive evidence for this assumption is lacking, because investigators are naturally reluctant to test the point at which reducing the dialysis "dose" produces clinical symptoms. Although current targets may indicate the minimum solute clearance targets required to achieve an acceptable long-term clinical outcome, some patients need more dialysis to overcome uremic symptoms. In addition, it must always be remembered that the term *dialysis adequacy* is restricted to the description of solute removal adequacy only and does not encompass the other aspects of care. Control of hypertension, correction of dyslipidemia, maintenance of fluid balance, maximal cardiovascular risk reduction, and management of comorbidities can hugely influence outcome in any dialysis patient, but even here, conclusive, randomized, prospective studies are lacking. Despite these issues, anuric patients can usually be adequately managed on peritoneal dialysis by appropriate prescription adjustments, including the use of APD regimens and icodextrin.

It is now well recognized that residual kidney function is extremely important in providing adequate solute clearance.

TABLE 55-3 **An Example of Urea Kt/V Calculation**

Patient

70-kg adult woman on CAPD (four exchanges/day)

Data to be obtained

24-hr dialysate volume (4 × 2 L infusion ++ 1 L net ultrafiltrate = 9 L)

D/P ratio for urea (0.9), determined by collecting the total drained dialysate for 24 hr

Residual kidney urea clearance, determined by dividing the 24-hr urine urea nitrogen by the BUN (20 L/wk, which corresponds to 2 mL/min)

Calculation

Peritoneal urea clearance/day (D/P × volume)	= 0.9 × 9 L = 8.1 L
Weekly peritoneal urea clearance	= 8.1 L/day × 7 days/wk = 56.7 L/wk
Residual kidney urea clearance	= 20 L/wk
Total urea clearance (Kt)	= 56.7 L/wk ++ 20 L/wk = 76.7 L/wk
Volume of urea distribution (V)*	= (0.55 × Weight in kg) = 38.5 L
Weekly Kt/V	= 76.7 L ÷ 38.5 L = 2.0

BUN, blood urea nitrogen; CAPD, continuous ambulatory peritoneal dialysis; D/P ratio, dialysate-to-plasma creatinine ratio.
*Volume of urea distribution (V) can be estimated as 0.60 (male) or 0.55 (female) times the body weight in kilograms. However, it is more accurate to use the formula of Watson and Watson, which takes into account weight (in kilograms), height (in centimeters), gender, and age (in years). For males, V(L) = 2.477 + (0.3362 × Weight) + (0.1074 × Height) − (0.09516 × Age). For females, V(L) = −2.097 + (0.2466 × Weight) + (0.1069 × Height). The data collection for creatinine clearance (CrCl) is similar to that for Kt/V. However, the urinary component of CrCl is usually corrected for creatinine secretion by averaging it with the urinary urea clearance. The peritoneal CrCl is simply calculated by dividing the creatinine content of the 24-hr dialysate by the serum creatinine concentration. The total CrCl (peritoneal + kidney) is normalized to 1.73 m^2 body surface area.

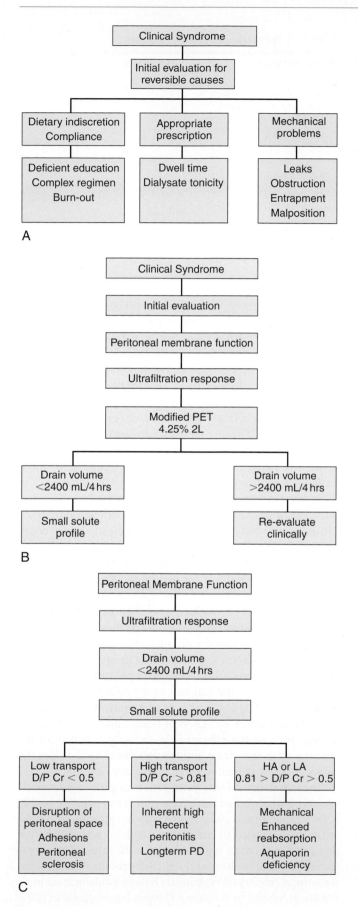

A

B

C

Most studies show that residual kidney function correlates with improved survival and less morbidity, and its preservation forms an important part of the management for a peritoneal dialysis patient. To preserve residual kidney function, nephrotoxic drugs such as aminoglycosides and nonsteroidal anti-inflammatory agents should be avoided whenever possible, and episodes of hypotension from any cause should be corrected as rapidly as possible. Residual kidney function is better preserved in patients receiving peritoneal dialysis than in those receiving hemodialysis, so peritoneal dialysis may be the better initial therapy option for end-stage renal failure.

Fluid Removal on Peritoneal Dialysis

Although peritoneal dialysis patients benefit from continuous daily fluid removal, it is generally accepted that most are mildly fluid overloaded to some extent. This reflects the fact that they undergo medical or nursing review only once every 2 to 3 months, rather than three times per week as in hemodialysis, and restoration of an appropriate "dry weight" is not in the hands of the dialysis provider. Whether this state of continuous mild overload is more or less harmful than the thrice-weekly rapid variation in fluid status experienced by a hemodialysis patient is unknown, but the problem tends to become more troublesome in the long term, when residual kidney function is lost and peritoneal dialysis ultrafiltration capacity is reduced. It appears that fluid removal has a more significant impact on outcome than solute clearance. Net ultrafiltration of at least 750 mL/day is associated with better survival in anuric patients, although the exact reason is unclear. Greater emphasis is now placed on optimizing fluid status, and algorithms are available that help the physician manage fluid overload in CAPD patients (**Fig. 55-5**). The use of icodextrin for the longest dwell achieves better fluid balance and results in improvement in left ventricular indices.

Nutrition in the Peritoneal Dialysis Patient

Up to 40% of peritoneal dialysis patients are believed to be protein-malnourished on the basis of anthropometric studies. This condition is in part due to losses of amino acids and protein in the dialysate, the loss of protein being approximately 8 to 12 g/day. Peritonitis markedly increases dialysate protein losses. The appetite of the patient may be suppressed by the absorbed dialysate glucose and also by uremia resulting in lower intake of protein and other nutrients. Both the Kt/V and the weekly CrCl correlate, albeit weakly, with

FIGURE 55-5 A, Evaluation of the clinical syndrome of fluid overload. This initially entails the evaluation and search for reversible causes. **B,** After reversible causes are excluded, it is appropriate to evaluate peritoneal membrane function using the modified peritoneal equilibration test (PET) with 2 L of 4.25% glucose. **C,** Algorithm for further evaluation and treatment based on the small solute profile. For high-transport patients, the therapy is outlined. For low-transport patients peritoneal dialysis may not be possible and peritoneal sclerosis should be excluded, especially encapsulating peritoneal sclerosis. D/P Cr, ratio of dialysate to plasma creatinine; HA, high-average transport; LA, low-average transport; PD, peritoneal dialysis.

dietary protein intake, suggesting that a certain minimum dose of dialysis is required for adequate protein intake. The serum albumin level is inversely related to both mortality and hospitalization in peritoneal dialysis patients, although it must be remembered that serum albumin is greatly influenced by inflammation and is a poor marker of nutritional status when used alone. Protein intake of at least 1.2 g/kg/day is recommended for peritoneal dialysis patients, but many ingest only 0.8 to 1.0 g/kg/day. The K/DOQI recommendations are that such patients should first receive dietary counseling and education; then, if protein intake remains inadequate, oral supplements should be prescribed. The use of amino acid dialysate (in which amino acids replace the glucose) has been tried on a limited basis as a means of correcting protein malnutrition, but proof of its long-term nutritional benefit is lacking. It is especially difficult to correct malnutrition related to inflammation and comorbidity. This "type II" malnutrition may well be cytokine mediated, and its correction necessitates establishing an underlying cause for the "inflammation." Type I malnutrition is more readily amenable to protein and calorie supplementation.

The amount of calories absorbed from dialysate glucose depends on the dextrose concentration used (1.50, 2.50, or 4.25 g/dL) and on the membrane permeability of the patient. The development of obesity is not unusual in patients undergoing peritoneal dialysis, especially in those who were already overweight at the start of dialysis. In addition, glucose absorption frequently results in hyperlipidemia, which may contribute to atherosclerotic cardiovascular disease.

COMPLICATIONS OF PERITONEAL DIALYSIS
Peritonitis

Peritonitis remains a major complication of peritoneal dialysis; it accounts for 15% to 35% of hospital admissions for these patients and is the major cause of catheter loss and technique failure resulting in transfer to hemodialysis. Entry of bacteria into the catheter during an exchange procedure (touch contamination) is the most common source, but organisms can also track along the external surface of the catheter or migrate into the peritoneum from another abdominal viscus.

Diagnosis of peritonitis requires the presence of two of the following criteria in any combination:

- Organisms identified on Gram staining or subsequent culture
- Cloudy fluid (white cell count >100/mm^3; >50% neutrophils)
- Symptoms and signs of peritoneal inflammation

Cloudy dialysate effluent is almost invariably present, and abdominal pain is present in about 80% to 95% of cases. Gastrointestinal symptoms, chills, and fever are present in as many as 25% of the cases, and abdominal tenderness 75%. Bacteremia is rare. Gram staining of the effluent is seldom helpful, except with fungal peritonitis, but cultures are usually positive. In many centers, 20% of peritonitis episodes

TABLE 55-4 Microorganisms Causing Peritonitis

MICROORGANISMS	FREQUENCY (%)
Gram-positive	
Staphylococcus epidermidis	30-40
Staphylococcus aureus	15-20
Streptococcus	10-15
Other gram-positive	2-5
Gram-negative	
Pseudomonas	5-10
Enterobacter	5-20
Other gram-negative	5-7
Fungi	2-10
Other organisms	2-5
Culture-negative	10-30

result in a "no growth" culture result, predominantly as a result of inadequate culture techniques.

The causes of peritonitis are given in **Table 55-4**, together with the frequency of infection with these organisms. The rate of peritonitis with *Staphylococcus epidermidis* has decreased since the introduction of the Y-set and the flush-before-fill technique, so *Staphylococcus aureus* and enteric organisms now account for a larger proportion of peritonitis episodes than in the past. Because patients infected with these organisms are more symptomatic than those with *S. epidermidis* peritonitis, peritonitis has become a less frequent but more severe complication, often requiring hospital admission.

Peritonitis rates, originally very high in the late 1970s and early 1980s, have decreased to less than one episode every 2 to 3 dialysis years, owing to improvements in the procedure for performing the dialysis tubing connections, which have decreased the risk of touch contamination (see **Fig. 55-3**). The catheter removal rate for peritonitis depends on the infecting microorganism. Peritonitis due to *S. epidermidis* is less likely to result in catheter loss than peritonitis due to *S. aureus* or *Pseudomonas aeruginosa*. If these more virulent organisms are associated with a catheter tunnel or exit-site infection, the catheter loss rate can be as high as 90%. Fungal peritonitis almost invariably requires catheter removal, because a medical cure can only rarely be achieved. There is no apparent difference in rates of peritonitis between CAPD and APD. However, detection of peritonitis on APD can be delayed because the effluent is less readily available for inspection after each drain and the volume of fluid dilutes the cells so that the patient may not notice any clouding.

The initial treatment of peritonitis is empiric and designed to cover both gram-positive cocci and gram-negative bacilli. A first-generation cephalosporin such as cefazolin or cephalothin may be used in conjunction with an aminoglycoside or a third-generation cephalosporin, with subsequent therapy tailored to the culture and sensitivity results. The latest International Society of Peritoneal Dialysis guidelines on peritonitis, published in *Peritoneal Dialysis International* in 2005, advocated the initial use of a cephalosporin or vancomycin to provide gram-positive coverage, plus ceftazidime or an aminoglycoside for gram-negative coverage, while bacteriologic identification and sensitivity studies are in process. There is the potential problem with the first-generation cephalosporins in that they may not adequately cover methicillin-resistant staphylococci, whereas widespread empiric use of vancomycin raises concerns about the promotion of resistance in staphylococci generally, which might then result in widespread methicillin and vancomycin resistance. The guidelines offer no specific guidance on this matter and advise regional variation depending on the local pattern of infections and sensitivities in the population. However, the long half-life of vancomycin in peritoneal dialysis patients makes it very simple to administer, and it is still quite widely used as a result. Aminoglycoside levels should be monitored to avoid accelerated loss of residual kidney function or ototoxicity; however, because these antibiotics also have a relatively long-half life in peritoneal dialysis patients, the traditional advice regarding peak and trough levels is invalid, and these values probably tell the physician nothing about intraperitoneal levels.

A listing of antibiotics and their dosing schedules is given in **Table 55-5**. Antibiotics are usually given intermittently once a day and administered intraperitoneally in the long-dwell exchange (overnight in CAPD and during the daytime long dwell in APD). They can also be given continuously in every exchange. The dosage may need adjustment if residual kidney function is significant. Duration of therapy depends on the organisms and the severity of the peritonitis; it is usually 14 days for *S. epidermidis* infections and 3 weeks for most other infections.

It should be possible (up to 80% of cases) to achieve complete cure without having to resort to catheter removal. Persistent symptoms beyond 96 hours can occur in 10% to 30% of episodes, and cure is then effected by removal of the catheter. Cure may be obtained if antibiotics alone are continued beyond 96 hours without catheter removal, but there is a high risk of damage to the peritoneum, and neither the short-term bacterial outcome nor the long-term peritoneal membrane effect is good. Therefore, if there is not clear evidence of improvement (i.e., reduction in abdominal pain, falling dialysis fluid cell count, visual clearing of the peritoneal dialysis effluent) after 96 hours of treatment with appropriate antibiotic therapy, the catheter should be removed as soon as possible. In a study in which antibiotics were continued for 10 days for "resistant" peritonitis without clearing of the fluid and without catheter removal, one third of the patients died; another one third lost ultrafiltration, necessitating discontinuation of peritoneal dialysis; and only one third were able to continue with peritoneal dialysis. Relapsing peritonitis is a feature in about 10% to 15% of episodes. Catheter removal is necessary in as many as 15% of these cases, and death has been reported in 1% to 3%.

Peritonitis results in a marked increase in acute peritoneal protein losses and a transient decrease in ultrafiltration due to the increased permeability to the dialysate dextrose. Although peritoneal membrane changes are usually transient and related to acute peritonitis, peritoneal fibrosis (often referred to as sclerosis) may be involved in severe episodes or as a cumulative effect of multiple episodes of peritonitis (see later discussion).

Peritoneal Catheter Infection

Peritoneal catheter infections can involve the exit site (erythema or purulent drainage), the tunnel (edema, erythema, or tenderness over the subcutaneous pathway), or both simultaneously. *S. aureus* is the most common cause of exit site and tunnel infections, with *Pseudomonas* being the next most frequent organism. *S. aureus* exit site infections are difficult to treat and frequently progress to tunnel infections and peritonitis, in which case catheter removal is required for resolution. *S. aureus* nasal carriage is associated with an increased risk of *S. aureus* catheter infection. Treatment of nasal carriers with intranasal mupirocin, twice daily for 5 days each month; mupirocin applied daily to the exit site regardless of carrier status; or oral rifampin 600 mg/day for 5 days every 12 weeks has been shown to be effective in

---

TABLE 55-5 Antibiotics and Dosing Schedules for Intraperitoneal Use Unless Otherwise Stated

| ANTIBIOTIC | INITIAL DOSE (mg/L)* | Subsequent Doses | |
		EACH EXCHANGE (mg/L)	ONCE DAILY (mg)
Ampicillin	125	125	No data
Aztreonam	1000	250	1000
Cefazolin	500	125	500
Ceftazidime	500	125	1000
Fluconazole	200 mg PO	—	200 PO
Aminoglycosides[†]	20	4	20
Metronidazole	500 mg PO/IV	—	500 PO/IV tid
Vancomycin	15-30 mg/kg	25	15-30 mg/kg q5-7d

*Once-daily antibiotic dosing with the long dwell is preferred to the addition of antibiotic to each exchange and has been shown to be efficacious for cefazolin, cephalothin, and ceftazidime. Patients receiving automated peritoneal dialysis (APD) may be changed to a continuous ambulatory peritoneal dialysis (CAPD) schedule; if they remain on an APD schedule, antibiotics are added to each exchange.
[†]This group includes gentamicin, tobramycin, and netilmicin (same doses for all).

reducing *S. aureus* catheter infections. The application of mupirocin at the exit site as part of routine exit site care has resulted in a dramatic reduction of exit site infections and peritonitis related to *S. aureus*. Bacteriologic monitoring of the peritoneal dialysis population for *S. aureus* carriage is unnecessary when this approach is adopted, but there is concern that it may in the future encourage growth of resistant organisms. *P. aeruginosa* catheter exit site infections are very difficult to resolve and frequently relapse. Ciprofloxacin is often used to treat such catheter infections, but if the infection does not resolve or if *P. aeruginosa* peritonitis develops, the catheter must be removed promptly.

Catheter Malfunctions, Hernias, and Fluid Leaks

The most important noninfectious complications during peritoneal dialysis are abdominal wall–related hernias, leakages of dialysis fluid, and inflow and outflow malfunctions. Before peritoneal dialysis treatment is started, all significant abdominal wall–related hernias should be corrected. With the presence of 2 to 3 L of dialysate in the abdominal cavity, there is an increased intra-abdominal pressure, and preexisting hernias will worsen during peritoneal dialysis treatment. The most frequently occurring hernias after commencement of peritoneal dialysis are incisional, umbilical, and inguinal hernias. Significant hernias should be repaired surgically, and IPD may be continued postoperatively using low dwell volumes in a supine position.

Leakage of peritoneal fluid is related to catheter implantation technique, trauma, or patient-related anatomic abnormalities. It can occur early (<30 days) or late (>30 days) after implantation and can have various clinical manifestations depending on whether the leak is external or subcutaneous. Early leakage is usually external, appearing as fluid through the wound or the exit site. Late leakage may develop at the site of any incision and entry into the peritoneal cavity. The exact site of the leakage can be determined by computed tomography after infusion of 2 L of dialysis fluid containing radiocontrast material. Scrotal or labial edema can be a sign of an early or late fluid leak, usually through a patent processus vaginalis. Therapy usually entails a period off peritoneal dialysis, during which the patient is maintained on hemodialysis or on limited, small-volume peritoneal dialysis in the supine position as necessary. For recurrent leaks, surgical repair is essential. Leakage of fluid into the subcutaneous tissue is sometimes occult and difficult to diagnose. It may manifest as diminished drainage, which might be mistaken for ultrafiltration failure. Computed tomography and abdominal scintigraphy may identify the leak.

Outflow/inflow obstruction is the most frequently observed early event, occurring within 2 weeks after implantation of the catheter, although it may also be seen later, during other problems such as peritonitis. One-way outflow obstruction is the most frequent problem and is characterized by poor flow and failure to drain the peritoneal cavity. Common causes include both intraluminal factors (blood clot, fibrin) and extraluminal factors (constipation, occlusion of catheter holes by adjacent organs or omental wrapping, catheter tip dislocation out of the true pelvis, incorrect catheter placement at implantation). A kidney, ureter, and bladder (KUB) radiographic study is useful in localizing the peritoneal dialysis catheter tip and evaluating for malposition. Depending on the cause, appropriate therapy may entail laxatives, heparinized saline flushes, urokinase instillation into the catheter, manipulation under fluoroscopy guidance (using a stiff wire or stylet combined with a "whiplash" technique), and laparoscopic revision or open replacement of the catheter.

Peritoneal Membrane Changes: Encapsulating Peritoneal Sclerosis and Ultrafiltration Failure

The peritoneum undergoing peritoneal dialysis reacts in response to the new environment. There is thickening of the peritoneal interstitium and basement membrane reduplication, both in the mesothelium and in the capillaries. These changes occur in response to the nonphysiologic composition of standard dialysis solutions and also from the direct actions of glucose and GDPs, which cause formation of advanced glycation end-products (AGEs) and related changes in the peritoneal membrane. Changes in peritoneal microvessels and neovascularization occur, analogous to those seen in diabetic retinopathy, with deposition of type IV collagen. Other conditions that are important in the pathogenesis of peritoneal thickening are recurrent acute peritonitis and chronic inflammatory reactions mediated by uremic or low-level bacterial activation of peritoneal macrophages and intraperitoneal production of pro-inflammatory and pro-fibrotic cytokines such as vascular endothelial growth factor, interleukin 6, and transforming growth factor-β.

Data from an international biopsy registry showed that thickening of the membrane usually occurs over a period of 4 to 5 years of peritoneal dialysis and is associated with increasing severity of vasculopathy, although there is considerable interpatient variability, and some patients show only relatively minor changes even after more than 5 years on dialysis. For patients who have been undergoing peritoneal dialysis for more than 5 years, it is prudent to be vigilant for signs of a sudden increase in peritoneal permeability, particularly in association with raised inflammatory markers or vague gastrointestinal symptoms. These signs may indicate development of the rare condition known as *encapsulating peritoneal sclerosis* (EPS), which is characterized by dense fibrosis and thickening of the peritoneum with bowel adhesions and encapsulation. The pathogenesis of EPS is complex, and no single etiologic factor has been identified; factors such as multiple episodes of peritonitis, use of high-glucose dialysis solutions, and genetic predisposition have been proposed, with little substantiating evidence. Although EPS is rare, its incidence rises significantly after 5 years of peritoneal dialysis therapy. EPS is a serious, life-threatening condition with variable reported mortality, which probably depends on severity at the time of diagnosis. One series reported a

60% death rate within 4 months after presentation with intestinal obstruction. Progressive loss of ultrafiltration and sudden development of high-transporter status may be early warning signs in some patients. However the designation "EPS" should be reserved for the point at which *encapsulation* has clearly occurred. Clinically, the features are those of ileus or frank intestinal obstruction. Diarrhea is also observed when partial obstruction spontaneously resolves. Gut motility is compromised as a result of binding of the intestinal loops to the parietal peritoneum and abdominal wall by an aggressive fibrotic process. Treatment consists of resting the bowel with total parenteral nutrition and surgical enterolysis for obstructive symptoms, which is best undertaken at specialist centers. Some advocate cessation of peritoneal dialysis and conversion to hemodialysis, but others suspect that such a change may exacerbate the fibrotic process. There are anecdotal reports of use of antifibrotic agents such as tamoxifen or immunosuppressive agents, with limited success.

Net ultrafiltration failure is the most important transport abnormality in patients undergoing long-term peritoneal dialysis. On the basis of clinical symptoms, its prevalence has been reported to increase from 3% after 1 year on CAPD to about 30% after 6 years. *Ultrafiltration failure* is defined as net ultrafiltration of less than 400 mL after a 4-hour dwell using 2 L of 4.25% glucose-containing dialysate. This condition is associated with a large peritoneal vascular surface area and impaired aquaporin channel–mediated water transport. It is best managed with frequent, short dwells and elimination of long dwells, such as with nocturnal APD, combined with daytime icodextrin. Because icodextrin is such a large molecule, its reabsorption is relatively unaffected by membrane permeability. It exerts colloid oncotic pressure and is able to maintain gradual but sustained ultrafiltration for 12 hours or longer. Improvement of peritoneal function can be brought about by minimizing glucose exposure (i.e., using glucose-free dialysate), providing peritoneal rest (being "dry" during the day on APD), using solutions that are low in GDPs, and using icodextrin, which has been shown to extend peritoneal dialysis therapy time in patients with loss of ultrafiltration. Mortality in this group is higher than for other patients on peritoneal dialysis, probably because of poor fluid control, which adds to the overall cardiovascular risk, as well as increased protein loss in the dialysate, which compromises nutrition.

Diabetic Patients on Peritoneal Dialysis

Diabetic glomerulosclerosis is the most common cause of kidney failure worldwide among peritoneal dialysis patients. Most diabetic patients require insulin while they are on peritoneal dialysis, even if they did not require it before the initiation of dialysis. This condition is partly the result of glucose absorption from the dialysate and associated weight gain. Insulin can be given to peritoneal dialysis patients via the intraperitoneal route (thought to be better because it is more physiologic, although evidence is lacking), the subcutaneous route, or a combination of both. If given intraperitoneally, the total daily dose of insulin required must be increased because insulin adsorbs onto the polyvinylchloride bags. Patients undergoing APD usually require long-acting subcutaneous insulin (with or without intraperitoneal regular insulin) for adequate glucose control. Injection of insulin into dialysis fluid bags confers a theoretical risk of bacterial contamination and subsequent peritonitis, although no evidence of this consequence has been reported. Nevertheless, it is not a widely used route of insulin administration for diabetic patients at present.

OUTCOMES OF PERITONEAL DIALYSIS

Survival of patients on peritoneal dialysis is similar to those on hemodialysis and is probably slightly better during the first 2 years of dialysis therapy. Underlying comorbidity very much dictates outcome, although several observational studies from Canada and Europe have suggested that there is a survival advantage in commencing dialysis therapy with peritoneal dialysis and then changing to hemodialysis when the therapy fails, rather than starting on hemodialysis first. Beginning with peritoneal dialysis maximizes the advantages that it confers during the first few years of dialysis, in terms of preservation of residual kidney function and better fluid control. If patient preference and medical conditions allow, peritoneal dialysis may well be the most appropriate initial dialysis therapy when a patient reaches chronic kidney disease stage 5.

Patient and technique survival are improving. Registry data from the 2007 United States Renal Data System showed almost identical 5-year actuarial patient survival (31%) with peritoneal dialysis and with hemodialysis. Risk factors for death among patients undergoing peritoneal dialysis include increasing age, presence of cardiovascular disease or diabetes mellitus, decreased serum albumin level, poor nutritional status as determined by anthropometric measurements, and inadequate dialysis. The leading causes of death are cardiovascular disease and infections.

Patients transfer from peritoneal dialysis to hemodialysis for a multitude of reasons, including peritonitis or exit site infection, catheter malfunction, inability to perform the dialysis procedure, and inadequate clearance or ultrafiltration (particularly with loss of residual kidney function) (see **Fig. 55-5**). In many cases, the patient who loses a catheter because of peritonitis or a catheter infection elects to switch to hemodialysis permanently. The increasing use of the Y-set and "flush-before-fill" systems is associated with improved technique survival on CAPD that is primarily due to lower peritonitis rates. It is hoped that long-term outcomes will improve with greater emphasis on maintenance of residual renal function, greater use of more physiologic peritoneal dialysis solutions, and the use of peritoneal dialysis in an integrated renal replacement treatment program, as an equally important modality to hemodialysis and perhaps as the first dialytic treatment for most patients with end-stage renal disease.

Transplantation is the goal for many patients undergoing dialysis. The allograft and patient survival rates of transplanted peritoneal dialysis patients are similar to those of transplanted hemodialysis patients, but there is reduced delayed graft function in the former group. Delayed graft function, in combination with graft rejection, is a strong predictor of graft survival. If the transplant does not initially function, peritoneal dialysis may be continued, provided that the peritoneal cavity was not entered during surgery. The peritoneal catheter is usually left in place for 2 to 3 months, until the graft is functioning well.

Use of Peritoneal Dialysis in an Integrated Renal Replacement Therapy Program

The utilization of peritoneal dialysis worldwide varies from 2% to 3% to more than 80% of the dialysis population in different countries. Such discrepancies cannot be explained by medical variables alone. The major reasons reside in nonmedical factors such as finance and reimbursement, as well as physician biases and prejudices, which have a serious impact on therapy options conveyed to patients. There is a decline in the use of peritoneal dialysis in many Western countries, partly related to lack of patient choice and information.

PERITONEAL DIALYSIS FOR ACUTE KIDNEY INJURY

IPD can be successfully used to manage acute kidney injury. Traditionally, a rigid peritoneal catheter was inserted percutaneously using a stylet, without a subcutaneous tunnel

and therefore with an increased risk of fluid leakage and peritonitis. However, bedside insertion of a Tenckhoff catheter using the Seldinger technique under local anesthesia is equally straightforward and carries a much smaller risk of infection. Rapid exchanges are performed to maximize clearance of small solutes—up to one exchange per hour, ideally, using an APD machine. More frequent exchanges are unlikely to improve solute clearance and introduce a large "down time," when the peritoneum is mostly empty in between dwells. The patient may be kept on APD for 48 hours or even longer, or IPD may be performed daily for 10 to 12 hours. Although these procedures are extremely effective for volume control and are better tolerated by hemodynamically unstable patients than hemodialysis, clearance of small solutes may be inadequate in catabolic patients or patients undergoing total parenteral nutrition who are receiving large protein loads. In addition, in the intensive care unit setting, the risk of peritonitis remains, although it should be remembered that central venous hemodialysis catheters also carry significant risks of bacteremia and other complications. Nevertheless, peritoneal dialysis has been largely replaced by hemodialysis and by continuous venovenous hemofiltration or hemodiafiltration for the management of acute kidney injury in hospitals with an active peritoneal dialysis program.

BIBLIOGRAPHY

Abu-Alfa AK, Burkart J, Piraino B, et al: Approach to fluid management in peritoneal dialysis: A practical algorithm. Kidney Int Suppl (81):S8-S16, 2002.

Brown EA, Davies SJ, Rutherford P, et al: Survival of functionally anuric patients on automated peritoneal dialysis: The European APD Outcome Study. J Am Soc Nephrol 14:2948-2957, 2003.

Chatoth DK, Golper TA, Gokal R: Morbidity and mortality in redefining adequacy of peritoneal dialysis: A step beyond the National Kidney Foundation Dialysis Outcomes Quality Initiative. Am J Kidney Dis 33:617-632, 1999.

Churchill DN, Thorpe KE, Nolph KD, et al: Increased peritoneal membrane transport is associated with decreased patient and technique survival for continuous peritoneal dialysis patients. The Canada-USA (CANUSA) Peritoneal Dialysis Study Group. J Am Soc Nephrol 9:1285-1292, 1998.

Coles GA, Williams JD: What is the place of peritoneal dialysis in the integrated treatment of renal failure? Kidney Int 54:2234-2240, 1998.

Davies SJ, Phillips L, Griffiths AM, et al: What really happens to people on long-term peritoneal dialysis? Kidney Int 54:2207-2217, 1998.

Davies SJ, Woodrow G, Donovan K, et al: Icodextrin improves the fluid status of peritoneal dialysis patients: Results of a double-blind randomized controlled trial. J Am Soc Nephrol 14:2338-2344, 2003.

Fenton SS, Schaubel DE, Desmeules M, et al: Hemodialysis versus peritoneal dialysis: A comparison of adjusted mortality rates. Am J Kidney Dis 30:334-342, 1997.

Flanigan M, Gokal R: Peritoneal catheters and exit-site practices toward optimum peritoneal access: A review of current developments. Perit Dial Int 25:132-139, 2005.

Gokal R: New strategies for peritoneal dialysis fluids. Nephrol Dial Transplant 12(Suppl 1):74-77, 1997.

Gokal R: Peritoneal dialysis in the 21st century: An analysis of current problems and future developments. J Am Soc Nephrol 13(Suppl 1):S104-S116, 2002.

Gokal R, Alexander S, Ash S, et al: Peritoneal catheters and exit-site practices toward optimum peritoneal access: 1998 Update. Official report from the International Society for Peritoneal Dialysis. Perit Dial Int 18:11-33, 1998.

Grassmann A, Gioberge S, Moeller S, Brown G: ESRD patients in 2004: Global overview of patient numbers, treatment modalities and associated trends. Nephrol Dial Transplant 20:2587-2593, 2005.

Grassmann A, Gioberge S, Moeller S, Brown G: End-stage renal disease: Global demographics in 2005 and observed trends. Artif Organs 30:895-897, 2006.

Hendriks PM, Ho-dac-Pannekeet MM, van Gulik TM, et al: Peritoneal sclerosis in chronic peritoneal dialysis patients: Analysis of clinical presentation, risk factors, and peritoneal transport kinetics. Perit Dial Int 17:136-143, 1997.

Lee HY, Choi HY, Park HC, et al: Changing prescribing practice in CAPD patients in Korea: Increased utilization of low GDP solutions improves patient outcome. Nephrol Dial Transplant 21:2893-2899, 2006.

Lo WK, Ho YW, Li CS, et al: Effect of Kt/V on survival and clinical outcome in CAPD patients in a randomized prospective study. Kidney Int 64:649-656, 2003.

Mistry CD, Gokal R, Peers E: A randomized multicenter clinical trial comparing isosmolar icodextrin with hyperosmolar glucose solutions in CAPD. MIDAS Study Group: Multicenter Investigation of Icodextrin in Ambulatory Peritoneal Dialysis. Kidney Int 46:496-503, 1994.

Mujais S, Nolph K, Gokal R, et al: Evaluation and management of ultrafiltration problems in peritoneal dialysis. International Society for Peritoneal Dialysis Ad Hoc Committee on Ultrafiltration Management in Peritoneal Dialysis. Perit Dial Int 20(Suppl 4): S5-S21, 2000.

Mupirocin Study Group: Nasal mupirocin prevents *Staphylococcus aureus* exit-site infection during peritoneal dialysis. Mupirocin Study Group. J Am Soc Nephrol 7:2403-2408, 1996.

Nakayama M, Kawaguchi Y, Yamada K, et al: Immunohistochemical detection of advanced glycosylation end-products in the peritoneum and its possible pathophysiological role in CAPD. Kidney Int 51:182-186, 1997.

National Kidney Foundation: NKF-K/DOQI clinical practice guidelines for peritoneal dialysis adequacy. National Kidney Foundation. Am J Kidney Dis 30:S67-136, 1997.

National Kidney Foundation. K/DOQI guidelines. 2007. Available at http://www.kidney.org/professionals/kdoqi/guidelines_updates/doqi_upex.html (accessed July 25, 2008).

Nissenson AR, Prichard SS, Cheng IK, et al: ESRD modality selection into the 21st century: The importance of non medical factors. ASAIO J 43:143-150, 1997.

Paniagua R, Amato D, Vonesh E, et al: Effects of increased peritoneal clearances on mortality rates in peritoneal dialysis: ADEMEX, a prospective, randomized, controlled trial. J Am Soc Nephrol 13:1307-1320, 2002.

Piraino B, Bailie GR, Bernardini J, et al: Peritoneal dialysis-related infections recommendations: 2005 Update. Perit Dial Int 25:107-131, 2005.

Stenvinkel P, Chung SH, Heimburger O, Lindholm B: Malnutrition, inflammation, and atherosclerosis in peritoneal dialysis patients. Perit Dial Int 21(Suppl 3):S157-S162, 2001.

Summers AM, Clancy MJ, Syed F, et al: Single-center experience of encapsulating peritoneal sclerosis in patients on peritoneal dialysis for end-stage renal failure. Kidney Int 68:2381-2388, 2005.

Uttley L, Vardhan A, Mahajan S, et al: Decrease in infections with the introduction of mupirocin cream at the peritoneal dialysis catheter exit site. J Nephrol 17:242-245, 2004.

Vardhan A, Zweers MM, Gokal R, Krediet RT: A solutions portfolio approach in peritoneal dialysis. Kidney Int Suppl (88):S114-S123, 2003.

Williams JD, Craig KJ, Topley N, et al: Morphologic changes in the peritoneal membrane of patients with renal disease. J Am Soc Nephrol 13:470-479, 2002.

CHAPTER 56

Outcome of End-Stage Renal Disease Therapies

Srinivasan Beddhu

According to the United States Renal Data System (USRDS), there were 485,012 prevalent patients with end-stage renal disease (ESRD) in December 2005. Of these, 29.6% had a functioning kidney transplant. Of the remainder, 91.4% were receiving in-center hemodialysis, 7.5% were performing peritoneal dialysis, and 0.6% were performing home hemodialysis. An additional 0.5% could not be classified. This chapter reviews the morbidity, mortality, and economic costs of ESRD; factors that influence survival in dialysis patients; and comparative outcomes of kidney replacement therapies.

MORBIDITY

The USRDS is a national registry of dialysis patients. U.S. Medicare regulations stipulate that all patients starting on chronic dialysis therapy must be reported to the USRDS, regardless of their insurance status. The outcomes of these patients are tracked by USRDS using the Medicare database and national Vital Statistics (maintained by the National Center for Health Statistics). Based on USRDS data, there are approximately 2 hospital admissions and 14.5 hospital days per patient-year of follow-up for dialysis patients. About one third of these hospitalizations are related to cardiovascular disease, and about one sixth are related to vascular access. Transplant patients have lower hospital admission rates (0.9 per patient-year) and fewer hospital days (5.7 days per patient-year).

Several studies have shown that the quality of life of dialysis patients is lower than that of the general population. In general, fatigue and lack of energy are the most common complaints of dialysis patients. Travel to the dialysis facility three times a week for several hours each session is a significant additional burden for in-center hemodialysis patients. Patients with ESRD often have significant comorbidities, such as hypertension, diabetes mellitus, peripheral vascular disease, infertility, and erectile dysfunction, that contribute to their burden of illness. Problems with vascular access further contribute to the frustrations of hemodialysis patients.

MORTALITY

Based on USRDS data, the 5-year survival rate of ESRD patients is only 39%. This is lower than that of stage IIIB breast cancer (54% survival at 5 years). The annual mortality rate of dialysis patients is approximately 23%, compared with less than 0.1% in the U.S. general population (**Fig. 56-1**). Even kidney transplant recipients have a substantially higher

mortality rate (approximately 7%) compared with the general population. Consequently, the life expectancy of dialysis and transplant populations is much lower than that of the general population (**Fig. 56-2**).

Survival in the ESRD population varies widely among patients and is strongly influenced by associated comorbid conditions, as illustrated in **Figure 56-3**. Although the 2-year survival rate for hemodialysis patients in the highest quartile of comorbidity scores was 40%, it was 95% in the quartile with the lowest comorbidity scores. The additional life expectancy of a 30-year old individual who received a kidney transplant with glomerulonephritis as the cause of kidney failure is almost 50 years (see **Fig. 56-2**). Therefore, nihilism toward ESRD, particularly in younger people with lower comorbidity scores, is not warranted. Most, if not all, patients with advanced kidney failure are apprehensive about their future, and they need to be educated on this important issue.

The all-cause, cardiovascular, and infectious disease mortality rates of ESRD patients have been steadily declining over the past decade, even as the comorbidity burden of the incident ESRD population has increased. It is difficult to assign this improved survival to any particular intervention. Of note, the mortality rates of other diseases, such as heart disease and cancer, are also declining in the United States.

ECONOMIC COSTS

The total Medicare costs for ESRD care in 2005 were $19.3 billion, which was 5.8% of the entire Medicare budget of $330 billion. Of these ESRD costs, 36% were for inpatient

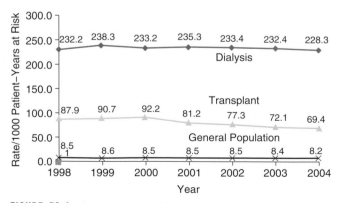

FIGURE 56-1 Mortality in the U.S. dialysis, transplant, and general populations. (Data from United States Renal Data System 2007 Annual Report and Centers for Disease Control.)

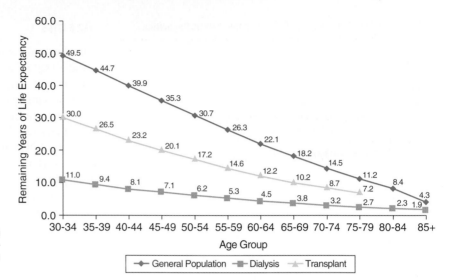

FIGURE 56-2 Expected remaining years of life in U.S. general and end-stage renal disease populations. (Data from United States Renal Data System 2007 Annual Report.)

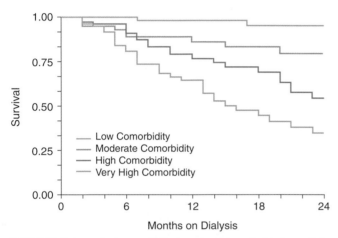

FIGURE 56-3 Impact of comorbidity on actuarial survival in hemodialysis patients. Lines show quartiles of Charlson Comorbidity Score. (Data from Beddhu S, Bruns FJ, Saul M, et al: A simple comorbidity scale predicts clinical outcomes and costs in dialysis patients. Am J Med 108:609-613, 2000.)

care, 37% for outpatient care, 21% for physician-supplier claims, and the rest were for skilled care, home care, and hospice care. Outpatient costs included $3.3 billion for hemodialysis, $0.26 billion for peritoneal dialysis, $1.9 billion for erythropoiesis-stimulating agents, $ 0.37 billion for intravenous Vitamin D, and $ 0.23 billion for intravenous iron.

In 2005, per patient-year costs for dialysis and functioning allograft were $68,585 and $17,273, respectively. The total costs for the year in which a transplant event or graft failure occurred were $102,637 and $79,704, respectively.

Medicare expenditures for ESRD care soared from $8.9 billion in 1995 to $19.3 in 2005. These increasing amounts reflected the increase in the number of ESRD patients as well as the entry to dialysis of an older and sicker population that required more nondialysis medical care. With continued growth of the ESRD population, these costs are likely to increase in the coming decades.

FACTORS INFLUENCING MORTALITY IN THE DIALYSIS POPULATION

Demographics

Table 56-1 summarizes the factors that might influence survival in dialysis patients. As expected, age is a strong predictor of death. Although African American race is associated with increased risk of death in the general population, it is associated with better survival in dialysis patients. The reasons for this are unclear but several have been suggested, including better nutritional status, a lower rate of transplantation that results in a healthier pool of African Americans staying on dialysis, and survival bias (i.e., African Americans who survive to dialysis are likely to be healthier). Hispanic ethnicity is also associated with better survival on dialysis, compared with white race.

Timing of Referral to Nephrologists

Compared with patients referred early to nephrologists, those who were referred late were more likely to have hypoalbuminemia, to have lower hemoglobin, to have received no erythropoietin supplementation, and not to have a functioning permanent vascular access at the initiation of dialysis. Late referral was also associated with increased mortality. One interpretation of these data is that early referral to nephrologists improves the care of patients with advanced chronic kidney disease. Alternatively, late referral could simply be a surrogate marker of poor access to health care.

Timing of Initiation of Dialysis

The National Kidney Foundation Kidney/Dialysis Outcomes Quality Initiative (K/DOQI) peritoneal dialysis guidelines previously recommended that patients should be advised to initiate some form of dialysis when their weekly native kidney Kt/V_{urea} (an index of urea clearance—see Chapter 54) fell to less than 2.0, which is equivalent to a

TABLE 56-1 Factors Influencing Survival in the Dialysis Population

Demographic factors
 Age
 Race
 Ethnicity

Dialysis-related factors
 Timing of referral and placement of vascular access
 Timing of initiation of dialysis
 Type of vascular access
 Type of dialysis modality
 Dialysis dose

Kidney disease–related factors
 Anemia
 Calcium-phosphorus, parathyroid hormone levels, and vascular
  calcification

Cardiovascular disease
 Atherosclerosis
 Cardiomyopathy
 Arrhythmias
 Valvular heart disease

Blood pressure

Nutritional status
 Body size
 Muscle mass
 Serum albumin

Metabolic disorders
 Inflammation
 Oxidative stress
 Insulin resistance
 Dyslipidemia

glomerular filtration rate (GFR) of approximately 10.5 mL/min/1.73 m². Data from observational studies did not support this recommendation, however. The current K/DOQI recommendation is that, when a patient reaches stage 5 of chronic kidney disease (GFR <15 mL/min/1.73 m²), the nephrologist should evaluate the benefits, risks, and disadvantages of beginning kidney replacement therapy. Individual clinical circumstances and certain complications of kidney failure such, as volume overload resistant to medical therapy or failure to thrive, may prompt initiation of therapy before stage 5. An ongoing randomized, controlled trial of early versus late initiation of dialysis in Australia and New Zealand may provide more definitive answers for this question.

The mean estimated GFR at initiation of dialysis in the United States, calculated by the Modification of Diet in Renal Disease (MDRD) equation, was 9.1 mL/min/ 1.73 m². However, caution is warranted when estimating GFR using the MDRD formula in patients with advanced kidney failure, because this equation might overestimate GFR in undernourished individuals and underestimate GFR in those with high muscle mass (see Chapter 2). Reliance on estimated GFR for initiation of dialysis could result in delayed initiation in malnourished patients.

Dialysis Dose

The effects of dialysis dose on mortality are discussed in Chapters 54 and 55.

Anemia

Observational studies have suggested better survival in hemodialysis patients with higher blood hemoglobin levels. In contrast, randomized, controlled trials in patients with chronic kidney disease and hemodialysis showed either no benefit or an increased mortality rate with higher hemoglobin levels (see Chapter 60). Therefore, the current (2007) NKF K/DOQI guidelines recommend a target hemoglobin level of 11 to 12 g/dL for dialysis patients receiving erythropoietin therapy. Although anemia management remains a rapidly evolving area, it is clear that both anemia and the use of erythropoiesis-stimulating agents affect clinical outcomes of dialysis patients.

Vascular Access

Use of a central venous catheter for hemodialysis access is associated with a greater risk of death than use of an arteriovenous graft or native fistula. The best survival rates are is seen in patients with arteriovenous fistulas. The causative factors for these associations have not been clearly established. It is possible that the worse outcome is a reflection of higher levels of comorbidity in patients who receive catheters or arteriovenous grafts. Nonetheless, complications such as infection and thrombosis are highest with catheters and lowest with arteriovenous fistulas. Therefore, to the extent that the establishment of an arteriovenous fistula can be readily accomplished, this form of vascular access is preferred (see Chapter 54).

FACTORS INFLUENCING CARDIOVASCULAR DISEASE IN THE DIALYSIS POPULATION

Cardiovascular disease is the primary cause of death in dialysis patients. The manifestations of cardiac diseases in dialysis patients are discussed in detail in Chapter 59. Although a number of factors associated with differences in outcome have been identified, data from interventional trials are limited. For many of these factors, no firm conclusion about appropriate interventions to improve outcome can be made. Several of the risk factors are discussed here.

Calcium-Phosphorus, Parathyroid Hormone Levels, and Vascular Calcification

Higher concentrations of serum phosphorus, higher calcium-phosphorus product, and both high and low levels of parathyroid hormone are associated with increased vascular calcification and mortality in dialysis patients. Interventional trials provide conflicting data. Several randomized, controlled trials showed that therapy with sevelamer, compared to calcium-containing phosphorus binders, was associated with decreased arterial calcification, particularly in patients who were older and had preexisting calcification. In one study that included 129 incident hemodialysis patients, sevelamer treatment was also associated with a lower mortality rate, although this was only a secondary end point. However, in a much larger, multicenter, randomized, open-label, parallel-design trial ($N = 2103$), all-cause mortality rates and cause-specific mortality rates were not significantly different between the sevelamer arm and the calcium-based binder arm. Only in patients older than 65 years of age was there a significant effect of sevelamer in lowering the mortality rate.

Blood Pressure

In a large observational study, predialysis systolic blood pressure of 150 to 180 mm Hg was not associated with a higher mortality risk, compared with the reference group of 120 to 149 mm Hg, but the relative mortality risk increased significantly as systolic pressures fell to less than 110 mm Hg. Another study noted a "U"-shaped relationship between predialysis systolic blood pressure and cardiovascular mortality in chronic hemodialysis patients, with worse outcomes at either extreme of blood pressure values. The likely explanation of the worse outcome in individuals with low blood pressure is that it is a marker for preexisting cardiac dysfunction. Independent of these results, hypertension is associated with concentric left ventricular hypertrophy on echocardiography, de novo cardiac failure, and de novo ischemic heart disease in dialysis patients. Furthermore, high pulse pressure, calculated as the difference between the systolic and diastolic blood pressures and an indicator of noncompliant blood vessels, has been shown to be a strong predictor of all-cause and cardiovascular death in hemodialysis patients.

Nutritional Status

In contrast to the association of high body mass index (BMI) with increased mortality in the general population, high BMI is associated with better survival in dialysis patients. Although it has been suggested that obesity is protective rather than harmful, high BMI or abdominal adiposity is associated with cardiovascular risk factors including insulin resistance, diabetes, inflammation, anemia, coronary calcification, and carotid atherosclerosis in dialysis patients. These apparently contradictory associations might be explained by the dual competing effects of adiposity on survival: a deleterious metabolic effect resulting in insulin resistance, dyslipidemia, hypertension, and inflammation may be outweighed by a protective nutritional effect in dialysis patients. In addition to large body size, the presence of other indicators of better nutritional status, such as high muscle mass and higher serum albumin concentration, is particularly associated with better survival in dialysis patients.

Inflammation and Oxidative Stress

Elevated serum concentration of C-reactive protein (CRP), a marker of inflammation, is a strong predictor of mortality in dialysis patients, as it is in the general population. Inflammation may decrease patient survival by promoting atherosclerosis and malnutrition. However, statistical adjustment for nutritional status only modestly attenuates the associations of inflammation with mortality, suggesting that the effects of inflammation on mortality are not largely mediated by deterioration in nutritional status.

In dialysis patients, oxidative stress is thought to play a major role in morbidity and mortality. Two antioxidants, acetylcysteine and vitamin E, were shown to reduce cardiovascular events in dialysis patients in two separate small, randomized, controlled trials. Larger randomized trials are required to confirm the usefulness of anti-inflammatory and antioxidant medications in improving cardiovascular outcomes in dialysis patients.

Dyslipidemias

Epidemiologic studies using large national databases showed increased risk of death with lower serum cholesterol levels in hemodialysis patients. However, low cholesterol may be a surrogate for inflammation and poor nutrition, which are common in this population. In a German randomized trial involving diabetic hemodialysis patients, the addition of atorvastatin had no statistically significant effect on the composite primary end point of cardiovascular death, nonfatal myocardial infarction, and stroke. It should be noted that, instead of hypercholesterolemia, the uremic dyslipidemia is characterized by elevated serum triglycerides and lipoprotein(a) and decreased high-density lipoprotein (HDL)-cholesterol concentrations that are largely unaffected by statin therapy. Therefore, the lack of effects of a statin does not rule out dyslipidemia as a potentially modifiable cardiovascular risk factor in dialysis patients.

COMPARISON OF KIDNEY TRANSPLANTATION WITH DIALYSIS THERAPY

As discussed earlier, kidney transplantation is associated with lower morbidity and mortality when compared with dialysis therapies. However, kidney transplant recipients are a select population, because very old and sick patients are not considered to be candidates for transplantation. This raises the question whether the survival advantages associated with kidney transplantation are a result of selection bias or whether kidney transplantation per se improves survival. A large randomized, controlled trial of kidney transplantation versus dialysis would be the way to answer this question directly, but such a trial is impossible, because most patients have strong preference for one form of kidney replacement therapy or another.

Observational studies comparing outcomes of dialysis patients who satisfied all of the screening criteria for transplantation but were still awaiting transplantation (waitlisted patients) with this of patients who actually received their allograft avoid many, albeit not all, of the issues associated with selection bias. In one such study comparing waitlisted dialysis patients with those who received a first cadaveric transplant between 1991 and 1997, the relative risk of death was 2.8 times higher during the first 2 weeks after transplantation than for patients on dialysis with equal lengths of follow-up since placement on the waiting list; however, at 18 months, the risk was 68% lower. The long-term mortality rates in the various subgroups were 48% to 82% lower in transplant recipients than in patients remaining on the waiting list. These data suggest that long-term survival after kidney transplantation is better than after continued dialysis therapy. Therefore, all patients needing kidney replacement therapy should be encouraged to undergo the procedure, provided they are suitable candidates (see Chapter 62).

A related issue is the timing of kidney transplantation. Preemptive transplantation (i.e., transplantation before a patient needs to initiate dialysis), has been suggested to improve survival, compared with transplantation after initiation on dialysis. Nonetheless, because of the potential acute and chronic complications associated with kidney transplantation (see Chapter 63), the appropriateness of preemptive transplantation in individuals with stable, relatively preserved kidney function (e.g., GFR >15 mL/min/1.73 m^2), who might not develop uremic symptoms for an extended period of time, is unclear. Further studies are warranted before any firm conclusions can be drawn concerning the optimal timing of kidney transplantation.

COMPARISONS AMONG DIALYSIS THERAPIES

Even though transplantation is considered superior to dialysis therapies, most ESRD patients must be maintained on dialysis because of the shortage of donor organs and because many of these patients are not candidates for transplantation. Hemodiafiltration (see Chapter 54) is used to a limited extent as a chronic outpatient therapy in Europe and Japan, but there is a paucity of data comparing the outcomes of this form of therapy with those of dialysis. In the United States, there are three principal options for dialysis: in-center hemodialysis, home hemodialysis, and home peritoneal dialysis. In addition, new data on hemodialysis at increased frequency are emerging. The following discussion focuses on comparisons of in-center hemodialysis versus peritoneal dialysis and conventional hemodialysis versus frequent hemodialysis.

In-center Conventional Hemodialysis Versus Peritoneal Dialysis

In contrast to the thrice-weekly schedule of standard hemodialysis, peritoneal dialysis can be performed continuously and therefore might be more physiologic. Fluid removal can be accomplished gently, without hypotension most of the time. Potassium removal is also better with peritoneal dialysis, permitting liberalization of the diet. In addition, the convenience of performing peritoneal dialysis at home is attractive to many patients.

On the other hand, the weekly dialysis dose delivered with peritoneal dialysis (Kt/V of approximately 2.0 for urea; see Chapter 55) is much lower than that delivered with in-center hemodialysis (approximately 3.6). Peritoneal dialysate contains high concentrations of glucose, resulting in higher blood glucose levels, weight gain with insulin resistance, and dyslipidemia. Whether each of these factors influences the long-term clinical outcomes of patients is unclear.

A randomized, controlled trial attempted to answer this question, but random assignment to a particular dialysis modality is difficult, because potential subjects typically have a preference. As might be expected, this trial did not enroll adequate numbers of patients, and definitive inferences could not be drawn. An adequately powered, randomized trial is not likely to be feasible, so comparative outcomes can only be inferred from observational studies, which have produced conflicting results. Canadian studies suggested a better survival advantage for peritoneal dialysis, but, once adjustment for comorbidity and lower burden of acute indications for initiating dialysis therapy were made, this apparent advantage disappeared. Analyses of prevalent dialysis patients in the early 1990s in the USRDS suggested a worse survival with peritoneal dialysis, but these differences were not seen when incident patients were included. More recent data from the USRDS showed that peritoneal dialysis was associated with a higher risk of death in diabetics but a lower risk of death in nondiabetics, compared with hemodialysis. Another study found that incident ESRD patients with a clinical history of congestive heart failure experienced poorer survival when treated with peritoneal dialysis compared with hemodialysis, despite the potential advantage of continuous volume removal via peritoneal dialysis.

In a prospective cohort study of 1041 patients starting dialysis, the risk for death after adjustment for comorbidity did not differ between patients undergoing peritoneal dialysis ($n = 274$) and those undergoing hemodialysis ($n = 767$) during the first year, but the risk became significantly higher (relative hazard, 2.34) among those undergoing peritoneal dialysis in the second year.

Taken together, these data suggest that, whereas in-center hemodialysis and peritoneal dialysis have similar outcomes in the aggregate, there are important subgroups for whom hemodialysis might be preferable: patients older than 45 years of age and patients with diabetes. For individuals with a history of heart failure, hemodialysis might be preferable for those who can tolerate this modality without hypotension. In younger patients with low comorbidity and better functional status, peritoneal dialysis might be preferable.

Conventional Hemodialysis Versus Frequent Hemodialysis

The current standard schedule for hemodialysis in the United States is three sessions per week of 3 to 4 hours each. This approach is highly unphysiologic, because uremic toxins and fluid build up on nondialysis days, and their removal occurs abruptly. Theoretically, a better approach would be to increase the frequency and dose of dialysis, using short (2-hour) dialysis sessions on 6 to 7 days per week or nocturnal dialysis with 4- to 8-hour sessions on 3 to 7 days per week. The short daily dialysis could be performed at home or in-center, whereas nocturnal hemodialysis is more suited to home therapy.

Preliminary studies on frequent dialysis have been promising. Observational studies suggested that frequent dialysis therapies result in lower blood pressure, higher hemoglobin, reduction in erythropoietin use, lower serum calcium, lower serum phosphorus, lower parathyroid hormone levels, and improved cognitive abilities, compared with conventional dialysis. A recent randomized, controlled trial of 56 patients found that those treated with frequent nocturnal hemodialysis had significantly reduced left ventricular mass compared with those remaining on a conventional hemodialysis schedule. Frequent nocturnal hemodialysis was also associated with lower systolic blood pressure and lower serum phosphorus levels, allowing a reduction in or discontinuation of antihypertensive medications and oral phosphate binders.

Therefore, frequent hemodialysis appears to be a promising modality that might substantially improve outcomes in dialysis patients. However, before frequent hemodialysis is widely adopted, more positive results from randomized. controlled trials, preferably with major clinical event end points, should be available to support the usefulness of these dialysis schedules. Two trials of daily short in-center hemodialysis and frequent nocturnal home hemodialysis are currently underway, sponsored by the National Institutes of Health.

In summary, ESRD is associated with significant morbidity, mortality, and economic costs. The high mortality rate observed in dialysis patients is multifactorial. Some risk factors such as age and race are not modifiable, but many, including anemia, vascular calcification, dialysis dose, and, potentially, hemodialysis frequency, can be modified to improve outcomes. Transplantation is the preferred form of kidney replacement therapy. Although hemodialysis and peritoneal dialysis are comparable in the aggregate, hemodialysis might be better for older patients with higher burdens of comorbidity including diabetes and congestive heart failure. The optimal timing for initiation of dialysis and for transplantation is unclear and requires investigation. Further research is needed to determine whether therapy targeted toward malnutrition, inflammation, oxidative stress, and uremic dyslipidemia could improve outcomes in the dialysis population.

BIBLIOGRAPHY

Beddhu S, Samore MH, Roberts MS, et al: Impact of timing of initiation of dialysis on mortality. J Am Soc Nephrol 14: 2305-2312, 2003.

Beddhu S, Cheung AK, Larive B, et al; and the HEMO Study Group. Inflammation and the inverse associations of body nass index and serum creatinine with mortality in hemodialysis patients. J Ren Nutr 17:372-380, 2007.

Besarab A, Bolton WK, Browne JK, et al: The effects of normal as compared with low hematocrit values in patients with cardiac disease who are receiving hemodialysis and epoetin. N Engl J Med 339:584-590, 1998.

Boaz M, Smetana S, Weinstein T, et al: Secondary prevention with antioxidants of cardiovascular disease in endstage renal disease (SPACE): Randomised placebo-controlled trial. Lancet 356:1213-1218, 2000.

Chertow GM, Burke SK, Raggi P; Treat to Goal Working Group: Sevelamer attenuates the progression of coronary and aortic calcification in hemodialysis patients. Kidney Int 62:245-252, 2002.

Culleton BF, Walsh M, Klarenbach SW, et al: Effect of frequent nocturnal hemodialysis vs conventional hemodialysis on left ventricular mass and quality of life: A randomized controlled trial. JAMA 298:1291-1299, 2007.

Foley RN, Parfrey PS, Harnett JD, et al: Impact of hypertension on cardiomyopathy, morbidity and mortality in end-stage renal disease. Kidney Int 49:1379-1385, 1996.

Ganesh SK, Stack AG, Levin NW, et al: Association of elevated serum PO(4), Ca x PO(4) product, and parathyroid hormone with cardiac mortality risk in chronic hemodialysis patients. J Am Soc Nephrol 12:2131-2138, 2001.

Jaar BG, Coresh J, Plantinga LC, et al: Comparing the risk for death with peritoneal dialysis and hemodialysis in a national cohort of patients with chronic kidney disease. Ann Intern Med 143: 174-183, 2005.

Kalantar-Zadeh K, Abbott KC, Salahudeen AK, et al: Survival advantages of obesity in dialysis patients. Am J Clin Nutr 81: 543-554, 2005.

Korevaar JC, Jansen MA, Dekker FW, et al: When to initiate dialysis: Effect of proposed US guidelines on survival. Lancet 358:1046-1050, 2001.

Kwan BC, Beddhu S: A story half untold: Adiposity, adipokines and outcomes in dialysis population. Semin Dial 20:493-497, 2007.

Singh AK, Szczech L, Tang KL, et al: Correction of anemia with epoetin alfa in chronic kidney disease. N Engl J Med 355: 2085-2098, 2006.

Stenvinkel P, Heimburger O, Paultre F, et al: Strong association between malnutrition, inflammation, and atherosclerosis in chronic renal failure. Kidney Int 55:1899-1911, 1999.

Suki WN, Zabaneh R, Cangiano JL, et al: Effects of sevelamer and calcium-based phosphate binders on mortality in hemodialysis patients. Kidney Int 72:1130-1137, 2007.

Tepel M, van der Giet M, Statz M, et al: The antioxidant acetylcysteine reduces cardiovascular events in patients with end-stage renal failure: A randomized, controlled trial. Circulation 107:992-995, 2003.

Vonesh EF, Snyder JJ, Foley RN, Collins AJ: Mortality studies comparing peritoneal dialysis and hemodialysis: What do they tell us? Kidney Int Suppl (103):S3-S11, 2006.

Wanner C, Krane V, Marz W, et al: Atorvastatin in patients with type 2 diabetes mellitus undergoing hemodialysis. N Engl J Med 353:238-248, 2005.

Wolfe RA, Ashby VB, Milford EL, et al: Comparison of mortality in all patients on dialysis, patients on dialysis awaiting transplantation, and recipients of a first cadaveric transplant. N Engl J Med 341:1725-1730, 1999.

Zager PG, Nikolic J, Brown RH, et al: "U" curve association of blood pressure and mortality in hemodialysis patients. Kidney Int 54:561-569, 1998.

the typical American dietary content of 160 mEq (4 g) per day. However, the decision to implement dietary sodium restriction depends on the individual patient's fluid status, urinary sodium excretion, and the presence or absence of hypertension.

During renal replacement therapy, urine output usually continues to decline in proportion to the decline in the GFR. Many patients become anuric. Fluid intake must be controlled and prescribed individually. Balance of both sodium and water is maintained by matching dietary intake to the removal by dialysis plus any losses incurred via residual kidney function.

Potassium

As kidney failure progresses, the ability of the tubules to secrete potassium decreases. Nephron adaptation occurs to maintain potassium balance by increasing the amount secreted by the tubules and by increasing the amount excreted into the stool. As much as 20% to 50% of ingested potassium can appear in the stool when the GFR is less than 5 mL/min/1.73 m^2. These two adaptations are sufficient to maintain potassium balance with normal potassium intake (100 mEq/day, or 3.9 g/day) if the GFR is greater than 10 mL/min/1.73 m^2 and the urine output is at least 1000 mL/day. Once the GFR drops below 10 mL/min/1.73 m^2 or the patient becomes oliguric, dietary potassium restriction is necessary to maintain serum levels in the normal range of 3.5 to 5.0 mEq/L.

Dietary potassium restriction for hemodialysis patients is required to avoid hyperkalemia. Potassium accumulates in the body between dialysis treatments unless the patient has gastrointestinal losses or a urine output greater than 500 mL/day. Hyperkalemia can be caused by eating potassium-dense foods or potassium supplements, or it can be secondary to catabolism, hemolysis, or acidemia. **Table 57-2** identifies a variety of high-potassium foods. When counseling patients about intake of potassium or other dietary components, it is important to use patient education materials that have been modified to incorporate culturally specific foods.

The recommended potassium intake for hemodialysis patients is 51 to 77 mEq/day (2 to 3 g/day). Hyperkalemia causes cardiac arrhythmias and neurologic disturbances such as muscle weakness and flaccid quadriplegia. Because of the number of exchanges and dwell times, peritoneal dialysis results in a more continuous potassium clearance than does intermittent hemodialysis. Therefore, patients receiving peritoneal dialysis therapy can tolerate a more liberal diet intake of potassium (77 to 102 mEq/day, or 3 to 4 g/day) or, in some cases, an unrestricted intake. Potassium requirements in CKD stages 1 through 4 are based on the

---

TABLE 57-2 **Sampling of Foods that Contain High Levels of Potassium and Should be Limited or Avoided to Prevent Hyperkalemia**

FRUITS	VEGETABLES	BEVERAGES AND OTHER FOODS
Apricots	Artichokes	Bran and bran products
Avocado	Beans, dried	
Banana	Broccoli	Chocolate
Cantaloupe	Brussels sprouts	Coconut
Casaba melon	Escarole	Granola
Dried fruits (dates, figs, raisins, prunes)	Endive	Low-sodium baking powder or soda
Honeydew	Greens (Swiss chard, collard, beet, dandelion, mustard)	Milk and milk products (ice cream, yogurt—2 cups)
Mango	Kale	Molasses
Nectarine	Kohlrabi	Nuts/seeds
Orange	Lentils	Peanut butter
Papaya	Legumes	Salt substitute or "lite" salt (containing potassium)
Rhubarb	Lima beans	Potassium chloride—DO NOT USE
Juice of fruits listed	Mushrooms	Snuff/chewing tobacco
Tangelo	Parsnips	
Watermelon	Potatoes (French fries, chips, baked, mashed, boiled, sweet potatoes, yams)	
	Pumpkin	
	Rutabaga	
	Spinach, Swiss chard	
	Salt-free vegetable juice (ALL vegetable juices)	
	Tomatoes	
	Winter squash (acorn, butternut, Hubbard)	

individual's disease, metabolism, serum potassium levels, and medications. Patients with type 4 renal tubular acidosis and those receiving drugs that interfere with the renin-angiotensin-aldosterone system may need more rigorous potassium restriction to avoid hyperkalemia.

Phosphorus, Calcium, and Vitamin D

The kidney filters approximately 7 g of phosphorus daily, of which 80% to 90% is reabsorbed by the renal tubules and the remainder is excreted in the urine. In early kidney failure, hyperphosphatemia is prevented by an adaptive decrease in tubular phosphate resorption. Not until the GFR falls to less than 20 mL/min does hyperphosphatemia usually become evident.

As kidney failure progresses, the damaged kidney does not respond to parathyroid hormone (PTH) with increased excretion. Phosphorus continues to accumulate as less is filtered by the kidney. Serum phosphorus levels rise, and dietary restriction becomes necessary. Dietary phosphorus restriction to 800 to 1000 mg/day, or 17 mg/kg of body weight per day, is commonly recommended. **Tables 57-3** and **57-4** provide examples of foods that are high in phosphorus content. Diet restriction alone is not sufficient to maintain normal serum levels, however. Phosphate-binding medications (e.g., calcium salts, sevelamer, lanthanum carbonate), which bind to dietary phosphorus and prevent its absorption in the gastrointestinal tract, are frequently required.

Bone resorption and impaired mineralization of newly formed bone are exacerbated by the decreased availability of the active form of vitamin D (1,25-dihydroxycholecalciferol). Careful monitoring of calcium, phosphorus, and PTH levels and subsequent titration of vitamin D, vitamin D analogues and calcimimetic agents is essential in the management of secondary hyperparathyroidism (see Chapters 56 and 58).

TABLE 57-3 Foods that Contain High Levels of Phosphorus and Should be Limited or Avoided to Prevent Hyperphosphatemia

LEGUMES, NUTS AND SEEDS, WHOLE GRAINS	MEAT AND OTHER FOODS	DAIRY AND BEVERAGES
Beans (navy, kidney, lima, pinto)	Chocolate	Beer
Soybeans	Dried fruit	Colas: Coke, RC, Pepsi, Dr. Pepper
Black-eyed peas	Molasses	Eggnog
Lentils	Beef liver, calf liver	Hot chocolate
Peanut Butter	Liver sausage	Milk
Nuts	Liverwurst	Casseroles
Coconuts	Beef, bottom round	Cheese
Pumpkin seeds	Pork, fresh	Cream soups
Sunflower seeds	Veal, cubes, rib roast	Custard
Bran, bran flakes, bran muffins		Ice cream
Brown rice		Pudding
Wheat germ		Yogurt
Raisin bran, 100% bran		
100% whole grain		

TABLE 57-4 Hidden Sources of Phosphorus and Alternatives*

HIDDEN SOURCES OF PHOSPHORUS	SUGGESTED ALTERNATIVES
Disodium phosphate	Use fresh meat products.
Monosodium phosphate	Use natural (not processed) cheeses, in very small amounts.
Sodium hexametaphosphate	Prepare pancakes, waffles, biscuits, and breads from raw ingredients, not ready-made mixes with unknown contents.
Potassium tripolyphosphate	Limit the obvious sources of phosphorus, such as dairy foods, colas, beans, nuts, and chocolate.
Trisodium triphosphate	
Sodium tripolyphosphate	
Tetrasodium pyrophosphate	
Phosphoric acid	

*It is important for both patients and clinicians to be familiar with the hidden sources of phosphorus in food products that are not typically identified on the nutrient food label. This table lists some forms of phosphorus that are included in the ingredient lists of many foods, as well as some suggestions for limiting the intake of foods that contain them.

Water and Fat-Soluble Vitamins

Adult dialysis patients usually have low blood levels of the water-soluble vitamins unless they take a vitamin supplement. The causes include losses into the dialysate; dietary restrictions of protein, potassium, and phosphorus; anorexia and reduced food intake; and alterations in metabolism. Supplementation is in order using the Dietary Reference Intakes (DRIs) established by the Food and Nutrition Board of the Institute of Medicine as a guide. Higher doses are recommended for the dialysis patient for pyridoxine (B_6), folate, and ascorbic acid. The recommended amounts for dialysis patients are 10 mg for vitamin B_6, 0.8 to 1 mg for folate, and 60 mg for ascorbic acid. The same amounts are recommended for patients in earlier stages of CKD, except that 5 mg of pyridoxine is recommended.

Increased requirement for vitamin B_6 by dialysis patients is evidenced by low plasma and red blood cell pyridoxine levels and low plasma levels of the vitamin's coenzyme, pyridoxine phosphate. Abnormal lymphocyte function, depressed immune response, and abnormal plasma leucine and valine levels in this patient population have been ameliorated by pyridoxine supplementation.

Reduced plasma and leukocyte ascorbic acid levels have been reported in dialysis patients and are most likely caused by restriction of fruits and vegetables necessary for control of potassium intake as well as by dialysis losses. Dietary supplementation in excess of 60 mg/day of ascorbic acid is not recommended, however, to avoid oxalosis.

Inadequate dietary intake, loss to the dialysate of approximately 37% per hemodialysis session, and altered metabolism are possible causes of folate deficiency. Low serum folate levels as well as inhibition in membrane transport of this vitamin by anions such as phosphate have been observed in dialysis patients.

Vitamin A and retinol-binding protein are normally cleared by the kidneys and therefore become elevated as kidney function deteriorates. Vitamin A supplementation should be avoided, to prevent vitamin A toxicity. Vitamin K replacement is not indicated unless intestinal flora are suppressed by antibiotic therapy. Vitamin E supplementation has not been shown to be cardioprotective.

Special vitamin supplements for dialysis patients that meet these requirements are available, depending on the formulation, either over the counter or by prescription.

Minerals and Trace Elements

The dietary requirements for trace elements are not known, and, with the exception of iron, supplementation is not usually recommended. Adequacy of diet, medications, and the nutritional and medical status of patients with any stage of CKD determine the need for supplementation of minerals.

Hypermagnesemia may be present, becausde magnesium is normally excreted primarily by the kidneys. Although the "renal diet" tends to contain less magnesium than a typical American diet, active restriction of dietary magnesium usually is not necessary to maintain normal serum levels. Hypermagnesemia has been induced by ingestion of magnesium-containing antacids, enemas, and laxatives.

The requirement for iron is affected by intake, dialysis-induced blood losses, frequent laboratory testing, impaired intestinal iron absorption, and occult gastrointestinal bleeding. All of these factors are likely to cause iron deficiency anemia. The monitoring of iron status and the intravenous administration of iron supplement is described in detail in Chapter 60.

For patients with CKD stages 1 through 4 who may require oral iron therapy, ferrous gluconate, ferrous fumarate, or ferrous sulfate may be recommended. Ferrous gluconate contains 12% elemental iron; ferrous fumarate, 33% elemental iron; and ferrous sulfate, 20% elemental iron. Ferrous gluconate is often better tolerated. Maximal absorptionoccurs if the supplement taken on an empty stomach, but individuals who experience gastric upset may take them with food. However, tea, coffee, milk, cereals, dietary fiber, eggs, and antacids should not be taken with iron, because absorption will be decreased. Intestinal iron absorption will be enhanced if iron is taken with vitamin C (200 mg vitamin C or more per 30 mg of elemental iron). Low plasma zinc levels observed in dialysis patients may be the result of dietary restriction of protein, impaired zinc absorption, redistribution of the body pool zinc, or a decrease in zinc binding to plasma protein. Uremic symptoms of hypogeusia, sexual impotence, and anorexia have been reported to improve after subjects were given zinc supplementation in clinical trials, but routine zinc replacement is not usually prescribed.

The effects of aluminum retention are a concern for dialysis patients. Accumulation of aluminum in cerebral gray matter may be responsible for the dialysis encephalopathy syndrome. Aluminum has also been noted to accumulate in bone and may play a role in CKD bone disease. These problems have largely disappeared since the use of aluminum-containing phosphate binders was abandoned. Nonetheless, medications containing aluminum should not be prescribed to patients with advanced CKD or ESRD.

Carnitine

L-Carnitine (1-3-hydroxy-4-*N*-trimethylaminobutyrate) is an amino acid whose main function is to transfer long-chain fatty acids from the cytoplasm through the inner membrane of the mitochondria for oxidation. Carnitine deficiency can result in inefficient energy production and impaired oxidation of long-chain fatty acids. The high prevalences of cardiomyopathy, skeletal myopathy, and dyslipidemia that characterize the dialysis patient population have prompted investigators to question whether carnitine deficiency contributes to these problems. Routine L-carnitine therapy is not currently recommended because of the lack of data demonstrating improvement in outcomes such as hypertriglyceridemia or (EPO) erythropoietin resistance. Carnitine supplementation may be indicated for patients who present with muscle weakness and fatigue associated with low plasma carnitine levels for which no other cause can be identified.

NUTRITION ASSESSMENT AND MANAGEMENT OF CHRONIC KIDNEY DISEASE

Current nutrition assessment and management in adult dialysis patients routinely relies on analysis of biochemical parameters as reflected by blood indices. These values are usually reported monthly for stable patients. Serum values commonly reviewed for nutritional evaluation are BUN, creatinine, total proteins, albumin, potassium, phosphorus, calcium, sodium, cholesterol, triglycerides, glucose, and alkaline phosphatase. Other important elements in the nutrition assessment include anthropometric measurements, physical and clinical evaluations, and food intake information. These data are incorporated with the patient's dry weight (i.e., the weight at which the patient is free of detectable peripheral edema and has normal blood pressure without postural hypotension), interdialytic fluid weight gains, and blood pressure measurements to evaluate nutrition and fluid status. These values, together and alone, are reviewed in the context of the patient's previous values and trends.

Blood Urea Nitrogen

A significant correlation between dietary protein intake and the predialysis BUN concentration has been observed when patients are clinically stable, and BUN can be used to indirectly monitor the patient's protein intake. Optimal BUN values for adult dialysis patients are in the range of 60 to 80 mg/dL. A BUN value higher than 100 mg/dL suggests excessive dietary protein intake, inadequate dialysis, catabolism, or gastrointestinal bleeding. A BUN value lower than 60 mg/dL suggests inadequate protein intake, anabolism, residual kidney function, or intense dialysis. Because the BUN is dependent on other factors in addition to dietary protein intake, other laboratory and clinical parameters should be considered in conjunction with BUN for nutrition management.

Decreases in serum albumin concentration and dry weight are important indicators of nutritional status, but there may be a lag of a few months between a compromised protein intake and these changes, preventing the dietitian from responding preemptively. The determination of protein intake can provide an earlier clue. One of the methods of assessing protein intake is the normalized protein catabolic rate (nPCR). In CKD stages 1 through 4, the nPCR is calculated by multiplying the BUN by the rate of urea nitrogen generation in milligrams per minute (equivalent to total body water) and adding urinary urea nitrogen. For CKD stage 5, nPCR is derived from predialysis and postdialysis BUN levels, because urinary urea nitrogen values are not typically available. This calculation assumes that the urea generation rate can be used to estimate nPCR because urea is the primary product of protein catabolism; it also assumes that nPCR equals dietary protein intake when the patient is in nitrogen balance. The desired range of nPCR for chronic dialysis patients and, hence, the necessary dietary protein intake, is 1.2 to 1.3 g/kg of dry body weight. If a patient is catabolic (as evidenced by weight loss, decreased serum albumin, or onset of medical illness), the nPCR is greater than dietary protein intake, whereas an anabolic patient's nPCR is less than protein intake.

Protein balance can be calculated from the difference between dietary protein intake and nPCR. This method is best used to monitor nitrogen balance of noncatabolic patients, because catabolized protein can be both exogenous (i.e., derived from the diet) and endogenous. The nPCR should be incorporated into the nutrition assessment procedure for all stages of CKD. For CKD stages 1 through 4, nitrogen balance should be determined if a patient presents with a deleterious change in nutritional status or appetite (e.g., hypoalbuminemia, weight loss); in stage 5, nPCR should be determined as part of the monthly Kt/V calculation.

Serum Proteins

Levels of serum total protein, transferrin, albumin, and prealbumin are all commonly used for nutrition assessment of visceral protein stores. In patients with CKD of any stage, the reliability of these parameters for nutritional status is questionable because of the metabolic and fluid derangements associated with the uremic state. All serum protein levels are affected by the hydration status. Serum transferrin becomes elevated with iron deficiency and depressed in the presence of iron overload.

Of these three serum proteins, albumin is currently the parameter most frequently used to assess visceral stores in CKD stages 1 through 5, probably because of the wide availability of the albumin assay and its association with outcome, although this association may be mediated by non-nutritional factors. Serum albumin levels have been extensively correlated with mortality in hemodialysis patients. A twofold increase in the relative risk of death has been reported for patients with serum albumin levels in the normal range of 3.5 to 4.0 g/dL, compared with the upper range of normal (4.0 to 4.5 g/dL); patients who had a serum albumin concentration of 2.5 g/dL had almost 20 times the risk of death of patients in the upper range of normal.

Serum albumin has a long half-life (18 to 20 days) and often is a late marker of malnutrition. However, low serum albumin levels are often accompanied by abnormal levels of other indices that reflect malnutrition (e.g., anthropometrics, total lymphocyte count, serum transferrin) and are usually interpreted to indicate a state of poor nutrition These other markers are influenced by such factors as fluid balance and anemia. so that no one marker can be relied upon to assess nutritional status. A panel of indices reflecting the various compartments is required to complete a nutrition assessment., In addition, non-nutritional factors that affect serum albumin metabolism in patients with CKD and their implications for the use of serum albumin as a marker of malnutrition have been identified. These factors include responses to inflammation (i.e., synthesis of acute phase reactant proteins such as C-reactive protein and cytokine release), acute metabolic acidosis, and the hormonal milieu. In states of inflammation, hepatic synthesis of C-reactive protein and other positive acute phase reactant proteins is prioritized over albumin synthesis. Hence, albumin is a negative acute phase reactive protein, and serum levels fall due to reduced hepatic albumin synthesis.

Serum prealbumin has shorter half-life (2 days) than albumin and for this reason has been considered to be a more sensitive nutritional measure. It may be falsely elevated in CKD due to decreased renal catabolism. Nonetheless, prealbumin levels lower than 30 mg/dL in dialysis patients are associated with increased mortality. In addition, because prealbumin has been directly correlated with changes in nutritional status, it can be useful for longitudinal monitoring of a patient with stable kidney function over time.

Insulin-like growth factor 1 (IGF-1), a serum protein with mitogenic properties and insulin-like activities, may be a sensitive biochemical indicator of nitrogen balance. A serum IGF-1 concentration lower than 200 ng/mL has been reported to indicate poor nutritional status. Moreover, current research suggests that treatment with recombinant human IGF-1 may induce an anabolic response in malnourished dialysis patients. Additional research is needed before definitive recommendations can be offered in regard to IGF-1 supplementation.

Sodium, Potassium, Phosphorus, and Calcium

Serum chemistry results, together with the patient's dry weight, blood pressure, and interdialytic weight gain, are typically monitored monthly for chronic hemodialysis patients. The nonserum parameters, such as interdialytic weight gain and predialysis and postdialysis blood pressure, are recorded at each dialysis treatment. Causes of fluctuations in these values must be determined and discussed with the patient in relation to potential nutritional interventions. For example, if the values for BUN, potassium, and phosphorus are all elevated, the cause might be tissue catabolism, inadequate dialysis, and/or excessive oral, enteral, or parenteral protein intake.

Isolated hyperphosphatemia can be controlled via diet, phosphate binders, decreased vitamin D supplementation, and, to some degree, adjustment of the dialysis prescription. In CKD patients with elevated PTH levels or elevated serum phosphorus levels (>5.5 mg/dL) or both, dietary phosphorus intake should be limited to 800 to 1000 mg/day (see **Tables 57-3** and **57-4**).

When providing nutrition therapy, the goal serum range for potassium is 3.5 to 5.5 mEq/L and that for phosphorus is 3.5 to 5.5 mg/dL. Recent data suggest improved outcomes when patients maintain serum calcium concentrations in the range of 8.4 to 10.2 mg/dL. Dietary calcium intake is one factor that affects serum calcium. However, the use of calcimimetics that lower serum calcium or vitamin D analogues that increase serum calcium levels must be considered when determining intervention for calcium. Stringent dietary control of calcium at 800 mg/day for a patient who has also been receiving a vitamin D analogue has not been demonstrated

to be successful in achieving calcium goals and may simply be imposing an additional dietary hardship unnecessarily. Further research is needed on the interrelationships between dietary calcium intake and alterations in calcium metabolism imposed by vitamin D analogues and calcimimetics.

Lipids

Although they are difficult to achieve, normal cholesterol and triglyceride values are the goal for patients with CKD stages 1 through 5. Whereas total fat intake as a percentage of calories is important, the fatty acid composition of dietary fat also plays a role in prevention of cardiovascular disease (CVD). Saturated and trans fatty acids are known to modify serum lipoprotein patterns toward those associated with CVD risk (i.e., elevated total cholesterol, low-density lipoproteins, and triglycerides plus decreased high-density lipoproteins). The exact percentage of calories that should be obtained from carbohydrates and fats varies according to nutritional status, level of kidney function, and presence of other comorbid conditions (e.g., diabetes) in an individual patient. In general, however, the recommendation for CKD patients is to keep fat calories to less than 30% of total calories. This is similar to the recommendation for the general population.

An abundance of literature supports a beneficial effect of omega-9 and particularly omega-3 fatty acids for the prevention and treatment of CVD. However, nutrient recommendations for these fatty acids in patients with CKD have not yet been established. The NKF-K/DOQI Clinical Guidelines for Cardiovascular Disease included a section reviewing these potentially beneficial effects without establishing a guideline. A reasonable recommendation based on opinion as included in the NKF-K/DOQI Clinical Guidelines for Diabetes and CKD is to distribute the 30% of fat calories as follows: 10% omega-3 fatty acids, 10% omega-9 fatty acids, 5% omega-6 fatty acids, and 5% saturated fatty acids. This would translate into a diet that used fats predominantly derived from canola and olive oils, with minimal use of butter, lard, and other vegetable oils.

Glucose

Abnormal carbohydrate metabolism is frequently observed in CKD patients, especially in those with infection or peripheral insulin resistance and in those who are approaching stage 5 because of uremia. On the other hand, patients with insulin-dependent diabetes may require a smaller insulin dose or discontinuation of insulin because of decreased insulin clearance by the kidneys. Therefore, close monitoring of insulin and diet is necessary in all stages of CKD. Ideally, normal glucose levels should be maintained in CKD patients with and without diabetes, to prevent the complications of hypoglycemia or hyperglycemia.

Patients undergoing peritoneal dialysis may develop glucose intolerance and gain weight because they absorb glucose from the dialysate. Calculation of energy requirements for peritoneal dialysis patients must take into consideration the amount of glucose absorbed during the procedure (see Chapter 56). To estimate the amount of calories obtained from the dialysis procedure, the total grams of dextrose used over 24 hours is multiplied by 3.4 kcal/g (or, for anhydrous dextrose, by 3.7 kcal/g); the result is then multiplied by the estimated absorption rate of 70%. For example, if a patients uses two 1-L bags of 1.5% dextrose, one 2-L bag of 4.25% dextrose, and one 2-L bag of 2.5% dextrose in 24 hours, the total grams of dextrose used is 30 + 85 + 50 = 165 g. The amount of calories absorbed from the dialysate is then calculated as follows: 165 g × 3.4 kcal/g × 70% = 393 kcal absorbed.

Anthropometry

Anthropometry includes measurements of body weight (estimated dry weight for dialysis patients), height, triceps skinfold, abdominal circumference, calf circumference, midarm muscle circumference, elbow breadth, and subscapular skinfold; these values provide information about the distribution of body fat and skeletal muscle mass. Over time, these measurements identify nutritional deficiencies or excesses in calorie and protein reserves compared to standardized percentiles. One of the problems with using anthropometric measurements to assess the nutrition status in CKD is that the reference values used are derived from measurements obtained from healthy individuals. This is a potential pitfall, given the known alterations in body composition associated with uremia and the presence of edema. Anthropometry is usually performed on the nondominant arm, but in hemodialysis patients the dominant arm is used if the contralateral arm has a vascular access in place. To minimize the interference of edema, measurements should be made during the last hour of dialysis. For routine care, anthropometric measurements are recommended every 3 to 6 months.

Other methods of assessing body composition include dual-energy x-ray absorptiometry (DEXA) and bioelectrical impedance. These techniques are accurate, but at present they are used principally for research purposes because of equipment availability, radiation dose, patient acceptance, and cost or reimbursement issues.

Physical and Clinical Evaluation

Wasting syndrome, a protein-calorie malnutrition state that is prevalent in the dialysis population, is sometimes seen in earlier CKD stages as well. It is characterized by decreased relative body weight (patient's body weight divided by "normal weight" for the same age range, height, gender, and skeletal frame size), skinfold thickness (adipose store), arm muscle mass, and total body nitrogen as well as signs of macronutrient and micronutrient deficiencies (e.g., hair loss; dry, flaky skin).

Another method used to assess protein-energy status is *subjective global assessment* (SGA). SGA requires evaluation of subjective and objective patient information, including the medical history and physical examination. Based on this

evaluation, the patient is classified into various nutritional status categories from well-nourished to severely malnourished. This technique was originally devised for nutrition assessment of general surgery patients, but it has been validated for use in peritoneal dialysis patients as well. The NKF-K/DOQI recommended the SGA as part of routine nutrition monitoring.

Patient-Reported Food Intake

Obtaining patient-reported food intake is an important component of the nutritional care of the patient with CKD. In addition to providing the opportunity to quantify food intake, food records reveal sources of problems related to food intake and tolerance, food habits, patterns, and allergies. The interactive nature of reported food intake provides the dietitian with an opportunity to establish rapport with each patient. All of this information can be used to formulate an individual meal plan to help the patient meet his or her nutritional needs. Reported food intake can be obtained in the form of a 24-hour recall, a multiple-day food record, diet history (retrospective general review of usual intake), or food frequency (how often foods from each food group are eaten and which specific foods within each group are included in the diet). The most valid method is currently unknown, because they have not been widely studied in the CKD patient population. Recently, a Food Frequency Questionnaire was found useful to evaluate the diet intake in a cohort of hemodialysis patients. More studies in this area are needed.

Regardless of the reporting method, the data should include current nutrient intake, factors that affect intake (e.g., difficulty chewing or swallowing, other physical impediments to adequate intake, nausea, vomiting, diarrhea, allergies), current medications, food preferences, cultural influences on food intake, meal patterns, meals eaten away from home, and portion sizes. Fluid intake, including solid foods with high water content, should be reported in the same detail. Whenever possible, diet information should be collected directly from the patient. Otherwise, family members or caregivers may be interviewed.

NUTRITION IN ACUTE KIDNEY INJURY

Data for nutrition therapy in acute kidney injury (AKI) are both limited and conflicting. If dialysis is initiated, the recommendations for protein are 1.2 to 1.5 g/kg/day. Calorie recommendations tend to be in the range of 35 to 40 kcal/kg. Patients who are not dialyzed are provided with protein and calories depending on their degree of catabolism. Large amounts of calories may not be provided Although AKI is generally believed to be a catabolic state, the magnitude of the required increase in protein and calorie intake in AKI patients is significantly dependent on the nature of the precipitating event. Not only must protein and calorie requirements be estimated, but altered intake of vitamins and electrolytes should be considered in view of the degree of kidney dysfunction. Continuous renal replacement therapy (see Chapter 55) generally allows for sufficient nutrition with tube feedings while mitigating fluid overload and electrolyte complications. Any form of dialysis intervention requires close monitoring and assessment to allow ongoing adjustment of the nutritional regimen. For example, AKI patients undergoing acute hemodialysis or continuous renal replacement therapy should receive water-soluble vitamin supplementation to compensate for dialytic losses.

Noncatabolic patients may not require dialysis therapy if normal fluid and electrolyte balance can be maintained and BUN does not exceed 80 mg/dL. This profile of AKI typically results from administration of contrast agents or nephrotoxic drugs. These patients are not usually nutritionally depleted and have lower urea generation rates. Oral and enteral feedings are preferred as long as the gastrointestinal tract is functioning normally. Catabolic AKI patients are most frequently encountered in the intensive care unit in the setting of multisystem organ failure. Such patients are frequently hypercatabolic and require total parenteral nutrition.

INTRADIALYTIC NUTRITION SUPPORT

In addition to being a means of nutritional support for patients with AKI, intravenous nutrition is sometimes used as an intervention for malnutrition in patients receiving maintenance hemodialysis or peritoneal dialysis. For the former group, intravenous amino acids, carbohydrates, and fats are infused directly into the venous drip chamber of the hemodialysis machine during treatment. This therapy is referred to as *intradialytic parenteral nutrition* (IDPN). The benefits of this therapy have not yet been studied in large, prospective, randomized trials. In peritoneal dialysis, amino acids can be used as a dialysis solution in rotation with dextrose-enriched dialysate exchanges (see Chapter 56). This approach is termed *intraperitoneal nutrition*. The data regarding benefits of this intervention for malnutrition and hypoalbuminemia as well as overall patient outcomes are to date inconclusive.

BIBLIOGRAPHY

Beddhu S, Cheung AK, Larive B, et al: Hemodiaysis (HEMO) Study Group. Inflammation and inverse associations of body mass index and serum creatinine with mortality in hemodialysis patients. J Ren Nutr 17:372-380, 2007.

Fouque D, Kalantar-Zadeh K Kopple J, et al: A proposed nomenclature and diagnostic criteria for protein-energy wasting in acute and chronic kidney disease. Kidney Int 73:391-398, 2007.

Friedman A, Moe S: Review of the effects of omega-3 supplementation in dialysis patients. Clin J Am Soc Nephrol 1:182-192, 2005.

Ikizler A: Effects of hemodialysis on protein metabolism. J Ren Nutr 15:39-43, 2005.

Moe S, Chen NX: Mechanisms of vascular calcification in chronic kidney disease. J Am Soc Nephrol 19:213-216, 2008.

National Kidney Foundation: NKF-K/DOQI clinical practice guidelines for nutrition in chronic renal failure. Am J Kidney Dis 35(Suppl 2):S1-S140, 2000.

National Kidney Foundation: NKF-K/DOQI clinical practice guidelines for chronic kidney disease: Evaluation, classification, and stratification. Am J Kidney Dis 39(Suppl 1):S1-S266, 2002.

National Kidney Foundation Kidney Disease Outcomes Quality Initiative: Clinical practice guidelines for cardiovascular disease in dialysis patients. State of the science: Novel and controversial topics in cardiovascular diseases. Am J Kidney Dis 45(Suppl 3): S90-S97, 2005.

National Kidney Foundation Kidney Disease Outcomes Quality Initiative: Clinical practice guide and clinical practice recommendations for diabetes and chronic kidney disease. Am J Kidney Dis 49(Suppl 2):S12-S154, 2007.

CHAPTER 58

Bone Disorders in Chronic Kidney Disease

Nadine D. Tanenbaum and L. Darryl Quarles

Chronic kidney disease (CKD) alters the regulation of calcium and phosphate homeostasis, leading to secondary hyperparathyroidism, metabolic bone disease, soft tissue calcifications, and other metabolic derangements that have a significant impact on morbidity and mortality. Although bone disease and abnormalities of parathyroid function are historically the main clinical focus of this disorder, cardiovascular diseases and extraskeletal calcifications are increasingly recognized as complications resulting from disordered phosphate metabolism and mineral homeostasis or from treatment with calcium and vitamin D sterols. Earlier interventions and stringent management guidelines have been proposed for subjects with CKD by the National Kidney Foundation (NKF) Kidney Disease Outcomes Quality Initiative (K/DOQI), with the hope of more effectively and safely treating this disorder. In addition, new treatments with calcimimetic drugs that target the calcium-sensing receptor in the parathyroid gland are now available. Finally, emerging knowledge of the role of the phosphaturic hormone fibroblast growth factor 23 (FGF-23) in disordered mineral metabolism in CKD and of the importance of vitamin D pathways in regulating innate immunity and organ function (in addition to its more traditional role in regulating mineral metabolism) has led to a re-examination of the pathogenesis and treatment of disordered mineral metabolism in CKD.

PATHOGENESIS OF ABNORMAL MINERAL METABOLISM AND SECONDARY HYPERPARATHYROIDISM IN CHRONIC KIDNEY DISEASE

An increase in circulating parathyroid hormone (PTH) concentrations is the hallmark of secondary hyperparathyroidism. The major metabolic abnormalities leading to the increase in PTH are diminished production of $1,25\text{-}(OH)_2D_3$ (calcitriol, the activated form of vitamin D), decreased serum calcium, and increased serum phosphorus. In normal subjects, PTH is responsible for maintaining the serum calcium concentration within a narrow range through direct actions on the distal tubule of the kidney to increase calcium resorption and on bone to increase calcium and phosphate efflux (**Fig. 58-1**). In addition, some PTH effects are mediated

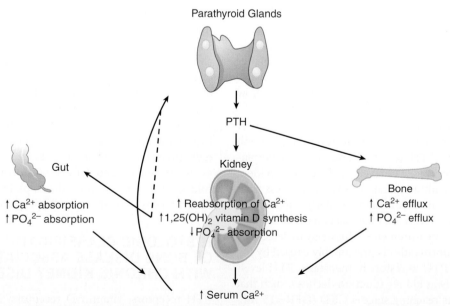

FIGURE 58-1 Regulation of systemic calcium homeostasis. Parathyroid hormone (PTH) is a calcemic hormone that targets the kidney to promote renal calcium conservation and the bone to increase efflux of calcium and phosphorus. PTH-mediated production of $1,25(OH)_2D_3$ (activated vitamin D) by the kidney increases gastrointestinal calcium and phosphate absorption. The phosphaturic actions of PTH on the kidney cause it to excrete the excess phosphate that accompanies calcium absorption by the intestines and calcium efflux from bone. Changes in calcium, $1,25(OH)_2D_3$, and phosphate levels exert feedback on the parathyroid glands (*dotted line*).

through its stimulatory effect on the production of calcitriol. Vitamin D_3 is formed when 7-dehydrocholesterol in the skin absorbs solar radiation. Vitamin D_3 is also found in oily fish such as salmon, in fish liver oils, in supplemented milk, and in eggs in lesser amounts. Vitamin D_3 undergoes hydroxylation in the liver to biologically inactive 25-hydroxyvitamin D, in a conversion that is not tightly regulated. Then, in the renal proximal tubule, 25-$(OH)D_3$ undergoes 1α-hydroxylation to its active form, calcitriol, in a step stimulated by PTH. Calcitriol increases gastrointestinal absorption of calcium and phosphate and promotes osteoclast maturation.

The net effect of PTH is to create the positive calcium balance that is necessary to maintain calcium homeostasis. To prevent a concomitant positive phosphate balance resulting from the skeletal effects of PTH and the gastrointestinal actions of calcitriol, PTH acts secondarily to increase renal phosphorus excretion, mostly by decreasing activity of the sodium phosphate cotransporter in the proximal renal tubule. PTH is probably not the primary phosphaturic hormone, however. Emerging data suggest that FGF-23 is a key regulator of phosphate homeostasis. Gene transcription of FGF-23 in mouse models is regulated both by systemic factors, such as hyperphosphatemia and elevated 1,25-$(OH)_2D_3$ levels, and by local bone-derived factors. FGF-23 knockout mice are hyperphosphatemic and display soft tissue and vascular calcifications, growth retardation, and bone mineralization abnormalities. FGF-23 is expressed mainly in osteocytes in bone and, to much a much lesser extent, in the bone marrow, the ventrolateral thalamic nucleus, the thymus, and lymph nodes. FGF-23 promotes phosphate excretion by inhibition of sodium-dependent phosphate resorption. It also inhibits 1α-hydroxylase activity in the proximal tubule, leading to a decrease in calcitriol synthesis. The actions of FGF-23 on the parathyroid gland remain to be further elucidated, but recent studies suggest that it may inhibit PTH secretion. In addition, FGF-23 has been implicated in the pathogenesis of kidney fibrosis. In any case, FGF-23 levels are increased early in CKD and correlate with the degree of hyperphosphatemia. Moreover, treatment with vitamin D analogues elevates FGF-23 levels. Further studies are needed to determine how to interpret the significance of FGF-23 levels in CKD.

Parathyroid disease in CKD is a progressive disorder characterized by both increased PTH secretion and growth in the number of the PTH-secreting chief cells (hyperplasia). Elevations in serum PTH levels first become evident when the glomerular filtration rate (GFR) falls to less than 60 mL/min/1.73 m^2. This occurs before hyperphosphatemia, reduction in calcitriol levels, or hypocalcemia is detectable by routine laboratory measurements. This delay in detectable serum chemistry abnormalities is presumably caused by the actions of increased PTH to restore homeostasis. PTH levels increase progressively as kidney function declines, such that all untreated subjects reaching stage 5 CKD (GFR <15 mL/min/1.73 m^2 or dialysis) would be expected to have elevated PTH levels.

Four molecular targets regulating parathyroid gland function have been identified. These are the G protein–coupled calcium-sensing receptor (CaSR), the vitamin D receptor (VDR), a putative extracellular phosphate sensor, and the FGF-23 receptor, which is the FGFR:Klotho complex. Calcium acting through the CaSR is the major regulator of PTH transcription, secretion, and parathyroid gland hyperplasia. Calcitriol, which acts on the VDR in the parathyroid gland to suppress PTH transcription, but not PTH secretion, has overlapping functions with the CaSR. It appears, however, that the physiologic role of the VDR in regulating parathyroid gland function may be subordinate to that of calcium. In this regard, secondary hyperparathyroidism and bone abnormalities in VDR-deficient mice can be corrected by normalizing the serum calcium concentration. Extracellular phosphate also has direct effects on parathyroid production, apparently through the regulation of PTH messenger RNA (mRNA) levels, possibly by increasing post-transcriptional PTH mRNA message stability. Hyperphosphatemia may also indirectly affect PTH production by lowering ionized calcium through chelation and by suppressing 1α-hydroxylase and, hence, calcitriol production by the kidney. All the effects of hyperphosphatemia favor PTH secretion. Although animal studies have indicated that phosphate restriction alone is sufficient to prevent the development of secondary hyperparathyroidism in early CKD, these studies do not necessarily implicate hyperphosphatemia in a primary role, because the increase in calcitriol production that accompanies dietary phosphate restriction can directly affect parathyroid gland function. Finally, FGF-23 has recently been shown to target the parathyroid gland via FGFR:Klotho complexes and to suppress PTH secretion. In summary, the pathogenesis of secondary hyperparathyroidism is complex and represents a compensatory response to reduced levels of serum calcium and 1,25$(OH)_2D_3$ and increased levels serum phosphorus.

Unless adequately treated, secondary hyperparathyroidism progresses inexorably, with the frequency of parathyroidectomy proportional to the number of years on dialysis. The difficulty in treating hyperparathyroidism is in part due to the massive hyperplasia and possibly adenomatous transformation of the parathyroid gland that occurs as a result of the chronic stimulation of PTH production in CKD. Enlarged, hyperplastic parathyroid glands retain some responsiveness to calcium-mediated PTH suppression in secondary hyperparathyroidism. As this responsiveness is lost due to reductions in extracellular CaSR and VDR expression as well as autonomous adenomatous transformation of the parathyroid gland, hypercalcemia develops in some patients. This occurrence is termed *tertiary* hyperparathyroidism.

HISTOLOGIC CLASSIFICATIONS OF BONE DISEASE ASSOCIATED WITH CHRONIC KIDNEY DISEASE

PTH receptors, vitamin D receptors, and calcium-sensing receptors are all present in osteoblasts. Osteoblast-mediated bone formation is coupled to osteoclast-mediated bone resorption through osteoblastic paracrine pathways. The circulating level of PTH is the primary determinant of bone turnover in CKD and is a major determinant of the type of bone disease present. The specific types of histologic changes also depend on the age of the patient, the duration and cause of kidney failure, the type of dialysis therapy used, the presence of acidosis, vitamin D status, accumulation of metals such as aluminum, and other conditions affecting mineralization of the extracellular matrix.

Bone disease associated with CKD (**Fig. 58-2**) has traditionally been classified histologically according to the degrees of abnormal bone turnover and impaired mineralization of the extracellular matrix. These histologic changes in bone have been best studied in dialysis patients. The current categories are as follows:

1. Secondary hyperparathyroidism or high-turnover bone disease or osteitis fibrosa
2. Mixed uremic bone disease (a mixture of high-turnover bone disease and osteomalacia)
3. Osteomalacia (defective mineralization)
4. Adynamic bone disease (decreased rates of bone formation without a mineralization defect)

High-turnover bone disease caused by excess PTH is characterized by greater number and size of osteoclasts and an increase in the number of resorption lacunae with scalloped trabeculae, as well as abnormally high numbers of osteoblasts. There is an increased amount of osteoid (unmineralized bone), which may have a woven appearance that reflects disordered collagen arrangement under conditions of rapid matrix deposition. The excess in osteoid surfaces that accompanies increased bone turnover has been described as mixed uremic bone disease, but it may reflect a normal response to increased turnover rather than superimposed defective mineralization. Peritrabecular fibrosis (and even marrow fibrosis), reflecting PTH stimulation of osteoblastic precursors, is observed in severe disease.

Osteomalacia is characterized by prolongation of the mineralization lag time as well as by increased thickness, surface area, and volume of osteoid. Osteomalacia was formerly linked to aluminum toxicity from both contamination of water in dialysates and use of aluminum-based phosphate binders (see Chapter 62). Other causes of osteomalacia that may

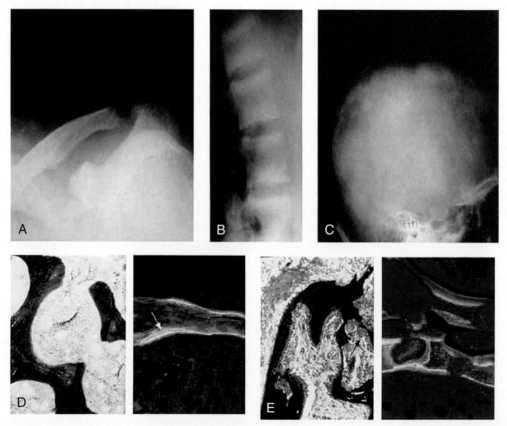

FIGURE 58-2 Radiographic and histologic features of bone disease associated with chronic kidney disease (CID). **A,** Radiographic findings of severe erosion of the distal clavicle resulting from secondary hyperparathyroidism. **B,** An example of "rugger-jersey spine" resulting from sclerosis of the end plates associated with hyperparathyroidism. **C,** A "pepper-pot skull" with areas of erosion and patchy osteosclerosis associated with hyperparathyroidism. **D,** Histologic appearance of normal bone. On the left, a section stained with Goldner Masson trichrome stain shows mineralized lamellar bone (*blue*) and adjacent nonmineralized osteoid surfaces (*red-brown*). On the right, a Villanueva-stained section viewed under fluorescent light shows tetracycline labeling of freshly formed bone. Double staining (*arrow*) indicates amount of new bone laid down during the interval between the two periods of tetracycline administration. **E,** Histologic appearance of osteitis fibrosa in a patient with stage 5 CKD and elevated parathyroid hormone levels. On the left, Goldner Masson trichrome stain reveals increased numbers of multinucleated osteoclasts at resorptive surfaces (*black arrow*) and extensive bone marrow fibrosis (as shown by light blue staining of marrow). On the right, tetracycline labeling reveals marked increases in the osteoid (*orange-red staining*) and in sites of new bone formation as measured by the yellow-green bands below the osteoid surfaces. (A-C, From Martin KJ, Gonzalez EA, Slatopolsky E: Renal osteodystrophy. In Brenner BM [ed]: Brenner and Rector's The Kidney, 7th ed. Philadelphia, Saunders, 2004, p 2280, with permission.)

be present in CKD patients include 25-hydroxyvitamin D deficiency (secondary to poor dietary vitamin D and calcium intake and lack of exposure to sunlight due to poor mobility and extended hospitalizations), metabolic acidosis (which inhibits both osteoblasts and osteoclasts), and hypophosphatemia (e.g., in Fanconi's syndrome).

Adynamic bone disease is a low-turnover bone state that has received increased attention. Bone mineralization is best assessed using tetracycline-labeled bone biopsies. Tetracycline is deposited in newly mineralized bone. Two doses of tetracycline spaced by a known time interval can be administered before bone biopsy. Subsequent measurement of the width of the mineralized bone deposited between the luminescent tetracycline bands on biopsy reflects the rate of bone mineralization. In bone biopsy series, as many as 40% of hemodialysis patients and 50% of peritoneal dialysis patients have adynamic bone disease. In this disorder, the amount of osteoid thickness is normal or reduced, and there is no mineralization defect. The main findings are decreased numbers of osteoclasts and osteoblasts and very low rates of bone formation as measured by tetracycline labeling. High serum calcium levels sometimes seen in adynamic bone disease may in part be secondary to high oral calcium loads and suppression of PTH when calcium-based phosphate binders are used. There may also be a decreased ability of bone to buffer calcium loads. The main risk factors for adynamic bone disease are peritoneal dialysis, older age, corticosteroid use, and diabetes. It is thought that adynamic bone disease represents a state of relative hypoparathyroidism in CKD.

This long-standing classification of CKD-associated bone disease has been questioned. One concern is that mixed uremic bone disease may not represent a distinct entity, because increased turnover is most often accompanied by variable degrees of reversible mineralization deficit. Another problem is the uncertainty about the existence of adynamic bone disease, which in reality represents a low rate of bone formation that overlaps the normal range and is probably caused by subnormal PTH secretion accompanying an excess of calcium and/or vitamin D treatment. Thus, adynamic bone disease may not be a naturally occurring separate disease but a consequence of overtreatment of hyperparathyroidism with calcium and calcitriol.

CLINICAL MANIFESTATIONS OF BONE DISEASES ASSOCIATED WITH CHRONIC KIDNEY DISEASE

Most patients with CKD and mildly elevated circulating levels of PTH are asymptomatic. When clinical features of bone disease are present, they can be classified into musculoskeletal and extraskeletal manifestations.

Musculoskeletal Manifestations

Fractures, tendon rupture, and bone pain due to metabolic bone disease, muscle pain and weakness, and periarticular pain are the major musculoskeletal manifestations associated with CKD. The most clinically significant effect of metabolic bone disease in CKD is hip fracture, which has a high incidence among stage 5 CKD patients and is associated with an increased risk for death. There is a roughly 4.4-fold increase in hip fracture risk in dialysis patients compared to the general population, but studies attempting to link the type of histologic bone disease or a specific level of PTH to increased fracture risk have been inconclusive. The utility of measurements of bone mineral density (BMD) as an indicator of fracture risk has not been established in CKD.

Extraskeletal Manifestations

The most important evolution in the understanding of the clinical significance of disordered bone and mineral metabolism in CKD has been the recognition that it is a systemic disorder affecting soft tissues, particularly vessels, heart valves, and skin. Cardiovascular disease accounts for approximately half of all deaths of dialysis patients (see Chapter 60). Coronary artery and vascular calcifications occur frequently in stage 5 CKD and increase as a function of the number of years on dialysis. In addition to traditional cardiovascular risk factors, patients with CKD have a number of nontraditional cardiovascular risk factors that are thought to predispose these patients to increased vascular calcifications. Gaining a better understanding of the etiology of increased vascular calcification and how it may influence clinical cardiovascular events is of critical importance.

Several patterns of vascular calcification have been described. The first occurs as focal calcification associated with lipid-laden foam cells seen in atherosclerotic plaques. These calcifications may increase both the fragility and the risk for rupture of plaques. Some have questioned the role of calcification in the pathogenesis of the atherosclerotic vascular lesions, raising the possibility that it is an epiphenomenon. The second pattern of vascular calcification is diffuse; it is not associated with atherosclerotic plaques and occurs in the media of vessels. This pattern is seen with aging, diabetes, and progressive kidney failure. This so-called Mönckeberg's sclerosis was thought to be of little clinical significance for many years, but its effects of increasing blood vessel stiffness and reducing vascular compliance, which result in a widened pulse pressure, increased cardiac afterload, and left ventricular hypertrophy, are potential mechanisms whereby vascular calcification could contribute to cardiovascular morbidity (**Fig. 58-3**). Coronary calcium load as detected by electron-beam computed tomography (EBCT) has not been shown to correlate in dialysis patients with the degree of coronary vessel stenosis, suggesting that medial calcification is a disease entity separate from atherosclerosis in these patients.

The exact mechanisms of vascular medial calcification are not clear but probably reflect the combined effects of decreased mineralization inhibitors, such as matrix Gla protein (a calcification inhibitor known to be expressed by smooth muscle cells and macrophages in the artery wall) and increased mineralization inducers. It is now clear that vascular calcification is an active, cell-mediated process. Accumulating

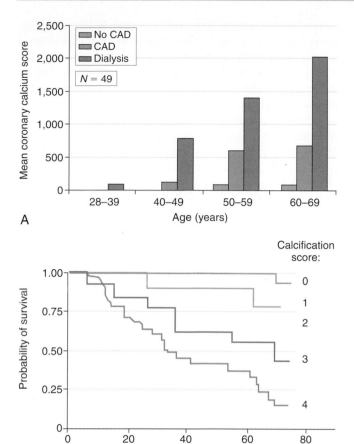

FIGURE 58-3 Increased risk of death and cardiovascular calcification in dialysis patients. **A,** A calcium score was determined by electron beam computed tomography (EBCT). The mean coronary artery calcium score was significantly higher in hemodialysis patients than in nondialysis patients with documented cardiovascular disease. **B,** Risk of death in hemodialysis patients increases as a function of a calcification score measured ultrasonographically. (P < .0001 for comparisons among all curves). (A, From Braun J, Oldendorf M, Moshage W, et al: Electron beam computed tomography in the evaluation of cardiac calcifications in chronic dialysis patients. Am J Kidney Dis 27:394-401, 1996, with permission from the National Kidney Foundation. B, From Blacher J, Guerin AP, Pannier B, et al: Arterial calcification, arterial stiffness, and cardiovascular risk in end-stage renal disease. Hypertension 38:938, 2001, with permission.)

evidence suggests that vascular smooth muscle cells undergo a phenotypic transition to an osteoblast-like cell that is important in driving the calcification process. Elevated serum phosphorus causes upregulation of a type III sodium-dependent phosphate cotransporter called Pit-1 (POU1F1) in smooth muscle cells. The resulting increased intracellular phosphorus upregulates core binding factor alpha 1 (Cbfa1/RUNX2), a transcription factor that is believed to be critical in mediating this phenotypic switch to osteoblast-like cells. Concomitantly, bone matrix proteins, such as osteopontin and osteocalcin, are found in calcified but not uncalcified vessels. Clinically, an increased calcium-phosphorus product (obtained by multiplying a patient's serum calcium concentration, preferably corrected for albumin, by the serum phosphorus level, both expressed in milligrams per deciliter) is associated with an increased risk of vascular and visceral calcification. Incremental elevations of serum phosphorus

are an independent risk factor for increased mortality in patients undergoing chronic maintenance hemodialysis. This has recently been shown to be true also in CKD patients not yet on dialysis, in whom incremental increases in serum phosphorus greater than 3.5 mg/dL were independently associated with an incremental risk for mortality.

An emerging area of study concerns how uremia may affect the vascular calcification process, independent of its effects on serum phosphorus. For example, the glycoprotein fetuin-A, which is downregulated during the acute phase response, is an important inhibitor of calcification. Patients on hemodialysis have lower serum fetuin-A levels than do controls. Higher cardiovascular mortality was associated in univariate analysis with lower fetuin-A levels in hemodialysis patients, but this association did not persist after correction for accompanying risk factors by multivariate analysis.

The contribution of vitamin D in vascular calcification is controversial and debated. Some studies suggest that calcitriol can modulate vascular smooth muscle growth and influence vascular calcification by upregulation of the VDR and increased calcium uptake into smooth muscle cells. Vitamin D treatment enhances the extent of artery calcification in animals that are also given warfarin to inhibit γ-carboxylation of the matrix Gla protein. On the other hand, in several large retrospective clinical studies, hemodialysis patients treated with active vitamin D analogues had lower mortality rates than patients not treated with active vitamin D compounds. However, these observational studies were potentially confounded by other variables, and prospective trials evaluating the role of vitamin D in survival in ESRD are needed to confirm this hypothesis—especially because all vitamin D analogues are associated with dose-dependent increases in serum calcium and serum phosphate, factors that are associated with vascular calcifications and increased mortality.

Calciphylaxis, or calcemic uremic arteriolopathy, is another form of vascular calcification that is observed primarily, although not exclusively, in stage 5 CKD. The prevalence is not well established, but it has been reported to occur in 1% to 4% of dialysis patients. Calciphylaxis manifests with extensive calcifications of the skin, muscles, and subcutaneous tissues. Most often, skin lesions occur on the breast, abdomen, and thighs. Unusual presentations, such as necrosis of the tongue and of the penis, as well as visceral involvement of the lungs, pancreas, and intestines, have been described. On examination, there may be seen not only a violaceous rash, skin nodules, skin firmness, and eschars, but also livedo reticularis and painful hyperesthesia of the skin. Nonhealing ulcerations of the skin and gangrene resistant to medical therapy often lead to amputation, uncontrollable sepsis, and death. Histologically, there is extensive medial calcification of small arteries, arterioles, capillaries, and venules, as well as intimal proliferation, endovascular fibrosis, and sometimes thrombosis. Whether the molecular pathogenesis of calciphylaxis is similar to that of Mönckeberg's sclerosis is not clear. Cases reported to be associated with very high PTH levels improved after parathyroidectomy. However, there are reported cases in which the PTH levels were only mildly elevated. Other risk factors for calciphylaxis are obesity, advancing age, female gender, diabetes mellitus, warfarin use, recent trauma, hypotension, and calcium ingestion. Anecdotal reports suggest that sodium thiosulfate, bisphosphonate therapy, daily hemodialysis, hyperbaric oxygen treatment, and normalization of serum phosphate levels may improve outcomes.

Musculoskeletal Abnormalities Not Related to Disordered Calcium and Phosphate Homeostasis: Amyloidosis

Patients who have been on dialysis for at least 7 years can develop osteoarticular amyloid depositions that consist of a protein called β_2-microglobulin (β_2M). This protein, which is found in the cell membrane and serves to stabilize the major histocompatibility complex (MHC) class I antigen on cell surfaces, is normally released into the plasma with cell turnover and cleared by the kidney. Severe forms of β_2M-deposition disease manifest as a destructive spondyloarthropathy, often in the cervical and lumbar spine, that can lead to spinal instability and vertebral compression. Magnetic resonance imaging (low signal intensity on both T1- and T2-weighted images) is important in distinguishing this entity from other destructive spinal processes. Carpal tunnel syndrome and arthritis are more frequent manifestations of β_2M amyloid deposition. β_2M deposits are found in periarticular areas, joints, and tendon sheaths. Bone cysts, especially in regions next to large joints where tendons insert (e.g., hip, proximal humerus, proximal tibia), can be seen on radiography. There is no effective treatment except for kidney transplantation to prevent ongoing bony damage from amyloidosis. High-flux hemodialysis or hemofiltration with increased clearance of β_2M compared to conventional dialysis may be beneficial (see Chapter 55).

DIAGNOSIS OF BONE DISEASES ASSOCIATED WTIH CHRONIC KIDNEY DISEASE

Biochemical Parameters

Abnormal parathyroid gland function is assessed by measurement of random circulating PTH levels. Full-length PTH has a half-life of 2 to 4 minutes. PTH is cleaved into an inactive C-terminal fragment, an active N-terminal fragment, and inactive midregion fragments in the peripheral tissues. These PTH fragments are normally excreted in the kidney and therefore have a prolonged half-life in kidney failure. A two-site immunoreactive assay is currently used to measure circulating PTH concentrations. This "intact PTH" assay uses two antibodies: one detects an epitope near the N-terminal end, and the other detects the C-terminal end. The assay actually detects the full-length bioactive PTH, called PTH(1-84) (i.e., amino acid residues 1 through 84) and PTH fragments such as PTH(7-84). The PTH fragment PTH(7-84) may lack biologic activity or may potentially have distinct biologic actions. It may have hypocalcemic effects in vivo, and it has been shown to inhibit osteoclastic bone resorption in vitro. Newer, second-generation immunoreactive PTH assays ("whole PTH" or "bio-intact PTH") have been developed that recognize amino acid residues 1 through 4 of the N-terminal region of PTH and specifically detect full-length PTH(1-84). PTH levels using the whole PTH assay are approximately 50% to 60% lower than those measured with the intact PTH assay. The best way of using this more specific assay has not been determined. The normal range of the intact PTH assay is 10 to 65 pg/mL in patients with normal kidney function. However, because of end-organ resistance to PTH that is more severe in the later stages of CKD, possibly mediated by a decrease in PTH receptors on osteoblasts, the recommended target PTH levels are twofold to threefold greater than the upper limit of the normal range in dialysis patients. The recommended target ranges for serum intact PTH are 35 to 70 pg/mL, 70 to 110 pg/mL, and 150 to 300 pg/mL for CKD stages 3, 4, and 5, respectively, reflecting the progressive resistance to PTH as CKD progresses (**Table 58-1**).

PTH levels are a direct measure of parathyroid gland function and an indirect measure of bone remodeling. PTH levels greater than 300 pg/mL correlate with the bony changes of secondary hyperparathyroidism and/or osteitis fibrosis. However, these observations are primarily derived from older studies in which patient demographics differed from those of today's dialysis population and before the widespread use of active vitamin D analogues. Patients with adynamic bone disease usually have intact PTH levels lower than 150 pg/mL, but these values also occur in subjects with normal bone.

PTH is only a crude, indirect measure of bone turnover, because factors other than PTH can affect bone. The

---

TABLE 58-1 K/DOQI Clinical Practice Guidelines for Bone Metabolism and Disease in Chronic Kidney Disease

		Recommended Target Serum Values			
CKD STAGE	GFR RANGE (mL/min/1.73 m²)	PHOSPHORUS (mg/dL)	CALCIUM (CORRECTED, mg/dL)	Ca × P (mg²/dL²)	INTACT PTH (pg/mL)
3	30-59	2.7-4.6	8.4-10.2	—	35-70
4	15-29	2.7-4.6	8.4-10.2	—	70-110
5	<15, dialysis	3.5-5.5	8.4-9.5	<55	150-300

CKD, chronic kidney disease; Ca × P, calcium-phosphorus product; GFR, glomerular filtration rate; K/DOQI, Kidney Disease Outcomes Quality Initiative; PTH, parathyroid hormone.

Modified from National Kidney Foundation: Kidney Disease Outcomes Quality Initiative. Clinical practice guidelines for bone metabolism and disease in chronic kidney disease. Am J Kidney Dis 43:S1-S201, 2004.

predictive power of PTH levels as a measure of bone turnover can be increased by assessment of bone-specific alkaline phosphatase levels, which correlate with the degree of osteoblastic activity. Other biochemical markers of bone turnover are being developed that may provide a more accurate assessment of osteoblast and osteoclast activity in bone. For example, serum tartrate-resistant acid phosphatase 5b levels correlate well with histologic indices of osteoclasts and may serve as a specific marker for osteoclastic activity in CKD patients with bone disease. Efforts to correlate the different subtypes of bone disease with various markers of bone remodeling in both dialysis and predialysis patients is an area of ongoing research.

Bone Biopsy

Although it is no longer frequently performed, the gold standard for assessing and diagnosing the various types of bone disease in patients with CKD is an iliac crest bone biopsy with double tetracycline labeling. Bone histomorphometric analysis of the biopsy specimen includes assessment of bone and fibrosis volumes, amount of osteoid and mineralization, and numbers of osteoblasts and osteoclasts seen on bony surfaces. Bone biopsies should be considered in the setting of nontraumatic fracture with no other clear underlying cause, suspected aluminum toxicity to confirm the presence of osteomalacia before chelation therapy or parathyroidectomy in patients with severe musculoskeletal symptoms and/or hypercalcemia with intermediate (100 to 500 pg/mL) intact PTH levels, and to confirm the diagnosis of adynamic bone disease.

Imaging

In general, radiographic studies are not indicated in the diagnosis of the bone disorders associated with CKD, although certain radiographic changes can be seen (see **Fig. 58-3A** through C). Increased osteoblast function, especially in the setting of severe elevations of PTH, can lead to increased trabecular bone volume and accounts for the sclerotic changes that manifest as a "rugger-jersey spine" on radiography. Osteoclast-mediated bone resorption of secondary hyperparathyroidism results in cortical thinning and the classic radiographic evidence of subperiosteal, intracortical, and endosteal bone resorption. Subperiosteal erosions are best seen at the distal ends of the phalanges and clavicles and at the sacroiliac joints. Radiographically, expansile lytic lesions (brown tumors) can be seen in severe osteitis fibrosis. Pseudofractures, which appear as wide, radiolucent bands perpendicular to the bone long axis, can be seen in osteomalacia.

There is currently no accurate correlation between BMD as measured by dual-energy x-ray absorptiometry (DEXA) and the type of CKD-associated bone disease present. Osteoporosis is defined as a BMD that is at least 2.5 standard deviations lower than the mean BMD of a young adult of the same gender. Although patients with CKD typically have lower BMDs than the general population, the interpretation of DEXA scans is further complicated in secondary hyperparathyroidism because of focal areas of osteosclerosis, the presence of extraskeletal calcifications, and the variable presence of osteomalacia. BMD may be considered in patients who have undergone kidney transplantation or who have known risk factors or previous fractures and are candidates for osteoporosis therapy.

TREATMENT OF DISORDERED BONE AND MINERAL METABOLISM IN CHRONIC KIDNEY DISEASE

The treatment of disordered mineral metabolism in CKD is directed toward normalizing serum calcium, phosphate, and PTH and metabolic acidosis while minimizing the risks associated with the therapies. In the United States, the types of treatment chosen are influenced by the economic constraints of the health care system, which reimburses for parenteral medications and limits the frequency of hemodialysis in most patients to three treatments per week. Clinical practice guidelines for bone metabolism and disease in CKD stages 3, 4, and 5 have been developed by the K/DOQI and are outlined in **Table 58-1.**

The K/DOQI recommendations are influenced by data linking an elevated serum phosphorus concentration or calcium-phosphorus product to increased mortality and by the growing concern that excessive calcium exposure may increase the risk of cardiovascular calcification. Although they are supported by retrospective studies, there are no prospective studies that establish the efficacy and safety of the specific recommendations for target biochemical ranges included in these guidelines. Moreover, achieving these targets with current treatment regimens is difficult. For example, in a survey of 288 facilities that included 749 dialysis patients treated with vitamin D therapy, only 29% had average intact PTH levels within the defined target range. When serum calcium, phosphorus, and calcium-phosphorus product were included, the number of stage 5 CKD patients currently achieving K/DOQI guidelines for all these parameters was even lower. Nonetheless, these guidelines are a first step in standardizing the approach to this difficult disorder.

The various tools for treating hyperphosphatemia and secondary hyperparathyroidism include dietary phosphorus restriction, calcium-based and non–calcium-based phosphate binders, calcitriol or other active vitamin D analogues, calcimimetics, daily or nocturnal hemodialysis, and parathyroidectomy.

Controlling Serum Phosphorus

Dietary phosphorus restriction (800 to 1000 mg/day) is difficult to attain but should be initiated for all subjects with stage 5 CKD. Dairy products, nuts, beer, and chocolate all have a high content of phosphorus (see Chapter 58). For patients who are undergoing thrice-weekly dialysis and are receiving adequate nutrition, dietary phosphate restriction will be inadequate to correct the positive phosphate balance, especially in the presence of concurrent active vitamin D therapy, which increases phosphorus absorption from the gut. More frequent and prolonged hemodialysis (see Chapter 55) has been associated with lower serum phosphorus levels, but with thrice-weekly hemodialysis,, phosphate binders are almost invariably required.

The choice of phosphate binder used (i.e., calcium-containing versus non-aluminum, non–calcium-containing) depends on many considerations, including the binder's efficacy, side effects, and cost. For many years, calcium-based phosphate binders were the mainstay of therapy to control serum phosphate levels. Commonly used calcium-based phosphate binders include calcium carbonate and calcium acetate. Calcium carbonate contains 500 mg of elemental calcium in a 1250-mg tablet, whereas calcium acetate contains 169 mg of elemental calcium in one 667-mg tablet. Calcium citrate should not be used as a phosphate binder, because citrate increases aluminum absorption from the gut. Calcium-based phosphate binders should be taken with meals to maximize binding of ingested phosphorus in the gut. When they are taken in the fasting state, more calcium is absorbed systemically and less phosphorus is bound. The concomitant use of active vitamin D sterols increases calcium absorption and the risk of hypercalcemia. Whereas the risk of calcium loading in relation to mortality remains to be established, the K/DOQI recommendations in stage 5 CKD are to limit the total dose of calcium-based phosphate binders to 1500 mg elemental calcium per day and the total intake of elemental calcium to 2000 mg/day. Calcium acetate has greater phosphorus-binding capacity than calcium carbonate, potentially allowing the use of lower doses of calcium binder. However, various small trials have not shown significant differences in the prevalence of hypercalcemia between these two compounds.

Vascular calcifications have been documented by EBCT to develop in the coronary arteries of dialysis patients before 30 years of age. This, taken with growing concern about the possible clinical consequences of vascular calcifications, has led to the greater use of non-calcium binders. Sevelamer is a non-calcium phosphate binder containing cross-linked poly-allylamine hydrochloride. It acts as an ion exchange polymer to bind phosphorus in the gut and is a less effective phosphate binder than calcium on a weight basis. However, in human trials, sevelamer, when titrated to meet serum phosphorus goals, appeared equal in efficacy to the calcium-containing binders. Sevelamer has also been shown to decrease serum cholesterol and low-density lipoproteins and increase high-density lipoproteins in stage 5 CKD patients. Sevelamer has been associated with fewer arterial calcifications than calcium-based phosphate binders in dialysis patients. Whether this effect is due to less calcium loading, the lipid-lowering effect, or mild acidosis induced by sevelamer has not been established. Sevelamer-induced acidosis has been attributed to the replacement of bicarbonate for chloride on the polymer and also to sevelamer's binding of short-chain fatty acids in the large intestines. The net effect of acidosis on vascular calcification

in vivo is not fully understood. Sevelamer is more costly than calcium binders and may be associated with gastrointestinal side effects at higher doses that can limit its use in some individuals. Nevertheless, regimens using vitamin D analogues to raise calcium and suppress PTH, along with sevelamer to lower phosphorus, are effective in controlling both the skeletal and extraskeletal complications of stage 5 CKD.

The effect of sevelamer on cardiovascular mortality remains a critical question. Recently, prospective trials comparing the effect of sevelamer versus calcium-containing phosphate binders on mortality produced equivocal results. One small, randomized trial with 127 new hemodialysis patients monitored for a mean of 44 months demonstrated a significant overall survival advantage for sevelamer, although specific cardiovascular mortality was not assessed. The larger, open-labeled Dialysis Clinical Outcomes Revisited (DCOR) trial, which randomly assigned 2103 patients to either sevelamer or calcium-containing binders with a mean follow-up of 20.3 months, failed to show a difference in cardiovascular mortality between the two groups. In subgroup analysis of the DCOR results, patients older than 65 years of age who were treated with sevelamer had a lower all-cause mortality, but not lower cardiovascular mortality. In addition, among patients who remained in the study for longer than 2 years those treated with sevelamer had a decrease in all-cause mortality. The short duration of follow-up, the high drop-out rate, and the fact that the study was not powered statistically to detect differences in specific causes of death are limitations of this study. Further investigations are needed to determine whether sevelamer in fact decreases cardiovascular events and cardiovascular mortality.

Although they are the most effective binders, aluminum-containing phosphate binders are not often used because of the potential for systemic absorption of aluminum and subsequent neurologic, hematologic, and bone toxicity (see Chapter 61). Absorption of aluminum is increased by the concomitant use of sodium citrate for metabolic acidosis. Because of the potential for long-term toxicity, aluminum-containing antacids should be used only for a short period (<4 weeks) and for severe hyperphosphatemia that is refractory to other treatments.

Another newer, non–calcium-based phosphate binder is lanthanum carbonate. Lanthanum, like aluminum, is a trivalent cation with an ability to chelate dietary phosphate, but it has low systemic absorption. In a phase III trial over a 1-year period, lanthanum carbonate controlled serum phosphorus levels to an extent comparable to high-dose calcium carbonate. Mild gastrointestinal symptoms were the most common side effect in the lanthanum group. Lanthanum, unlike sevelamer, is an effective binder even in acidic environments in the gut and does not bind bile acids. Adherence may be better than with calcium-based binders or sevelamer as a result of lower pill burden. Because there is accumulation of small amounts of lanthanum in bone, it is important to continue to assess its side effects in long-term studies. Polynuclear iron compounds that form insoluble complexes with phosphate are under early investigation.

Activating the Calcium-Sensing and Vitamin D Receptors to Suppress Parathyroid Hormone Hyperfunction

Vitamin D Analogues

Treatment with $1,25\text{-}(OH_2)D_3$ (calcitriol) or an active vitamin D analogue (paricalcitol, doxercalciferol, alfacalcidol, or 22-oxacalcitrol) is also a means of controlling secondary hyperparathyroidism. By binding to the VDR on parathyroid tissues, the vitamin D analogue suppresses PTH production. There is not uniform agreement about the route, dose, and type of active vitamin D analogue that should be given. Some of the available vitamin D analogues cause less hypercalcemia than calcitriol, possibly because of decreased intestinal calcium absorption. The "second-generation" analogue paricalcitol has generated interest, because studies suggest that it leads to less elevation of serum calcium and phosphorus as well as a greater PTH suppression than calcitriol. When paricalcitol was compared to calcitriol in a large prospective, nonrandomized, 3-year trial in hemodialysis patients, in resulted in statistically significantly lower mortality rates. Although this study initially raised questions about the extent to which efforts to control secondary hyperparathyroidism with vitamin D analogues might cause harm, subsequent retrospective studies suggested improved survival in dialysis patients treated with active vitamin D analogues, compared with patients who did not receive vitamin D at all. However, a Recent analysis of a large international dialysis database supported the possibility that the effect of vitamin D may represent a patient selection bias. Prospective clinical trials are needed to determine whether vitamin D therapy offers a survival advantage in dialysis patients.

The current recommendations are to administer active vitamin D sterols to all patients undergoing hemodialysis or peritoneal dialysis who have serum intact PTH values greater than 300 pg/mL, provided that their serum phosphorus is less than 5.5 mg/dL and their total serum calcium, corrected for serum albumin, is less than 9.5 mg/dL. Equipotent intravenous doses of calcitriol, paricalcitol, and doxercalciferol for PTH suppression are 0.5, 2.5, and 5.0 μg, respectively, for PTH suppression. Whereas intermittent intravenous administration of active vitamin D analogues is common in the United States, in other countries daily oral therapy is more common. It remains to be established which approach is more effective in lowering serum PTH and reducing toxicity. Typical doses of calcitriol are 0.5 to 4.0 μg intravenously after each hemodialysis session. Calcitriol can also be given intraperitoneally. Typical oral doses are 0.25 to 1.0 μg/day. No data support the use of higher doses of vitamin D, which are associated with elevations of calcium and phosphorus.

Stage 5 CKD patients whose PTH levels drop to less than 150 pg/mL during treatment for secondary hyperparathyroidism require a reduction in their active vitamin D analogue or possibly in their phosphate binders. In patients with suspected osteomalacia, the risk for aluminum toxicity should be assessed. In patients with presumed adynamic bone disease, vitamin D analogues or phosphate binders can

be decreased enough to allow the intact PTH level to drift up to levels within the target range. Individuals who develop hypercalcemia while taking vitamin D analogues can be switched to a lower calcium dialysate bath and their vitamin D dose decreased or stopped.

Treatment with $25\text{-}(OH)D_3$ is recommended in the K/DOQI guidelines for stage 5 CKD patients who have levels of $25\text{-}(OH)D_3$ lower than 30 ng/mL. However, the utility of this treatment is not well-established, because these patients would not be expected to be able to convert this intermediate to calcitriol. Also, recent studies have suggested that it is difficult to normalize serum $25\text{-}(OH)D_3$ levels in patients with ESRD with typical replacement doses of ergocalciferol.

Calcimimetics

A newer class of drugs called calcimimetics offers a novel approach to treating secondary hyperparathyroidism without using active vitamin D analogues or raising serum calcium levels. Calcimimetics are CaSR agonists that act on the parathyroid gland by allosterically increasing the sensitivity of the receptor to calcium. Cinacalcet, the first available drug of this group, was approved by the U.S. Food and Drug Administration (FDA) in 2004 to treat secondary hyperparathyroidism in patients with stage 5 CKD. Treatment with cinacalcet causes significant decreases in PTH without elevating serum calcium or phosphorus concentrations. In fact, there is usually a reduction in serum calcium and a tendency to reduced serum phosphorus with calcimimetics. In one study, the use of cinacalcet resulted in approximately 41% of patients' attaining the PTH and calcium-phosphorus product goals recommended by the K/DOQI guidelines, compared with fewer than 10% achieving these targets in the group treated with phosphate binders and vitamin D analogues alone. Additional studies are needed to evaluate the effect of cinacalcet in altering the natural history of parathyroid gland hyperplasia. An ongoing prospective trial is examining the impact of lowering the calcium-phosphorus product with this drug on vascular calcifications and cardiovascular mortality (**Fig. 58-4**).

Parathyroidectomy

As an option remaining for patients with uncontrolled hyperparathyroidism, parathyroidectomy should be considered for persistently elevated intact PTH levels (>800 pg/mL) associated with hypercalcemia and/or hyperphosphatemia despite medical management, and for calciphylaxis or severe bone pain and fractures in the presence of elevated intact PTH levels. Either a subtotal parathyroidectomy or a total parathyroidectomy with forearm gland implantation can be performed. Some surgeons favor the latter procedure to avoid the need for repeated invasive neck surgery if hyperparathyroidism recurs. Glands can be removed from the forearm if necessary. Both subtotal and total parathyroidectomy with implantation are effective methods, and there are no studies comparing these approaches. Nonetheless, there is a 15% to 30% recurrence rate of hyperparathyroidism after complete or partial parathyroidectomy. Percutaneous

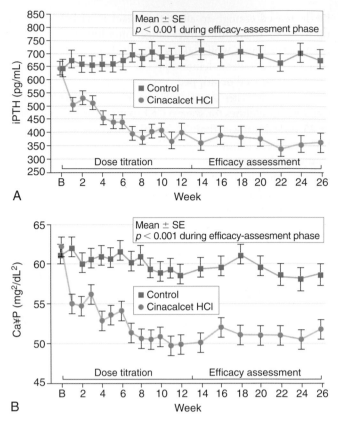

FIGURE 58-4. Suppression of serum parathyroid hormone (PTH) levels (**A**) by cinacalcet without elevation of the serum calcium-phosphorus (Ca × P) product (**B**) in hemodialysis patients with secondary hyperparathyroidism not adequately controlled by treatment with phosphate binders and vitamin D analogues. SE, standard error. (From Block GA, Martin KJ, de Francisco AL, et al: Cinacalcet for secondary hyperparathyroidism in patients receiving hemodialysis. N Engl J Med 350:1516-1525, 2004, with permission.)

ethanol injection into the gland as an ablation procedure for hyperparathyroidism refractory to medical management is performed in some centers, in lieu of surgical parathyroidectomy. "Hungry bone" syndrome is a frequent complication of parathyroidectomy, especially when markedly elevated PTH values are acutely reduced. This syndrome is characterized by hypocalcemia, hypophosphatemia, and hypomagnesemia secondary to increased bone uptake of these three ions after removal of the resorptive influence of PTH. For unclear reasons, hyperkalemia is occasionally seen. If severe or symptomatic hypocalcemia develops, treatment with a continuous calcium infusion is necessary. Concomitant treatment with oral calcitriol before and after parathyroidectomy may mitigate the hungry bone syndrome.

Patients with Stage 3 and Stage 4 Chronic Kidney Disease

Treatment of patients with stage 3 and stage 4 CKD who are not yet on dialysis has not been well studied; however, the early development of parathyroid gland hyperplasia due to chronic stimulation suggests that treatment should focus on prevention of parathyroid gland hyperplasia early in CKD. Phosphate restriction, phosphate binders, and calcium

supplementation are the mainstays of treatment in stages 3 and 4 CKD. Metabolic acidosis causes an efflux of calcium from bone, because bone buffers hydrogen ions with carbonate release. Chronic metabolic acidosis should be corrected with sodium bicarbonate supplementation. The need for and timing of therapy with active vitamin D analogues in stages 3 and 4 CKD have not been firmly established. Treatment with active vitamin D analogues, ideally with those that are less calcemic than calcitriol (e.g., paricalcitol), should be used only for persistently elevated intact PTH levels after administration of phosphate binders.

CKD patients are at increased risk for low levels of 25-hydroxyvitamin D for several potential reasons, including lack of sunlight if chronically ill or bedridden, poor oral intake of foods containing vitamin D, lower skin production of vitamin D_3 in elderly patients secondary to lower skin content of 7-dehydrocholesterol, and the presence of nephrotic syndrome causing loss of 25-hydroxyvitamin D and vitamin D–binding protein in the urine. Although the level of 25-hydroxyvitamin D in CKD that is diagnostic of hypovitaminosis D has not been firmly established, levels less than 30 ng/mL are associated with rising PTH levels. Stage 3 and 4 CKD patients with vitamin D levels lower than 30 ng/mL should be supplemented with ergocalciferol (vitamin D_2) or cholecalciferol (vitamin D_3). In patients without CKD, correction of vitamin D deficiency increases BMD and decreases the incidence of fractures. Cinacalcet has not been well studied in patients with CKD stages 3 and 4 and is not approved by the FDA for these patients.

Bisphosphonates

The use of bisphosphonates in patients with ESRD is poorly studied, and these agents are not widely prescribed in this setting because of concern that their use may exacerbate adynamic bone disease. Limited recent data suggest that use of the bisphosphonates alendronate and risedronate is safe and effective in reducing fracture incidence in osteoporotic patients with CKD.

Kidney Transplantation

The bony changes of secondary hyperparathyroidism improve after transplantation; however, in patients with severe hyperparathyroidism before transplantation, elevated serum levels of PTH can persist for as long as 10 years. The incidence of parathyroidectomy remains high after kidney transplantation, probably reflecting the irreversible hyperplasia of parathyroid glands that occurs during the course of CKD. It is not uncommon for patients to develop hypophosphatemia after kidney transplantation. This reduction in serum phosphorus may be mediated by persistent hyperparathyroidism and by other variables unrelated to PTH, such as increased levels of FGF-23 that also reduce renal tubular reabsorption of phosphate. Typically, phosphate supplementation is reserved for severe hypophosphatemia (<1.5 mg/dL). More aggressive use of phosphate supplementation may exacerbate secondary hyperparathyroidism. Transplantation also prevents, but does not reverse, bone damage from amyloidosis caused by β_2M deposition. Symptoms of amyloidosis frequently abate after transplantation, perhaps because of concomitant steroid therapy.

Although successful kidney transplantation corrects many of the conditions that lead to disordered mineral metabolism associated with kidney failure, the prednisone used to prevent rejection results in increased bone fragility, osteoporosis, and increased fracture rates. Other risk factors for fractures in this population include the presence of pretransplantation fracture, diabetes mellitus, and older age. In fact, the risk of fractures is greater in kidney transplant recipients than in patients on dialysis. There is an early rapid decrease in BMD during the first year after transplantation, as measured by DEXA scan, and then a slower, ongoing BMD loss that is similar to that in the general aging population. DEXA scans have been recommended in kidney transplant patients at the time of the transplantation and then yearly, at least for the first several years. In contrast to the general population, however, there is no clear evidence that low BMD by DEXA correlates with increased fracture risk in kidney transplant recipients. Calcium and vitamin D supplementation may be effective in counteracting the effects of glucocorticoids to reduce gastrointestinal calcium absorption. Studies have shown that calcium supplementation used with active vitamin D compounds preserves BMD at least early in the post-transplant period, but data showing that such treatment reduces fracture incidence are lacking. Intravenous bisphosphonate given at the time of transplantation and periodically within the first year thereafter appears to decrease the rate of bone loss as measured by BMD. However, given the concern for bisphosphonate-induced adynamic bone disease in this population and the lack of data on reduced facture incidence with this approach, there are currently no consensus recommendations on the use of bisphosphonates in kidney recipients. Decisions should be individualized, and caution should be maintained.

Avascular necrosis is another complication of kidney transplantation. It most typically occurs in the femoral heads or other weight-bearing joints and is characterized by the collapse of surface bone and cartilage. The pathogenesis of this disorder is not clear, but it is probably related to prednisone therapy. Magnetic resonance imaging is the most sensitive technique for evaluating patients with hip pain after transplantation for the presence of avascular necrosis. Surgical therapies include core decompression and hip replacement.

Post-transplantation distal limb syndrome is characterized by an often severe bilateral pain in the feet, ankles, or knees that begins within 3 months after transplantation. It is associated with elevated alkaline phosphatase levels and evidence of bone marrow edema and/or hemorrhage by magnetic resonance imaging of the affected areas. The condition, which is thought to result from intraosseous hypertension and has been associated with calcineurin inhibitors, is usually self-limited, resolving spontaneously within 6 months. Some patients have pain relief after the calcineurin inhibitor dose is lowered or a calcium channel blocker is added.

BIBLIOGRAPHY

Block GA: Association of serum phosphorus and calcium × phosphate product with mortality risk in chronic hemodialysis patients: A national study. Am J Kidney Dis 31:607-617, 1998.

Block GA, Klassen PS, Lazarus JM, et al: Mineral metabolism, mortality, and morbidity in maintenance hemodialysis. J Am Soc Nephrol 15:2208-2218, 2004.

Block GA, Martin KJ, de Francisco AL, et al: Cinacalcet for secondary hyperparathyroidism in patients receiving hemodialysis. N Engl J Med 350:1516-1525, 2004.

Block GA, Raggi P, Bellasi A, et al: Mortality effect of coronary calcification and phosphate binder choice in incident hemodialysis patients. Kidney Int 71:438-441, 2007.

Bricker NS, Fine LG: Uremia: Formulations and expectations. The trade-off hypothesis: Current status. Kidney Int 8:S5-S8, 1978.

Brown EM, Gamba G, Riccardi D, et al: Cloning and characterization of an extracellular Ca^{2+}-sensing receptor from bovine parathyroid. Nature 366:575-580, 1993.

Chertow GM, Burke SK, Raggi P, et al: Sevelamer attenuates the progression of coronary and aortic calcification in hemodialysis patients. Kidney Int 62:245-252, 2002.

D'Haese PC, Spasovski GB: A multicenter study on the effects of lanthanum carbonate (Fosrenol) and calcium carbonate on renal bone disease in dialysis patients. Kidney Int 85:S73-S78, 2003.

Drueke TB: β_2-Microglobulin and amyloidosis. Nephrol Dial Transplant 15:17-24, 2000.

Goodman WG, Coburn JW, Slatopolsky E, et al: Renal osteodystrophy in adults and children. In Favus MJ (ed): Primer on the Metabolic Bone Diseases and Disorders of Mineral Metabolism. 5th ed. Washington, DC, American Society for Bone and Mineral Research, 2003, pp 430-447.

Goodman WG, Goldin J, Kuizon BD, et al: Coronary-artery calcification in young adults with end-stage renal disease who are undergoing dialysis. N Engl J Med 342:1478-1483, 2000.

Indridason OS, Heath H III, Khosla S, et al: Non-suppressible parathyroid hormone secretion is related to gland size in uremic secondary hyperparathyroidism. Kidney Int 50:1664-1671, 1996.

Ketteler M, Bongartz P, Westenfeld R, et al: Association of low fetuin-A (AHSG) concentrations in serum with cardiovascular mortality in patients on dialysis: A cross-sectional study. Lancet 361:827-833, 2003.

Liu S, Quarles LD: How fibroblast growth factor 23 works. J Am Soc Nephrol 18:1637-1647, 2007.

Moe SM, Chen NX: Pathophysiology of vascular calcification in chronic kidney disease. Circ Res 17:560-567, 2004.

Parfitt AM: Renal bone disease: A new conceptual framework for the interpretation of bone histomorphometry. Curr Opin Nephrol Hypertens 12:387-403, 2003.

Price PA, Faus SA, Williamson MK: Warfarin-induced artery calcification is accelerated by growth and vitamin D. Arterioscler Thromb Vasc Biol 20:317-327, 2000.

Quarles LD, Lobaugh B, Murphy G: Intact parathyroid hormone overestimates the presence and severity of parathyroid-mediated osseous abnormalities in uremia. J Clin Endocrinol Metab 75:145-150, 1992.

Quarles LD, Sherrard DJ, Adler S, et al: The calcimimetic AMG 073 as a potential treatment for secondary hyperparathyroidism of end-stage renal disease. J Am Soc Nephrol 14:575-583, 2003.

Sprague SM, Llach F, Amdahl M, et al: Paricalcitol versus calcitriol in the treatment of secondary hyperparathyroidism. Kidney Int 63:1483-1490, 2003.

Stehman-Breen CO, Sherrard DJ, Alem AM, et al: Risk factors fractures for hip fracture among patients with end-stage renal disease. Kidney Int 58:2200-2205, 2000.

Sugarman JR, Frederick PR, Frankenfield DL, et al: Developing clinical performance measures based on the Dialysis Outcomes Quality Initiative Clinical Practice Guidelines: Process, outcomes and implications. Am J Kidney Dis 42:806-812, 2003.

Suki WN, Zabaneh R, Cangiano JL, et al: Effects of sevelamer and calcium-based phosphate binders on mortality in hemodialysis patients. Kidney Int 72:1130-1137, 2007.

Teng M, Wolf M, Lowrie E, et al: Survival of patients undergoing hemodialysis with paricalcitol or calcitriol therapy. N Engl J Med 349:446-456, 2003.

Teng M, Wolf M, Ofsthun MN, et al: Activated injectable vitamin D and hemodialysis survival: A historical cohort study. J Am Soc Nephrol 16:1115-1125, 2005.

Weisinger JR, Carlini RG, Rojas E, et al: Bone disease after renal transplantation. Clin J Am Soc Nephrol 6:1300-1313, 2006.

CHAPTER 59

Cardiac Function and Cardiovascular Disease in Chronic Kidney Disease

Daniel E. Weiner and Mark J. Sarnak

Cardiovascular disease (CVD) represents the leading cause of mortality throughout the spectrum of chronic kidney disease (CKD), with increased risk seen in individuals with microalbuminuria as well as in those with reduced kidney function. The risk of CVD outcomes increases as kidney function declines, reaching levels of 10 to 20 times that of the general population in dialysis patients.

EPIDEMIOLOGY OF CARDIOVASCULAR DISEASE IN CHRONIC KIDNEY DISEASE

Chronic Kidney Disease, Stages 3 and 4

Manifesting with cardiac ischemia, heart failure, and arrhythmia, CVD is overwhelmingly the leading cause of morbidity and mortality in individuals with CKD. Among patients with reduced kidney function, there is a progressive increase in the age-standardized rate of cardiovascular events as kidney function declines. Compared with an age-standardized baseline rate of 21 cardiovascular events per 1000 person-years in individuals with an estimated glomerular filtration rate (eGFR) higher than 60 mL/min/1.73 m^2, the number of events increase to 37, 113, 218, and 366 per 1000 person-years as eGFR decreases to 45 to 59 mL/min/1.73 m^2 (early stage 3 CKD), 30-44 mL/min/1.73 m^2 (late stage 3), 15-29 mL/min/1.73 m^2 (stage 4) and less than 15 mL/min/1.73 m^2 (stage 5), respectively. Even in analyses that adjust for demographic and socioeconomic risk factors as well as cardiovascular risk factors such as diabetes, hypertension, and dyslipidemia, the risk of a cardiovascular event increases dramatically as kidney function declines (**Fig. 59-1**). This relationship is independent of preexisting CVD (**Fig. 59-2**).

Population screening programs administered by the National Kidney Foundation have also noted a high prevalence of CVD, with 12% to 20% of individuals with an eGFR between 30 and 59 mL/min/1.73 m^2 (stage 3 CKD) stating that they had had a prior "heart attack or stroke," compared with 5% to 10% of those with an eGFR of 60 mL/min/1.73 m^2 or greater. In analyses adjusted for risk factors similar to those already mentioned, both reduced eGFR and microalbuminuria were independently associated with prevalent CVD. Similar results were appreciated in pooled community

cohorts, where, in unadjusted analysis, CVD was prevalent in 31.3% of individuals with an eGFR between 15 and 60 mL/min/1.73 m^2 (stage 3 to 4 CKD), compared with 14.4% of those with an eGFR greater than 60 mL/min/1.73 m^2.

Although few studies have evaluated incidence rates of left ventricular hypertrophy (LVH), this condition is highly prevalent and frequently develops before the need for kidney replacement therapy, most likely as a result of both pressure and volume overload. In one cross-sectional study of 175 patients with CKD, LVH was present in 27% of patients with creatinine clearance greater than 50 mL/min, in 31% of those with creatinine clearance between 25 and 49 mL/min, and in 45% of those with creatinine clearance of less than 25 mL/min. This finding contrasts with a prevalence of LVH of less than 20% in patients of similar age in the general population.

Both the incidence and the prevalence of heart failure are also high in CKD. In the Atherosclerosis Risk in

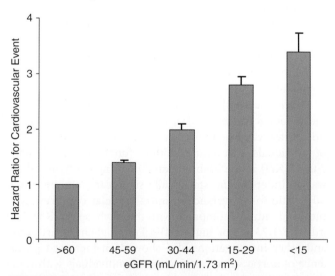

FIGURE 59-1 Hazard ratios for cardiovascular events according to the baseline estimated glomerular filtration rate (eGFR), adjusted for baseline age, gender, income, education, coronary disease, chronic heart failure, stroke or transient ischemic attack, peripheral artery disease, diabetes, hypertension, dyslipidemia, cancer, hypoalbuminemia, dementia, liver disease, proteinuria, prior hospitalizations, and subsequent dialysis requirement.
(Data from Go AS, Chertow GM, Fan D, et al: Chronic kidney disease and the risks of death, cardiovascular events, and hospitalization. N Engl J Med 351: 1301, 2004.)

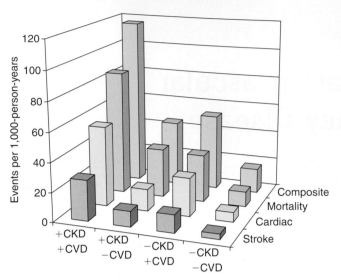

FIGURE 59-2 Unadjusted event rates for individuals with (+) and without (−) chronic kidney disease (CKD) and cardiovascular disease (CVD) at baseline. CKD was defined as an estimated glomerular filtration rate (eGFR) of 15 to 59 mL/min/1.73 m². Cardiac events included myocardial infarction and fatal coronary disease. Stroke included both fatal and nonfatal stroke events. Mortality included all causes of death, and the composite outcome included any cardiac, stroke, or mortality event. (From Weiner DE, Tabatabai S, Tighiouart H, et al: Cardiovascular outcomes and all-cause mortality: Exploring the interaction between CKD and cardiovascular disease. Am J Kidney Dis 48:396, 2006, with permission.)

Communities study, individuals with an eGFR of less than 60 mL/min/1.73 m² at baseline had twice the risk of incident heart failure hospitalization and death of those with an eGFR of 90 mL/min/1.73 m² or higher, regardless of the presence of baseline coronary disease. Similarly, heart failure is highly prevalent in CKD. Among adult members of a large group model health maintenance organization in the northwestern United States, 6.0% of individuals with predominantly early stage 3 CKD had a diagnostic code for heart failure compared with 1.8% of individuals in an age- and sex-matched population.

Other structural heart diseases seen commonly in CKD include aortic valve, mitral valve, and mitral annular calcification. Mitral valve or annular calcification was present in 20% of individuals with reduced kidney function (roughly stage 3 to 4 CKD) in the Framingham Offspring Study, and there was an independent, statistically significant 60% increased odds ratio for prevalence of mitral annular calcification in these individuals, compared with those whose eGFR was 60 mL/min/1.73 m² or higher. The Framingham Heart Study and other investigations also showed an increased prevalence of aortic valve calcification in individuals with CKD that was attenuated after adjustment for other risk factors. Microalbuminuria was not described in these studies.

Chronic Kidney Disease, Stage 5 and Dialysis

Among dialysis patients, CVD is common, with similar cardiovascular mortality rates in a 20-year-old dialysis patient and an 80-year-old member of the general population

(**Fig. 59-3**). This most likely reflects both a high prevalence of CVD (22.5% of individuals initiating dialysis in the United States in 2006 had known coronary disease) and a high case-fatality rate as compared to the general population. Even in the absence of clinically apparent coronary disease, subclinical coronary disease may be highly prevalent. In a study of 30 incident asymptomatic dialysis patients with no known coronary disease history, cardiac catheterization revealed significant coronary disease in 16 patients (10 of whom had diabetes mellitus), including 5 with luminal narrowing greater than 90%. Of note, only 2 of these 5 patients had dipyridamole thallium scintigraphy results suggestive of ischemia. The import of this small but provocative report will be better understood if the findings are repeated in a larger, more generalizable population.

Heart failure rates are also extremely high. Based on administrative data from the United States Renal Data System (USRDS), approximately 25% of patients undergoing hemodialysis and 18% of those undergoing peritoneal dialysis are diagnosed with heart failure annually, whereas approximately 55% of prevalent hemodialysis patients are identified as having a history of heart failure.

A study of prevalent hemodialysis patients also revealed high rates of valvular calcification; 45% of subjects had calcification of the mitral valve, and 34% had calcification of the aortic valve, compared with an expected prevalence of 3% to 5% in the general population. Overall, studies have demonstrated rates of mitral annular calcification ranging from 30% to 50% in hemodialysis patients. Disorders of mineral metabolism, potentially associated with incident and progressive CVD via vascular and valvular calcification as well as vitamin D deficiency and hyperparathyroidism independent of calcification, are covered in Chapters 13 and 58.

TYPES OF CARDIOVASCULAR DISEASE

CVD in CKD patients has a variety of manifestations, chiefly comprising atherosclerosis, arteriosclerosis, and cardiomyopathy/valvular disease (**Table 59-1**). In most cases, clinically apparent CVD reflects the interplay among these manifestations. *Atherosclerosis* is defined as an occlusive disease of the vasculature that occurs as a result of the deposition of lipid-laden plaques, and *arteriosclerosis* is defined as nonocclusive remodeling of the vasculature accompanied by a loss of arterial elasticity. Both of these conditions may manifest with ischemic heart disease and heart failure. Certain risk factors, including dyslipidemia, primarily predispose an individual to development and progression of atherosclerosis, and others, including elevated calcium-phosphorus product, may predispose one to arteriosclerosis. Other risk factors, including volume overload and anemia, may primarily predispose an person to cardiac remodeling and LVH. Over time, the interplay among these manifestations may yield both segmental

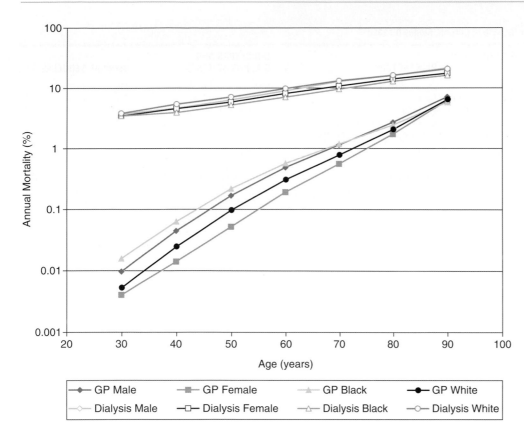

| ◆ GP Male | ■ GP Female | ▲ GP Black | ● GP White |
| ◇ Dialysis Male | □ Dialysis Female | △ Dialysis Black | ○ Dialysis White |

FIGURE 59-3 Cardiovascular disease mortality rates (including death from arrhythmia, cardiomyopathy, cardiac arrest, myocardial infarction, atherosclerotic heart disease, or pulmonary edema) in the general population (GP) and in patients with chronic kidney failure treated by dialysis.

(From Foley RN, Parfrey PS, Sarnak MJ: Clinical epidemiology of cardiovascular disease in chronic renal disease. Am J Kidney Dis 32(5 Suppl 3):S112-S119, 1998, with permission)

perfusion defects due to larger coronary artery disease and insufficient subendocardial perfusion secondary to cardiac hypertrophy (causing increased demand). The end result is myocyte death.

RISK FACTORS FOR CARDIOVASCULAR DISEASE

Much of the increased burden of CVD in CKD results from the increased prevalence of both traditional and nontraditional CVD risk factors. Traditional risk factors are those factors identified in the Framingham Heart Study as conferring increased risk of CVD in the general population. Nontraditional risk factors are those factors not identified in the initial reports of the Framingham Heart Study that increase in prevalence as kidney function declines and that have been hypothesized to be CVD risk factors in patients with CKD (**Table 59-2**). All CKD stages, even stages 1 and 2, in which microalbuminuria is present but GFR is preserved, have been independently associated with CVD in epidemiologic studies. Although CKD may directly contribute to the development of CVD through various mechanisms (e.g., retention of salt and water, anemia, abnormal mineral metabolism), it is also probable that CKD represents a risk state in which factors associated with the development of CKD (including diabetes, hypertension, and possibly dyslipidemia) account for the enhanced CVD risk. In the latter hypothesis, the presence of CKD is a measure of the severity of these other risk factors.

ISCHEMIC HEART DISEASE
Prediction of Ischemic Heart Disease

The Framingham coronary heart disease prediction equations utilized traditional risk factors including age, gender, diabetes, blood pressure, and lipid levels to estimate cardiac risk in a general U.S. population. However, use of these well-accepted prediction equations to assign cardiac risk to patients with CKD may be problematic, because risk factors that are at least in part dependent on intact nutrition (e.g., serum cholesterol) and cardiac health (e.g., systolic and diastolic blood pressure) appear to have different relationships with adverse outcomes in these patients. Accordingly, although many of the same traditional risk factors that predict coronary heart disease in the general population (e.g., diabetes, hypertension) are also important risk factors in the predialysis CKD population, the relative importance of each risk factor may be different. In particular, diabetes in individuals with CKD is a more powerful marker of cardiac risk than it is in the general population, perhaps reflecting the fact that diabetes severe enough to cause kidney damage is also capable of causing systemic vascular disease.

In dialysis patients, the Framingham equations fail altogether, although older individuals and those with diabetes do have higher rates of cardiovascular events. In patients undergoing hemodialysis, there is little increase in mortality risk at even the highest systolic blood pressures, whereas lower systolic blood pressures (<120 mm Hg) are associated with the highest risk of mortality. These altered risk factor relationships do not

TABLE 59-1 Types of Cardiovascular Disease in Chronic Kidney Disease

CVD TYPE	PATHOLOGIC OR STRUCTURAL MANIFESTATION	RISK FACTORS	INDICATORS AND DIAGNOSTIC TESTS	CLINICAL SEQUELAE
Arterial disease	Atherosclerosis (luminal narrowing of arteries due to plaques)	Dyslipidemia Diabetes mellitus Hypertension Other traditional and nontraditional risk factors	Inducible ischemia on nuclear imaging Cardiac catheterization	MI Angina Sudden cardiac death Heart failure
	Arteriosclerosis (diffuse dilatation and wall hypertrophy of larger arteries with loss of arterial elasticity)	Hypertension Volume overload Hyperparathyroidism Hyperphosphatemia Medial calcification	Vascular calcification Increased pulse pressure Aortic pulse wave velocity Cardiac CT Other arterial imaging	MI Angina Sudden cardiac death Heart failure LV hypertrophy
Cardiomyopathy	LV hypertrophy (adaptive hypertrophy to compensate for increased cardiac demand)	Pressure overload (increased afterload due to hypertension, valvular disease, arteriosclerosis) Volume overload (volume retention due to progressive kidney disease ± anemia)	Echocardiography Cardiovascular MRI	MI Angina Sudden cardiac death Heart failure
	Decreased LV contractility	Ischemic heart disease Hypertension LV hypertrophy Other traditional and nontraditional risk factors	Echocardiography	Cardiorenal syndrome Sudden cardiac death Heart failure MI Angina
	Impaired LV relaxation	Hypertension Anemia and volume overload Abnormal mineral metabolism Other arteriosclerosis risk factors Other traditional and nontraditional risk factors	Echocardiography	Heart failure MI Angina Sudden cardiac death
Structural Disease	Pericardial disease	Delayed or insufficient dialysis	Echocardiography	Heart failure Hypotension
	Aortic and mitral valve disease	CKD stage 3 to 5 Abnormal metabolism of calcium, phosphate, PTH Aging Dialysis vintage	Echocardiography	Aortic stenosis Endocarditis Heart failure
	Mitral annular calcification	CKD stage 3 to 5 Abnormal metabolism of calcium, phosphate, PTH	Echocardiography (uniform echodense, rigid band located near the base of the posterior mitral leaflet)	Arrhythmia Embolism Endocarditis Heart failure
	Endocarditis	Valvular disease Chronic venous catheters	Echocardiography	Arrhythmia Heart failure Embolism
Arrhythmia	Atrial fibrillation	Ischemic heart disease Cardiomyopathy	Electrocardiography	Hypotension Embolism
	Ventricular arrhythmia	Ischemic heart disease Cardiomyopathy Electrolyte abnormalities	Electrocardiography Electrophysiology study	Sudden cardiac death

CKD, chronic kidney disease; CVD, cardiovascular disease; CT, computed tomography; LV, left ventricle; MI, myocardial infarction; MRI, magnetic resonance imaging; PTH, parathyroid hormone.

speak to therapeutic options but probably reflect patients' current health status and cardiac and nutritional reserve.

Diagnosis of Ischemic Heart Disease

No single diagnostic test has proved optimal for identifying ischemic heart disease in patients with CKD, and each has pitfalls specific to CKD that may affect sensitivity and specificity. Currently, a functional assessment of perfusion that includes cardiac imaging is probably the best initial option to identify cardiac ischemia. These assessments include exercise or pharmacologic nuclear stress tests as well as exercise or pharmacologic stress echocardiography. Importantly, the ability to perform exercise stress testing is often limited by comorbid conditions in the CKD population. There is, at best, a very limited role for stress electrocardiography (ECG) in this population given the high prevalence of baseline ECG abnormalities and CVD. As a single test, stress echocardiography, with exercise or with pharmacologic stimulation if exercise is not feasible, is useful because it also provides information on valvular and other structural disease. There is no absolute contraindication to cardiac catheterization in patients

TABLE 59-2 Traditional and Nontraditional Cardiovascular Risk Factors in Chronic Kidney Disease

TRADITIONAL RISK FACTORS	NONTRADITIONAL RISK FACTORS
Older age	Albuminuria
Male gender	Lipoprotein(a) and apo(a) isoforms
Hypertension	Lipoprotein remnants
Higher LDL cholesterol	Anemia
Lower HDL cholesterol	Abnormal mineral metabolism
Diabetes	Extracellular fluid volume overload
Smoking	Electrolyte imbalance
Physical inactivity	Oxidative stress
Menopause	Inflammation
Family history of CVD	Malnutrition
Left ventricular hypertrophy	Thrombogenic factors
	Sleep disturbances
	Altered nitric oxide/endothelin balance

CVD, cardiovascular disease; HDL, high-density lipoprotein; LDL, low-density lipoprotein.

Revised from Sarnak MJ, Levey AS, Schoolwerth AC, et al: Kidney disease as a risk factor for development of cardiovascular disease: A statement from the American Heart Association Councils on Kidney in Cardiovascular Disease, High Blood Pressure Research, Clinical Cardiology, and Epidemiology and Prevention. Circulation 108:2154-2169, 2003.

with CKD, including those already on dialysis, although preservation of existing kidney function is an important consideration in all stages of kidney disease. With careful management and conservative use of iodinated contrast material (see Chapter 34), most individuals with stage 3 or 4 CKD can avoid significant contrast nephropathy.

Treatment of Ischemic Heart Disease

Chronic Kidney Disease, Stages 3 and 4

In the earlier stages of CKD, there is a moderate body of data, predominantly comprising subgroup analyses derived from larger clinical trials, that demonstrates benefits with interventions that are favorable in the general population. Therefore, currently accepted treatment strategies for primary prevention of cardiac disease in individuals with all stages of CKD mirror those seen in the general population, with specific attention to avoidance of common adverse effects associated with cardiac therapies in later stages of CKD. Specifically, in individuals with stage 3 or 4 CKD, dyslipidemia, hypertension, and diabetes should be aggressively treated, because therapies directed to these conditions are likely to reduce not only the risk of cardiac disease but also the risk of progression to kidney failure. Challenges with therapy include the risk of hyperkalemia with blockade of the renin-angiotensin-aldosterone system, and the risks and benefits of aggressive blockade need to be assessed on an individual basis. Other concerns in CKD include an increased risk of rhabdomyolysis seen with dual statin and fibrate therapy; this combination should be avoided in advanced CKD. Low-dose

aspirin use in individuals with cardiac risk factors is probably beneficial. Blood pressure management is discussed in detail in Chapter 65, and diabetes and diabetic nephropathy in Chapter 26.

There are minimal trial data on secondary prevention strategies in CKD; however, in the absence of active or chronic gastrointestinal bleeding, there is no specific contraindication to chronic antiplatelet therapy. However, individuals with CKD are less likely to receive appropriate medications after myocardial infarction, including aspirin, β-blockers, angiotensin-converting enzyme (ACE) inhibitors, lipid-lowering agents and revascularization therapies such as coronary artery bypass grafting and percutaneous angioplasty with stenting, despite suggestive evidence that these therapies are associated with improved survival regardless of level of kidney function.

Chronic Kidney Disease, Stage 5 and Dialysis

To date, there are essentially no clinical trials that demonstrate a significant survival benefit with accepted CHD therapies in the dialysis population, and current practice is chiefly based on observational data and extrapolations from the non-CKD population. Whether this paucity of data has caused or is a consequence of a degree of therapeutic nihilism prevalent in the cardiac care of CKD patients is uncertain. The overall failure to find interventions that significantly reduce the CVD burden in individuals on chronic dialysis most likely reflects the fact that there are numerous competing causes of death in these patients, and addressing only one at a time may not make a significant impact in reducing mortality.

Interventions directed at blood pressure and diet are challenging given the difficulty of maintaining blood pressure in a narrow range as well as the catabolic nature of the dialysis milieu. Moreover, some risk factors associated with adverse events in the general population appear to be protective in the dialysis population. For example, higher blood pressure and obesity are associated with better survival in dialysis patients, probably because they reflect, respectively, greater cardiac and nutritional reserves. Other challenges with risk factor management include difficulty with ascertainment. For example, blood pressure measurements are often unreliable due to the presence of dialysis access and arterial calcification, and glycated hemoglobin measurements may not accurately reflect diabetes control given the reduced half-life of red blood cells in hemodialysis patients. Despite a lack of definitive supporting evidence, the following targets are reasonable based predominantly on clinical practice guidelines extracting data from the nondialysis population: (1) predialysis blood pressure goal of less than 140/90 mm Hg, optimally accomplished by achieving appropriate dry weight and then with pharmacologic therapy, provided there is no substantial orthostatic hypotension or symptomatic intradialytic hypotension; (2) serum LDL cholesterol goal of less than 100 mg/dL in individuals with known atherogenic disease; and (3) reasonably tight diabetes control based on frequent glucose assessments.

Finally, smoking cessation efforts are essential in all stages of CKD. As with earlier stages of CKD, ischemic heart disease can be treated invasively in dialysis patients. Several observational studies have shown that dialysis patients with coronary artery disease benefit from coronary revascularization, and that revascularization, if appropriate, is favorable to medical management; however, selection bias is always a concern when interpreting these reports, because randomized trials are lacking.

LEFT VENTRICULAR HYPERTROPHY AND HEART FAILURE

Diagnosis of Left Ventricular Hypertrophy and Heart Failure

Diagnosis of LVH is readily accomplished with echocardiography. Cardiac function should be assessed in the euvolemic state, because significant volume depletion and overload both reduce left ventricular inotropy. Accordingly, in dialysis patients, two-dimensional echocardiogram results are likely to be most meaningful on the interdialytic day. Three-dimensional echocardiography may be useful to assess left ventricle structure, because it avoids the use of geometric assumptions of shape that are required to estimate left ventricle mass and volume. Magnetic resonance imaging may be more precise for assessing structure than echocardiography, but this technique is not yet widely available, and the costs may be prohibitive. Screening echocardiography is currently recommended for incident dialysis patients; however, there is no evidence to date that this results in any improvement in clinical outcomes.

Heart failure is defined as a clinical syndrome characterized by specific symptoms, including dyspnea and fatigue, and signs, including edema and rales. Although this constellation of signs and symptoms may be consistent with heart failure, it is also present in many individuals with CKD and may simply reflect volume overload. Regardless of the specific cause, individuals with persistent or recurrent volume overload have poor clinical outcomes overall. Importantly, in hemodialysis, where preload is rapidly changing and fluid overload is managed with ultrafiltration, hypotension may be the only manifestation of heart failure.

Treatment of Left Ventricular Hypertrophy and Heart Failure

Potentially modifiable risk factors for LVH include anemia, hypertension, extracellular volume overload, abnormal mineral metabolism including hyperphosphatemia and secondary hyperparathyroidism, and, on rare occasions, arteriovenous fistulas that are causing high-output heart failure. However, definitive clinical trials evaluating the effect on mortality of modification of these risk factors for development and persistence of LVH are not currently available, leading to reliance on surrogate outcomes. Whereas ACE inhibitor and angiotensin receptor blocker (ARB) therapy may result in a favorable surrogate outcome, namely left ventricular mass reduction, in CKD, randomized trials in CKD targeting higher hemoglobin levels with recombinant human erythropoietin had no effect on the similar surrogate outcome of LVH or left ventricular mass. Critically, no trials have demonstrated a reduction in nonsurrogate outcomes (i.e., cardiac or mortality outcomes) with these interventions when used for the purpose of treating or preventing LVH.

Heart failure therapy differs by CKD stage, because diuretics are a mainstay of therapy in predialysis patients whereas acute fluid overload in dialysis patients is treated with ultrafiltration. Chronic therapy for heart failure in CKD stages 3 through 5 has not been adequately studied; most recommendations are either extrapolated from the general population or based on small trials. ACE inhibitors and ARBs probably have both cardiac and kidney benefits independent of their blood pressure–lowering effects in all CKD stages, with limited data suggesting some improvement in left ventricular geometry associated with these medications. Potential further benefits associated with aldosterone blockade (e.g., spironolactone) are currently being studied, with a major limitation being hyperkalemia, especially when these agents are used in conjunction with ACE inhibitors or ARBs. β-Blocking agents, another mainstay of heart failure therapy in the general population, are also beneficial in patients with CKD, with evidence supporting the use of carvedilol to reduce mortality risk in dialysis patients with left ventricular dysfunction. Cardiac glycosides (e.g., digoxin) are frequently used to treat heart failure in the general population, where they decrease morbidity but not mortality. Although there are no specific studies of cardiac glycosides in CKD, they should be used judiciously if at all, and with careful attention to dosage, drug levels, and potassium balance.

ARRHYTHMIA AND SUDDEN CARDIAC DEATH

Arrhythmias are extremely common in individuals with CKD, most likely reflecting the high prevalence of structural heart disease, ischemic heart disease, and electrolyte abnormalities. Atrial fibrillation is the most common arrhythmia, with prevalence estimates for paroxysmal and permanent atrial fibrillation as high as 30%. Ventricular arrhythmias probably are also exceedingly common, although true rates cannot be determined. Prevalent dialysis patients have a mortality rate of 62 per 1000 person-years attributable to cardiac arrest (cause unknown) or arrhythmia, according to 2003-2005 USRDS data. Similar results were seen in the HEMO study, in which a consensus committee determined cause of death. In HEMO, death rates directly attributable to arrhythmia and to ischemic heart disease (most commonly defined by sudden death in individual with prior coronary disease) were 11 and 40 per 1000 person-years, respectively.

There are few data on prevention and treatment of arrhythmia and sudden cardiac death in the CKD population, and most current treatment recommendations mirror those seen in the general population. Of note, there are no trial data for use of antiarrhythmic agents in dialysis patients or for use of warfarin to prevent embolic stroke in dialysis patients with atrial fibrillation. The number of dialysis patients who have received an implantable cardioverter defibrillator (ICD) to prevent sudden cardiac death has increased exponentially over the past decade. In 2005, 1723 dialysis patients (0.6% of all dialysis patients) received an ICD. ICD use has not been rigorously studied in the dialysis population, and there have been no assessments of the cost to society per quality adjusted life-year gained with this procedure.

BIBLIOGRAPHY

Cice G, Ferrara L, D'Andrea A, et al: Carvedilol increases two-year survival in dialysis patients with dilated cardiomyopathy: A prospective, placebo-controlled trial. J Am Coll Cardiol 41:1438-1444, 2003.

deFilippi CWS, Rosanio S, Tiblier E, et al: Cardiac troponin T and C-reactive protein for predicting prognosis, coronary atherosclerosis, and cardiomyopathy in patients undergoing long-term hemodialysis. JAMA 290:353-359, 2003.

Fox CS, Larson MG, Vasan RS, et al: Cross-sectional association of kidney function with valvular and annular calcification: The Framingham heart study. J Am Soc Nephrol 17:521-527, 2006.

Go AS, Chertow GM, Fan D, et al: Chronic kidney disease and the risks of death, cardiovascular events, and hospitalization. N Engl J Med 351:1296-1305, 2004.

Herzog CA, Ma JZ, Collins AJ: Comparative survival of dialysis patients in the United States after coronary angioplasty, coronary artery stenting, and coronary artery bypass surgery and impact of diabetes. Circulation 106:2207-2211, 2002.

Keeley EC, Kadakia R, Soman S, et al: Analysis of long-term survival after revascularization in patients with chronic kidney disease presenting with acute coronary syndromes. Am J Cardiol 92:509-514, 2003.

Lubowsky ND, Siegel R, Pittas AG: Management of glycemia in patients with diabetes mellitus and CKD. Am J Kidney Dis 50:810-823, 2007.

Ohtake T, Kobayashi S, Moriya H, et al: High prevalence of occult coronary artery stenosis in patients with chronic kidney disease at the initiation of renal replacement therapy: An angiographic examination. J Am Soc Nephrol 16:1141-1148, 2005.

Raggi P, Boulay A, Chasan-Taber S, et al: Cardiac calcification in adult hemodialysis patients: A link between end-stage renal disease and cardiovascular disease? J Am Coll Cardiol 39:695-701, 2002.

Sarnak MJ: Cardiovascular complications in chronic kidney disease. Am J Kidney Dis 41(5 Suppl):11-17, 2003.

Sarnak MJ, Levey AS, Schoolwerth AC, et al: Kidney disease as a risk factor for development of cardiovascular disease: A statement from the American Heart Association Councils on Kidney in Cardiovascular Disease, High Blood Pressure Research, Clinical Cardiology, and Epidemiology and Prevention. Circulation 108:2154-2169, 2003.

Umana E, Ahmed W, Alpert MA: Valvular and perivalvular abnormalities in end-stage renal disease. Am J Med Sci 325:237-242, 2003.

Weiner DE, Sarnak MJ: Chronic kidney disease and cardiovascular disease: A bi-directional relationship? Dial Transplantation 36:113-120, 2007.

Weiner DE, Tabatabai S, Tighiouart H, et al: Cardiovascular outcomes and all-cause mortality: Exploring the interaction between CKD and cardiovascular disease. Am J Kidney Dis 48:392-401, 2006.

Weiner DE, Tighiouart H, Elsayed EF, et al: The Framingham predictive instrument in chronic kidney disease. J Am Coll Cardiol 50:217-224, 2007.

Wright RS, Reeder GS, Herzog CA, et al: Acute myocardial infarction and renal dysfunction: A high-risk combination. Ann Intern Med 137:563-570, 2002.

CHAPTER 60

Hematologic Manifestations of Chronic Kidney Disease

Jay B. Wish

ANEMIA

Epidemiology and Pathogenesis

Anemia is defined by the World Health Organization as a hemoglobin (Hb) concentration of less than 13.0 g/L in adult men and nonmenstruating women and less than 12.0 g/dL in menstruating women. The incidence of anemia in patients with chronic kidney disease (CKD) increases as the glomerular filtration rate (GFR) declines. Population studies such as the National Health and Nutrition Examination Survey (NHANES) by the National Institutes of Health and the Prevalence of Anemia in Early Renal Insufficiency (PAERI) study suggest that the incidence of anemia is less than 10% in CKD stages 1 and 2, 20% to 40% in CKD stage 3, 50% to 60% in CKD stage 4, and more than 70% in CKD stage 5.

The pathogenesis of anemia in patients with CKD is multifactorial (**Table 60-1**), but the contribution of erythropoietin (EPO) deficiency becomes greater as GFR declines. Hypoxia inducible factor (HIF), which is produced in the kidneys and other tissues, is a substance whose spontaneous degradation is inhibited in the presence of decreased oxygen delivery due to anemia or hypoxemia. The sustained presence of HIF leads to signal transduction and the synthesis of EPO. In normal patients, plasma EPO levels increase dramatically in response to anemia. Because of their loss of functioning mass, the kidneys in patients with CKD fail to increase EPO production in response to anemia or other conditions that decrease oxygen delivery.

TABLE 60-1 **Factors That Cause or Contribute to Anemia in Patients with Chronic Kidney Disease**

Insufficient production of endogenous erythropoietin

Iron deficiency

Acute and chronic inflammatory conditions

Severe hyperparathyroidism

Aluminum toxicity

Folate deficiency

Decreased survival of red blood cells

The kidneys produce about 90% of circulating EPO, so loss of EPO production in the setting of CKD is the primary cause of anemia in these patients. EPO binds to receptors on erythroid progenitor cells in the bone marrow, specifically the burst-forming units (BFU-E) and colony-forming units (CFU-E). The absence of EPO causes these cells to undergo programmed death or apoptosis, which is mediated by the Fas antigen. In the presence of EPO, these erythroid progenitors differentiate into reticulocytes and red blood cells (RBCs).

Figure 60-1 demonstrates the complex interactions among EPO; pro-inflammatory cytokines such as interleukin 1 (IL-1), tumor necrosis factor-α (TNF-α), IL-6, and interferon-γ (IFN-γ); hepcidin; and iron in the production of RBCs. Hepcidin is a recently discovered peptide, produced by the liver, that interferes with RBC production by decreasing iron availability for incorporation into erythroblasts. Hepcidin gene expression is upregulated by IL-6 and iron overload and downregulated by TNF-α and iron deficiency. At the cell surface of macrophages and jejunal cells (and probably other cells), hepcidin binds to ferroportin, the membrane-embedded iron exporter, resulting in internalization and degradation of the complex. This inhibits iron transport across the cell membrane, trapping it in macrophages and preventing it from being absorbed from the intestine. Hepcidin activity is probably the basis for most of the "anemia of chronic disease" syndromes, and it contributes to the anemia in patients with CKD when inflammation and infection are present. However, in anemic CKD patients without inflammation or infection, EPO deficiency plays a much greater role than hepcidin.

The evidence for inhibition of RBC production by uremic toxins in patients with CKD is poor, because most of these patients have an appropriate erythropoietic response to endogenously administered EPO if they are iron replete and free of inflammation or infection. It has been demonstrated that RBC survival is decreased in patients with CKD to 60 to 90 days, compared with 120 days in normal individuals. This may be a result of RBC trauma due to microvascualar disease as well as decreased resistance to oxidative stress. The lack of EPO in patients with CKD also contributes to neocytolysis, a physiologic process that

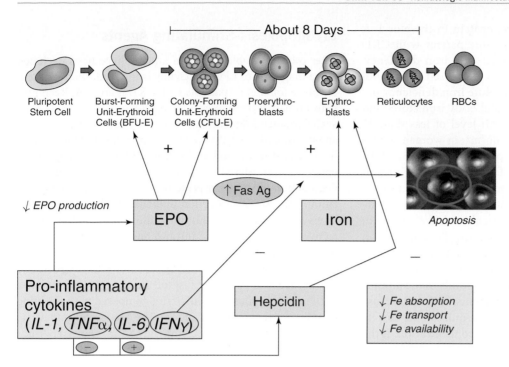

| About 8 Days |

Pluripotent Stem Cell — Burst-Forming Unit-Erythroid Cells (BFU-E) — Colony-Forming Unit-Erythroid Cells (CFU-E) — Proerythro-blasts — Erythro-blasts — Reticulocytes — RBCs

↑ Fas Ag

↓ EPO production

EPO

Iron

Apoptosis

Pro-inflammatory cytokines (IL-1, TNFα, IL-6, IFNγ)

Hepcidin

↓ Fe absorption
↓ Fe transport
↓ Fe availability

FIGURE 60-1 Erythropoiesis in chronic kidney disease. Ag, antigen; EPO, erythropoietin; Fe iron; IFN, interferon; IL, interleukin; RBCs, red blood cells; TNF, tumor necrosis factor. (Courtesy of Iain Macdougall, MD.)

leads to hemolysis of the youngest RBCs in the circulation. Hemolysis induced by hemodialysis is discussed in Chapter 54.

Clinical Manifestations

The major clinical manifestations of anemia in patients with or without CKD are fatigue (both with exercise and at rest), decreased cognitive skills, loss of libido, and decreased sense of well-being. These symptoms tend to occur when the Hb is less than 10 g/dL and are more severe at lower Hb levels. More insidious are the cardiac complications of anemia, which may occur when the patient is otherwise asymptomatic and which may contribute to the adverse cardiovascular morbidity and mortality outcomes observed among patients with CKD. In patients with underlying coronary artery disease, anemia may lead to an exacerbation of angina symptoms because of decreased myocardial oxygen delivery. Decreased peripheral oxygen delivery due to anemia leads to peripheral vasodilation, increased sympathetic nervous system activity, increased heart rate and stroke volume, and, ultimately, left ventricular hypertrophy (LVH). It has been demonstrated that LVH strongly correlates with adverse outcomes (hospitalization and mortality) in patients with CKD. A decrease in Hb of 0.5 g/dL below normal correlates with a 32% increase in LVH risk, whereas a 5 mm Hg increase in systolic blood pressure correlates with only an 11% increase in LVH risk. Most anemic CKD patients treated with erythropoiesis-stimulating agents (ESAs) report a decrease in subjective symptoms and improved quality of life, but evidence supporting regression of LVH, fewer clinical cardiac events, or decreased mortality with ESA treatment is not compelling (see later discussion).

Laboratory Evaluation

Because the prevalence of anemia even among patients with stages 1 and 2 CKD is as high as 10%, the consequences of anemia are severe, and its treatment is straightforward, the 2006 National Kidney Foundation (NKF) Kidney Disease Outcomes Quality Initiative (K/DOQI) clinical practice guidelines and clinical practice recommendations for anemia in CKD recommended annual screening of all patients with CKD (regardless of stage) for anemia. If anemia is present (defined as Hb <13.5 g/dL in adult men and Hb <12.0 g/dL in adult women), then further evaluation should be undertaken to determine the cause of the anemia. This evaluation should include a complete blood count including RBC indices, reticulocyte count, serum ferritin concentration, and transferrin saturation (TSAT) or reticulocyte hemoglobin content (CHr). The anemia of EPO deficiency is normocytic (normal mean corpuscular volume, or MCV) and normochromic (normal mean corpuscular hemoglobin concentration, or MCHC). A low MCV (microcytosis) is suggestive of iron deficiency but may be seen in hemoglobinopathies such as thalassemia. A high MCV (macrocytosis) is suggestive of vitamin B_{12} or folate deficiency. If the MCV is elevated, vitamin B_{12} and folate levels should be assessed.

The serum ferritin level correlates with iron bound to tissue ferritin in the reticuloendothelial system. Serum ferritin does not carry or bind to iron, and its function is unknown. Serum ferritin is also an acute phase reactant, and it increases in the setting of acute or chronic inflammation, independent of tissue iron stores. The TSAT is a measure of circulating iron available for delivery to the erythroid marrow and is calculated by dividing the serum iron concentration by the total iron binding capacity (TIBC). The TIBC correlates with the serum level of transferrin, which is the major iron-carrying protein in the blood. A TSAT of less than 16% in an anemic patient with CKD is consistent with absolute or functional iron deficiency, both of which are characterized by decreased delivery of iron to the erythroid marrow. Absolute iron deficiency occurs in the setting of decreased total body iron stores and is accompanied by a serum ferritin level of less than 25 ng/mL in men and less than 12 ng/mL in women. Functional iron deficiency is seen in patients with a low TSAT and a normal or elevated serum ferritin. It may be a result of the pharmacologic stimulation of RBC production by ESAs, which causes iron demand by the erythroid marrow to outstrip the ability of the reticuloendothelial system to release iron to circulating transferrin. Functional iron deficiency may also result from the action of hepcidin in the setting of inflammation or infection. The hallmark of functional iron deficiency is that it responds to the administration of intravenous iron supplements, with an increase in Hb level and/or a decrease in ESA requirements despite the normal or elevated serum ferritin concentration. If the anemic patient with a low TSAT and a normal or high serum ferritin level does not respond to intravenous iron, the presumptive diagnosis is reticuloendothelial blockade, meaning that hepcidin has completely prevented the release of iron from macrophages to circulating transferrin. It should be noted that, although the diagnosis of iron depletion is based on a serum ferritin concentration of less than 25 ng/mL and that of iron deficient erythropoiesis is based on a TSAT of less than 16%, anemic CKD patients with considerably higher serum ferritin and TSAT levels have been shown to respond to iron supplements (see "Iron Therapy").

The reticulocyte count is a useful and inexpensive test to distinguish anemia caused by underproduction of RBCs from that caused by RBC loss or destruction. In the setting of EPO deficiency, RBC production is decreased, so most anemic patients with CKD would be expected to have a decreased absolute reticulocyte count (<40,000 to 50,000 cells per microliter of whole blood). An elevated reticulocyte count is inconsistent with EPO deficiency, and an evaluation for hemolysis and blood loss should be undertaken.

Although it would seem that demonstration of a decreased blood EPO level would secure the diagnosis of EPO deficiency, routine testing for EPO level in anemic patients with CKD is not recommended. The reason is that patients who respond to exogenous ESAs may have a normal or even an elevated EPO concentration, which may nevertheless be inappropriately low for the severity of their anemia, and the test is expensive. Therefore, it is recommended that EPO deficiency be a diagnosis of exclusion (i.e., negative evaluation for other treatable causes of anemia) in the anemic CKD patient. However, a cause other than EPO deficiency should also be considered if the severity of the anemia is disproportionate to the degree of reduction in kidney function or if leukopenia and/or thrombocytopenia is present.

Erythropoiesis-Stimulating Agents

After other treatable causes of anemia have been excluded and a diagnosis of EPO deficiency is inferred, the treatment of choice for anemic patients with CKD is an ESA. Recombinant human erythropoietin (rHuEPO, or epoetin) has been available since 1989 and has revolutionized the treatment of anemia in patients with CKD, who previously depended on blood transfusions and androgens. Although absorption of epoetin administered subcutaneously is incomplete, with degradation of some the protein before it reaches the circulation, the slower absorption and sustained serum epoetin levels make this route of administration 20% to 30% more effective than a comparable intravenously administered dose. Nonetheless, more than 95% of patients undergoing hemodialysis patients in the United States receive their epoetin by the intravenous route because of the painless convenience of the extracorporeal blood circuit compared with the sting of subcutaneous administration. The U.S. Food and Drug Administration (FDA) recommends intravenous ESA administration in hemodialysis patients because of the risk of pure red cell aplasia (discussed later) that is associated with the subcutaneous route for all currently available ESAs. In other parts of the world, epoetin is typically administered subcutaneously to hemodialysis patients because of the 20% to 30% dosage reduction compared with the intravenous route.

Patients with CKD who are not yet on dialysis and patients undergoing peritoneal dialysis usually receive epoetin subcutaneously. The package insert for epoetin recommends thrice-weekly dosing, because the clinical trials that were submitted for approval by the FDA involved hemodialysis patients who received the drug thrice weekly, with each dialysis. For CKD patients not on dialysis and peritoneal dialysis patients, thrice-weekly dosing is not practical; it is more painful because of the subcutaneous route, and it is not necessary, because clinical trials in these patients have shown epoetin to be effective without a dosing penalty when given every 1 to 2 weeks. Epoetin is effective in maintaining target Hb levels in 76% of CKD patients not on dialysis when administered as infrequently as every 4 weeks. It is recommended that the dose of ESAs be titrated by 25% once monthly to achieve the target Hb level. If the Hb concentration exceeds the target range, ESA doses should be decreased but not always discontinued or held. As indicated in **Figure 60-1**, the erythroid maturation cycle exceeds 8 days, so interruption of this pipeline with BFU-E and CFU-E apoptosis in the absence of an ESA will turn off RBC production long enough to possibly decrease the level of Hb to below the target range.

Darbepoetin-alfa is a bioengineered epoetin molecule with two additional N-linked carbohydrate side chains. It has a longer half-life and duration of action than epoetin. As with epoetin, recent studies have demonstrated that darbepoetin is effective in maintaining target Hb levels when administered as infrequently as every 4 weeks in selected patients. There appears to be no difference in subcutaneous versus intravenous administration in terms of efficacy. The side effect profile of darbepoetin is virtually identical to that of epoetin; both agents are associated with the development or exacerbation of hypertension in 20% to 30% of patients. The mechanism for the hypertension is multifactorial and is related to increased RBC mass, attenuation of the peripheral vasodilation associated with anemia, and, perhaps, a direct inhibitory effect on vascular endothelial vasodilatory mediators such as nitric oxide and prostaglandins. The existence or exacerbation of hypertension is not a contraindication to ESA therapy; rather, the hypertension should be treated with more aggressive pharmacologic therapy, increased ultrafiltration on dialysis, and/or a decrease in the ESA dose to slow the rate of Hb rise and allow for physiologic vasomotor adaptation. There is no evidence that the rate of vascular access thrombosis is increased in hemodialysis patients when ESA treatment is employed to maintain Hb levels within the currently recommended target range. All other side effects reported with ESA therapy are no greater than with placebo.

Pure Red Cell Aplasia

Pure red cell aplasia (PRCA) is a form of aplastic anemia that is caused by the production of anti-erythropoietin antibodies induced by administration of exogenous ESAs. The diagnosis of PRCA should be suspected in a patient with a sudden weekly drop in Hb of approximately 1 g/dL or a weekly transfusion requirement and low reticulocyte count (<20,000 cells/μL) despite a high dose of ESA for several months. In contrast to classic aplastic anemia, the white blood cell and platelet counts are preserved in PRCA. A definitive diagnosis of PRCA is made by the demonstration of anti-erythropoietin antibodies in the blood or a bone marrow examination revealing normal cellularity and less than 4% erythroblasts. Treatment includes discontinuation of the ESA and immunosuppressive therapy (e.g., cyclophosphamide); most patients respond after several months and do not relapse after the immunosuppressive therapy is discontinued. An episode of PRCA in Europe was traced almost exclusively to subcutaneous administration of a form of epoetin-alfa stabilized with Tween 80. This additive was never used in the United States, where PRCA has always been rare. With removal of this preparation from the European market, the incidence of PRCA fell dramatically.

Target Hemoglobin Level

The target Hb level for anemic patients with CKD treated with ESAs has been a subject of considerable controversy, because observational studies have disagreed with the results of interventional trials. Based on studies of epoetin efficacy in the early 1990s which compared outcomes in untreated patients with hematocrit (Hct) values in the mid-20s with those in treated patients with Hct values in the mid-30s, the first version of the NKF-K/DOQI anemia guidelines (1997) had an opinion-based recommendation that the target Hct

for epoetin-treated patients should be 33% to 36%. However, a number of observational studies from the United States Renal Data System (USRDS) and from large dialysis chain databases suggested that the benefits of higher Hct or Hb levels extend to levels greater than 39% and 13 g/dL, respectively, with quality of life increasing directly across the spectrum of Hct/Hb levels. In 1998, results from the Normal Hematocrit Study, which randomized 1223 hemodialysis patients with underlying cardiac disease receiving epoetin to a target Hct of 30% versus a target Hct of 42%, became available. The study was terminated early because of the low likelihood that the patients randomized to the higher Hct would show better outcomes. The patients in the higher Hct group had a relative risk of 1.3 (confidence interval, 0.9 to 1.9) for the primary end point, death or myocardial infarction. Furthermore, patients in the higher Hct group had a significantly greater incidence of vascular access thrombosis. Based on this study, the 2001 version of the NKF-K/DOQI anemia guidelines recommended a target Hb of 11 to 12 g/dL in ESA-treated anemic patients with CKD.

The Cardiovascular Risk Reduction by Early Anemia Treatment with Epoetin Beta (CREATE) study randomly assigned 603 patients with GFR of 15 to 35 mL/min/1.73 m^2 and a baseline Hb of 11 to 12.5 g/dL to one of two groups. Group 1 patients were immediately treated with epoetin-beta to a target Hb of 13 to 15 g/dL. Group 2 patients were treated only when their Hb fell to less than 10.5 g/dL to a target Hb of only 10.5 to 11.5 g/dL. There was no difference between the two groups in the primary end point, time to first cardiovascular event. Although there was no difference in the rate of decline in GFR between the two groups, patients in group 1 required dialysis more often. Patients in group 1 also had better general health and improved physical function, based on standard survey instruments. There was no difference between the two groups in combined adverse events.

The Correction of Hemoglobin and Outcomes in Renal Insufficiency (CHOIR) study was a much larger study in which 1432 patients with stage 4 CKD were randomized to a target Hb of 11.3 g/dL versus 13.5 g/dL. The average follow-up period was 16 months, and the study was terminated early due to safety concerns in the higher Hb group. The primary end point was a composite of death, myocardial infarction, hospitalization for congestive heart failure (without renal replacement therapy), and stroke. The patients in the higher Hb group had a significantly higher incidence of composite end point, congestive heart failure, death, and hospitalization (cardiovascular and all-cause). There was no difference between the groups in rates of stroke, myocardial infarction, or renal replacement therapy or in quality of life.

Based on the results of the CHOIR and CREATE studies, the FDA changed the package insert for epoetin and darbepoetin to state that the physician should "individualize dosing to achieve and maintain hemoglobin levels within the range of 10 to 12 g/dL" in patients with CKD. The FDA recommendations not withstanding, in 2007 the NKF- K/DOQI anemia workgroup published an updated recommendation that the Hb target for ESA-treated CKD patients should be 11.0 to 12.0 g/dL and a guideline (moderately strong evidence) that the Hb target should not exceed 13 g/dL.

Iron Therapy

Iron deficiency frequently coexists with EPO deficiency as a cause of anemia in patients with CKD who are not undergoing hemodialysis, and it almost universally develops in patients on hemodialysis because of blood losses in the extracorporeal circuit, frequent blood testing, oozing from vascular access sites after the dialysis needles are withdrawn, and vascular access surgical procedures. CKD patients not on hemodialysis may develop iron deficiency because of inadequate oral iron intake due to dietary protein restriction or loss of taste for red meat. Even if iron deficiency is not present at the time of initial anemia evaluation, it often develops after the initiation of ESA therapy, because the stimulation of new RBC production exhausts existing iron stores. Therefore, it is important to regularly monitor iron status with serum ferritin and TSAT levels monthly during initiation of ESA therapy and every 3 months after a stable Hb level has been achieved. As mentioned earlier, the target serum ferritin and TSAT levels for patients receiving ESAs are higher than those used to diagnose iron deficiency in the general population because of the phenomenon of functional iron deficiency induced by ESA-stimulated bone marrow RBC production. The target serum ferritin level recommended by the 2006 NKF-K/DOQI anemia guidelines is 200 ng/mL or greater for hemodialysis patients and 100 ng/mL or greater for non-hemodialysis patients receiving ESAs. The target TSAT level is 20% or greater in patients receiving ESAs with or without hemodialysis.

Supplemental iron can be administered orally or intravenously. Oral iron may be sufficient to achieve target iron parameters in non-hemodialysis CKD patients, because they do not have the ongoing blood losses of patients undergoing hemodialysis. However, even in non-hemodialysis CKD patients, oral iron may be ineffective because of compliance issues, side effects, and the magnitude of iron deficit. Commonly prescribed oral ferrous iron salts (sulfate, fumarate, gluconate) must be oxidized by stomach acid to the ferric form before they can be absorbed by the small intestine. This step may be impaired if stomach acid is buffered by food or an antacid or if the patient is taking a histamine–2 blocker or proton pump inhibitor. Therefore, oral iron salts should be administered 1 hour before or 2 hours after a meal. The minimal effective oral iron dose to repair iron deficiency is 200 mg of elemental iron daily, but each 325-mg tablet of ferrous sulfate contains only 65 mg of elemental iron, meaning that an iron-deficient patient must take at least three tablets daily in divided doses. The bioavailability of oral iron salts is only 1% to 2% of the administered dose in patients with elevated serum ferritin, so even a compliant patient may be unable to repair an iron deficit with an oral agent. Finally, oral iron salts are associated with gastrointestinal side effects

such as epigastric pain and constipation that may further limit compliance.

For non-hemodialysis patients with iron deficiency unresponsive to oral iron and for all hemodialysis patients receiving ESAs whose iron parameters are at or below target levels, intravenous iron therapy is recommended. Intravenous iron is currently available in the United States in three forms: iron dextran, iron sucrose, and iron gluconate. Iron dextran is the least expensive type, but it has been associated with fatal anaphylactic reactions, leading to a "black box" warning by the FDA and the need for a test dose of 25 mg at the time of the first administration. The absence of a reaction to the test dose makes it less likely, but does not guarantee, that the patient will not have an anaphylactic reaction to a therapeutic dose of iron dextran. An advantage of iron dextran is that it can be administered in doses as high as 1000 mg in a single session. This may be a consideration for non-hemodialysis patients who must travel a long distance to a health care facility to receive intravenous iron, and it saves veins for future hemodialysis vascular access because fewer infusions are required. Iron sucrose and iron gluconate have never been associated with a fatal anaphylactic reaction and do not require a test dose. However, they can be administered to a maximum of only 250 to 300 mg per session, so a non-hemodialysis patient with severe iron deficiency will require several infusions to replete iron stores. Iron sucrose and iron gluconate are preferred in hemodialysis patients whose regular visits and access to the circulation through the extracorporeal circuit make smaller and more frequent dosing appropriate. Iron sucrose and iron gluconate have been associated with nonfatal anaphylactic reactions, hypotension, and nausea/vomiting. For all of the currently available intravenous iron agents, the slower the infusion rate, the lower the incidence of side effects.

There are two intravenous iron preparations, ferumoxytol and ferric carboxymaltose, that can be given in rapid infusion doses of 500 to 1000 mg and are currently undergoing clinical trials. They have potential appeal to non-hemodialysis CKD patients with iron deficiency because they would allow decreased frequency and duration of clinic visits to receive intravenous iron therapy and would preserve veins for hemodialysis vascular access.

The Dialysis Patients' Response to IV Iron with Elevated Ferritin (DRIVE) study examined the efficacy of intravenous iron administration in hemodialysis patients who had Hb less than 11 g/dL on adequate ESA therapy, TSAT less than 25%, and a serum ferritin concentration of 500 to 1200 ng/mL. The study found that administration of eight 125-mg doses of iron gluconate resulted in more efficient erythropoiesis, with a more frequent rise in Hb levels, a decrease in ESA requirements, and adverse events comparable to those in a control group that received no intravenous iron. These findings suggest that there is a spectrum of responsiveness to intravenous iron which extends to patients with serum ferritin levels as high as 1200 ng/mL.

A number of concerns have been raised about the potential toxicity of intravenous iron supplements, including cellular and vascular damage resulting from oxidative stress and impaired white blood cell function based on in vitro studies. There has been evidence of increased urinary excretion of markers of tubular injury, but not increased albuminuria, in CKD patients receiving intravenous iron sucrose. However, observational studies have not demonstrated increased hospitalizations or mortality in hemodialysis patients receiving less than an average of 400 mg of intravenous iron per month, and intravenous iron therapy was not identified as a risk factor for bacteremia in hemodialysis patients in a multivariate analysis. Serial liver biopsies in patients with hemochromatosis revealed no significant organ injury when the serum ferritin level was less than 2000 ng/mL. The 2006 K/DOQI anemia guidelines suggested that decisions regarding intravenous iron therapy in patients with serum ferritin levels greater than 500 ng/mL should weigh ESA responsiveness, Hb concentration, TSAT level, and the patient's clinical status.

Resistance to Erythropoiesis-Stimulating Agents and Adjuvant Therapy

ESA resistance is defined as failure to achieve a Hb level greater than 11 g/dL despite an epoetin dose of more than 500 units/kg/wk or the equivalent of another ESA. The causes of ESA resistance are the same as the causes of anemia in CKD (see **Table 60-1**), with the obvious exception of erythropoietin deficiency and with the addition of PRCA. After iron deficiency, the most common cause of ESA resistance in patients with CKD is inflammation/infection. This is often associated with high levels of acute phase reactants such as serum ferritin and C-reactive protein and a high erythrocyte sedimentation rate, but the source of the inflammation/infection may not be readily apparent. It has been demonstrated that hemodialysis patients who use catheters for vascular access have lower mean Hb levels and higher mean ESA doses, which probably reflects the inflammatory state induced by the presence of the catheter and its biofilm even in the absence of positive cultures for pathogens.

There is insufficient evidence to support the use of adjuvants to ESA therapy, such as l-carnitine and vitamin C, in the management of anemia in patients with CKD. Although androgens were widely used to increase Hb levels in dialysis patients in the pre-ESA era, their use is not recommended because of insufficient evidence to support their efficacy in patients receiving adequate doses of ESAs and because of the potential for long-term toxicity.

Despite the use of adequate doses of ESA and iron therapy, transfusions with RBCs are sometimes required in the setting of ESA resistance or acute blood loss. Transfusion therapy is considered a last resort because of the potential for development of sensitization affecting future transplantation and the small risk of bloodborne infections. There is no single Hb concentration that necessitates transfusion, and the decision of whether and when to transfuse should be made based on the patient's individual situation, including comorbid illnesses, symptoms, acuity of Hb decrease, and potential for future transplantation as well as the Hb level.

OTHER HEMATOLOGIC MANIFESTATIONS OF KIDNEY DISEASE

Abnormalities of Hemostasis

Patients with advanced stages of CKD typically have normal results on coagulation studies and normal platelet counts, yet they exhibit an increased bleeding tendency because of defects in platelet function. This is manifested by a prolonged bleeding time, abnormal studies of platelet aggregation and adhesiveness, and decreased release of platelet factor 3. There may also be an abnormal interaction between platelets and vascular endothelium, mediated by decreased activity of von Willebrand's factor (vWF) as well as increased release of endothelial nitric oxide and prostacyclin in uremia. The clinical manifestations of these abnormalities include an increased tendency and increased duration of bleeding after trauma and in the setting of serosal inflammation. This often manifests as epistaxis, bleeding with tooth brushing, and easy bruisability, but it can result in life-threatening gastrointestinal hemorrhage or hemorrhagic pericarditis. The bleeding diathesis is only partially corrected by dialysis, and larger molecules that accumulate in the setting of renal failure, such has parathyroid hormone, have also been implicated. The anemia may also contribute to the bleeding diathesis of uremia, because higher RBC counts push platelets closer to the vessel wall, making them more effective. Treatment of anemia with RBC transfusion and/or ESAs to a Hb concentration greater than 10 g/dL has been shown to improve the bleeding diathesis. Platelet function has been shown to improve after the initiation of ESA therapy before the Hb rises, suggesting that ESAs may improve platelet function directly.

The treatment of choice for bleeding episodes in uremic patients is to provide adequate dialysis with minimal or no anticoagulation and to initiate ESA therapy. If bleeding continues or if the patient is at risk for bleeding from an invasive procedure, then treatment with desmopressin (dDAVP) should be considered. dDAVP is a synthetic form of antidiuretic hormone that has minimal vasopressor activity and is used in the treatment of diabetes insipidus. The mechanism of its action in the setting of uremic bleeding is thought to be related to the release of vWF from endothelial cells and platelets. The dose of dDAVP is 0.3 µg/kg intravenously or 3 µg/kg intranasally and can be repeated 1 to 2 times before tachyphylaxis develops. The onset of action is immediate, and the duration of action is 4 to 8 hours. More than half of patients treated with dDAVP respond with an improvement in bleeding time, and the reason for the lack of response in other patients is unknown. Because of the tachyphylaxis, it is recommended that dDAVP be given only once, immediately before an invasive procedure (and not the day before), to test its ability to correct the bleeding time. dDAVP tachyphylaxis appears to abate after 48 hours, and twice-weekly therapy has been shown to be effective in some patients with chronic bleeding.

Conjugated estrogens (Premarin) provide a duration of action up to 14 days, but the onset of action takes 6 hours.

The dose is 0.6 mg/kg daily for 5 consecutive days, and this regimen has been effective in controlling gastrointestinal bleeding associated with ateriovenous malformations in uremic patients. The mechanism of action is thought to be related to inhibition of vascular nitric oxide production.

Like dDAVP, cryoprecipitate provides vWF, but it is less convenient to use and carries the risk of bloodborne infections. The onset of action of cryoprecipitate is 1 hour, and its effect is maximal at 12 hours; the dose is 10 units and can be repeated as necessary. The response to cryoprecipitate is highly variable, and it should be reserved for life-threatening hemorrhage.

The platelet hemostatic defect in uremia does not appear to protect against vascular access thrombosis, which is a common problem in hemodialysis patients. The use of antiplatelet agents such as aspirin and clopidogrel to preserve vascular access may be associated with an unacceptably high rate of bleeding and is not recommended. Use of these agents for conventional indications, such as coronary artery and cerebrovascular disease, is not contraindicated in patients with CKD, although the benefit must be weighed against risk. Similarly, heparin and warfarin are frequently needed for conventional indications in patients with CKD, but the use of these agents superimposes a risk of bleeding on the underlying abnormalities of platelet function. It is estimated that the incidence of venous thrombotic and thromboembolic disease (exclusive of vascular access thrombosis) in patients with CKD is twice that of the general population. This is attributed to the complications of nephrotic syndrome with increased plasma fibrinogen and decreased plasma antithrombin III levels, the presence of systemic lupus with circulating "anticoagulants" such as antiphospholipid antibodies, elevated levels of homocysteine, venous injury from previous catheter placement, and the continued presence of intravascular "foreign bodies" such as dialysis catheters and arteriovenous grafts. Increased experience with enoxaparin in patients with CKD has simplified anticoagulation in certain settings, because monitoring of the partial thromboplastin time is not required. The dose of enoxaparin for CKD patients with GFR less than 30 mL/min/1.73 m^2 is 1 mg/kg SC daily for deep venous thrombosis (DVT) and acute coronary syndromes or 30 mg daily SC for DVT prophylaxis.

Abnormalities of Leukocytes

Except for a transient decrease in circulating granulocytes during the first 15 to 30 minutes of hemodialysis when older, unmodified cellulosic membranes are used, the white blood cell count of patients with uremia tends to be normal. The decrease in circulating granulocytes during unmodified cellulosic membrane hemodialysis is caused by alternative complement pathway activation, which leads to microleukoagglutination and margination of granulocytes in the pulmonary circulation. This may be responsible for the transient hypoxia that is sometimes observed during hemodialysis, and it is completely reversed by the end of the dialysis treatment. The function of granulocytes, including chemotaxis, adherence, phagocytosis, and production of reactive oxygen species is altered in uremia; these changes also may be exacerbated by exposure to unmodified cellulosic membranes. Impaired granulocyte function is associated with increased susceptibility to infection with encapsulated bacteria such as *Staphylococcus,* contributing to the high incidence of these types of infections in dialysis patients.

Monocyte and lymphocyte function are also impaired in uremia, leading to a decrease in cellular-type immunity. This can be manifested by an increased susceptibility to viral infections such as influenza, decreased response to vaccinations, and anergy to immunologic skin testing. The latter phenomenon makes it important to place control skin tests (e.g., mumps, streptokinase/streptodornase) when evaluating the response to tuberculosis skin tests. The activity of autoimmune diseases such as systemic lupus erythematosus may be attenuated after uremia supervenes. An impairment of cytokine release decreases the febrile response to pathogens in uremic patients, so that infections may go unnoticed and may become more serious before diagnosis. The clinical implication is that symptoms suggestive of infection must trigger an aggressive diagnostic and therapeutic response in this vulnerable population.

BIBLIOGRAPHY

Aronoff GR: Safety of intravenous iron in clinical practice: Implications for anemia management protocols. J Am Soc Nephrol 15(Suppl 2):S99-S106, 2004.

Berns JS, Mesenkis A: Pharmacologic adjuvants to epoetin in the treatment of anemia in patients on hemodialysis. Hemodialysis Int 9:7-22, 2005.

Besarab A, Amin N, Ahsan M, et al: Optimization of epoetin therapy with intravenous iron therapy in hemodialysis patients. J Am Soc Nephrol 11:530-538, 2000.

Besarab A, Bolton WK, Browne JK, et al: The effects of normal as compared with low hematocrit values in patients with cardiac disease who are receiving hemodialysis and erythropoietin. N Engl J Med 339:584-590, 1998.

Besarab A, Reyes CM, Hornberger J: Meta-analysis of subcutaneous versus intravenous epoetin in maintenance treatment of anemia in hemodialysis patients. Am J Kidney Dis 40:439-446, 2002.

Collins AJ, Li S, St. Peter W, et al: Death, hospitalization and economic associations among incident hemodialysis patients with hematocrit values of 36% to 39%. J Am Soc Nephrol 12:2465-2473, 2001.

Coyne DW, Kapoian T, Suki W, et al: DRIVE Study Group: Ferric gluconate is highly efficacious in anemic hemodialysis patients with high serum ferritin and low transferrin saturation: Results of the Dialysis Patients' Response to IV Iron with Elevated Ferritin (DRIVE) Study. J Am Soc Nephrol 18:975-984, 2007.

Drueke TB, Locatelli F, Clyne N, et al: Normalization of hemoglobin level in patients with chronic kidney disease and anemia. N Engl J Med 355:2071-2984, 2006.

Fishbane S, Berns JS: Hemoglobin cycling in dialysis patients treated with recombinant human erythropoietin. Kidney Int 68:1337-1343, 2005.

Horl WH: Clinical aspects of iron use in the anemia of kidney disease. J Am Soc Nephrol 18:382-393, 2007.

Jadoul M, Vanrenterghem Y, Foret M, et al: Darbepoetin alfa administered once monthly maintains haemoglobin levels in stable dialysis patients. Nephrol Dial Transplant 19:898-903, 2004.

National Kidney Foundation: K/DOQI clinical practice guidelines and clinical practice recommendations for anemia in chronic kidney disease. Am J Kidney Dis 47(Suppl 3):S1-S145, 2006.

National Kidney Foundation: K/DOQI clinical practice guidelines and clinical practice recommendations for anemia in chronic kidney disease: 2007 Update of hemoglobin target. Am J Kidney Dis 50:471-530, 2007.

McClellan W, Aronoff SL, Bolton WK, et al: The prevalence of anemia in patients with chronic kidney disease. Curr Med Res Opin 20:1501-1510, 2004.

Phrommintkul A, Haas SJ, Elsik M, et al: Mortality and target hemoglobin concentrations in anaemic patients with chronic kidney disease treated with erythropoietin: A metaanalysis. Lancet 369:318-388, 2007.

Provenzano R, Bhaduri S, Singh AK; PROMPT Study Group: Extended epoetin alfa dosing as maintenance treatment for the anemia of chronic kidney disease: The PROMPT study. Clin Nephrol 64:113-123, 2005.

Singh AK, Szczech L, Tang KL, et al: Correction of anemia with epoetin alfa in chronic kidney disease. N Engl J Med 355:2085-2098, 2006.

Wish JB: Assessing iron status: Beyond serum ferritin and transferrin saturation. Clin J Am Soc Nephrol 1(Suppl 1):54-58, 2006.

Wish JB, Coyne DW: Use of erythropoiesis-stimulating agents in patients with chronic kidney disease: Overcoming the pharmacological and pharmacoeconomic limitations of existing therapies. Mayo Clin Proc 82:1371-1380, 2007.

CHAPTER 61

Endocrine and Neurologic Manifestations of Chronic Kidney Disease

Jean-Paul Kovalik and Eugene C. Kovalik

ENDOCRINE MANIFESTATIONS

Chronic kidney disease (CKD), end-stage renal disease (ESRD), and kidney transplantation all affect the endocrine system. Alterations in signal-feedback mechanisms and in production, transport, metabolism, elimination, and protein binding of hormones occur, as do a variety of drug interactions (Tables 61-1 and 61-2). As a result, the levels of some hormones, including growth hormone, prolactin, and catecholamines, are elevated in CKD. In addition, hormonal assays may give aberrant results in patients with kidney disease if the assays cross-react with inactive metabolites that are excreted by the normal kidney but accumulate with a falling glomerular filtration rate (GFR). Glucagon and calcitonin are two examples.

Hypothalamic-Hypophyseal Axes

Thyroid Hormones

Thyroid abnormalities have been well documented in CKD patients. The prevalence of goiter as determined by thyroid ultrasound is close to 100% in renal transplant recipients, 50% in hemodialysis patients, and 25% in peritoneal dialysis patients. Plasma levels of total thyroxine (T_4) are normal or decreased, and triiodothyronine (T_3) levels are depressed. Plasma levels of free T_4 may be low without obvious clinical hypothyroidism. The use of plasma reverse T_3 (rT_3) to differentiate hypothyroid states from the euthyroid sick state is not helpful in patients with CKD, because rT_3 levels are often normal. These abnormalities tend to worsen with the progression of CKD, and they are normalized with renal transplantation. Plasma concentrations of thyroid-stimulating hormone (TSH) tend to be normal despite the abnormalities in thyroid hormone levels, and they are therefore the best indicator of thyroid function for the diagnosis of hypothyroidism or hyperthyroidism, especially with the use of ultrasensitive TSH assays. The basal metabolic rate, a reflection of thyroid status, is usually normal in patients with CKD.

TABLE 61-1 Pathogenetic Mechanisms of Endocrine Dysfunction in Chronic Kidney Disease

Increased Circulating Hormone Levels

Impaired renal or extrarenal clearance (e.g., insulin, glucagon, PTH, calcitonin, prolactin)

Increased secretion (e.g., PTH, aldosterone)

Accumulation of hormone protein fragments that may lack bioactivity (e.g., glucagon, PTH, calcitonin, prolactin)

Decreased Circulating Hormone Levels

Decreased secretion by diseased kidney (e.g., EPO, renin, 1,25(OH)$_2$ vitamin D$_3$)

Decreased secretion by other endocrine glands (e.g., testosterone, estrogen, progesterone)

Decreased Sensitivity to Hormones

Altered target tissue response (e.g., insulin, glucagon, 1,25(OH)$_2$ vitamin D$_3$, EPO, PTH)

EPO, erythropoietin; PTH, parathyroid hormone.

From Mooradian AD: Endocrine dysfunction due to renal disease. In Becker KL (ed): Principles and Practice of Endocrinology and Metabolism. Philadelphia, Lippincott, 1995, p 1759.

TABLE 61-2 Directional Changes of Hormones in Chronic Kidney Disease

Hypothalamopituitary Axis

GH ↑ prolactin ↑

Thyroid

TT$_4$ N or ↓, FT$_4$ N or ↓

TT$_3$ ↓, FT$_3$ ↓, rT$_3$ N, TSH N

Gonads

Testosterone ↓, spermatogenesis ↓

Estrogen N or ↓, progesterone ↓

LH N or ↑, FSH N

Pancreas

Insulin ↑, glucagon ↑

Adrenal Glands

Aldosterone N or ↓, cortisol N or ↑

ACTH N or ↑

Catecholamines N or ↑

Kidney

EPO ↓, renin ↓, 1,25(OH)$_2$ vitamin D$_3$ ↓

ACTH, adrenocorticotropic hormone; EPO, erythropoietin; FSH, follicle-stimulating hormone; FT$_3$, free triiodothyronine; FT$_4$, free thyroxine; GH, growth hormone; LH, luteinizing hormone; N, no change; rT$_3$, reverse triiodothyronine; TT$_3$, total triiodothyronine; TT$_4$, total thyroxine; TSH, thyroid-stimulating hormone.

From Lim VS: In Greenberg A (ed): Primer on Kidney Diseases. San Diego, Academic Press, 1994, p 315.

Although TSH levels are normal in patients with CKD, subtle abnormalities exist in the hypothalamic-hypophyseal axis. Exogenous thyrotropin-releasing hormone (TRH) stimulation produces a blunted TSH response. This reduced response is seen even in patients with a 50% reduction in the GFR. The usual nocturnal TSH surge is absent. Despite this blunted response to TRH, CKD patients who develop true hypothyroidism display an appropriate elevation of the TSH level. Peripheral conversion of T_4 to the more biologically active T_3 is diminished in persons with CKD. In experimental models using uremic rats, tissue T_3 levels are reduced, suggesting that peripheral organs are in a hypothyroid state. This is thought to be an adaptive response to protect against protein loss because administering T_3 to patients on maintenance hemodialysis resulted in worsened nitrogen balance. After kidney transplantation, thyroid function tests normalize, although some patients may still have an abnormal TSH response to TRH due to glucocorticoid suppression of TSH secretion.

Growth Hormone

Plasma levels of growth hormone (GH) are elevated in patients with CKD and ESRD, because of increased secretion and impaired clearance of the hormone. GH action is mediated primarily through insulin-like growth factor (IGF), a polypeptide hormone released by GH-responsive tissues. Total plasma levels of IGF are normal in CKD. However, patients with CKD have elevated levels of IGF-binding proteins and a decrease in levels of free bioactive IGF. Dynamic testing of the GH axis reveals several abnormalities. Oral glucose loading does not suppress GH levels, whereas intravenous glucose, glucagon, or TRH paradoxically increase GH levels. GH-releasing hormone (GHRH) and L-dopa infusions also cause prolonged and exaggerated responses in GH secretion. However, insulin-induced hypoglycemia does not stimulate GH secretion. Correction of anemia with erythropoietin corrects the paradoxic response of GH secretion to TRH and insulin-induced hypoglycemia, although the prolonged GHRH response remains. Several small trials of recombinant human growth hormone (rhGH) therapy have enrolled hemodialysis patients. Compared with placebo controls, patients receiving rhGH replacement showed improvement in nitrogen balance, increased lean body mass, and decreased fat mass.

In children, uremia results in growth retardation despite normal or elevated plasma levels of GH and IGF. Circulating levels of IGF-binding protein are elevated in children with CKD, resulting in decreased availability of free bioactive IGF. Contributing variables include protein malnutrition, chronic acidosis, recurrent infections, and hyperparathyroidism. Adequate nutrition, dialysis, and correction of acidosis and hyperparathyroidism improve but do not normalize growth. Kidney transplantation does not reverse the abnormal growth patterns observed in children, probably because of the effects of exogenous glucocorticoids used for immunosuppression. The availability and use of rhGH has greatly improved the well-being of children with CKD, restoring growth velocity and increasing muscle mass without adversely affecting epiphyseal closure. Use of rhGH does not affect glucose tolerance in children but does tend to aggravate preexisting hyperinsulinemia. The use of rhGH after kidney transplantation in children also significantly improves growth without increasing adverse events.

Prolactin

Prolactin secretion is normally inhibited by prolactin inhibitory factor (PIF), which is controlled by dopaminergic neurons. Basal plasma levels of prolactin are elevated up to six times normal in patients with CKD because of decreased dopaminergic activity. Many medications that have antidopaminergic effects also contribute to increased prolactin levels by decreasing the tonic inhibitory effects of dopamine. The major effects of increased prolactin levels are reflected in the reproductive abnormalities observed in CKD and ESRD patients: gynecomastia, impotence, and amenorrhea. Most of these effects are indirect and related to the inhibitory effect of prolactin on gonadotrophin release. Bromocriptine can reduce prolactin levels, but its effectiveness in relieving symptoms has not been well established. Side effects such as nausea and gastrointestinal upset lead to discontinuation of therapy in one third of patients. Erythropoietin therapy can normalize prolactin levels and may improve sexual dysfunction in men and menstrual regularity in women, although the mechanism of these effects is not well established.

Any medications (i.e., α-methyldopa, phenothiazines, neuroleptics, metoclopramide, and histamine$_2$-blockers, especially cimetidine) that can increase prolactin levels should be minimized or avoided if possible, particularly if gynecomastia becomes painful or cosmetically displeasing for male patients. As observed in pubertal boys, gynecomastia in men with CKD may be related in part to the increased estrogen-to-androgen ratio that commonly occurs in this setting. Mammography should be performed for patients with true gynecomastia (i.e., firm subareolar tissue rather than fat deposition), because breast cancer does occur, although rarely, in men. Alternative therapies for gynecomastia in men include subcutaneous mastectomies or breast bud irradiation.

Glucocorticoids

Patients with CKD exhibit normal to elevated levels of adrenocorticotropic hormone (ACTH) without clinical significance. The ACTH response to corticotropin-releasing hormone (CRH) can be blunted or normal. Correction of anemia with erythropoietin can lead to an exaggerated ACTH response to CRH. The standard ACTH stimulation test for diagnosing hypocortisolism is not affected by the uremic state.

Basal cortisol levels in CKD patients are normal. Circadian rhythm of cortisol secretion remains intact. The usual 1-mg oral low-dose overnight or 2-day dexamethasone suppression tests used to evaluate hypercortisolism do not suppress cortisol levels in patients with CKD, partly because of decreased oral absorption of the drug and an altered set point of the axis. The 1-mg intravenous or 8-mg oral high-dose overnight dexamethasone test can suppress cortisol levels in

CKD patients. Although insulin-induced hypoglycemia fails to raise plasma cortisol levels, the response to major stress such as surgery is preserved.

Gonadotropins

Effects in Male Patients

Loss of libido, impotence, testicular atrophy, gynecomastia, and infertility may occur in male patients with CKD or ESRD. Plasma testosterone is decreased, and testosterone-binding globulin levels are normal. Levels of luteinizing hormone (LH), which controls testosterone production, are increased. Plasma levels of follicle-stimulating hormone (FSH) are elevated, indicating that spermatogenesis feedback is impaired, and testicular biopsies confirm abnormal sperm maturation. Prolonged stimulation with human chorionic gonadotropin (hCG) can result in increased testosterone levels, suggesting some preservation of testicular reserve. The response to administration of LH-releasing hormone (LHRH) is unpredictable; blunted, normal, and exaggerated, prolonged responses have all been observed. It appears that a central hypothalamic insensitivity and peripheral testicular failure exist in men with CKD or ESRD. Hyperprolactinemia and elevated parathyroid hormone (PTH) levels may contribute to the combined central and peripheral defects in the hypothalamic-pituitary-gonadal axis.

Testosterone replacement therapy was a standard treatment for anemia resulting from kidney disease before the advent of recombinant erythropoietin. Past studies on testosterone therapy in hypogonadal men receiving hemodialysis showed up to a 24% improvement in hemoglobin values and increased dry weights and serum albumin values. A later study of hypogonadal male hemodialysis patients receiving erythropoietin found no benefit of testosterone therapy on erythropoietin dose, lean body mass, or sexual function. Patients in the treatment arm of the study failed to achieve therapeutic serum testosterone levels, suggesting issues with drug delivery or poor medication compliance. Treatment with erythropoietin can improve symptoms of fatigue, lack of energy, and decreased sexual function without affecting testosterone levels. Zinc deficiency was thought to contribute to hypogonadism, although replacement therapy has yielded various results. A trial of zinc supplementation can be attempted for those with documented zinc deficiency. Although kidney transplantation reverses many of the symptoms, the hypogonadism may worsen as a consequence of glucocorticoid administration.

Although impotence in the CKD population is related to impairments in testosterone secretion, it may also be caused by neuropathies or vasculopathies. Drugs that can contribute to impotence (i.e., β-blockers) should be discontinued or reduced in dose, unless there is a specific and compelling indication for the drug. Sildenafil and its newer analogues have significantly improved the ability to treat impotence and should be used as first-line agents. Because of their vasoconstrictor effects, cavernous injections should be used with caution in severely hypertensive patients. Unfortunately, many patients fail to respond to these measures and require vacuum erector devices or penile implants. **Figure 61-1** outlines an approach to sexual dysfunction in the male patient.

Effects in Female Patients

Women with CKD and ESRD may have diminished libido or an inability to achieve orgasms. Approximately one half of postpubertal women on dialysis become amenorrheic, and those who still have menses find their menstrual cycles progressively irregular and become anovulatory as kidney function declines. Fewer than 10% of women on dialysis have regular menses. Plasma levels of estradiol, estrone, progesterone, and testosterone are normal to low. FSH levels are normal with mildly elevated LH levels, resulting in an increased LH/FSH ratio that is similar to prepubertal patterns and in those with a defect in the positive hypothalamic feedback mechanism in response to estrogen. Without positive feedback, the midcycle LH and FSH surge fails to occur, and anovulation results. Nonetheless, women who have some residual kidney function and who are well dialyzed may become pregnant and carry to term, although the fetus tends to be premature and small for gestational age (see Chapter 50). Unlike premenopausal women, postmenopausal women with CKD or ESRD have the expected increases in LH and FSH. They also may have hyperprolactinemia. Hormone replacement therapy in postmenopausal women should follow the recommendations for women with normal kidney function.

Transplantation rapidly restores fertility to premenopausal women. Ovulation can start within a month of transplantation. Appropriate counseling should be undertaken to stress the need for contraception. Current guidelines call for women who wish to become pregnant to wait 2 years with stable renal function, no evidence of rejection, serum creatinine concentration less than 1.8 mg/dL with minimal immunosuppression, and normal or readily controlled blood pressure. Good data on the use of oral contraceptives in the transplant patient group are lacking. Referral to a gynecologist should be made if this mode of contraception is considered because of the possible increased risk of thromboembolic disease. **Figure 61-2** outlines an approach to sexual dysfunction in uremic women. The evaluation focuses on menstrual irregularities and decreased libido. The latter is more difficult to treat because it can be caused by a variety of factors, including systemic illness, psychological problems such as depression or anxiety disorders, relationship conflicts, partner performance, and fatigue. Besides hormonal evaluation that includes thyroid, prolactin, estrogen, and androgen profiles, mechanical issues such as dyspareunia should be addressed. Referral to a gynecologist or endocrinologist is useful.

Carbohydrate Metabolism

Patients with CKD can develop what has been called *pseudodiabetes*. The condition results from a combination of peripheral resistance to insulin, circulating inhibitors of insulin action, and decreased islet cell insulin release. Dialysis corrects these defects by improving tissue sensitivity to insulin and enhancing pancreatic insulin secretion. In contrast, diabetics with CKD and ESRD often find that their need for

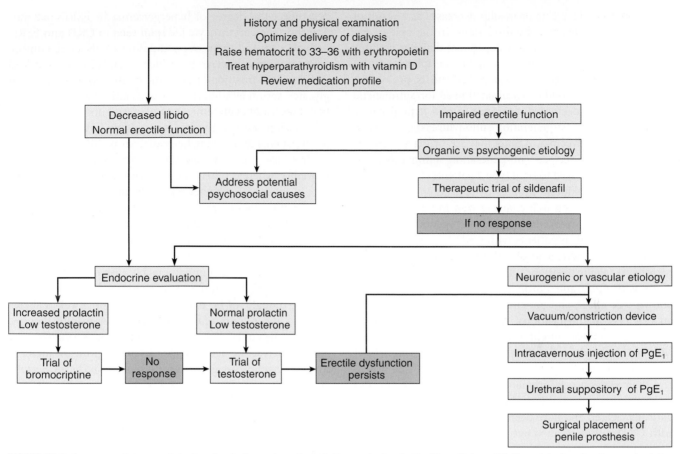

FIGURE 61-1 An approach to sexual dysfunction in the male patient. PgE$_1$, prostaglandin E$_1$. (From Palmer BF: Sexual dysfunction in uremia. J Am Soc Nephrol 10:1384, 1999.)

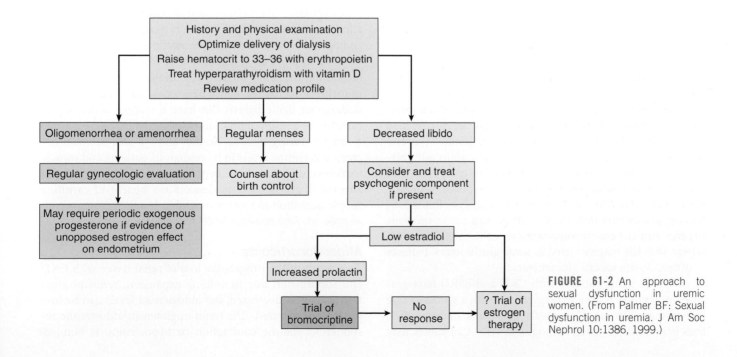

FIGURE 61-2 An approach to sexual dysfunction in uremic women. (From Palmer BF: Sexual dysfunction in uremia. J Am Soc Nephrol 10:1386, 1999.)

oral hypoglycemic agents or insulin decreases as a result of reduced insulin clearance by the kidney. In the case of patients with type 2, non–insulin-dependent diabetes mellitus (NIDDM), a condition mostly caused by peripheral insulin resistance, the endogenous insulin half-life is prolonged, resulting in a decreased or eliminated need for antidiabetic medication. The decreased clearance of oral hypoglycemic agents (i.e., most first-generation sulfonylureas) can lead to prolonged hypoglycemia. Agents that are primarily hepatically metabolized (i.e., second-generation sulfonylureas) or insulin should be used to treat type 2 patients.

The pharmacokinetic profiles of various insulin preparations have not been well characterized in CKD, and care should be used when employing these agents. Metformin is contraindicated in patients with CKD because of the increased risk for lactic acidosis. Thiazolidinediones decrease peripheral insulin resistance and appear safe to use in patients with CKD and ESRD, although fluid retention is a known side effect, and patients should be monitored while on this class of medications. Acarbose is not significantly absorbed, whereas miglitol can accumulate in patients with reduced kidney function. The clinical effectiveness of α-glucosidase inhibitors in CKD has not been established, and their use is not recommended. The short-acting insulin secretagogues repaglinide and nateglinide are primarily hepatically cleared and have been used successfully in patients with CKD, although an active metabolite of nateglinide accumulates in patients with impaired kidney function and can lead to hypoglycemia. Several newer agents act through glucagon-like peptide 1 (GLP-1), a gut-derived hormone that enhances physiologic pancreatic insulin release. Exenatide is a long-lasting GLP-1 analogue that is administered by subcutaneous injection. Exenatide is cleared renally, and its use is not recommended in patients with diminished kidney function. Sitagliptin is an oral inhibitor of dipeptidyl peptidase IV (DPP-IV), an enzyme that breaks down GLP-1. Although sitagliptin is primarily excreted by the kidneys, pharmacokinetic studies show that it can be used in a dose-reduced fashion in patients with CKD.

Type 1, insulin-dependent diabetes mellitus (IDDM) patients may need their insulin dose reduced, but never discontinued, because their underlying problem is a lack of endogenous insulin production. Glycemic control can worsen in peritoneal dialysis patients as a result of the glucose load absorbed from the peritoneal dialysis fluid. Results of several small studies suggest that intraperitoneal insulin administration leads to improved glycemic control compared with subcutaneous insulin injection but at the expense of slightly higher rates of peritonitis. New peritoneal dialysis fluids containing icodextrins instead of dextrose can cause spurious hyperglycemia, because some of the absorbed metabolites interfere with the reagents used in some glucometers. Patients may need to use special glucometers.

Although many patients with CKD and ESRD have glucose intolerance, fasting hyperglycemia with a glucose value higher than 126 mg/dL suggests that frank diabetes mellitus is present. Glycated hemoglobin (Hb A_{1C}) values may not reflect the degree of hyperglycemia in ESRD patients. The shortened erythrocyte life span seen in CKD and ESRD patients can lead to an overestimation of glycemic control, whereas uremia, hypertriglyceridemia, and acidosis may lead to an underestimation of glycemic control. Measurement of glycated serum albumin (i.e., fructosamine) levels may be a better indicator of glycemic control in patients with CKD. The relationship between glycated hemoglobin levels and mortality in patients undergoing hemodialysis is still unclear. Many studies have found no association between A_{1C} levels and mortality, whereas others found a paradoxic survival advantage in those with a higher A_{1C}. A recent retrospective study of a large dialysis database showed that after adjustment for comorbidities such as malnutrition and anemia, a higher A_{1C} value was associated with an increased risk for death.

Transplantation often reveals an underlying abnormality of glucose metabolism in patients because of the high doses of steroids used for immunosuppression. Patients not previously thought to be diabetic can develop frank diabetes mellitus and require oral hypoglycemic or insulin therapy. Those known to be diabetic may require conversion from an oral hypoglycemic agent to insulin or a significant increase in their insulin dosage because of steroid-induced peripheral resistance to insulin action. Calcineurin inhibitors can be diabetogenic, with tacrolimus use associated with higher rates of post-transplant diabetes compared with cyclosporine. Studies suggest that the incidence of de novo diabetes 2 years after kidney transplantation among cyclosporine users is 17.9%, compared with 29.7% for those patients taking tacrolimus.

Spontaneous and fasting hypoglycemia can occur in CKD and ESRD patients because of malnutrition, impaired glycogenolysis, carnitine deficiency, and reduced renal gluconeogenesis. Besides nutritional evaluation and supplementation, plasma carnitine levels should be measured, and a trial of supplementation should be attempted if levels are decreased and hypoglycemia persists despite efforts to improve inadequate nutrition. Carnitine is a quaternary ammonium compound synthesized from the amino acids lysine and methionine. It plays an essential role in energy metabolism by facilitating the entry of fatty acid molecules into the inner mitochondrial matrix, where beta oxidation occurs. Patients undergoing hemodialysis can have a relative deficiency of carnitine as a result of poor nutrition and increased carnitine clearance during dialysis. Studies show a link between decreased carnitine levels in hemodialysis patients and muscle weakness, dialysis-related hypotension, hyperlipidemia, and anemia. There is some evidence for a benefit of carnitine supplementation to raise hemoglobin levels in patients with anemia who are resistant to erythropoietin.

Mineralocorticoids

As a result of the progressive loss of renal tissue with CKD and suppression due to volume expansion, renin production usually is decreased, but aldosterone levels can be low, normal, or elevated. The renin-angiotensin-aldosterone response to volume contraction or hypotension is blunted.

Measurements of plasma renin levels are not particularly useful in evaluating hypertension in CKD patients. With low renin levels, hyperkalemia becomes the most important stimulus for aldosterone secretion, and aldosterone stimulates colonic loss of potassium, an often-overlooked means of potassium removal in CKD patients. The elevated serum levels of aldosterone may play a role in the progression of kidney disease because of their enhancement of high blood pressure and direct effects on mesangial and vascular collagen synthesis. Urinary aldosterone secretion is a strong predictor of urinary albumin secretion.

It is difficult to diagnose hyperaldosteronism in CKD patients as kidney disease progresses. Elevated 24-hour levels of urine aldosterone in the setting of new-onset hypertension should prompt adrenal imaging, followed by adrenal vein sampling if an aldosterone-producing adrenal adenoma is suspected.

Adrenal Medulla

Basal levels of catecholamines in CKD and dialysis patients are elevated because of several factors, including decreased degradation and decreased neuronal reuptake of catecholamines. Hemodialysis treatments remove catecholamines, although not in sufficient amounts to cause intradialytic hypotension in most patients. The diagnosis of pheochromocytoma is difficult in patients with CKD. Clonidine suppression testing has not been validated in this setting. The observation of high plasma levels of catecholamines should be combined with appropriate radiologic studies to make the diagnosis.

Lipids and Atherogenesis

In the absence of nephrotic syndrome, patients with CKD and ESRD infrequently have hypercholesterolemia or elevated levels of low-density lipoprotein (LDL) cholesterol, but hypertriglyceridemia is observed in one half of these patients. Conversely, levels of intermediate-density lipoprotein (IDL) and small, dense LDL cholesterol are increased partly as a result of decreased lipoprotein and hepatic lipase activities. Heparin administration during hemodialysis causes the release of hepatic and endothelial lipases, further depleting these enzymes and impairing the removal of plasma triglycerides. Low levels of high-density lipoprotein (HDL), which facilitates reverse cholesterol transport from peripheral tissues, are common. These changes lead to a qualitative difference in the lipid profile of patients with CKD and ESRD, with accumulation of atherogenic IDL and small, dense LDL and lowering of levels of protective HDL cholesterol. Nephrotic patients are an exception; they have elevated levels of LDL, IDL, and very-low-density lipoprotein (VLDL) cholesterol, whereas the level of HDL cholesterol is unchanged or lower. The lipid profile improves as the nephrotic syndrome improves. When kidney disease is active, these abnormalities are often resistant to treatment with statins.

Elevated levels of plasma lipoprotein(a) [Lp(a)] and homocysteine are considered to be independent risk factors for atherosclerosis in the general population. Studies of Lp(a) demonstrate increased levels in CKD and ESRD patients, but the isoform distribution is similar to that of patients without kidney failure. Production rates of Lp(a) are unchanged in CKD and ESRD patients, but plasma clearance is diminished. Plasma levels of homocysteine are elevated in 75% to 90% of peritoneal dialysis and hemodialysis patients. Isotope studies suggest that in hemodialysis patients, hyperhomocysteinemia is caused by a decrease in homocysteine remethylation to methionine rather than defects in the transsulfuration pathway. The hyperhomocysteinemia seen in hemodialysis patients has been associated with an increased risk of vascular access thrombosis. Lowering homocysteine levels through the use of folic acid and vitamin B_6 and B_{12} supplements did not improve survival or reduce the incidence of vascular disease in patients with CKD or ESRD.

Treatment of lipid disorders in CKD should follow the general guidelines used for patients with normal kidney function, because subgroup analysis from several major statin intervention trials has demonstrated cardiovascular benefit for patients with stage 1 through 3 CKD. Evidence for lipid-lowering therapy in ESRD is less clear. A large-scale trial of statin therapy to lower LDL cholesterol in hemodialysis patients with type 2 diabetes showed no benefit on the rates of cardiovascular death, nonfatal myocardial infarction, or all-cause mortality. Patients randomized to statin therapy had a slightly increased rate of fatal stroke. The results of the trial suggest that the pathogenesis of vascular disease in patients with type 2 diabetes who are on maintenance hemodialysis may be different from patients without ESRD. Patients with elevated LDL levels should be started on therapeutic lifestyle modifications and then advanced to pharmacologic therapy. Bile acid resin binders, such as cholestyramine and colestipol, should be avoided, because they may worsen hypertriglyceridemia. Fibric acid derivatives, such as gemfibrozil and clofibrate, are effective in lowering triglyceride levels but should be used with careful monitoring in CKD and ESRD patients, because they are cleared primarily by the kidney and their accumulation increases the risk of rhabdomyolysis, especially when used in combination with a statin. The safest agents are statins. High doses of statins may increase the risk of myalgias and rhabdomyolysis, and administration requires close patient follow-up. Because of its many side effects, such as insulin resistance and gastric irritation, nicotinic acid is not a good lipid-lowering agent in the CKD population. Experience with its use is limited, but it can be used with close follow-up.

Although initial studies demonstrated the possible protective effects of the antioxidant vitamin E on cardiovascular mortality in the general population, later randomized trials found no benefit of vitamin E in preventing cardiovascular events. A subgroup analysis found no benefit of vitamin E supplementation on cardiovascular outcomes in people with mild to moderate impairment of kidney function. However, a small clinical trial found that high-dose (800 IU/day) vitamin E supplementation in hemodialysis patients with preexisting cardiovascular disease resulted in a decreased incidence of myocardial infarction. Vitamin C also acts as an antioxidant, but its use in CKD and ESRD patients is relatively contraindicated. Vitamin C is metabolized into oxalate, which is excreted by the kidney. Consequently, patients with CKD and ESRD have decreased urinary oxalate excretion, and vitamin C supplementation can result in elevated serum oxalate levels or hyperoxaluria and stone formation.

In kidney transplant recipients, plasma total levels of cholesterol, triglycerides, LDL, oxidized LDL, Lp(a), and homocysteine are elevated, whereas HDL levels vary. In addition to the increased cardiovascular risks, post-transplantation lipid abnormalities may contribute to chronic graft rejection. Treatment of lipid abnormalities in transplant recipients is similar to that of CKD patients. Bile resin binders should be avoided because they interfere with cyclosporine absorption from the gastrointestinal tract. Fibrates increase the risk for rhabdomyolysis with a decreased GFR, particularly when used in combination with cyclosporine. Statins have been safely used in transplant recipients without major side effects. At least one study has shown a reduction in acute rejection episodes with the use of pravastatin. Patients receiving antioxidant therapy should have careful monitoring of immunosuppressant levels, because several small studies have demonstrated decreased blood trough levels of cyclosporine in transplant recipients taking supplements.

NEUROLOGIC MANIFESTATIONS

Nervous system dysfunction commonly occurs in CKD patients. The spectrum of abnormalities includes mild to severe alterations in the sensorium, cognitive dysfunction, generalized weakness, and peripheral neuropathies. These problems can occur before the initiation of dialytic therapy and can progress despite ostensibly adequate renal replacement therapy with dialysis.

Uremic Encephalopathy

Symptoms and Signs
The term *uremic encephalopathy* refers to the central nervous system (CNS) signs and symptoms that result from a decline in kidney function. The threshold for development of uremic encephalopathy is a fall in the GFR to a level below 10% of normal. Symptoms are more severe and abrupt in onset when associated with an acute rather than a chronic loss of kidney function. Psychomotor behavior, cognition, memory, speech, perception, and emotion can be affected. In this respect, uremic encephalopathy resembles and can be difficult to differentiate from organic brain syndromes due to other causes. Patients with kidney disease can develop hypertensive encephalopathy characterized by encephalopathic symptoms and severe hypertension. Rapid recognition and treatment with antihypertensive medications can lead to reversal of the neurologic dysfunction.

Fluid and electrolyte disturbances are common in patients with kidney disease and can mediate central nervous system depression. Drug clearance is altered in patients with kidney disease and can result in drug toxicity that leads to encephalopathy.

In patients with advanced liver and kidney disease, particularly those with hepatorenal syndrome, it is often difficult to determine whether the encephalopathy results from hepatic or renal causes, or both. In such patients, the blood urea nitrogen (BUN) and serum creatinine levels do not always reflect the degree of renal functional impairment. Mildly elevated levels of BUN and creatinine may underestimate the magnitude of the loss of kidney function due to malnutrition or a diminished capacity to generate urea and creatinine. The diagnosis of uremic encephalopathy in an acutely ill patient with hepatic failure may be made by exclusion of other causes, such as hypercalcemia, hypernatremia, hyponatremia, hyperglycemia, hypoglycemia, hypoxia, and hypercapnia, or made in retrospect after improvement is observed in response to dialysis or other specific therapy, such as treatment of hepatic encephalopathy or discontinuation of narcotics, benzodiazepines, or other medications that can affect the sensorium.

The initial neurologic presentation of patients with severe acute kidney injury may include signs of psychosis, lassitude, and lethargy, with disorientation and confusion occurring later. Physical findings may include cranial nerve signs, nystagmus, dysarthria, abnormal gait, and motor signs manifested by symmetrical and asymmetrical weakness, fasciculations, and asymmetrical variation in deep tendon reflexes. These findings may progress to asterixis and hyperreflexia with unsustained clonus at the ankle. Patients may have spontaneous myoclonus, and it has the same significance as asterixis. If uremia is left untreated and allowed to progress, seizures and coma often supervene.

Electroencephalograms (EEGs) in patients with severe acute kidney injury usually are grossly abnormal initially and are not improved by dialysis during the first few weeks of treatment. The EEG may remain abnormal for as long as 6 months despite apparently adequate renal replacement therapy. Completely normal tracings may not be reached until the patient receives a kidney transplant or recovers kidney function. Despite the presence of these abnormalities, the EEG is not useful for diagnosing uremic encephalopathy, because similar findings can be seen in other toxic and metabolic encephalopathies.

Pathogenesis
Although many influences may contribute to uremic encephalopathy, no precise correlation exists between the degree of encephalopathy and any of the commonly measured blood chemical components associated with kidney dysfunction (i.e., BUN, creatinine, bicarbonate, or pH). There are numerous potential or putative uremic toxins, including PTH and other nitrogenous wastes (see Chapter 52). Unfortunately, levels of these agents do not reliably correlate with the severity of symptoms.

Uremic Polyneuropathy

Neuropathy of some degree is probably present in about 65% of patients with CKD or ESRD. The findings may be subtle, and abnormal nerve conduction may occur in the absence of symptoms or physical findings. Specific questions about paresthesias, diminished sensation, sexual dysfunction, or presyncope may elicit a history of sensory or autonomic neuropathy that can be confirmed by careful physical examination. Uremic polyneuropathy is a distal, symmetrical, mixed polyneuropathy and is associated with a secondary demyelinating process in the posterior columns of the spinal cord and the CNS. Motor and sensory modalities usually are affected, and the lower extremities are more severely involved than the upper extremities. Dysfunction is usually maximal distally and is characterized by mixed motor and sensory abnormalities, resulting in weakness and wasting in the arms and legs with sensory changes in a glove and stocking distribution.

Like uremic encephalopathy, the pathophysiology of uremic polyneuropathy has not been well established, although many uremic toxins have been implicated. PTH and β_2-microglobulin have been associated with uremic polyneuropathy. More recent nerve excitability studies implicate the elevated potassium levels seen in CKD as a cause of neuropathy. Uremic neuropathy may in part be related to structural nerve damage of unknown origin and to the cumulative effects of multiple toxic agents over months to years.

Symptoms and Signs

The restless leg syndrome is a common early manifestation of kidney failure in patients with CKD. Clinically, patients experience sensations such as crawling, prickling, and pruritus in their lower extremities. The sensations are generally worse distally and are usually more prominent in the evening. Patients are awakened because they cannot find a comfortable sleeping position. The burning foot syndrome, which occurs in less than 10% of patients with kidney failure, represents swelling and tenderness of the distal lower extremities. The physical signs of peripheral nerve dysfunction often begin with loss of deep tendon reflexes, particularly in the ankle and knee. Sensory modalities that are lost include pain, light touch, vibration, and pressure. Clinically, uremic polyneuropathy cannot easily be distinguished from the neuropathies associated with diabetes mellitus, chronic alcoholism, and other nutritional deficiency states. The occurrence of uremic polyneuropathy bears no relationship to the type of underlying kidney disease. However, some disorders, including amyloidosis, multiple myeloma, systemic lupus erythematosus, polyarteritis nodosa, diabetes mellitus, and hepatic failure, can cause peripheral neuropathy and kidney disease.

Diagnosis and Treatment

Motor nerve conduction velocity has limited utility in detecting moderately impaired peripheral nerve function in CKD and ESRD patients because of a daily test variability of as much as 20%. Sensory nerve conduction velocity testing is more sensitive, but its performance can be painful.

No single treatment appears to be uniformly effective, probably because of the multifactorial causes of the neuropathies. Analgesics (e.g., nonsteroidal agents, cyclooxygenase 2 inhibitors), opiates, quinine, muscle relaxants, anticonvulsants (e.g., gabapentin, carbamazepine), antidepressants (e.g., tricyclics), anxiolytics (e.g., benzodiazepines), and antiarrhythmics have produced various results. Dopaminergic agents (e.g., ropinirole) and L-dopa may have specific benefit for restless leg syndrome. Often, a trial-and-error method is the only way to find the best therapy for an individual. There is no reliable evidence to suggest that increasing the intensity of dialysis in ESRD patients beyond the current standard ameliorates symptoms. Kidney transplantation leads to improvement in uremic neuropathy, although recovery may be slow and limited.

Uremic Mononeuropathy

Isolated or multiple isolated lesions of the peripheral nerves are designated as *mononeuropathies*, and they occur with increased frequency in patients with CKD and ESRD. The most common mononeuropathies involve the ulnar and median nerves. Damage to the ulnar nerve at the level of the wrist can lead to weakness of the intrinsic hand muscles and sensory loss along the hypothenar eminence. The presumed cause is compression of the nerve along Guyon's canal resulting from calcium deposition or ischemia from small-vessel vascular disease. Carpal tunnel syndrome develops when the median nerve is entrapped within the carpal tunnel. Symptoms and signs include pain and paresthesia along the ventral surface of the hand and first three fingers and thenar muscle atrophy. In patients with ESRD, median nerve entrapment in the carpal tunnel can be a result of calcium deposition, dialysis-associated amyloidosis, or placement of an arteriovenous shunt, which can increase venous pressure in the distal limb or cause ischemia of the nerve due to stealing of blood flow. Nerve conduction studies are useful in confirming the diagnosis.

Treatment involves conservative measures such as splinting the hand and use of anti-inflammatory medications. Local injection with corticosteroids can help with carpal tunnel syndrome, and surgical decompression is used to treat more refractory cases of ulnar and median nerve neuropathy. An acute femoral neuropathy occurs in up to 2% of patients after kidney transplantation and is a result of compression of the nerve during the procedure. Patients report weakness, pain, and sensory deficits in the thigh that frequently improve over time.

Autonomic and Cranial Nerve Dysfunction

Autonomic dysfunction is common in CKD and is usually associated with postural hypotension, impaired sweating, impotence, and gastrointestinal motility disturbances. Hemodialysis-associated hypotension is often associated with autonomic insufficiency, especially in patients with diabetes or amyloidosis. Heart rate response to the Valsalva maneuver, beat-to-beat heart rate respiratory variability, and vascular response to norepinephrine infusion can be used to evaluate autonomic dysfunction.

Cranial nerve involvement in uremia often manifests as transient nystagmus, miosis, heterophoria (i.e., tendency for the eyes to deviate from parallel), and facial asymmetry. Involvement of cranial nerve VIII, including auditory and vestibular functions, can occur and must be differentiated from deafness due to hereditary nephritis and drug ototoxicity such as that caused by aminoglycosides or high-dose furosemide regimens.

Cognitive Dysfunction

Cognitive dysfunction is not well characterized and has no distinctive anatomic lesions. On the basis of psychological testing, progressive loss of kidney function is associated with loss of cognitive function. Because CKD patients are often older, they are also susceptible to other conditions that can cause a decline in intellectual function, such as Alzheimer's disease, multi-infarct dementia, and chronic alcoholism. It is often difficult to clearly establish a cause for the declining intellectual function.

Complications of Dialysis Therapy

Dialysis Disequilibrium Syndrome

Several CNS disorders may occur as a consequence of dialytic therapy. One such disorder is dialysis disequilibrium syndrome (DDS), which can occur acutely in patients who have recently initiated hemodialysis, usually during or after the first several treatments. The symptom complex varies and may include muscle cramps, anorexia, restlessness, dizziness, headache, nausea, emesis, blurred vision, muscular twitching, disorientation, hypertension, tremors, seizures, and obtundation. It occurs most often in the elderly and in children. The syndrome usually is associated with intense initiation of hemodialysis, but it is rarely seen today because of a more gradual and earlier initiation of hemodialysis. DDS has not been described in peritoneal dialysis patients.

It is thought that DDS results from overly rapid correction of plasma osmolality, causing cerebral edema. As kidney function declines, the brain increases intracellular osmolality to protect itself from the associated extracellular hyperosmolality. If brain osmolality did not increase, the brain would lose water and shrink. Such a reduction in brain volume is undesirable, because it can lead to intracranial hemorrhage. The brain increases intracellular osmolality by generating intracellular amino acids, methylamines, and polyols, collectively called the *idiogenic osmoles*. A similar process occurs with hyperglycemia and hypernatremia. Any treatment, such as hemodialysis, that acutely lowers plasma osmolality without allowing adequate time for the internal removal of neuronal intracellular idiogenic osmoles generates a brain-to-plasma osmolar gradient, which can result in water uptake by the brain and cerebral edema.

To avoid DDS, nephrologists typically select an initial dialysis prescription that is deliberately inefficient (i.e., shortened treatment time and a dialyzer with a low blood flow rate and small surface area) to permit a gradual lowering of the plasma-to-CNS osmolar gradient and allow the brain to dissipate the idiogenic osmoles. During subsequent treatments, the duration of dialysis and the blood flow rate and surface area of the dialyzer are increased. Other measures to prevent DDS include ultrafiltration to remove fluid without altering serum osmolality, followed by dialysis and the intravenous bolus administration of mannitol or glucose during dialysis.

Dialysis Dementia

Dialysis dementia is a progressive, frequently fatal neurologic disease that is seen almost exclusively in patients who are chronically treated with hemodialysis. Dialysis dementia can occur in isolation or in association with osteomalacia, proximal myopathy, and anemia, and it occurs in three settings: an epidemic form, a sporadic form, and with childhood kidney disease. Initial symptoms of this disorder include dysarthria, apraxia, and slurring of speech with stuttering and hesitancy. Later in the course of the disease, symptoms progress to personality changes, psychosis, myoclonus, seizures, and eventually dementia and death within 6 months after the onset of symptoms. The diagnosis of dialysis dementia depends on the presence of the typical clinical picture, the characteristic electroencephalographic findings (i.e., multifocal bursts of high-amplitude delta activity with spikes and sharp waves), and most importantly, exclusion of other causes of CNS dysfunction.

The epidemic form of dialysis dementia, which occurred mainly in the 1970s, has been clearly linked to aluminum. Aluminum content in the brain is more than threefold greater in patients with dialysis dementia than in those on chronic hemodialysis without dementia. Aluminum sources include drinking water, cooking pots, and medications such as aluminum-containing antacids and sucralfate. Coadministration of citrate increases aluminum absorption from the gastrointestinal tract. Before deionization of the water used in hemodialysis became routine, most of the aluminum in dialysis patients came from dialysate water. Numerous patients in units that did not remove aluminum from source water developed dialysis dementia along with painful fracturing osteomalacia as a result of aluminum toxicity on the bone. This epidemic form of dialysis dementia disappeared after its relationship to aluminum exposure was established and water purification standards were upgraded accordingly. The sporadic form occurred in patients who had been on chronic hemodialysis for more than 2 years, and it was thought to be caused by long-term exposure to aluminum-based phosphate binders and aluminum in drinking water. Deionization of dialysate water removes aluminum, cadmium, mercury, lead, manganese, copper, nickel, thallium, boron, and tin. In addition to aluminum, several other trace elements and minerals may be involved in the pathogenesis of dialysis dementia. Fortunately, with improved water treatment and the elimination of routine use of aluminum-containing antacids, dialysis dementia has become rare. Yearly testing is recommended for aluminum overload in dialysis patients. Those with elevated serum levels can undergo the low-dose deferoxamine test to diagnose aluminum overload. Infusion of deferoxamine results in liberation of aluminum stored in tissues. Aluminum overload is diagnosed when post-treatment serum aluminum levels rise above a predefined threshold.

Dialysis dementia has been reported in children with kidney failure. Many received high doses of oral aluminum-containing phosphate binders, but some were neither on dialysis nor exposed to aluminum. In post-transplantation pediatric patients with neurodevelopmental deficits, serum aluminum levels were no different from levels found in patients with normal school performance. Encephalopathy in children with CKD and ESRD therefore cannot be ascribed to aluminum alone and may represent developmental neurologic defects resulting from exposure of the growing brain to the uremic milieu.

Treatment of Dialysis Complications

Although diazepam and clonazepam appear to be useful in controlling initial seizure activity associated with dialysis dementia, the drugs usually become ineffective and do not appear to alter the usually fatal outcome. Intravenous administration of deferoxamine chelates aluminum and promotes its removal during hemodialysis. Improvement in symptoms has been reported for several patients treated with deferoxamine.

BIBLIOGRAPHY

Andreoli SP, Bergstein JM, Sherrard DJ: Aluminum intoxication from aluminum containing phosphate binders in children with azotemia not undergoing dialysis. N Engl J Med 310:1079-1084, 1984.

Arieff AI: Dialysis disequilibrium syndrome: Current concepts on pathogenesis and prevention. Kidney Int 45:629-635, 1994.

Blackhall ML, Fassett RG, Sharman JE, et al: Effects of antioxidant supplementation on blood cyclosporine A and glomerular filtration rate in renal transplant recipients. Nephrol Dial Transplant 20:1970-1975, 2005.

Boaz M, Smetana S, Weinstein T, et al: Secondary Prevention with Antioxidants of Cardiovascular Disease in Endstage Renal Disease (SPACE): Randomized placebo-controlled trial. Lancet 356:1213-1218, 2000.

Bostom AG, Gohh RY, Tsai MY, et al: Excess prevalence of fasting and postmethionine-loading hyperhomocysteinemia in stable renal transplant recipients. Atheroscler Thromb Vasc Biol 17:1894-1900, 1997.

Brockenbrough AT, Dittrich MO, Page ST, et al: Transdermal androgen therapy to augment EPO in the treatment of anemia of chronic renal disease. Am J Kidney Dis 47:251-262, 2006.

Brouns R, DeDeyn PP: Neurological complications in renal failure: A review. Clin Neurol Neurosurg 107:1-16, 2004.

Deck KA, Fischer B, Hillen H: Studies on cortisol metabolism during hemodialysis. Eur J Clin Invest 9:203-207, 1979.

Dember LM, Jaber BL: Dialysis-related amyloidosis: Late finding or hidden epidemic. Semin Dial 19:105-109, 2006.

D'Haese PC, Couttenye MM, Goodman WG, et al: Use of the low-dose desferrioxamine test to diagnose and differentiate between patients with aluminum-related bone disease, increased risk for aluminum toxicity, or aluminum overload. Nephrol Dial Transplant 10:1874-1884, 1995.

Fraser CL, Arieff AI: Nervous system complications in uremia. Ann Intern Med 109:143-153, 1988.

Frystyk J, Ivarsen P, Skjaerbaek C, et al: Serum-free insulin-like growth factor I correlates with clearance in patients with chronic renal failure. Kidney Int 56:2076-2084, 1999.

Grundy SM: Management of hyperlipidemia of kidney disease. Kidney Int 37:847-853, 1990.

Haffner D, Nissel R, Wuhl E, et al: Metabolic effects of long-term growth hormone treatment in pubertal children with chronic renal failure and after kidney transplantation. Pediatr Res 43:209-215, 1998.

Hansen TB, Gram J, Jensen PB, et al: Influence of growth hormone on whole body and regional soft tissue composition in adult patients on hemodialysis: A double-blind, randomized, placebo-controlled study. Clin Nephrol 53:99-107, 2000.

Holdsworth S, Atkins RC, Kretser DM: The pituitary-testicular axis in men with chronic renal failure. N Engl J Med 296:1245-1249, 1977.

Hostetter T, Ibrahim H: Aldosterone in chronic kidney and cardiac disease. Kidney Int 14:2395-2401, 2003.

Inaba M, Okuno S, Kumeda Y, et al: Glycated albumin is a better glycemic indicator than glycated hemoglobin values in hemodialysis patients with diabetes: Effect of anemia and erythropoietin injection. J Am Soc Nephrol 18:896-903, 2007.

Jamison RL, Hartigan P, Kaufman JS, et al: Effect of homocysteine lowering on mortality and vascular disease in advanced chronic kidney disease and end-stage renal disease. JAMA 298:1163-1170, 2007.

Joy MS, Cefalu WT, Hogan SL, et al: Long-term glycemic control measurements in diabetic patients receiving hemodialysis. Am J Kidney Dis 39:297-307, 2002.

Kalantar-Zadeh K, Kopple JD, Regidor DL, et al: Hemoglobin A_{1c} and survival in maintenance hemodialysis patients. Diabetes Care 30:1049-1055, 2007.

Kalantar-Zadeh K, Kovesdy CP, Derose SF, et al: Racial and survival paradoxes in chronic kidney disease. Nature Clin Pract Nephrol 3:493-506, 2007.

Katznelson S, Wilkinson AH, Kobashigawa JA, et al: The effect of pravastatin on acute rejection after kidney transplantation: A pilot study. Transplantation 61:1469-1474, 1996.

Kokot F, Wiecek A, Grzeszczak W, et al: Influence of erythropoietin treatment on function of the pituitary-adrenal axis and somatotropin secretion in hemodialyzed patients. Clin Nephrol 33:241-246, 1990.

Krishnan AV, Kiernan MC: Uremic neuropathy: Clinical features and new pathophysiological insights. Muscle Nerve 35:273-290, 2007.

Kwan BCH, Kronenberg F, Beddu S, et al: Lipoprotein metabolism and lipid management in chronic kidney disease. J Am Soc Nephrol 18:1246-1261, 2007.

Lebkowska U, Malyszko J, Mysliwiec M: Thyroid function and morphology in kidney transplant recipients, hemodialyzed and peritoneally dialyzed patients. Transplant Proc 35:2945-2948, 2003.

Lim VS: Reproductive function in patients with renal insufficiency. Am J Kidney Dis 9:363-367, 1987.

Lim VS, Flanigan MJ, Zavala DC, et al: Protective adaptation of low serum triiodothyronine in patients with chronic renal failure. Kidney Int 28:541-549, 1985.

Mann JF, Lonn EM, Yi Q, et al: Effect of vitamin E on cardiovascular outcomes in people with mild-to-moderate renal insufficiency: Results of the HOPE study. Kidney Int 65:1375-1380, 2004.

Massey ZA, Kasiske BL: Post-transplant hyperlipidemia: Mechanisms and management. J Am Soc Nephrol 7:971-977, 1996.

Moustapha A, Gupta A, Robinson K, et al: Prevalence and determinants of hyperhomocysteinemia in hemodialysis and peritoneal dialysis. Kidney Int 55:1470-1475, 1999.

Nakao T, Matsumoto H, Okada T, et al: Influence of erythropoietin treatment on hemoglobin A_{1c} levels in patients with chronic renal failure on hemodialysis. Intern Med 37:826-830, 1998.

Nevalainen PI, Lahtela JT, Mustonen J, et al: Subcutaneous and intraperitoneal insulin therapy in diabetic patients on CAPD. Perit Dial Int 16:S288-S291, 1996.

N'Gankam V, Uehlinger U, Dick B, et al: Increased cortisol metabolites and reduced activity of 11β-hydroxysteroid dehydrogenase in patients on hemodialysis. Kidney Int 61:1859-1866, 2002.

Palmer BF: Sexual dysfunction in uremia. J Am Soc Nephrol 10:1381-1388, 1999.

Ponticelli C, Campise MR: Neurological complications in kidney transplant recipients. J Nephrol 18:521-528, 2005.

Pupim LB, Flakoll PJ, Yu C, et al: Recombinant human growth hormone improves muscle amino acid uptake and protein metabolism in chronic hemodialysis patients. Am J Clin Nutr 82:1235-1243, 2005.

Qvist E, Pihko H, Fagerudd P, et al: Neurodevelopmental outcome in high-risk patients after renal transplantation in early childhood. Pediatr Transplant 6:53-62, 2002.

Ramirez G: Abnormalities in the hypothalamic-hypophyseal axes in patients with chronic renal failure. Semin Dial 7:138-146, 1994.

Ramirez G, Butcher DE, Newton JL, et al: Bromocriptine and the hypothalamic hypophyseal function in patients with chronic renal failure on chronic hemodialysis. Am J Kidney Dis 6:111-118, 1985.

Schaefer RM, Kokot F, Geiger H, et al: Improved sexual function in hemodialysis patients on recombinant erythropoietin: A possible role for prolactin. Clin Nephrol 31:1-5, 1989.

Sechi LA, Zingaro L, Catena C, et al: Lipoprotein(a) and apolipoprotein(a) isoforms and proteinuria in patients with moderate renal failure. Kidney Int 56:1049-1057, 1999.

Shemin D, Lapane KL, Bausserman L, et al: Plasma homocysteine and hemodialysis access thrombosis: A prospective study. J Am Soc Nephrol 10:1095-1099, 1999.

Snyder RW, Berns JS: Use of insulin and oral hypoglycemic medications in patients with diabetes mellitus and advanced kidney disease. Semin Dial 17:365-370, 2004.

Tonelli M, Isles C, Curhan GC, et al: Effect of pravastatin on cardiovascular events in people with chronic kidney disease. Circulation 110:1557-1563, 2004.

Van Guldener C, Kulik W, Berger R, et al: Homocysteine and methionine metabolism in ESRD: A stable isotope study. Kidney Int 56:1064-1071, 1999.

Vanholder R, De Smet R, Glorieux G, et al: Review on uremic toxins: Classification, concentration, and interindividual variability. Kidney Int 63:1934-1943, 2003.

Wanner C, Krane V, Marz W, et al: Atorvastatin in patients with type 2 diabetes mellitus undergoing hemodialysis. N Engl J Med 353:238-248, 2005.

Woodward RS, Schnitzler MA, Baty J, et al: Incidence and cost of new onset diabetes mellitus among US wait-listed and transplant renal allograft recipients. Am J Transplant 3:590-598, 2003.

Wrone EM, Hornberger JM, Zehnder JL, et al: Randomized trial of folic acid for prevention of cardiovascular events in end-stage renal disease. J Am Soc Nephrol 15:420-426, 2004.

CHAPTER 62

Selection of Prospective Kidney Transplant Recipients

Bertram L. Kasiske and Jeffrey J. Connaire

Compared with patients awaiting kidney transplantation, patients who have received a kidney transplant usually survive longer and have a better quality of life. This is true regardless of age, gender, race or ethnicity, or cause of kidney disease. Therefore, transplantation is probably the treatment of choice for most patients with end-stage renal disease (ESRD). Nevertheless, not all patients are suitable for transplantation, and a patient's nephrologist usually performs the initial evaluation to decide if and when to refer a patient to a transplantation center.

WHO IS A CANDIDATE FOR KIDNEY TRANSPLANTATION?

There are few absolute contraindications for kidney transplantation. No absolute age precludes transplantation, and patients older than 50 years of age are the most rapidly growing segment of the waiting list for deceased-donor transplants (**Fig. 62-1**). However, physiologic age and overall health status should be carefully considered, especially in individuals who are older than 60 years. Probably the most common reason to decline referral is that the patient's overall condition is so poor that the patient is not expected to survive, even with a transplant, for more than 2 years. This group may include patients who are severely debilitated, patients with incurable cancer, and patients with severe cardiovascular disease that is not amenable

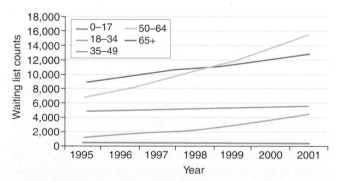

FIGURE 62-1 Growth in the deceased-donor kidney transplantation waiting list count in United Network for Organ Sharing, 1995-2005, by recipient age in years.

(Data from United States Renal Data System: USRDS 2007 Annual Data Report: Atlas of End-Stage Renal Disease in the United States. Bethesda, MD, National Institutes of Health, National Institute of Diabetes and Digestive Kidney Diseases, 2007.)

to treatment. In questionable cases, it is best to refer the patient to the transplantation center and to make it clear to the center and the patient that the purpose of the referral is to consider whether transplantation is suitable and that the referral will not necessarily result in the patient's approval for transplantation.

EARLY REFERRAL

Early referral to a transplantation center is important. Patient and allograft survival rates are better for patients who undergo transplantation before they begin chronic maintenance dialysis (i.e., pre-emptive transplantation) than for patients who receive transplants after they initiate dialysis. It is equally important to be sure that the transplantation candidate has ESRD. A small percentage of patients presenting with presumed ESRD (e.g., patients with renal vascular disease or interstitial nephritis) may regain function. Knowing the cause of kidney disease (e.g., type 1 diabetes typically progresses inexorably) and the rate of decline in estimated kidney function can help to determine when a patient should be referred to a transplantation center. The rate of decline can be ascertained in the clinic by plotting time versus the reciprocal of serum creatinine concentration or estimated glomerular filtration rate (GFR), as determined by the Modification of Diet in Renal Disease (MDRD) equation (see Chapter 2).

Patients with stage 3 or 4 chronic kidney disease (CKD) should be referred to a nephrologist, and patients with stage 4 CKD should be referred by their nephrologist to a transplantation center, unless they are clearly not candidates for the procedure. Stage 3 refers to patients with an estimated GFR of 30 to 59 mL/min/1.73 m^2. Stage 4 refers to patients with an estimated GFR of 15 to 29 mL/min/1.73 m^2. In the United States, patients can begin accumulating waiting time on the United Network for Organ Sharing (UNOS) waiting list for a deceased-donor transplant when the measured or estimated GFR is 20 mL/min or lower. In general, it is better to refer too early than too late.

WHO IS A CANDIDATE FOR PANCREAS TRANSPLANTATION?

Patients whose quality of life is poor because they have diabetes that is difficult to control may wish to consider pancreas transplantation. Pancreas transplantation undertaken before kidney transplantation may be appropriate for some, but it may accelerate the decline in native kidney function by the use of immunosuppressive agents such as calcineurin inhibitors. Simultaneous deceased-donor kidney and pancreas transplantation usually requires that the patient spend time waiting for an available kidney. Because the waiting time for a deceased-donor pancreas is much shorter than the waiting time for a kidney, many patients choose to have a living-donor kidney followed by a deceased-donor pancreas transplantation. In one analysis of UNOS and Organ Procurement and Transplantation Network (OPTN) data, this strategy, compared with wait-listed individuals, was associated with a higher mortality rate than simultaneous pancreas and kidney transplantation. A subsequent analysis refuted this finding. In a 2004 retrospective analysis of 47 pancreas-after-kidney transplantations, the corrected iothalamate GFR declined from 63 mL/min/1.73 m² before to 36 mL/min/1.73 m² after transplantation. The GFR was significantly worse than in the simultaneous pancreas and kidney transplantation reported in that series. Pancreas-after-kidney transplantation must weigh the potential of effects on the kidney allograft against the improved glycemic control and quality of life offered by pancreas transplantation.

Although pancreas transplantation may prevent recurrence of diabetic nephropathy, recurrent diabetic nephropathy is rarely the cause of kidney graft failure. Stabilization or improvement of diabetic retinopathy has been reported after pancreas transplantation and after kidney and pancreas transplantation in case-control series, but pancreas transplantation has not been compared with intensive efforts to medically optimize glycemic control. Patients should understand that the reason for pancreas transplantation is to improve the quality of life, not to prevent chronic diabetic complications. It has never been shown that the additional risk of pancreas transplantation outweighs any benefits with regard to long-term complications. Moreover, diabetes control may be improved, and some long-term complications may be reduced by kidney transplantation alone.

RISK OF RECURRENT KIDNEY DISEASE

Many kidney diseases other than diabetes recur after transplantation, but rarely does the risk of recurrence prohibit transplantation. Recurrent disease and its association with allograft loss were carefully studied in an Australian series of 1505 patients with biopsy-proven glomerulonephritis as a cause of their original kidney failure. The rate of allograft loss due to recurrent disease at 10 years was low, with only 8.4% being lost to recurrent disease. The 10-year allograft loss rate was not different for patients with glomerulonephritis as a cause of kidney failure versus patients with other causes of kidney failure, but recurrent disease did supersede acute rejection as a cause of late graft loss.

The most common cause of recurrence that results in graft failure is idiopathic focal segmental glomerulosclerosis (FSGS). The risk of recurrence in the first kidney transplant is probably about 25% to 30%. However, patients who have lost a transplanted kidney because of recurrent FSGS have at least a 50% chance of losing the second transplant to FSGS, and these odds probably increase with each subsequent transplant. Therapy with plasma exchange may reduce proteinuria from recurrent FSGS and may prolong the life of the graft. Plasma exchange is thought to act by removing a glomerular permeability factor that causes proteinuria in some patients with idiopathic FSGS.

Patients with nondiarrheal hemolytic uremic syndrome or thrombotic thrombocytopenic purpura may have recurrence of the disease after transplantation. However, the true rate of recurrence is difficult to ascertain, because the syndrome can also be caused by the immunosuppressive agents cyclosporine, tacrolimus, and probably sirolimus.

Type 1 membranoproliferative glomerulonephritis (MPGN) recurs in 20% to 30% of transplant recipients, whereas type 2 MPGN (i.e., dense-deposit disease) recurs in 90% to 100%. Type 2 MPGN is an example of how recurrent disease may not always equate with poor allograft outcome. None of 18 allografts in the Australian series was lost to recurrent disease at 10 years. Membranous nephropathy recurs in approximately 25% of transplant recipients.

Immunoglobulin A (IgA) nephropathy and Henoch-Schönlein purpura frequently cause IgA deposition in the transplanted kidney, but they infrequently cause graft failure. The estimated recurrence rate of clinically apparent IgA nephropathy (associated with elevated serum levels of creatinine or proteinuria) is approximately 30%.

Antineutrophil cytoplasmic antibody (ANCA)–associated vasculitis may recur in as many as 20% of transplant recipients. Unfortunately, the presence or absence of ANCA at the time of transplantation does not appear to predict recurrence. Antiglomerular basement membrane (anti-GBM) disease recurs in 10% to 25% of patients, but there is no effective way to predict when this will happen. Patients with Alport's syndrome lack GBM antigens. Approximately 10% of these patients develop de novo anti-GBM disease after transplantation because of the production of antibodies against GBM antigens that their immune systems encounter for the first time after transplantation. Systemic lupus erythematosus recurs infrequently, and recurrence rarely results in graft failure.

Primary oxalosis is rare, but without treatment, oxalate deposition quickly recurs in the transplanted kidney. Fortunately, intensive treatment with orthophosphate and pyridoxine, with or without liver transplantation to provide a source of the deficient enzyme, is often successful.

Secondary amyloidosis, with the deposition of amyloid AA fibrils, frequently recurs in the allograft if the underlying cause of the disease is still present. Patients with secondary amyloidosis often have severe, progressive cardiovascular disease caused by amyloid deposition. Nevertheless, the course of secondary amyloidosis may be slow enough to allow transplantation. Death from amyloidosis remains the major limiting factor in transplanting these patients, with 5-year patient survival rates ranging from 30% to 80% in published series. Early death of amyloidosis patients after transplantation usually is caused by cardiac complications or infection. In surviving patients, 5-year graft survival rates are generally acceptable (about 80%), and they have been reported to be as high as 100%. Patients with primary (AL) amyloidosis should have any underlying plasma cell dyscrasias treated and controlled before transplantation. The treatment may include bone marrow or stem cell transplantation, which may reduce the requirement for long-term immunosuppression.

Patients with sickle cell nephropathy can be successfully transplanted if their overall condition does not preclude surgery. Graft survival has generally been reported to be about 75% at 1 year, compared with 90% to 95% in other types of kidney diseases.

Polyomavirus nephropathy, a recently identified cause of allograft failure, usually occurs in the setting of more intense immunosuppression. Clinical experience with retransplantation in the patient who has lost a graft to polyomavirus is limited, but with lower-intensity immunosuppression, the recurrence rate seems to be low.

CANCER

Immunosuppression usually favors the growth of malignant tumors, and an active malignancy is usually an absolute contraindication to transplantation. Exceptions are locally invasive basal cell or squamous cell skin carcinomas. Some authorities have argued that applying guidelines for cancer screening that have been designed for use in the general population to transplantation candidates may not be warranted because of the shorter life expectancy of patients with ESRD compared with that of the general population. However, the chance of detecting cancers with screening seems to be higher among transplantation candidates than the general population. The cost-effectiveness of screening may be greater for the kidney transplant recipient, because detecting cancer may enable better survival for the kidney recipient and may prevent kidneys from being transplanted into patients with occult cancer. Most transplantation physicians recommend that all patients undergo routine screening with a physical examination, chest radiograph, and age-appropriate screening for colon cancer. Women should have mammography, a pelvic examination, and a Pap test, following the guidelines established for the general population.

Immunosuppression probably increases the risk of cancer recurrence. Data from registries, although imperfect, provide some guidance about the chances of recurrence of different malignant tumors. The overall recurrence rate for malignancies treated before transplantation is 20% to 25%. Because more than one half of these recurrences are in patients treated within 2 years before transplantation, many centers recommend a 2-year, disease-free interval before kidney transplantation. However, a waiting period of as long as 5 years may be prudent for lymphomas; breast, prostate, and colon cancers; and symptomatic renal cell carcinomas, especially if the renal cell carcinoma is greater than 5 cm in diameter. It is probably not necessary to delay transplantation for smaller, incidentally discovered, asymptomatic renal cell carcinomas and adequately treated in situ carcinomas of the skin or uterine cervix.

INFECTIONS

Immunosuppression greatly increases the risk for life-threatening infections. Immunizations for influenza (yearly), pneumococcus, and hepatitis B are mandatory for transplantation candidates. The effectiveness of these vaccinations is not well documented in patients with ESRD, but their potential benefits outweigh their negligible risks. Patients should be screened for infections that may become problematic with immunosuppression. Sites of occult infection include the lung, urinary tract, and hemodialysis and peritoneal dialysis catheters. Dialysis-related peritonitis within 3 to 4 weeks is a relative contraindication to transplantation.

Patients should be screened for human immunodeficiency virus (HIV). Before the era of highly effective antiretroviral therapy, HIV was considered an absolute contraindication to kidney transplantation. However, some centers are reporting encouraging results among patients who were HIV positive but without active disease at the time of transplantation. Interactions between antiretroviral drugs and immunosuppressive agents make it mandatory that HIV-positive transplantation patients be managed in centers with appropriate expertise.

Tuberculosis is common in the ESRD population. Screening should include a high index of suspicion, a chest radiograph, and a purified protein derivative skin test, unless the patient has a history of a positive skin test result. High-risk individuals are those with a history of active disease, those from a high-risk population (e.g., from endemic areas, immunocompromised in addition to having ESRD), and patients with an abnormal chest radiographic finding that is consistent with active or inactive tuberculosis. High-risk individuals should receive prophylactic therapy if they have not already had documented treatment. Most investigators recommend prophylaxis for 6 to 12 months, but it probably is not necessary to delay transplantation after therapy has begun.

Although cytomegalovirus (CMV) infection is common and is often transmitted with the transplanted organ, the presence of CMV antibodies in donors and recipients should not preclude transplantation. Most centers routinely use prophylactic therapy (e.g., ganciclovir, valganciclovir) for CMV-seronegative recipients of kidneys from CMV-seropositive donors. Some centers also use prophylaxis for CMV-seropositive recipients of kidneys from CMV-seropositive or seronegative donors. However, few use prophylaxis if both donor and recipient are seronegative. Potential recipients who are seronegative for the varicella-zoster virus are at risk for disseminated infection and should be identified before transplantation. Patients from tropical regions should be screened for *Strongyloides stercoralis*, and transplantation should occur only if response to treatment is satisfactory.

Particularly difficult to evaluate are patients who are being evaluated for another kidney transplantation and who have had a viral infection that might have caused the first graft to fail. However, second transplants have been successful in patients who have had Epstein-Barr virus–associated B-cell lymphomas. Similarly, patients who have lost a kidney transplant because of BK virus nephropathy can have successful kidney transplantations, with or without removal of the failed allograft.

LIVER DISEASE

Liver failure is a major cause of morbidity and mortality after kidney transplantation, and kidney transplantation candidates should be carefully screened for liver disease. The hepatitis A and E viruses do not cause chronic liver disease, whereas hepatitis B virus (HBV) and hepatitis C virus (HCV) can cause chronic active hepatitis after transplantation. Recipients who are positive for hepatitis B surface antigen (HBsAg) are at increased risk for dying of liver disease in the post-transplantation period; however, HBsAg positivity per se is not a contraindication to transplantation. Patients who are HBsAg positive and have serologic evidence of viral replication detected by polymerase chain reaction assay or the presence of hepatitis B early antigen (HBeAg) should probably forgo transplantation pending effective treatment. Likewise, HBsAg-positive patients who also have hepatitis D, which is rare, often develop severe liver disease and therefore should not receive a transplant. Otherwise, HBsAg-positive patients with elevated levels of liver enzymes should undergo biopsy, and those with chronic active hepatitis may be candidates for antiviral therapy (e.g., lamivudine). The decision about whether such patients should undergo transplantation or remain on dialysis is often difficult. Patients with liver disease that is severe may be candidates for simultaneous liver and kidney transplantation. Fortunately, the incidence of HBV is declining in the ESRD population, largely because of effective vaccination and isolation procedures.

Although the natural history of HCV is less well defined, patients who test positive for HCV antibodies should be considered for liver biopsy if enzyme levels are elevated and possibly even if enzyme levels are not elevated, because clinically significant hepatitis may occur without enzyme elevation in ESRD. Patients with HCV and evidence of viral replication identified by polymerase chain reaction or chronic active hepatitis confirmed on biopsy are probably at increased risk for progressive liver disease after transplantation. Antiviral therapy, such as interferon-alfa or ribavirin, has been used to induce remission of HCV disease before transplantation; however, the long-term results of antiviral therapy in patients with ESRD are unclear.

ISCHEMIC HEART DISEASE

Ischemic heart disease (IHD) is a major cause of death after kidney transplantation. Patients with CKD are considered to be in the highest-risk category (i.e., equivalent to someone with diabetes or preexisting IHD) for risk factor management. Risk factors should be optimized before and after transplantation. The concentration of low-density lipoprotein

cholesterol should be less than 100 mg/dL. Blood pressure ideally should be less than 130/80 mm Hg in patients on peritoneal dialysis or not on dialysis and 140/90 mm Hg before dialysis for patients on chronic hemodialysis. Patients should be strongly encouraged to abstain from cigarette smoking. To control blood pressure, perioperative β-blockade should be considered in high-risk patients (e.g., underlying cardiovascular disease, diabetes, multiple risk factors) unless contraindicated. Aspirin prophylaxis should also be considered.

With the increased risk of perioperative IHD events, most centers screen for asymptomatic IHD, although firm evidence for the cost-effectiveness of this approach is lacking. The Coronary Artery Revascularization Prophylaxis (CARP) trial, in which high-risk patients from the general population were randomized to coronary artery revascularization before undergoing aortic or peripheral arterial surgery, showed no benefit from revascularization. Nevertheless, most centers select high-risk patients (i.e., patients with known cardiovascular disease, diabetes, age older than 45 to 50 years, or multiple risk factors) for a noninvasive cardiac stress test. However, noninvasive stress tests are often less sensitive in patients with ESRD than in the general population. Nevertheless, patients whose stress test is positive for reversible ischemia usually undergo coronary angiography with angioplasty or bypass surgery if there are significant lesions. Long waiting times for a deceased-donor kidney mean that cardiovascular disease in high-risk patients may progress, and periodic rescreening (i.e., annually in patients with diabetes and biannually in other patients) is recommended based on consensus. Prospective investigations of the utility of rescreening have not been performed, and in one retrospective study, adherence to periodic screening guidelines did not correlate with perioperative cardiac events.

CEREBROVASCULAR DISEASE

Patients are at increased risk for atherosclerotic cerebrovascular disease events after kidney transplantation compared with pretransplantation patients or the general population. Patients with a history of transient ischemic attacks or other cerebral vascular disease events should be evaluated for possible treatment and should be free of symptoms for at least 6 months before transplantation surgery. Whether asymptomatic patients should undergo screening with a carotid ultrasound examination is unclear. In the general population, controlled trials have shown that the success of prophylactic carotid endarterectomy depends on the center and on the selection of patients. However, all patients should be managed with appropriate intervention for risk factors.

OBESITY

Obesity, an increasingly important problem in patients with ESRD, carries an increased risk of postoperative complications, particularly wound infections and type 2 diabetes. Obesity also is associated with an increased risk for graft failure. Although few studies have examined the safety and efficacy of a weight-reduction diet in patients with ESRD, obese patients who have a body mass index of 30 to 39 kg/m^2 should be encouraged to lose weight. A 10% reduction in body weight is usually achievable by diet. Patients with body mass indices of 40 kg/m^2 or higher may need bariatric surgery to lose weight before transplantation. Although these strategies are frequently employed before transplantation, an analysis of wait-listed patients showed that a decline in BMI while on the waiting list was not protective for post-transplantation mortality or graft loss and was associated with rapid regain of the weight after transplantation.

PSYCHOSOCIAL EVALUATION

Transplantation candidates should be screened for cognitive or psychologic impairments that may interfere with their ability to give informed consent. Failure to adhere to immunosuppressive therapy is a major cause of kidney allograft failure, and the psychological assessment should attempt to identify patients who are at risk. However, reliably identifying patients who will not adhere to therapy is difficult at best, and care should be exercised to avoid unjustifiably refusing transplantation. Most centers require that patients with a history of chemical dependency undergo treatment and demonstrate a period of abstinence, usually 6 months, before transplantation. Major psychiatric disorders are usually apparent during the routine pretransplantation evaluation, and appropriate psychiatric care can be sought.

UROLOGIC EVALUATION

In the absence of a history of chronic urinary tract infection or bladder dysfunction, urologic evaluation and a voiding cystourethrogram are probably unnecessary. High-risk patients, such as those with diabetes, can be screened by obtaining a postvoid residual urine volume. If the postvoid urine volume is greater than 100 mL, a voiding cystourethrogram and urologic evaluation should be obtained. In patients with a dysfunctional bladder, every effort should be made to avoid urinary diversion, such as ureteroileostomy. A few patients may need to use intermittent self-catheterization for optimal bladder drainage.

Pretransplantation native kidney nephrectomies are indicated in patients with reflux associated with chronic infection, polycystic kidneys that are symptomatic or too large to accommodate the allograft, severe nephrotic syndrome, nephrolithiasis associated with infection, renal carcinoma, and hypertension that is difficult to control.

GASTROINTESTINAL EVALUATION

Patients with symptomatic, recurrent cholecystitis should undergo cholecystectomy, because cholecystitis in an immunocompromised transplant recipient may be more severe and more difficult to diagnose and treat. However, most centers do not routinely screen patients with for gallbladder disease, and most do not perform cholecystectomy for asymptomatic cholelithiasis. Similarly, patients with symptomatic diverticulitis may be considered for partial colectomy, but most centers do not conduct screening and surgery for asymptomatic diverticular disease. Peptic ulcer disease is common in the post-transplantation period. However, it can usually be managed medically, and most centers do not routinely perform endoscopy as part of the pretransplantation evaluation. Patients with potential or established malabsorption conditions, such as short gut, sprue, or a history of gastric bypass, may have decreased absorption of immunosuppressive medications. They should be considered for pretransplantation pharmacokinetic evaluation with trough plasma drug levels or area-under-the curve assessment.

PULMONARY EVALUATION

Patients with chronic obstructive lung disease are at increased risk for surgical complications and postoperative pneumonia. Patients with a history of cigarette smoking and dyspnea on exertion should undergo pulmonary function testing to allow better assessment of this surgical risk. Patients should be offered one or more of several therapies that have been shown to be effective in smoking cessation, and if possible, they should be offered a formal smoking cessation program. It is reasonable to refuse transplantation until patients demonstrate abstinence from smoking for some period.

BLOOD AND TISSUE TYPING

Three major immunologic barriers to transplantation need to be addressed. First, transplants should be ABO blood group compatible. Second, the degree of matching at the major histocompatibility complex (MHC) loci A, B, and DR correlates with long-term graft survival and is used in the UNOS system for allocating deceased-donor kidneys. Third, the presence of preformed antibodies and how broadly they react to a random panel of antigens from the general population correlate directly with the likelihood of a positive cross-match when an organ becomes available, and these standards are used in the UNOS kidney allocation scheme.

Blood and MHC tissue types are determined when it is apparent that the patient is a suitable transplantation candidate. Serum is collected at the initial evaluation and at least quarterly thereafter to measure preformed antibodies. An estimate of the number of preformed antibodies is made by reacting the potential recipient's blood against a panel of lymphocytes from a random sample of the general population. The percentage of cells that react with the antibodies is called the percent panel-reactive antibody (PRA). A high PRA value suggests that it will be more difficult to find a donor with a negative cross-match for that recipient. A high PRA also is associated with decreased graft survival, even if the final cross-match is negative. Patients usually develop a high PRA value as a result of prior blood transfusion, transplantation, or pregnancy. A recipient's PRA value may fall over time, especially if blood transfusions are avoided. Some centers have been using flow cytometry and single-antigen beads (i.e., flow PRA) to identify antibodies to single MHC antigens. These techniques identify preformed antibodies against donor antigens (i.e., donor-specific antibodies). These antibodies may be detected at low levels, even with a negative cross-match result, and they are associated with antibody-mediated rejection. Even in the absence of antibody-mediated rejection, the presence of a donor-specific antibody is associated with allograft loss.

As a final screen, the recipient's most recent serum sample is tested against donor antigens, because a positive cross-match indicates the presence of preformed antibodies that can cause hyperacute rejection (see Chapter 63). Because not all reacting antibodies cause hyperacute rejection, other laboratory tests are performed to determine whether the recipient's reacting antibody should preclude transplantation. Usually, the serum with the highest previous PRA value is tested at the time of final cross-matching. Recipients with a negative cross-match but a positive historical cross-match result may undergo transplantation, but they are at higher risk for antibody-mediated rejection.

Some centers use plasmapheresis and the infusion of large doses of polyclonal intravenous immunoglobulin (IVIG) to overcome ABO blood group incompatibility and positive cross-matches. Plasma exchange removes preformed antibodies, and IVIG suppresses subsequent antibody production. These procedures, sometimes combined with splenectomy and rituximab therapy, have allowed a number of patients to receive kidney transplants from blood group–incompatible donors or from donors with a positive cross-match result. The risks of antibody-mediated rejection and graft failure are nevertheless increased. As an alternative, some centers are exploring innovative organ exchange programs, whereby kidneys from live donors that are immunologically incompatible with the targeted recipients are exchanged for kidneys from other live donors that are immunologically compatible.

ALLOCATION OF DECEASED-DONOR KIDNEYS IN THE UNITED STATES

A patient who is medically ready for transplantation can be placed on the UNOS waiting list to receive a deceased-donor kidney. Kidneys are allocated by UNOS (under contract from the U.S. government) according to a priority system that is designed to balance equity with efficiency. The following sections provide a brief version of the much more complex UNOS allocation scheme. A complete description can be found in the UNOS policies (available at http://www.unos.org/policiesandbylaws/policies.asp?resources=true [accessed July 30, 2008]). The final decision to accept an organ rests with the transplantation surgeon and physician responsible for the care of the candidate.

Expanded Criteria Donors

To reduce the time it takes to find a recipient for kidneys that may be refused at multiple centers, UNOS allows transplantation candidates to indicate whether they are willing to accept an expanded criteria donor (ECD) kidney. An ECD kidney is from a deceased donor at least 60 years old or from a donor 50 to 59 years old plus at least two of the following criteria: cerebral vascular accident as the cause of death; hypertension at any time; and most recent serum creatinine level greater than 1.5 mg/dL. An ECD kidney is first offered to someone who has agreed to accept an ECD kidney, using the allocation rules that are similar to those used for standard donor kidneys (described later). Candidates for ECD kidneys are also eligible for standard donor kidneys.

Blood Group Priorities

Waiting times vary for different blood groups. Some blood types, such as types O and B, have the longest waiting times, and other blood types, such as types A and AB, have much shorter waiting times. Because of these disparities in waiting times, kidneys from blood type O donors are allocated only to blood type O candidates, and kidneys from blood type B donors are allocated only to blood type B candidates, with an exception for zero antigen–mismatch candidates (discussed later).

Mandatory Sharing of Zero Antigen–Mismatched Kidneys

ABO blood type–compatible candidates are preferentially offered available donor kidneys that have no human leukocyte antigen (HLA)-A, -B, or -DR antigens that the candidate does not also have. In this instance, the candidate may not have an antibody to any donor HLA-A, -B, or -DR antigen. Exceptions to this rule include deceased-donor kidneys procured for simultaneous kidney and non-kidney organ transplantation and kidneys procured during a donation after cardiac death (DCD). These kidneys do not have to be shared unless the zero antigen–mismatched candidate is local.

Donation after Cardiac Death

DCD donors are *controlled* or *uncontrolled*. A controlled donor is one whose life support is withdrawn and whose family has given written consent for organ donation in the controlled environment of the operating room. An uncontrolled donor is one who dies before the consent for organ donation has been obtained, and catheters are placed in the femoral vessels and peritoneum to cool the organs until consent can be obtained from the family.

Geographic Sequence of Deceased Kidney Allocation

With the exception of kidneys that are shared as a result of a zero antigen mismatch, offered as "payback," or allocated according to a voluntary organ sharing arrangement, kidneys are allocated first locally, then regionally, and then nationally according the UNOS allocation polices.

Double Kidney Offers

Kidneys from adult donors are offered singly (i.e., one kidney to one recipient) unless the donor meets at least two of the following conditions: age older than 60 years; estimated creatinine clearance rate higher than 65 mL/min based on the serum creatinine level on admission to the terminal hospitalization; rising serum creatinine level (>2.5 mg/dL) at the time of organ retrieval; history of long-standing hypertension or diabetes mellitus; and moderate to severe glomerulosclerosis (15% to 49%) on biopsy. Kidneys offered for double kidney allocation are allocated first locally, then regionally, and then nationally.

The Point System for Kidney Allocation

All potential recipients who have an ABO blood type that is compatible with that of the deceased donor are prioritized according to waiting time, quality of antigen mismatch, calculated PRA value, age, history of donation, and prospective cross-matching.

Waiting Time

Waiting time begins when a candidate is placed on the waiting list and the estimated GFR, as determined by creatinine clearance, Cockroft-Gault estimation, or MDRD estimation, is 20 mL/min or less. For candidates younger than 18 years, waiting time begins with placement on the waiting list, regardless of the level of kidney function. Patients can be on the waiting list and receive a zero antigen–mismatch kidney transplant at any level of estimated GFR. One point is assigned to the candidate waiting for the longest period, with fractions of points being assigned proportionately to all other candidates. An additional 1 point is assigned for each full year of waiting time. Points are calculated separately for each geographic (i.e., local, regional, and national) level of kidney allocation.

Quality of Antigen Mismatch

Points are assigned to a candidate based on the number of mismatches between the candidate's antigens and the donor's antigens at the DR locus. Two points are assigned if there are no DR mismatches, and 1 point is assigned if there is one DR mismatch.

Sensitized Wait List Candidates: Calculated Panel-Reactive Antibody Value

The calculated panel-reactive antibody (CPRA) value is the percentage of donors expected to have one or more unacceptable antigens indicated on the waiting list for the candidate. Unacceptable antigens are defined by laboratory detection of HLA-specific antibodies using a solid-phase immunoassay with purified HLA molecules. The transplantation center establishes criteria for additional unacceptable antigens, such as repeat transplant mismatches. The CPRA value is calculated automatically when the unacceptable antigens are listed or updated on the waiting list. The CPRA is derived from HLA antigen or allele group and haplotype frequencies for the different racial or ethnic groups in proportion to their representations in the national deceased-donor population. Sensitized candidates on the waiting list with a CPRA value of 80% or higher receive 4 points.

Children

Candidates younger than 11 years of age receive 4 points, and those between 11 and 17 years old receive 3 points for allocation of kidneys from donors with zero antigen mismatches. Kidneys from donors younger than 35 years (e.g., those not subject to mandatory sharing for 0 HLA mismatching) are offered first to transplantation candidates younger than 18 years at the time of listing, regardless of the number of points assigned to the candidate relative to candidates 18 years old or older. Exceptions are adult candidates assigned 4 points for PRA levels of 80% or greater who otherwise rank higher than all other listed candidates.

History of Donation

A candidate receives 4 points for ever having donated an organ or segment of an organ for transplantation within the United States.

Prospective Cross-matching

A prospective cross-match is mandatory for all candidates, except when clinical circumstances support its omission.

LIVING DONORS

The number of new transplantations has not kept pace with the growth in the number of patients developing ESRD (**Fig. 62-2**), and there has been a growing shortage of deceased-donor kidneys. With this shortage, a greater emphasis has been placed on transplants from living donors (**Fig. 62-3**). Kidneys from living donors usually survive longer than deceased-donor kidneys. The mean duration of graft survival is longest if the donor kidney is from an identical twin, followed by a two-haplotype–matched sibling, followed by a one-haplotype–matched sibling or parent, which has the same graft survival as a zero-haplotype–matched sibling and a distantly related or unrelated (emotionally related) living donor. Mean survival rates of deceased-donor kidneys are lower than all these living-donor categories. Living-donor kidneys have the added advantages of more easily allowing pre-emptive transplantation and sparing more deceased-donor kidneys for individuals who do not have suitable living donors.

Potential living (blood-related and emotionally related) donors should be counseled about the short-term and long-term risks of donation. A survey of 171 transplantation centers found that in the period from 1999 to 2001, the mortality rate was 0.03%, and the complication rate requiring reoperation was 0.4%, principally for bleeding, bowel obstruction, or incisional hernia. Laparoscopic nephrectomy has substantially reduced the morbidity of kidney donation, without compromising long-term outcomes for the recipient. A meta-analysis of 48 studies, including 3124 donors and 1703 controls, found little evidence of progressive kidney

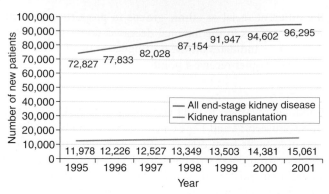

FIGURE 62-2 Number of new end-stage kidney disease patients (including kidney transplant patients) and number of new kidney transplantations in the United States, 1988-2004. (Data from United States Renal Data System: USRDS 2007 Annual Data Report: Atlas of End-Stage Renal Disease in the United States. Bethesda, MD, National Institutes of Health, National Institute of Diabetes and Digestive Kidney Diseases, 2007.)

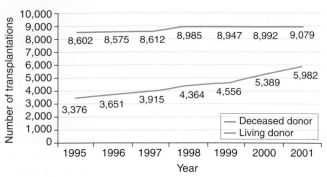

FIGURE 62-3 The number of deceased donor and living donor transplantations in the United States by donor type, 1988-2004. (Data from United States Renal Data System: USRDS 2007 Annual Data Report: Atlas of End-Stage Renal Disease in the United States. Bethesda, MD, National Institutes of Health, National Institute of Diabetes and Digestive Kidney Diseases, 2007.)

dysfunction among the donors over an average of 6 years. The estimated mean residual GFR of the donors was 86 mL/min/1.73 m². Although there was a small mean increase in blood pressure (5 mm Hg) in the donors after kidney donation, this increase was not enough to raise the prevalence of hypertension in these individuals. There was also a statistically significant increase in proteinuria, but the increase (mean weighted difference of 66 mg/day) was probably too small to be of clinical relevance.

Proteinuria greater than 150 mg/24 hr should be considered a contraindication to donation. Microscopic hematuria and pyuria should be investigated to rule out underlying kidney disease that would preclude donation. Kidney function should be normal after adjusting for gender, age, and possible dietary influences on the GFR.

Blood typing and cross-matching are often the first steps in evaluating a living donor. If a potential donor and recipient are blood group compatible and cross-match negative, further evaluation can be carried out. This should include a psychological evaluation to ensure that the donation is truly voluntary and that the donor can give informed consent. A complete medical evaluation should be carried out to uncover conditions that would increase the risk of surgery. Potential

donors should be screened for conditions such as hypertension that may be made worse by having only one kidney. A controversial issue involves the extent to which possible incipient diabetes in donors with a positive family history or other risk factors for diabetes should be tested, because the effect of the solitary kidney on the rate of progression of diabetic nephropathy (if diabetes occurs) is uncertain. It is reasonable to screen with a fasting and 2-hour postprandial blood glucose test. Consideration should be given to the risk of inherited kidney diseases, such as autosomal dominant polycystic kidney disease. The medical evaluation should ensure that the donor is free of diseases that could be transmitted with the kidney, including malignancies, HIV infection, viral hepatitis, and tuberculosis.

If there is more than one potential living donor, selection should be based on medical and nonmedical criteria, and good matching need not be the only determinant of donor choice. Although the best donor is usually a member of the recipient's immediate family, most centers consider an emotionally related donor, such as the spouse. After a potential donor has been selected and evaluated, the final step is usually contrast arteriography or an equivalent imaging technique to define the renal vasculature and to look for potential anatomic abnormalities.

BIBLIOGRAPHY

Andresdottir MB, Assmann KJ, Hoitsma AJ: Recurrence of type I membranoproliferative glomerulonephritis after renal transplantation. Transplantation 63:1628-1633, 1997.

Artero M, Biava C, Amend W, et al: Recurrent focal glomerulosclerosis: Natural history and response to therapy. Am J Med 92:375-383, 1992.

Birkeland SA, Hamilton-Dutoit S, Bendtzen K: Long-term follow-up of kidney transplant patients with posttransplant lymphoproliferative disorder: Duration of posttransplant lymphoproliferative disorder-induced operational graft tolerance, interleukin-18 course, and results of retransplantation. Transplantation 76:153-158, 2003.

Boudville N, Ramesh Prasad GV, Knoll G, et al: Meta-analysis: Risk for hypertension in living kidney donors. Ann Intern Med 145:185-196, 2006.

Bumgardner GL, Amend WC, Ascher NL, Vincenti FG: Single-center long-term results of renal transplantation for IgA nephropathy. Transplantation 65:1053-1060, 1998.

Çelik A, Saglam F, Dolek D, et al: Outcome of kidney transplantation for renal amyloidosis: A single-center experience. Transplant Proc 38:435-439, 2006.

Conlon PJ, Brennan DC, Pfaf WW, et al: Renal transplantation in adults with thrombotic thrombocytopenic purpura/hemolytic-uraemic syndrome. Nephrol Dial Transplant 11:1810-1814, 1996.

Couchoud C, Pouteil-Noble C, Colon S, Touraine JL: Recurrence of membranous nephropathy after renal transplantation. Transplantation 59:1275-1279, 1995.

Droz D, Nabarra B, Noel LH, et al: Recurrence of dense deposits in transplant kidneys. Kidney Int 15:386-395, 1979.

Frohnert PP, Donadio JV Jr, Velosa JA, et al: The fate of renal transplants in patients with IgA nephropathy. Clin Transplant 11:127-133, 1997.

Garg AX, Muirhead N, Knoll G, et al: Proteinuria and reduced kidney function in living kidney donors: A systematic review, meta-analysis, and meta-regression. Kidney Int 70:1801-1810, 2006.

Giannarelli R, Coppelli A, Sartini M, et al: Effects of pancreas-kidney transplantation on diabetic retinopathy. Transplant Int 18:619-622, 2005.

Gill JS, Ma I, Landsberg D, Johnson, et al: Cardiovascular events and investigation in patients who are awaiting cadaveric kidney transplantation. J Am Soc Nephrol 16:808-816, 2005.

Ginevri F, Pastorino N, de Santis R, et al: Retransplantation after kidney graft loss due to polyoma BK virus nephropathy: Successful outcome without original allograft nephrectomy. Am J Kidney Dis 42:821-825, 2003.

Gruessner RW, Suterland DE, Guressner AC: Mortality assessment for pancreas transplants. Am J Transplant 4:2018-2026, 2004.

Kasiske BL, Cangro CB, Hariharan S, et al: The evaluation of renal transplant candidates: Clinical practice guidelines. Am J Transplant 2:5-95, 2002.

Kasiske BL, Ma JZ, Louis TA, Swan SK: Long-term effects of reduced renal mass in humans. Kidney Int 48:814-819, 1995.

Kasiske BL, Ravenscraft M, Ramos EL, et al: The evaluation of living renal transplant donors: Clinical practice guidelines. J Am Soc Nephrol 7:2288-2313, 1996.

Kasiske BL, Snyder JJ, Matas AJ, et al: Preemptive kidney transplantation: The advantage and the advantaged. J Am Soc Nephrol 13:1358-1364, 2002.

Knoll G, Cockfield S, Blydt-Hansen T, et al: Canadian Society of Transplantation consensus guidelines on eligibility for kidney transplantation. Can Med Assoc J 10:1181-1184, 2005.

Larson LS, Bohorquez H, Rea DJ, et al: Pancreas-after-kidney transplantation: An increasingly attractive alternative to simultaneous pancreas-kidney transplantation. Transplantation 77:838-843, 2004.

Lefaucheur C, Suberbielle-Boissel C, Hill GS, et al: Clinical relevance of preformed HLA donor-specific antibodies in kidney transplantation. Am J Transplant 8:324-331, 2008.

Matas AJ, Bartlett ST, Leichtman AB, et al: Morbidity and mortality after living kidney donation, 1999-2001: Survey of United States transplant centers. Am J Transplant 3:830-834, 2003.

McFalls EO, Ward HB, Moritz TE, et al: Coronary artery revascularization before major vascular surgery. N Engl J Med 351:2795-2804, 2004.

Penn I: Evaluation of transplant candidates with pre-existing malignancies. Ann Transplant 2:14-17, 1997.

Roland ME, Stock PG: Review of solid-organ transplantation in HIV-infected patients. Transplantation 75:425-429, 2003.

Sherif AM, Refaie AJ, Sobh MA, et al: Long-term outcome of live donor kidney transplantation for renal amyloidosis. Am J Kidney Dis 42:370-375, 2003.

Schold JD, Srinivas TR, Guerra G, et al: A "weight-listing" paradox for candidates of renal transplantation? Am J Transplant 7:550-559, 2007.

Trofe J, Hisrch HH, Ramos E: Polyomavirus-associated nephropathy: Update of clinical management in kidney transplant patients. Transpl Infect Dis 8:76-85, 2006.

Venstrom JM, McBride MA, Rother KI, et al: Survival after pancreas transplantation in patients with diabetes and preserved kidney function. JAMA 290:2817-2823, 2003.

United States Renal Data System: USRDS 2007 Annual Data Report: Atlas of End-Stage Renal Disease in the United States. Bethesda, MD, National Institutes of Health, National Institute of Diabetes and Digestive Kidney Diseases, 2007.

CHAPTER 63

Post-transplantation Monitoring and Outcomes

Roslyn B. Mannon

POSTSURGICAL MANAGEMENT

The transplantation procedure requires meticulous surgical technique, with care to create viable anastomoses to blood vessels and the urinary tract. The typical approach includes a donor renal artery anastomosed end-to-end on a Carrel aortic patch to the recipient external iliac artery and the donor vein anastomosed to the external iliac vein. A ureteroneocystostomy is created by enveloping the donor ureter in the bladder musculature to prevent reflux. A stent may be placed to maintain patency of the ureteral anastomosis, and it should be removed by 4 weeks after transplantation. The kidney is placed in the iliac fossa in an extraperitoneal location.

After transplantation, the patient's recovery often is swift and marked by significant changes in fluid and electrolyte status if the allograft functions well. Hypotension must be avoided. Because of significant post-transplantation diuresis, care must be taken in the first 24 hours to monitor urine output hourly for replacement of fluids. Hypocalcemia and hypomagnesemia may accompany this diuresis. Immediate allograft function is seen almost uniformly with living donors, whereas allografts from deceased donors may have significant dysfunction and produce oliguria, necessitating the continuation of dialysis. Serum chemistry values must be obtained every 12 to 24 hours or more frequently as indicated to identify the extent of dysfunction and need for dialytic intervention. Immediate perioperative complications include bleeding and thrombosis of the renal artery or renal vein, which require surgical exploration and repair.

Delayed graft function, historically defined as the need for dialysis during the week of transplantation, can manifest as primary nonfunction or initial function followed by decline in function. Risks for delayed graft function include prolonged cold ischemia time (>24 hours), prolonged warm ischemia time (>20 minutes), older donor age (>50 years), traumatic brain injury of the donor, and other donor comorbidities, including hypertension. Postoperative radionuclide scanning can determine the presence of acute tubular necrosis, vascular abnormality, urinary leak, or ureteral obstruction. Coupled with a kidney ultrasound study, which can identify perinephric fluid collections, such as lymphocele, hematoma, or urinoma; vascular complications; and urinary obstruction, a diagnosis and management plan can be quickly formulated. Renal biopsy is appropriate for evaluating early post-transplantation graft dysfunction if there are no obvious surgical abnormalities.

Early histologic findings may include calcineurin inhibitor (CNI) toxicity, acute cellular rejection, and acute tubular necrosis. The prognosis of delayed function is based on the severity of dysfunction and on any accompanying immunologic response against the allograft.

THE ALLOIMMUNE RESPONSE AND REJECTION

Rejection is triggered when the host immune system engages foreign antigens and activates cellular and humoral (antibody) effector responses, leading to graft injury and destruction. These foreign antigens are called major histocompatibility (MHC) proteins, and their genes are located on chromosome 6. They consist of class I antigens expressed on all cells and class II antigens expressed only on antigen-presenting cells (APCs) and on inflamed tissue cells. Critical responders in this process are T lymphocytes. CD8-positive T cells (i.e., cytotoxic cells) engage class I MHC molecules and function by directly lysing cells in the donor graft, but they are not essential for the rejection. CD4-positive T cells are important first responders that engage class II MHC molecules and are thought to be absolutely required for rejection. These cells produce a variety of cytokines, resulting in amplification of the immune response and acting in an autocrine fashion. The process of allorecognition was believed to occur primarily in the graft, but studies now suggest that secondary lymphoid sites are required for this activation.

T-cell activation requires two signals: *signal one*, the engagement of recipient T-cell receptor (TCR) with APCs and MHC molecules resulting in signaling by means of CD3 protein, and a costimulatory *signal two*. Although there are numerous costimulatory molecules on T cells, the focus of clinical transplantation has been on CD28, binding CD80 (B7-1) and CD86 (B7-2) on activated APCs, and CD154 (CD40 ligand), binding CD40 expressed on APCs and B cells. Blockade of these signals leads to death of antigen-specific T cells or specific inactivation of such cells, and it may provide a potential avenue to tolerance. T cells also possess CTLA4, a protein that is a negative regulator of the immune response that can compete for binding with CD80 and CD86. Studies in human transplant recipients with LEA29Y (belatacept), a second-generation humanized fusion protein that binds CTLA4, have shown significant clinical promise in suppressing rejection and facilitating graft survival.

IMMUNOSUPPRESSION

Immunosuppressive medications usually are required for the lifetime of the transplant to prevent allograft rejection. With current therapies, acute rejection rates are as low as 6% to 11%, with graft and patient survival rates higher than 90% at 1 year. Standard therapy includes *induction agents,* which are agents given perioperatively, and *maintenance therapy,* which is continued for the lifetime of the kidney.

Induction therapy typically consists of methylprednisolone intravenously administered at the time of engraftment, followed by orally administered prednisone that is tapered over the first 3 months. The intensity of therapy and duration of the steroid are at the discretion of the transplantation center. Since 1995, induction therapy has frequently included monoclonal, non–lymphocyte-depleting therapy with basiliximab or daclizumab. These antibodies block CD25, the interleukin 2 (IL-2) receptor on T cells, thereby limiting cell proliferation. Both agents have been associated with a marked decline in acute rejection rates compared with an era when these agents were not available. Both agents are well tolerated because they are chimeric or humanized, respectively. For higher-risk patients and donors, induction therapy may include polyclonal antibody therapy, such as rabbit anti-thymocyte globulin (ATG). This antibody cocktail contains multiple specificities to T-cell surface antigens and to common specificities on B cells, monocytes, and some adhesion and costimulatory molecules. Treatment begins during the engraftment period with appropriate steroid preparation or antihistamine plus acetaminophen, or both, to prevent any allergic symptoms. Side effects include fever, tachycardia, hypertension, itching, shortness of breath, and urticaria. The therapeutic effect may be monitored by the extent of lymphocyte depletion, and dose-limiting toxicities include absolute neutrophil counts below 1000 cells/μL and platelet counts below 100,000/μL.

Other monoclonal induction strategies include murine anti-CD3 antibody, which is used infrequently because of its potential allergic symptoms and its toxicity due to cell lysis and third spacing. Alemtuzumab (i.e., anti-CD52 monoclonal antibody) has gained favor as a potent agent for induction, facilitating so-called prope or near-tolerance in some patient populations. With a rapid onset of lymphocyte depletion, potency higher than that of other therapies, and requirement for less frequent administration, this agent is being used more often. Side effects include neutropenia, particularly of lymphocytes and monocytes. Other toxicities are less common because this monoclonal antibody is humanized, but pretreatment should include steroids and antihistamines to prevent infusion-related reactions. The use of this agent in routine kidney transplantation is still being intensely studied. Induction therapies are quite potent, and they may facilitate early and long-term avoidance of maintenance therapy. For example, in the setting of delayed graft function, avoidance of CNIs or mammalian target of rapamycin (mTOR) inhibitors can prevent unnecessary prolongation of acute tubular injury. In long-term settings, the use of antibody induction

to facilitate avoidance of steroids or CNIs has been analyzed in several studies, with mixed results.

Maintenance therapy typically involves three classes of agents. Oral corticosteroid therapy usually consists of prednisone started postoperatively at a dose of 1.0 mg/kg/day, tapering over 3 months down to 0.2 mg/kg/day, with a standard dose of 10 mg/day for most adult patients. Significant side effects include cataracts, increased risk of infection, bone loss and fractures, avascular necrosis, hypertension, weight gain, hypercholesterolemia, glucose intolerance, and acne. These side effects have led to a strong interest in avoidance and withdrawal protocols.

The second class of agents is the antimetabolites. Azathioprine, which is a derivative of 6-mercaptopurine, suppresses de novo purine synthesis. Dosing is 1 to 2 mg/kg/day, and side effects include thrombocytopenia, macrocytosis, and marrow depression. Use of this drug is associated with increased susceptibility to cancer and infection, cholestatic hepatitis, and pancreatitis. Because this agent is metabolized by xanthine oxidase, concurrent use of allopurinol can cause severe leukopenia. The use of azathioprine in many transplantation programs has been replaced during the past decade by mycophenolate mofetil, based on several pivotal studies demonstrating a significant reduction in early acute rejection. Mycophenolate mofetil inhibits inosine monophosphate dehydrogenase, the key enzyme in de novo purine synthesis, thereby blocking DNA and RNA synthesis. Clinically, this drug inhibits T- and B-lymphocyte and monocyte proliferation. Dose is limited by bone marrow toxicity, particularly leukopenia and anemia. Other side effects include gastric reflux and ulceration, pancreatitis, and diarrhea. Mycophenolate mofetil has a complex metabolism within the liver, and drug activity may be monitored by measuring the active metabolite mycophenolic acid.

The third component of triple immunosuppressive therapy consists of the CNIs cyclosporine and tacrolimus. Cyclosporine binds to cyclophilin and tacrolimus to FK-binding protein. After binding, these complexes inhibit the phosphatase calcineurin, blocking migration of nuclear factor of activated T cells (NF-AT) from the cytoplasm to the nucleus, limiting the transcription of IL-2, IL-4, interferon-γ, and tumor necrosis factor-α. Drug dosing is based on trough (C_0) levels, with cyclosporine dosage of 3 to 8 mg/kg/day and tacrolimus dosage of 0.05 to 0.2 mg/kg/day, each divided at 12-hour intervals. Both agents are metabolized by the cytochrome P-450 CYP3A4 enzyme. Consequently, any drug that induces or inhibits this cytochrome action may increase or decrease drug dose, respectively. Common drug interactions are given in **Table 63-1**.

CNIs have multiple toxicities, particularly acute and chronic nephrotoxicity. In acute nephrotoxicity, graft dysfunction results from renal vasoconstriction, which is typically reversible by discontinuing the drug. Thrombotic microangiopathy may occur in acute and chronic settings, which may be ameliorated by discontinuing the agent. Over months to years of treatment, chronic injury is manifested by elevated serum creatinine levels, which may be associated

TABLE 63-1 **Selected Common Drug Interactions with Calcineurin Inhibitors**

INCREASES CNI LEVEL (INHIBITS ENZYME)*	DECREASES CNI LEVEL (STIMULATES ENZYME)*

Calcium channel blockers
  Diltiazem
  Verapamil
	Antibiotics
	  Rifabutin
	  Rifampin

Antiarrhythmics
  Amiodarone
	Antiepileptics
	  Phenobarbital
	  Phenytoin
	  Carbamazepine

HIV protease inhibitors
  Ritonavir
  Saquinavir
  Indinavir
	Herbal substances
	  St. John's wort

Azole antifungal agents
  Ketoconazole
  Clotrimazole
  Itraconazole
  Voriconazole	

Antibiotics
  Erythromycin base
  Clarithromycin
  Synercid (quinupristin and
    dalfopristin)	

Antidepressants Fluvoxamine	
Other agents Grapefruit juice	

*Listed drugs interact with the calcineurin inhibitors (CNI) cyclosporine and tacrolimus because they are metabolized by the cytochrome P-450 CYP3A4 isoenzyme.

HIV, human immunodeficiency virus.

with modest proteinuria and hypertension. Transplant biopsy may demonstrate a striped pattern of interstitial fibrosis, accompanied by arteriolar hyalinosis and isometric tubular epithelial cell vacuolization. Management includes reducing or discontinuing the CNI. Accompanying hypertension can be treated with dihydropyridine calcium channel blockers, which reduces arteriolar vasoconstriction. Chronic toxicity in many cases is not reversible, but in some cases, discontinuation of the CNI followed by institution of mycophenolate mofetil has been associated with amelioration in the decline of graft function.

CNIs have been associated with many metabolic toxicities, including hypomagnesemia, hyperkalemia, and hyperuricemia. Tacrolimus is associated with diabetes, and risk factors for diabetes include African American lineage, older recipient age, hepatitis C infection, and an a body mass index (BMI) greater than 30 kg/m². Cyclosporine is also associated with physically disfiguring adverse effects, including gingival hyperplasia and hirsutism. Both drugs may be associated with neurotoxicity characterized by tremor, dysesthesias, insomnia, or headache. However, the dramatic improvement in acute rejection rates and short-term outcomes has led to their widespread use.

The mTOR inhibitor sirolimus is a macrolide antibiotic derived from *Streptomyces* that binds FK-binding protein; the complex then binds mTOR, a molecule that is critical to RNA transcription and translation of cell cycle proteins and growth factors blocking cell cycle. Preclinical studies suggested that the use of sirolimus may facilitate donor-specific tolerance. Metabolized by CYP3A4 in the liver with a prolonged half-life of 62 hours, dosing is daily and based on 24-hour trough blood levels. The pivotal studies that used sirolimus with cyclosporine were associated with significantly lower rates of acute rejection, graft loss, and patient death compared with cyclosporine and azathioprine. Moreover, combining sirolimus with tacrolimus facilitated steroid avoidance in solid organ transplantation and in islet cell transplantation. Side effects include delayed wound healing and lymphocele formation, a particular problem in the early postoperative period; oral ulceration, which is dose dependent; hypertriglyceridemia, which often is worse in the first 6 months of use; and bone marrow suppression, including thrombocytopenia, leukopenia, and anemia. Sirolimus has been associated with other serious toxicities, including peripheral edema, pneumonitis, pleural effusions, ascites, and reflex sympathetic dystrophy. Although sirolimus is not believed to be directly nephrotoxic, it may prolong delayed graft function as described earlier. Thrombotic microangiopathy has also been reported. Coupled with cyclosporine, a slowly rising serum creatinine level has been reported, which may be related to exacerbation of CNI toxicity. Sirolimus also has been associated with proteinuria that may be in the nephrotic range. Biopsy of some of these grafts has shown focal glomerulosclerosis, although not consistently. Proteinuria may resolve with discontinuation of sirolimus.

The most common maintenance regimen in current use is corticosteroids, mycophenolate mofetil, and tacrolimus. Maintenance is often coupled to induction therapy with anti-CD25 monoclonal antibody or depletional induction therapy. The choice of therapy depends on the immunologic risks of the donor and recipient. Considerable debate has been placed on withdrawal of CNIs in the late posttransplantation period or conversion to alternative agents in an effort to minimize long-term nephrotoxicity. The results of these studies have been mixed. Moreover, even in the absence of CNIs, atrophy and fibrosis have been observed in kidney allografts.

POST-TRANSPLANTATION LABORATORY MONITORING

The risk of acute rejection is highest during the first 6 months after transplantation, and it then diminishes over time. Late acute rejection often results from nonadherence or a decline in immunosuppressant levels due to altered metabolism. Monitoring of the patient includes physical examination and a standard serum metabolic panel, complete blood cell count, trough serum CNI level, and urinalysis twice weekly for the first month. The random urine protein-to-creatinine ratio is monitored periodically. The frequency of visits and blood tests decreases over time, depending on the graft function and other comorbidities. The care team must emphasize to patients that adherence is a constant necessity and that, if illness prevents taking medication, they should contact the physician for an alternative plan. The use of serum creatinine and drug levels constitutes typical immune monitoring after transplantation, but these methods are relatively insensitive for detecting rejection. Alternative methods of immune system monitoring being studied include in vitro measures of T-cell activation in blood and urine samples. Many centers have advocated the use of surveillance or protocol kidney graft biopsies that are performed at specified intervals. Histologic rejection can often be seen before changes in serum creatinine levels, but the impact of interventions guided by surveillance biopsy findings is not clear. In a landmark study, surveillance kidney biopsies demonstrated the almost universal development of CNI toxicity in monitored kidney transplants. Surveillance biopsies have provided novel genomic information regarding graft disease pathogenesis and may potentially be used as end points in clinical trials.

ALLOGRAFT DYSFUNCTION AND HISTOPATHOLOGY

Kidney graft dysfunction is defined as an increase in serum creatinine of 15% from baseline, which is often the primary indicator for biopsy. Other indicators for biopsy include oliguria and proteinuria. The Banff criteria (**Table 63-2**) have standardized the criteria for allograft pathology. The parenchyma of each biopsy is analyzed, including tubules, glomeruli, and vessels. The severity of interstitial inflammation with lymphocytes (i) is scored from 0 (absent) to 3 (severe). Because tubules are the target of acute cellular rejection, lymphocyte infiltration into tubules or tubulitis (t) is the basis of the diagnosis. Vessel wall infiltration (v) or arteritis increases the rank of acute rejection to grade II. Borderline rejection is diagnosed when the tubulitis score is mild or t1, but interstitial inflammation severity may range from mild to severe. The extent of infiltration does not affect the response to therapy. Treatment for acute rejection includes bolus methylprednisolone, ATG, and intensification of maintenance immunosuppression. Rejection that is resistant to steroids and ATG has been treated with some success with intravenous immune globulin (IVIG) or anti-CD20 antibody, or both. Even successfully reversed, acute rejection has been associated with shortened graft survival, although it has been appreciated that a return to baseline function indicates a more positive prognosis. Lymphocyte infiltration in glomeruli (g) may accompany acute rejection, but it is not a criterion of rejection.

Antibody-mediated rejection (AMR) may be characterized several different pathologies, including acute tubular necrosis, vasculitis, and peritubular capillary inflammation. After antibody binds to its target antigen, it promotes the binding of cytotoxic cells and induces the binding of complement components, leading to target cell death. Immunostaining of activated complement component C4d in peritubular capillaries of kidney transplants indicates the presence of alloantibody within the graft. AMR may occur days to

TABLE 63-2 Banff 2007 Criteria for Allograft Pathology

1. **Normal**

2. **Antibody-mediated changes (may coincide with categories 3, 4, and 5)**
   C4d deposition without morphologic evidence of active rejection
   C4d+, presence of circulating antidonor antibody, no signs of acute or chronic TCMR or ACMR.
   Acute antibody-mediated rejection
   C4d+, presence of circulating antidonor antibodies, morphologic evidence of acute tissue injury such as (Type/Grade):
   I. ATN-like minimal inflammation
   II. Capillary and glomerular inflammation (ptc/g>0) and/or thromboses
   III. Arterial -v3*
   Chronic active antibody-mediated rejection
   C4d+, presence of circulating antidonor antibodies, morphologic evidence of chronic tissue injury such as glomerular double contours and/or peritubular capillary basement membrane multilayering and/or interstitial fibrosis/tubular atrophy and/or fibrosis.

3. **Borderline Changes**
   Suspicious for acute T cell mediated rejection. No intimal arteritis, but foci of tubulitis (t1, t2, or t3) with minor interstitial inflammation (i0 or i1) or interstitial infiltration (i2, i3) with mild (t1) tubulitis (t1, i1 or greater)

4. **T cell-mediated rejection (TCMR; may coincide with 2, 5 and 6)**
   Acute T cell mediated rejection (Type/Grade)
   IA. Significant interstitial infiltration (i2; >25% of parenchyma affected) and foci of moderate tubulitis (t2; >4 mononuclear cells/tubular cross section or group of 10 tubular cells)
   IB. Significant interstitial infiltration (i2; >25% of parenchyma affected) and foci of Severe tubulitis (t3; >10 mononuclear cells/tubular cross-section or group of 10 tubular cells)
   IIA. Mild-to-moderate intimal arteritis (v1)
   IIB. Severe intimal arteritis comprising >25% of the luminal area (v2)
   III. Transmural arteritis and/or arterial fibrinoid change and necrosis of medial smooth muscle
   Chronic active T-cell-mediated-rejection
   Chronic allograft arteriopathy (arterial intimal fibrosis with mononuclear cell infiltration)

5. **Interstitial fibrosis and tubular atrophy, no evidence of any specific etiology (Grade)**
   I. Mild interstitial fibrosis (ci1) and tubular atrophy (ct1) < 25% of cortical area affected
   II. Moderate interstitial fibrosis (ci2) and tubular atrophy (ct2); 26-50% of cortical area affected
   III. Severe interstitial fibrosis (ci3) and tubular atrophy (ct3) > 50% of cortical area affected

6. **Other changes not considered to be due to rejection—** acute and/or chronic (may coincide with categories 2, 3, 4, and 5)

*Degrees of lymphocyte infiltration are scored 0 (absent) to 3 (severe) ATN, acute tubular necrosis; C4d+, activated complement component C4d; ci interstial fibrosis; ct, tubular atrophy; i, interstitial infiltration; t, tubulitis; v, vessel wall infiltration or arteritis; ptc, peritubular capillaritis; g, glomerulitis; cg, glomerulopathy.

weeks after transplantation. Because of pretransplantation cross-matching, hyperacute AMR is rarely seen. Treatment of acute AMR includes plasmapheresis, IVIG to downregulate antibody production, and in some centers, anti-CD20 antibody to deplete B cells. Alloantibody should be characterized, quantified, and monitored by the histocompatibility laboratory. Although most cases of AMR may be seen in the early posttransplantation period, chronic and continuous antibody deposition may be associated with chronic graft failure.

CNI toxicity may mediate allograft dysfunction, which is histologically characterized by isometric tubular vacuolization or arteriolar hyalinosis, or both. When toxicity is persistent and chronic, interstitial fibrosis and tubular atrophy also occur. BK polyomavirus nephropathy (discussed later) is a cause of graft injury and loss. Initial histologic descriptions included findings consistent with acute cellular rejection, such as tubulitis and interstitial inflammation. However, tubular epithelial viral cytopathic changes and immunostaining for the large T viral antigen indicate nephropathy. Interstitial infiltration with B cells may indicate post-transplantation lymphoproliferative disorder (PTLD), and it is confirmed by in situ hybridization for the Epstein-Barr Virus (EBV) genome, which is the causative agent for PTLD. Other potential lesions include acute interstitial nephritis, pyelonephritis, and ischemic changes, whose management predominantly is independent of immunosuppressives. Because of the relative safety of a transplant biopsy, it may be the most useful strategy in settings of acute allograft dysfunction, rather than empiric intensification of immunosuppression.

CHRONIC AND LONG-TERM GRAFT DYSFUNCTION

Despite dramatic declines in acute rejection rates and improvement in short-term graft survival, long-term graft survival continues to be problematic. For example, adjusted 5-year graft survival rates for 2005 were only 69.2% for deceased donors and only 80.1% for living donors. The leading cause of late graft loss is death with a functioning graft, most commonly due to cardiovascular disease (discussed later). The second most common cause of loss of graft function is chronic allograft nephropathy, a disorder histologically characterized by interstitial fibrosis (Banff ci) and tubular atrophy (Banff ct). Chronic allograft nephropathy may occur months to years after transplantation, and it is accompanied by hypertension or proteinuria, or both. Immunologic (e.g., chronic rejection, immune response to infection or injury) and nonimmunologic factors have been implicated in the pathogenesis of chronic allograft nephropathy. Histologically, ci and ct are graded from 1 (mild) to 3 (severe), and chronic allograft nephropathy severity is based on a combination of these changes (see **Table 63-2**). Biopsy is important to delineate the cause of late graft failure, which may include uncontrolled hypertension, CNI toxicity, BK polyomavirus infection, transplant glomerulopathy, and recurrent kidney disease. Therapy includes the typical strategies for chronic kidney disease, including the control of blood pressure, glucose concentration, and lipid levels.

Chronic transplant glomerulopathy is a disorder histologically characterized by widespread involvement of all glomeruli, with enlargement and duplication of the glomerular basement membrane and endothelial cell activation. Electron microscopy reveals subendothelial accumulation of electron lucent material, reduplication of the basement membrane, and interposition of mesangial cells into the capillary wall. Clinically, nephrotic proteinuria and accelerated graft failure are seen. Associated risk factors for development include the presence of anti-HLA antibodies at the time of transplantation and late acute rejection. Glomerular and endothelial C4d deposition may be associated with chronic transplant glomerulopathy. Effective therapy is not known, but empiric management includes intensification of maintenance immunosuppression and the use of angiotensin-converting enzyme (ACE) inhibitors and, in some centers, IVIG.

Recurrent glomerular disease is potential contributor to late graft loss, accounting for approximately 8% of allografts lost during a 10-year period. Focal segmental glomerulosclerosis recurs commonly and can do so immediately after transplantation in association with nephrotic-range proteinuria and a rapid decline in graft function. Allograft loss is most common in recipients with focal segmental glomerulosclerosis and mesangiocapillary type I glomerulonephritis. Although IgA nephropathy, pauci-immune glomerulonephritis, and membranous nephropathy also recur, they do so later in the transplantation course and are less likely to cause graft loss. De novo glomerulonephritis may also occur in renal allografts and may be caused by transplant glomerulopathy, hemolytic uremic syndrome, membranous glomerulonephritis, membranoproliferative disease, or hepatitis C infection. Consequently, recipients with proteinuria, hematuria, or a decline in allograft function should undergo a diagnostic approach that includes protein quantitation, graft biopsy including immunofluorescence and electron microscopy, and serologic evaluation. Treatment for recurrent de novo glomerulonephritis remains limited (see Chapter 62).

LONG-TERM MEDICAL MANAGEMENT OF THE KIDNEY TRANSPLANT RECIPIENT
Cardiovascular Disease

As for other patients with chronic kidney disease, cardiovascular disease is the leading cause of death for transplant recipients. Risk factors include hypertension, diabetes, and graft dysfunction. The relative risk of cardiovascular death increases significantly when the serum creatinine level is greater than 1.5 mg/dL. Based on limited specific information about transplant recipients, recommendations for management include dietary modification, discontinuing smoking, and control of blood pressure, lipid levels, and glucose levels. Screening for cardiovascular disease begins with the initial transplantation evaluation, although substantial time might have elapsed for recipients of deceased-donor grafts since the initial assessment. For asymptomatic patients, it is not clear that screening for coronary artery disease leads to a reduction in mortality rates. Low-dose aspirin may be used to prevent clinical events in those with underlying cardiovascular disease and those who are without proven disease but are at high risk for cardiovascular events.

Hypertension

Hypertension is seen in 60% to 80% of all transplant recipients, and it confers a significant negative impact on long-term kidney graft survival. Consequently, blood pressure targets should be a systolic pressure below 130 mm Hg and a diastolic pressure below 80 mm Hg. There is insufficient clinical evidence to recommend one class of antihypertensive drugs over another. Dihydropyridine calcium channel blockers may be useful in controlling hypertension associated with CNIs, and their use has been associated with improved graft outcome. There is conflicting evidence about whether ACE inhibitors are associated with improved graft and patient survival.

Dyslipidemia

Dyslipidemia is defined as a serum total cholesterol level greater than 240 mg/dL, low-density lipoprotein (LDL) cholesterol level greater than 130 mg/dL, high-density lipoprotein (HDL) cholesterol level less than 40 mg/dL, or triglyceride level greater than 200 mg/dL, and about 60% of recipients meet this definition. The pathogenesis is multifactorial, including preexisting dyslipidemia, weight gain, diabetes, and the use of corticosteroids, sirolimus, and CNIs. Importantly, dyslipidemia is associated with an increased risk for cardiovascular death in kidney transplant recipients. Statins constitute primary treatment, with a target total cholesterol level less than 200 mg/dL and LDL level less than 100 mg/dL. Triglyceride management often entails the use of fibrates. A landmark study in kidney transplant recipients demonstrated that fluvastatin was safe and effective in lowering cholesterol and that it significantly reduced rates of myocardial infarction and cardiac death. A fasting lipid panel should be obtained at least quarterly in the first year. Patients should be monitored for rhabdomyolysis because the concomitant use of statins with CNIs (especially cyclosporine) is associated with an increased risk of myopathy that is augmented by fibrate use.

New-Onset Diabetes after Transplantation

The prevalence of new-onset diabetes after transplantation (NODAT) has been estimated at 9% at 3 months, 16% at 1 year, and about 25% at 3 years after transplantation, with the greatest risk of development occurring in the first 6 months after transplantation, depending on immunosuppressive strategy used. Diabetes may be detected by fasting plasma glucose levels greater than 126 mg/dL or 2-hour plasma glucose levels of 200 mg/dL in a glucose tolerance test. Impaired glucose tolerance is indicated by plasma glucose levels of 100 to 125 mg/dL or a 2-hour glucose level grater than 140 mg/dL in a glucose tolerance test. Risk factors include recipient age older than 60 years, obesity, African American race, use of tacrolimus, and hepatitis C infection (e.g., possible effect on B cells, increased insulin resistance, decreased hepatic glucose uptake).

NODAT is characterized by insulin resistance, which may accompany obesity, and ketoacidosis is rare. The impact of NODAT is considerable, because patient survival and graft survival are decreased, in part because of the increased rate of cardiovascular events. Management of NODAT should emphasize modifiable factors, such as weight reduction, exercise, and use of antihyperglycemic agents. Modification of immunosuppression is also a consideration.

Obesity

Obesity often is associated with NODAT. As many as 60% of kidney transplant recipients are obese at the time of surgery, and this trend is increasing with each decade. Average weight gain is about 3 kg in the first year after transplantation, and risk factors include female sex, African American lineage, and diabetes. An elevated BMI has been associated with significantly higher rates of graft loss, chronic graft injury, and delayed graft function, although these results have not been consistent. Avoidance of steroids has produced mixed results in preventing additional weight gain after transplantation. Diet and physical exercise are important in the management of these patients.

Hematologic Complications

Anemia, defined as a hemoglobin level less than 13 g/dL, occurs in 20% to 40% of transplant recipients. The cause is multifactorial and may include inadequate erythropoietin production (possibly related lack of synthesis by the graft), iron deficiency, and medications including, ACE inhibitors, angiotensin receptor blockers (ARBs), mycophenolate mofetil, and sirolimus. Systemic viral infections such as cytomegalovirus (CMV) may cause anemia. Parvovirus B19 may lead to pure red cell aplasia that responds to IVIG treatment. The benefits of anemia correction in transplant recipients are being studied. Supplementation using an erythropoiesis-stimulating agent should be guided by the cause and extent of anemia, with a maximal hemoglobin target of 12 g/dL. In contrast, erythrocytosis, defined as a hemoglobin level grater than 17 g/dL, may occur in only 10% to 20% of recipients. It should be treated because it has been linked to thromboembolic disease. Treatment includes ACE inhibitors or ARBs, which block erythroid precursor development, and if they are ineffective, phlebotomy can be used.

Leukopenia is frequently seen after transplantation. A differential cell count should be obtained to identify the cell type affected. Lymphopenia should be expected after depletional induction therapy with ATG or alemtuzumab, and it may take 6 to 12 months to resolve. Infection with CMV is associated with lymphopenia, as is the use of ganciclovir to treat CMV. Immunosuppression by mycophenolate and sirolimus is associated with leukopenia, which tends to be dose related. Severe neutropenia should be managed with granulocyte colony-stimulating factor and monitored closely.

Metabolic Abnormalities and Bone Disease

Metabolic bone disease is common, in part because of secondary hyperparathyroidism and preexisting bone disease, and it is complicated by electrolyte disorders such as hypokalemia, hypomagnesemia, and hypophosphatemia. Elevated calcium levels may occur because of high serum parathormone (PTH) levels. Although serum PTH levels often normalize over the first year after transplantation, recipients with persistent hypercalcemia may require cinacalcet therapy or parathyroidectomy. Vitamin D deficiency is often overlooked, and replacement therapy may assist in reducing PTH levels.

Osteoporosis may occur in more than 60% of transplant recipients and may be exacerbated by the use of steroid therapy and CNIs. The risk of fracture is about 10% after kidney transplantation, and the foot and ankle are common sites. Bone density should be measured at the time of transplantation, at 6 months after transplantation, and yearly thereafter. Osteopenia should be managed with vitamin D and calcium supplementation. Progression to osteoporosis is an indication for bisphosphonates (although they should be avoided with adynamic bone histology). Aseptic necrosis, typically of the femoral head, occurs in about 5% of recipients and is associated with steroid use. Magnetic resonance imaging (MRI) is diagnostic, and therapy involves femoral head decompression or total hip replacement.

Gout occurs in about 10% of recipients, and hyperuricemia may occur after transplantation, in part because of reduced kidney function, diuretics, and volume depletion. Cyclosporine inhibits the proximal tubular secretion of uric acid. Acute gout attacks are amenable to steroids or colchicine, or both. In chronic suppression, colchicine has been associated with myopathy with cyclosporine treatment. The role of hyperuricemia in graft dysfunction in transplant recipients remains unknown.

Malignancy

The incidence of malignancy after kidney transplantation has been rising during the past decade, affecting about 10% of recipients in the first 3 years after transplantation. Cancers are increasingly the cause of patients' deaths, and recipients with cancer have a higher rate of mortality than their noncancer counterparts. Compared with the general population, the risk of nonmelanoma skin cancer, Kaposi's sarcoma, and non-Hodgkin's lymphoma is 20-fold higher, and for renal cell cancer in the native kidney, the risk is 15-fold higher.

Risk factors for cancer in transplant recipients include older recipient age, white race, male sex, and prior cancer. Recipients with prior cancers must be disease free for established times before transplantation. The immunosuppressive burden, rather than a specific agent, has been associated with post-transplantation malignancy. Viral infection also affects the prevalence of certain malignancies. Specifically, hepatitis B and C infections are associated with hepatobiliary cancer. Human papillomavirus infection mediates epithelial cancers, affecting the cervix, perineum, vulva, lip, and mouth. Human herpesvirus 8 mediates Kaposi's sarcoma.

Finding the balance between sufficient immunosuppression and cancer risk is an important task for all clinicians. Cancer surveillance guidelines used in the general population are the current care standard, but their adequacy is being reviewed. Some studies have indicated sirolimus has an antitumor effect in Kaposi's sarcoma. This may be related to inhibition of vascular endothelial growth factor. Clinical trials using sirolimus have also indicated a reduction in de novo cancers in recipients compared with those not on sirolimus. Additional studies are designed to understand the mechanism of the effect of sirolimus and specific efficacy.

PTLD accounts for about 10% of all malignancies after transplantation. About 93% are non-Hodgkin's lymphomas. The disease is caused by EBV-infected B cells, and tumors may be polymorphic and polyclonal or monoclonal and highly malignant. PTLD manifests frequently in the kidney allograft with diffuse involvement of lymph nodes, spleen, and liver, and in about 25% of recipients, PTLD involves the brain. Hemophagocytic syndrome, a disorder in which macrophages ingest all marrow precursors and cause severe pancytopenia, fever, and splenomegaly, is a rare but fatal complication. Risk factors for development include EBV mismatch with seropositive donor organs transplanted into seronegative recipients, particularly in the context of lymphocyte depletional therapy.

Prophylactic antiviral agents such as ganciclovir and acyclovir have been effective in preventing PTLD. In children, monitoring for the EBV genome may detect early infection and allow monitored immunosuppressive withdrawal. Therapy for PTLD includes reduction or withdrawal of immunosuppression and, if unresponsive, chemotherapy. Radiation therapy is reserved for disease affecting the central nervous system. Remission is not uncommon, but more than 50% of patients die of their tumor or complications of treatment.

Infection

The risk of infection after transplantation is related to the net state of recipient immunosuppression and epidemiologic factors, such as donor-derived infection, recipient infection, nosocomial infection, and community exposures. Donor-derived disease can be avoided by appropriate screening for disseminated infections such as human immunodeficiency virus (HIV) infection and hepatitis and by recognition of CMV and EBV serostatus. Unrecognized fungemia or bacteremia may add to morbidity. Recipients' infections are assessed at the time of listing and managed before transplantation, including appropriate vaccinations. Nosocomial exposures occur during hospitalization and may be further complicated by colonization of the recipient. Community exposures include viral disease and geographically related infections. In the first month after transplantation, nosocomial infections may include methicillin-resistant *Staphylococcus aureus*, *vancomycin-resistant Enterococcus* and *Candida* infections,

Clostridium difficile colitis, urinary tract infections, and hemodialysis or peritoneal dialysis catheter-related infections.

During the first year after transplantation, viral infections are common, with CMV and EBV of greatest concern, followed by herpes simplex virus, hepatitis B and C, and BK polyomavirus. Opportunistic infections derived from donors or recipient exposures, also contribute. After the first year, community-acquired infection is of primary concern and includes pneumonia, urinary tract infections, *Aspergillus*, and CMV.

BK polyomavirus nephropathy is a key cause of late graft loss. Infection may be recipient or donor derived and harbored quiescently in the uroepithelium. After institution of immunosuppression, the virus may reactivate and begin replicating. Left unchecked, viral infection in the renal tubular epithelium evokes an inflammatory response not unlike that seen in acute rejection, resulting ultimately atrophy and fibrosis. Treatment involves reduction or withdrawal of immunosuppression. Specific anti-BK agents are not available, but some investigators have found success using IVIG or cidofovir. The latter is highly nephrotoxic. The use of leflunomide as an antiviral and immunosuppressive agent has had limited success. Early diagnosis with early reduction in immunosuppression may avert graft loss. Monitoring by urine cytology is inexpensive but not sensitive for nephropathy. Viral genome DNA of more than 10,000 copies/mL detected in plasma by polymerase chain reaction (PCR) positively predicts nephropathy in 50% to 85%. Prospective viral genome monitoring holds the most promise in identifying patients at risk for disease.

Transplant recipients receive antimicrobial prophylaxis to minimize infection. This includes trimethoprim-sulfamethoxazole for the first 6 months after transplantation to prevent urinary tract infection and *Pneumocystis* infection. As do all other herpesviruses, CMV becomes latent after primary infection, exposing transplant recipients to reactivation of their own virus or virus transplanted with the donor kidney. CMV prophylaxis is instituted if there is evidence of prior infection in the recipient or seropositivity of the donor. The highest risk of CMV disease is in seronegative recipients of a kidney from a seropositive donor. Seropositive recipients of kidneys of seropositive or seronegative donors are at intermediate risk. Patients in the highest risk groups should receive ganciclovir or valganciclovir for at least the first 3 months after transplantation. Many centers extend the time of prophylaxis in the setting of lymphocyte depletion to 6 months or until the absolute lymphocyte count exceeds 500 cells/mm^3. The use of prophylactic therapy and monitoring for CMV has reduced post-transplantation infections dramatically. Many centers employ surveillance strategies with serial measurements of CMV in plasma by PCR, and treat only if a significant titer of virus copies is detected. Low-risk seronegative recipients of kidneys from seronegative donors typically do not receive prophylaxis. Fungal prophylaxis using clotrimazole or oral nystatin should be prescribed.

Evaluation for fever should take into account any presenting signs and symptoms and the time after transplantation. Workup should include culture of blood and urine, and it should include sputum and stool if relevant. Nasal pharyngeal washes with enzyme-linked immunosorbent assay (ELISA) testing for respiratory viruses are useful for recipients with upper respiratory symptoms without localization. Radiographic studies should include a chest radiograph and kidney-ureter-bladder (KUB) radiograph if indicated to identify other abdominal pathology. PCR should be considered for the detection of CMV and EBV. After appropriate cultures have been obtained and the white blood cell count and differential cell count assessed, patients should be closely observed and placed on broad-spectrum antimicrobials. Pulmonary infiltrates should be assessed quickly by inducing sputum or using bronchoscopy. It is important to note that immunosuppressed patients often lack fever and other symptoms, and, even in the absence of a particular symptom, the differential diagnosis should remain broad. Further testing is indicated based on the patient's presenting features. An early infectious disease consultation should be considered to guide evaluation and therapy.

BIBLIOGRAPHY

Briganti EM, Russ GR, McNeil JJ, et al: Risk of renal allograft loss from recurrent glomerulonephritis. N Engl J Med 347:103, 2002.

Danovitch G: Handbook of Kidney Transplantation, 4th ed. Philadelphia, Lippincott Williams & Wilkins, 2004.

Davidson J, Wilkinson A, Dantal J, et al: New-onset diabetes after transplantation: 2003 International consensus guidelines. Proceedings of an international expert panel meeting. Transplantation 75:S3, 2003.

Djamali A, Samaniego M, Muth B, et al: Medical care of kidney transplant recipients after the first posttransplant year. Clin J Am Soc Nephrol 1:623, 2006.

Fishman JA: Infection in solid-organ transplant recipients. N Engl J Med 357:2601, 2007.

Halloran PF: Immunosuppressive drugs for kidney transplantation. N Engl J Med 351:2715, 2004.

Health Resources and Services Administration, Healthcare Systems Bureau, Division of Transplantation: 2006 Annual Report of the U.S. Organ Procurement and Transplantation Network and the Scientific Registry of Transplant Recipients: Transplant Data 1996-2005. Rockville, MD, HRSA, 2007.

Holdaas H, Fellstrom B, Jardine AG, et al: Effect of fluvastatin on cardiac outcomes in renal transplant recipients: A multicentre, randomised, placebo-controlled trial. Lancet 361:2024, 2003.

Kasiske BL: Clinical practice guidelines for managing dyslipidemias in kidney transplant patients. Am J Transplant 5:1576, 2005.

Kasiske BL, Snyder JJ, Gilbertson DT, Wang C: Cancer after kidney transplantation in the United States. Am J Transplant 4:905, 2004.

Kasiske BL, Vazquez MA, Harmon WE, et al: Recommendations for the outpatient surveillance of renal transplant recipients. American Society of Transplantation. J Am Soc Nephrol 11(Suppl 15):S1, 2000.

Mannon RB, Kirk AD: Beyond histology: Novel tools to diagnose allograft dysfunction. Clin J Am Soc Nephrol 1:358, 2006.

Meier-Kriesche HU, Baliga R, Kaplan B: Decreased renal function is a strong risk factor for cardiovascular death after renal transplantation. Transplantation 75:1291, 2003.

Meier-Kriesche HU, Schold JD, Srinivas TR, Kaplan B: Lack of improvement in renal allograft survival despite a marked decrease in acute rejection rates over the most recent era. Am J Transplant 4:378, 2004.

Nankivell BJ, Borrows RJ, Fung CL, et al: The natural history of chronic allograft nephropathy. N Engl J Med 349:2326, 2003.

Nankivell BJ, Chapman JR: The significance of subclinical rejection and the value of protocol biopsies. Am J Transplant 6:2006, 2006.

Ojo AO: Cardiovascular complications after renal transplantation and their prevention. Transplantation 82:603, 2006.

Racusen LC, Colvin RB, Solez K, et al: Antibody-mediated rejection criteria: An addition to the Banff '97 classification of renal allograft rejection. Am J Transplant 3:708, 2003.

Solez K, Colvin RB, Racusen LC, et al: Banff of Classification of Renal Allograft Pathology: Updates and future direction. AM J Transplant 8:753, 2008.

Tang IY, Meier-Kriesche HU, Kaplan B: Immunosuppressive strategies to improve outcomes of kidney transplantation. Semin Nephrol 27:377, 2007.

Wilkinson A, Davidson J, Dotta F, et al: Guidelines for the treatment and management of new-onset diabetes after transplantation. Clin Transplant 19:291, 2005.

Hypertension

CHAPTER 64

Pathogenesis of Hypertension

Christopher S. Wilcox

Hypertension implies an increase in either cardiac output or total peripheral resistance (TPR). Essential hypertension developing in young adults is often initiated by an increase in cardiac output, associated with signs of overactivity of the sympathetic nervous system; the blood pressure (BP) is labile, and the heart rate is increased. Later, the BP increases further because of a rise in TPR, with consequent restoration of a normal cardiac output. Most patients with sustained hypertension who are encountered in clinical practice have an elevated TPR. This is accompanied by vasoconstriction of resistance vessels, but, over time, vascular remodeling contributes a structural component to increased vascular resistance.

Left ventricular systole creates a shock wave that is reflected back from the peripheral resistance vessels. During early diastole, this wave reaches the ascending aorta, where it is visible as the dicrotic notch in tracings of aortic pressure. With aging, there is loss of elasticity and an increase in the tone of the resistance vessels; as a result, the pressure wave is transmitted more rapidly to and fro within the arterial tree. Eventually, this shock wave in the aorta coincides with the upstroke of the aortic systolic pressure wave, leading to an abrupt increase in the height of the systolic BP. This accounts for the frequent finding of isolated, or predominant, systolic hypertension in the elderly. In contrast, systolic hypertension in the young usually reflects an enhanced cardiac contractility and output.

PATHOPHYSIOLOGY OF HYPERTENSION

When a normal person arises, there is an abrupt fall in venous return. An ensuing drop in cardiac output elicits a baroreflex response, as resistance vessels contract to buffer the immediate fall in BP and as capacitance vessels contract to restore venous return. The outcome is only a small drop in the systolic BP, with a modest rise in diastolic BP and heart rate. During prolonged standing, increased renal sympathetic nerve activity enhances the reabsorption of sodium chloride (NaCl) and fluid by the renal tubules, as well as the release of renin from the juxtaglomerular apparatus, with the subsequent generation of angiotensin II and aldosterone, which maintain the BP and the volume of the circulation. In contrast, the BP of patients with autonomic insufficiency declines progressively on standing, often to the point of syncope. These patients with autonomic failure illustrate vividly the crucial importance of a stable BP for efficient function of the brain, heart, and kidneys. Therefore, it is no surprise that

evolution has provided multiple, coordinated BP-regulatory processes. The understanding of the cause for a sustained change in BP, such as hypertension, requires knowledge of a number of interrelated pathophysiologic processes. The most important and best understood of these are discussed in this chapter.

Renal Mechanisms and Salt Balance

The kidney has a unique role in BP regulation. Renal salt and water retention sufficient to increase the extracellular fluid (ECF) volume, blood volume, and mean circulatory filling pressure enhances venous return, cardiac output, and BP. The kidney is so effective in excreting excess NaCl and fluid during periods of surfeit, or retaining them during periods of deficit, that the ECF and blood volumes normally vary less than 10% with changes in salt intake. Consequently, the role of body fluids in hypertension is subtle. For example, a 10-fold increase in daily NaCl intake in normal subjects increases ECF volume by less than 1 L (about 7%) and normally does not increase BP. Conversely, a diet with no salt content leads to the loss of approximately 1 L of body fluid over 3 to 5 days and only a trivial fall in BP. Very different effects are seen in patients with chronic kidney disease (CKD), whose BP often increases with the level of salt intake. This "salt-sensitive" component to BP increases progressively with loss of kidney function in patients with vascular or glomerular kidney disease. Among normotensive subjects, a salt-sensitive component to BP is apparent in about 30% and appears to be genetically determined. Salt sensitivity is almost twice as frequent in patients with hypertension and is particularly common among African Americans, the elderly, and those who develop CKD. It is generally associated with a lower level of plasma renin activity (PRA).

What underlies salt sensitivity? The normal kidneys are exquisitely sensitive to BP. A rise in mean arterial pressure (MAP) of as little as 1 to 3 mm Hg elicits a subtle increase in renal NaCl and fluid elimination. This "pressure natriuresis" also works in reverse and conserves NaCl and fluid during decreases in BP. It is rapid, quantitative, and fundamental for normal homeostasis. It is primarily a result of changes in tubular NaCl reabsorption rather than total renal blood flow or glomerular filtration rate (GFR). This autoregulatory mechanism accurately adjusts salt excretion and body fluids in healthy kidneys across a wide range of BPs. Two primary mechanisms of pressure natriuresis have been identified.

First, in some studies in rats, a rise in renal perfusion pressure increases blood flow selectively through the medulla, which is not autoregulated. This increase in pressure and flow enhances renal interstitial hydraulic pressure throughout the kidney, which impairs fluid uptake into the bloodstream. Therefore, net NaCl and fluid reabsorption is diminished. Second, the degree of stretch of the afferent arteriole regulates the secretion of renin into the bloodstream, and hence the generation of angiotensin II. Therefore, an increase in BP that is transmitted to this site reduces renin secretion. Angiotensin II coordinates the body's salt and fluid retention mechanisms by stimulating thirst and enhancing NaCl and fluid reabsorption in the loop and distal nephron segments. By stimulating secretion of aldosterone and arginine vasopressin and inhibiting atrial natriuretic peptide (ANP), angiotensin II further enhances reabsorption in the distal nephron. Thus, during normal homeostasis, an increase in BP is matched by a decrease in PRA. It follows that a normal or elevated value for PRA in hypertension is effectively "inappropriate" for the level of BP and is thereby contributing to the maintenance of hypertension.

The relationships between long-term changes in salt intake, the renin-angiotensin-aldosterone system (RAAS) and BP are shown diagrammatically in **Figure 64-1**. Normal human subjects regulate the RAAS closely with changes in salt intake. A challenge in the form of an increase in salt intake brings about only a modest and transient rise in MAP, because the RAAS is suppressed and the highly effective pressure natriuresis mechanism rapidly increases renal NaCl and fluid elimination sufficiently to restore a normal blood volume and BP. Expressed quantitatively in **Figure 64-1**, the slope of the increase in NaCl excretion with BP is almost vertical. The steepness of this slope, or the gain of the pressure natriuresis relationship, reflects reciprocal changes in the RAAS with BP that dictate appropriate changes in salt handling by the kidney. Therefore, when the RAAS is artificially fixed, the slope

of the pressure natriuresis relationship flattens, leading to salt sensitivity, and the set point is displaced, leading to a change in ambient BP. For example, an infusion of angiotensin II into a normal subject raises the BP. Because angiotensin II is being infused, the kidney cannot reduce angiotensin II levels appropriately by reducing renin secretion. Therefore, the pressure natriuresis mechanism is prevented, and the BP elevation is sustained without an effective and complete renal compensation. In contrast, normal subjects treated with an angiotensin-converting enzyme (ACE) inhibitor to block angiotensin II generation or with an angiotensin receptor blocker (ARB) to block AT_1 receptors have a fall in BP. Again, the kidney cannot dictate an appropriate rise or action of angiotensin II and aldosterone that would be required to retain sufficient NaCl and fluid to buffer the fall in BP. Therefore, when the RAAS is fixed, the BP changes as a function of salt intake and becomes highly "salt sensitive" (see **Fig. 64-1**). These studies demonstrate the unique role of the RAAS in long-term BP regulation and its importance in isolating BP from NaCl intake.

Some recent findings add complexity to these simple relationships. Renin also is generated within the connecting tubule and collecting ducts. This renal renin may contribute to the very high level of angiotensin within the kidney that does not share the same relationship with dietary salt. Animal models of diabetes mellitus demonstrate an increase in local angiotensin generation and action in the kidneys that may contribute to the beneficial effects of ACE inhibitor and ARB therapy despite low circulating renin levels. Other studies have shown that prorenin, although not active itself, becomes activated after binding to a renin receptor in the tissues, where novel signaling adds another component to the effects of the RAAS. This is important, because these actions may not be blocked by conventional RAAS antagonists. It is presently controversial whether the novel renin inhibitors block this renin receptor.

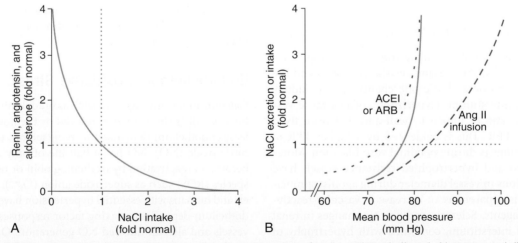

FIGURE 64-1 A, Normal, steady-state relationship between plasma concentrations of renin, angiotensin II, and aldosterone and dietary salt intake. **B,** Relationships between sodium excretion, relative to intake and mean arterial blood pressure in normal subjects (*solid line*), in subjects given an angiotensin-converting enzyme inhibitor (ACEI) or angiotensin receptor blocker (ARB) (*short dashes*), and in subjects given an infusion of angiotensin II (Ang II) (*long dashes*) to prevent adaptive changes in Ang II levels. (Modified from Guyton AC et al: In Laragh JH, Brenner BM [eds]: Hypertension, Pathophysiology, Diagnosis and Management. New York, Raven, 1995, pp 1311-1326 with permission.)

Three compelling lines of evidence implicate the kidney and RAAS in long-term BP regulation. First, transplantation studies between genetically hypertensive and normotensive rat strains showed that a normotensive animal that receives a kidney from a hypertensive animal become hypertensive, and vice versa. Similarly, human kidney transplant recipients frequently become hypertensive if they receive a kidney from a hypertensive donor. Apparently, the kidney in hypertension is programmed to retain salt and water inappropriately for a normal level of BP, thereby resetting the pressure natriuresis to a higher level of BP and dictating the appearance of hypertension in the recipient even if the neurohumoral environment is that of normotension. Nevertheless, recent studies in gene deleted or transgenic mice subjected to renal transplantation concluded that the increase in BP during prolonged infusion of angiotensin II was mediated by combined effects within the kidney and the systemic circulation, most likely involving the brain. A second observation was that BP is normally reduced 5% to 20% by an ACE inhibitor, an ARB, an aldosterone receptor antagonist, or a renin inhibitor. The fall in BP was greatest in those with elevated PRA values and was enhanced by dietary salt restriction or concurrent use of diuretic drugs (see **Fig. 64-1**). Third, almost 90% of patients approaching end-stage renal disease (ESRD) have hypertension.

Total-Body Autoregulation

An increase in cardiac output necessarily increases peripheral blood flow. However, each organ has intrinsic mechanisms that adapt blood flow to its metabolic needs. Therefore, over time, an increase in cardiac output is translated into an increase in TPR. The outcome is that organ blood flow is maintained, but hypertension becomes sustained. This total-body autoregulation is demonstrated in human subjects given salt-retaining mineralocorticosteroid hormones. An initial rise in cardiac output is translated in most into sustained hypertension and a raised TPR over 5 to 15 days.

Structural Components to Hypertension

Hypertension causes not only hypertrophic or eutrophic remodeling in the distributing and resistance vessels and the heart but also fibrotic and sclerotic changes in the kidney glomeruli and interstitium. Hypertrophy of resistance vessels limits the ratio of lumen to wall and dictates a fixed component to TPR. This is evidenced by a higher TPR of hypertensive subjects during maximal vasodilatation. Moreover, thickened and hypertrophied resistance vessels have greater reductions in vessel diameter during agonist stimulation, and this is apparent as an increase in vascular reactivity to pressor agents. Sclerotic and fibrotic changes in renal glomeruli and interstitium, combined with hypertrophy of the afferent arterioles, limit the sensing of BP in the juxtaglomerular apparatus and interstitium of the kidney. This blunts renin release and pressure natriuresis, thereby contributing to salt sensitivity and sustained hypertension. Rats receiving

intermittent weak electrical stimulation of the hypothalamus initially have an abrupt increase in BP followed by an abrupt reduction after the cessation of the stimulus; however, after about 6 weeks, the baseline BP increases in parallel with the appearance of hypertrophy of the resistance vessels. These structural components may explain why it often takes some weeks or months to achieve maximal antihypertensive action from a drug, a reduction in salt intake, or correction of a renal artery stenosis. Vascular and left ventricular hypertrophy is largely, but not completely, reversible during treatment of hypertension, whereas fibrotic and sclerotic changes are not.

Sympathetic Nervous System, Brain, and Baroreflexes

A rise in BP elicits a baroreflex-induced reduction in tone of the sympathetic nervous system and an increase in tone of the parasympathetic nervous system. Paradoxically, human hypertension is often associated with an increase in heart rate, maintained or increased plasma catecholamine levels, and an increase in directly measured sympathetic nerve discharge despite the stimulus to the baroreceptors. What is the cause of this inappropriate activation of the sympathetic nervous system in hypertension? Studies in animals show that the baroreflex "resets" to the ambient level of BP after 2 to 5 days. It no longer continues to "fight" the elevated BP but defends it at the new elevated level. Much of this adaptation occurs within the baroreceptors themselves. Additionally, animal models have identified central mechanisms that alter the gain of the baroreflex process, and therefore the sympathetic tone, in hypertension. The importance of central mechanisms in human hypertension is apparent from the effectiveness of drugs, such as clonidine, that act within the brain to decrease the sympathetic tone. Finally, with aging and atherosclerosis, the walls of the carotid sinus and other baroreflex sensing sites become less distensible. Therefore, the BP is less effective in stretching the afferent nerve endings, and the sensitivity of the baroreflex is diminished. This may contribute to the enhanced sympathetic nerve activity and increased plasma catecholamines that are characteristic of elderly hypertensive subjects.

Endothelium and Oxidative Stress

Calcium-mobilizing agonists such as bradykinin or acetylcholine, as well as shear forces produced by the flow of blood, release endothelium-dependent relaxing factors, predominantly nitric oxide (NO). NO has a half-life of only a few seconds because of inactivation by oxyhemoglobin or reactive oxygen species (ROS) such as superoxide anion ($O_2^{\bullet-}$). Animal models and humans with essential hypertension have defects in endothelium-dependent relaxing factor responses of peripheral vessels and also diminished NO generation. One underlying mechanism is oxidative stress. Excessive $O_2^{\bullet-}$ formation inactivates NO, leading to a functional NO deficiency. Another mechanism is the appearance of inhibitors of nitric oxide synthase (NOS), including asymmetric dimethyl arginine

(ADMA). Finally, atherosclerosis, prolonged hypertension, or the development of malignant hypertension causes structural changes of the endothelium that limit NO generation further. In the kidney, NO inhibits renal NaCl reabsorption in the loop of Henle and collecting ducts. Therefore, NO deficiency not only induces vasoconstriction but also diminishes renal pressure natriuresis. Functional NO deficiency in large blood vessels contributes to vascular inflammation and atherosclerosis.

Genetic Contributions

The heritability of human hypertension can be assessed from differences in the concordance of hypertension between identical twins (who share all genes and a similar environment) versus nonidentical twins (who share only a similar environment). These studies suggest that genetic factors contribute less than half to the development of hypertension in modern humans. Studies in mice with targeted disruption of individual genes or insertions of extra copies of genes provided direct evidence for critical regulatory roles for certain gene products in hypertension. Deletions of the genes for endothelial NOS or ANP lead to salt-dependent hypertension in mice. The BP of mice with deletion or insertion of the gene encoding ACE decreases with the number of copies of the gene. These are compelling examples of circumstances in which a single gene can sustain hypertension. However, there is increasing recognition of the complexity and importance of gene–gene interactions and the crucial effects of the genetic background on the changes in BP that accompany insertion or deletion of a gene.

Presently, compelling evidence for individual gene defects in most subjects with human essential hypertension is lacking. However, certain rare forms of hereditary hypertension are caused by single-gene defects. For example, dexamethasone-suppressible hyperaldosteronism is caused by a chimeric rearrangement of the gene encoding aldosterone synthase that renders the enzyme responsive to adrenocorticotropic hormone. Liddle's syndrome is caused by a mutation in the gene encoding one component of the endothelial sodium channel that is expressed in the distal convoluted tubule. The mutated form has lost its normal regulation, leading to a permanent "open state" of the sodium channel that dictates inappropriate renal NaCl retention and salt-sensitive, low-renin hypertension (see Chapters 9, 40, and 66).

AGENTS IMPLICATED IN HYPERTENSION

Alterations in the synthesis, secretion, degradation, or action of numerous substances are implicated in certain categories of hypertension. The most important of these are described in the following paragraphs.

Renin, Angiotensin II, and Aldosterone

The PRA is not appropriately suppressed in most patients with essential hypertension and is increased above normal values in approximately 15%. Subjects with normal or high PRA have a greater antihypertensive response to single-agent therapy with an ACE inhibitor, an ARB, or a β-blocker than patients with low-renin hypertension, who respond especially to salt restriction and diuretic therapy. The RAAS is particularly important in the maintenance of BP in patients with renovascular hypertension, although its importance wanes during the chronic phase, when structural alterations in blood vessels or damage in the kidney dictate a RAAS-independent component to the hypertension.

Sympathetic Nervous System and Catecholamines

Pheochromocytoma is a catecholamine-secreting tumor, often occurring in the adrenal medulla, that increases plasma catecholamines 10- to 1000-fold. However, even such extraordinary increases in pressor amines are rarely fatal, because an intact renal pressure natriuresis mechanism reduces the blood volume, thereby limiting the rise in BP. Indeed, such patients can have orthostatic hypotension between episodes of catecholamine secretion (see Chapter 66).

An increased sympathetic nerve tone of resistance vessels in human essential hypertension causes α_1-receptor–mediated vasoconstriction of the blood vessels and β_1-receptor–mediated increases in contractility and output of the heart that are only modestly offset by β_2-receptor–mediated vasorelaxation of peripheral blood vessels. Increased sympathetic nerve discharge to the kidney leads to α_1-mediated enhancement of NaCl reabsorption and β_1-mediated renin release.

Dopamine

Dopamine is synthesized in the brain and renal tubular epithelial cells independent of sympathetic nerves. Dopamine synthesis in the kidney is enhanced during volume expansion and contributes to decreased reabsorption of NaCl, especially in the proximal tubule. Defects in tubular dopamine responsiveness are apparent in genetic models of hypertension. Recent evidence relates single nucleotide polymorphisms of genes that regulate dopamine receptors to human salt-sensitive hypertension.

Arachidonate Metabolites

Arachidonate is esterified as a phospholipid in cell membranes. It is released by phospholipases that are activated by agents such as angiotensin II. Arachidonate is metabolized principally by three enzymes. Cyclooxygenase (COX) generates unstable intermediates whose subsequent metabolism by specific enzymes yields prostaglandins that are either vasodilative (e.g., prostaglandin I_2 [PGI_2]), vasoconstrictive (e.g., thromboxane), or of mixed effect (e.g., PGE_2). COX-1 is expressed in many tissues, including platelets, resistance vessels, glomeruli, and cortical collecting ducts. COX-2 is induced by inflammatory mediators. However, the normal kidney is unusual in expressing substantial COX-2, which is located in macula densa cells, tubules, renal medullary interstitial cells, and arterioles. The net effect of blocking COX-1 in some studies is to cause fluid and NaCl retention, leading to a modest salt-sensitive increase in BP. COX-2 is implicated in renin secretion and renovascular hypertension. Blockade of COX-2 has little effect on normal BP but can increase BP in those with essential hypertension. Nonsteroidal anti-inflammatory agents exacerbate essential hypertension, blunt the antihypertensive actions of most commonly used agents, predispose to acute renal failure during volume depletion or hypotension, and blunt the natriuretic action of loop diuretics. In contrast, aspirin reduces blood pressure in patients with renovascular hypertension, testifying to the prohypertensive actions of thromboxane and other prostanoids that active the thromboxane-prostanoid receptor in this condition. Metabolism of arachidonate by cytochrome P-450 monooxygenase yields 19,20-hydroxyeicosatetraenoic acid (HETE), which is a vasoconstrictor of blood vessels but inhibits tubular NaCl reabsorption. Metabolism by epoxygenase leads to epoxyeicosatrienoic acids (EETs), which are powerful vasodilators and natriuretic agents. Arachidonate metabolites act primarily as modulating agents in normal physiology; however, their role in human essential hypertension remains elusive.

L-Arginine-Nitric Oxide Pathway

NO is generated by three isoforms of NOS that are widely expressed in the body. NO interacts with many heme-centered enzymes. Activation of guanylyl cyclase generates cyclic guanosine monophosphate, which is a powerful vasorelaxant and inhibits NaCl reabsorption in the kidney. Defects in NO generation in the endothelium of blood vessels in human essential hypertension may contribute to increased peripheral resistance, vascular remodeling, and atherosclerosis, whereas defects in renal NO generation may contribute to inappropriate renal NaCl retention and salt sensitivity. There is a profound reduction in NOS activity in hypertensive human subjects and in those with CKD.

Reactive Oxygen Species

The incomplete reduction of molecular oxygen, either by the respiratory chain during cellular respiration or by oxidases such as nicotinamide adenine dinucleotide phosphate (NADPH) oxidase yields ROS including $O_2^{\bullet-}$ and generates peroxynitrite ($ONOO^-$), which has long-lasting effects through oxidizing and nitrosylating reactions. Reaction of ROS with lipids yields oxidized low-density lipoprotein (LDL), which promotes atherosclerosis, and isoprostanes, which cause vasoconstriction, salt retention, and platelet aggregation. ROS are difficult to quantitate, but indirect evidence suggests that hypertension, especially in the setting of CKD, is a state of oxidative stress. Drugs that effectively reduce $O_2^{\bullet-}$ reduce BP in animal models of hypertension, but they are largely unexamined in human hypertension.

Endothelins

Endothelins are produced especially in cells of the vascular endothelium and collecting tubules. Discrete receptors mediate either increased vascular resistance (type A) or the release of NO and inhibition of NaCl reabsorption in the collecting ducts (type B). Endothelin type A receptors potentiate the vasoconstriction accompanying angiotensin II infusion or blockade of NOS. Endothelin is released by hypoxia, specific agonists such as angiotensin II, salt loading, and cytokines. Nonspecific blockade of endothelin receptors lowers BP in models of volume-expanded hypertension. The role of endothelin in human essential hypertension is unclear.

Atrial Natriuretic Peptide

ANP is released from the heart during atrial stretch. It acts on receptors that increase GFR, decrease NaCl reabsorption in the distal nephron, and inhibit renin secretion. ANP is released during volume expansion and contributes to the natriuretic response. Its role in essential hypertension is unclear. Endopeptidase inhibitors that block ANP degradation are natriuretic and antihypertensive; but they also inhibit the metabolism of kinins. Although an increase in kinins may contribute to the fall in BP with endopeptidase or ACE inhibitors, kinins can cause an irritant cough or a more serious anaphylactoid reaction.

PATHOGENESIS OF HYPERTENSION IN CHRONIC KIDNEY DISEASE

As CKD progresses, the prevalence of salt-sensitive hypertension increases in proportion to the fall in GFR. Hypertension is almost universal in patients with CKD due to primary glomerular or vascular disease, whereas those with primary tubulointerstitial disease are often normotensive or, occasionally, salt losing.

With declining nephron number, CKD limits the ability to adjust NaCl excretion rapidly and quantitatively during changes in intake. The role of ECF volume expansion is apparent from the ability of hemodialysis to lower BP, often to normotensive levels, in patients with ESRD.

Additional mechanisms besides primary renal fluid retention contribute to the increased TPR and hypertension in patients with CKD. The RAAS is often inappropriately stimulated. The ESRD kidney generates abnormal renal afferent nerve impulses, which entrain an increased sympathetic nerve discharge that is reversed by bilateral nephrectomy. Plasma levels of endothelin increase with kidney failure. CKD induces oxidative stress, which contributes to vascular disease and impaired endothelium-dependent relaxing factor responses. A decreased generation of NO from L-arginine follows the accumulation of ADMA, which inhibits NOS. The thromboxane prostanoid receptor is activated and contributes to vasoconstriction and structural damage.

Clearly, hypertension in CKD is multifactorial, but volume expansion and salt sensitivity are predominant. Pressor mechanisms mediated by angiotensin II, catecholamines, endothelin, or thromboxane prostanoid receptors become more potent during volume expansion. This fact may underlie the importance of these systems in the ESRD patients. Finally, many of the pathways that contribute to hypertension in ESRD, such as impaired NO generation and excessive production of endothelin, ROS, and ADMA, also contribute to atherosclerosis, cardiac hypertrophy, and progressive renal fibrosis and sclerosis. Indeed, in poorly treated hypertension, kidney damage leads to additional hypertension, which itself engenders further kidney damage, generating a vicious spiral culminating in accelerated hypertension, progressively diminishing kidney function, and the requirement for renal replacement therapy. Therefore, rational management of hypertension in CKD first entails vigorous salt-depleting therapy with a salt-restricted diet and diuretic therapy. Patients frequently require additional therapy to combat the enhanced vasoconstriction and to attempt to slow the rate of progression.

BIBLIOGRAPHY

DiBona GF: Sympathetic nervous system and the kidney in hypertension. Curr Opin Nephrol Hypertens 11:197-200, 2002.

Guyton AC, Hall JE, Coleman TG, Manning RD: The dominant role of the kidneys in the long-term regulation of arterial pressure in normal and hypertensive states. In Laragh JH, Brenner BM (eds): Hypertension: Pathophysiology, Diagnosis and Management. New York, Raven, 1990, pp 1029-1052.

Navar LG: The role of the kidneys in hypertension. J Clin Hypertens 7:542-549, 2005.

Wilcox CS: Oxidative stress and nitric oxide deficiency in the kidney: A critical link to hypertension? Am J Physiol Regul Integr Comp Physiol 289:R913-R935, 2005.

Wilcox CS (ed): Therapy in Nephrology and Hypertension, 3rd ed. Philadelphia, WB Saunders, 2007.

CHAPTER 65

Evaluation and Management of Hypertension

Nitin Khosla and George L. Bakris

Hypertension is the most common disease-specific reason for Americans to visit a physician. High blood pressure, especially systolic elevation, is an important risk factor that increases the likelihood of cardiovascular outcomes such as stroke, myocardial infarction (MI), and heart failure, which are the most common causes of death in people with kidney disease. Moreover, the financial burden of treating cardiovascular disease is a staggering $400 billion per year. Despite expanded knowledge and understanding of approaches to achieve guideline blood pressure goals, the 2003-2004 Nutritional Health and Nutrition Examination Survey showed that only 37% of patients achieved the target blood pressure.

The National High Blood Pressure Education Program of the National Heart, Lung, and Blood Institute impaneled the Joint National Committee on Prevention, Detection, Evaluation, and Treatment of High Blood Pressure (JNC) to provide recommendations on these important topics, based on the latest scientific research, using a consensus process. The Seventh Joint National Committee (JNC7) report redefined the approach to high blood pressure by making the diagnostic criteria simple and easy to relate to risk and treatment. This categorization and treatment model is presented in **Table 65-1**. Whereas normal blood pressure is less than 120/80 mm Hg, a new category called *prehypertension* is introduced and encompasses the blood pressure range between 120 to 139 mm Hg systolic and/or 80 to 89 mm Hg diastolic. The motivation for this designation was to draw the attention of providers and patients to the definite increase in cardiovascular risk of individuals with prehypertension compared to those with normal blood pressure (**Fig. 65-1**). However, recent analyses have demonstrated a higher cardiovascular risk in those with prehypertension.

EVALUATION OF THE HYPERTENSIVE PATIENT

Six key issues must be addressed during the evaluation of a person with an elevated blood pressure reading:

1. Documenting an accurate diagnosis of hypertension (requires two separate readings 1 to 2 months apart that are obtained after the patient has been seated quietly for 5 minutes with the feet flat on the floor and arm relaxed at the level of the heart)
2. Defining the presence or absence of target organ damage related to hypertension
3. Screening for other cardiovascular risk factors that often accompany hypertension
4. Stratifying the risk for cardiovascular disease
5. Assessing whether the patient is likely to have an identifiable cause of hypertension (i.e., secondary causes)
6. Integrating lifestyle, clinical information, and laboratory data that may be helpful in the initial or subsequent choice of therapy

ROUTINE EVALUATION IN ALL HYPERTENSIVE PATIENTS

The approach to assessing possible target organ damage includes a thorough history, physical examination, and laboratory analysis, including determinations of blood urea nitrogen (BUN), creatinine, and electrolytes; a lipid panel; a urinalysis; and an electrocardiogram (ECG). A spot urine test for albumin-to-creatinine ratio should be part of every annual checkup for individuals with diabetes or kidney disease or patients at high risk for cardiovascular disease.

The physical examination should be focused on clues to identify secondary causes of hypertension, such as a continuous abdominal or flank bruit, which may be a sign of renal arterial disease; an abdominal or flank mass that is consistent with polycystic kidney disease; or a thyroid abnormality that is consistent with a diagnosis of thyroid dysfunction. Visualization of the optic fundi is important but often overlooked. The optic fundus is the only site in the body where blood vessels can be examined directly. The impact of controlling hypertension on ophthalmic end points, such as visual loss, retinal hemorrhages, and laser photocoagulation procedures, is clinically relevant, particularly for diabetic hypertensive patients.

Cardiac Evaluation

One of the most important features of the physical examination of hypertensive patients is the cardiac examination. An atrial (S_4) gallop is a common finding that may suggest hypertensive heart disease, although it is not a very sensitive or specific indicator. The ECG is currently recommended as a part of the initial evaluation of all persons with hypertension. It is useful in documenting previously undetected MI, myocardial ischemia, and cardiac rhythm disturbance, and it is the least expensive and possibly most cost-effective way to diagnose or exclude left ventricular hypertrophy (LVH). Electrocardiographic evidence of LVH is associated with a more

TABLE 65-1 JNC7 Staging and Recommended Treatment of Hypertension to Prevent Cardiovascular Events

| | | | | Initial Drug Therapy | |
BP CLASSIFICATION	SBP* (mm Hg)	DBP* (mm Hg)	LIFESTYLE MODIFICATION	WITHOUT COMPELLING INDICATIONS	WITH COMPELLING INDICATIONS
Normal	<120	and <80	Encourage		
Prehypertension	120-139	or 80-89	Yes	No antihypertensive drug indicated	Drugs for compelling indications[†]
Stage 1 hypertension	140-159	or 90-99	Yes	Thiazide-type diuretics for most; may consider ACEI, ARB, BB, CCB, or combination	Drugs for the compelling indications[†]
Stage 2 hypertension	≥160	or ≥100	Yes	Two-drug combination for most[‡] (usually thiazide-type diuretic and ACEI or ARB or BB or CCB)	Other antihypertensive drugs (diuretics, ACEI, ARB, BB, CCB) as needed

ACEI, angiotensin-converting enzyme inhibitor; ARB, angiotensin receptor blocker; BB, β-blocker; BP, blood pressure; CCB, calcium channel blocker; DBP, diastolic blood pressure; JNC7, Seventh Joint National Committee on Prevention, Detection, Evaluation, and Treatment of High Blood Pressure; SBP, systolic blood pressure.

*Treatment is determined by highest BP category.

[†]Treat patients with chronic kidney disease or diabetes to BP goal of less than 130/80 mm Hg.

[‡]Initial combined therapy should be used cautiously in those at risk for orthostatic hypotension.

From Chobanian AV, Bakris GL, Black HR, et al: Seventh Report of the Joint National Committee on Prevention, Detection, Evaluation, and Treatment of High Blood Pressure. Hypertension 42:1206-1252, 2003, with permission.

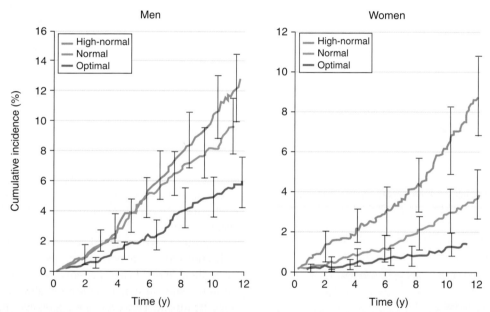

FIGURE 65-1 Impact of high-normal blood pressure (BP) on cumulative incidence of cardiovascular disease. Optimal BP: <120/80 mm Hg; normal BP: 120-129/80-84 mm Hg; high-normal BP: 130-139/85-89 mm Hg. Definitions from the Sixth Joint National Committee (JNC6) report were used in this analysis. The JNC7 redefined the optimal group as normal and the other two groups as prehypertensive. (From Vasan RS, Larson MG, Leip EP, et al: Impact of high-normal blood pressure on the risk of cardiovascular disease. N Engl J Med 345:1291-1297, 2001, with permission.)

than threefold increase in the incidence of cardiovascular events. LVH can be associated with intimal hyperplasia of the epicardial coronary arteries, increased coronary vascular resistance, and reduced diastolic relaxation, in some cases resulting in symptoms of heart failure with preserved systolic function.

Kidney Evaluation

Current recommendations for the evaluation of kidney function in the general population include measurement of BUN and serum creatinine levels and a dipstick test for proteinuria. For evaluation of albuminuria in individuals with suspected kidney disease, the guidelines of the National Institutes of Health (NIH) and National Kidney Foundation (NKF) consensus panel should be followed (see Fig. 53-3 in Chapter 53). In patients with diabetes or kidney disease at any stage, a spot urine test of the albumin-to-creatinine ratio is recommended by the NKF, the JNC7, and the American Diabetes Association. Microalbuminuria, defined as a urine albumin-to-creatinine ratio between 30 and 299 mg/g of creatinine, is a significant risk marker for cardiovascular events in patients, regardless of diabetes status.

The prevalence of microalbuminuria in type 2 diabetes is 20%, with a range of 12% to 36%, and it is more common (about 30%) in those older than 55 years. The prevalence of microalbuminuria ranges from 5% to 40% in nondiabetic hypertensives. In addition to measurement of albuminuria, an estimated glomerular filtration rate (GFR) should be used to define kidney function. The GFR can be calculated using the methods described in Chapters 3 and 53.

Evaluation of Identifiable Causes of Hypertension

There are many identifiable causes of nonidiopathic (secondary) hypertension (**Table 65-2**). In patients with some of these causes, the elevation of blood pressure can be ameliorated or eliminated with specific treatment, such as angioplasty, surgery, or avoidance of the ingested agent that caused the hypertension. Other causes, such as specific enzyme deficiencies, coarctation of the aorta, and Ask-Upmark kidney, are rare. Secondary causes of hypertension are discussed in Chapter 66.

TREATMENT OF HYPERTENSION

After the diagnosis has been established in a patient, hypertension is best managed through an integrated approach that combines lifestyle modifications with a treatment regimen that takes into account comorbid conditions. Age and ethnic background play important roles in the selection of antihypertensive drugs. JNC7 provided guidelines for initiation of hypertensive agents that were primarily based on outcome trials, the largest of which was the Antihypertensive and Lipid-Lowering Treatment to Prevent Heart Attack Trial (ALLHAT).

TABLE 65-2 Identifiable Causes of Secondary Hypertension

Obesity

Chronic kidney disease

Coarctation of the aorta

Cushing's syndrome and other glucocorticoid excess states, including chronic steroid therapy

Drug-induced or drug-related
  Nonsteroidal anti-inflammatory drugs; cyclooxygenase 2 inhibitors
  Cocaine, amphetamines, other illicit drugs
  Sympathomimetics (e.g., decongestants, anorectics)
  Oral contraceptive hormones
  Adrenal steroid hormones
  Cyclosporine and tacrolimus
  Erythropoietin
  Licorice, including some chewing tobacco
    Selected over-the-counter dietary supplements and medicines
    (e.g., ephedra, ma huang, bitter orange)

Obstructive uropathy

Pheochromocytoma

Primary aldosteronism and other mineralocorticoid excess states

Renovascular hypertension

Sleep apnea

Thyroid or parathyroid disease

The ALLHAT was a randomized, prospective study of 33,357 hypertensive patients at high risk for cardiovascular events. The purpose of this trial was to evaluate differences among four drug classes on the primary end point of fatal coronary heart disease or nonfatal MI. There was no difference in the primary end point among the drug classes. Secondary outcomes included all-cause mortality, stroke, and combined cardiovascular disease events. There were differences between groups favoring a risk reduction for those randomized to chlorthalidone (a thiazide-like diuretic) compared with the other three agents: amlodipine (a dihydropyridine calcium channel blocker), lisinopril (an angiotensin-converting enzyme [ACE] inhibitor), or doxazosin (an α-adrenergic blocker). Because chlorthalidone was the reference group against which the other agents were compared and because it was a *superiority* rather than an *equivalence* trial, the principal findings indicated that diuretics were superior to the other classes tested, because the other classes did not have fewer coronary heart disease deaths or nonfatal MIs. These results apply to people with demographic characteristics similar to the individuals enrolled in the trial (i.e., age older than 55 years with high cardiovascular risk). The JNC7 therefore used the wording that thiazide-like diuretics are first-line treatment for "most people."

Lifestyle Modifications

The JNC7 report built on an advisory from the National High Blood Pressure Education Program to recommend weight loss for overweight hypertensive patients, modification of dietary sodium intake to 100 mmol/day or less, and modification of alcohol intake to no more than two drinks per day. In addition, all recommendations for lifestyle modifications include smoking cessation to maximize overall cardiovascular risk reduction.

For those with stage 1 hypertension and no compelling indications for antihypertensive medicines (i.e., <15% of the 72 million hypertensive patients), consideration should be given to using lifestyle modification alone before pharmacologic treatment. However, the aggressive lifestyle modifications achieved in clinical trials are very difficult to achieve in clinical practice. Moreover, it has been repeatedly shown that drug therapy leads to sooner and greater reductions in blood pressure and a greater likelihood of achieving blood pressure goals compared with lifestyle modifications alone. For those with stage 2 hypertension, pharmacologic treatment should be initiated along with lifestyle modifications (see **Table 65-1**). According to JNC7 and the 2007 European Hypertension Guidelines, treatment for stage 2 hypertension should be initiated with combination (two-drug) antihypertensive therapy if blood pressure is more than 20/10 mm Hg above the goal.

Pharmacologic Therapy

Antihypertensive medications should be initiated if, on two separate occasions, the systolic pressure is persistently 140 mm Hg or higher or the diastolic pressure is 90 mm Hg or higher in the office; for those with diabetes or chronic kidney disease (CKD), therapy should be initiated at blood pressure levels higher than 130/80 mm Hg. **Table 65-3** lists a selection of the approved antihypertensive drugs available in the United States.

Patients with prehypertension pose a special dilemma. Although the Trial of Preventing Hypertension (TROPHY) showed that treatment of prehypertensive patients with an intermediate dose of an angiotensin receptor blocker (ARB) delayed the onset of frank hypertension while the patient was taking the medication, there are no data to indicate whether such treatment leads to a reduction in cardiovascular outcomes. Based on the current data, pharmacologic therapy is *not* recommended for prehypertension; lifestyle modification is the mainstay of therapy for this stage of hypertension.

Initial Drug Therapy

The JNC7 recommended that a thiazide-like diuretic be the initial choice for most patients. The word *most* refers to the category of patients in whom diuretics have reduced cardiovascular events in trials (usually individuals ≥55 years of age). Special consideration should be given, however, to the specific thiazide chosen. Chlorthalidone is superior to hydrochlorothiazide in terms of blood pressure reduction; however, there has been no head-to-head outcome trial to evaluate differences. Also, thiazide diuretics should not be the initial agents used in all patients. The crucial point is achievement of blood pressure goals using agents with the lowest side effect profiles. As stated in the 2007 European Guidelines, "It is not so important how treatment is started but very important that blood pressure goals are achieved."

If compelling indications are present (i.e., diabetes or kidney disease), all guidelines recommend that an ACE inhibitor or ARB be used as initial therapy and titrated to the maximal dose, with a diuretic or calcium antagonist used as an add-on drug if needed to achieve the blood pressure goal. If the blood pressure goal is not achieved within 2 to 3 months with monotherapy that is appropriately uptitrated to doses used in trials, then a second agent should be added. For those patients with a blood pressure more than 20/10 mm Hg above the goal and a GFR higher than 60 mL/min, an ARB or ACE inhibitor in combination with either a thiazide diuretic or a calcium antagonist is advised as initial therapy.

Sequence of Additional Drugs

The results of many trials, including ALLHAT, have shown that only about 25% of people with hypertension can achieve their target blood pressure level with monotherapy. Moreover, in individuals with stage 2 hypertension (i.e., 20/10 mm Hg above the goal), initiation of combination therapy is recommended, because virtually all of these patients will require two or more drugs to reach their blood pressure goal. In these circumstances, if a thiazide diuretic was the initial agent, then an ACE inhibitor, ARB, or calcium channel blocker can be used as the second agent to attain the blood pressure goal, depending on the concomitant conditions. In the Study of Trandolapril/Verapamil SR and Insulin Resistance (STAR),

TABLE 65-3 Oral Antihypertensive Drugs that Positively Influence Cardiovascular or Renal Outcomes

DRUG (TRADE NAME)	USUAL DOSE RANGE (mg/DAY)	USUAL DAILY FREQUENCY*
Thiazide Diuretics		
Chlorthalidone[†]	12.5-25	1
Hydrochlorothiazide[†]	12.5-50	1
Loop Diuretics		
Furosemide[†]	20-80	2
Aldosterone Receptor Blockers		
Eplerenone	50-100	1
Spironolactone[†]	25-50	1
β-Blockers		
Bisoprolol[†]	2.5-10	1
Metoprolol[†]	50-100	1-2
Propranolol[†]	40-160	2
Combined α- and β-Blockers		
Carvedilol[†]	12.5-50	2
Carvedilol CR (Coreg CR)	10-80	1
Angiotensin-Converting Enzyme Inhibitors		
Benazepril[†]	10-40	1
Captopril[†]	25-100	2
Enalapril[†]	5-40	1-2
Fosinopril	10-40	1
Perindopril	4-8	1
Ramipril	2.5-20	1
Trandolapril	1-4	1
Angiotensin (AT1) Receptor Blockers		
Candesartan	8-32	1
Eprosartan	400-800	1-2
Irbesartan	150-300	1
Losartan	25-100	1-2
Telmisartan	20-80	1
Valsartan	80-320	1-2
Calcium Channel Blockers—Nondihydropyridines		
Diltiazem extended release (Cardizem CD, Dilacor XR, Tiazac[†])	180-420	1
Diltiazem extended release (Cardizem LA)	120-540	1
Verapamil immediate release (Calan, Isoptin[†])	80-320	2
Verapamil long-acting (Calan SR, Isoptin SR[†])	120-480	1-2
Verapamil (Coeur, Covera HS, Verelan PM)	120-360	1
Calcium Channel Blockers—Dihydropyridines		
Amlodipine[†]	2.5-10	1
Nisoldipine	10-40	1

(Continued)

TABLE 65-3 Oral Antihypertensive Drugs that Positively Influence Cardiovascular or Renal Outcomes—cont'd

DRUG (TRADE NAME)	USUAL DOSE RANGE (mg/DAY)	USUAL DAILY FREQUENCY*
Central α$_2$-Agonists and Other Centrally Acting Drugs		
Methyldopa†	250-1000	2
Direct Vasodilators		
Hydralazine†	25-100	2

*In some patients treated once daily, the antihypertensive effect diminishes toward the end of the dosing interval (i.e., trough effect). Blood pressure should be measured just before dosing to determine whether satisfactory control is obtained. An increase in dosage or frequency may need to be considered. These dosages may vary from those recommended in the package inserts.

†Available now or soon to become available in generic preparations. Trade names can vary by preparation when dosing.

From Chobanian AV, Bakris GL, Black HR, et al: Seventh Report of the Joint National Committee on Prevention, Detection, Evaluation, and Treatment of High Blood Pressure. Hypertension 42:1206-1252, 2003, with permission.

people with impaired fasting glucose levels and normal kidney function had a lower incidence of new-onset diabetes when treated with a renin-angiotensin blocker combined with a calcium antagonist versus one combined with a thiazide diuretic. In this 1-year trial of more than 250 people, the incidence of new-onset diabetes was almost fourfold higher at 1 year among those randomized to a fixed dose of an ARB combined with a thiazide diuretic versus an ACE inhibitor combined with a calcium antagonist. The STAR results showed that a blocker of the renin-angiotensin system, when used in concert with a thiazide diuretic, can protect against development of new-onset diabetes in the setting of impaired glucose tolerance. This is a further consideration in those with impaired fasting glucose and obesity who need combination therapy. The Avoiding Cardiovascular Events through Combination Therapy in Patients Living with Systolic Hypertension (ACCOMPLISH) trial was scheduled to be completed in early 2008. It is expected to provide cardiovascular outcome data for 12,000 people at high risk for events randomized to receive either a fixed-dose combination of an ACE inhibitor plus a diuretic or an ACE inhibitor plus a calcium antagonist.

Achievement of Blood Pressure Goal

The blood pressure goal should be achieved within 6 months after the initiation of therapy. This is important, because in all clinical trials, events start to separate the groups at 6 months, and almost always this separation reflects differences in blood pressure.

One of the perceived limitations to achieving the goal of less than 130/80 mm Hg in individuals with kidney disease or diabetes is the fear that lowering diastolic blood pressure excessively may lead to a J-curve effect, increasing cardiovascular mortality. A post hoc analysis of trials enrolling patients with kidney disease randomized to different levels of blood pressure control refuted this view. However, although post-hoc analyses of the Reduction of Endpoints in NIDDM with the Angiotensin II Antagonist Losartan (RENAAL) study and the Irbesartan Diabetic Nephropathy Trial (IDNT)

showed no J-curve effect for cardiovascular mortality related to diastolic blood pressure, they did reveal an increased risk in the IDNT when systolic pressure was lowered to less than 115 mm Hg in patients in whom the presence of heart failure, rather than MI, drove the events. Therefore, diastolic pressures down to the 60s should not be a deterrent from achieving a low systolic pressure in older people without angina or symptomatic coronary artery disease, because in individuals older than 50 years, systolic pressure is a much stronger predictor of cardiovascular events than diastolic pressure.

Factors to Consider in Building an Antihypertensive Drug Regimen

Several issues, including comorbidities, specific risks, and safety, should be considered when antihypertensive drug therapy is chosen.

Comorbidities and Other Risk Factors

The JNC7 recognized two possible influences that may alter the choice of initial treatment in an individual hypertensive patient: (1) comorbid conditions such as osteoporosis, for which thiazide diuretics are useful, and angina pectoris, for which β-blockers and nondihydropyridine calcium channel blockers are useful; and (2) compelling conditions, defined as the presence of other medical conditions that are commonly associated with hypertension.

Specific Risk Factors

Dyslipidemia

With the exception of β-blockers and diuretics, all other classes of antihypertensive agents are considered lipid neutral. β-Blockers and diuretics have been repeatedly shown to reduce adverse cardiovascular outcomes, and their potential to raise lipid levels therefore does not translate into a major clinical issue, at least over 5 years' duration, as noted in trials. Moreover, the shift to pharmacologic treatment of dyslipidemia in concert with treatment of hypertension avoids management issues arising from the use of these agents.

New-Onset Diabetes Mellitus

Peripheral α-blockers, ACE inhibitors, and ARBs generally improve insulin sensitivity. Although calcium antagonists are neutral in their effects on insulin sensitivity, thiazides and vasoconstricting β-blockers worsen insulin sensitivity and increase the risk of frank diabetes. However, meta-analysis have clearly demonstrated that vasodilating β-blockers (i.e. carvedilol and nebivolol) do not worsen glucose tolerance. Moreover, the STAR trial provided evidence that use of an ACE inhibitor does not protect against diuretic-related development of new-onset diabetes in patients with impaired fasting glucose tolerance. Although no trial has continued long enough to assess the effects of new-onset diabetes on outcome, there are data to suggest that the benefits of blood pressure lowering may be diminished albeit not significantly if new-onset diabetes occurs with either diuretics or β-blockers.

The β-blocker atenolol was not better than placebo in clinical trials and is no longer considered first-line therapy for uncomplicated hypertension.

Left Ventricular Hypertrophy

LVH is a robust independent risk factor for cardiovascular mortality, probably because it reflects the degree of blood pressure control over the long term. LVH results from chronic elevations in arterial pressure that cause cardiac myocyte hypertrophy and remodeling of the coronary resistance vessels, which ultimately leads to increased ventricular wall stiffness and diastolic dysfunction. There is a direct relationship between LVH and CKD stage, because most patients with stage 3 or higher CKD and virtually all patients with end-stage renal disease (ESRD) have LVH. A meta-analysis revealed that ACE inhibitors were the most efficacious for regressing LVH, followed by calcium antagonists, diuretics, and β-blockers. In contrast, direct vasodilators do not to reduce LVH.

Heart Failure

Hypertension is a major risk factor for the development of both systolic and diastolic heart failure, typically occurring many years later. Distinguishing between the two subtypes of heart failure is done most easily by estimating the left ventricular ejection fraction, and the results dictate therapy. Patients with systolic heart failure improve their blood pressure and long-term prognosis with ACE inhibitors and diuretics, to which can be added β-blockers, aldosterone receptor antagonists, and other drugs as needed. Treatment of hypertension in patients with diastolic dysfunction has not been well studied, but most authorities recommend using drugs that reduce heart rate, increase diastolic filling time, and allow the heart muscle to relax more fully: β-blockers or nondihydropyridine calcium channel blockers. Although these suggestions make physiologic sense, there are no clinical trial data to support them.

The Spectrum of Albuminuria

The normal rate of albumin excretion is less than 20 mg/day. Persistent values between 30 and 299 mg/day define the range for microalbuminuria. Several studies in different patient populations support the concept that microalbuminuria is an important risk factor for cardiovascular disease and associated early cardiovascular mortality in patients with and without diabetes, regardless of the presence of hypertension. The risk of an adverse cardiovascular event grows progressively as absolute levels of microalbuminuria increase. Unfortunately, there is no conclusive evidence from outcome trials to establish that reducing microalbuminuria results in less cardiovascular risk independent of blood pressure lowering. ACE inhibitors and ARBs have the most consistent data showing reduction in microalbuminuria and delaying its progression to macroalbuminuria (i.e., proteinuria). These agents reduce albuminuria by reducing intraglomerular pressure and altering membrane permeability at the level of the podocyte.

Conversely, retrospective analyses of clinical trials enrolling patients with advanced CKD demonstrated that reducing proteinuria (macroalbuminuria >300 mg/day) by 30% to 35% below baseline is associated with marked slowing in disease progression to ESRD, an effect not totally related to blood pressure reduction. In two specific trials, the African-American Study of Kidney Disease (a nondiabetic cohort) and the IDNT, the randomized groups of patients in whom proteinuria was not reduced did not experience the same magnitude of slowing of progression of CKD as did those in whom proteinuria declined, despite similar blood pressure control. **Figure 65-2** integrates the recommendations of the JNC7, the American Diabetes Association, the NKF and updated 2008 American Society of Hypertension to provide an approach to achieving the blood pressure goal and reducing the risk of kidney disease progression. Achievement of the goal blood pressure (<130/80 mm Hg) is particularly important, especially in people with more than 1g/day of proteinuria (**Fig. 65-3**).

Coronary Artery Disease

The American Heart Association recently changed the blood pressure target for patients with carotid artery disease (CAD), a CAD risk equivalent (e.g., carotid artery disease, peripheral arterial disease, abdominal aortic aneurysm), or a 10-year Framingham risk of more than 10% to less than 130/80 mm Hg. Although no trial has looked at whether a lower target in those patients with CAD reduces poor outcomes, this recommendation was extrapolated from other clinical data. Results for the subset of patients with CAD in the Comparison of AMlodipine versus Enalapril to Limit Occurrences of Thrombosis (CAMELOT) study demonstrated a regression of atheroma volume at blood pressures less than 120/80 mm Hg and no change in the prehypertensive range. This recommendation also stems from data showing that cardiovascular risk in the general population doubles for every increase in blood pressure of 20/10 mm Hg over 115/75 mm Hg. Although the target for blood pressure has changed, the antihypertensive agents used in those with CAD have not. β-Blockers and nondihydropyridine calcium channel blockers are effective antihypertensive agents with major antianginal efficacy. In the ALLHAT trial, amlodipine was equal in its protection against heart attack to chlorthalidone and lisinopril.

Blood Pressure Management after Stroke

In the immediate setting of acute stroke (within 72 hours), most neurologists avoid antihypertensive drugs unless blood pressure is very high (>185/110 mm Hg). If treatment is necessary at this time, an intravenously administered, short-acting drug is preferred, because it can be discontinued quickly if the patient's neurologic condition deteriorates acutely. After this period, the use of a combination of an ACE inhibitor or ARB with a thiazide diuretic has been shown to reduce recurrent events.

Safety: Adverse Reactions and Side Effects

The two primary types of adverse reactions and side effects that occur with antihypertensive drugs are clinical and biochemical. The clinical side effects are more evident to the

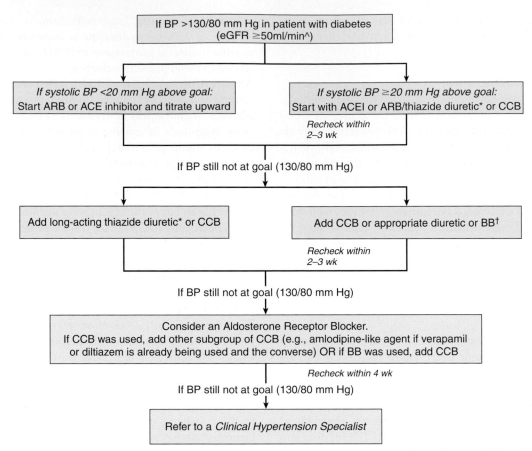

FIGURE 65-2 Integrated approach to achieving blood pressure goal in patients with kidney disease or diabetes. *Doses of 12.5 or 25 mg/day should be used; doses of 50 mg/day and higher have not demonstrated cardiovascular risk reduction. Thiazides are not useful in individuals with serum creatinine values higher than 2 mg/dL. Loop diuretics should be substituted. **β-Blockers are preferred if the patient has coronary disease or has recently suffered a myocardial infarction. Once-daily β-blocker dosing is preferred. Verapamil may be substituted for a β-blocker in patients with coronary disease, because it was shown to be as efficacious as the β-blockers for reducing mortality in large outcome trials. ACEI, angiotensin-converting enzyme inhibitor; ARB, angiotensin receptor blocker; BB, β-blocker; BP, blood pressure; CCB, calcium channel blocker.

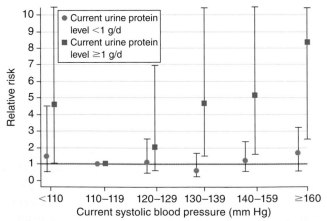

FIGURE 65-3 Relative risk of kidney disease progression in relation to blood pressure and level of proteinuria. The reference group for each level of proteinuria is the systolic blood pressure interval of 110 to 119 mm Hg. With proteinuria of less than 1g/day, the blood pressure recommendation of less than 130 mm Hg for those with nondiabetic kidney disease is appropriate. If proteinuria is greater than 1g/day, systolic blood pressure should be less than 120 mm Hg, if possible. The National Kidney Foundation K/DOQI Clinical Practice Guidelines should be consulted. (From Jafar TH, Stark PC, Schmid CH, et al: Progression of chronic kidney disease: The role of blood pressure control, proteinuria, and angiotensin-converting enzyme inhibition: A patient-level meta-analysis. Ann Intern Med 139:244-252, 2003, with permission.)

patients and are perceived by them or by the clinician to be related to the drug. The appearance of these adverse reactions requires that the drug be stopped or the dose reduced or that the patient be willing to remain on therapy until the side effect becomes tolerable or disappears. Weight gain, erectile dysfunction, depression, bronchospasm, and bradycardia are common with β-blockers. Calcium channel blockers may cause constipation, headache, dizziness or lightheadedness, flushing, and peripheral edema, especially at higher doses. ACE inhibitor–related cough develops in about 15% to 20% of patients in the United States, but it is very common in the Asian population and can occur in up to 50% of Asian people. Cough is class specific and usually occurs within 1 to 2 weeks after the initiation of the treatment, but its onset may occur after as long as 6 months. It is more common in women and resolves within 1 week after discontinuation of the offending agent. The mechanism for the associated cough and angioedema with ACE inhibitors is unknown, although it may be related to inhibition of bradykinin degradation. If cough is the main presenting symptom, switching to an ARB commonly alleviates the problem. However, if patients develop angioedema on an ACE inhibitor, changing to an ARB is advised with caution, because no reliable data are available regarding the risk of recurrent angioedema, although it is thought to be low.

Biochemical side effects consist of alterations in electrolyte balance and lipid profiles, which may or may not be perceived by the patient or the provider. These abnormalities are usually detected by laboratory analysis or other diagnostic tests (e.g., ECG). The widespread use of thiazide diuretics is not free of risk; although lower doses in the range of 12.5 to 25 mg/day may be associated with fewer side effects, individual variation is seen in clinical practice. A higher dose of thiazide diuretics (>25 mg/day) is associated with hyperuricemia and may result in gouty arthritis. The other electrolyte abnormalities seen with thiazide diuretics are hypokalemia, hyponatremia, hypercalcemia, and hypomagnesemia. Long-term use of thiazide diuretics also predisposes to hyperglycemia and diabetes. In two very large trials, about 11% of people taking thiazide diuretics who had a body mass index greater than 30 and were older than 55 years of age developed new-onset diabetes. This was s significantly higher proportion than in those taking ACE inhibitors or calcium channel blockers.

Lipid abnormalities are seen with certain antihypertensive agents. High doses of thiazide diuretics (>25 mg/day) produce an elevation of total and low-density lipoprotein cholesterol. β-Blockers have little effect on cholesterol level, but their use leads to increases in triglyceride levels and an associated drop in cardioprotective high-density lipoprotein cholesterol. Carvedilol, a newer β-blocker, is a combined non-selective β- and α_1-blocker that prevents lipid peroxidation and is not associated with lipid abnormalities.

Hyperkalemia is a common abnormality in patients treated with agents such as spironolactone, ACE inhibitors, and ARBs. The overall incidence of hyperkalemia (plasma potassium concentration >5.5 mEq/L) is approximately 5% with ACE inhibitors. More prominent hyperkalemia may be seen in patients with impaired kidney function. Among those with stage 3 or higher CKD (GFR ≤30 mL/min), limited evidence suggests that increases in serum potassium may be less pronounced with an ARB than with an ACE inhibitor. Although short-term discontinuation of an ACE inhibitor or ARB may be appropriate until an elevated potassium level is controlled, hyperkalemia is not a reason to permanently discontinue therapy in patients with CKD. Other measures, such as avoidance of nonsteroidal anti-inflammatory agents, reduction in dietary potassium, and addition of kaliuretic diuretics such as loop diuretics in appropriate doses, should be tried first.

Special Circumstances

Hypertension occurs in about 10% of pregnancies and is a major cause of perinatal morbidity and mortality in most developing countries (see Chapter 50). Other special circumstances include hypertensive emergencies and drug interactions.

Hypertensive Emergencies and Urgencies

Hypertensive emergency, as defined by JNC7, is a severely elevated blood pressure (>180/120 mm Hg) with signs and symptoms of acute end-organ damage. Patients must be hospitalized and treated immediately with parenteral drug therapy. Patients sometimes present with very high blood pressures but without evidence of acute target organ damage; this situation is considered as *hypertensive urgency* and need not be treated in the hospital setting or using intravenous medication. A physician caring for a patient with elevated blood pressures needs to be able to distinguish between these two situations for two major reasons. The route of administration of drug therapy is different (i.e., parenteral therapy for emergencies and oral therapy for urgencies), and hospitalization (usually in the intensive care unit) is necessary for hypertensive emergencies but is not required for hypertensive urgencies.

If symptomatic with either severe headache, visual changes, or chest pain, admission to hospital and possibly ICU is manatory. In hypertensive emergency a patient with elevated blood pressure who is totally a symptomatic and has no physical signs of increased cravial pressure like papilledema, out patient management is adequate.

Most authorities suggest that in most true hypertensive emergencies (with the exception of aortic dissection and some neurologic crises), the mean arterial pressure should be reduced only 10% to 15% during the first hour and by about 25% over the first 2 to 3 hours. Reductions of blood pressure too rapidly to less than 90 mm Hg diastolic or even by as little as 35% of the initial mean arterial pressure have been associated with major organ dysfunction, coma, and death. Oral antihypertensive therapy should be instituted after 6 to 12 hours of parenteral therapy. Evaluation of secondary causes of hypertension may be considered after transfer from the intensive care unit. A general approach to the treatment of patients with hypertensive emergencies is summarized in **Table 65-4**.

The choice of medications to treat a hypertensive emergency depends on the clinical situation. However, the drug used should be effective in reducing blood pressure and should have a short half-life, so that consequences, if they occur, are easier to overcome. Sodium nitroprusside has been considered the standard intravenously administered drug for all hypertensive crises. However, limitations of nitroprusside therapy include the need for invasive monitoring (i.e., an arterial line is required in most hospitals), its effect in abolishing cerebral autoregulation, and its metabolic products (i.e., thiocyanate and cyanide). These ions accumulate when nitroprusside is used in patients with renal or hepatic dysfunction and contraindicate the use of nitroprusside in pregnancy. Two newer agents, nicardipine and the dopamine 1–selective agent fenoldopam, have gained popularity because they have no toxic metabolites, do not interfere with cerebral autoregulation, and have been used safely outside the intensive care unit, although the major reasons for the latter have more to do with hospital staffing and clinical practice than a difference in specific safety issues between the drugs.

Hypertensive emergency may result in malignant nephrosclerosis, with hematuria, proteinuria, and acute renal failure. Within the kidney, fibrinoid necrosis in arterioles

TABLE 65-4 Types of Hypertensive Crises with Suggested Drug Therapy and Blood Pressure Targets

TYPE OF CRISIS	DRUG OF CHOICE	BLOOD PRESSURE TARGET
Neurologic		
Hypertensive encephalopathy	Nitroprusside*	25% reduction in MAP over 2-3 hr
Intracranial hemorrhage or acute stroke in evolution	Nitroprusside* (controversial)	0-25% reduction in MAP over 6-12 hr (controversial)
Acute head injury or trauma	Nitroprusside*	0-25% reduction in MAP over 2-3 hr (controversial)
Subarachnoid hemorrhage	Nimodipine	Up to 25% reduction in MAP in previously hypertensive patients
Cardiac		
Ischemia or infarction	Nitroglycerin or nicardipine	Reduction in ischemia
Heart failure	Nitroprusside* or nitroglycerin	Improvement in failure (typically 10-15% decrease in BP)
Aortic dissection	β-blocker plus nitroprusside*	120 mm Hg systolic in 30 min (if possible)
Renal		
Hematuria or acute renal failure	Fenoldopam	0-25% reduction in MAP over 1-12 hr

Catecholamine excess states
  Pheochromocytoma
  Abrupt drug withdrawal
	
	Phentolamine
	Withdrawn drug
		
		To control paroxysms
		Typically, only one dose necessary

Pregnancy-Related		
Eclampsia	Methyldopa, hydralazine, MgSO$_4$	Typically, less than 90 mm Hg diastolic, but often lower

BP, blood pressure; MAP, mean arterial pressure.
*Some physicians prefer an intravenous infusion of fenoldopam or nicardipine, neither of which has potentially toxic metabolites, over nitroprusside. Studies have shown improvements in kidney function during therapy with the former compared with nitroprusside.
Adapted from Elliott WJ: Hypertensive emergencies. Crit Care Clin 17:435-451, 2001.

and capillaries is observed. The renal vascular disease in this circumstance results in glomerular ischemia and activation of the renin-angiotensin system, which leads to further deterioration of blood pressure. Lowering blood pressure is the most important aspect of the management of this condition, and it should be the main objective, even if it leads to a worsening of kidney function. Over time, renal function may recover. Some physicians prefer fenoldopam to nicardipine or nitroprusside in this setting because of its specific renal-vasodilating effects. This has not been shown to affect outcomes in clinical trials. Depending on the height of the initial systolic pressure, the goal is to reduce the systolic blood pressure by about 20% to 25% within the first 2 to 3 hours, because it will reduce the risk of stroke. After the blood pressure reaches this level, additional lowering should be pursued with agents that block the renin-angiotensin system. This level of reduction is especially important in poststroke patients, for whom attempts to get the blood pressure to levels of less than 140 mm Hg should take months to achieve, in order to preserve circulation to the penumbra of the brain.

Hypertensive emergencies resulting from catecholamine-excess states (e.g., pheochromocytoma, monoamine oxidase inhibitor crises, cocaine intoxication) are best managed with long-acting α-blockade, such as with phenoxybenzamine. In patients with pheochromocytoma, acute bouts of hypertension may occur before or during surgical intervention, and they should be treated with intravenous phentolamine.

Phentolamine is a short-acting, nonselective, α-adrenergic blocker. Effective α-adrenergic blockade permits expansion of blood volume, which is usually severely decreased because of excessive adrenergic vasoconstriction. A β-blocker may then be added to overcome tachycardia, but it should never begin the regimen because blockade of vasodilatory peripheral β-adrenergic receptors with unopposed α-adrenergic receptor stimulation can lead to an additional elevation in blood pressure.

Drug Interactions

The most commonly used antihypertensive agents do not have any serious interactions with anticoagulants, platelet inhibitors, or antibiotics. Nondihydropyridine calcium channel blockers, β-blockers, and telmisartan (an ARB) must be used with care if prescribed with digoxin. The nodal blocking effect of the nondihydropyridine calcium channel blockers and the β-blockers can be additive with that of digoxin. These calcium channel blockers and telmisartan reduce digoxin elimination, potentially leading to digoxin toxicity.

Nonsteroidal anti-inflammatory agents may raise blood pressure and interfere with the activity of all antihypertensive agents. The newer cyclooxygenase 2 inhibitors also increase blood pressure, but the magnitude of the rise is less marked with celecoxib because of its shorter half-life than all other agents in this class (see Chapter 38). Use of multiple antihypertensive agents may be problematic under certain circumstances. β-Blockers in concert with nondihydropyridine calcium antagonists are warranted if the patient has a hyperdynamic circulation, such as a young person with elevated blood pressure and tachycardia. In contrast, in older people, this combination should be used with caution. An ECG should be checked first because this combination is contraindicated in the presence of second-degree heart block. Moreover, β-blockers or verapamil should not be used with clonidine in the presence of any type of heart block because of the risk of precipitating complete heart block and profound orthostatic hypotension due to baroreceptor inhibition.

The combination of ACE inhibitors or ARBs with spironolactone or eplerenone may precipitate hyperkalemia, particularly in patients with CKD. However, significant clinical benefits can result from using this combination in certain situations. In the Eplerenone Post-Acute Myocardial Infarction Heart Failure Efficacy and Survival Study (EPHESUS), this combination resulted in a 13% further risk reduction of cardiovascular death among individuals with systolic heart failure who were already receiving an ACE inhibitor or an ARB and a β-blocker. This benefit existed until the serum potassium concentration reached 5.6 mEq/L.

The addition of eplerenone to an ACE inhibitor can be done safely and can lead to significant reductions in proteinuria. It can be beneficial to use these combinations, although patients should be counseled on how to avoid hyperkalemia. Potassium levels should be checked within 1 to 2 weeks after the institution of this combination.

CONCLUSIONS

Even though treating hypertension can be costly and sometimes can seem unrewarding, the benefits to individual patients and to society make the effort worthwhile. Physicians must be careful not to become apathetic about hypertension. This important public health problem has not been solved and will not be solved until all hypertensive patients are able to avail themselves of what has been among the most successful examples of preventive medicine. For prevention of hypertension-related kidney disease and in individuals with diabetes, it is essential to reduce systolic blood pressure to at least 130 mm Hg with agents that reduce proteinuria (i.e., ACE inhibitors, ARBs, and aldosterone antagonists).

BIBLIOGRAPHY

American Association of Clinical Endocrinologists: Medical guidelines for clinical practice for the management of diabetes mellitus. Endocr Pract 13(Suppl 1):1-68, 2007.

Bakris GL, Weir MR: Angiotensin-converting enzyme inhibitor-associated elevations in serum creatinine: Is this a cause for concern? Arch Intern Med 160:685-693, 2000.

Bakris GL, Weir MR, Secic M, et al: Differential effects of calcium antagonist subclasses on markers of nephropathy progression. Kidney Int 65:1991-2002, 2004.

Black HR, Bakris GL, Elliott WJ: Hypertension: Epidemiology, pathophysiology, diagnosis and treatment. In Fuster V, Alexander W, O'Rourke R, et al (eds): Hurst's The Heart. New York, McGraw-Hill, 2001, pp 1553-1604.

Chobanian AV, Bakris GL, Black HR, et al: Seventh Report of the Joint National Committee on Prevention, Detection, Evaluation, and Treatment of High Blood Pressure. Hypertension 42:1206-1252, 2003.

de Simone G, Verdecchia P, Pede S, et al: Prognosis of inappropriate left ventricular mass in hypertension: The MAVI study. Hypertension 40:470-476, 2002.

Elliott WJ: Hypertensive emergencies. Crit Care Clin 17:435-451, 2001.

Epstein M, Williams GH, Weinberger M, et al: Selective aldosterone blockade with eplerenone reduces albuminuria in patients with type 2 diabetes. Clin J Am Soc Nephrol 1:940-951, 2006.

Jacobsen P, Andersen S, Jensen BR, Parving HH: Additive effect of ACE inhibition and angiotensin II receptor blockade in type I diabetic patients with diabetic nephropathy. J Am Soc Nephrol 14:992-999, 2003.

Jafar TH, Stark PC, Schmid CH, et al: Progression of chronic kidney disease: The role of blood pressure control, proteinuria, and angiotensin-converting enzyme inhibition—A patient-level meta-analysis. Ann Intern Med 139:244-252, 2003.

Jones CA, Francis ME, Eberhardt MS, et al: Microalbuminuria in the US population: Third National Health and Nutrition Examination Survey. Am J Kidney Dis 39:445-459, 2002.

Julius S, Nesbitt SD, Egan BM, et al: Feasibility of treating prehypertension with an angiotensin-receptor blocker. N Engl J Med 354:1685-1697, 2006.

Khosla N, Chua DY, Elliott WJ, Bakris GL: Are chlorthalidone and hydrochlorothiazide equivalent blood-pressure-lowering medications? J Clin Hypertens (Greenwich) 7:354-356, 2005.

Khosla N, Sarafidis PA, Bakris GL: Microalbuminuria. Clin Lab Med 26:635-653, 2006.

Levy D, Larson MG, Vasan RS, et al: The progression from hypertension to congestive heart failure. JAMA 275:1557-1562, 1996.

Mancia G, De Backer G, Dominiczak A, et al: 2007 Guidelines for the Management of Arterial Hypertension: The Task Force for the Management of Arterial Hypertension of the European Society of Hypertension (ESH) and of the European Society of Cardiology (ESC). J Hypertens 25:1105-1187, 2007.

Nathan S, Pepine CJ, Bakris GL: Calcium antagonists: Effects on cardio-renal risk in hypertensive patients. Hypertension 46:637-642, 2005.

National Kidney Foundation: K/DOQI Clinical Practice Guidelines on Hypertension and Antihypertensive Agents in Chronic Kidney Disease. Am J Kidney Dis 43(Suppl 2):1-290, 2004.

National Kidney Foundation: K/DOQI clinical practice guidelines and clinical practice recommendations for diabetes and chronic kidney disease. Am J Kidney Dis 49(Suppl 2):S12-S154, 2007.

Rosendorff C, Black HR, Cannon CP, et al: Treatment of hypertension in the prevention and management of ischemic heart disease: A scientific statement from the American Heart Association Council for High Blood Pressure Research and the Councils on Clinical Cardiology and Epidemiology and Prevention. Circulation 115:2761-2788, 2007.

P. A. Sarafidis and G. L. Bakris. Antihypertensive therapy and the risk of new-onset diabetes. *Diabetes Care* 29 (5):1167-1169, 2006.

P. A. Sarafidis and G. L. Bakris. Renin-angiotensin blockade and kidney disease. *Lancet* 372 (9638):511-512, 2008.

Thom T, Haase N, Rosamond W, et al: Heart disease and stroke statistics: 2006 update. A report from the American Heart Association Statistics Committee and Stroke Statistics Subcommittee. Circulation 113:e85-e151, 2006.

Vasan RS, Larson MG, Leip EP, et al: Impact of high-normal blood pressure on the risk of cardiovascular disease. N Engl J Med 345:1291-1297, 2001.

Voyaki SM, Staessen JA, Thijs L, et al: Follow-up of renal function in treated and untreated older patients with isolated systolic hypertension. Systolic Hypertension in Europe (Syst-Eur) Trial Investigators. J Hypertens 19:511-519, 2001.

CHAPTER 66

Secondary Hypertension

Rory McQuillan and Peter Conlon

Hypertension is the second most common cause of consultation to primary care physicians in the developed world, and accounts for many millions of visits every year. Although most cases constitute essential or idiopathic hypertension, about 10% reflect an underlying pathophysiology and are considered secondary hypertension. It is important that physicians can identify patients for whom screening for secondary hypertension is appropriate, so as to minimize overinvestigation of essential hypertension while not failing to diagnose the readily treatable underlying conditions that may be present. Many of the causes of secondary hypertension are reversible, and specific treatment may allow significant improvement in or normalization of the blood pressure.

Table 66-1 lists some clinical clues that may suggest the presence of secondary hypertension. Categorized in **Table 66-2** are the many causes of secondary hypertension. This chapter provides a concise overview of these conditions and suggests a practical clinical approach to the diagnosis and treatment of the patient with suspected secondary hypertension.

RENAL CAUSES OF SECONDARY HYPERTENSION

Renovascular Hypertension

Renovascular disease is the most common correctable cause of secondary hypertension. Its prevalence varies according to the clinical circumstances; it is relatively uncommon in patients with mild hypertension but quite common (incidence of 10% to 45%) in patients with severe or refractory hypertension. Although it was previously thought to be much less common in the African American population, some studies suggest that the prevalence is similar to that among whites, particularly when clinical situations similar to those in **Table 66-3** are present.

Renal artery stenosis consists of narrowing of the renal artery by more than 50%, and it may be unilateral or bilateral. Associated clinical syndromes include renovascular hypertension, ischemic renal function impairment, and otherwise unexplained recurrent episodes of acute pulmonary edema. Renovascular hypertension is mediated by activation of the renin-angiotensin-aldosterone system (RAAS) as a result of renal underperfusion resulting from unilateral or bilateral renal artery stenosis. Patients with renal artery stenosis can be classified as those with fibromuscular dysplasia (FMD) and those with atherosclerotic renal artery stenosis (ARAS). Rarely, renal artery stenosis may be caused by extrinsic renal

TABLE 66-1 Clues to the Presence of Secondary Hypertension

Young age at onset (< 40 yrs.)
Sudden onset of hypertension
Uncontrolled or refractory hypertension
Malignant hypertension
Features of a recognized underlying cause

TABLE 66-2 Causes of Secondary Hypertension

Renal Causes
Renovascular hypertension
Renal parenchymal hypertension
Endocrine Causes
Primary hyperaldosteronism
Cushing's syndrome
Pheochromocytoma
Hyperreninism
Hypothyroidism
Hyperparathyroidism
Cardiovascular or Cardiopulmonary Causes
Coarctation of the aorta
Obstructive sleep apnea
Drugs
Glucocorticoids
Nonsteroidal anti-inflammatory drugs
Combined oral contraceptive pill
Calcineurin inhibitors
Phenylephrine, caffeine
Licorice
Inherited Causes
Glucocorticoid–remediable aldosteronism
Syndrome of apparent mineralocorticoid excess (SAME)
Gordon's syndrome (i.e., type 2 pseudohypoaldosteronism)
Liddle's syndrome
Congenital adrenal hyperplasia

TABLE 66-3   Clinical Clues to the Presence of Renovascular Disease

Abrupt onset of or accelerated hypertension at any age

Episodes of flash pulmonary edema with normal ventricular function

Acute, unexplained rise in the serum creatinine level after use of an angiotensin-converting enzyme inhibitor or angiotensin receptor blocker

Elevated serum creatinine level in patients with severe or refractory hypertension

Asymmetrical renal size

Moderate to severe hypertension in a patient with diffuse atherosclerotic disease

---

artery compression, neurofibromatosis type 1, or Williams' syndrome.

FMD is a nonatherosclerotic, noninflammatory vascular disease that causes stenosis in medium-size and small arteries, most commonly the renal and carotid arteries. Renovascular hypertension is the most common manifestation, usually occurring in 30- to 50-year-old women. The progression of stenosis is slow, and renal function is usually well preserved. The most common subtype of the disease causes medial dysplasia of the affected artery, with multiple contiguous stenoses creating the appearance of a string of beads on imaging. FMD has an estimated prevalence among hypertensive patients of less than 1%, but this may be an underestimation because of the probable high rate of undetected cases. It can be a familial disease. Diagnosis of renal artery FMD should prompt screening of the carotid arteries for associated lesions. Revascularization with percutaneous angioplasty is usually successful in improving the associated hypertension.

ARAS usually is found in patients older than 50 years who are cigarette smokers and who often have other cardiovascular risk factors. It constitutes more than 85% of all renovascular disease. Lesions tend to progress, and there is often coexistent renal function impairment. The treatment of these patients, which is not well defined, is discussed later.

Diagnosis

The several, well-recognized clinical situations that suggest the presence of renovascular disease are summarized in **Table 66-3**. Clinical examination may reveal evidence of systemic atherosclerotic disease, such as carotid or femoral bruits or absent pedal pulses. The presence or absence of abdominal bruits is not particularly useful. The urine sediment is usually bland, with mild to moderate proteinuria.

The gold standard diagnostic investigation for renal artery stenosis is conventional arteriography (**Fig. 66-1**). Most centers do not proceed directly to arteriography because of the risk of contrast nephrotoxicity, cholesterol embolization, and damage to the renal or femoral arteries. Whereas captopril renography was formerly used extensively, the most popular screening tests currently are magnetic resonance angiography (MRA), duplex ultrasonography, or computed tomography (CT) spiral angiography with contrast.

MRA has been the screening investigation of choice for renal artery stenosis in most centers (**Fig. 66-2**). MRA is noninvasive, avoids ionizing radiation, and uses a nonnephrotoxic contrast agent (i.e., gadolinium). Meta-analyses comparing MRA, with or without gadolinium, with conventional angiography show that gadolinium-enhanced MRA is 97% sensitive and 93% specific for identifying renal artery stenosis and is considerably better at depicting accessory renal arteries than nongadolinium scans. However, nephrogenic systemic fibrosis (NSF), a recently described condition, has been linked to gadolinium exposure in patients with a GFR below 30 mL/min. The causal link is based on research showing gadolinium in skin biopsies of patients with NSF. NSF is a rapidly progressive, debilitating condition that causes cutaneous and visceral fibrosis for which there

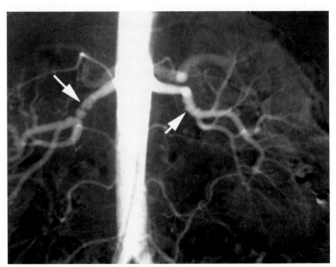

FIGURE 66-1 Conventional renal angiography demonstrates the classic beadlike appearance of fibromuscular dysplasia in both renal arteries. (Courtesy of Professor Mick Lee, Beaumont Hospital, Dublin, Ireland.)

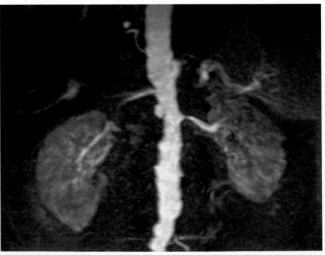

FIGURE 66-2 Magnetic resonance angiography of the aorta and renal arteries shows diffuse atherosclerotic disease of the aorta and right renal artery and a tight ostial stenosis of the left renal artery. (Courtesy of Professor Mick Lee, Beaumont Hospital, Dublin, Ireland.)

is no well-defined treatment. Gadolinium should therefore be avoided in patients with a GFR less than 30 mL/min (see Chapter 5).

Spiral CT with CT angiography is highly sensitive and specific compared with conventional angiography. Accuracy is reduced in patients with serum creatinine levels above 2 mg/dL, probably because of reduced renal blood flow. The need for a significant contrast load in patients with coexistent impairment of kidney function is a limitation.

Duplex ultrasonography of the renal arteries also reliably detects renal artery stenosis. With an experienced ultrasonographer, the sensitivity and specificity has been as high as 97% to 99% in one trial enrolling patients who later underwent conventional angiography. This method is time consuming, but is the preferred screening test at a number of institutions, where the considerable expertise required is available. The sensitivity and specificity of Doppler ultrasonography is estimated at best at about 80% to 85% in most published trials.

Performing an isotope renogram (DTPA scan) after administration of an angiotensin-converting enzyme (ACE) inhibitor is no longer popular. Although the sensitivity and specificity of this method in high-risk populations may be greater than 90% for high-grade lesions, they are much reduced in low-risk patients and in patients with bilateral disease of equal severity. It is also more cumbersome to perform than the other available screening tests.

Treatment

All patients with renal artery stenosis should be on appropriate antihypertensive therapy. Treatment with lipid-lowering drugs and antiplatelet agents should be used as indicated. These drugs are particularly likely to be of benefit in older patients with atherosclerotic lesions.

Hypertensive patients with FMD should initially be treated with an ACE inhibitor or angiotensin receptor blocker (ARB). If they remain hypertensive, the treatment of choice is revascularization with percutaneous transluminal renal angioplasty (PTRA). PTRA in patients with FMD is almost always technically successful, with a low restenosis rate, minimal risk, and usually an improvement or complete cure of the associated hypertension (see **Fig. 66-1**). There is sparse literature addressing the use of stenting in this disease, presumably because of the high rate of prolonged success with angioplasty alone. Stenting is an option in cases of restenosis, although in view of the young age of many of these patients, surgical revascularization is usually the best long-term option.

Management of ARAS is not so straightforward. Nonselective correction of stenotic lesions has led to disappointing results, and it is clear that not all lesions are functionally significant. It is helpful to decide before recommending revascularization procedures whether the indication for intervention is for treatment of renovascular hypertension or preservation of kidney function, or both. Another group in whom revascularization may be considered is patients presenting with flash pulmonary edema.

Treatment of Renovascular Hypertension

Renovascular hypertension typically manifests as an abrupt onset of severe hypertension or a marked deterioration from a previously stable baseline. Chronic stable hypertension present for many years is unlikely to be caused by progressive renal artery stenosis and is therefore unlikely to respond to intervention. Some useful criteria can help to predict whether a patient with suspected renovascular hypertension will or will not respond to revascularization. First, data suggest that angioplasty, with or without stenting, cannot improve blood pressure in patients who have already lost more than 60% of kidney function. Second, evaluation of the renal resistance index with Doppler ultrasonography or captopril scintigraphy in centers with appropriate expertise has emerged as an excellent method to prospectively classify patients as responders or nonresponders. A renal resistance index value of 80 or more reliably predicts patients in whom revascularization will not improve kidney function, blood pressure, or kidney survival. Evaluation of the renal resistance index has not been part of the routine assessment for patients with FMD. A recent large meta-analysis of studies comparing balloon angioplasty with medical management of patients with uncontrolled hypertension and renal artery stenosis suggested that angioplasty has at least a significant but modest effect on blood pressure but that complete cure of hypertension is rare.

Preservation of Kidney Function

The issue of revascularization for preservation of kidney function, particularly in patients with well-controlled or normal blood pressure, is controversial. The same meta-analysis mentioned previously suggested no benefit of PTRA over medical therapy for preservation or improvement of kidney function. It is well established that ARAS tends to progress in a large percentage of patients, usually within only a few years of diagnosis, and that this progression has been associated with a progressive decline in kidney function. It is estimated that at least 10% to 15% of patients entering dialysis programs have atherosclerotic renal artery disease as the primary cause of their renal failure. The problem seems to be that patients, particularly those with serum creatinine levels of 2.5 mg/dL or higher, already have significant, irreversible renal parenchymal disease. The abnormal renal function is unlikely to be affected by revascularization unless there is a coincident improvement in associated renovascular hypertension, if present. There must also be signs of salvageability of the kidney or of kidneys being revascularized. Signs of poor salvageability include kidney size less than 9 cm, reduced function detected on a renal flow scan, a renal resistive index greater than 80 on Doppler ultrasonography, serum creatinine level greater than 2.5 mg/dL, significant proteinuria, evidence of an alternative renal diagnosis, or findings of marked chronicity on kidney biopsy.

In patients with known renal artery stenosis greater than 60%, a good policy seems to be following serial kidney function over time to identify those who are progressively losing function but who still have evidence of salvageability.

There is some evidence that this group responds better to intervention than those with chronic, stable kidney function impairment.

After the decision has been made to intervene, most centers then proceed to PTRA rather than surgical repair. Because of the high rate of initial failure or early restenosis, current evidence suggests that angioplasty with stenting is the treatment of choice for ostial renal artery stenosis, producing a better technical success rate and better long-term patency than angioplasty alone. The role of primary stenting in nonostial lesions is unclear. Stenting has been used when the results of angioplasty were suboptimal and in restenotic lesions. The Cardiovascular Outcomes in Renal Artery Lesions (CORAL) trial is an ongoing, randomized trial that seeks to determine whether stenting is superior to medical management in terms of controlling hypertension, arresting the decline in renal function, and preventing cardiovascular events.

Surgery is reserved for patients with restenotic or technically difficult lesions. In centers with dedicated renovascular surgeons, referral may be earlier and even may be the primary recommendation, particularly in young fit patients with ostial lesions.

Contrast nephrotoxicity, atheroembolism to the kidneys and distal vasculature (see Chapter 35), and local damage to the femoral artery are complications of PTRA that occur in as many as 20% of patients. **Figure 66-3** shows a stent in the left renal artery after percutaneous intervention.

Treatment of Flash Pulmonary Edema
ARAS may manifest as recurrent episodes of flash pulmonary edema. There is evidence from small, nonrandomized trials that this subgroup of patients benefits from renal artery stenting, and treatment is strongly recommended by the American college of Cardiology.

Renal Parenchymal Hypertension

Hypertension is a common feature of much of acute and chronic kidney disease (CKD), particularly in glomerular and vascular disorders. Hypertension results from a combination

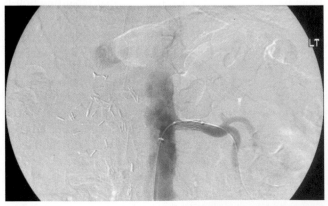

FIGURE 66-3 A stent can be seen in the ostium of the left renal artery. (Courtesy of Professor Mick Lee, Beaumont Hospital, Dublin, Ireland.)

of a positive salt balance, increased activity of the RAAS, and hyperstimulation of the sympathetic system. Treatment of hypertension in CKD consists of dietary salt restriction and promotion of salt excretion with diuretics, inhibition of the RAAS system with ACE inhibition and ARBs, and inhibition of the sympathetic nervous system. Clues to the presence of renal parenchymal disease in hypertensive patients are elevated serum creatinine levels and abnormal urinalysis results. A kidney ultrasonogram is a useful noninvasive screening test to assess kidney size and asymmetry and to rule out major renal structural abnormalities or obstructive lesions. The varied disorders have many treatments available, and a discussion of each is beyond the scope of this chapter.

ENDOCRINE CAUSES OF SECONDARY HYPERTENSION

Hypertension is a feature of several endocrine conditions (see **Table 66-2**). However, the best-characterized associations are those with primary hyperaldosteronism, Cushing's syndrome, and pheochromocytoma.

Primary Hyperaldosteronism

Primary hyperaldosteronism is the most common cause of hypertension due to an endocrinopathy. Its incidence increases with the severity of hypertension. Among patients with resistant hypertension, the prevalence of primary hyperaldosteronism is estimated to be 17% to 20%.

As a group, African American patients tend to have lower renin levels, but no ethnic differences in the prevalence of primary hyperaldosteronism have been described. No difference between the sexes has been reported.

Primary hyperaldosteronism may be caused by bilateral adrenal hyperplasia (65% of cases), aldosterone producing adenoma (30% of cases), or rarely, a secretory adrenal carcinoma or inherited endocrinopathies (discussed later). Patients with adrenal adenomas tend to be younger and have a more severe clinical picture than those with adrenal hyperplasia.

Clinical Syndrome
Conn first described the clinical syndrome in 1955 in a 34-year-old woman with hypertension, episodic paralysis, hypokalemia, and metabolic alkalosis. She was subsequently cured by the removal of an adrenal adenoma.

Diagnosis
Although hypokalemia may arouse suspicions of a diagnosis of hyperaldosteronism, it is not present in most cases. Testing for hyperaldosteronism should be considered in any of the following circumstances: hypertension and spontaneous hypokalemia or hypokalemia induced by a low-dose diuretic, severe hypertension (i.e., systolic pressure of 160 mm Hg or diastolic pressure of 100 mm Hg, or both); a patient requiring three or more antihypertensive drugs; hypertension manifesting at a young age (<40 years); patients with an adrenal

incidentaloma; and hypertensive relatives of a patient with primary hyperaldosteronism.

Ratio of Plasma Aldosterone Concentration to Plasma Renin Activity

Measurement of the ratio of plasma aldosterone concentration (PAC) to plasma renin activity (PRA) is the screening test of choice for patients with suspected primary hyperaldosteronism. A PAC/PRA ratio greater than 20 in combination with a PAC greater than 15 ng/dL or 416 pmol/L is considered a positive screening test result. The test is performed in the morning on an ambulatory patient. Hypokalemia, if present, should be corrected first, because hypokalemia reduces the secretion of aldosterone. Aldosterone antagonists and amiloride should be stopped 6 weeks before testing. ACE inhibitors, ARBs, and diuretics can falsely elevate the PRA value. Therefore, if the patient is taking an ARB, an ACE inhibitor, or a diuretic, the presence of a detectable PRA or a low PAC/PRA ratio does not exclude a diagnosis of primary hyperaldosteronism. However, if the PRA is undetectable in a patient taking an ACE or ARB, then a diagnosis of primary hyperaldosteronism should be considered, and the ACE inhibitors or ARB does not need to be stopped. Adrenergic inhibitors (i.e., β-blockers and, to a lesser extent, α_2-agonists) suppress renin and reduce aldosterone levels, although to a lesser degree, in normal individuals. The PAC/PRA ratio may be increased in hypertensive patients without hyperaldosteronism who are taking adrenergic antagonists, but the PAC will not be more than 416 pmol/L, and the diagnostic power of the test is therefore not affected.

Confirmatory Tests

The PAC/PRA ratio is a screening tool, and confirmatory tests are necessary to confirm autonomous adrenal production of aldosterone. The hallmark of this disorder is nonsuppressible aldosterone secretion with nonstimulatable renin secretion. In principle, administration of a sodium load should result in suppression of aldosterone in normal individuals, whereas in patients with hyperaldosteronism, suppression will not occur. This may be achieved by means of oral sodium chloride load over several days or by delivery of intravenous saline over several hours.

An alternative is the fludrocortisone suppression test, in which fludrocortisone acetate is given at a dosage of 0.1 mg every 6 hours for 4 days together with a high-sodium diet. In the normal individual, aldosterone is suppressed.

These tests are not without risk, particularly for patients with poor left ventricular function. An alternative is the captopril suppression test, in which oral administration of captopril does not suppress aldosterone levels below 416 pmol/L in patients with primary hyperaldosteronism. This test has the advantage of avoiding salt loading in individuals in whom this is contraindicated, but it may cause profound hypotension in some patients.

All of these tests are cumbersome and time consuming. Many centers now directly proceed to imaging after a positive biochemical screening test result.

Radiology

The adrenal glands are imaged with CT or magnetic resonance imaging (MRI) to determine the cause of the primary hyperaldosteronism. Adenomas that are 10 mm in diameter and sometimes even smaller can be detected.

The relative merits of CT and MRI are not entirely clear. One study showed MRI to be much more sensitive than CT for adrenal adenoma detection but to have a higher rate of false-positive scans. It is estimated that with CT alone, as many as 40% of adenomas may be missed. Radionuclide scintigraphy with [131I]iodocholesterol is sensitive for adenomas, but it is not widely available, and there are several case reports of missed lesions.

A major problem is the high incidence of radiologically detected, nonfunctioning adenomas (4% of the general population on CT; 7% on autopsy), particularly after the age of 40 years. For a patient younger than 40 years with profound hyperaldosteronism (e.g., PAC > 30 ng/dL), an adenoma found on CT that is larger than 1 cm of uniform diameter and hypodense (<10 Hounsfield units), and a contralateral adrenal gland that appears normal on scanning, it is reasonable to proceed to adrenalectomy, because the chance of an aldosterone-producing adenoma is high. In older people, adrenal vein sampling should be performed whenever possible if an adenoma is detected, because aldosterone-producing adenomas become increasingly uncommon with advancing age. If the adrenal glands are normal on scanning, patients should proceed directly to adrenal vein sampling. This technique can strongly predict a successful result of unilateral adrenalectomy. It must be performed by an experienced radiologist and is more accurate when performed after adrenocorticotropic hormone (ACTH) stimulation. The position in the adrenal vein is confirmed by simultaneously measuring adrenal vein and peripheral vein cortisol levels. A greater than fivefold increase in PAC compared with the contralateral side should be demonstrated on the side of an adenoma. In adrenal hyperplasia, there should be little difference between the two adrenal values. Occasionally, the adenoma may be extra-adrenal, and the result of adrenal vein sampling is normal. If imaging and adrenal vein sampling are negative, the rare diagnosis of glucocorticoid-remediable aldosteronism (discussed later) should be considered.

Treatment

Patients with adenomas should be referred for unilateral laparoscopic adrenalectomy. Removal of well-localized unilateral lesions is very successful. There are some case reports of embolization of adenomas with ethanol in patients medically unfit for surgery. Selective hypoaldosteronism may occur for some months after surgery, and potassium supplementation should be cautious during this period. The drugs of choice for medical management of adrenal hyperplasia and preoperative management of adenomas in the past have been spironolactone, amiloride, and ACE inhibitors. Eplerenone, a newer selective aldosterone receptor antagonist, is popular because it causes much less gynecomastia than spironolactone.

Hyper-reninism

Renin-secreting tumors are rare. Patients are hypertensive and hypokalemic, with high PRA along with elevated aldosterone levels and urinary potassium excretion. These tumors usually originate from the juxtaglomerular apparatus in the kidney, but renin production has been reported with other malignancies, including teratomas and ovarian tumors.

Cushing's Syndrome

Cushing's syndrome is a clinical condition resulting from excess effects of exogenous or endogenous glucocorticoids. Patients develop a characteristic clinical appearance, with the classic cushingoid *moon facies* related to facial fat deposition, along with truncal obesity, abdominal striae, hirsutism, and kyphoscoliosis. Patients have various degrees of multiorgan involvement with diabetes mellitus, cataracts, neuropsychiatric disorders, proximal myopathy, avascular necrosis of humeral and femoral heads, osteoporosis, and secondary hypertension, among the more prominent of the manifold possible complications. The original syndrome described by Cushing related to a patient with pituitary ACTH excess driving excess cortisol production. As a consequence, pituitary-dependent disease is known as Cushing's disease. Hypertension, resulting from the mineralocorticoid effect of the glucocorticoids, is a common feature. Causes of Cushing's syndrome are listed in **Table 66-4**. The most common cause of endogenous excess is a pituitary adenoma.

Diagnosis

The presence of cortisol excess must be confirmed biochemically. This can be achieved with the low-dose dexamethasone suppression test, measurement of 24-hour urinary free-cortisol levels, or assessment of circadian pattern of cortisol secretion.

Overnight, Low-Dose Dexamethasone Suppression Test

A 2-mg dose of dexamethasone is taken at 11 PM, and a plasma cortisol sample is drawn at 9 AM the next morning. Suppression is defined as a cortisol level of less than 5 mg/dL.

Circadian Testing of Cortisol Secretion

Cortisol levels are measured at 9 AM and 11 PM. They are usually high in the morning and lowest at night.

Other causes of abnormally high cortisol secretion should be considered, such as stress, endogenous depression, and

---

TABLE 66-4 Causes of Cushing's Syndrome

Exogenous glucocorticoid administration

Endogenous glucocorticoid excess
   Adrenocorticotropic hormone (ACTH)
     Ectopic production
     Pituitary secretory adenoma (Cushing's disease)
   Cortisol
   Adrenal cortical adenoma or carcinoma

---

chronic excess alcohol consumption. A normal response to an insulin suppression test suggests endogenous depression.

When cortisol excess is confirmed, further testing to elucidate a pituitary, adrenal, or ectopic source should follow. Extremely high plasma or urinary cortisol levels suggest adrenal carcinoma or ectopic ACTH secretion. An adrenal carcinoma often causes marked virilization and a severe hypokalemic metabolic alkalosis.

Plasma Adrenocorticotropic Hormone

If there is an adrenal source of glucocorticoids, ACTH levels should be suppressed below the normal range. A normal or moderately raised level suggests pituitary disease. High levels suggest ectopic disease.

High-Dose Dexamethasone Suppression Test

Dexamethasone (2 mg every 6 hours) is given for 2 days. Cortisol levels are measured at 9 AM on day 1 and day 3. Suppression of cortisol to less than 50% of the day 1 level is defined as suppression. Pituitary-dependent Cushing's disease should respond in this way, whereas ectopic ACTH production should not.

Imaging

CT or MRI of the adrenals or the pituitary, depending on the clinical suspicion, should be performed. If ectopic ACTH is diagnosed, a bronchial neoplasm should be aggressively ruled out.

Treatment

If the cause is exogenous steroid use, efforts should be made to withdraw the medication dose carefully and slowly if the patient can do so or if the clinical condition being treated allows. Steroid-sparing agents may help.

Endogenous Cushing's syndrome is best treated by surgical excision. If imaging does not reliably demonstrate a pituitary lesion, radiation may be used. If there is adrenal overactivity and tumor localization is not possible or there is symptomatic ectopic ACTH activity, symptoms may be relieved by suppressing the adrenal gland with medications such as metyrapone, aminoglutethimide, or mitotane.

Pheochromocytoma

Pheochromocytoma is a secretory tumor of neurochromaffin cells in the adrenal medulla. It is a rare condition that causes less than 0.2% of all hypertension cases. Symptoms result from catecholamine hypersecretion.

Patients classically present with the triad of episodic headache, sweating, and tachycardia; most have at least two of these. Pallor, paroxysmal hypotension, orthostatic hypotension, visual blurring, papilledema, high erythrocyte sedimentation rate, weight loss, polyuria, polydipsia, psychiatric disorders, hyperglycemia, dilated cardiomyopathy, and rarely, secondary erythrocytosis are less common clinical features. About one half of patients have paroxysms of hypertension, whereas most of the remainder have apparently essential hypertension. Many have no symptoms and are detected serendipitously with abdominal radiology, at surgery, or at postmortem examination.

When referring to these tumors, the "10% rule" is often cited and is still clinically useful: approximately 10% of cases are extra-adrenal, 10% are malignant, and 10% are bilateral; 10% are associated with familial syndromes, and the remaining cases are sporadic. There are two main familial syndromes associated with pheochromocytoma:

1. In patients with von Hippel-Lindau syndrome, pheochromocytoma occurs in 10% to 20%.
2. Multiple endocrine neoplasia syndrome type 2 is associated with medullary thyroid carcinoma and hyperparathyroidism. Pheochromocytoma occurs in 20% to 50% of affected individuals.

Pheochromocytoma is found in less than 5% of patients with neurofibromatosis type 1. Genetic screening is recommended if the patient is younger than 21 years of age, has extra-adrenal or bilateral disease, or has multiple paragangliomas.

Diagnosis

A classic history of the typical triad of symptoms or a family history may suggest the diagnosis. The screening tests used are measurements of urinary and plasma catecholamines or their metabolites.

Urinary and Plasma Catecholamine Levels

A study based on prospective data collected from 152 consecutive patients with pheochromocytoma compared the relative diagnostic sensitivities of the various catecholamine and catecholamine metabolite levels. It found that the most sensitive tests were urinary normetanephrine and platelet norepinephrine levels, with sensitivities of 96.9% and 93.8%, respectively. For patients in whom a pheochromocytoma is clinically suspected but cannot be confirmed by urinary, plasma, or platelet catecholamine levels, a ^{131}I-labeled metaiodobenzylguanidine (MIBG) radioisotope scan may be performed. MIBG is an analogue of epinephrine. It improves the sensitivity of platelet epinephrine to 100%. When combined with an MIBG plasma norepinephrine assay, it has a sensitivity of 97.1 % in predicting the presence of pheochromocytoma. The reason for the increased sensitivity of platelet epinephrine is likely that the neurosecretory granules in the platelets concentrate the catecholamines that are intermittently secreted by the pheochromocytoma. Measurement of platelet epinephrine should be part of the standard screening for pheochromocytoma.

Clonidine Suppression Test

The clonidine suppression test is an alternative way of confirming a diagnosis when catecholamine levels are suggestive but not diagnostic of pheochromocytoma. Clonidine is given after all antihypertensives have been withheld for at least 12 hours; plasma catecholamines are measured 3 hours later and should fall to less than 500 pg/mL in normal individuals. This test is 90% sensitive for pheochromocytoma.

Radiology

Imaging should be performed after biochemical confirmation of the diagnosis using the assays already described. Ninety-five percent of pheochromocytomas are intra-abdominal, with 90% located in the adrenal glands. CT or MRI is the initial modality of choice (**Fig. 66-4**); both are up to 98% sensitive but are only about 70% specific because of the high prevalence of nonfunctional adrenal adenomas, particularly with increasing age.

If the result of CT or MRI is negative despite positive screening assays, the diagnosis should be reconsidered. If pheochromocytoma is still strongly suspected, an MIBG or total-body MRI should be performed. In addition to their role previously described, MIBG scans can be used to detect pheochromocytomas when the result of CT or MRI is negative or to detect extra-adrenal or metastatic disease. Positron emission tomographic (PET) scanning may have a future role in detecting metastatic disease.

Treatment

The definitive treatment for a pheochromocytoma is surgical excision, but medical treatment to control the effects of the catecholamine excess is crucial preoperatively. There are several accepted approaches. The most widely used is administration of the α-blocker phenoxybenzamine, starting at a dose of 10 mg once daily and increasing the dose every few days until blood pressure and symptoms are controlled. A β-blocker may then be added to control tachycardia. Using this approach, a patient should be ready for surgery in 10 to 14 days.

A β-blocker should never be given first, because the subsequent unopposed α-agonist vasoconstrictive action can precipitate markedly worse hypertension. A hypertensive crisis precipitated by a β-blocker may be a clue to the presence of a pheochromocytoma in a patient with hypertension.

Surgery for pheochromocytoma has a perioperative mortality rate of 2.4% and a morbidity rate of 24%. If there are

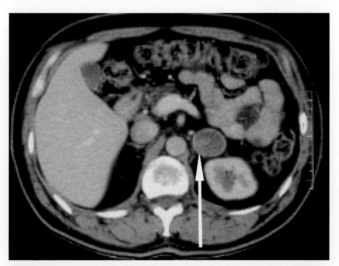

FIGURE 66-4 Computed tomogram shows a pheochromocytoma arising from the left adrenal gland (*arrow*). (Courtesy of Professor Mick Lee, Beaumont Hospital, Dublin, Ireland.)

metastases, they should be resected if possible. Skeletal lesions may be irradiated. Chemotherapy may be used in selected patients.

Prognosis

Long-term follow-up is indicated in all patients, because there is a high incidence of recurrent hypertension even with complete tumor removal, especially in older patients with a family history of hypertension. The tumor recurs in about 10% of patients, and recurrences usually are seen in familial cases. A significant proportion of recurrences are malignant.

CARDIOVASCULAR AND CARDIOPULMONARY CAUSES OF SECONDARY HYPERTENSION

Coarctation of the Aorta

Coarctation is a congenital narrowing of the aortic lumen, occurring most commonly just distal to the origin of the left subclavian artery. Clinically, the patient has hypertension when measured in the upper limbs, with reduced or unmeasurable blood pressure in the legs. If the coarctation is proximal to the origin of the left subclavian artery, the blood pressure and brachial pulsation in the left upper limb may be reduced. The femoral pulses may be delayed or diminished compared with the radial or brachial pulses, and there may be an audible bruit over the patient's back. Diagnosis is confirmed with aortic imaging, and treatment is surgical.

Sleep Apnea Syndrome

The association of obesity, obstructive sleep apnea, and hypertension has long been recognized. Although the pathophysiology is not clear, the apneic syndrome itself seems to contribute directly to the hypertension, along with other comorbid conditions such as obesity. Many cases of obstructive sleep apnea go undiagnosed unless the physician is alert to the possibility. In most studies of patients with sleep apnea and hypertension, daytime and nighttime levels of blood pressure were improved significantly after treatment with continuous positive airway pressure (CPAP) or related modalities.

INHERITED CAUSES OF SECONDARY HYPERTENSION

Several mendelian disorders are associated with hypertension. Although all are probably significantly underdiagnosed, each is rare. They are all associated with upregulation of sodium reabsorption in the distal nephron, with accompanying expansion of extracellular volume. The PRA is uniformly suppressed. These conditions may be divided into primary disorders of the distal nephron and primary adrenal disorders.

Distal Nephron Disorders

Liddle's Syndrome

Reabsorption of sodium in the collecting duct depends on the activity of the amiloride-sensitive epithelial sodium channel (ENaC), which consists of three subunits encoded by different genes. Mutations in the β and γ subunits result in increased ENaC-mediated sodium flux. The activity of the channel is based on recycling of the transporter between the apical membrane and the subapical vesicles. Mutations result in deletion of the binding site necessary for degradation or recycling, leading to an increased number of functional sodium transport channels.

Hypertension usually begins in childhood but may not be diagnosed until early adulthood. The presence of metabolic alkalosis and hypokalemia varies. PRA and PAC are suppressed. Treatment involves a low-salt diet and an agent that directly inhibits ENaC, such as amiloride or triamterene. Mineralocorticoid receptor antagonists do not have an effect, because the defective sodium transport is independent of aldosterone.

Gordon's Syndrome: Type 2 Pseudohypoaldosteronism

Gordon and colleagues first described this syndrome of hypertension and hyperkalemia in 1970. It has since been characterized as an autosomal dominant disorder caused by mutations in two members of the WNK (with no lysine [K]) family of serine-threonine kinases, a group of enzymes involved in regulating the activity of the thiazide-sensitive Na-Cl cotransporter (NCCT) molecule in the distal convoluted tubule.

WNK4 phosphorylates NCCT, which prevents incorporation of the transporter into the apical membrane. Missense mutations in the WNK4 gene (chromosome 17) produce mutant proteins that allow increased NCCT expression, a lesion complementary to the deficiency of NCCT expression in Gitelman's syndrome. WNK1 is predominantly a cytoplasmic protein that inhibits WNK4 function. Large deletions in the WNK1 gene (chromosome 12) increase WNK1 production, leading to excess WNK4 inhibition and to increased NCCT expression. Both WNK kinase mutations cause overactivity of the NCCT, with resultant excess salt reabsorption. This causes volume-dependent hypertension and suppression of the RAAS. Augmented absorption at this site reduces collecting duct sodium delivery, which leads to potassium and acid retention and hyperkalemic metabolic acidosis. The hyperkalemia may be exacerbated by the fact that the same mutation in WNK4 that releases NCCT from suppression has an opposite, inhibitory effect on the secretory renal outer medullary potassium channels (ROMKs), thereby inhibiting potassium secretion. The PRA value is low. Aldosterone levels vary and may be increased by hyperkalemia, although not enough to correct it. The metabolic abnormalities hyperkalemia and hyperchloremic metabolic alkalosis tend to precede the onset of hypertension, which often does not manifest until adult life. Spitzer-Weinstein syndrome, which consists of hyperkalemia, metabolic acidosis, and growth failure but not hypertension, is thought to be an early manifestation of Gordon's syndrome.

Treatment typically involves a combination of dietary salt restriction with a low-dose thiazide or loop diuretics, and it is usually very effective. WNK kinases and their targets may offer novel targets for future antihypertensive agents.

Syndrome of Apparent Mineralocorticoid Excess

Apparent mineralocorticoid excess (AME) is a rare autosomal recessive disorder in which the enzyme 11β-dehyroxysteroid dehydrogenase type 2 (11HD2) is inactive. In aldosterone-sensitive tissues, this enzyme usually converts cortisol to inactive metabolites and thereby prevents it from attaching to the mineralocorticoid receptor. In AME, cortisol acts on the mineralocorticoid receptor, causing apparent hyperaldosteronism despite suppressed aldosterone levels. Because of the lack of 11HD2, the conversion of cortisol to cortisone is impaired, resulting in an abnormal ratio of cortisol metabolites (i.e., tetrahydrocortisol and allotetrahydrocortisol) to cortisone metabolites (e.g., tetrahydrocortisone) in the urine. The disease was thought to be invariably present from childhood, with patients presenting with low birth weight, failure to thrive, hypokalemia, and metabolic alkalosis, and it has been associated with end-organ damage and a high mortality rate if untreated. However, milder phenotypes with only partial inactivation of 11HD2 have been described. Mineralocorticoid receptor blockers, potassium supplementation, and dietary sodium restriction are the mainstays of treatment. A mild acquired variant may be encountered in patients with excessive licorice intake. To produce an inherent weak mineralocorticoid effect, the principal metabolite of licorice (i.e., glycyrrhizic acid) inhibits the same enzyme that is deficient in AME. An old treatment for peptic ulcers, carbenoxolone, was associated with hypertension for similar reasons.

Hypertension Exacerbated by Pregnancy

Hypertension exacerbated by pregnancy is a recently described and rare genetic condition in which an activating mutation of the mineralocorticoid receptor renders it especially sensitive to nonmineralocorticoid steroids such as progesterone, which increases 100-fold during pregnancy, although affected individuals are hypertensive before pregnancy. The mineralocorticoid receptor in these patients can also be activated by spironolactone.

Adrenal Disorders

Glucocorticoid-Remediable Aldosteronism: Familial Hyperaldosteronism Type 1

Glucocorticoid-remediable aldosteronism is a rare subtype of primary hyperaldosteronism in which the hyperaldosteronism can be reversed with steroid administration. Glucocorticoid-remediable aldosteronism is inherited and should be suspected in patients with an early onset of hypertension and a family history positive for early hypertension or intracerebral hemorrhage. Individuals are otherwise usually phenotypically normal.

Glucocorticoid-remediable aldosteronism is inherited as an autosomal dominant trait. It may be suspected from a positive family history and early onset of hypertension before the age of 21 years. The plasma potassium concentration may be low but is often normal. One clue is severe hypokalemia after administration of a thiazide diuretic (due to increased sodium delivery to the aldosterone-sensitive potassium-secretory site in the cortical collecting tubule). As many as 18% of patients suffer a cerebrovascular complication, mainly hemorrhage from ruptured berry aneurysms. The incidence of aneurysm is similar to that among patients with adult polycystic kidney disease. Surveillance MRA has been recommended, but the benefit of this approach has not been proved. Mean age of onset of cerebral hemorrhage if an aneurysm is present is 32 years.

Pathogenesis

In the adrenal cortex, aldosterone is normally synthesized in the zona glomerulosa, whereas glucocorticoids are predominantly synthesized in the adjacent zona fasciculata. Two isozymes of the enzyme 11β-hydroxylase, encoded by chromosome 8, are responsible for the synthesis of aldosterone and cortisol. The isozyme in the zona glomerulosa (aldosterone synthase or CYP11B2) mediates aldosterone production under the influence of potassium and angiotensin II, whereas that in the zona fasciculata (CYP11B1) encodes cortisol production under the influence of ACTH. In glucocorticoid-remediable aldosteronism, the promoter region for CYP11B1 fuses with the coding sequences of the aldosterone synthase enzyme, CYP11B2, resulting in ACTH-dependent aldosterone synthesis in the zona fasciculata.

Diagnosis

Diagnosis may be achieved by dexamethasone suppression testing demonstrating the production of 18-carbon oxidation products of cortisol. However, a genetic test demonstrating the pathologic chimeric gene is recommended, because there is a significant false-positive rate for patients with primary hyperaldosteronism when tested with dexamethasone. This test can be obtained from the International Registry for Glucocorticoid-Remediable Aldosteronism (http://www.brighamandwomens.org/gra/).

Treatment

Corticosteroids suppress ACTH and lower the blood pressure to normal. The target dose should be enough to suppress aldosterone levels sufficiently without causing debilitating side effects.

Familial Hyperaldosteronism Type II

In familial hyperaldosteronism type II, excess mineralocorticoid production is responsible for hypertension, but it is not suppressible by dexamethasone. Autosomal dominance suggests a single gene mutation, and the locus has been narrowed to a band on chromosome 7. Familial hyperaldosteronism type II is clinically and biochemically indistinguishable from noninherited primary hyperaldosteronism and can be detected only by a positive family history.

Congenital Adrenal Hyperplasia

Congenital adrenal hyperplasia is an autosomal recessive disorder. Patients cannot synthesize cortisol. In this condition, defects in the final steps of steroid biosynthesis result in excess mineralocorticoid and androgen effects, with coincident signs of glucocorticoid deficiency. The most common forms, 17α-hydroxylase deficiency and 11β-hydroxylase deficiency, may cause hypertension due to overproduction of excess cortisol precursors that are or are metabolized to mineralocorticoid agonists.

BIBLIOGRAPHY

Conlon PJ, O'Riordan E, Kalra PA: New insights into the epidemiologic and clinical manifestations of atherosclerotic renovascular disease. Am J Kidney Dis 35:573-587, 2000.

Conn JW: Presidential address. I. Painting background. II. Primary hyperaldosteronism, a new clinical syndrome. J Lab Clin Med 45:3-17, 1955.

Guller U, Turek J, Eubanks S, et al: Detecting pheochromocytoma: Defining the most sensitive test. Ann Surg 243:102-207, 2006.

Mattson C, Young WF Jr: Primary aldosteronism: Diagnostic and treatment strategies. Nat Clin Pract Nephrol 2:198-208, 2006.

Nadar S, Lip GY, Beevers DG: Primary hyperaldosteronism. Ann Clin Biochem 40(Pt 5):439-452, 2003.

Nordmann AJ, Woo K, Parkes R, et al: Balloon angioplasty or medical therapy for hypertensive patients with atherosclerotic renal artery disease? A meta-analysis of randomized-controlled trials. Am J Med 114:44-50, 2003.

Pohl MA: Renal artery stenosis, renal vascular hypertension and ischemic nephropathy. In Schrier RW, Gottschalk CW (eds): Diseases of the Kidney, 6th ed. Boston, Little, Brown, 1997, pp 1367-1425.

Radermacher J, Chavan A, Bleck J, et al: Use of Doppler ultrasonography to predict the outcome of therapy for renal artery stenosis. N Engl J Med 344:410-417, 2001.

Radermacher J, Weinkove R, Haller H: Techniques for predicting a favourable response to renal angioplasty in patients with renovascular disease. Curr Opin Nephrol Hypertens 10:799-805, 2001.

Ramos F, Kotliar C, Alvarez D, et al: Renal function and outcome of PTRA and stenting for atherosclerotic renal artery stenosis. Kidney Int 63:276-282, 2003.

Safian RD: Atherosclerotic renal artery stenosis. Curr Treat Options Cardiovasc Med 5:91-101, 2003.

Slovut DP, Olin JW: Fibromuscular dysplasia. N Engl J Med 350:1862-1871, 2004.

Tan KT, van Beek EJ, Brown PW, et al: Magnetic resonance angiography for the diagnosis of renal artery stenosis: A meta-analysis. Clin Radiol 58:257, 2003.

Vehaskari VM: Heritable forms of hypertension. Pediatr Nephrol Jul 24, 2007 [Epub ahead of print].

Wilson FH, Disse-Nicodeme S, Choate KA, et al: Human hypertension caused by mutations in WNK kinases. Science 293:1107-1112, 2001.

Index

Page numbers followed by *f* indicate figure(s); *t*, table(s).